PULMONARY AND PERIPHERAL GAS EXCHANGE IN HEALTH AND DISEASE

LUNG BIOLOGY IN HEALTH AND DISEASE

Executive Editor

Claude Lenfant
Director, National Heart, Lung and Blood Institute
National Institutes of Health
Bethesda, Maryland

1. Immunologic and Infectious Reactions in the Lung, *edited by C. H. Kirkpatrick and H. Y. Reynolds*
2. The Biochemical Basis of Pulmonary Function, *edited by R. G. Crystal*
3. Bioengineering Aspects of the Lung, *edited by J. B. West*
4. Metabolic Functions of the Lung, *edited by Y. S. Bakhle and J. R. Vane*
5. Respiratory Defense Mechanisms (in two parts), *edited by J. D. Brain, D. F. Proctor, and L. M. Reid*
6. Development of the Lung, *edited by W. A. Hodson*
7. Lung Water and Solute Exchange, *edited by N. C. Staub*
8. Extrapulmonary Manifestations of Respiratory Disease, *edited by E. D. Robin*
9. Chronic Obstructive Pulmonary Disease, *edited by T. L. Petty*
10. Pathogenesis and Therapy of Lung Cancer, *edited by C. C. Harris*
11. Genetic Determinants of Pulmonary Disease, *edited by S. D. Litwin*
12. The Lung in the Transition Between Health and Disease, *edited by P. T. Macklem and S. Permutt*
13. Evolution of Respiratory Processes: A Comparative Approach, *edited by S. C. Wood and C. Lenfant*
14. Pulmonary Vascular Diseases, *edited by K. M. Moser*
15. Physiology and Pharmacology of the Airways, *edited by J. A. Nadel*
16. Diagnostic Techniques in Pulmonary Disease (in two parts), *edited by M. A. Sackner*
17. Regulation of Breathing (in two parts), *edited by T. F. Hornbein*
18. Occupational Lung Diseases: Research Approaches and Methods, *edited by H. Weill and M. Turner-Warwick*
19. Immunopharmacology of the Lung, *edited by H. H. Newball*
20. Sarcoidosis and Other Granulomatous Diseases of the Lung, *edited by B. L. Fanburg*
21. Sleep and Breathing, *edited by N. A. Saunders and C. E. Sullivan*
22. *Pneumocystis carinii* Pneumonia: Pathogenesis, Diagnosis, and Treatment, *edited by L. S. Young*
23. Pulmonary Nuclear Medicine: Techniques in Diagnosis of Lung Disease, *edited by H. L. Atkins*
24. Acute Respiratory Failure, *edited by W. M. Zapol and K. J. Falke*
25. Gas Mixing and Distribution in the Lung, *edited by L. A. Engel and M. Paiva*

26. High-Frequency Ventilation in Intensive Care and During Surgery, *edited by G. Carlon and W. S. Howland*
27. Pulmonary Development: Transition from Intrauterine to Extrauterine Life, *edited by G. H. Nelson*
28. Chronic Obstructive Pulmonary Disease: Second Edition, *edited by T. L. Petty*
29. The Thorax (in two parts), *edited by C. Roussos and P. T. Macklem*
30. The Pleura in Health and Disease, *edited by J. Chrétien, J. Bignon, and A. Hirsch*
31. Drug Therapy for Asthma: Research and Clinical Practice, *edited by J. W. Jenne and S. Murphy*
32. Pulmonary Endothelium in Health and Disease, *edited by U. S. Ryan*
33. The Airways: Neural Control in Health and Disease, *edited by M. A. Kaliner and P. J. Barnes*
34. Pathophysiology and Treatment of Inhalation Injuries, *edited by J. Loke*
35. Respiratory Function of the Upper Airway, *edited by O. P. Mathew and G. Sant'Ambrogio*
36. Chronic Obstructive Pulmonary Disease: A Behavioral Perspective, *edited by A. J. McSweeny and I. Grant*
37. Biology of Lung Cancer: Diagnosis and Treatment, *edited by S. T. Rosen, J. L. Mulshine, F. Cuttitta, and P. G. Abrams*
38. Pulmonary Vascular Physiology and Pathophysiology, *edited by E. K. Weir and J. T. Reeves*
39. Comparative Pulmonary Physiology: Current Concepts, *edited by S. C. Wood*
40. Respiratory Physiology: An Analytical Approach, *edited by H. K. Chang and M. Paiva*
41. Lung Cell Biology, *edited by D. Massaro*
42. Heart–Lung Interactions in Health and Disease, *edited by S. M. Scharf and S. S. Cassidy*
43. Clinical Epidemiology of Chronic Obstructive Pulmonary Disease, *edited by M. J. Hensley and N. A. Saunders*
44. Surgical Pathology of Lung Neoplasms, *edited by A. M. Marchevsky*
45. The Lung in Rheumatic Diseases, *edited by G. W. Cannon and G. A. Zimmerman*
46. Diagnostic Imaging of the Lung, *edited by C. E. Putman*
47. Models of Lung Disease: Microscopy and Structural Methods, *edited by J. Gil*
48. Electron Microscopy of the Lung, *edited by D. E. Schraufnagel*
49. Asthma: Its Pathology and Treatment, *edited by M. A. Kaliner, P. J. Barnes, and C. G. A. Persson*
50. Acute Respiratory Failure: Second Edition, *edited by W. M. Zapol and F. Lemaire*
51. Lung Disease in the Tropics, *edited by O. P. Sharma*
52. Exercise: Pulmonary Physiology and Pathophysiology, *edited by B. J. Whipp and K. Wasserman*
53. Developmental Neurobiology of Breathing, *edited by G. G. Haddad and J. P. Farber*
54. Mediators of Pulmonary Inflammation, *edited by M. A. Bray and W. H. Anderson*
55. The Airway Epithelium, *edited by S. G. Farmer and D. Hay*

56. Physiological Adaptations in Vertebrates: Respiration, Circulation, and Metabolism, *edited by S. C. Wood, R. E. Weber, A. R. Hargens, and R. W. Millard*
57. The Bronchial Circulation, *edited by J. Butler*
58. Lung Cancer Differentiation: Implications for Diagnosis and Treatment, *edited by S. D. Bernal and P. J. Hesketh*
59. Pulmonary Complications of Systemic Disease, *edited by J. F. Murray*
60. Lung Vascular Injury: Molecular and Cellular Response, *edited by A. Johnson and T. J. Ferro*
61. Cytokines of the Lung, *edited by J. Kelley*
62. The Mast Cell in Health and Disease, *edited by M. A. Kaliner and D. D. Metcalfe*
63. Pulmonary Disease in the Elderly Patient, *edited by D. A. Mahler*
64. Cystic Fibrosis, *edited by P. B. Davis*
65. Signal Transduction in Lung Cells, *edited by J. S. Brody, D. M. Center, and V. A. Tkachuk*
66. Tuberculosis: A Comprehensive International Approach, *edited by L. B. Reichman and E. S. Hershfield*
67. Pharmacology of the Respiratory Tract: Experimental and Clinical Research, *edited by K. F. Chung and P. J. Barnes*
68. Prevention of Respiratory Diseases, *edited by A. Hirsch, M. Goldberg, J.-P. Martin, and R. Masse*
69. *Pneumocystis carinii* Pneumonia: Second Edition, *edited by P. D. Walzer*
70. Fluid and Solute Transport in the Airspaces of the Lungs, *edited by R. M. Effros and H. K. Chang*
71. Sleep and Breathing: Second Edition, *edited by N. A. Saunders and C. E. Sullivan*
72. Airway Secretion: Physiological Bases for the Control of Mucous Hypersecretion, *edited by T. Takishima and S. Shimura*
73. Sarcoidosis and Other Granulomatous Disorders, *edited by D. G. James*
74. Epidemiology of Lung Cancer, *edited by J. M. Samet*
75. Pulmonary Embolism, *edited by M. Morpurgo*
76. Sports and Exercise Medicine, *edited by S. C. Wood and R. C. Roach*
77. Endotoxin and the Lungs, *edited by K. L. Brigham*
78. The Mesothelial Cell and Mesothelioma, *edited by M.-C. Jaurand and J. Bignon*
79. Regulation of Breathing: Second Edition, *edited by J. A. Dempsey and A. I. Pack*
80. Pulmonary Fibrosis, *edited by S. Hin. Phan and R. S. Thrall*
81. Long-Term Oxygen Therapy: Scientific Basis and Clinical Application, *edited by W. J. O'Donohue, Jr.*
82. Ventral Brainstem Mechanisms and Control of Respiration and Blood Pressure, *edited by C. O. Trouth, R. M. Millis, H. F. Kiwull-Schöne, and M. E. Schläfke*
83. A History of Breathing Physiology, *edited by D. F. Proctor*
84. Surfactant Therapy for Lung Disease, *edited by B. Robertson and H. W. Taeusch*
85. The Thorax: Second Edition, Revised and Expanded (in three parts), *edited by C. Roussos*

86. Severe Asthma: Pathogenesis and Clinical Management, *edited by S. J. Szefler and D. Y. M. Leung*
87. *Mycobacterium avium*–Complex Infection: Progress in Research and Treatment, *edited by J. A. Korvick and C. A. Benson*
88. Alpha 1–Antitrypsin Deficiency: Biology • Pathogenesis • Clinical Manifestations • Therapy, *edited by R. G. Crystal*
89. Adhesion Molecules and the Lung, *edited by P. A. Ward and J. C. Fantone*
90. Respiratory Sensation, *edited by L. Adams and A. Guz*
91. Pulmonary Rehabilitation, *edited by A. P. Fishman*
92. Acute Respiratory Failure in Chronic Obstructive Pulmonary Disease, *edited by J.-P. Derenne, W. A. Whitelaw, and T. Similowski*
93. Environmental Impact on the Airways: From Injury to Repair, *edited by J. Chrétien and D. Dusser*
94. Inhalation Aerosols: Physical and Biological Basis for Therapy, *edited by A. J. Hickey*
95. Tissue Oxygen Deprivation: From Molecular to Integrated Function, *edited by G. G. Haddad and G. Lister*
96. The Genetics of Asthma, *edited by S. B. Liggett and D. A. Meyers*
97. Inhaled Glucocorticoids in Asthma: Mechanisms and Clinical Actions, *edited by R. P. Schleimer, W. W. Busse, and P. M. O'Byrne*
98. Nitric Oxide and the Lung, *edited by W. M. Zapol and K. D. Bloch*
99. Primary Pulmonary Hypertension, *edited by L. J. Rubin and S. Rich*
100. Lung Growth and Development, *edited by J. A. McDonald*
101. Parasitic Lung Diseases, *edited by A. A. F. Mahmoud*
102. Lung Macrophages and Dendritic Cells in Health and Disease, *edited by M. F. Lipscomb and S. W. Russell*
103. Pulmonary and Cardiac Imaging, *edited by C. Chiles and C. E. Putman*
104. Gene Therapy for Diseases of the Lung, *edited by K. L. Brigham*
105. Oxygen, Gene Expression, and Cellular Function, *edited by L. Biadasz Clerch and D. J. Massaro*
106. Beta$_2$-Agonists in Asthma Treatment, *edited by R. Pauwels and P. M. O'Byrne*
107. Inhalation Delivery of Therapeutic Peptides and Proteins, *edited by A. L. Adjei and P. K. Gupta*
108. Asthma in the Elderly, *edited by R. A. Barbee and J. W. Bloom*
109. Treatment of the Hospitalized Cystic Fibrosis Patient, *edited by D. M. Orenstein and R. C. Stern*
110. Asthma and Immunological Diseases in Pregnancy and Early Infancy, *edited by M. Schatz, R. S. Zeiger, and H. N. Claman*
111. Dyspnea, *edited by D. A. Mahler*
112. Proinflammatory and Antiinflammatory Peptides, *edited by S. I. Said*
113. Self-Management of Asthma, *edited by H. Kotses and A. Harver*
114. Eicosanoids, Aspirin, and Asthma, *edited by A. Szczeklik, R. J. Gryglewski, and J. R. Vane*
115. Fatal Asthma, *edited by A. L. Sheffer*
116. Pulmonary Edema, *edited by M. A. Matthay and D. H. Ingbar*
117. Inflammatory Mechanisms in Asthma, *edited by S. T. Holgate and W. W. Busse*
118. Physiological Basis of Ventilatory Support, *edited by J. J. Marini and A. S. Slutsky*

119. Human Immunodeficiency Virus and the Lung, *edited by M. J. Rosen and J. M. Beck*
120. Five-Lipoxygenase Products in Asthma, *edited by J. M. Drazen, S.-E. Dahlén, and T. H. Lee*
121. Complexity in Structure and Function of the Lung, *edited by M. P. Hlastala and H. T. Robertson*
122. Biology of Lung Cancer, *edited by M. A. Kane and P. A. Bunn, Jr.*
123. Rhinitis: Mechanisms and Management, *edited by R. M. Naclerio, S. R. Durham, and N. Mygind*
124. Lung Tumors: Fundamental Biology and Clinical Management, *edited by C. Brambilla and E. Brambilla*
125. Interleukin-5: From Molecule to Drug Target for Asthma, *edited by C. J. Sanderson*
126. Pediatric Asthma, *edited by S. Murphy and H. W. Kelly*
127. Viral Infections of the Respiratory Tract, *edited by R. Dolin and P. F. Wright*
128. Air Pollutants and the Respiratory Tract, *edited by D. L. Swift and W. M. Foster*
129. Gastroesophageal Reflux Disease and Airway Disease, *edited by M. R. Stein*
130. Exercise-Induced Asthma, *edited by E. R. McFadden, Jr.*
131. LAM and Other Diseases Characterized by Smooth Muscle Proliferation, *edited by J. Moss*
132. The Lung at Depth, *edited by C. E. G. Lundgren and J. N. Miller*
133. Regulation of Sleep and Circadian Rhythms, *edited by F. W. Turek and P. C. Zee*
134. Anticholinergic Agents in the Upper and Lower Airways, *edited by S. L. Spector*
135. Control of Breathing in Health and Disease, *edited by M. D. Altose and Y. Kawakami*
136. Immunotherapy in Asthma, *edited by J. Bousquet and H. Yssel*
137. Chronic Lung Disease in Early Infancy, *edited by R. D. Bland and J. J. Coalson*
138. Asthma's Impact on Society: The Social and Economic Burden, *edited by K. B. Weiss, A. S. Buist, and S. D. Sullivan*
139. New and Exploratory Therapeutic Agents for Asthma, *edited by M. Yeadon and Z. Diamant*
140. Multimodality Treatment of Lung Cancer, *edited by A. T. Skarin*
141. Cytokines in Pulmonary Disease: Infection and Inflammation, *edited by S. Nelson and T. R. Martin*
142. Diagnostic Pulmonary Pathology, *edited by P. T. Cagle*
143. Particle–Lung Interactions, *edited by P. Gehr and J. Heyder*
144. Tuberculosis: A Comprehensive International Approach, Second Edition, Revised and Expanded, *edited by L. B. Reichman and E. S. Hershfield*
145. Combination Therapy for Asthma and Chronic Obstructive Pulmonary Disease, *edited by R. J. Martin and M. Kraft*
146. Sleep Apnea: Implications in Cardiovascular and Cerebrovascular Disease, *edited by T. D. Bradley and J. S. Floras*
147. Sleep and Breathing in Children: A Developmental Approach, *edited by G. M. Loughlin, J. L. Carroll, and C. L. Marcus*

138. Asthma's Impact on Society: The Social and Economic Burden, *edited by K. B. Weiss, A. S. Buist, and S. D. Sullivan*
139. New and Exploratory Therapeutic Agents for Asthma, *edited by M. Yeadon and Z. Diamant*
140. Multimodality Treatment of Lung Cancer, *edited by A. T. Skarin*
141. Cytokines in Pulmonary Disease: Infection and Inflammation, *edited by S. Nelson and T. R. Martin*
142. Diagnostic Pulmonary Pathology, *edited by P. T. Cagle*
143. Particle–Lung Interactions, *edited by P. Gehr and J. Heyder*
144. Tuberculosis: A Comprehensive International Approach, Second Edition, Revised and Expanded, *edited by L. B. Reichman and E. S. Hershfield*
145. Combination Therapy for Asthma and Chronic Obstructive Pulmonary Disease, *edited by R. J. Martin and M. Kraft*
146. Sleep Apnea: Implications in Cardiovascular and Cerebrovascular Disease, *edited by T. D. Bradley and J. S. Floras*
147. Sleep and Breathing in Children: A Developmental Approach, *edited by G. M. Loughlin, J. L. Carroll, and C. L. Marcus*
148. Pulmonary and Peripheral Gas Exchange in Health and Disease, *edited by J. Roca, R. Rodriguez-Roisen, and P. D. Wagner*
149. Lung Surfactants: Basic Science and Clinical Applications, *edited by R. H. Notter*
150. Nosocomial Pneumonia, *edited by W. R. Jarvis*

ADDITIONAL VOLUMES IN PREPARATION

Environmental Asthma, *edited by R. K. Bush*

Fetal Origins of Cardiovascular and Lung Disease, *edited by D. J. P. Barker*

Long-Term Mechanical Ventilation, *edited by N. S. Hill*

Airway Remodeling, *edited by P. Howarth, J. Wilson, J. Bousquet, and R. Pauwels*

Asthma and Respiratory Infections, *edited by D. P. Skoner*

Respiratory-Circulatory Interactions in Health and Disease, *edited by S. M. Scharf, M. R. Pinsky, and S. Magder*

The opinions expressed in these volumes do not necessarily represent the views of the National Institutes of Health.

PULMONARY AND PERIPHERAL GAS EXCHANGE IN HEALTH AND DISEASE

Edited by

Josep Roca
Roberto Rodriguez-Roisin

*Hospital Clínic
University of Barcelona
Barcelona, Spain*

Peter D. Wagner

*University of California, San Diego
La Jolla, California*

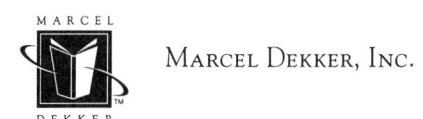

Marcel Dekker, Inc. New York · Basel

ISBN: 0-8247-0335-9

This book is printed on acid-free paper.

Headquarters
Marcel Dekker, Inc.
270 Madison Avenue, New York, NY 10016
tel: 212-696-9000; fax: 212-685-4540

Eastern Hemisphere Distribution
Marcel Dekker AG
Hutgasse 4, Postfach 812, CH-4001 Basel, Switzerland
tel: 41-61-261-8482; fax: 41-61-261-8896

World Wide Web
http://www.dekker.com

The publisher offers discounts on this book when ordered in bulk quantities. For more information, write to Special Sales/Professional Marketing at the headquarters address above.

Copyright © 2000 by Marcel Dekker, Inc. All Rights Reserved.

Neither this book nor any part may be reproduced or transmitted in any form or by any means, electronic or mechanical, including photocopying, microfilming, and recording, or by any information storage and retrieval system, without permission in writing from the publisher.

Current printing (last digit):
10 9 8 7 6 5 4 3 2 1

PRINTED IN THE UNITED STATES OF AMERICA

Introduction

> In the tidal flux, the lobed pair avidly
>   grasp the invisible ...
> Braids of vessels and cartilage descend
>   in vanishing smallness,
> to grape clusters of alveoli, the sheerest
>   of membranes, where oxygen
> crosses the infinite cellular web, where air turns
>   to blood, spirit to flesh ...
>
> *Alice Jones* (1)

These verses from the poem "The Lungs" capture the essence of this book. Just see the last verse:

> according to need, so even the cells in the darkest
>   corners can breathe.

Gas exchange, first in the lung and then in the tissues, has been, and is, the most critical function of the lung in health and disease. Over the past quarter-century, we have witnessed an amazing explosion of knowledge about the biology of cells and subcellular elements in the lung and elsewhere. Genes that regulate physiological processes have been uncovered and sometimes manipulated to correct their malfunction. This is truly wonderful!

But let us never forget that if it were not for the "invisible"—the oxygen that flows through "braids of vessels"—the "darkest corners" would remain dark forever and would not be the source of life.

This series of monographs has frequently reported on gas exchange since its inaugural book in 1976, but never as comprehensively as now. Indeed, in this volume, pulmonary gas exchange is coupled with gas exchange in the periphery. Malfunctions in one of these two sites and how each site impacts on the other are fully explored and discussed.

The reader need only see the list of contributors and editors to be assured of the authoritativeness of this book. Some may believe that integrative physiology and pathophysiology are outdated. This book shows how vibrant this field is and how critical it is to a full and practical understanding of human pathology.

As the Executive Editor of this series, I am grateful to Drs. Roca, Rodriguez-Roisin, and Wagner, and their chapter authors for the opportunity to present this volume to the readership.

Claude Lenfant, M.D.
Bethesda, Maryland

Reference

1. Jones A. Verse and Universe. In: Brown K, ed. Poems About Science and Mathematics. Minneapolis, Minnesota: Milkweed Publications, 1998.

Preface

Survival depends on availability of oxygen to all body tissues and cells. Research has revealed the detailed pathways for oxygen transport between the environment and the tissues, but virtually all work has examined just individual parts of this pathway. For example, we know much about how lung diseases disturb gas exchange in the lung, and we are learning more every year about oxygen transport to and within specific organs and tissues such as brain, heart, gut, and muscle.

However, the body works as an integrated system. For oxygen, this means that, for example, disturbed gas exchange in damaged lungs will have a potentially negative effect on oxygen transport to the various organs and tissues. Conversely, abnormal function of body tissues may affect the composition of the venous blood returning to the lungs and the distribution of blood flow among organs. This will in turn affect the way in which the lungs are able to take up oxygen.

The overarching theme of this book is therefore to take gas exchange to this integrated level—to better understand how abnormalities in any one organ's ability to transport and utilize oxygen affect the function and oxygen exchange characteristics of the other organs. The rationale for this theme should be evident in that understanding oxygen availability in such a complex system as the whole organism requires examination of how the oxygen transport system works integratively—how all the parts come together even under duress—to permit continued survival.

In this volume, we have consciously used examples from the world of normal physiology—exercise and altitude, in particular—to illustrate the integrative principles at work in health. Application to disease is also addressed, but it becomes evident that, in disease at least, we have a long way to go before we can comfortably say we understand how the body does (or does not) make sufficient O_2 available for survival. This compendium clearly lays out current physiological thinking, showcases our best attempts at understanding disease processes as they affect O_2 transport, and, most importantly, indicates the direction for future research.

Josep Roca
Roberto Rodriguez-Roisin
Peter D. Wagner

Contributors

Alvar G. N. Agustí, M.D.   Head and Director of Research, Department of Pulmonary Medicine, Hospital Universitari Son Dureta, Palma de Mallorca, Spain

Joan Albert Barberà, M.D.   Department of Respiratory Medicine, Hospital Clínic, University of Barcelona, Barcelona, Spain

Ainat Beniaminovitz, M.D.   Department of Medicine, New York Presbyterian Hospital, Columbia University, New York, New York

Mayer Brezis, M.D.   Professor of Medicine, The Hebrew University Medical School, and Department of Medicine, Hadassah University Hospital, Mount Scopus, Jerusalem, Israel

Stephen M. Cain, Ph.D.   Department of Physiology and Biophysics, University of Alabama at Birmingham, Birmingham, Alabama

A. B. Hamish Crawford, M.B., Ch.B., F.R.A.C.P.   Department of Respiratory Medicine, Liverpool and Westmead Hospitals, Sydney, Australia

Scott E. Curtis, M.D.[*]   Associate Professor of Pediatrics, Physiology, and Biophysics, Department of Pediatrics, University of Alabama at Birmingham, Birmingham, Alabama

Charles G. Gallagher   Department of Respiratory Medicine, St. Vincent's University Hospital, Dublin, Ireland

Robb Glenny   Division of Pulmonary and Critical Care Medicine, Department of Medicine, Washington University, Seattle, Washington

---

[*]*Current affiliation*: Department of Pediatric Critical Care, DeVos Children's Hospital, Grand Rapids, Michigan.

Göran Hedenstierna, M.D., Ph.D. Professor/Chairman, Department of Medical Sciences, Clinical Physiology, Uppsala University, Uppsala, Sweden

Samuel Noam Heyman, M.D. Associate Professor of Medicine, The Hebrew University Medical School, and Department of Medicine, Hadassah University Hospital, Mount Scopus, Jerusalem, Israel

Peter W. Hochachka, O.C., Ph.D., D.Sc., F.R.S.C. Professor, Departments of Zoology, Radiology, and Sports Medicine, University of British Columbia, Vancouver, British Columbia, Canada

Robert L. Johnson, Jr., M.D. Professor of Medicine, Department of Internal Medicine, University of Texas Southwestern Medical Center, Dallas, Texas

Donna M. Mancini, M.D. Associate Professor of Medicine, Department of Medicine, New York Presbyterian Hospital, Columbia University, New York, New York

Christian Mélot, M.D., Ph.D., M.Sci. Biostat. Department of Intensive Care, Erasme Hospital, Free University of Brussels, Brussels, Belgium

Geoffrey E. Moore, M.D. Assistant Professor of Medicine, Department of Internal Medicine, University of Pittsburgh, Pittsburgh, Pennsylvania

Timothy I. Musch, Ph.D. Departments of Kinesiology, Anatomy, and Physiology, Kansas State University, Manhattan, Kansas

Robert Naeije, M.D., Ph.D. Professor of Physiology and Medicine, Departments of Physiology and Intensive Care, Erasme Hospital, Free University of Brussels, Brussels, Belgium

Claude A. Piantadosi, M.D. Professor of Medicine, Department of Medicine (Pulmonary and Critical Care), Duke University Medical Center, Durham, North Carolina

David C. Poole, Ph.D. Professor, Departments of Kinesiology, Anatomy, and Physiology, Kansas State University, Manhattan, Kansas

Christian Putensen, M.D. Professor of Anesthesiology and Intensive Care Medicine, Director of Intensive Care Medicine, Division of Intensive Care Medicine, Department of Anesthesiology and Intensive Care Medicine, University of Bonn, Bonn, Germany

Josep Roca, M.D. Associate Professor of Medicine and Chief of Section, Department of Respiratory Medicine, Hospital Clínic, University of Barcelona, Barcelona, Spain

Roberto Rodriguez-Roisin, M.D., F.R.C.P.(E) Professor and Chairman of Medicine, Chief of Service, Department of Respiratory Medicine, Hospital Clínic, University of Barcelona, Barcelona, Spain

James A. Russell, A.B., M.D., F.R.C.P.(C) Professor and Chair, Department of Medicine, St. Paul's Hospital, Vancouver, British Columbia, Canada

Robert B. Schoene, M.D. Professor of Medicine, Department of Medicine, University of Washington, Seattle, Washington

Paul T. Schumacker, Ph.D. Professor, Department of Medicine, The University of Chicago, Chicago, Illinois

Steven S. Segal, Ph.D. The John B. Pierce Laboratory and Department of Cellular and Molecular Physiology, Yale University School of Medicine, New Haven, Connecticut

Ari Uusaro, M.D., Ph.D., M.H.Sc. (Epid) Senior Attending Specialist, Division of Intensive Care, Department of Anesthesiology and Intensive Care, Kuopio University Hospital, Kuopio, Finland

Peter D. Wagner, M.D. Professor of Medicine and Bioengineering, Department of Medicine, University of California, San Diego, La Jolla, California

Keith R. Walley, M.D. Professor of Medicine, Department of Medicine, University of British Columbia, Vancouver, British Columbia, Canada

John B. West, M.D., Ph.D., D.Sc. Professor of Medicine and Physiology, Department of Medicine, University of California, San Diego, La Jolla, California

Robert M. Winslow, M.D. Sangart, Inc., San Diego, California

Iven H. Young, M.B., B.S., Ph.D., F.R.A.C.P. Clinical Associate Professor and Head, Department of Respiratory Medicine, Royal Prince Alfred Hospital, Sydney, Australia

Contents

Introduction Claude Lenfant		*iii*
Preface		*v*
Contributors		*vii*

Part One. BASIC PRINCIPLES

1. Pulmonary and Peripheral Gas Exchange and Their Interactions — **1**

Josep Roca, Roberto Rodriguez-Roisin, and Peter D. Wagner

I.	Introduction	1
II.	The Gas Transport Pathway: Environment to Mitochondria	2
III.	Mechanisms of O_2 Transport Impairment in the Lungs and Tissues	22
IV.	Integration of Lungs and Tissues in Gas Transport and Exchange	23
V.	Conclusion	25
	References	25

2. Oxygen and Metabolic Homeostasis During Large-Scale Change in Tissue Work Rates — **29**

Peter W. Hochachka

I.	Contrasting Requirements of Homeostasis and Tissue Work	29
II.	Human Muscle Metabolism During Work	30
III.	Widespread Stability of Metabolites During Changes in Metabolic Rates	36
IV.	Demands of Homeostasis Take Precedence During Changes in Work Rates of Tissues	37
V.	Oxygen Delivery and Metabolic Regulation	39
VI.	Transducing the Oxygen Signal in Working Tissue	39

VII.	An Unsolved Regulatory Problem	40
VIII.	Summary	41
	References	41

3. Experimental Approaches to the Study of Gas Exchange   45

Robert L. Johnson, Jr., and Scott E. Curtis

I.	Introduction	45
II.	Total Respiratory Gas Exchange	46
III.	Gas Exchange in the Lung	49
IV.	Peripheral Gas Exchange	88
V.	Summary	107
	References	108

Part Two. PULMONARY GAS EXCHANGE

4. Gas Exchange in Health: Rest, Exercise, and Aging   121

Robb Glenny, Peter D. Wagner, Josep Roca, and Roberto Rodriguez-Roisin

I.	Heterogeneity of Pulmonary Gas Exchange at Rest	122
II.	Determinants of O_2 and CO_2 Exchange at Rest	136
III.	Pulmonary Gas Exchange During Exercise	137
IV.	Effects of Aging on Pulmonary Gas Exchange	138
V.	Summary	143
	References	143

5. Gas Exchange in Health: Altitude and Microgravity   149

John B. West

I.	Introduction	149
II.	High Altitude	149
III.	Microgravity	162
	References	171

6. Anesthesia and Gas Exchange   177

Göran Hedenstierna

I.	Introduction	177
II.	Oxygenation and Venous Admixture	178
III.	Distributions of Ventilation and Perfusion	179
IV.	Alveolar Hypoventilation and Diffusion Limitation	181
V.	Morphologic Correlates of Shunt and Low $\dot{V}_A/\dot{Q}$	182

VI.	Prevention of Atelectasis During Anesthesia	185
VII.	Hypoxic Pulmonary Vasoconstriction	189
VIII.	Obstructive Lung Disease	190
IX.	One-Lung Ventilation	191
X.	Postoperative Lung Function	192
XI.	Conclusion	193
	References	193

7. Asthma — 199

Iven H. Young and A. B. Hamish Crawford

I.	Introduction	199
II.	Arterial Blood Gas Abnormalities	201
III.	Topographical Distribution of Ventilation and Blood Flow	206
IV.	Functional Maldistribution of Ventilation	208
V.	Functional Distributions of $\dot{V}_A/\dot{Q}$ Ratios	210
VI.	Summary and Conclusions	221
	References	223

8. Chronic Obstructive Pulmonary Disease — 229

Joan Albert Barberà

I.	Introduction	229
II.	Physiological Basis of Abnormal Gas Exchange in COPD	230
III.	Structure and Function Correlations	237
IV.	Gas Exchange in the Natural History of COPD	241
V.	Gas Exchange During Exercise	246
VI.	Effect of Therapeutic Interventions on Gas Exchange	250
VII.	Conclusions	256
	References	256

9. Interstitial Lung Diseases — 263

Alvar G. N. Agustí

I.	Introduction	263
II.	Resting Pulmonary Gas Exchange	264
III.	Pulmonary Gas Exchange During Exercise	265
IV.	Integrated View: The Mechanisms of Abnormal Exercise Performance in ILD	271
V.	Relationship Between Diffusing Capacity for Carbon Monoxide and the Mechanisms of Abnormal Pulmonary Gas Exchange in ILD	278

	VI. Conclusions	280
	References	280

10. Pulmonary Vascular Diseases   285

Christian Mélot and Robert Naeije

I.	Introduction	285
II.	Acute Pulmonary Arterial Obstruction: Pulmonary Embolism	286
III.	Chronic Pulmonary Vascular Obstruction	296
IV.	Conclusions	299
	References	300

11. Acute Lung Injury   303

Christian Putensen

I.	Introduction	303
II.	Acute Injury of the Lungs	304
III.	Pulmonary Gas Exchange in ARDS	305
IV.	Therapeutic Concepts to Improve $\dot{V}_A/\dot{Q}$ Matching in ARDS	313
V.	Conclusion	322
	References	323

Part Three.   **GAS EXCHANGE IN THE PERIPHERY: ORGANS AND SYSTEMS**

12. Whole-Body Oxygen Transport and Use   331

Stephen M. Cain and Scott E. Curtis

I.	Introduction	331
II.	The Interrelationship Between Oxygen Transport and Use in Health	332
III.	Matching of Oxygen Transport to Use in Health	337
IV.	Matching of Oxygen Transport to Use in Disease	347
V.	Summary	352
	References	353

13. Gas Exchange in the Heart   359

Keith R. Walley

I.	Introduction	359
II.	Coronary Circulation	362

III.	Determinants of Myocardial Oxygen Demand	363
IV.	Determinants of Myocardial Oxygen Supply	368
V.	Myocardial Oxygen Extraction	371
VI.	Relationship of Blood Flow Heterogeneity to Oxygen Extraction	373
VII.	Myocardial Oxygen Extraction in Sepsis	374
VIII.	Myocardial Oxygen Extraction in Coronary Occlusive Disease	375
IX.	Summary	376
	References	376

14. Localization and Dispersion of Oxygen Demand and Supply in Skeletal Muscle — 383

Steven S. Segal

I.	Introduction	383
II.	Muscle Blood Flow and Oxygen Uptake	385
III.	Oxygen Flux Within Muscle Fibers	387
IV.	Oxygen Flux from Microvessels to Muscle Fibers	389
V.	Intramuscular Dispersion of Metabolic Demand	396
VI.	Conclusions	400
	References	401

15. The Gut: Oxygen Transport and Gas Exchange Function — 409

Paul T. Schumacker

I.	Introduction	409
II.	Structure and Function of the Gut Vascular Anatomy	410
III.	Vascular Models of the Gut Microcirculation	411
IV.	Role of Extrinsic Autonomic Neurohumoral Control of Gut Blood Flow	412
V.	Metabolic Control of the Gut Microcirculation	413
VI.	Oxygen Delivery—Consumption Relationships	414
VII.	Physiological Shunting of Oxygen in the Gut Microcirculation	416
VIII.	Perfusion Heterogeneity in the Gut Microcirculation	420
IX.	Pathophysiology of Gas Transport	423
X.	Mechanisms of Impaired Tissue Oxygen Extraction	425
XI.	Pathological Oxygen Supply Dependency in Critical Illness and Sepsis	427
XII.	Summary	429
	References	430

16. The Brain — 435

Claude A. Piantadosi

I.	Cerebral Blood Flow and Metabolism	435
II.	Neurovascular Coupling: The Link Between Cerebral Blood Flow, Metabolism, and Function	437
III.	Cerebral Hypoxia	443
IV.	Summary	444
	References	445

17. The Kidney — 447

Samuel Noam Heyman and Mayer Brezis

I.	Introduction	447
II.	The Renal Circulation	448
III.	Intrarenal Oxygen Gradient	451
IV.	Outer Medullary Oxygen Balance	451
V.	Control of Medullary Oxygen Balance	453
VI.	Acute Tubular Necrosis and Distal Tubular Injury in Humans	457
VII.	Distal Tubular Injury: Experimental Evidence for Oxygen Insufficiency	457
VIII.	Medical Conditions Predisposing to Acute Tubular Necrosis: Implications for Medullary Oxygen Imbalance	458
IX.	Animal Models of Acute Renal Failure with Hypoxic Outer Medullary Necrosis	460
X.	Disparate Mechanisms for Hypoxic Injury in Different Nephron Segments	462
XI.	Medullary Hypoxia and Chronic Tubulointerstitial Disease	462
XII.	Medullary Oxygen Balance and the Prevention/Treatment of Acute Tubular Necrosis	463
XIII.	Control of Erythropoietin Production: A Role for Renal Parenchymal Oxygen Insufficiency	464
	References	465

Part Four. INTEGRATED GAS EXCHANGE RESPONSES

18. Pulmonary and Peripheral Gas Exchange During Exercise — 469

David C. Poole and Timothy I. Musch

I.	Introduction	469
II.	Pulmonary and Muscle Gas Exchange	470

III.	Cardiovascular System	488
IV.	Muscle Microcirculation	495
V.	Maximum Oxygen Consumption in Health and Disease	509
VI.	Summary and Conclusions	516
	References	517

19. Gas Exchange in Lung and Muscle at High Altitude 525

Robert B. Schoene

I.	Introduction	525
II.	The Problem	526
III.	The Lung	526
IV.	Gas Exchange in the Tissues	535
V.	High Altitude	536
VI.	Blood Flow	537
VII.	The Role of Hemoglobin	540
VIII.	Oxygen-Hemoglobin Affinity	542
IX.	Diffusion of Oxygen from Blood to the Tissue	543
X.	Summary	546
	References	547

20. Systemic Gas Exchange and Exercise Performance in Chronic Pulmonary Disease 553

Charles G. Gallagher

I.	Introduction	553
II.	Respiratory Responses	555
III.	Cardiovascular Responses	565
IV.	Skeletal Muscle Responses	566
V.	Exercise Limitation	567
VI.	Conclusion	573
	References	573

21. Cardiopulmonary and Peripheral Vascular Alterations in Chronic Congestive Heart Failure 581

Donna M. Mancini and Ainat Beniaminovitz

I.	Introduction	581
II.	Pathophysiology of Heart Failure: Cardiac Adaptations	582
III.	Peripheral Vascular and Skeletal Muscle Adaptations in Congestive Heart Failure	585
IV.	Pulmonary Adaptation in Congestive Heart Failure	594

	V. Exercise Training in Congestive Heart Failure	602
	References	606
22.	**Role of Hemoglobin in the Delivery of Oxygen to Tissues**	**617**
	Robert M. Winslow	
	I. Introduction	617
	II. Autoregulation of Tissue Oxygen Delivery	629
	III. Nitric Oxide as the Endothelium-Derived Relaxing Factor	632
	IV. Cell-Free Hemoglobin: New Tools to Study Oxygen Transport	634
	V. Summary and Hypothesis: The OEC Is a Critical Link in Oxygen Signal Transduction	640
	References	641
23.	**Integrated Gas Exchange Response: Chronic Renal Failure**	**649**
	Geoffrey E. Moore	
	I. Introduction	649
	II. Oxygen Transport Factors Affecting Aerobic Capacity	653
	III. Integrated Oxygen Transport	662
	IV. Interactions Between Systems	667
	V. Systemic Factors	668
	VI. Conclusions	673
	References	676
24.	**Multiple Organ Failure**	**685**
	Ari Uusaro and James A. Russell	
	I. Introduction	685
	II. Definitions and Epidemiology of Multiple Organ Dysfunction/Failure	685
	III. Hypothesis	687
	IV. Mechanisms of Imbalance Between Oxygen Delivery and Consumption that Could Cause Multiple System Organ Failure	689
	V. The Oxygen Delivery/Consumption Relationship: Physiology	695
	VI. Evidence for Occult Tissue Hypoxia as a Cause of Multiple System Organ Failure	697
	VII. Evidence Against Occult Tissue Hypoxia as a Cause of Multiple System Organ Failure	708

VIII.	Alternative Mechanisms of Multiple Organ Failure	723
IX.	Facilitative Role for Tissue Hypoxia in MSOF	725
X.	Summary	725
	References	727

Author Index   *743*
Subject Index   *805*

PULMONARY AND PERIPHERAL GAS EXCHANGE IN HEALTH AND DISEASE

1

Pulmonary and Peripheral Gas Exchange and Their Interactions

JOSEP ROCA and
ROBERTO RODRIGUEZ-ROISIN

Hospital Clínic, University of Barcelona
Barcelona, Spain

PETER D. WAGNER

University of California, San Diego
La Jolla, California

I. Introduction

Perhaps nothing is as critical to survival as the successful transport of O_2 from the air we breathe to the various tissue mitochondria that use O_2 for energy production. There is an abundance of evidence to support the argument that limits to O_2 transport define maximal organismal function during many forms of exercise in health: An endurance athlete cannot become elite without extraordinary O_2 transport capacity; maximal exercise is severely curtailed with increasing altitude during mountain climbing. Evidence is also emerging to support the criticality of O_2 transport at the other end of the metabolic scale: Poor organismal function in many disease states is also, at least in part, a result of interference to O_2 transport. In particular, in critically ill patients with severe acute disease affecting usually several key organs, O_2 use is found to vary with O_2 supply. This is poorly understood, largely because of a lack of adequate tools to study the problem. Explanations could lie in O_2 transport (via diffusion-limited O_2 unloading in the tissues or via nonuniform distribution of blood flow between or within organs). Alternatively, tissues could regulate their O_2 consumption in response to O_2 availability.

Thus, there still remains considerable uncertainty in the basic understanding of the mechanisms of O_2 transport limitation and in the relation between O_2 transport, O_2 use, and other aspects of metabolism such as enzyme function and substrate/metabolite transport. Consequently, understanding the overall process of gas exchange between the environment and the mitochondria is complex and integrative. Integration is manifest within the many steps of the O_2 (and CO_2) transport pathways between air and mitochondria. Another axis of integration relates to distribution of blood flow and O_2 supply, among as well as within, different tissues. Yet another axis of integration requires biochemical processes of cell metabolism to be coupled with biophysical processes of O_2 and CO_2 transport and metabolite exchanges.

The purpose of this chapter is to provide some integrative insight into the workings of the O_2 transport system in health and disease. Here we illustrate how it is no longer tenable to analyze gas exchange in the lungs without regard for gas exchange in the tissues. When considering tissue gas exchange in any organ, it is just as important to allow simultaneously for pulmonary gas exchange. Furthermore, when O_2 transport is the constraint on oxygen consumption per unit time ($\dot{V}O_2$), all components of the O_2 transport pathway are linked such that a change in any one component would affect $\dot{V}O_2$. Thus, there is no single limiting factor to $\dot{V}O_2$ in such circumstances (1).

If the reader can achieve a clear understanding of these mutually dependent gas exchange processes, the reasons for their interdependence, and the concepts that link the components of the O_2 transport pathway, this chapter will have achieved its objective. The major emphasis is on the transport of O_2 because most is known about this gas compared with CO_2. Because the transport pathways for these two gases are in essence the same, the same general concepts should apply to both gases. However, there are differences in their behavior and control largely because of the intimate relation between CO_2 and H^+ regulation, the larger tissue storage capacity for CO_2 compared with O_2, and the generally greater dependence of CO_2 transport on ventilation.

We begin with a description of the structural and functional components of the transport pathway, indicate their workings under resting conditions in health, and then use the paradigm of exercise to dissect the maximal function of each component and show their interactions. Finally, the spectrum of aberrations in gas transport in disease is addressed and analyzed on the framework of understanding gained from these exercise-based studies in health.

This approach clearly touches on many of the topics addressed in the chapters that make up the bulk of this book. However, here they are used illustratively to define principles, whereas in subsequent chapters they are the focal point of the discussion and are explored in much greater detail.

II. The Gas Transport Pathway: Environment to Mitochondria

The transport pathway has been described frequently and is well defined. Perhaps the most readable account is that of Weibel (2). Our version is shown in Figure 1,

STRUCTURE   FUNCTION

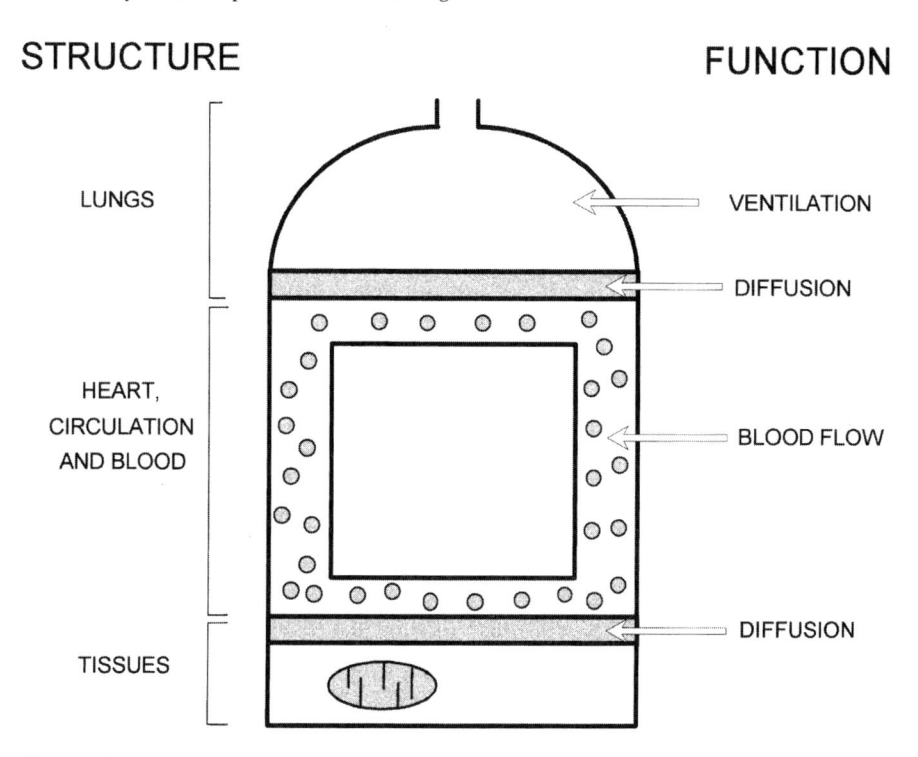

```
LUNGS                                    VENTILATION
                                         DIFFUSION

HEART,
CIRCULATION                              BLOOD FLOW
AND BLOOD

                                         DIFFUSION
TISSUES
```

Figure 1 Major elements of the oxygen transport pathway. To move oxygen from the air to the mitochondria requires the integrated efforts of several tissues or organs, as indicated, and several major convective and diffusive processes as well. Note that for simplicity, nonuniformity of ventilation/perfusion ratios in the lung and/or metabolism/perfusion ratios in the tissues has been omitted, although perhaps in health, and certainly in disease, nonuniformity in both locations may be of considerable importance.

which depicts several organs and tissues connected by the circulation. The lungs are the interface between the air and blood. The heart and vascular tree pump and distribute that blood to the various tissues of the body, and then the blood is returned to the lungs to be renewed by giving up CO_2 and taking on O_2. In addition to showing these structures, Figure 1 illustrates the principal functional activities at each step. The following sections define the different steps O_2 undergoes from the environment to the tissue mitochondria.

A. Ventilation

Ventilation delivers O_2 from the air to the alveoli and simultaneously transports CO_2 from the alveoli to the air. Ventilation is a transport process that is fueled by two mechanisms: convection and diffusion. Movement of air from the mouth along the first 17 or so airway generations to the alveolated gas exchange region is dominated by convective flow of air along a hydrostatic pressure gradient: Ohm's law, in effect. Because the volume of this part of the airway system is generally much less than the volume of air inhaled with each breath, this so-called anatomical dead-space volume is well washed out with each breath. In contrast, beyond airway generation 17 or so, and onward to the alveoli at generation 23 (3), diffusion becomes increasingly important as a transport process. Although convective air movement still occurs here, the net forward convective velocity is very low because of the exponential increase in total airway cross-sectional area (caused, in turn, by the essentially dichotomous branching of the airways). Moreover, each breath does not completely empty and then fill the alveoli: End-expiratory lung volume is 3 to 4 L in humans, whereas tidal volume is usually only approximately 500 mL. Thus, each breath must be considered as 'topping up'' alveolar O_2 stores such that the air from each breath must mix with air already present in the alveolar spaces. This combination (low convective forward velocity and the requirement to mix some 500 mL into a much larger gas volume with each breath) means that the convective process no longer suffices for transport and diffusive mixing becomes necessary. Current experimental evidence supports the conclusion that gas mixing by diffusion is sufficiently rapid to assure virtually perfect mixing each breath, at least in health (4).

To be fair, measurable effects of noninstantaneous diffusive mixing at the alveolar level have been demonstrated (5), principally by comparing gases of different molecular weight inhaled together. Such studies show the lighter molecules mixing faster than the heavier ones, but when considering how much of an effect would this have on lowering arterial partial pressure of oxygen (Po_2; compared with perfect diffusive mixing), the answer is only a few millimeters of mercury (6).

The most important mechanism of ventilatory gas transport is, therefore, the convective component. The branching airway structure then immediately raises the question of how inhaled air is distributed among the 300 million or so alveoli. Despite many processes that would tend to disperse ventilation in a nonuniform manner, and as a result impair overall pulmonary gas exchange, it remains a remarkable finding that in health, ventilation distribution and its counterpart, blood flow, are sufficiently well distributed and well matched to one another that arterial Po_2 is usually within approximately 5 mm Hg of that expected from a perfect lung (7). However, in disease, ventilation/perfusion matching is important.

B. Ventilation/Perfusion Inequality

Ventilation/perfusion ($\dot{V}_A/\dot{Q}$) inequality is the term that is used to describe the degree to which ventilation and blood flow are not similarly distributed to the same alveoli. When $\dot{V}_A/\dot{Q}$ inequality exists, some alveoli may receive less ventilation than average, whereas others receive more. Alternatively (or in addition), blood flow may be unevenly distributed. The end result is that instead of all alveoli having the same $\dot{V}_A/\dot{Q}$ ratio (that would equal the ratio of alveolar ventilation to cardiac output for the whole lung), some have a V̇A/Q̇ ratio that is lower than average, whereas others have one that is higher than average. V̇A/Q̇ mismatching, no matter what its pathological basis, impairs gas exchange in the lungs, increasingly so the more uneven the distribution. Although arithmetically complex, the degree of interference to gas exchange can be studied in computer models (8). Because of differences in the shapes and slopes of the O_2 and CO_2 dissociation curves, the effects are generally greater for O_2 than CO_2, but both gases suffer. This V̇A/Q̇ inequality causes the arterial P_{O_2} to decrease while the average alveolar P_{O_2} increases. Similarly, arterial partial pressure of carbon dioxide (P_{CO_2}) increases while average alveolar P_{CO_2} decreases. These changes are illustrated by the simplest possible model of the problem, dividing the lungs into two "compartments." Figure 2 shows how arterial P_{O_2} would change as the distribution of ventilation is made more and more uneven between the two compartments. Importantly for these calculations, total lung ventilation and blood flow are held constant to permit the pure effects of V̇A/Q̇ inequality to be described. In most cases, patients will respond to the development of V̇A/Q̇ inequality by increasing total ventilation, cardiac output, or both in an effort to restore O_2 and CO_2 transport. Also held constant are the inspired gas O_2 and CO_2 composition and the O_2 and CO_2 levels of mixed venous

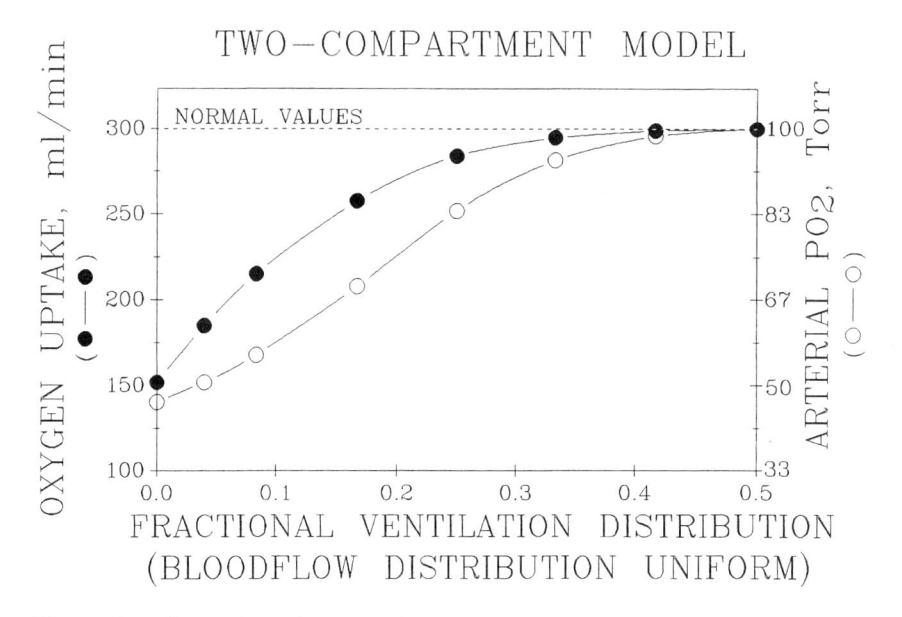

Figure 2 Effects of ventilation/perfusion inequality on gas exchange in the lungs. In this simplest case of a two-compartment lung, the distribution of ventilation is made progressively less uniform from initially equal (0.5) to completely unilateral (0.0). The oxygen uptake of the two-compartment model decreases progressively with increasingly nonuniform distribution and is mirrored by progressive arterial hypoxemia.

blood. Figure 2 also shows, under these constraints, how overall O_2 uptake by the lung must decrease as arterial blood gases deteriorate with increasing $\dot{V}_A/\dot{Q}$ mismatch. Most lung diseases can and do cause considerable $\dot{V}_A/\dot{Q}$ mismatch. If there were not ways for the body to compensate, the result would prove fatal because of the inability to provide sufficient O_2 uptake (and CO_2 removal) for metabolic requirements.

Therefore, it is important to understand how the body compensates, a remarkable process that underlies the theme of this book. The first line of defense is a passive process that intimately depends on the interaction between peripheral tissues and the lungs in the gas exchange process. As arterial P_{O_2} is reduced by $\dot{V}_A/\dot{Q}$ mismatch, the tissues still attempt to extract the required amount of O_2 from the hypoxemic blood. Unless $\dot{V}_A/\dot{Q}$ mismatch is extremely severe, this is feasible, but there is a price to pay: Venous blood returning from the tissues must have a subnormal P_{O_2} if the normal amount of O_2 is removed from hypoxemic arterial blood supplying the tissues. Accordingly, the lungs now are faced with oxygenating mixed venous blood that is more depleted of O_2 than usual and must do this in the face of continuing $\dot{V}_A/\dot{Q}$ inequality. Clearly, arterial P_{O_2} must decrease further under such circumstances (than if venous P_{O_2} had remained normal). Luckily, because mixed venous blood in health still contains 75% of the O_2 present in arterial blood, the reductions in venous P_{O_2} can be tolerated. Furthermore, as arterial and venous P_{O_2} both undergo this process, the arteriovenous difference in O_2 concentration usually can be restored to normal. This critical process then allows O_2 uptake to be restored to normal levels and accordingly permits survival. Therefore, the end result of a disease that causes $\dot{V}_A/\dot{Q}$ inequality is a decrease in both arterial and venous P_{O_2} but restoration of O_2 uptake. Correspondingly, arterial and mixed venous P_{CO_2} are both increased, and CO_2 output also can be restored to normal.

Figure 3 exemplifies the reduction in O_2 uptake and in venous and arterial P_{O_2} that occurs after development of $\dot{V}_A/\dot{Q}$ inequality, and how further reduction in arterial and venous P_{O_2} permit restoration of O_2 uptake, although the price is more severe hypoxemia than was noted from $\dot{V}_A/\dot{Q}$ mismatch alone. The importance of this passive, pulmonary-peripheral tissue interaction in gas exchange surfaces again and again in subsequent chapters.

Finally, when such events occur, several stimuli are produced that can increase both total ventilation and cardiac output. Central and peripheral chemoreceptors are important here, and the adjustment to total ventilation and cardiac output serve to improve arterial P_{O_2} and P_{CO_2}, moving them closer to normal.

All of the aforementioned arguments lead to the conclusion that the major influence of ventilation on gas transport in health is simply based on convection and, therefore, reduces rather simply to the question of the magnitude of alveolar ventilation and cardiac output in liters per minute. Other aspects of ventilation—diffusive mixing, nonuniform convective distribution—can be considered quantitatively unimportant in health. Of course, in diseases of the lungs, convective maldistribution of ventilation and blood flow often becomes a major factor in impairing

RESTORATION OF $\dot{V}O_2$ BY REDUCTION IN ARTERIAL AND MIXED VENOUS PO_2

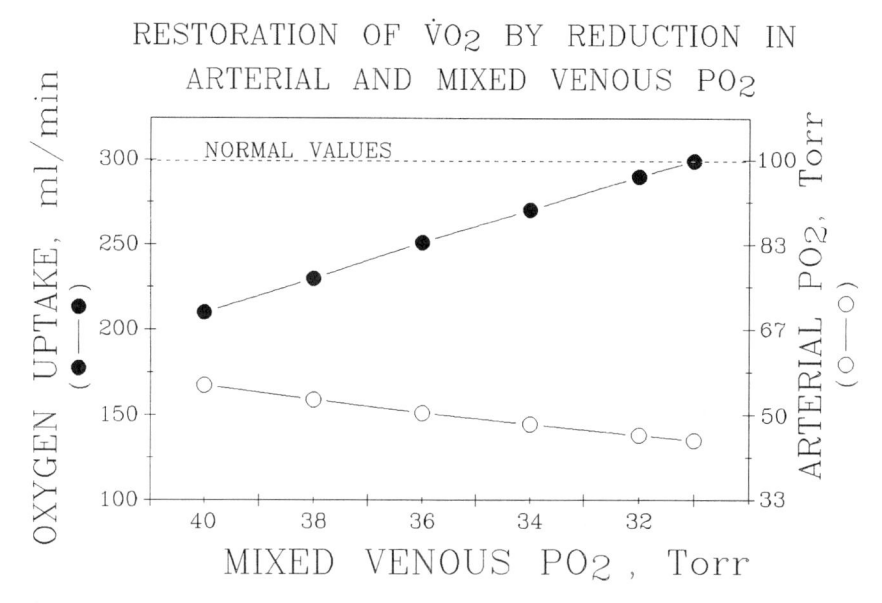

Figure 3 Compensatory value of increased O_2 extraction (reduction in mixed venous Po_2) in restoring oxygen uptake. In this case, ventilation/perfusion inequality before reduction in mixed venous Po_2 ($P\bar{v}_{O_2}$) = 40 mm Hg; left side of graph is approximately 200 mL/min, about one third below normal. Progressive reduction in mixed venous Po_2 from 40 to 31 mm Hg allows restoration of oxygen uptake (●) by using the steep portion of the oxyhemoglobin dissociation curve. However, as a consequence, arterial Po_2 (○) decreases further.

gas transport such that even if total alveolar ventilation and cardiac output are normal (or even increased), gas transport can be considerably impaired.

C. Diffusion

Diffusion of gases between alveolar gas and pulmonary capillary blood is the next major gas transport process after ventilation has delivered O_2 molecules from the air to the alveoli.

In healthy subjects at rest, the average time available to a single red cell flowing through pulmonary capillaries is 0.75 seconds, whereas it requires no more than approximately 0.25 seconds for Po_2 in the red cell to increase by diffusion from mixed venous to alveolar values (9). Thus, diffusion equilibration is normally complete at rest, with a large margin of safety. The evolutionary reason for this apparent structural excess likely lies in the survival value of exercise, where the time a red cell spends in the pulmonary capillary is greatly reduced, to approximately 0.25 seconds, similar to the time just necessary for complete exchange. Thus, during peak exercise, diffusion equilibration may or may not be complete in any given individual, depending on whether time available for gas exchange exceeds that necessary for exchange. In general, the more fit the healthy subject is, the higher the cardiac output is such that red cell transit time is reduced and diffusion equilibration can become incomplete (10). As a result, arterial P_{O_2} is less than alveolar P_{O_2}. Even when this happens, the consequences for O_2 transport are not large because arterial P_{O_2} is usually high enough to assure nearly normal hemoglobin (Hb) O_2 saturation.

In contrast, in hypoxia (i.e., at altitude), essentially all normal subjects will show significant reduction in arterial P_{O_2} less than alveolar values during exercise because of diffusion limitation (10). The reason for this effect of altitude is that gas exchange is forced to take place along the steeper portion of the O_2 Hb dissociation curve, thus reducing the driving O_2 pressures for the diffusive process compared with what is observed at sea level.

The question of whether diffusion limitation is observed in lung diseases has been studied extensively (and is discussed in subsequent chapters). In summary, it is not observed in lung diseases such as acute respiratory distress syndrome (ARDS), nor in chronic obstructive lung diseases such as asthma, emphysema, or bronchitis (see Chapter 8), even during exercise (11). However, in interstitial lung diseases, diffusion limitation sometimes may occur even at rest and is usually in evidence during exercise, accounting for part of the commonly observed decrease in arterial P_{O_2} under such conditions (see Chapter 9).

To understand better the reasons why diffusion limitation may or may not develop, it is necessary to examine the factors responsible for diffusive equilibration. The process of alveolar–capillary gas exchange has long been established to be passive diffusion along a concentration gradient (12), and the net gas flux or transport rate by diffusion is given by the product of the concentration difference (between alveolar gas and capillary blood) and a parameter reflecting diffusional conductance of the alveolar–capillary membrane. This is Fick's law of diffusion. The diffusional conductance (D) is itself a function of several factors: (1) It is directly proportional to the alveolar–capillary surface area available for exchange; (2) it is proportional to the physical solubility of the gas in the (blood-free) water of the alveolar–capillary wall tissue through which the gas must pass physically dissolved; (3) it is inversely proportional to the thickness of the alveolar–capillary tissue membrane; (4) it is inversely proportional to the square root of the molecular weight of the gas; and (5) D also depends on the basic nature of the alveolar–capillary membrane as a medium for diffusion (per unit area and thickness). For O_2, CO, and CO_2, D has also traditionally included a component that reflects the noninstantaneous reaction rates of these gases binding to Hb in the red cell (O_2, CO) (13) or reacting with water to form HCO_3^- ions (CO_2) (9).

Although diffusive conductance is therefore somewhat complex in its makeup, what is much more important in understanding the role of alveolar–capillary diffusion in affecting gas exchange is the following: For any given value of D, whether diffusional equilibration across the alveolar–capillary membrane is complete or not depends only partly on D. As previously defined, D does not depend on the make-up of the blood (i.e., its capacity to carry O_2 or any other gas) or the rate of flow of blood through the pulmonary capillaries ($\dot{Q}$), the vascular volume of those capillaries (VC), and, hence, the red cell transit time (VC/$\dot{Q}$). Thus, for any given value of D, blood with a high O_2-carrying capacity (i.e., high [Hb]) requires more time to allow diffusion of O_2 to fill these O_2 Hb binding sites than would blood with a lesser number of O_2 binding sites. Basically, the number of binding sites can be expressed as a term [often described in the literature as β (14)] that reflects both the [Hb] and just where along the nonlinear O_2 Hb dissociation curve O_2 exchange is occurring. Thus, β is in effect the slope of the O_2 Hb dissociation curve. However, β does not address red cell transit time through the capillaries— this depends on $\dot{Q}$. The higher the $\dot{Q}$, the less will be the red cell transit time. The important bottom line is that whether the process of diffusion between alveolar gas and capillary blood is complete depends on the compound ratio: $D/(\beta\dot{Q})$.

This principle was developed thoroughly by Piiper and Scheid (14) and is critical to understanding the role of diffusion in pulmonary gas exchange. For example, if D is reduced but $\dot{Q}$ is also similarly subnormal, the ratio $D/(\beta\dot{Q})$ may remain normal, and the diffusive process is complete. On the contrary, a situation that pairs a high value of β with a high cardiac output (e.g., exercise at high altitude) will likely produce hypoxemia from alveolar–capillary diffusion limitation even though D may well be normal (or even greater than normal), because $D/(\beta\dot{Q})$ is reduced.

As Piiper and Scheid (14) showed, an expression for quantifying the (in)completeness of pulmonary diffusion limitation can be derived as follows:

$$\frac{(P_A - Pc')}{(P_A - P\overline{v})} = e^{-D/(\beta\dot{Q})} \quad (1)$$

where P_A is the alveolar gas partial pressure, $P\overline{v}$ is the pulmonary arterial (mixed venous) gas partial pressure, and Pc' is end pulmonary capillary gas partial pressure. Thus, if D, β, and $\dot{Q}$ can be determined, $e^{-D/(\beta\dot{Q})}$ reflects the completeness of equilibration on a scale from zero (complete equilibration) to 1.0 (total absence of gas exchange by diffusion).

The compound ratio $D/(\beta\dot{Q})$ is useful in another context—it clearly defines the integrative roles played by the three organ/tissue systems involved: D reflects pulmonary parenchymal structure, β reflects the [Hb] and thus blood composition, whereas $\dot{Q}$ depends on cardiac function. Diffusive exchange of all gases is thus an integrated function of the lungs, the blood, and the heart.

This ratio also allows an understanding of why some gases (CO, O_2) are much more vulnerable to diffusion limitation than are others (e.g., inert gases). Recall that the numerator D contained a term proportional to the water solubility of the gas. However, β on the denominator is equivalent to the blood solubility of the gas. Despite the presence of Hb only in the latter, for essentially all inert gases, water and blood solubility are very similar. For O_2, however, the water solubility is 0.003 mL/100 mL/mm Hg, whereas β, the blood O_2 "solubility," or slope of the

O_2–Hb dissociation curve, is much greater at approximately 0.083 mL/100 mL/mm Hg (breathing air at sea level at rest). This figure comes from dividing the normal arteriovenous [O_2] difference of 5 mL/100 mL by the corresponding 60 mm Hg P_{O_2} difference between arterial blood (100 mm Hg) and mixed venous blood (40 mm Hg). Thus, β for O_2 is some 30 times greater than its water solubility. Other factors equal, O_2 is therefore some 30-fold more vulnerable to diffusion limitation in the lung than any inert gas. This calculation is even more remarkable for CO, where, on the steep part of its CO–Hb dissociation curve, β is some 8000-fold greater than the solubility of CO in water. It comes as no surprise, then, that CO is always diffusion-limited in its capillary uptake, not because D is low (it compares with that of O_2), but because $D/(\beta \dot{Q})$ is so low due to the extremely high value of β in relation to the solubility of CO in water.

Finally, the $D/(\beta \dot{Q})$ ratio explains a very important aspect of interaction between the lungs and the tissues in O_2 exchange: how the value of the mixed venous P_{O_2} affects the time required for pulmonary O_2 exchange by diffusion. Returning to Eq. (1), one would at first sight predict that any failure of diffusion equilibration, manifest by a positive alveolar-end capillary P_{O_2} difference ($P_A - P_{c'}$), would not change in a relative sense if $P\bar{v}$ were to decrease: assuming that a change in $P\bar{v}_{O_2}$ does not affect $D/(\beta \dot{Q})$, $(P_A - P_{c'})/(P_A - P\bar{v})$ would remain constant [from Eq. (1)]. However, as Figure 4 shows, for a constant alveolar and arterial P_{O_2}, as $P\bar{v}_{O_2}$ decreases, the mean value of β increases, so that $D/(\beta \dot{Q})$ decreases. The consequences are also shown in Figure 4 (lower panel), where Eq. (1) has been evaluated for O_2 using values of β corresponding to the points in the upper panel, keeping alveolar P_{O_2} and all other factors constant. The message here is that, all other factors unchanged, as mixed venous P_{O_2} decreases, the pulmonary O_2 uptake process by diffusion becomes increasingly compromised (15).

D. Circulation: Cardiovascular Function

The next step in O_2 transport is convective movement of O_2 bound to Hb in red cells through the systemic arterial tree to the tissues and organs of the body. O_2 transport ($\dot{Q}_{O_2}$) to the entire body is the product of cardiac output ($\dot{Q}_T$) and arterial O_2 concentration (Ca_{O_2}) (Eq. 2).

$$\dot{Q}_{O_2} = \dot{Q}_T * Ca_{O_2} \tag{2}$$

Arterial O_2 concentration, in turn, is determined by [Hb], arterial O_2 saturation (Sa_{O_2}), and arterial P_{O_2}:

$$\dot{Q}_{O_2} = 1.39 * \dot{Q}_T * [Hb] * Sa_{O_2} + 0.003 * P_{O_2} * \dot{Q}_T \tag{3}$$

The second term, reflecting physically dissolved O_2, is normally less than 2% of the total and may be neglected, so that:

$$\dot{Q}_{O_2} = 1.39 * \dot{Q}_T * [Hb] * Sa_{O_2} \tag{4}$$

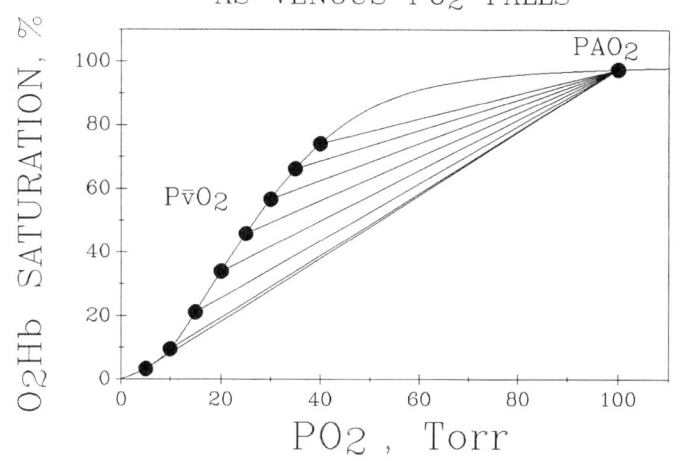

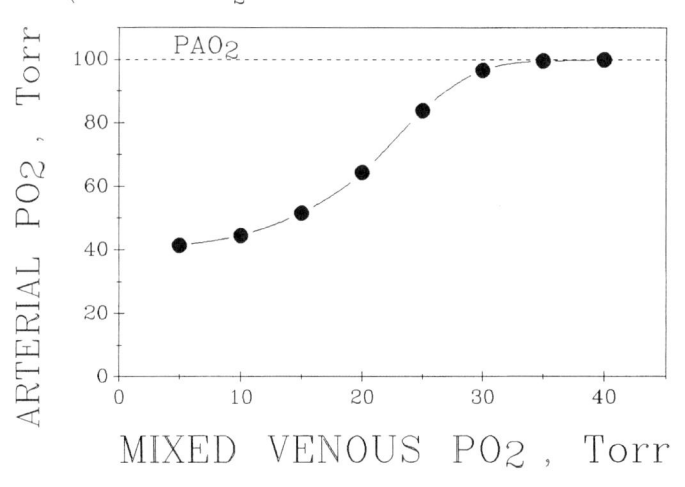

Figure 4 Importance of mixed venous P_{O_2} when diffusion limitation of oxygen uptake in the lung is present. In the example, when $P\bar{v}_{O_2}$ is 40 mm Hg and Pa_{O_2} is 100 mm Hg, arterial P_{O_2} equals alveolar P_{O_2} (upper panel). As Pv_{O_2} is progressively reduced, without any change in lung diffusing capacity or alveolar P_{O_2}, arterial hypoxemia develops (lower panel). The reason for the dependence of arterial P_{O_2} on mixed venous P_{O_2} in this situation is the progressive increase in average slope of the oxyhemoglobin dissociation curve between the alveolar and mixed venous values, as shown in the top panel by the straight lines joining Pa_{O_2} and Pv_{O_2}.

This concept is readily applied to each tissue or organ, so that tissue O_2 transport is the product of local tissue blood flow and arterial O_2 concentration.

Equation (4) points out a well-known level of integration in the O_2 transport process: O_2 transport depends on adequate cardiac function ($\dot{Q}_T$); adequate [Hb]; and adequate pulmonary function (Sa_{O_2}). At the local tissue level, tissue blood flow distribution must also be adequate. In critically ill patients, any of these factors may be abnormal. But even if $\dot{Q}_T$, [Hb], and Sa_{O_2} are normal, the distribution of blood flow among tissues and organs can be disturbed. Under such circumstances, undersupplied tissues may be critically deprived of O_2, whereas oversupplied tissues reap little or no additional benefit of the extra O_2.

Accordingly, adequate transport of O_2 to tissues requires several components of the O_2 transport system to work harmoniously and within normal or near-normal limits—not only the heart, lungs, and blood, but also the complex system that regulates blood flow distribution between and within organs and tissues—a system that depends on the autonomic nervous system as well as local factors such as local P_{O_2}, H^+ concentration, metabolites such as adenosine, and a host of other molecules such as prostaglandins and nitric oxide.

However, this addresses the transport of O_2 only into the microcirculation of tissue beds. It is not sufficient simply to get O_2 from the environment to such a microcirculation. The final step of O_2 transport from microvascular red cells to tissue mitochondria must be established or the entire O_2 transport process will be compromised. This tissue unloading of O_2 is, as in the lungs, a passive process of diffusion (16) and is addressed in Sec. II.E of this chapter. However, at the outset, a fundamental dilemma should be pointed out: In the process of O_2 transport to mitochondria, blood flow plays dual, opposing roles: (1) As previously discussed at length for the lungs (and as is discussed later in the context of tissue gas exchange), blood flow plays a direct role in determining how well O_2 is taken up by diffusion in the lungs and also how well it can be off-loaded by diffusion in the tissue microvasculature. This occurs as a result of the influence of blood flow rate on microvascular red cell transit time. Thus, with high blood flow, there is less time both to load O_2 in the lungs and unload it in the tissues. Therefore, a high blood flow rate may impair O_2 transport via diffusion limitation (2). However, because the rate of O_2 transported by the circulation to the tissues is proportional to the blood flow rate [see Eq. (4)], a high cardiac output will increase O_2 transport via increased convective flow of O_2-loaded red cells. These two effects of blood flow are clearly opposing in overall O_2 transport (17).

Examples of such situations are common and include hypoxia. Acutely, hypoxia may lead to an increase in cardiac output ($\dot{Q}_T$) that partly compensates for the hypoxically induced decrease in Sa_{O_2}. Chronic hypoxia causes further responses by leading to erythropoeisis and a higher [Hb]. Yet another example is observed in anemia, where blood flow generally increases to compensate partly for the decrease in [Hb]. In ARDS, cardiac output is often elevated, whereas arterial oxygenation is reduced. In all of these examples, O_2 unloading may be impaired if blood flow is elevated.

The discussion of cardiovascular function to this point has focused on overall principles of mass transport, distribution of flow, and diffusive exchange. However, at the level of a single organ, or even tissue within an organ, blood flow distribution in accordance with metabolic needs is the next key concept. Thus, the amount of O_2 transported to an organ or tissue or part of a tissue, as given by Eq. (4), may or may not be adequate for the required metabolic rate of the tissue. This concept is conveniently expressed by the well-known Fick principle:

$$\dot{V}O_2 = \dot{Q} * [CaO_2 - C\bar{v}O_2] \tag{5}$$

Here, the rate of O_2 consumption, $\dot{V}O_2$, is (in a steady state) expressed by the above mass balance equation. $\dot{Q}$ is again blood flow rate, and CaO_2 and $C\bar{v}O_2$ are the concentrations of O_2 in systemic arterial and organ (or tissue) venous blood, respectively. Clearly, the O_2 delivered to an organ or tissue [$\dot{Q} * CaO_2$ of Eq. (2) or (5)] must at least equal the required metabolic rate ($\dot{V}O_2$) or this metabolic rate could not be achieved. One can rarely, if ever, completely extract all O_2 from blood perfusing an organ; therefore, $C\bar{v}O_2$ is rarely, if ever, zero. Thus, O_2 transport generally must exceed $\dot{V}O_2$, not just equal it, to sustain the necessary metabolic rate.

When rearranged, Eq. (5) provides useful further insight into O_2 transport and use:

$$C\bar{v}O_2 = CaO_2 - \dot{V}O_2/\dot{Q} \tag{6}$$

Whether considering flow distribution between organs or within a single organ, Eq. (6) gives fundamental information about O_2 transport: The amount of unextracted, residual O_2 in venous blood ($C\bar{v}O_2$) depends on the ratio of metabolic rate to blood flow ($\dot{V}O_2/\dot{Q}$) because all tissues and organs receive the same arterial blood (i.e., the same CaO_2). This simple equation should also be kept in mind when interpreting the clinical significance of changes in mixed venous oxygenation, particularly in the intensive care setting. Thus, if the mixed venous [O_2] is found to increase in a patient, one should search for the explanation from the three component variables: arterial [O_2], metabolic rate ($\dot{V}O_2$) and cardiac output ($\dot{Q}$). An increase in arterial [O_2] or cardiac output, or a decrease in $\dot{V}O_2$, could individually produce the increase in $C\bar{v}O_2$. Decisions on whether an increase in venous [O_2] were clinically related to patient improvement or deterioration would naturally follow from knowing the physiological reason for the $C\bar{v}O_2$ change. As a corollary, interpreting venous [O_2] changes requires knowledge of all the determining variables: arterial [O_2], $\dot{V}O_2$, and $\dot{Q}$.

This analysis reflects only a physiological approach for considering the meaning of mixed venous [O_2]. The next set of questions—why has CaO_2, $\dot{V}O_2$, and/or $\dot{Q}$ changed—would have to be posed to understand the mechanistic basis of changes to the patient. However, the physiological basis leads the way to this more important question set and allows the clinician to focus on the relevant variables.

The Fick principle, and particularly its rewriting as Eq. (6), brings to the surface a closely related and complex issue: the ratio $\dot{V}_{O_2}/\dot{Q}$ in Eq. (6) is presented as a global ratio for the particular tissue, organ, or system under consideration. However, the possibility exists, especially in disease, that despite adequate overall blood flow, its distribution may be nonuniform (18). This nonuniformity may impair O_2 transport to mitochondria whose metabolic rate is higher in relation to blood flow, while providing needlessly excess O_2 to mitochondria of other cells that are better perfused. In this context, it is critical to keep in mind that what counts here is the distribution of blood flow in relation to metabolic rate [$\dot{V}_{O_2}/\dot{Q}$, as in Eq. (6)]. There is currently no method that can measure this distribution within intact tissues or organs. Regional $\dot{V}_{O_2}/\dot{Q}$ ratios could be calculated from Eq. (6) if regional venous O_2 levels could be measured, but that possibility remains to be developed. Various O_2 electrodes (surface, needle) are available but do not measure just venous O_2 levels and in many cases cause severe local damage that must disturb cell function and thus the very O_2 levels one wishes to measure. Hemoglobin or myoglobin spectroscopy also has been used but requires invasive surgical preparations and, for some methods, freezing of the tissue for in vitro spectroscopy (19). Near-infrared spectroscopy averages arterial, capillary, and venous blood. Myoglobin saturation can be measured by magnetic resonance spectroscopy (20), but without the spatial resolution required to assess heterogeneity; this approach can work only for muscle. Phosphorescence quenching is a newer, relatively less invasive approach for plasma P_{O_2} measurement, but it also has limitations as an extracellular probe and cannot yet be applied to humans (21).

Although the distribution of blood flow can be measured locally using microspheres or gas washout (e.g., Xenon) (18), both of these methods are unable to assess the distribution of $\dot{V}_{O_2}$. Consequently, today we are left in the inadequate position of not being able to assess $\dot{V}_{O_2}/\dot{Q}$ heterogeneity even in experimental animals. Despite this state of affairs, some consideration of the problem shows that as distinct from ventilation/perfusion heterogeneity in the lungs, tissue $\dot{V}_{O_2}/\dot{Q}$ heterogeneity, up to a point, does not impair O_2 transport [see Eq. (5)].

Suppose a tissue consisted of two compartments with equal values of $\dot{V}_{O_2}$ (150 mL/min), $\dot{Q}$ (3 l/min), C_{aO_2} (20 mL/dL), and, therefore, $C\bar{v}_{O_2}$ (Fig. 5A). Each compartment supports half the total metabolic rate, and venous [O_2] from each (and thus mixed venous [O_2]) is 15.0 mL/100 mL. If blood flow were redistributed (by changing F from 0.5 progressively down to zero), each compartment's venous [O_2] would change, but as long as flow is adequate in the low-flow unit, overall tissue $\dot{V}_{O_2}$ and mixed venous [O_2] would be completely undisturbed (Fig. 5B). In fact, flow in the poorly perfused compartment could theoretically decrease from 3.0 to 0.75 L/min and still, via Eq. (5) or (6), maintain the unit metabolic rate of 150 mL/min, although this would require complete O_2 extraction and thus a venous [O_2] of zero. Even at that point, total tissue $\dot{V}_{O_2}$ would be sustained at 300 mL/min, and mixed venous [O_2] would be undisturbed at 15 mL/100 mL. Only if blood flow decreased further to less than 0.75 L/min (or <25% of baseline) in this case would $\dot{V}O_2$ of the unit have to decrease, and only then would mixed venous [O_2] increase. Thus, a considerable degree of $\dot{V}O_2/\dot{Q}$ inhomogeneity can be "absorbed" by the reserve in the O_2 transport system.

Whether $\dot{V}O_2/\dot{Q}$ heterogeneity is physiologically and/or clinically important to O_2 transport is a key question that remains, for the most part, unanswerable given current technical limitations. Solving this problem would greatly enhance our understanding of tissue gas exchange in health and disease. What controls matching of $\dot{V}O_2$ to $\dot{Q}$ is (between and within organs) very complex and well beyond the scope of this chapter. Suffice it to say that $\dot{V}O_2/\dot{Q}$ heterogeneity is a potentially important factor in impairing tissue O_2 transport, especially in disease states typified by multiple organ failure; that we have no methods to measure it; and that a certain level of $\dot{V}O_2/\dot{Q}$ heterogeneity can exist and not perturb tissue gas exchange or metabolic rate.

E. Tissue O_2 Transport and O_2 Extraction

The fifth and final major step in the transport of O_2 from the air to the mitochondria is moving O_2 from the microvascular red cells to the mitochondria. Just as in the lungs, this is a passive process based on diffusion, but the pathway is more complex than in the lungs, where O_2 simply has to pass through a 0.5-μ-thick tissue sheet made up of thin cellular cytoplasmic elements separated by a basement membrane (3). In tissues, after O_2 is unloaded from the red cell Hb and diffuses out of the red cell, the plasma, and the capillary wall, it must enter the target cell and diffuse many microns (on average) to reach the mitochondria. It should come as no surprise, then, that in contrast to the lungs, the diffusive process is challenged, even in health. Although tissue diffusive conductances throughout the body may normally be adequate at rest, even light exercise produces evidence of incomplete equilibration. Thus, although microvascular Po_2 remains, on average, 40 to 50 mm Hg, intracellular Po_2 (in muscle) decreases to single-digit levels (19, 20) indicating a large Po_2 difference over the few microns separating the muscle microvascular red cells from the myocyte cell wall. In turn, this implies substantial impedance to the diffusion of O_2 of this region, and physiological evidence points to the amount of capillary surface area as the critical variable (22). Whether the capillary is also the principal site of diffusive impedance in tissues other than muscle remains to be determined, but this must await development of an appropriate noninvasive method for measuring intracellular Po_2 in myoglobin-free tissues. Whether such problems are important in diseased tissues is also currently unknown.

The important message to be taken from evidence of incomplete diffusive unloading of O_2 and the associated large red cell to sarcolemma Po_2 difference in muscle is that a substantial pressure head of O_2 must be maintained inside the microvasculature to allow the high O_2 flux rates required for metabolism. Put

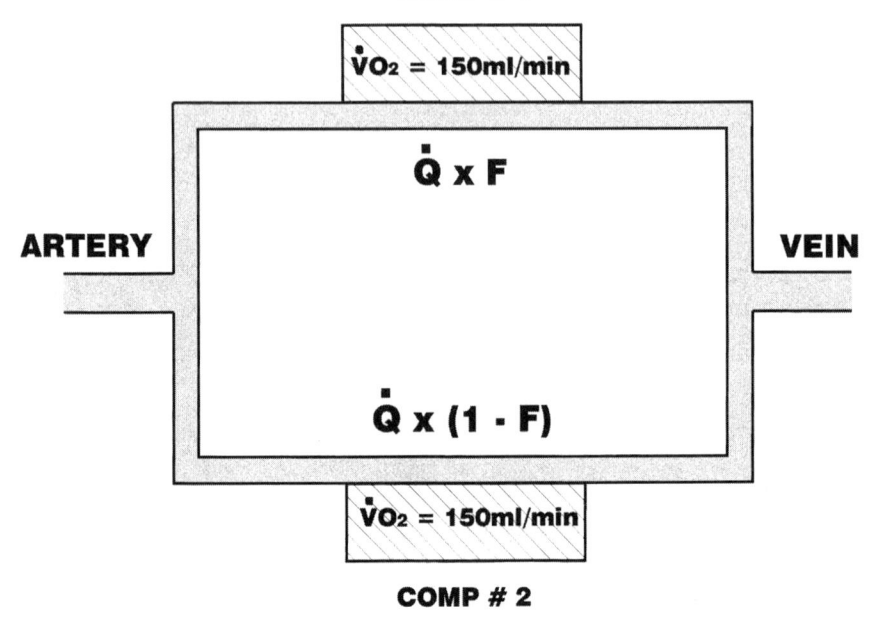

TWO COMPARTMENT MODEL
UNIFORM O₂ REQUIREMENTS
UNEVEN DISTRIBUTION OF BLOOD FLOW

COMP # 1

$\dot{V}O_2 = 150\,ml/min$

ARTERY

$\dot{Q} \times F$

VEIN

$\dot{Q} \times (1 - F)$

$\dot{V}O_2 = 150\,ml/min$

COMP # 2

TWO–COMPARTMENT MODEL

FRACTIONAL BLOODFLOW DISTRIBUTION
(O₂ REQUIREMENTS UNIFORM)

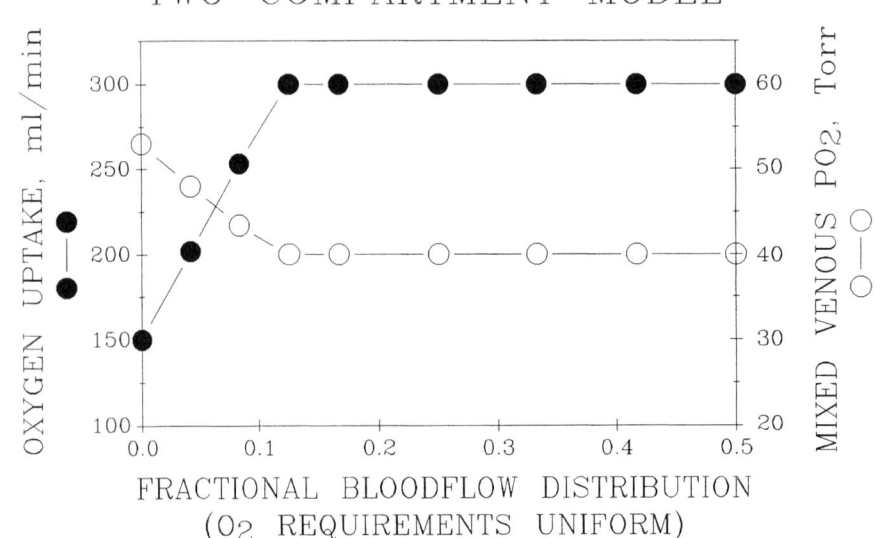

another way, the limited diffusive conductance prevents complete O_2 extraction and means that sometimes substantial amounts of O_2 must be returned from the tissues in the venous blood as the price paid for adequate rates of diffusion from the red cell to the mitochondria, at least in muscle. This is evident from the laws of diffusion, as embodied in Eq. (7):

$$\dot{V}_{O_2} = D_{TO_2}(\overline{P_{CAPO_2}} - \overline{P_{MITOO_2}}) \tag{7}$$

where $\dot{V}_{O_2}$ is the required diffusive flux rate of O_2 to support metabolism, D_{TO_2} is the diffusive conductance from red cell to mitochondria, and $\overline{P_{CAPO_2}}$ and $\overline{P_{MITOO_2}}$ are average capillary and mitochondrial P_{O_2} values, respectively. Thus, if D_{TO_2} is limited by the microvascular and tissue structure, and because $\overline{P_{MITOO_2}}$ cannot possibly be less than zero, $\overline{P_{CAPO_2}}$ must be maintained to supply enough O_2—yet maintaining capillary P_{O_2} requires "holding O_2 back," which also results in a limit to O_2 efflux. This conflict is conveniently depicted diagramatically by charting both Eq. (5) and Eq. (7) on the same diagram (1). In doing so, the ordinate is $\dot{V}_{O_2}$ and the abscissa is venous P_{O_2} [inferred from C_{VO_2} in Eq. (5) and from $\overline{P_{CAPO_2}}$ in Eq. (7). In fact, in Eq. (7), for graphical purposes, it can be assumed that $\overline{P_{CAPO_2}}$ and $P_{\bar{v}O_2}$ for a tissue are linearly related and proportional to one another, such that $\overline{P_{CAPO_2}} = k.P_{\bar{v}O_2}$. It is further assumed that under diffusion-limited conditions, mitochondrial P_{O_2} is within 1 or 2 mm Hg of zero (and can thus be neglected). Equation (7) becomes:

$$\dot{V}_{O_2} = D_{TO_2} * k * P_{\bar{v}O_2} \tag{8}$$

Figure 6 shows Eq. (5) and (8) on the same graph. Both express O_2 flux ($\dot{V}_{O_2}$): Eq. (5) simply as a mass balance system, and Eq. (8) as the diffusion equation. The shape and positions of these two equations are indicated in Figure 6, as is their single point of intersection, the only place where $\dot{V}_{O_2}$ is equal from both equations. Because both represent the O_2 flux rate, this point of intersection

---

Figure 5 A two-compartment model of nonuniform flow distribution in a peripheral tissue. In this example, metabolic rate is equal and, therefore, half of the total in the two compartments. The effect of progressive inequality of blood flow distribution on oxygen uptake and effluent tissue (venous) P_{O_2} is shown in the bottom panel. In the uniform state, where fractional blood flow distribution (F) is 0.5, metabolic requirements are easily satisfied, and mixed venous P_{O_2} is 40 mm Hg. Unlike the effect of nonuniformity in the lung (see Fig. 3), oxygen uptake is maintained at normal values, and mixed venous P_{O_2} is similarly conserved until blood flow distribution has become extremely nonuniform (approximately 0.12 in the aforementioned example). Only when less than 12% of the blood flow perfuses one compartment (and, therefore, >88% perfuses the other) is total oxygen transport inadequate to meet metabolic demands so that $\dot{V}_{O_2}$ decreases and venous P_{O_2} increases. The tissues, therefore, in contrast to the lungs are less susceptible to heterogeneity of blood flow and can sustain substantial abnormality without compromising tissue metabolism.

```
                  O₂ DELIVERY = Q̇ × CaO₂
  OXYGEN UPTAKE
                           ← V̇O₂MAX

                                  FICK PRINCIPLE LINE:
                                  V̇O₂ = Q̇ [CaO₂ − Cv̄O₂]
                      FICK LAW LINE:
                      V̇O₂ = DO₂ × k × Pv̄O₂

                  0                                    ARTERIAL
                         MUSCLE VENOUS PO₂
```

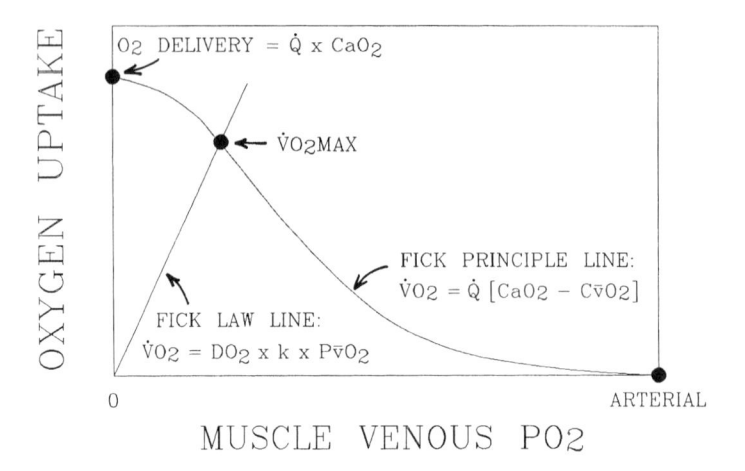

Figure 6 The relationship between oxygen uptake and muscle venous P_{O_2} is given by two different equations. One equation reflects mass conservation (Fick principle line), whereas the other represents diffusion of oxygen from the capillary to the mitochondria (Fick law line). The single point of intersection indicates the maximal rate of oxygen transport to the mitochondria allowed by the particular diffusive conductance of the tissue in the presence of the given convective oxygen delivery. See text for further explanation.

indicates the only feasible O_2 use rate under the given conditions that the governing O_2 transport variables will allow. These O_2 transport variables are, from Eq. (5): (1) the blood flow rate ($\dot{Q}$); (2) [Hb]; (3) Sa_{O_2}; and from Eq. (8) (4) the tissue O_2 conductance, D_{TO_2}.

Changes in any one of these four variables would, on its own, alter one of the two lines in Figure 6, and thus their point of intersection and, hence, maximal $\dot{V}_{O_2}$. This is a critical concept: Alteration in any of the governing variables that represent pulmonary, cardiac, hematological, and tissue O_2 transport capacities will affect the maximal rate at which O_2 can reach the mitochondria. It immediately suggests that the conventional question, "What is the limiting factor to O_2 transport?," must be replaced by a better posed question: "What are the relative (quantitative) roles of all of the above limiting factors to maximal O_2 transport?" Thus, there is no one limiting factor—all are simultaneously responsible for setting maximal $\dot{V}_{O_2}$ in a highly integrated fashion ($\dot{Q}$).

This construct and analysis is very useful for another purpose: separating the contributions of "central" and "peripheral" factors as limiting O_2 transport. In Figure 6, the curved line corresponding to Eq. (5) represents the "central" factors of blood flow, Sa_{O_2}, and [Hb] whereas the straight line depicts the "peripheral" factor representing O_2 conductance from red cells to mitochondria. Figure 7 shows how changes in central and peripheral factors would differently affect the points of intersection of the two lines and allow clear distinction of central from peripheral

Pulmonary and Peripheral Gas Exchange

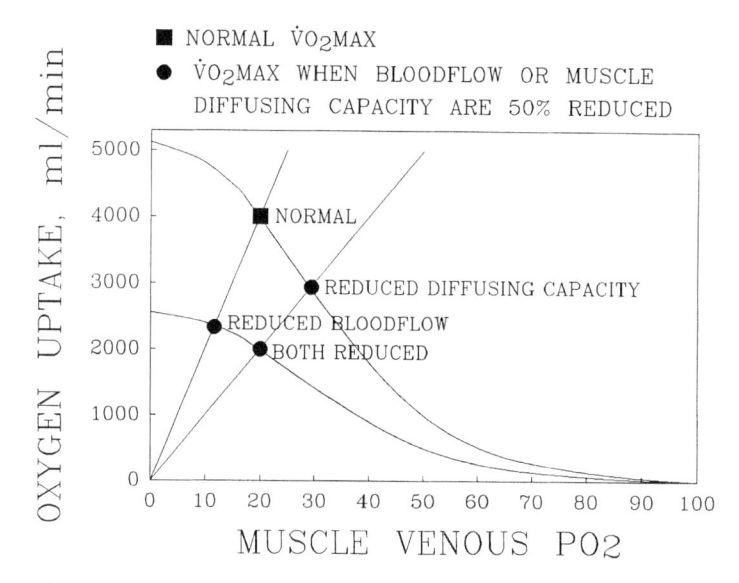

Figure 7 Diagram indicating how reducing diffusive transport within muscle, reducing blood flow to muscle, or reducing both together will affect maximal oxygen transport and use. The clear interaction between the convective transport of oxygen in the circulation and the subsequent diffusive unloading is shown.

factors. In this context, it needs to be pointed out that the well-known manipulation of Eq. (5) that has been applied traditionally to the same task of separating central and peripheral factors is conceptually flawed. From Eq. (5), it follows that:

$$\dot{V}_{O_2} = \dot{Q} \cdot C_{aO_2} \left[1 - \frac{C_{\bar{v}O_2}}{C_{aO_2}}\right] \quad (9)$$

Equation 9 thus separates $\dot{V}_{O_2}$ into O_2 transport ($\dot{Q} \cdot C_{aO_2}$) and O_2 extraction $\left(1 - \frac{C_{\bar{v}O_2}}{C_{aO_2}}\right)$ components. The former has usually been labeled central, whereas the latter traditionally defines peripheral factors. The former is adequate and does not differ from the application of this equation to Figures 6 and 7. However, extraction $\left(= 1 - \frac{C_{\bar{v}O_2}}{C_{aO_2}}\right)$ is not a pure function of the tissue O_2 conductance. Precisely the same concept as applied to alveolar–capillary diffusion in the lungs (14) is appropriate in the tissues: the degree to which extraction by diffusion is complete is a function of the compound ratio $D_{TO_2}/(\beta \dot{Q})$, with the symbols as defined previously. The equation that defines extraction as a function of $D_{TO_2}/(\beta \dot{Q})$ is as follows:

$$\text{Extraction} = 1 - e^{-D_{TO_2}/(\beta \dot{Q})} \quad (10)$$

Thus, just as in the lungs, extraction is a function of not only the tissue O_2 conductance (D_{TO_2}), but also of the slope of the O_2–Hb dissociation curve (β) and the tissue blood flow ($\dot{Q}$). These last two variables reflect what is classically a part of the central group of transport factors.

As a result, the approach offered in Figures 6 and 7 would be preferable should it be desired to separate central and peripheral factors in limiting O_2 transport. O_2 extraction, on the other hand, must be interpreted carefully: It reflects much more than peripheral or tissue transport function.

Just as importantly, the preceding analysis points out that using the term $\dot{Q}O_2 = \dot{Q} \cdot CaO_2$ to indicate total O_2 delivery must be used with care. $\dot{Q}O_2$ as so defined indicates the O_2 transport rate into the systemic arterial supply of the tissues. This is not the same as the maximal rate of O_2 transport to the mitochondria, which must be less than $\dot{Q}O_2$ to the extent that tissue O_2 extraction limitation exists (because of heterogeneity or limited diffusive conductance). Thus, $\dot{Q}O_2$ may be high, but if O_2 diffusional transport is compromised, mitochondrial O_2 delivery may also be compromised.

The entire preceding analysis has its foundation in normal exercising muscle physiology whose maximal $\dot{V}O_2$ can usually be shown to be dependent on O_2 supply. Only under such conditions would mitochondrial PO_2 be low enough to disregard in the analysis. If O_2 transport were not limiting O_2 consumption, mitochondrial O_2 levels presumably would be higher, and the diagrams shown in Figures 6 and 7 would be inadequate. Experimentally, this could be established by altering the fraction of inspired oxygen (FIO_2), for example, and assessing its effect on maximal $\dot{V}O_2$. When this was performed in athletes (23), the expected increase in $\dot{V}O_2$ in proportion to increases in capillary PO_2 was found. However, in unfit normal subjects, no such O_2 supply dependence of $\dot{V}O_2$ is observed (24), suggesting that mitochondrial oxidative capacity, and not O_2 transport, sets the limit to maximal $\dot{V}O_2$. It is interesting that in chronic diseases such as renal failure (25) and chronic obstructive pulmonary disease (26), maximal $\dot{V}O_2$ is again found to be O_2-supply–dependent, although with lower $\dot{V}O_2$ than in even unfit normal subjects. This may reflect a rarefied muscle capillary network (27) as well as reduced convective O_2 transport from anemia in the case of renal disease. However, the message is that the drive to determine what parts of the O_2 transport system have the greatest influence on maximal $\dot{V}O_2$ under any given conditions is only a relevant goal if that $\dot{V}O_2$ can be shown to be O_2-supply–dependent.

Can the aforementioned concepts apply to the other end of the metabolic spectrum (at low $\dot{V}O_2$ values at rest)? As shown in Figure 8, the answer is potentially yes. Suppose in a resting patient, $\dot{V}O_2$ is O_2-supply–independent above some critical value of O_2 transport (O_2 transport defined as $\dot{Q} \cdot CaO_2$). From this critical value on down, as O_2 transport is further reduced, the concepts behind the diagrams shown in Figures 6 and 7 can be applied and show that a linear decrease in $\dot{V}O_2$ with decreases in O_2 transport would be expected. The solid circles in Figure 8 thus trace the expected behavior of $\dot{V}O_2$ as O_2 transport is reduced from high to low values. This nonlinear relationship is precisely what experimental evidence shows (see Chapter 27). However, compatibility with such data does not prove the concept correct.

Pulmonary and Peripheral Gas Exchange

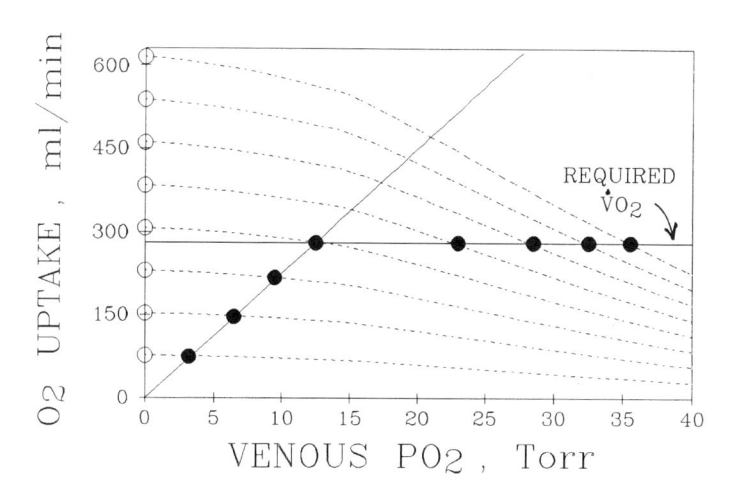

• ACTUAL $\dot{V}O_2$ AS O_2 DELIVERY (○) IS REDUCED

Figure 8 Extension of the concepts in Fig. 6 provides a model for how oxygen uptake in the resting state in syndromes of multiple organ failure become dependent on oxygen supply. As long as convective oxygen delivery in this example exceeds approximately 300 mL/min, the tissue metabolic requirements for oxygen can be met. However, if convective oxygen delivery decreases below this value, the diffusive conductance for oxygen is insufficient to permit a high enough extraction to meet metabolic requirements. Hence, oxygen use decreases, with further reduction in delivery. The dashed lines represent the mass conservation lines of Fig. 6, each for a different level of convective oxygen delivery into the tissue.

Two other competing hypotheses should be considered because they would produce identical relationships. These possibilities are as follows: (1) heterogeneity of the $\dot{V}O_2/\dot{Q}$ relation without any O_2 diffusional transport limitation; and (2) reduction in cellular metabolic rate in response to reduced O_2 availability as $\dot{Q}O_2$ is reduced. These complex possibilities remain to be resolved.

F. Overall Summary

Two important concepts have emerged at different points in this chapter and require underlining and reinforcing:

1. the close similarity of mechanisms impairing O_2 transport in the lungs and in the tissues; and
2. the integrative nature of pulmonary and tissue gas exchange where the exchange behavior of one directly modulates the exchange behavior of the other.

III. Mechanisms of O_2 Transport Impairment in the Lungs and Tissues

The four causes of arterial hypoxemia are well known in respiratory physiology: (1) hypoventilation; (2) diffusion limitation; (3) shunting; and (4) ventilation/perfusion ($\dot{V}_A/\dot{Q}$) inequality (28). We wish to point out that precisely similar mechanisms are potentially present in tissues, albeit with some differences in emphasis or detail.

1. The analog of alveolar hypoventilation in the lungs impairing lung O_2 uptake is tissue hypoperfusion failing to deliver enough O_2 in the reduced blood flow to support metabolism. The consequences are rather similar—reduced P_{O_2} and increased P_{CO_2} in the blood draining the lungs (arterial blood) or tissues (venous blood). The Fick principle in either case [Eq. (5); or more accurately the analysis of Figs. 6 and 7] will dictate the critical value of $\dot{Q}$ below which $\dot{V}_{O_2}$ cannot be sustained.

2. Diffusion limitation seems to be important in both pulmonary and tissue exchange and is governed by the same processes in each site, as expressed in the previously defined ratio $D/(\beta\dot{Q})$. In the lungs, it takes maximum exercise to see such limitations, unless one ascends to altitude. On the other hand, the tissues are more vulnerable to this problem even at sea level. This difference can be explained by two factors: first, the generally greater diffusion distances for O_2 in tissues than in the lungs; and second, the nonlinear shape of the O_2–Hb dissociation curve. This shape facilitates diffusive loading in the lungs but, conversely, impairs diffusive unloading in the tissues ($\dot{Q}$). Tissue diffusion limitation likely explains why O_2 extraction is rarely, if ever, complete and seems to be accounted for by a limited capillary surface area for diffusion of O_2 out of the microvasculature, at least in muscle.

3. Heterogeneity of $\dot{V}_A/\dot{Q}$ ratios in the lung has its counterpart in heterogeneity of $\dot{V}_{O_2}/\dot{Q}$ ratios in the tissues. In the lung, this progressively impairs O_2 transport, but in the tissues, $\dot{V}_{O_2}/\dot{Q}$ heterogeneity will diminish O_2 transport only after blood flow in the highest $\dot{V}_{O_2}/\dot{Q}$ regions has decreased below levels that would require 100% O_2 extraction. Before that, considerable $\dot{V}_{O_2}/\dot{Q}$ heterogeneity could be present without any external evidence of impaired O_2 transport and with maintenance of $\dot{V}_{O_2}$ at normal levels. Although $\dot{V}_A/\dot{Q}$ inequality can be measured (4, 29), $\dot{V}_{O_2}/\dot{Q}$ heterogeneity cannot yet be assessed. It is important to note perfusion heterogeneity measured with microspheres says little about $\dot{V}_{O_2}/\dot{Q}$ heterogeneity because regional $\dot{V}_{O_2}$ cannot be measured to go with microsphere-based blood flow estimates. If blood flow is tightly regulated to match $\dot{V}_{O_2}$, there might be little or no $\dot{V}_{O_2}/\dot{Q}$ heterogeneity despite considerable perfusion heterogeneity per se.

4. Shunting is a concept applicable to both lungs and tissues and describes the passage of blood directly from inflowing to outflowing arms of the circulation, thus bypassing gas exchange completely. Shunts are rarely observed in normal lungs but may occur to some extent in normal tissues. Such shunts are based on vascular channels and convection of blood through them. So-called diffusional

shunts may occur in tissues but not in lungs. These shunts allow direct flow of O_2 by diffusion from arterioles to nearby venules, effectively reducing O_2 availability to cells. However, evidence for their functional significance is not strong, at least in muscle tissue (30).

IV. Integration of Lungs and Tissues in Gas Transport and Exchange

It is appropriate to conclude this chapter with a closer and more quantitative look at its major theme: that how the lungs exchange gas affects how the tissues exchange gas, and vice versa. The lungs and tissues affect one another's performance because, in each case, the blood departing one is the blood entering the other; it is well known that the composition of the blood entering the lungs affects pulmonary gas exchange (8,15), and so, too, the make-up of the blood entering the tissues affects gas exchange there. This can be analyzed as follows:

If one returns to the basic diffusion equations governing gas exchange in the lungs, Eq. (1), we have for any gas:

$$\frac{(P_A - Pa)}{(P_A - P\bar{v})} = e^{-D_L/(\beta \dot{Q})} \tag{11}$$

The corresponding equation for the tissues is:

$$P\bar{v} = Pa * e^{-D_T/(\beta \dot{Q})} \tag{12}$$

These equations were developed by Piiper and Scheid (14). D_T and D_L are the O_2 diffusional conductances of the tissues and lungs, respectively.

From the Fick principle:

$$\dot{V}_{GAS} = \dot{Q} * (Ca - C\bar{v}) \tag{13}$$

we can write:

$$\dot{V}_{GAS} = \dot{Q} * \beta * (Pa - P\bar{v}) \tag{14}$$

because β is the solubility of the gas, and concentration is partial pressure times solubility.

Eliminating Pa and $P\bar{v}$ by combining Eq. (11), (12), and (14) yields:

$$\dot{V}_{GAS} = P_A * \beta * \dot{Q} * [1 - e^{-D_T/(\beta \dot{Q})}][1 - e^{-D_L/(\beta \dot{Q})}]/$$
$$[1 - e^{-D_T/(\beta \dot{Q})} * e^{-D_L/(\beta \dot{Q})}] \tag{15}$$

Equation (15) shows that for a given level of ventilation (which, in turn, will define P_A), maximal $\dot{V}_{GAS}$ will be a function of the gas solubility (β), blood flow ($\dot{Q}$), and the two diffusional conductances of the lung (D_L) and tissue (D_T). This construct assumes that ventilation/perfusion inequality in the lung and perfusion/metabolism heterogeneity in the tissues are negligible. Moreover, $\beta \dot{Q}$ always

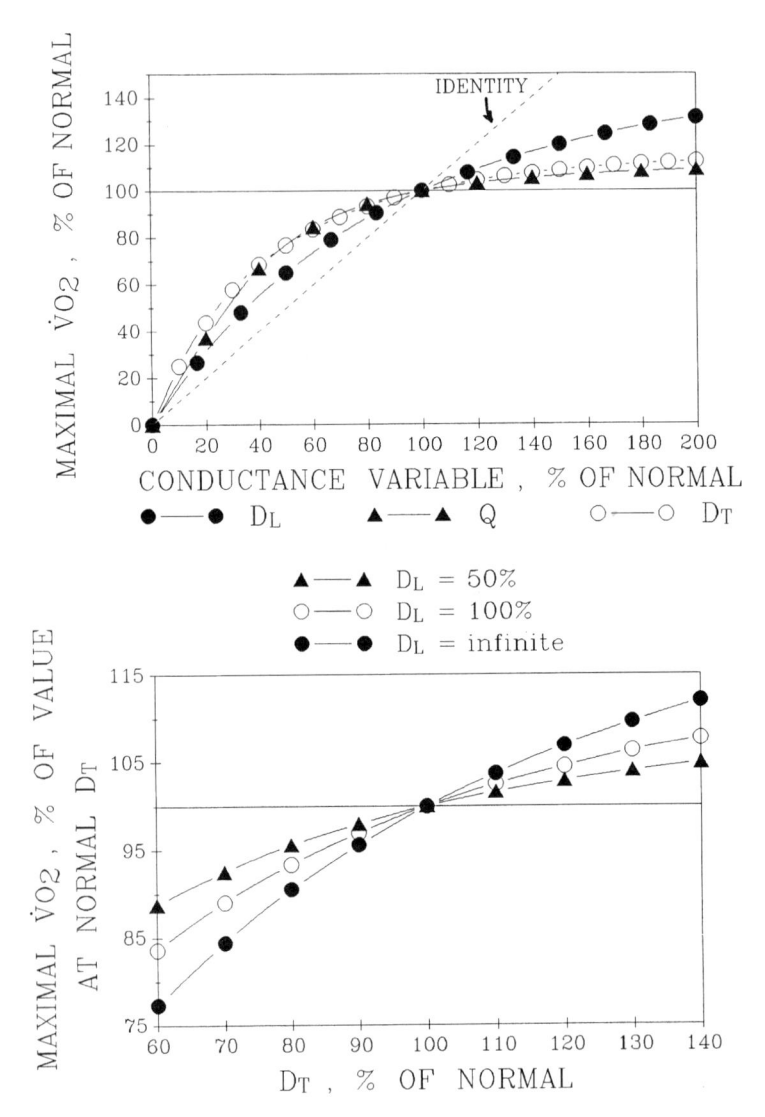

Figure 9 Calculations showing how maximal oxygen consumption during exercise depends on individual components of the oxygen transport pathway, indicated by their conductances (D_L, pulmonary diffusive conductance; $\dot{Q}$, muscle blood flow; D_T, muscle oxygen diffusing conductance). Variation in any of the three conductances yields rather similar effects on maximal $\dot{V}O_2$. The relationships are not linear and show more sensitivity to reduction in each variable than to an increase in each variable. In the lower panel, interaction between conductance variables is shown. In this example, the sensitivity of maximal $\dot{V}O_2$ to muscle oxygen-diffusing conductance is indicated at three different levels of pulmonary oxygen diffusion conductance. When pulmonary diffusion conductance is high, variations in tissue conductance have a greater effect on increasing or decreasing maximal $\dot{V}O_2$ than when the pulmonary diffusing conductance is reduced. See text for further details.

appears as a product—the individual variables β and $\dot{Q}$ do not appear separately, indicating that effects of similar relative changes in β and $\dot{Q}$ would be identical.

Figure 9 (top panel) plots Eq. (15) as a function of $\dot{Q}$, D_L, and D_T. Data for these plots come from measurements in normal subjects made just before a simulated ascent of Mount Everest (31), where at sea level, at $\dot{V}_{O_2}$max, $\beta = 2.5$ mL O_2/L blood per mm Hg, $\dot{Q} = 25$ L/min, $D_L = 60$ mL/min/mm Hg, $D_T = 100$ mL/min/mm Hg, and $P_A = 100$ mm Hg.

These are approximate numbers, rounded off for presentation purposes. They are applied to Eq. (15) with the knowledge that the O_2–Hb curve is nonlinear such that a constant value of β is not strictly accurate; however, the point of this exercise is to show the individual influences of each part of the O_2 transport pathway. Maximal O_2 use is a nonlinear function of each conductance: $\dot{V}_{O_2}$ is hardly increased by large increases in any conductance variable but will decrease more sharply as conductances are reduced. Note, in particular, that the three conductances (D_L, D_T, and $\dot{Q}$) have numerically similar effects over a wide range.

In the lower panel of Figure 9, the interdependence of conductance for O_2 at difference points in the O_2 pathway is illustrated for one case: how $\dot{V}_{O_2}$max would be affected by tissue O_2 conductance (D_T) under conditions of different pulmonary O_2 conductance (D_L). When D_L is normal, the influence of D_T is less than when D_L is infinitely great. As D_L is reduced below normal, variation in D_T is less influential. This illustrates the general principle that the organ with lowest conductance relative to normal will dominate limits to O_2 transport and lessen the dependence of $\dot{V}_{O_2}$max on conductance values of other parts of the system.

V. Conclusion

The O_2 transport pathway is a complex system of convective and diffusive steps, each of which possesses a definable conductance for O_2. These steps act together to provide an integrated overall maximal capacity that depends on each of the component conductances. In so doing, any one of the steps has the power to change maximal transport. Moreover, how the lungs exchange gas is affected by how the tissues exchange gas, and vice versa. As a result, each transport step exerts its modulating influence on maximal transport in more than one way, often with opposing results. These concepts of O_2 transport should replace the older approach of considering the ill-posed question of which one transport step limits O_2 use. Although developed and most widely applied to exercise in health, the basic principles are fundamental and will still govern gas transport and exchange at rest in disease when the supply of O_2 is limiting the metabolic rate of the tissues.

References

1. Wagner PD. Determinants of maximal oxygen transport and utilization. Annu Rev Physiol 1996; 58:21–50.

2. Weibel ER. The Pathway for Oxygen: Structure and Function in the Mammalian Respiratory System. Cambridge: University Press, 1984.
3. Weibel ER. Morphometry of the Human Lung. Berlin: Springer, 1963.
4. Wagner PD, West JB. Ventilation-perfusion relationships. In: West JB, ed. Pulmonary Gas Exchange. Vol. 1. New York: Academic Press, 1980, pp 219–262.
5. Okubo T, Piiper J. Intrapulmonary gas mixing in excised dog lung lobes studies by simultaneous wash-out of two inert gases. Respir Physiol 1974; 21:223–239.
6. Hlastala MP, Scheid P, Piiper J. Interpretation of inert gas retention and excretion in the presence of stratified inhomogeneity. Respir Physiol 1981; 46:247–259.
7. Cardús J, Burgos F, Diaz O, Roca J, Barberà JA, Marrades RM, Rodriguez-Roisin R, Wagner PD. Increase in pulmonary ventilation/perfusion inequality with age in healthy individuals. Am J Respir Crit Care Med 1997; 156:648–653.
8. West JB. Ventilation/perfusion inequality and overall gas exchange in computer models of the lung. Respir Physiol 1969; 7:88–110.
9. Wagner PD. Diffusion and chemical reaction in pulmonary gas exchange. Physiol Rev 1977; 57:257–312.
10. Wagner PD, Gale GE, Moon RE, Torr-Bueno J, Stolp BW, Saltzman HA. Pulmonary gas exchange in humans exercising at sea level and simulated altitude. J Appl Physiol 1986; 60:260–270.
11. Wagner PD, Dantzker DR, Dueck R, Clausen JL, West JB. Ventilation/perfusion inequality in chronic obstructive pulmonary disease. J Clin Invest 1977; 59:203–216.
12. Barcroft J, Cooke A, Hartridge H, Parsons TR, Parsons W. The flow of oxygen through the pulmonary epithelium. J Physiol 1920; 53:450–472.
13. Roughton FJW, Forster RE. Relative importance of diffusion and chemical reaction rates in determining rate of exchange of gases in the human lung, with special reference to true diffusing capacity of pulmonary membrane and volume of blood in the lung capillaries. J Appl Physiol 1957; 11:290–302.
14. Piiper J, Scheid P. Model for capillary-alveolar equilibration with special reference to O_2 uptake in hypoxia. Respir Physiol 1981; 46:193–208.
15. Wagner PD. Influence of mixed venous P_{O_2} on diffusion of O_2 across the pulmonary blood:gas barrier. Clin Physiol 1982; 2:105–115.
16. Krogh A. The number and distribution of capillaries in muscle with calculations of the pressure head necessary for supplying the tissue. J Physiol 1919; 52:409–415.
17. Wagner PD. A theoretical analysis of factors determining $\dot{V}_{O_2 MAX}$ at sea level and altitude. Resp Physiol 1996; 106:329–343.
18. Cerretelli P, Marconi C, Pendergast D, Meyer M, Heisler N, Piiper J. Blood flow in exercising muscles by xenon clearance and by microsphere trapping. J Appl Physiol 1984; 56:24–30.
19. Honig CR, Gayeski TEJ, Federspiel WJ, Clark A Jr, Clark P. Muscle O_2 gradients from hemoglobin to cytochrome: new concepts, new complexities. Adv Exp Med Biol 1984; 169:23–38.
20. Richardson RS, Noyszewski EA, Kendrick KF, Leigh JS, Wagner PD. Myoglobin O_2 desaturation during exercise: evidence of limited O_2 transport. J Clin Invest 1995; 96:1916–1926.
21. Wilson DF, Vinogradov SA. Recent advances in oxygen measurements using phosphorescence quenching. In: Oxygen Transport to Tissue XVI. New York: Plenum Press, 1994, pp 61–66.

22. Bebout DE, Hogan MC, Hempleman SC, Wagner PD. Effects of training and immobilization on $\dot{V}O_2$ and DO_2 in dog gastrocnemius muscle *in situ*. J Appl Physiol 1993; 74:1697–1703.
23. Knight DR, Schaffartzik W, Poole DC, Hogan MC, Bebout DE, Wagner PD. Effects of hyperoxia on maximal leg O_2 supply and utilization in humans. J Appl Physiol 1993; 75:2586–2594.
24. Cardús J, Marrades RM, Roca J, Barberà JA, Diaz O, Masclans JR, Rodriguez-Roisin R, Wagner PD. Effect of F_{IO_2} on leg $\dot{V}O_2$ during cycle ergometry in sedentary subjects. Med Sci Sports Exerc 1998; 30:697–703.
25. Marrades RM, Roca J, Campistol J, Diaz O, Barberà JA, Torregrosa JV, Masclans JR, Cobos A, Rodriguez-Roisin R, Wagner PD. Effects of erythropoietin on muscle O_2 transport during exercise in patients with chronic renal failure. J Clin Invest 1996; 97:2092–2100.
26. Mitlehner W, Kerb W. Exercise hypoxemia and the effects of increased inspiratory oxygen concentration in severe chronic obstructive pulmonary disease. Respiration 1994; 61:255–262.
27. Diesel W, Emms M, Knight BK, Noakes TD, van Zyl Smit R, Kaschula ROC, Sinclair-Smith CC. Morphologic features of the myopathy associated with chronic renal failure. Am J Kidney Dis 1993; 22:677–684.
28. West JB. Respiratory Physiology: The Essentials. 3rd ed. Baltimore: Williams & Wilkins, 1984.
29. Evans JW, Wagner PD. Limits on $\dot{V}_A/\dot{Q}$ distributions from analysis of experimental inert gas elimination. J Appl Physiol 1977; 42:889–898.
30. Honig CR, Gayeski TEJ, Clark A Jr, Clark PAA. Arteriovenous oxygen diffusion shunt is negligible in resting and working gracilis muscles. Am J Physiol 1991; 261:H2031–2043.
31. Cymerman A, Reeves JT, Sutton JR, Rock PB, Groves BM, Malconian MK, Young PM, Wagner PD, Houston CS. Operation Everest II: maximal oxygen uptake at extreme altitude. J Appl Physiol 1989; 66:2446–2453.

2

Oxygen and Metabolic Homeostasis During Large-Scale Change in Tissue Work Rates

PETER W. HOCHACHKA

University of British Columbia
Vancouver, British Columbia, Canada

I. Contrasting Requirements of Homeostasis and Tissue Work

As originally envisaged, the term *homeostasis* refers to the constancy of the internal milieu in the face of external perturbations that may be caused by extracellular factors, or in the case we shall consider, by change in intracellular biological function (1). All tissues in the vertebrate body are able to sustain routinely changes in work and metabolic rates, but the absolute magnitude of such change varies greatly tissue by tissue. Compared with modest 1.5- to 2-fold differences in metabolic rates between resting metabolic rates (RMRs) and activated states, which are common to many tissues such as liver and brain, skeletal muscles in humans must be able to sustain up to, or even more than, 100-fold changes in adenosine triphosphate (ATP) turnover rates. Among vertebrate endotherms, cardiac muscle typically must sustain 3- to 10-fold changes in work rate. The highest muscle metabolic rate (in the range of 600 μmol ATP/g/min) seems to be that of hummingbird breast muscle during hovering flight—a rate more than 500 times muscle RMR (2–4). During muscle ischemia, hypoxemia, or hypoxia, the metabolism of muscle, like that of many other tissues under oxygen-lacking conditions, may need to sustain a suppression of metabolism even below resting rates (5), thus even further extending the enormous range between lowest and highest sustainable ATP turnover rates of this remarkable tissue. This review focuses mainly on skeletal and cardiac muscles, with the hope of teasing out principles applicable to tissues in general.

Most recent popular interpretations of how these kinds of large-scale differences in steady-state energy turnover are regulated assume cybernetic feedback control circuitry. The standard theory is summarized in numerous publications (6–14). Activation signals arriving at the muscle cell increase ATP demand by "turning on" cell ATPases whose catalytic function serves to increase product (adenosine diphosphate [ADP] Pi, H^+) concentrations; the latter then play roles as substrates and as positive feedback signals for accelerating ATP supply pathways. These models usually assume that metabolites such as ADP and Pi are pivotal in mitochondrial metabolic control, but powerful activation of cell work also demands a proportional activation of some 30 or so other catalytic functions (enzymes, transporters, exchangers, pumps) at essentially every step involved in ATP-supply and -demand pathways. Hence, if substrate, product, and modulator concentration changes are to be the main mediators of large (up to 100-fold) change in ATP turnover rate, one would anticipate equally large perturbations in pool sizes of numerous intermediates. This would be especially true for regulation processes based on Michaelis-Menten kinetics, where the kinetic order cannot exceed 1 (15,16). That is, a given percent change in catalytic rate (ATP turnover rate) cannot exceed the percent change in substrate concentration driving the metabolic change (17,18). Homeostasis demands constancy of the internal milieu, whereas muscle work would seem to require drastic changes in intracellular conditions, the degree of perturbation being somehow related to the intensity of work. The problem (and paradox) we wish to assess here is how the conflicting demands of homeostasis versus metabolic regulation are resolved during different work and metabolic states, i.e., how tissues sustain both metabolic homeostasis and metabolic regulation.

II. Human Muscle Metabolism During Work

A recent study (19) using noninvasive magnetic resonance spectroscopy (MRS) technology illustrates the situation well. In the present analysis, our ^{31}P MRS protocol simultaneously interrogated two muscles, the gastrocnemius (mainly fast-twitch fibers) and the soleus (mainly slow-twitch fibers), at rest and during graded exercise. Muscle [H^+] was calculated from the exchange-averaged or time-averaged chemical shift difference between monoprotonated and diprotonated phosphate. The concentrations of free ADP ([ADP]) were calculated from the equilibrium constant for creatine phosphokinase (CPK), assumed to be 1.77×10^9, with free Mg^{++} taken to be 1 mmol/L and unchanging with exercise; this calculation takes into account the effects of pH on the calculated [ADP]. In addition, for these calculations, we assumed a resting [ATP] of 6 mmol/L and a total creatine pool ([PCr] + [Cr]) of 24 mmol/L, 75% phosphorylated (values well within the range expected for muscles of humans and other mammals). Any error in these estimates would change the calculated value of [ADP] but would not alter the fractional changes in concentrations during rest–work–recovery transitions; the latter information is most relevant to this analysis. To reduce between-subject variations, relative PCr concentrations were calculated as {PCr}, defined as the area under the PCr peak divided by the combined areas under the PCr, β-phosphate of ATP, and Pi peaks. ATP turnover rates during different metabolic states could not be determined directly in these studies; instead, the ATP turnover rates were treated as a percentage of the maximum sustainable rate, analagous to percent of maximum voluntary exercise. However, we should mention that it is known that (i) the ATP turnover rate during sustained submaximal muscle exercise is a direct function of the work rate (2), which is why the latter can be used as an index of the former (21); and (ii) during work protocols involving small muscle masses in humans (22,23), the maximum ATP turnover is high (because cardiac output can be preferentially directed to a small working area). Assuming a similar maximum rate of approximately 100 μmol/g/min for these studies indicates muscle exercise intensities equivalent to ATP turnover rates of 20, 30, and 40 μmol/g/min in each of the three work episodes; these are approximately 20, 30, and 40 times muscle RMRs (approximately 0.5 to 1.5 μmol/g/min for both slow-twitch and fast-twitch muscles).

The data on PCr, ATP, ADP, Pi, and H^+ (Figs. 1A through 1D) for the gastrocnemius were similar to those previously found (24) for exercising muscles: declining {PCr} during exercise (maximally down to approximately one-fourth resting values) with concomitant increase in {Pi} to work-related new steady states, followed by rapid recoveries during each subsequent rest interval. The chemical shift for Pi also showed modest adjustment, indicating modest change in the equilibrium between diprotonated and monoprotonated phosphate caused by H^+ accumulation (Fig. 1A). In contrast, the three ATP peaks remained stable throughout the protocol (data for the β peak are shown in Fig. 1A). For soleus, all [metabolites] seemed more stable during exercise than in gastrocnemius (Figs. 1D and 2A).

We also analyzed the data using ATP turnover rate (assumed proportional to muscle exercise intensity) as the independent parameter. In the gastrocnemius, the change in ATP demand or in the work rate was linearly reflected in decreasing PCr concentrations (Fig. 2B). Because change in {Pi} is essentially stochiometric with change in {PCr}, a good relationship was also observed between {Pi} and ATP turnover rate (Fig. 3A). However, it is important to note that the relationship extended far beyond the apparent K_M for Pi of mitochondrial metabolism (20); as with the {PCr} data, a kinetic order of 1 was not observed. For these reasons, it seems that both {PCr} and {Pi} reliably reflect the ATP turnover rate demanded by the imposed exercises but do not regulate the ATP turnover rate through effects on mitochondrial metabolism.

In contrast to the simple linear relationships between PCr and Pi concentrations and ATP turnover rates, the relationships with [ADP] and gastrocnemius work intensities were complex (Fig. 3B). Although changes in ADP concentration are consistent with some role in metabolic activation (13), the increase in [ADP] was not a simple and direct (1:1) function of work rate, as would be required

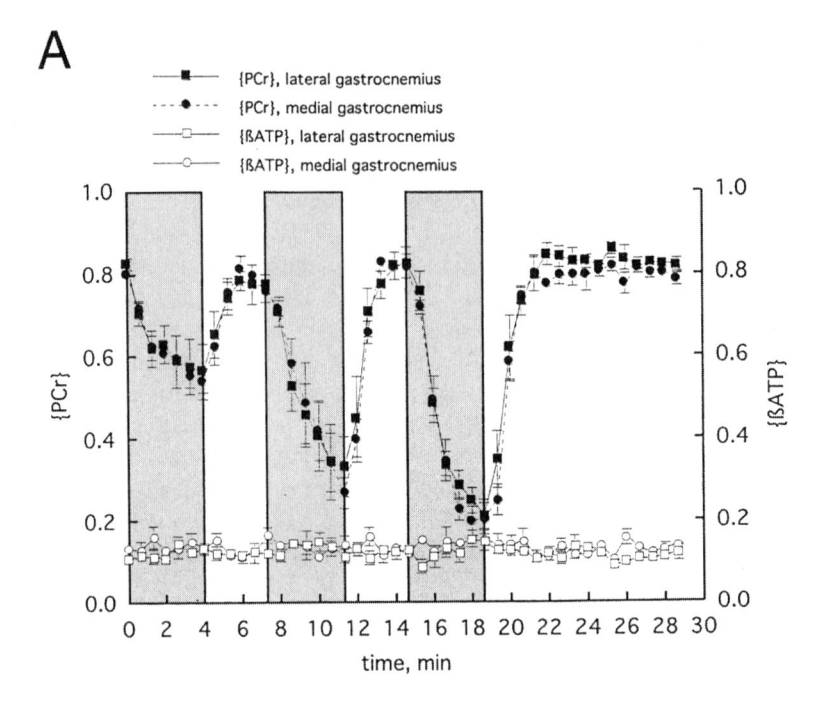

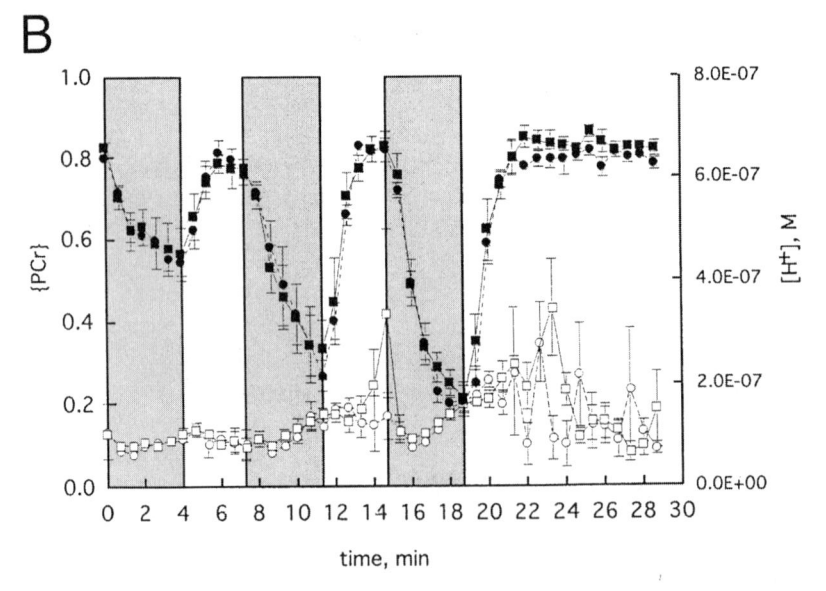

Figure 1 (A, upper left) Rest, exercise, and recovery effects on PCr and ATP in human medial and lateral gastrocnemius (n = 4). Exercise periods shaded were, from left to right, 20%, 30%, and 40% of the ramped maximum. Bars are SEs. (B, lower left). Same patterns for H^+ with PCr data replotted for reference. The concentrations of PCr and Pi are given as a fraction of the sum of [PCr] + [Pi] + [ATP]; the notations, {PCr} and {Pi}, were introduced by Matheson et al. (24). (Modified from Ref. 19.)

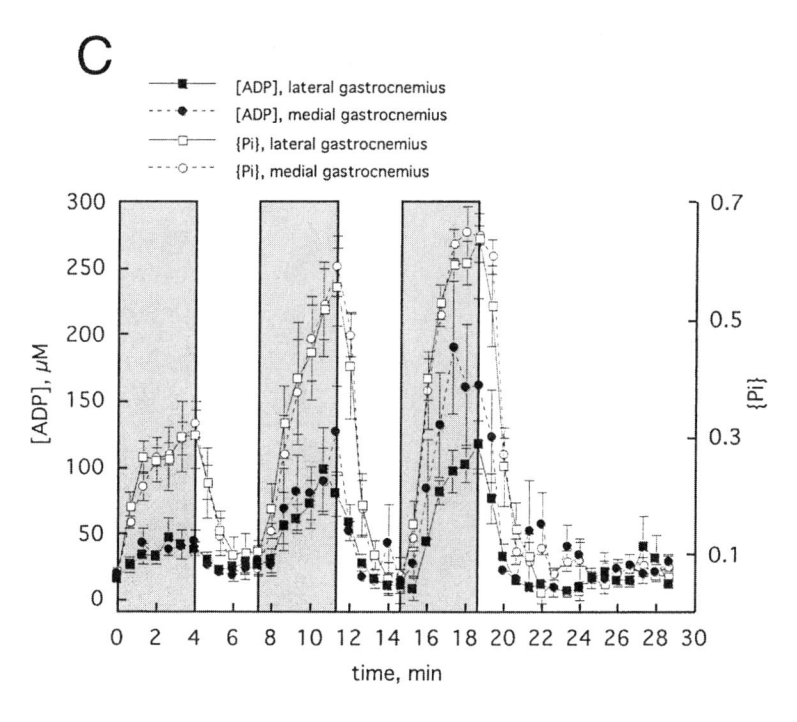

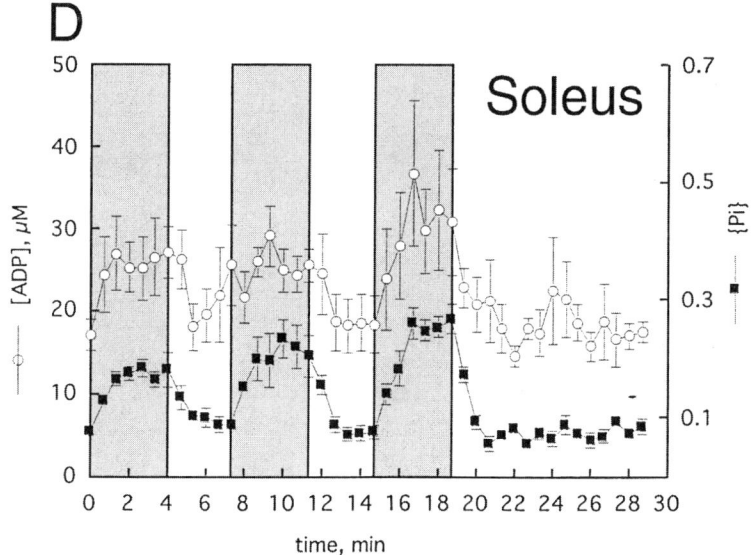

Figure 1 (C, upper right) Same patterns for ADP and Pi. (D) Same patterns for ADP and Pi in the soleus muscle. (Modified from Ref. 19.)

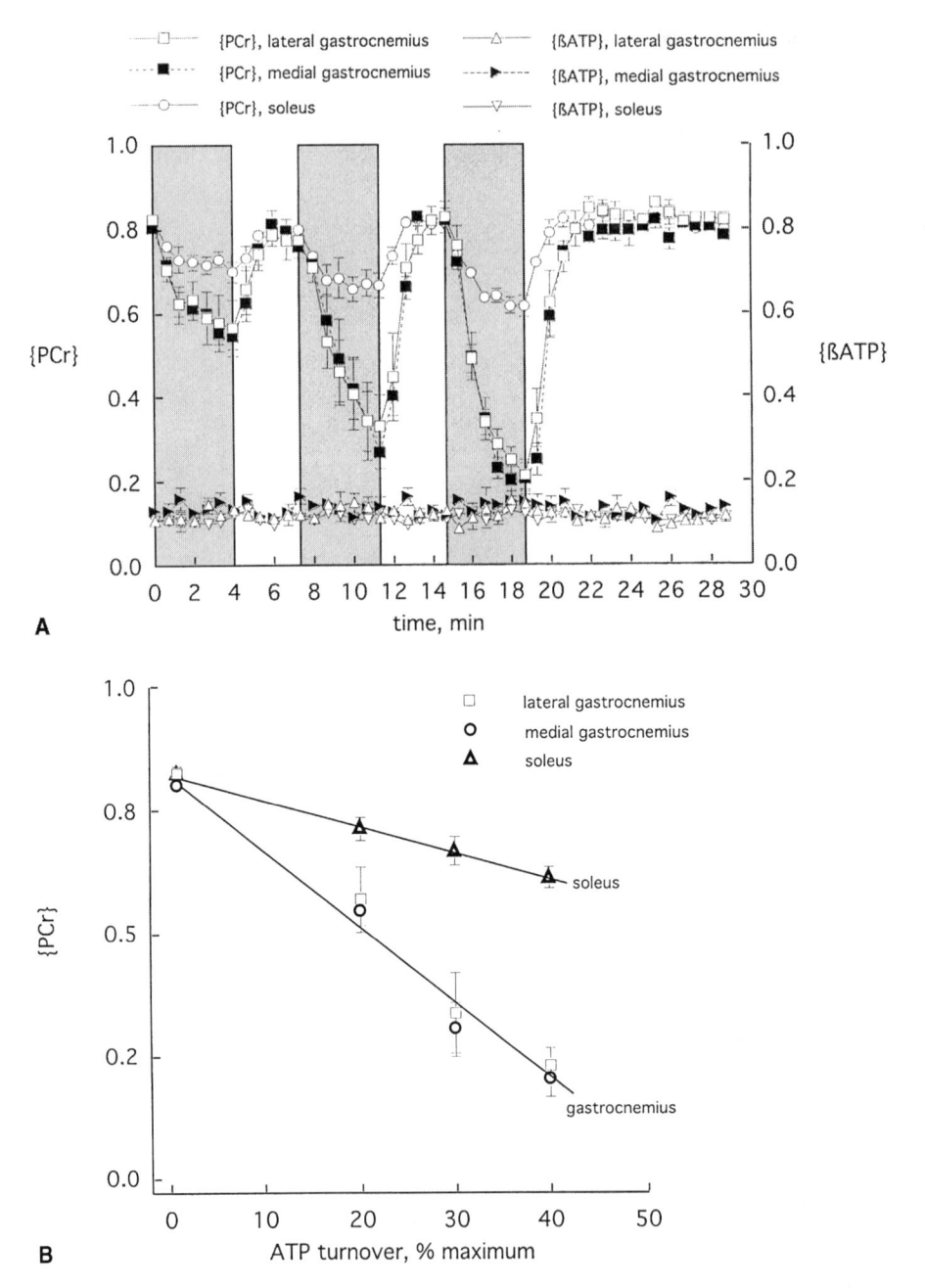

Figure 2 (A, upper panel) Rest, exercise, and recovery effects on PCr and ATP in soleus compared with the gastrocnemius (the latter data are the same as in Fig. 1A). (B, lower panel) Change in muscle ATP turnover rate (as percent sustained maximum) is plotted as the independent parameter versus {PCr} as the dependent parameter. (Modified from Ref. 19.)

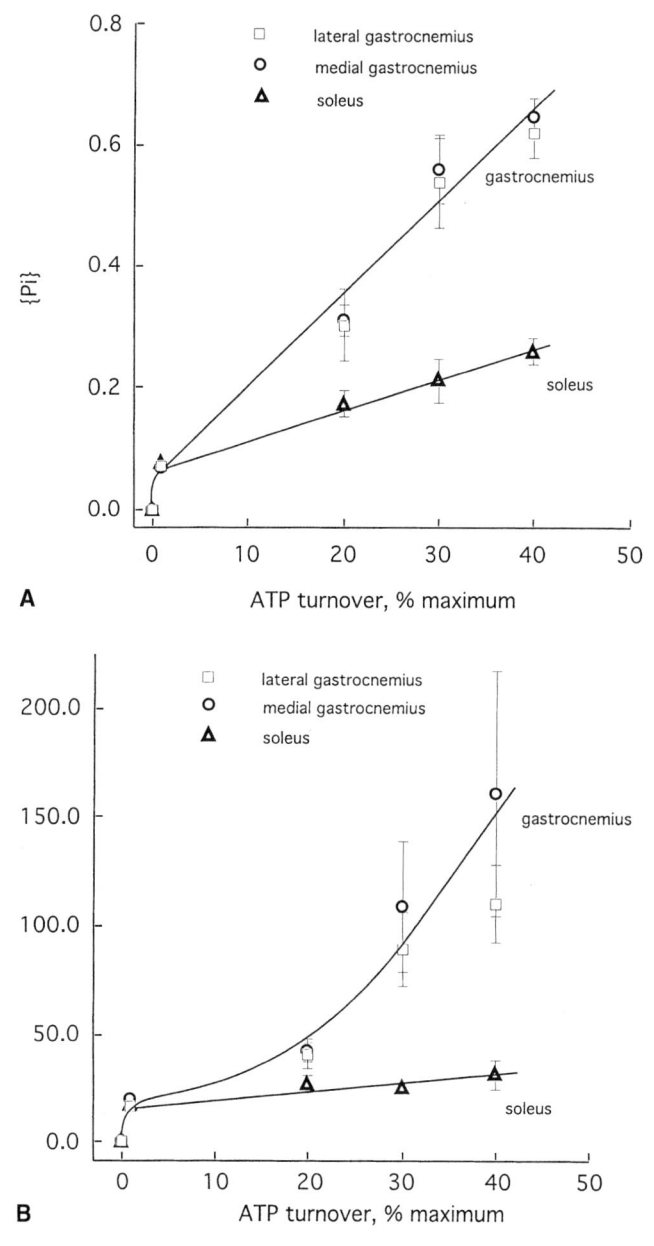

Figure 3 (A, upper panel) Change in muscle ATP turnover rate (as percent sustained maximum) is plotted as the independent parameter versus {Pi} as the dependent parameter. At zero {Pi}, the ATP turnover rate is assumed to be necessarily zero. (B, lower panel) Change in muscle ATP turnover rate (as percent of sustained maximum) is plotted as the independent parameter versus [ADP] as the dependent parameter. At zero [ADP], the ATP turnover rate is again assumed to be necessarily zero. (Modified from Ref. 19.)

by the Michaelis-Menten models of ADP control that are popular in this field. This difficulty with ADP as a primary regulator of ATP turnover rate is also noted elsewhere (6,18,20,25,26). Even if we assume signoidal ADP saturation kinetics (18,27), such rest–work comparisons mean that the fractional changes in ADP concentrations seem to be much less than that required for the fractional changes in ATP turnover rates in gastrocnemius muscle. Therefore, it is unlikely that the former could "drive" the latter; again, it may be more realistic to view changes in [ADP] as reflecting changes in ATP demand by muscle ATPases (17,25). Be that as it may, the data clearly emphasize that in the case of the gastrocnemius, no simple causal relations exist between imposed exercise (ATP turnover rates) and ADP concentration changes, and the same applies to {PCr} and {Pi}.

For the soleus, the case for regulation of ATP turnover rate by any of these metabolites is even weaker than for the gastrocnemius (Figs. 2B and 3). The kinetic order is further from 1 in the case of PCr and Pi—even if both PCr and Pi consistently reflect the differing exercise intensities. With regard to [ADP], the soleus sustains the three exercise intensities at essentially constant ADP concentrations (Fig. 3B).

Taken together, these results can be interpreted to mean that, in muscles formed mainly of fast-twitch fibers, ADP and Pi may play fine-tuning roles in regulating ATP turnover rates, but that some other (currently unknown) course-control mechanisms must be operative in controlling large-scale changes in ATP turnover rates during muscle work (18). In contrast, in slow-twitch oxidative fibers (which dominate soleus muscle), neither ADP nor Pi seems to be of any particular regulatory significance—a situation rather reminiscent of the heart of large mammals (6), including humans (26), and in agreement with those few animal studies that have examined this issue in slow-twitch muscle noninvasively (13). In earlier studies (18,24,25), the coupling patterns between ATP-demand and ATP-supply pathways in cardiac and slow-twitch muscles were described as "tighter" than those in fast-twitch muscles because large changes in ATP turnover rates could be sustained with modest (or immeasurable) changes in these key high-energy phosphate metabolites.

III. Widespread Stability of Metabolites During Changes in Metabolic Rates

The reason we discuss the aforementioned results for human muscle in detail is because they are in no way unusual. Similar observations for the adenylates, phosphagen, Pi, and H^+ arise from studies of a wide assortment of preparations, including invertebrates (28), fishes and other ectothermic vertebrates (29), mammals and birds (see Ref. 18 for literature in this area). Furthermore, some of these studies have also analyzed many of the intermediates in specific ATP-supply pathways, including glycolysis (25,30) and the Krebs cycle (31). Here, too, changes in [pathway intermediates] are minute (0.5- to 3-fold) compared with the large changes in pathway fluxes that are simultaneously sustained by the working tissue.

IV. Demands of Homeostasis Take Precedence During Changes in Work Rates of Tissues

The implications emerging from the analysis to this point are interesting. Although on first glance it may seem that the requirements for sustaining large changes in work would disrupt homeostasis, the data indicate just the opposite. Namely, it seems clear that (i) [ATP] is almost perfectly homeostatic under most conditions (except under very extreme fatigue conditions not considered in this analysis)—empirically this has been known for three decades or more; and (ii) other intermediates in pathways of ATP supply or demand are also stabilized but within less rigorously controlled concentration ranges. Nevertheless, they sustain much smaller percent change than that in overall flux through enzyme-catalyzed reactions in ATP-supply and -demand pathways. For convenience, the latter may be considered to be held in a "relatively" homeostatic condition because the percent changes in concentrations of intermediates are far less than those in metabolic rates with which they correlate.

In tissues such as liver, the difference between RMR and maximally activated metabolism is much more modest. A popular model used to explain stable concentrations of adenylates (and other intermediates) at varying ATP turnover rates assumes coordinate control by Ca^{++} of both ATP-supply and -demand pathways (see Ref. 32 and literature therein). For muscle and heart, these kinds of mechanisms seem inadequate to account for the rate changes observed (6). We have argued (17,18) that the simplest model to account for these observations of unanticipated metabolic homeostasis assumes regulation of the concentrations of catalytically active enzymes in pathways of both ATP demand and supply (e_o regulation); this would achieve changes in ATP turnover rates proportional to the k_{cat} of the enzymes involved with no required change in substrate or product concentrations (see Refs. 33 and 34 for a possible example of this kind of regulation). Another model for enzymes that operate under near-equilibrium conditions assumes that very high catalytic capacities assure sensitive responses to small changes in substrate/product ratios (see Refs. 18 and 35 for literature in this area). Such near-equilibrium function of CPK is the accepted explanation for the especially precise regulation of [ATP] during rate transitions—the traditional ATP "buffering" role of CPK (Fig. 4, upper panel). Still, for models assuming key regulatory roles for pathway intermediates, the relative homeostasis of most metabolites consistently presents a disturbing difficulty: the percent change in [putative regulatory intermediate] is always very much less than that in flux required to match the change in ATP turnover rate. In Atkinson's (15,16) terms, the kinetic order is usually less than 1, too low to be "driving" the observed flux or metabolic rate changes. The only metabolite that seems to be an exception is oxygen.

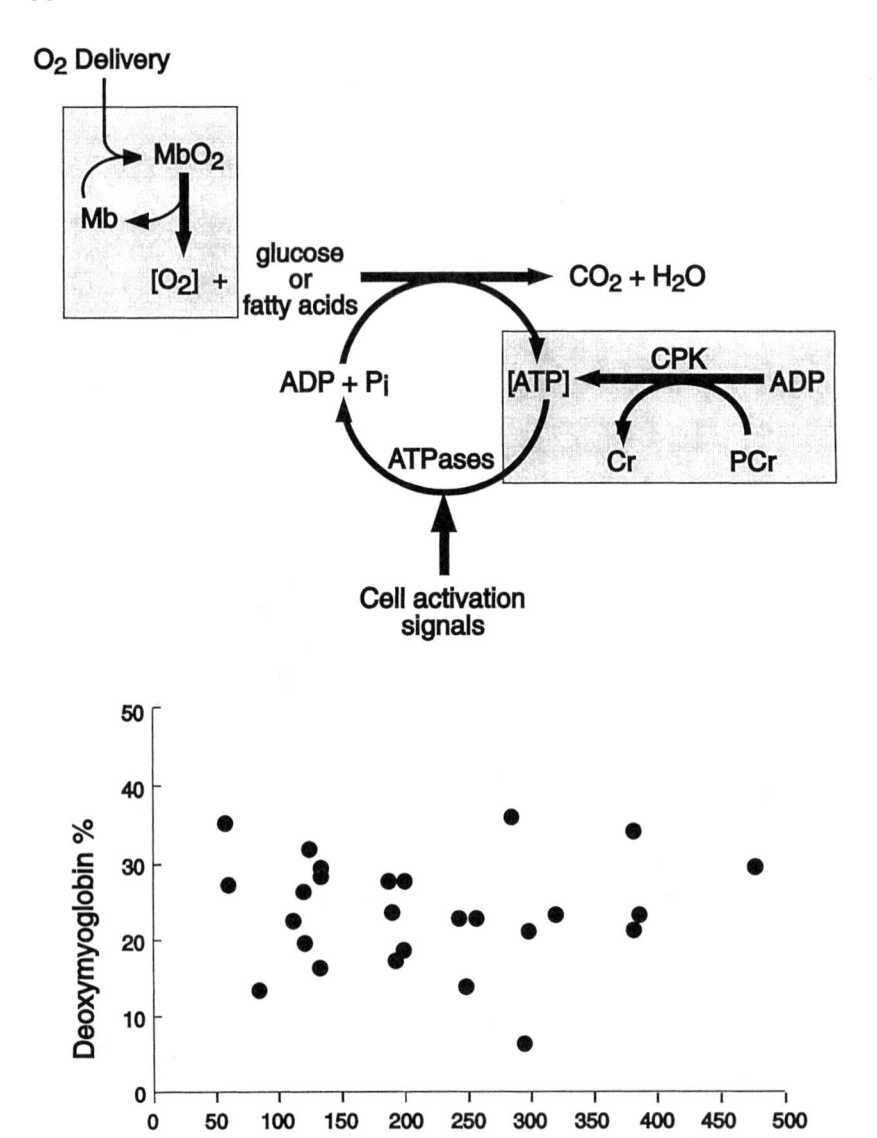

Figure 4 Schematic diagram illustrating the buffering roles of the CPK and of Mb in skeletal and cardiac muscles. The diagram is simplified and does not include the possibility for localized CPK buffering and transport functions within the cell, for which there is convincing evidence (46–48). Evidence for a myoglobin buffering role in skeletal and cardiac muscle comes from recent MRS data, which are consistent with earlier theoretical considerations in showing that %Mbo$_2$ remains constant over broad ranges of O$_2$ flux to mitochondrial metabolism. (From Refs. 40,43,44.)

V. Oxygen Delivery and Metabolic Regulation

There is a large literature on how oxygen functions as a substrate and as a potential regulator of metabolic rates of tissues, too large to review comprehensively in this chapter (see Refs. 36 and 37). For working muscle, suffice to emphasize that numerous studies have found relatively good 1:1 relationships between oxygen delivery and tissue work. For example, recent studies (20,38) using a dog gastrocnemius preparation showed such a relationship between oxygen delivery and work over more than an 18-fold change in ATP turnover rate. Hogan et al. (39) used the same preparation to analyze subtle submaximal work changes. These work transitions were sustained with immeasurable change in [phosphocreatine] and [ATP]; therefore, other [metabolites] were also presumably stable. However, through these transitions, a 1:1 relation between change in work and change in oxygen delivery was maintained. Such results are qualitatively similar to those found in many other studies, which is why many investigators in the field accept that oxygen plays a key role in regulating change in ATP turnover (18). The question then arises, how is the oxygen signal transduced within the cell?

VI. Transducing the Oxygen Signal in Working Tissue

The issue of how oxygen delivery translates into effects on metabolism within the cell requires quantitative information on intracellular oxygen concentrations. For most tissues, it has not been possible to quantify this key parameter, and it thus remains unknown. Fortunately, in cardiac and skeletal muscles, myoglobin (Mb) supplies a direct intracellular "monitor" of oxygen concentration. Because Mb is apparently freely diffusible in the cytosol (40) and the reaction Mb + O_2 ↔ MbO_2 is always in equilibrium (41), with a K_D of approximately 0.1 mmol/L (P50 of approximately 2 to 3 mm Hg), %MbO_2 measurements supply a direct and accurate window on intracellular [oxygen]. Earlier attempts at such measurements with working muscle preparations almost exclusively relied on near-infrared spectroscopy (see Ref. 42 for literature and an application of this technique in evaluation of muscle oxygenation status during voluntary diving in Weddell seals). More recently, workers have used MRS to take advantage of a histidine H being ^{1}H MRS "visible" in deoxyMb (which is paramagnetic) but being MRS "invisible" in oxyMb (40), thus allowing %MbO_2 quantification. Alternately, with water suppression (43), a Val E11 τ-methyl H, MRS visible in oxyMb but not in deoxyMb, can be monitored (chemical shift of approximately −3 ppm) to estimate intracellular %MbO_2. With this technology, workers in the field now have a noninvasive means to unequivocally detect the oxygenation state of Mb-containing muscles in different work and metabolic states.

The application of this technology to both working human skeletal muscles (44) and to perfused rat heart (40,43) leads to the same striking observation: namely, remarkably constant %MbO_2 despite large changes in work rate. An example of such data for the perfused rat heart (40) is shown in Figure 4 (lower panel). (This implies that in both heart and skeletal muscle, the %MbO$_2$ (and intracellular [oxygen]) is held essentially constant up to the maximum sustainable aerobic metabolic rate of the tissue (44). Just as CPK serves to buffer ATP concentrations during changes in muscle work, so Mb serves to buffer intracellular oxygen concentrations in different metabolic states (Fig. 4). In our context, under normoxic conditions, oxygen is thus perfectly homeostatic in the sense that its concentration is stable even while its flux to cytochrome oxidase can change by orders of magnitude.

Because the general reader may not appreciate how startling these new data actually are, it is worth emphasizing some key features. First, because of the buffering role of Mb, oxygen concentrations are low, in the P50 or K_D range. Second, because Mb is freely diffusible, is randomly distributed throughout the cytosol, and displays "on" and "off" rate constants that far exceed O$_2$ flux rates to the mitochondria (40,43), intracellular [oxygen] gradients are necessarily shallow. As emphasized by Connett et al. (9) and Gayeski and Honig (45), who discuss this point more fully, O$_2$ experiences a sharp gradient on entry into the muscle cell but not within the muscle cell per se. Once inside the cell, a randomly distributed, freely diffusible, partially saturated pool of Mb assures that intracellular [oxygen] is powerfully buffered and remains essentially stable throughout large changes in work and metabolic rates. Under these conditions, increasing O$_2$ consumption rates with increasing work could be achieved by increasing the catalytic activity of cytochrome oxidase (allosteric regulation), by increasing the availability of cytochrome oxidase (e_o regulation), or by locally generating steeper diffusion gradients from cytosol to O$_2$ binding sites in cytochrome oxidase. On pure geometric arguments, as well as empircal measurements, Connett et al. and Gayeski and Honig consider that they can rule out the latter alternative; i.e., the only steep gradient O$_2$ encounters occurs on entry into the muscle cell (see, for example, Ref. 45,49). Once inside the cell, gradients and concentrations are both low.

In our analysis of other metabolites, stable metabolite concentrations during changes in work rate were taken to indicate modest roles in regulation. The situation with O$_2$ is different: despite the data implying stable intracellular [O$_2$] through wide changes in work rate, oxygen delivery and V̇O$_2$ are closely related, suggesting a key role for oxygen in metabolic regulation, a final problem that still needs to be addressed.

VII. An Unsolved Regulatory Problem

The funademantal insight that oxygen delivery, not intracellular [oxygen], correlates with work rate creates a problem that molecular physiologists have yet to resolve; namely, the problem of how the oxygen signal "gets through" to the machinery of cell metabolism. At this time, it is clear that there is no widely accepted answer. From our analysis of the evidence, it seems safe, at least tentatively, to conclude that the required controlling signal for turning mitochondrial metabolism up or down is not cytosolic oxygen concentration. From the %MbO$_2$ studies available thus far (indicating stable [O$_2$] at differing work levels), one way to account for the apparent regulatory relationship between O$_2$ delivery and metabolic rate is to postulate an oxygen-sensing system presumably located in the cell membrane (or even more distally) and signal transduction pathways or mechanisms for informing the cell metabolic machinery when to respond to changing availability of oxygen (18). At this time, the properties of any such putative sensing and signal transduction systems remain to be elucidated. Indeed, further evidence for their actual existence is highly desirable.

VIII. Summary

Traditionally, the term *homeostasis* is defined as the maintenance of relatively constant internal milieu in the face of changing environmental conditions or changing physiological function. Tissues such as skeletal and cardiac muscles must sustain very large-scale changes in ATP turnover rate during equally large changes in work. In many skeletal muscles, these changes can exceed 100-fold. In unique biological circumstances (e.g., during periods of oxygen limitation, vasoconstriction, and hypometabolism), tissues such as skeletal muscles may be obliged to sustain further decreases in ATP turnover rates and operate for varying time periods at seriously suppressed ATP turnover rates. Examination of a number of cell and whole-organism level systems identifies ATP concentration as a key parameter of the interior milieu that is nearly universally homeostatic; it is common to observe no change in ATP concentration even while change in its turnover rate can increase or decrease by two orders of magnitude. A large number of other intermediates of cellular metabolism are also regulated within narrow concentration ranges, but none seemingly as precisely as [ATP]. Indeed, the only other metabolite in aerobic energy metabolism that is seemingly as homeostatic is oxygen, at least in working muscles. The central regulatory question is how to accomodate such homeostasis of intracellular O$_2$ with the often-observed close relationship between O$_2$ delivery and tissue energy requirements during changes in work rates.

Acknowledgment

These studies were supported by NSERC (Canada).

References

1. Hochachka PW, Somero GN. Biochemical Adaptation. Princeton: Princeton University Press, 1984, pp 1–521.
2. Suarez RK. Hummingbird flight: sustaining the highest mass-specific metabolic rates among vertebrates. Experientia 1992; 48:565–570.

3. Suarez RK, Lighton JRB, Moyes CD, Brown GS, Gass CL, Hochachka PW. Fuel selection in rufous hummingbirds: ecological implications of metabolic biochemistry. Proc Natl Acad Sci USA 1990; 87:9207–9210.
4. Suarez RK, Lighton JRB, Brown GS, Mathieu-Costello OA. Mitochondrial respiration in hummingbird flight muscle. Proc Natl Acad USA 1991; 88:4870–4873.
5. Hochachka PW, Guppy M. Metabolic Arrest and the Control of Biological Time. Cambridge, MA: Harvard University Press, 1987, pp. 1–237.
6. Balaban RS. Regulation of oxidative phosphorylation in the mammalian cell. Am J Physiol 1990; 258:C377–C389.
7. Chance B, Leigh JS Jr, Kent J, McCully K. Metabolic control principles and 31P NMR. Federation Proc 1986; 45:2915–2920.
8. Connett RJ. Analysis of metabolic control: new insights using scaled creatine kinase model. Am J Physiol 1988; 254:R949–959.
9. Connett RJ, Gayeski TE, Honig CR. Energy sources in fully aerobic rest-work transitions: a new role for glycolysis. Am J Physiol 1985; 248:H922–H929.
10. Connett RJ, Honig CR. Regulation of Vo_2max: do current biochemical hypothesis fit *in vivo* data? Am J Physiol 1989; 256:R898–R906.
11. From AHL, Zimmer SD, Michurski SP, Mohanakrishnan P, Ulstad VK, Thomas WJ, Ugurbil K. Regulation of oxidative phosphorylation in the intact cell. Biochemistry 1990; 29:3733–3743.
12. Funk CI, Clark A Jr, Connett RJ. A simple model of metabolism: applications to work transitions in muscle. Am J Physiol 1990; 258:C995–C1005.
13. Kushmerick MJ, Meyer RA, Brown TR. Regulation of oxygen consumption in fast- and slow-twitch muscle. Am J Physiol 1992; 263:C598–C606.
14. Rumsey WL, Schlosser C, Nuutinen EM, Robiollo M, Wilson DF. Cellular energetics and the oxygen dependence of respiration in cardiac myocytes is dated from adult rat. J Biol Chem 1990; 265:15392–15402.
15. Atkinson DE. Cellular Energy Metabolism and Its Regulation. New York: Academic Press, 1977.
16. Atkinson DE. In: Cornish-Bowden A, Cardenas ML, eds. Control of Metabolic Processes. New York: Plenum Press, 1990, pp 11–27.
17. Hochachka PW, Matheson GO. Regulation of ATP turnover over broad dynamic muscle work ranges. J Appl Physiol 1992; 73:570.
18. Hochachka PW. Muscles and Molecular and Metabolic Machines. Boca Raton: CRC Press, 1994, pp 1–157.
19. Allen PS, Matheson GO, Zhu G, Gheorgiu D, Dunlop RS, Falconer T, Stanley C, Hochachka PW. Simultaneous 31P magnetic resonance spectroscopy of the soleus and gastrocnemius in Sherpas during graded calf muscle exercise. Am J Physiol 1997; 273:R999–R1007.
20. Arthur PG, Hogan MC, Wagner PD, Hochachka PW. Modelling the effects of hypoxia on ATP turnover in exercising muscle. J Appl Physiol 1992; 73:737–760.
21. Nioka S, Argov Z, Dobson GP, Forster RE, Subramanian HV, Veech RL, Chance B. Substrate regulation of mitochondrial oxidative phosphorylation in hypercapnic rabbit muscle. J Appl Physiol 1991; 72:521–528.
22. Saltin B. Malleability of the system in overcoming limitations: Functional elements. J Exp Biol 1985; 115:45–345.

23. Andersen P, Saltin B. Maximal perfusion of skeletal muscle in man. J Physiol 1985; 366:233–249.
24. Matheson GO, Allen PS, Ellinger DC, Hanstock CC, Gheorghiu D, McKenzie DC, Stanley C, Parkhouse WS, Hochachka PW. Skeletal muscle metabolism and work capacity: a ^{31}P-NMR study of Andean natives and lowlanders. J Appl Physiol 1991; 70:1963–1976.
25. Hochachka PW, Bianconcini M, Parkhouse WS, Dobson GP. Role of actomyosin ATPase in metabolic regulation during intense exercise. Proc Natl Acad Sci USA 1991; 88:5764–5768.
26. Hochachka PW, Clark CM, Holden JE, Stanley C, Ugurbil K, Menon RS. 31P MRS of the Sherpa heart: a PCr/ATP signature of metabolic defense against hypobaric hypoxia. Proc Natl Acad Sci USA 1996; 93:1215–1220.
27. Jeneson JAL, Wiseman RW, Westerhoff HV, Kushmerick MJ. The signal transduction function for oxidative phosphorylation is at least second order in ADP. J Biol Chem 1996; 271:27995–27998.
28. Wegener G, Bolas NM, Thomas AAG. Locust flight metabolism studied in vivo with 31P NMR spectroscopy. J Comp Physiol B 1991; 161:247–256.
29. Dobson GP, Hochachka PW. Role of glycolysis in adenylate depletion and repletion during work and recovery in teleost white muscle. J Exp Biol 1987; 129:125–140.
30. Dobson GP, Parkhouse WS, Weber JM, Stuttard E, Harman J, Snow DH, Hochachka PW. Metabolic changes in skeletal muscle and blood in greyhounds during 800 m track sprint. Am J Physiol 1988; 255:R513–R519.
31. Rowan AN, Newsholme EA. Changes in the contents of adenine nucleotides and intermediates of glycolysis and the citric acid cycle in flight muscle of the locust upon flight and the relationship to the control of the cycle. Biochem J 1979; 178:209–216.
32. McCormack JG, Denton RM. The role of Ca^{++} transport and matrix Ca in signal transduction in mammalian tissues. Biochim Biophys Acta 1990; 1018:287–291.
33. Blum H, Nioka S, Johnson RG Jr. Activation of the Na+K+ ATPase in *Narcine brasiliensis*. Proc Natl Acad Sci USA 1990; 87:1247–1251.
34. Blum H, Balschi JA, Johnson RG Jr. Coupled *in vivo* activity of the membrane band Na^+K^+ ATPase in resting and stimulated electric organ of the electric fish *Narcine brasiliensis*. J Biol Chem 1991; 266:10254–10259.
35. Betts DF, Srivastava DK. The rationalization of high enzyme concentrations in metabolic pathways such as glycolysis. J Theoret Biol 1991; 151:155–167.
36. Hochachka PW. Patterns of O_2 dependence of metabolism. Adv Exp Med Biol 1988; 222:143–149.
37. Hochachka PW, Emmett B, Suarez RK. Limits and constraints in the scaling of oxidative and glycolytic enzymes in homeotherms. Can J Zool 1988; 66:1128–1138.
38. Hogan MC, Arthur PG, Bebout DE, Hochachka PW, Wagner PD. The role of O_2 in regulating tissue respiration in dog muscle working *in situ*. J Appl Physiol 1992; 73:728.
39. Hogan MC, Kurdak SS, Arthur PG. Effect of gradual reduction in O_2 delivery on intracellular homeostasis in contracting skeletal muscle. J Appl Physiol 1996; 80:1313–1321.
40. Jelicks LA, Wittenberg BA. 1H NMR studies of sarcoplasmic oxygenation in the red cell perfused rat heart. Biophys J 1995; 68:2129–2136.

41. McGilvery RW. Biochemistry: A Functional Approach. Philadelphia: Saunders, 1983.
42. Guyton GP, Stanek KS, Schneider RC, Hochachka PW, Hurford WE, Zapol DG, Liggins GC, Zapol WM. Myoglobin saturation in free-diving Weddell seals. J Appl Physiol 1996; 79:1148–1155.
43. Kreutzer U, Jue T. Critical intracellular O_2 in myocardium as determined by 1H nuclear magnetic resonance signal of myoglobin. Am J Physiol 1995; 268:H1675–H1681.
44. Richardson RS, Noyszewski EA, Kendrick KF, Leigh JS, Wagner PD. Myoglobin O_2 desaturation during exercise: evidence of limited O_2 transport. J Clin Invest 1996; 96:1916–1926.
45. Gayeski TEJ, Honig CR. O_2 gradients from sarcolemma to cell interior in red muscle at maximal Vo_2. Am J Physiol 1986; 251:H789–H799.
46. Bessman SP, Geiger PJ. Transport of energy in muscle: the phosphorylcreatine shuttle. Science 1981; 211:448–452.
47. Wallimann T, Schlosser T, Eppenberger HM. Function of the M-line bound creatine kinase as intramyofibrillar ATP regenerator at the receiving end of the phosphorylcreatine shuttle in muscle. J Biol Chem 1984; 259:5238–5246.
48. Wallimann T, Wyss M, Brdiczka D, Nicolay K, Eppenberger HM. Intracellular compartmentation, structure, and function of creatine kinase isozymes in tissues with high and fluctuating energy demands: the "phosphocreatine circuit" for cellular energy homeostasis. Biochem J 1992; 281:21–40.
49. Connett RJ, Honig CR, Gayeski TEJ, Brooks GA. Defining hypoxia. J Appl Physiol 1990; 63:833–842.

3

Experimental Approaches to the Study of Gas Exchange

ROBERT L. JOHNSON, JR.

University of Texas Southwestern
 Medical Center
Dallas, Texas

SCOTT E. CURTIS*

University of Alabama at Birmingham
Birmingham, Alabama

I. Introduction

Experimental approaches to the study of limits and efficiency of gas exchange in the lung include methods for measuring not only magnitudes of the major transport functions, i.e., ventilatory capacity, diffusing capacity, and cardiac output, but also how these transport functions are recruited and matched to one another from rest to maximal exercise. Similarly, in the periphery, experimental approaches include methods for measuring distribution of cardiac output and regional diffusing capacity and how these transport functions are recruited and regionally matched to metabolic requirements for each organ. In both lung and periphery, anatomical studies and mathematical modeling are often essential for understanding structure–function relationships and how anatomy, distorted by disease, can affect these relationships. This chapter surveys methods currently available and their development and rationale. The chapter is subdivided into three major sections: total gas exchange, gas exchange in the lung, and gas exchange in the periphery.

Current affiliation: DeVos Children's Hospital, Grand Rapids, Michigan.

II. Total Respiratory Gas Exchange

A. Open-Circuit Techniques

Measurement of Expired Ventilation and Gas Concentrations

Open-circuit techniques are based on the principle of conservation of mass. The difference between the inhaled and exhaled volumes of O_2 (or CO_2) must equal systemic O_2 consumption (CO_2 production). Thus, $\dot{V}_{O_2} = (\dot{V}_I \cdot F_{IO_2}) - (\dot{V}_E \cdot F_{EO_2})$ and $\dot{V}_{CO_2} = (\dot{V}_E \cdot F_{ECO_2}) - (\dot{V}_I \cdot F_{ICO_2})$. Precise measures of inspiratory and expiratory minute volumes ($\dot{V}_I$ and $\dot{V}_E$, respectively) and inhaled and exhaled gas fractions (F_I and F_E, respectively, measured dry) with volumes corerected from ambient to standard conditions of temperature and pressure, dry, must be made (1). To avoid the necessity of measuring the potentially small but important differences in inspiratory and expiratory volumes, a Haldane transformation can be applied and rewritten as:

$$\dot{V}_{O_2} = \dot{V}_E \left[F_{IO_2} \cdot \frac{F_{EN_2}}{F_{IN_2}} - F_{EO_2} \right] \tag{1}$$

where it is assumed that gas exchange is in a steady state, that only O_2, CO_2, and N_2 are present, and that inspired CO_2 (F_{ICO_2}) is negligible. F_{N_2} is estimated indirectly as $1 - (F_{O_2} + F_{CO_2})$, representing the fractional concentration of all inert gases, primarily $A_r + N_2$ when breathing air. When inspired O_2 is much greater than 50%, both the numerator and denominator become small. In that situation, small errors in the measurement of F_{IO_2}, F_{EO_2}, or F_{ECO_2} produce large errors in $\dot{V}_{O_2}$, precluding its use (2). Because F_{ICO_2} is generally negligible, $\dot{V}_{CO_2}$ can be calculated simply as: $\dot{V}_{CO_2} = \dot{V}_E \cdot F_{ECO_2}$. Exhaled volumes can be measured using a pneumotachometer or by collection into bags or spirometers. Gas leaks in the system may cause significant errors. Adequate mixing and drying of exhaled gas must be assured. The device used for measurement of inhaled and exhaled O_2 fractions may include Clark-type (polarographic) electrodes, fuel cells, mass spectrometers, paramagnetic analyzers, or hot oxygen electrode (zirconium oxide) analyzers. CO_2 is generally measured with a mass spectrometer or infrared absorption analyzer. Choice of the many measuring systems available depends on whether the subject is breathing spontaneously or is ventilated, the F_{IO_2}, subject size, frequency of measurements required, and system cost and stability (for a review see Refs. 1, 3, and 4).

Breath-by-Breath Measurements of Gas Exchange

Methods have been developed for measuring breath-by-breath gas exchange at the mouth, using on-line computer acquisition and an algorithm that corrects for breath-by-breath changes in lung volume and intrapulmonary gas stores. These techniques are valuable for studying transients in gas exchange that occur at the beginning and end of exercise or after step changes in work load (5).

Open Circuit with Bias Flow

In many circumstances it is not possible or practical to design a mask or mouthpiece with a valving system for measuring expired ventilation. Seeherman et al. (6) designed a bias flow technique for measuring O_2 uptake up to maximal exercise in a wide range of mammals, from pygmy mice (7 g) to horses (105 kg). Large mammals were exercised on a motor-driven treadmill wearing a loose-fitting mask that allowed air to be drawn past the nose and mouth at a bias flow rate four to five times that of the expired ventilation; all expired volume was entrained past the gas analyzers. Small mammals were exercised on a motor-driven treadmill covered by a plastic canopy above the moving belt through which airflow was entrained past the analyzers. Expired ventilation cannot be measured with this system. However, if bias flow is used with a tight-fitting mask coupled with a three-way valve with both inspiratory and expiratory pneumotachometers, inspired and expired ventilation can be monitored continuously as the difference in flow between the two pneumotachometers (7).

B. Closed-Circuit Spirometry

Closed-circuit spirometry is a popular method of measuring $\dot{V}_{O_2}$ that in many ways is technically simpler than open-circuit methods. The subject is connected by mouthpiece, occlusive face mask, or endotracheal tube and breathes to and from a water-sealed spirometer filled with the desired F_{IO_2}, usually 1.0. The CO_2 is removed from exhaled gas before its return to the spirometer, so that changes in spirometer volume directly reflect O_2 consumption (1). It allows minute-to-minute measurements, works well with an F_{IO_2} of 1.0, and does not require measurement of gas flows or fractions. It does not provide an online measurement of $\dot{V}_{CO_2}$ ($\dot{V}_{CO_2}$ can be estimated crudely from the final weight change of the CO_2-absorbing granules), and as with all of these techniques, leaks can cause significant errors. It should be noted that respiratory gas analysis methods include all of the body's O_2 consumption, whereas the Fick method, described in the following section, fails to measure gas exchange across the bronchial and thebesian circulations.

C. Cardiac Output and the Fick Principle

The Fick principle is another application of the law of conservation of mass and can be applied to systemic or regional measures of $\dot{V}_{O_2}$ and $\dot{V}_{CO_2}$. It states that the steady-state consumption or production of a bloodborne substance by a tissue is equal to the arteriovenous content difference of the substance times the tissue blood flow. For systemic O_2 consumption, the equation is: $\dot{V}_{O_2} = CO(Ca_{O_2} - C\bar{v}_{O_2})$. Different methods are available to measure cardiac output (CO) and arterial and mixed venous O_2 contents (Ca_{O_2}, $C\bar{v}_{O_2}$). In laboratory animals, extravascular flow meters (discussed in Sec. II.B) may be placed surgically on the pulmonary artery or aorta. More often, a balloon-tipped catheter is floated into a pulmonary artery via a large vein. This permits collection of an adequately mixed systemic venous sample as well as the injection of material for dye or thermal dilution analysis. Thermal dilution is used almost exclusively and involves the rapid injection of a known volume of crystalloid, generally 3 to 10 mL, at a known temperature below body temperature, usually iced or at room temperature, at a known distance proximal to the catheter tip's thermistor (8). The area under the thermal dilution curve is measured at the thermistor and extrapolated to infinity from the exponential downslope; this area is inversely proportional to the CO, which is automatically calculated by computer. Results may vary significantly when injection occurs at different times in the respiratory cycle, particularly in the presence of hypovolemia or large tidal volumes. Errors in measurement of injectate volume and temperature also affect the results. Under the best of circumstances, a coefficient of variation (SD/mean) of 10% to 15% is observed. Placement may be difficult in low-output states or in small subjects, and although complications are infrequent, they may include such significant events as arrhythmias, vascular or cardiac wall rupture, pulmonary infarction, and bloodstream infection. In patients with congenital heart disease and intracardiac shunts, thermal dilution CO will not reflect systemic blood flow accurately.

Use of the Fick method requires measurement of blood O_2 content, which equals the sum of O_2 dissolved in the blood plus that bound to hemoglobin (Hb). The rarely used Van Slyke manometric method is the gold standard for measurement of blood O_2 and CO_2 content (9). Blood O_2 and CO_2 are chemically released then sequentially absorbed out of a closed system, and the resultant pressure changes are related to the blood O_2 and CO_2 contents. Although equations are available for estimating total blood CO_2 (10), the Van Slyke apparatus offers the only practical way to accurately investigate total CO_2 transport. Still in use in many research laboratories is the Lex-O_2-Con (Lexington Instruments, Waltham, Mass.), which approximates the Van Slyke apparatus in measurement accuracy of blood total O_2 content and is less demanding technically, but does not measure CO_2 content. Similar to the Van Slyke and in contrast to CO oximetry, Lex-O_2-Con measurements are very time consuming. Use of the Van Slyke method or Lex-O_2-Con remains necessary in studies in which O_2 is carried by substances other than Hb and plasma, e.g., perfluorocarbon. Most blood gas laboratories now rely on CO oximetry to measure oxyhemoglobin (O_2Hb) saturation and a blood gas analyzer to measure P_{O_2}, P_{CO_2}, and pH. Blood O_2 content is then calculated as %Sat · Hb (g/dL) · 1.39 (mL/g) + 0.003 [(mL/mm Hg)/dL] · P_{O_2} (mm Hg). Most CO oximeters measure light absorbance of the blood sample (after lysis of red blood cells) at five or six wavelengths of light and routinely estimate total Hb as well as the percentages of oxyHb, metHb, and carboxyHb present. Errors may be introduced when the wavelengths used are inappropriate to the type of Hb present, e.g., with fetal or animal Hb, although some CO oximeters can be customized to measure these samples accurately. A less rigorous method is to estimate saturation using P_{O_2} and a standard oxyHb dissociation curve. Failure to account for the effects of in vivo pH, P_{CO_2}, and red blood cell 2,3-diphosphoglycerate (DPG) levels on the dissociation curve will introduce errors in estimating oxyHb. The field of O_2 and CO_2 electrode design is beyond the scope of this chapter, but the interested reader can refer to several comprehensive reviews (11,12).

Many studies have compared the Fick and respiratory gas methods with variable results (3,8). The majority suggest that the Fick gives higher values of $\dot{V}_{O_2}$ than respiratory gas methods, perhaps secondary to the known tendency of thermal dilution methods to overestimate CO when CO is decreased. The respiratory gas methods are generally taken as more accurate, but they often are more technically challenging to perform properly. Regardless of any technical limitations, a significant deficiency of systemic $\dot{V}_{O_2}$ measures lies in their interpretation, because they cannot speak to whether regional or even total O_2 demand is being met adequately.

III. Gas Exchange in the Lung

A. Approaches to Structure–Function Relationships in Gas Exchange

Distribution of Ventilation

For convenience, the bronchial system is often described as a regular dichotomous branching tree. Twenty-three generations are numbered from the trachea (as generation 0) down to terminal alveolar sac (as generation 23) (13). Airway diameters and lengths decrease at successive generations in a constant ratio ($\approx 2^{-1/3}$ and $2^{-1/4}$, respectively) down to bronchi with approximately 1-mm diameter; at the same time, total cross-sectional area of successive generations increase. All path lengths to gas exchange units are equal. This description simplifies estimates of laminar and turbulent flow resistances and distribution of anatomical dead space to alveoli during breathing. The major drawback of this approach is that it fails to explain anatomically why alveolar ventilation is not uniformly distributed in a normal lung or how this dichotomously branching tree can fit into the thorax to fill completely the available asymmetrical space.

Calculations Based on Dimensions of Airways Measured by
Calibrated Bougies

In 1915, Rohrer (14) was the first to model comprehensively the effects of normal airway anatomy on distribution of airway resistance and ventilation based on postmortem measurements on the right lung of a 48-year-old man; he used calibrated bougies to measure the numbers, lengths, and diameters of the airways down to a 1-mm diameter, which he called lobular bronchioles. Based on his anatomical measurements, he modeled flow dynamics in the human lung for an irregularly dichotomous branching tree from hilum to the lobular bronchioles. Anatomy of lobules supplied by these 1-mm bronchioles were assumed to be a regular dichotomous tree based on a description by von Recklinghausen from which resistance to flow could be calculated. When bronchial segment lengths along pathways from the tracheal carina to lobules in different regions were summed, it was found that path lengths to lobules located centrally were shorter than those to peripheral lobules. The expected pressure decrease caused by laminar flow in each airway was calculated as the product of laminar flow resistance (K_1) based on Poisuelle's law and volume velocity ($K_1 \cdot \dot{V}$). Pressure decrease at branch points was calculated as combined energy losses from local changes in cross-sectional area and flow direction; these losses are proportional to gas density times $\dot{V}^2$. When critical velocity ($\dot{V}_k$), is exceeded in an air passage, pressure decrease from the resulting turbulent flow was estimated as $K_2 \cdot \dot{V}^2$ in that branch, where $K_2 = K_1/\dot{V}_k$. Total pressure decrease across airways (ΔP_{AW}) becomes the sum of a term in $\dot{V}$ and a term in $\dot{V}^2$, shown below:

	Laminar	Turbulent
Upper airways	$\Delta P_{AW} = 0.426 \cdot \dot{V}$	$+ 0.714 \cdot \dot{V}^2$
Lower airways		
Bronchial	$\Delta P_{AW} = 0.106 \cdot \dot{V}$	$+ 0.080 \cdot \dot{V}^2$
Lobular	$\Delta P_{AW} = 0.258 \cdot \dot{V}$	$+ 0.006 \cdot \dot{V}^2$
Total	$\Delta P_{AW} = 0.790 \cdot \dot{V}$	$+ 0.800 \cdot \dot{V}^2$

Internal flow resistances of lobules were assumed to be the same based on regular dichotomous branching. Regional lower airway laminar resistance varied depending on path length from the carina to a given lobule, ranging from 8 cm for a central lobule to 14 cm for a peripheral lobule, with corresponding resistances of 0.218 cm H_2O/(L/s) and 0.436 cm H_2O/(L/s), respectively. Based on his calculations, he concluded that the primary sites of variability in resistance to flow among lobules were located in bronchi, ranging from more than 1 and ≤ 3 mm in diameter. This is an early example of using anatomical measurements to predict and explain physiologic responses.

Calculations Based on Measurements of a Casted Bronchial Tree in Dogs

Ross (15) made similar measurements and calculations as those of Rohrer from polystyrene plastic casts of dog lungs down to terminal bronchial diameters of 1.5 mm and described another potential source of uneven alveolar ventilation even when total ventilation is uniform. As in Rhorer's results, branching in the dog lung was irregular; summed bronchial path lengths, from tracheal carina to a terminal bronchus, varied from 2 cm centrally to 13.7 cm peripherally. There were corresponding differences in anatomical dead-space volume between the tracheal carina and different terminal bronchi. For all bronchial pathways at the same path length (ΣL) from the carina there was a linear relationship between total dead-space volume of those pathways (V_D) and ΣL as follows:

$$V_D = 8.27 \cdot \Sigma L - 10.8 \quad (r = 0.98) \tag{2}$$

where L is in centimeters and V_D is in cubic centimeters. Adding the dead space of the upper airways to the right side of Eq. (2) (approximately 48 mL), he obtained $V_D = 8.27 \cdot \Sigma L + 37.2$; thus, the longer the distance of a terminal bronchus from the carina, the larger the dead space volume that must be displaced before fresh inspired air arrives at that terminal bronchus. Assuming that tidal volume is distributed uniformly among terminal units and that the fraction of total terminal units located at a given distance from the carina is given by N/N_T, dead-space ventilation to different terminal units becomes a function of distance (ΣL) from the carina:

$$\dot{V}_D = f \cdot \frac{N}{N_T}(8.27 \cdot \Sigma L + 37.2)$$

where f is frequency. Alveolar ventilation of lobules at a known distance (ΣL) from the carina becomes:

$$\dot{V}_{AL} = f \cdot \frac{N}{N_T}(V_T - 8.27 \cdot \Sigma L - 37.2) \tag{3}$$

where V_T is tidal volume. Ross used his measurements to estimate the expected effect of irregular branching on distribution of inspired dead space in a normal dog lung (Fig. 1). Hence, as distance of terminal units from the carina increases, dead space ventilation increases and alveolar ventilation decreases, creating uneven alveolar ventilation even if total ventilation is uniform.

Horsfield and Cumming (16,17) devised a method of ordering the airway generations from the periphery toward the trachea (a "division up" system) as being more functionally relevant when irregular branching exists (Horsefield method) than when ordering from the trachea down. Their initial system of ordering was subsequently modified to a similar "division up" ordering system designed originally for use by geomorphologists to describe branching rivers (Strahler method). Thus, if branching order by the Horsfield or Strahler numbering method is plotted with respect to the log of the number of respiratory bronchioles supplied, a straight line results, indicating that for successive increases in the branching order there is a fixed proportional increase in the number of respiratory bronchioles supplied, even though members of the same segment order are not all at the same distance from the carina. In fact, the lobule with the shortest path length was reached after only 8 dichotomous branchings and the longest after 25 branchings, similar to the findings of Roher (14) and of Ross (15) (Fig. 2).

Modeling Optimal Branching of the Acinar Tree and Comparison with Morphometric Measurements

The acinus usually is described as a regularly branching dichotomous system, but, in fact, the acinus also branches irregularly. Path lengths within the alveolar ducts of a morphometric reconstruction of the rat acinus by Mercer and Crapo varied

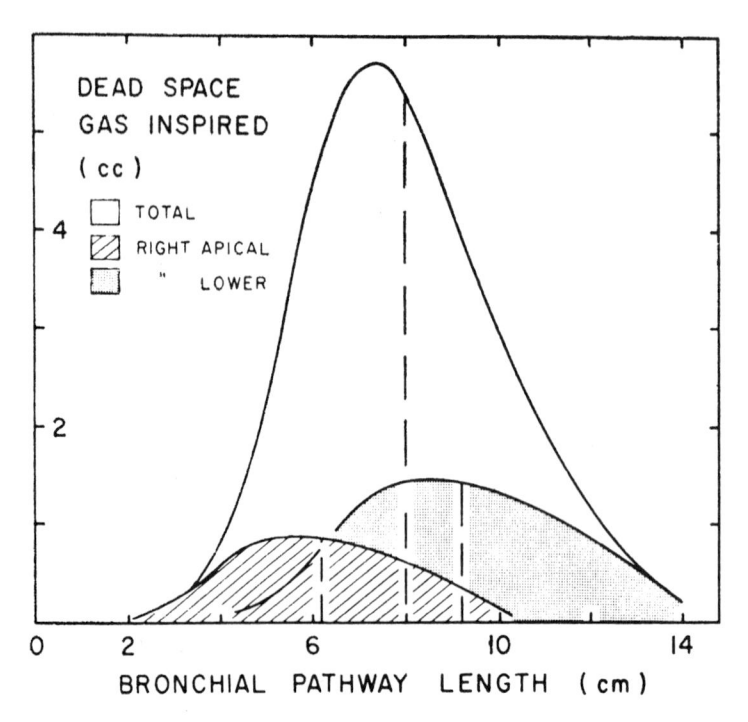

[Figure: Graph showing dead space gas inspired (cc) vs bronchial pathway length (cm), with three curves labeled Total, Right Apical, and Lower]

Figure 1 Estimated distribution of dead-space gas among alveoli of a normal dog at the end of inspiration based on anatomical measurements of airway dimensions and path lengths (15). The two lower curves represent distributions of dead space in lobes with mean bronchial path lengths, which are longer and shorter than the overall mean. Area under each curve represents total dead-space volume inspired into alveoli of each segment.

over a range of 500 to 2000 μm (18). Fung (19) modeled alveoli and ducts supplied by a respiratory bronchiole as space-filling tetrakaidecahedrons (14-hedrons) packed together; in Fung's model, alveolar mouths and ducts were generated by removing walls between adjacent 14-hedrons starting at the connecting bronchiole. Denny and Schroter (20) used Fung's space-filling model to estimate which walls must be removed to optimize gas exchange by reducing ductal path lengths to a minimum while increasing alveolar surface area to a maximum. The optimal distribution of gas-exchange pathways generated by the computational model closely mimicked the distribution of path lengths measured by Mercer and Crapo (18) (Fig. 3). It becomes apparent that, because of space-filling constraints imposed on the bronchoalveolar system, irregular branching in the bronchial tree becomes necessary to pack the largest alveolar surface area into a limited space with the least power requirements for distribution; the trade-off for this optimization is uneven ventilation.

Experimental Approaches to the Study of Gas Exchange 53

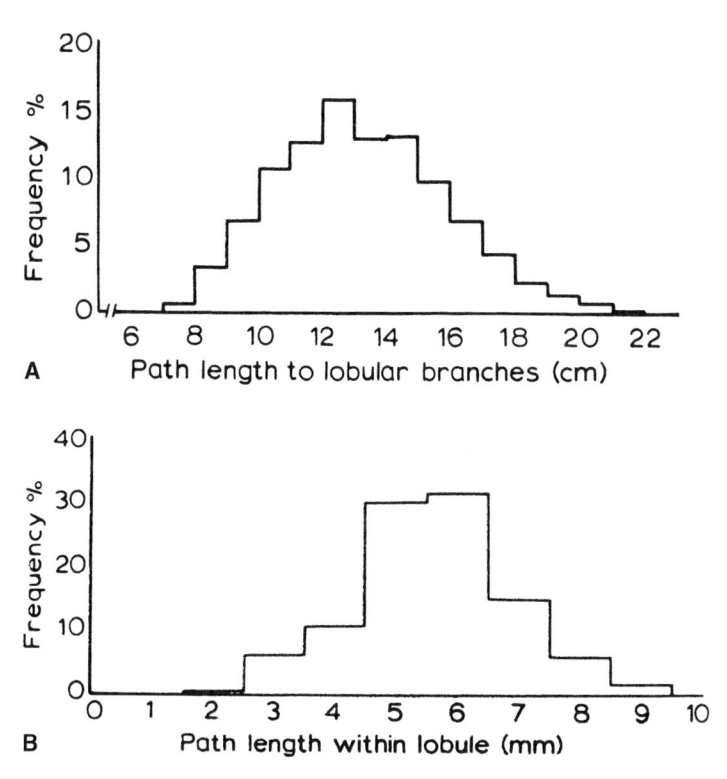

Figure 2 (A) Frequency distribution of path lengths (ΣL) to lobular branches in the human lung (17). There is a suggestion of bimodal distribution, possibly caused by difference in length between the right and left main bronchi. (B) Frequency distribution of path length (ΣL) from the lobular branches to the distal respiratory bronchioles (17).

Distribution of Perfusion

The Strahler ordering system has been used to describe the different generations of arteries and veins as well as airways (21–23). The pulmonary arterial and venous trees are also irregular dichotomous branching systems with variable path lengths to alveolar capillaries (24). Because branching of the arterial tree follows closely the branching of the bronchial tree to a given region, regions with long pathways and high resistance to ventilation should have correspondingly long pathways and high resistance to perfusion, tending to keep ventilation and perfusion matched; however, this kind of matching of total ventilation with respect to perfusion does not take into account nonuniform distribution of dead-space ventilation. Furthermore, there are different ratios of segment diameters between daughter and parent segments in the arterial and bronchial tree. Diameter of daughter branches in the bronchial tree are approximately $2^{-1/3}$ of the parent to 1-mm diameter bronchi, which theo-

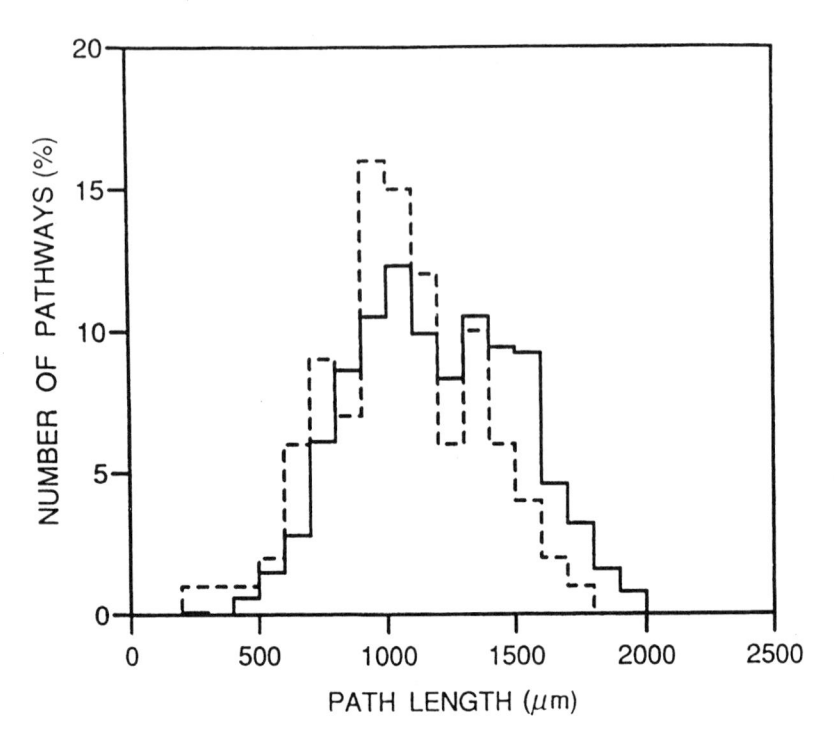

Figure 3 The average distribution for gas exchange pathways from the bronchiole–alveolar duct junction to the end of the alveolar sacs. Comparison of results of the computational model by Denny and Schroter (20) (—) and morphometric measurements by Mercer and Crapo (18) (---).

retically minimizes power requirements for alveolar ventilation (25,26); however, diameter of daughter branches in the arterial tree are approximately $2^{-1/2.3}$ (21), which is suboptimal for the power requirements of laminar blood flow. Effects of normal anatomy on ventilation-perfusion ratio ($\dot{V}/\dot{Q}$) matching has not been explored systematically.

Noninvasive Imaging Techniques to Describe Airway and Vascular Anatomy

Radiological techniques using computed tomography and magnetic resonance imaging are becoming increasingly important in describing anatomy in vivo and anatomical relationships to respiratory function (27,28). Thus, Wood et al. (28) described the dimension and branching patterns of both the airways and vascular system in dogs. Such techniques are widely applicable to a range of animals, including humans.

Anatomical Determinants of Diffusive Gas Exchange

Morphometry of Gas Exchange at the Alveolar Capillary Membrane

Most of the work in describing anatomical determinants of diffusive gas exchange in the lung has been performed by Weibel et al. (29,30) in humans as well as other mammals. In a deeply anesthetized, tracheostamized animal, a pneumothorax is introduced followed by rapid intratracheal instillation of 2.5% buffered gluteraldehyde at a fixed pressure head of 25 cm H_2O while the lung is still perfused in situ. After removal of the fixed lungs, a four-level stratified sampling technique is used for gross, low- and high-power light microscopic and electron microscopic stereologic analysis (30). Total alveolar and capillary surface areas, capillary blood volumes, and mean harmonic thickness of the alveolar capillary membrane are determined using randomly applied grids for linear intercept and point counting. Diffusing capacity of the lung (DL) is a measure of the rate at which a gas (usually O_2, CO_2, CO, or NO) can diffuse across the alveolar capillary membrane in milliliters per minute per mean gas tension difference in millimeters-mercury between alveolar air and Hb in capillary red blood cells. Roughton and Forster (31) indicated that the total resistance to diffusive gas exchange (1/DL) is the sum of the resistances offered by the membrane and plasma barriers to diffusion (1/DM) and the resistance offered by capillary red blood cells ($1/\Theta V_c$), where Θ is the rate of O_2, CO, or NO uptake by red blood cells expressed as (milliliter per minute)/millimeter mercury per milliliter of blood with a normal hematocrit, and Vc is the total pulmonary capillary blood volume in milliliters:

$$\frac{1}{D_L} = \frac{1}{DM} + \frac{1}{\Theta V_c} \cdot \frac{45}{\text{Hematocrit}} \tag{4}$$

Membrane diffusing capacity (DM) is estimated morphometrically from the total alveolar and capillary surface areas (S$_A$ and Sc, respectively):

$$DM = \frac{60 \cdot \alpha \cdot d}{760} \cdot \frac{S_A + S_c}{2 \cdot \tau_h} \tag{5}$$

where S$_A$ and Sc are alveolar and capillary surface areas, respectively, in square centimeters, α is the Bunsen solubility coefficient in standard atmosphere^{-1}, τ_h is the harmonic mean thickness of the membrane and plasma barrier in centimeters, 60 is seconds per minute, and 760 is millimeters mercury per standard atmosphere. Surface areas are estimated from random morphometric determinations of mean linear intercepts, and pulmonary capillary plasma and red blood cell volumes are estimated by point counting. Random linear distances (l) between alveolar and red blood cell surfaces are measured as the distance between intercepts of these surfaces by lines on a randomly oriented grid overlaid on electron micrographs. Reciprocals of these intercept interval lengths are weighted and averaged in accordance with

Table 1 Krogh Diffusion Coefficients for Different Gases Relative to CO and Θ for Different Gases from Multiple Sources

Gas	K_G/K_{CO}	Θ_G	Reference
O_2	1.13	2.8	Staub et al. (100)
		3.9	Yamaguchi et al. (122)
CO_2	20.0	5.1	Constantine et al. (123)
		1.84	Wagner and West (53)
NO	2.32	5.17	Carlsen and Comroe (124)

the following equation to estimate the randomly oriented mean harmonic diffusion path length across the tissue–plasma barrier to the red blood cell:

$$l_h = (\text{magnification})^{-1} \cdot \frac{\Sigma_i n_i}{\Sigma_i n_i / l_i} \tag{6}$$

where n_i is the number of measured intercept intervals with length, l_i. Mean harmonic barrier thickness is estimated from l_h as follows:

$$\tau_h = \frac{2}{3} \cdot l_h \tag{7}$$

where 2/3 is a correction factor based on stereologic principals to correct for the angle that the intercepting grid line makes with the normal to the membrane surface; the correction factor translates l_h to τ_h, which approximates the mean perpendicular distance from the red blood cell surface to the adjacent red blood cell surface; more recently, finite element modeling suggests that l_h provides a more accurate estimate of DM than τ_h in Eq. (5) (32) and that Weibel's previous estimates of DM are approximately 50% too high. Using appropriate values of Θ, α, and d for O_2, CO_2, CO, and NO (Table 1), DL for each of these gases can be estimated by morphometry and compared with physiological measurements.

Finite Difference and Finite Element Modeling of Diffusive Gas Exchange at the Capillary Level

Finite difference and finite element modeling techniques have been used to estimate the effects of changes in spacing between red blood cells in lung capillaries and changes in red blood cell shapes on diffusive gas exchange (32–38) (Fig. 4). These kinds of numerical analytical techniques have helped to clarify potential sources of error in both morphometric and physiological measurements of diffusing capacity. Finite difference modeling of diffusive gas exchange in a symmetrical model is performed by solving Fick's differential equation for diffusion by substituting small finite differences for the infinitesimal differentials in time, concentration, and distance; changes in concentration are calculated in small discreet steps of time and space and summed. When the geometry is more complex, finite element modeling is required in which the geometric components are subdivided into multiple small, nonoverlapping geometrical elements (e.g., quadrilaterals in two dimensions or tetrahedrons in three dimensions); given the concentration of the gas of interest at each corner of an element (a node), equations based on Fick's law of diffusion are set up for each node to solve for the net direction and magnitude of flux in or out of that element, based on the known solubility and diffusivity of the gas of interest in air, plasma, and tissue. A similar set of equations is set up for each element; a computer must be used to solve the multiple equations (usually thousands) simultaneously to provide the distribution of gas tensions and flux from alveolar air to each capillary red blood cell.

Finite element techniques were developed by engineers to calculate the distribution of stresses in a building or bridge in response to different loads to determine the strengths and elasticity of materials required or to estimate temperature gradients and heat flux in an engine caused by energy transfer. Only relatively recently have these techniques been applied to biology; nevertheless, these techniques can provide important insights into biological processes.

Modeling of Gas Phase Diffusion and Convection in the Acinus

Beyond the segmental bronchi and down to bronchi of about 1 mm in diameter, the cross-sectional area of the bronchial tree increases by a factor of approximately 1.26 at each dichotomous branch point. Beyond this point, in accordance with Weibel's model, there is a progressive increase in this factor to between 1.6 to 1.8 at each branch point in the lung acinus. As a consequence, the linear velocity of flow during inspiration progressively declines (linear velocity = volume velocity/total cross-sectional area). At a peak inspiratory flow of 250 mL/s during quiet breathing, linear velocity in a third-generation respiratory bronchiole would be approximately 0.16 cm/s, and for a given concentration gradient for oxygen at the convective interface, the oxygen flux by diffusion would be approximately three times the flux from convection; hence, in the respiratory unit of the lung, gas phase diffusion often is more important than convection in mixing (39). There is still controversy over whether there is sufficient time during a breath for complete mixing in the acinus (40–43).

Direct Visualization of Alveolar Capillary Perfusion

Wagner et al. (44–50) have implemented techniques for visualizing and recording by video camera the flow in subpleural alveolar capillaries of the lung in intact animals or in isolated perfused lungs. Using fluorescent dye injections in the pulmonary artery, dye-dilution curves can be recorded for a feeding arteriole and collecting venule to estimate mean transit time of plasma through the microcirculation; distribution of capillary transit times are estimated by deconvolution of the inlet and outlet dye-dilution curves (51). Capillary recruitment is quantified by

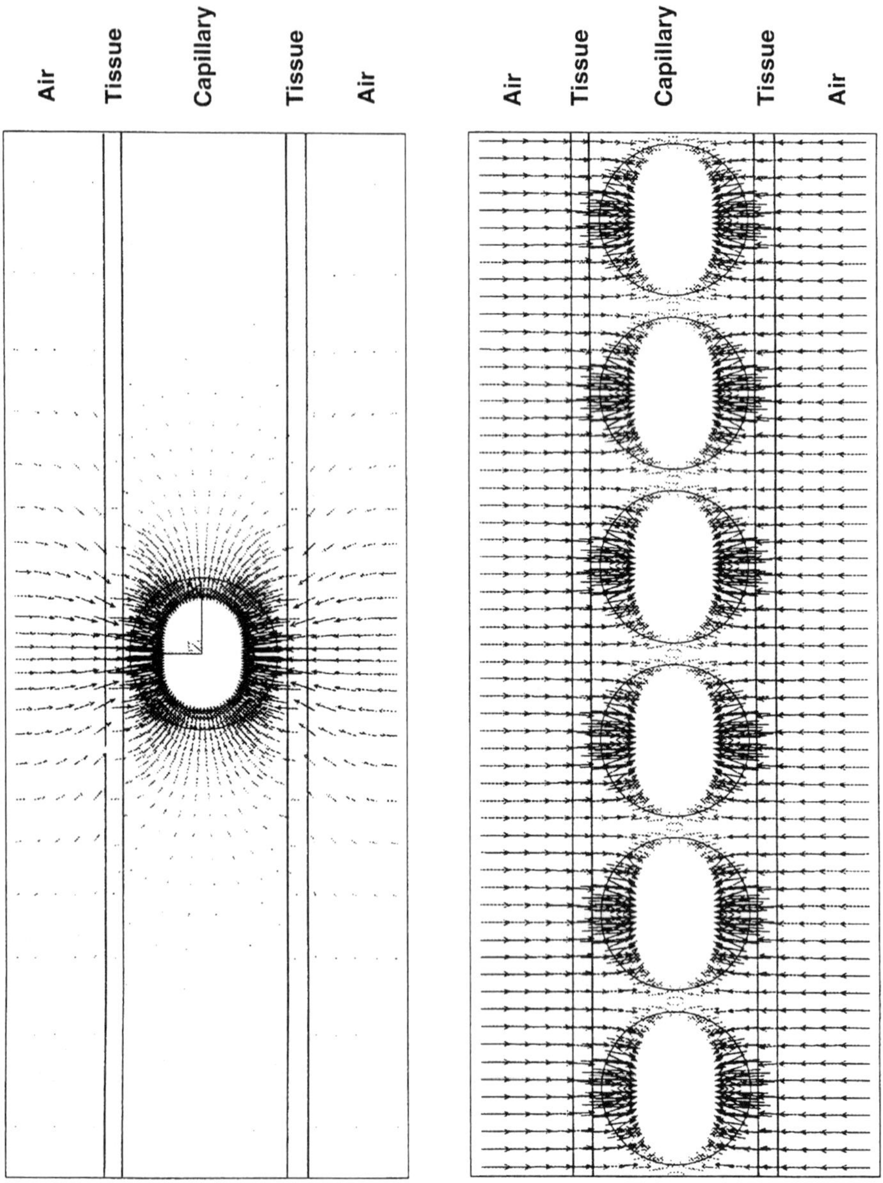
Air
Tissue
Capillary
Tissue
Air
Air
Tissue
Capillary
Tissue
Air

A

B

Figure 4 Finite element modeling (FEM) of the distribution of CO flux into a single red blood cell (A) and by closely packed red blood cells (B) as they pass through a lung capillary; direction and magnitude of local flux is indicated by direction and length of local arrows. The capillary membrane is not fully used for gas exchange by an isolated cell but becomes more completely used by closely packed cells. FEM has shown that efficient use of the alveolar capillary membrane in the lung is determined not only by the number of perfused capillaries but also by red blood cell shape and spacing between cells.

DATA FROM 10 DOGS

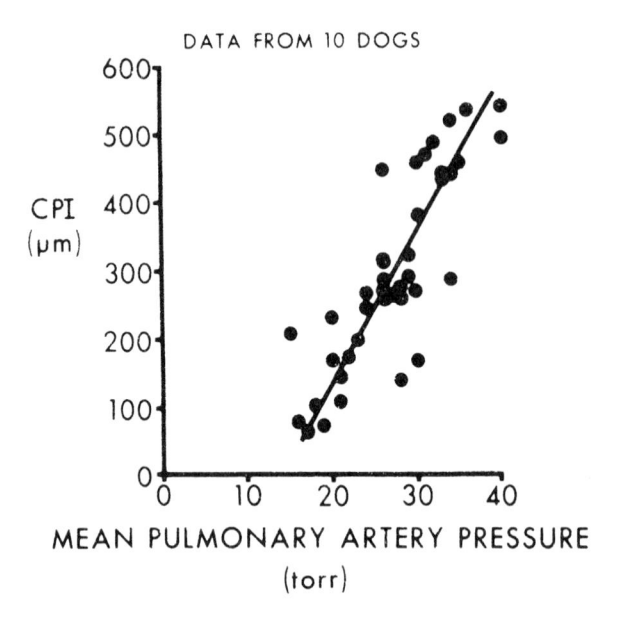

Figure 5 Relationship between capillary perfusion index (CPI) and pulmonary artery pressure in subpleural alveoli of zone II in the anesthetized dog as PA pressure is varied by alveolar hyperoxia, alveolar hypoxia, and infusion of prostaglandin E_1 (PGE_1). The microcirculation was observed directly through a transparent intercostal window (52).

measuring changes in a capillary perfusion index, i.e., the total length of perfused capillaries per unit area at alveolar wall. Such data can provide information on how and why capillaries are recruited in response to changes in pulmonary blood flow, pressure, hypoxia, or pharmacological intervention, and how such changes affect time spent by red blood cells in lung capillaries (52) (Fig. 5).

B. Measuring the Efficiency of Gas Exchange

Alveolar Arterial Oxygen Tension Difference as an Index of Gas Exchange Efficiency

The difference between mean alveolar and arterial Po_2 ($A-aPo_2$) is a simple index of efficiency of alveolar gas exchange. Arterial O_2 tension is easily measured; however, estimating the relevant mean alveolar Po_2 for the $A-aPo_2$ is conceptually more difficult and is discussed in the following sections.

Equilibrium Relationships Between Blood and Gas Tensions

Basic Equations. The lung can be likened to a tonometer. If we place a volume of air (initial V_A) and of venous blood (Q) at 37°C in a tonometer connected

Experimental Approaches to the Study of Gas Exchange

to a small bag that allows the final volume to expand or contract, gas tensions in the two phases will equilibrate over time; blood volume remains constant during approach to equilibrium, but volume of the gas phase may change depending on the relative volumes of gases that enter and leave the blood. Final gas tensions at equilibrium between blood and gas and final volume of the gas phase (final V_A) are determined by the following set of simultaneous mass balance equations:

$$Q[\text{initial } C_{CO_2} - \text{final } C_{CO_2}]$$
$$= \frac{\text{initial } P_{CO_2} \cdot \text{initial } V_A - \text{final } P_{CO_2} \cdot \text{final } V_A}{P_B} \cdot C_f \quad (8)$$

$$Q[\text{initial } C_{O_2} - \text{final } C_{O_2}]$$
$$= \frac{\text{initial } P_{O_2} \cdot \text{initial } V_A - \text{final } P_{O_2} \cdot \text{final } V_A}{P_B} \cdot C_f \quad (9)$$

$$Q[\text{initial } C_{CO_2} - \text{final } C_{CO_2}] - Q[\text{initial } C_{O_2} - \text{final } C_{O_2}]$$
$$= \text{final } V_A - \text{initial } V_A \quad (10)$$

CO_2 dissociation curve of blood:

$$P_{CO_2} = f(C_{CO_2}, \text{pH}, HCO_3) \text{ at equilibrium} \quad (11)$$

O_2 dissociation curve of blood:

$$P_{O_2} = f(C_{O_2}, \text{pH}, P_{CO_2}) \text{ at equilibrium} \quad (12)$$

where C_{CO_2} and C_{O_2} refer to blood contents of CO_2 and of O_2, respectively, in liters of gas under standard conditions (STP) / l blood; P_{CO_2} and P_{O_2} are tensions of CO_2 and O_2, respectively, in the gas phase, expressed in millimeters mercury; initial and final V_A are volumes of the gas phase at the ambient barometric pressure, saturated with water vapor at body temperature (BTPS). C_f is a conversion factor that converts volume at body temperature (t) and ambient barometric pressure (PB) to standard temperature (0°C) and pressure (760 mm Hg) = $(P_B/760) \cdot (273/273 + t)$. Eq. (11) and (12) are the CO_2 and O_2 dissociation curves and vary with acid base balance in accordance with the computer algorithms of Wagner and West (53) and Kelman (54,55).

If, in a completely homogeneous lung, blood remains in capillaries long enough to reach equilibrium with alveolar air, equilibrium equations [Eq. (8) to (12)] are equally valid for the lung as for a tonometer; the static air and blood volumes in the tonometer are equivalent to alveolar ventilation ($\dot{V}_A$) and pulmonary capillary blood flow ($\dot{Q}_c$), respectively; initial gas concentrations in the blood and gas phases in the tonometer are equivalent to those in inspired air, and mixed venous blood and final gas concentrations in the tonometer are equivalent to those in expired alveolar air and end-capillary blood. Substituting standard respiratory symbols for these equivalencies into equations [Eq. (8) to (10)], the revised equations become:

$$\dot{V}_{CO_2} = \dot{Q}c[C\bar{v}_{CO_2} - Ca_{CO_2}] = \frac{P_{ICO_2} \cdot \dot{V}_{A_{insp}} - P_{ACO_2} \cdot \dot{V}_{A_{exp}}}{P_B} \cdot C_f \qquad (13)$$

$$\dot{V}_{O_2} = \dot{Q}c[Ca_{O_2} - C\bar{v}_{O_2}] = \frac{P_{IO_2} \cdot \dot{V}_{A_{insp}} - P_{AO_2} \cdot \dot{V}_{A_{exp}}}{P_B} \cdot C_f \qquad (14)$$

$$\dot{V}_{CO_2} - \dot{V}_{O_2} = \dot{V}_{A_{exp}} - \dot{V}_{A_{insp}} \qquad (15)$$

Equations (11) to (15) are central to understanding steady-state exchange of respiratory gases as well as exchange of inert soluble gases; equations describing exchange of inert soluble gases in the lung are the same as those for CO_2 and O_2 except that Eq. (11) and (12) become linear relationships between inert gas tension and concentration in solution rather than the more complex nonlinear dissociation curves for CO_2 and O_2 in blood. These five equations are all that are necessary to describe equilibrium conditions in the lung.

The normal lung is not a homogeneous tonometer; the lung is made up of many regional tonometers with different ratios of $\dot{V}_A/\dot{Q}c$. Assuming equilibrium between alveolar and end-capillary blood in each tonometer, if mixed venous blood gases, inspired gas tensions, and $\dot{V}_A/\dot{Q}c$ ratios for each tonometer are known, the remaining five unknowns can be estimated using Eq. (11) to (15). Expired alveolar air from regions with different $\dot{V}_A/\dot{Q}c$ ratios are mixed in conducting airways to become expired alveolar ventilation ($\dot{V}_{A_{exp}}$); alveolar CO_2 and O_2 tensions in the mixture are averages weighted with respect to the fraction of the total $\dot{V}_A$ contributed from each region. End-capillary blood leaving these same regions is mixed with extra-alveolar bronchial and thebesian shunts in the left atrium and ventricle; the arterial blood CO_2 and O_2 contents are averages weighted with respect to the fraction of total $\dot{Q}c$ contributed from each region. The CO_2 and O_2 tensions in mixed expired alveolar air and the CO_2 and O_2 contents in mixed end-capillary blood still satisfy Eq. (12) to (15), but because of the different ways that the averages are weighted for alveolar air and arterial blood, arterial blood and mixed alveolar air are systematically different, i.e., now P_{AO_2} is greater than Pa_{O_2} and Pa_{CO_2} is greater than P_{ACO_2}; furthermore, less O_2 will have been taken up by the blood and less CO_2 will have been excreted in exhaled air than would have occurred in a homogeneous lung with the same ratio of pulmonary blood flow to alveolar ventilation.

Graphic Solutions. Equilibrium gas tensions between alveolar air and end-capillary blood can be estimated in any region of lung by solving Eq. (10) to (15) if the regional $\dot{V}_A/\dot{Q}c$ ratio is known and if mixed venous blood gases are known; this can be done by numerical techniques using a computer or by graphic methods. Computer methods are faster and more precise, but graphic techniques provide an understanding unavailable from looking at a matrix used to solve five simultaneous

Experimental Approaches to the Study of Gas Exchange

equations; hence, here we illustrate how solutions are achieved graphically using the basic five equations. For simplicity, we neglect P_{ICO_2}, assuming it to be zero.

Alveolar CO_2 and O_2 tensions in equilibrium with end-capillary blood gas contents can be estimated from the following relationships derived from Eq. (13) to (15) when plotted on the same graph with their respective CO_2 and O_2 dissociation curves if mixed venous contents, inspired gas tensions, and the $\dot{V}_A/\dot{Q}_c$ ratio are known [Eq. (11) and (12)] (Figs. 6A and B):

$$P_{ACO_2} = \frac{P_B}{\dot{V}_A/\dot{Q}} \cdot \frac{(C\bar{v}_{CO_2} - Cc'_{CO_2})}{C_f} \tag{16}$$

$$P_{AO_2} = [P_{IO_2} - P_{ACO_2} \cdot F_{IO_2}] - \frac{P_B F_{IN_2}}{\dot{V}_A/\dot{Q}c} \cdot \frac{(C\bar{v}_{CO_2} - Cc'_{CO_2})}{C_f} \tag{17}$$

Equation (16) is a linear relationship between alveolar CO_2 tension (P_{ACO_2}) and the difference between mixed venous and end-capillary CO_2 contents with a slope of ($863 \dot{N}_A/\dot{Q}c$); its intersection with the CO_2 dissociation curve is an equilibrium solution (56) (Fig. 6A). Equation (17) is a linear relationship between alveolar oxygen tension and the difference between end-capillary and mixed venous O_2 contents with a slope of ($863 \cdot F_{IN_2}/\dot{V}_A/\dot{Q}c$); its intersection with the O_2 dissociation curve is an equilibrium solution (56) (Fig. 6B).

Two additional linear relationships derived from Eq. (13) to (15) can be used to solve graphically for P_{ACO_2} and P_{AO_2} in a lung region if mixed venous blood contents and the respiratory quotient (R) are known (57,58):

$$P_{AO_2} = P_{IO_2} - P_{ACO_2} \cdot \left(F_{IO_2} - \frac{F_{IN_2}}{R} \right) \tag{18}$$

$$Cc'_{O_2} = C\bar{v}_{O_2} + \frac{C\bar{v}_{CO_2} - Cc'_{CO_2}}{R} \tag{19}$$

Using the CO_2 and O_2 dissociation curves [Eq. (11) and (12)] to convert mixed venous and end-capillary contents to tensions, Eq. (18) and (19) can be plotted together in a $P_{CO_2}-P_{O_2}$ diagram (Fig. 7). For the same mixed venous blood gases and whole-body R as that shown in Figure 6, the intersections of Eq. (18) and (19) should provide the same solution for the P_{CO_2} and P_{O_2} at alveolar capillary equilibrium in a homogeneous lung as that found graphically in Figure 6. Riley and Cournand (57) pointed out that the intersection of the two R lines represents the ideal alveolar gas composition that would have existed if $\dot{V}_A/\dot{Q}c$ ratios had been uniform; measured arterial O_2 and CO_2 tensions must fall on the blood R line to the left of the intersection.

Alveolar Arterial Oxygen Tension Difference

The difference between oxygen tension estimated in ideal alveolar gas and that measured in arterial blood is the $A-aD_{O_2}$ or $A-aP_{O_2}$ as shown in Figures 6B and 7. Riley and Cournand (57) also pointed out that a close approximation to

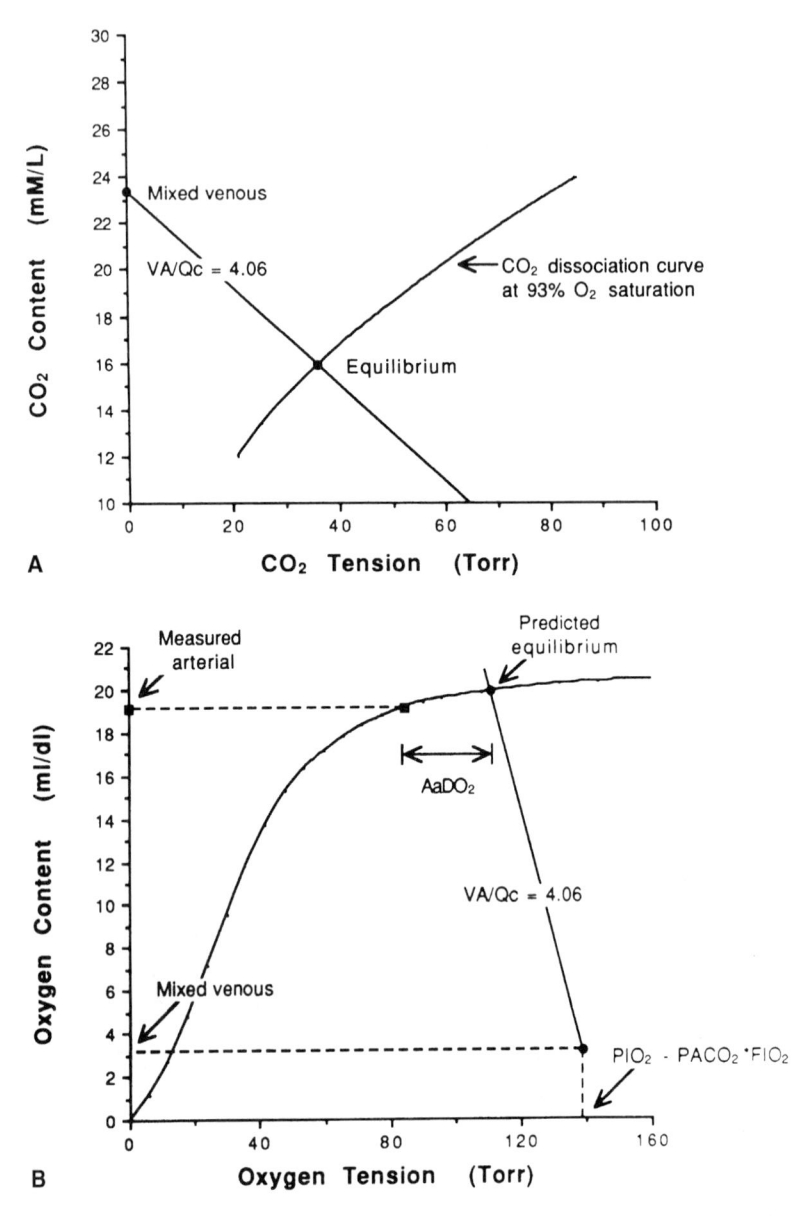

Figure 6 (A) Graphic solution for CO_2 content and tension at equilibrium between alveolar air and blood during exercise at a $\dot{V}/\dot{Q}$ ratio of 4.06. The solution is at the intersection of Eq. (16) and the CO_2 dissociation curve [Eq. (11)]. (B) Graphic solution for O_2 content and tension at equilibrium between alveolar air and blood. The solution is at the intersection of Eq. (17) and the O_2 dissociation curve. (Reproduced with permission from Ref. 56.)

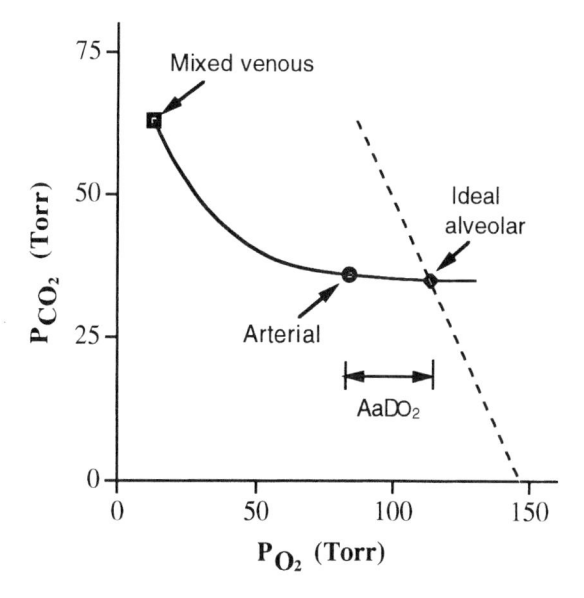

Figure 7 Simultaneous solution of Eq. (18) and (19) for the same data as in Figure 6 during heavy exercise. The whole body R was 1.05. Equation (18) is represented by the straight dashed line and Eq. (19) by the curved solid line. The solution is represented by the point of intersection which represents ideal alveolar air.

"ideal" alveolar gas is obtained more conveniently and without requiring mixed venous blood composition by assuming that measured arterial P_{CO_2} (Pa_{CO_2}) is equivalent to alveolar P_{CO_2} (P_{ACO_2}) in Eq. (18). Then, the following modification of Eq. (18) is used to approximate alveolar oxygen tension in "ideal" alveolar air:

$$P_{AO_2} = P_{IO_2} - Pa_{CO_2} \cdot \left(F_{IO_2} - \frac{F_{IN_2}}{R} \right) \tag{20}$$

The difference between this approximation to mean alveolar O_2 tension and measured arterial O_2 tension (A–aP_{O_2} or A–aD_{O_2}) is a useful and practical clinical index of the efficiency of oxygen exchange. In addition, the difference between arterial P_{CO_2} and mixed end-tidal or alveolar P_{CO_2} (A–aP_{CO_2}) becomes an index of the efficiency of CO_2 exchange. In an "ideal" lung where $\dot{V}_A/\dot{Q}c$ ratios are uniform and alveolar end-capillary gas tensions are in equilibrium with alveolar air in all units, both A–aP_{O_2} and A–aP_{CO_2} should be zero. Neither index defines mechanism of inefficiency. Other kinds of measurement are required to clarify mechanisms of exchange impairment.

Another useful equation based on the assumption that measured arterial P_{CO_2} is a good approximation of "ideal" alveolar P_{CO_2} is the following modification of Eq. (16):

$$\dot{V}_A = \frac{P_B}{P_{ACO_2}} \cdot \frac{\dot{V}_{CO_2}}{C_f} \qquad (21)$$

Substituting arterial P_{CO_2} for alveolar P_{CO_2} provides an estimate of effective alveolar ventilation:

$$\dot{V}_{A_{eff}} = \frac{P_B}{P_{aCO_2}} \cdot \frac{\dot{V}_{CO_2}}{C_f} \qquad (22)$$

If P_{ACO_2} is end-tidal mixed alveolar P_{ACO_2} used in Eq. (21), then $\dot{V}_A - \dot{V}_{A_{eff}}$ is an estimate of equivalent alveolar dead-space ventilation. This is not necessarily true alveolar dead space, but represents the magnitude of alveolar dead-space ventilation necessary to explain the A−aP_{CO_2} difference.

Distribution of Ventilation

Conventional Inert Gas Techniques

Single Breath. The alveolar plateau (general considerations): How does inspired air displace dead space in conducting airways to mix with alveolar air? This question has been a source of investigation since early in this century (39,58–60). After a single inspiration of oxygen followed by a slow exhalation, patterns of change in N_2 concentration in the expirate plotted with respect to expired volume can be divided into four phases: The initial part of the expirate is devoid of N_2 (phase I), followed by a rapid sigmoidal increase in N_2 concentration with respect to volume exhaled (phase II), followed by a slow increase along an almost constant slope (phase III, or the alveolar quasiplateau), and, if the exhalation is carried down below functional residual capacity (FRC), a terminal sharp increase in N_2 concentration occurs along a steeper slope (phase IV).

Alveolar plateau for gases of different molecular weight: If an inert insoluble gas such as helium or hydrogen is inspired, followed by slow exhalation, the same patterns are seen in mirror image to N_2 elimination curve with negative slopes of the inert gas concentrations. There is still disagreement among investigators about how much of these sloping concentration gradients in phase III are caused by (1) stratified inhomogeneity in the lung caused by incomplete penetration of the inspired gas by convection and diffusion into the terminal gas exchange units so that gas in deeper units is diluted less with inspired air and empty late during exhalation, or (2) parallel inhomogeneity caused by uneven convective distribution of inspired air among terminal gas exchange units so that poorly ventilated regions receive less inspired air and empty late during exhalation. More recently, gases with widely different molecular weights have been used as test gases, e.g., helium (molecular weight = 4; diffusion coefficient in alveolar air = 0.739 cm^2/s) and sulfur hexafluoride (molecular weight = 146; diffusion coefficient in alveolar air = 0.103 cm^2/s) (61). Stratified inhomogeneity should be minimized for a low-molecular-weight gas with a high coefficient of diffusion, whereas parallel inhomogeneity should not be affected by the molecular weight as long as laminar flow predominates. Results to date suggest that both mechanisms are involved in determining the mixing of inert gases in the lung, but the importance of diffusive resistance in the gas phase to oxygen and CO_2 exchange remains unclear (62,63).

Closing volume: The lung volume at the intersection between phase III and phase IV of the single-breath N_2 dilution curve previously described has been called *closing volume*, representing closure of small acinar units predominantly located at the base of the lung with the expression of gas having a high respiratory quotient (R). This has been used as a test of early small airways disease (64,65). Actual closure of small airways in the dependent regions of the lungs occurs even in normal subjects at lung volumes below FRC and has been demonstrated by other techniques, i.e., by nitrogen trapping when switching from room air to 100% O_2 breathing at low lung volumes (66) and by an ingenious combination of a radioactive xenon (^{133}Xe) gas bolus technique combined with a preceding inspiration of 80% N_2O (67). Inspiration and mixing of the N_2O in the lung is followed by breath-holding at a predetermined lung volume with the glottis held open; the radioactive bolus is introduced at the mouth. The N_2O is rapidly taken up by blood flow distal to patent airways and distributes the ^{133}Xe bolus from the mouth to different lung regions in proportion to their accessible blood flow; radioactivity is followed by scintillation probes distributed over the chest. Distribution of the ^{133}Xe after an airway bolus is compared under similar conditions wih regional distribution of ^{33}Xe in the lung after an intravenous bolus. If ^{133}Xe is distributed to a region in high concentration by an intravenous bolus but in low concentration or absent when introduced by airway bolus, airway closure in that region is indicated.

Multiple Breath Washin-Washout. A common technique for assessing the uniformity of ventilation in the lung is to measure the rate at which an inert gas can be washed in or out during normal ventilation, i.e., how fast inspired gas can mix with resident gas (68,69). The general equation applies to any inert gas whether used for washin or washout. If, for a homogeneous lung, V_A is alveolar volume at FRC and ΔV_A is tidal volume reaching the alveoli, then the dilution ratio of resident alveolar gas by each breath is given by:

$$R = \frac{V_A}{V_A + \Delta V_A} = \frac{1}{1 + \dot{V}_A/V_A} \tag{23}$$

where $\dot{V}_A$ is alveolar ventilation.

If FA_0 is the initial fractional concentration of the inert gas in the lung, FA_n is the fractional concentration after n breaths, and FA_∞ is the concentration after an infinite number of breaths, then:

$$\frac{(FA_n - FA_\infty)}{(FA_0 - FA_\infty)} = R^n \qquad (24)$$

If the inert gas is being washed out, $FA_\infty = 0$; if inert gas is being washed in, FA_∞ is the final equilibrium concentration and $FA_0 = 0$. Taking the logarithm of both sides of Eq. (24) and simplifying the equation by examining a washout in which FA_∞ is equal to zero:

$$\log FA_n = \log FA_0 + n \cdot \log R \qquad (25)$$

For a homogeneous lung, this indicates a linear relationship between $\log FA_n$ and the number of breaths (n) with a slope $= R$ and an intercept $\log FA_0$. For an inhomogeneous lung, the washout or washin semilogarithmic relationship is curvilinear (Fig. 8); in such a lung there is one linear relationship described by Eq. (25) for each region with a different $\dot{V}A/VA$ ratio. When $\dot{V}A_i \cdot FA_{in}$ from each such region (i) are mixed together in the expirate, the mixed $\log FA_n$ declines along a curvilinear relationship with respect to n; regions are washed out sequentially at rates determined by the regional $\dot{V}A_i/VA_i$ ratio until only the region with the slowest washout (i.e., lowest slope) remains, now being diluted by ventilation from regions with negligible amounts of the inert gas remaining. A straight line is typically fit to the semilogarithmic washout relationship from this slowest ventilated region and extrapolated back to the y intercept. This slowly washed out region is called region 1. Then the antilog of the slope of this line is $R_1 = 1/(1 + \dot{V}A_1/VA_1)$. The ratio of the intercept, FA_{int_1}, to the initial fractional concentration of the inert gas, FA_0, indicates the dilution of the inert gas from this region by alveolar air from regions that have already been washed out, i.e., $(FA_{int_1}/FA_0) = \dot{V}A_1/\dot{V}A_T$, where $\dot{V}A_T$ represents alveolar ventilation from all regions added together. The total volume of inert gas estimated to be washed out from region 1 divided by the initial inert gas concentration (FA_0) yields the volume of region 1 (VA_1). If each point on the linear washout estimated for region 1 (i.e., $\log FA_{1n}$) corresponding to breath n of the original washout curve is subtracted from $\log FA_n$, then a series of new points are generated, i.e., $\log FA_n - \log FA_{1n} = \log FA_{2n}$, which represents the washout from the rest of the lung. This has been referred to as "peeling off exponentials." From the logarithmic decline of FA_{n2}, $\dot{V}A_2/VA_2$, $\dot{V}A_2/\dot{V}A_T$, and VA_2 may be calculated. If the latter washout is not linear, a third disappearance curve may be generated. It is usually not worth peeling off more than three. Two logarithmic decays have been peeled off of the original washout curve in Fig. 8. The major problem with the technique is that its application can resolve only a limited number of ventilatory compartments. Its major advantage is simplicity.

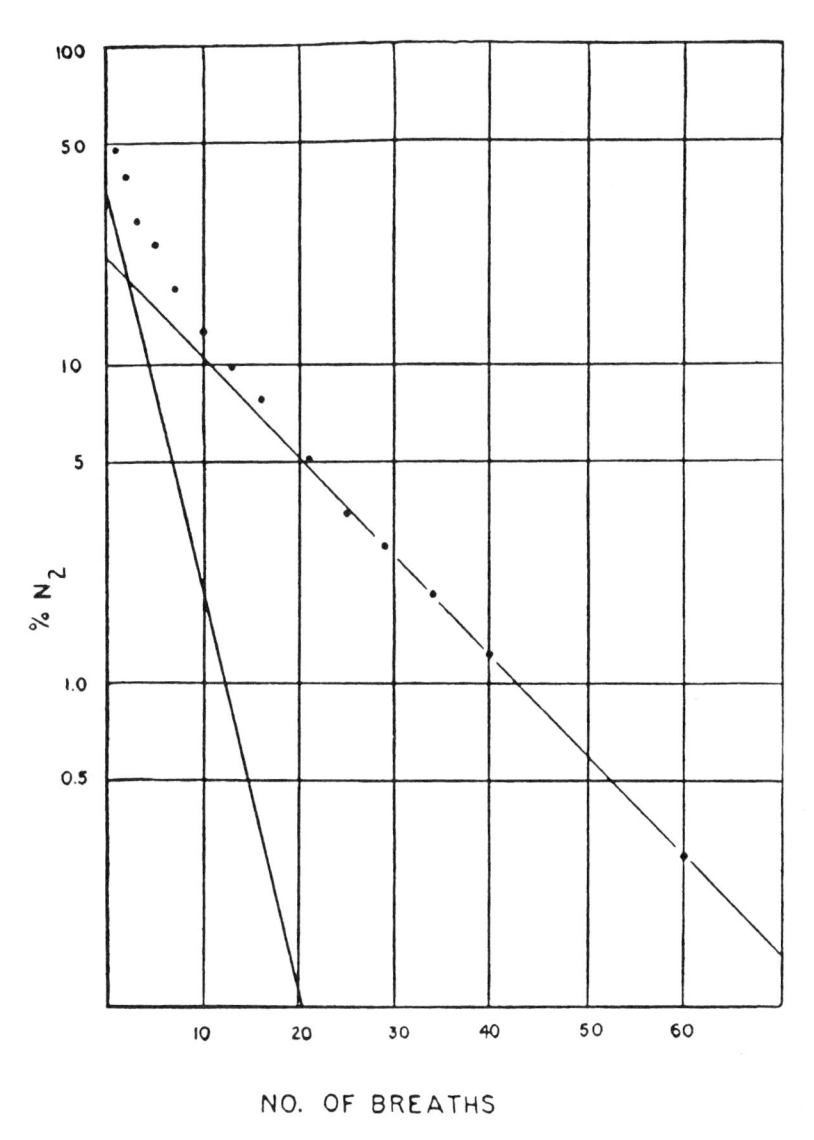

Figure 8 Graphic analysis of open-circuit nitrogen washout data from a healthy 53-year-old man. The data can be described by a two-compartment lung, a slowly ventilated compartment represented by the straight line fitted to the terminal data points, and a more rapidly ventilated compartment represented by the steeper line, which was obtained by subtracting the data on the first line from the corresponding discreet data points lying above it, i.e., often referred to as "peeling off exponentials." (From Ref. 68.)

Radioactive Gas Methods

Single Breath Distribution. If an insoluble radioactive gas that emits gamma radiation is inspired at a known concentration (FI) from a reservoir and the breath is held, the regional anatomical distribution of the gamma emitter can be measured from regional radioactive count rates (CR_r) obtained by a gamma camera or by gamma-counting probes placed at different locations over the chest. Then, by rebreathing the radioactive gas in a closed circuit until the gas concentration in the lung is in equilibrium with that in the reservoir $(FI)_{eq}$, the equilibrium count rates over each region $(CR_r)_{eq}$ provide local calibration factors:

$$\frac{(FI)_{eq}}{(CR_r)_{eq}} = \frac{(F_r)_{eq}}{(CR_r)_{eq}} = K_r = \frac{F_r}{CR_r} \tag{26}$$

where $(FI)_{eq}$ and $(F_r)_{eq}$ are the fractional concentrations of the radioactive gas in the reservoir and lung at equilibrium. If F_r is the fractional concentration of the gas in the same region after the first inspiration, and CR_r is the corresponding count rate over the region, then:

$$F_r = K_r \cdot CR_r \tag{27}$$

Because the count rate from a regional probe (CR_r) is dependent on the regional volume (V_r) included in the counting field times radioactive gas concentration (F_r) in the counting field, there is a different regional calibration factor (K_r) for each gamma-counting probe. Hence, a stepwise increase of inspired volume from the reservoir can be taken, for example, from residual volume (RV) to FRC and then to total lung capacity (TLC) with a breath-holding pause for determining count rates between each sequential step. This is followed by rebreathing of the inspired radioactive gas in a closed system until its concentration is the same in all regions; then count rates repeated at each previously measured lung volume to obtained the appropriate calibration factors, i.e., $(K_r)_{FRC}$ and $(K_r)_{TLC}$. Estimates of regional RV and FRC volumes with respect to regional TLC can then be calculated as follows:

$$\frac{RV_r}{FRC_r} = 1 - \frac{(K_r)_{FRC} \cdot (CR_r)_{FRC}}{FI} \tag{28}$$

$$\frac{RV_r}{TLC_r} = 1 - \frac{(K_r)_{TLC} \cdot (CR_r)_{TLC}}{FI} \tag{29}$$

$$\frac{FRC_r}{TLC_r} = \frac{FI - (K_r)_{TLC} \cdot (CR_r)_{TLC}}{FI - (K_r)_{FRC} \cdot (CR_r)_{FRC}} \tag{30}$$

Ball et al. (70) introduced these techniques using ^{133}Xe, which is relatively insoluble. The method was later modified by Dollfuss et al. (205) to measure topological distribution of a small bolus of ^{133}Xe introduced at the mouth during inspiration from different starting volumes. The technique has allowed sophisticated measurements of the effects of gravity on how inspired air is distributed between upper and dependent regions of the lung in different body positions.

Experimental Approaches to the Study of Gas Exchange 71

Multiple Breath Washin-Washout. An inert and insoluble radioactive gas is washed into the lung from a reservoir until equilibrium is achieved between reservoir and lung concentration; washout curves while breathing room air are followed by measuring the decrease in regional count rates with each successive breath. Washout is analyzed using Eq. (25).

Distribution of Perfusion

Single Breath of Radioactively Labeled CO_2

West and Dollery (78) used pairs of gamma-counting probes oriented front to back over the thorax to measure gamma radiation from a cylindrical core of lung between them; in seated subjects, four pairs of probes were stacked from lung base to apex over both right and left lungs to measure the distribution and clearance of radiation during breath-holding after a single breath of radioactively labeled CO_2. The CO_2 was labeled with ^{15}O prepared on-site with a cyclotron because the half-life is only 2 minutes. A liter of 3% CO_2 containing the label was rapidly inspired, and the breath was held approximately 15 seconds for gamma counting. Regional blood flow per unit lung volume ($\dot{Q}_r/V_r$) was calculated from the decrease in regional count rates (CR_r) with time of breath-holding as follows:

$$\frac{\dot{Q}_r}{V_r} = \frac{60 \cdot 760}{\alpha(Pb - 47)} \cdot \left[\frac{\Delta \ln(CR_r)}{\Delta t} - k\right] \qquad (31)$$

where $\dot{Q}_r/V_r$ is in minutes^{-1}, 60 is seconds per minute, 760 is millimeters mercury per standard atmosphere, α is the apparent Bunsen solubility coefficient for CO_2 in blood in standard atmosphere^{-1}, Pb is barometric pressure in millimeters mercury, 47 is water vapor tension at 37°C, $\Delta \ln(CR_r)/\Delta t$ is the logarithmic slope of the decay of regional count rate in seconds^{-1}, and k is the rate constant for the radioactive decay of ^{15}O. This technique demonstrated the decline in regional blood flow per unit volume from base to apex of the lung. Disappearance of labeled CO_2 from the lung is blood-flow limited and lends itself well to this technique. Interpretation of regional radioactivity after inhalation of O_2 or CO labeled with ^{15}O is more complex because regional decay of count rates from these labeled gases are limited partly by diffusion and partly by blood flow.

Intravenous Bolus of a Relatively Insoluble Radioactive Gas

Ball et al. (70) and Anthonisen (206) have used ^{133}Xe to measure blood flow during breath-holding at a preselected lung volume after an intravenous bolus injection of a known concentration dissolved in saline. The infused bolus was distributed in proportion to regional blood flow, and because of its low partition coefficient between air and blood, most was partitioned into the gas phase during a single pass. Regional count rates (CR_r) were measured with appropriately positioned probes during breath-holding; the subject then took a full inspiration of room air to TLC, and count rates were again measured followed by washout. After this the subject breathed again from a reservoir with a known concentration of ^{133}Xe until equilibration was achieved; regional count rates were again made during breath-holding at the same lung volumes used for blood flow measurements to obtain calibration factors (K_r). Then at each lung volume, the fractional concentration of ^{133}Xe can be calculated as $F_r = K_r \cdot CR_r$. A regional blood flow index is calculated as follows:

$$\frac{\dot{Q}_r/V_r}{\dot{Q}/V} = \frac{F_r}{\text{Xe infused}/V} \tag{32}$$

which is the regional blood flow expressed as a fraction of the total blood flow. Because alveolar diameters at FRC normally decrease from apex to base of an upright human, a given $\dot{Q}_r/V_r$ in the lung base may reflect less blood flow per alveolus than a similar $\dot{Q}_r/V_r$ in the apex. Inspiring to TLC reduces the disparity in alveolar diameters between apex and base; hence, final radioactive count rates are repeated at TLC to obtain a regional perfusion index more reflective of regional perfusion per alveolus:

$$\frac{\dot{Q}_r/TLC_r}{\dot{Q}/TLC} = \frac{(F_r)_{TLC}}{\text{Xe infused}/TLC} \tag{33}$$

These studies again indicated a progressive increase in perfusion index from lung apex to lung base in upright humans. Similarly, in the decubitus position, the lower lung has a higher perfusion index than the upper lung.

Radionuclide-Labeled Macroaggregated Albumin Particles (10 to 30 µm in Diameter)

Clinically, the most common technique for measuring regional distribution of perfusion is with technetium-99m (^{99m}Tc)-labeled macroaggregated albumin particles 10 to 30 µm in diameter, which are trapped in the microvasculature of the lungs. Approximately 100,000 to 300,000 particles labeled with approximately 2 µC of ^{99m}Tc are injected as a bolus through a central venous catheter, and regional scintillation count rates are measured with a gamma camera. If the study is for diagnosis of pulmonary embolism, the injection is made with the patient in the supine position to provide a more uniform distribution pattern free of apex-to-base gravitational effects. Perfusion studies are usually preceded by a ^{133}Xe equilibration and washout with images at various time intervals of washout to determine whether perfusion defects coincide with regions of impaired ventilatory washout (7). Generally, the data are not quantified, but symmetry and uniformity of perfusion and ventilation images are evaluated by eye for the presence of a region of reduced or absent perfusion. However, single-proton emission computed tomography after bolus infusions of labeled macroaggregated albumin can be quantified just as a radiodensity computed tomograph can be quantified, using regional/total count rates as an estimate of regional/total blood flow. Single-proton emission computed tomography has been used to define the spatial distribution of blood flow throughout the lungs of humans and dogs (72,73). The biological half-life for removal of the albumin particles is 4 to 6 hours.

Plastic Microspheres Labeled with Radionuclides or Colored Dye

Plastic microspheres (15 to 25 μm in diameter) labeled with a radionuclide emitting gamma radiation or with colored dye have been used to measure spatial distribution of blood flow in the lungs of animals (74–76). The microspheres are injected as a bolus through a catheter threaded into a central vein followed by a flush of saline sufficient to clear the catheter several times. Microspheres are trapped in the lung microvasculature in proportion to regional blood flow. By using a range of microspheres labeled with different radionuclides that emit gamma radiation of different energy levels or labeled with different colored dyes, multiple blood flow measurements can be performed in the same animal during multiple interventions, using a different label for each intervention. Gamma radiation with different energies can be separated with appropriate energy windows, and different colored dyes can be separated spectrophotometrically. After studies are completed, the animal is killed and the lungs are removed and blown dry with air delivered at 25 cm H_2O inflation pressure. The lung is placed in a cuboidal box and imbedded in urethane foam, which, when dry, provides a rigid support. The cuboidal form can be used to establish a three-dimensional coordinate system that is used to slice the lung parallel to the established coordinate planes into cubes, each with an x, y, z coordinate to define its position. Regional blood flow with respect to total blood flow can be determined for each cube. Thus, the blood flow distribution can be reconstructed spatially for a given set of experimental conditions.

Ventilation–Perfusion Relationships

Measuring Gas Concentrations in End-Tidal Alveolar Air

In 1953, Martin et al. (77) sampled end-tidal alveolar air from the upper and lower lobes in upright humans using small plastic catheters and found that R in the upper lobes, based on Eq. (18), was significantly higher than in the lower lobe, indicating a significantly higher $\dot{V}/\dot{Q}$ ratio in the upper relative to lower lobes. Using a flexible fiberoptic bronchoscope, the same kind of measurements can be made.

Regional $\dot{V}/\dot{Q}$ Ratios Using Radioactive Gases

As previously described, West and Dollery (78) measured regional perfusion and ventilation at four locations over each lung, extending from apex to base. Measurements were made after a single breath of a gas mixture containing CO_2 labeled with ^{15}O. Regional perfusion was estimated from the exponential decline in regional count rates [Eq (31)]; relative distribution of the inspired air was estimated from the same breath by the differences in the initial count rates with respect to the estimated volume within the counting field of each pair of probes. The first estimations of how $\dot{V}/\dot{Q}$ ratios decline from apex to base in upright humans were

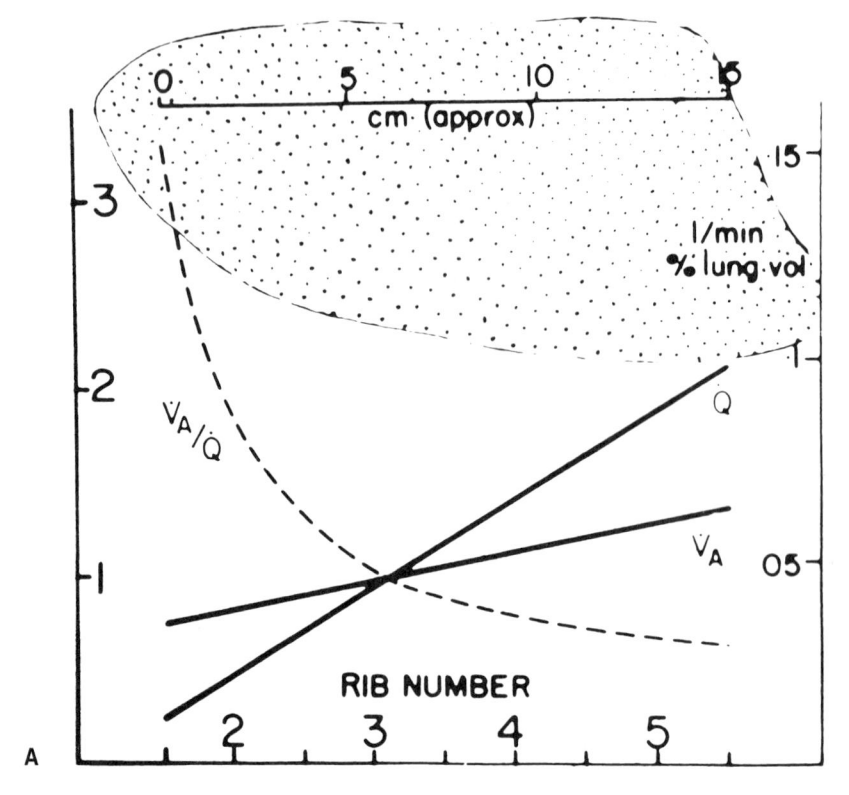

Figure 9 (A) Changes in blood flow (Q) and ventilation (VA) per unit lung volume down the lung (right-hand scale). The ratio ($\dot{V}_A/\dot{Q}$) is also shown (left-hand scale) (79).

obtained from these data (79). Taking the measured gradient of $\dot{V}/\dot{Q}$ down the lung in nine vertical compartments and assuming a mean resting CO, ventilation, and mixed venous blood gases, West (79) used Eq. (11) to (15) to calculated equilibrium gas tensions in each compartment and the resulting $A-aP_{O_2}$ and $A-aP_{CO_2}$ that should result (Fig. 9A). Similar estimates have been made for the distribution of Q_c/V_A and D_{LCO}/V_A using a bolus technique (80) (Fig. 9B).

Anthonisen et al. (81) later developed a steady-state technique for $\dot{V}/\dot{Q}$ measurements in which a constant intravenous infusion of ^{133}Xe dissolved in saline was maintained until a steady state was reached between perfusion delivery and ventilatory excretion and regional count rates for perfusion (CR_p) became constant. If CO is known or assumed, mixed venous concentration of Xe during infusion (Cv) expressed in millicuries per liter can be calculated from the infusion rate in millicuries per minute. The steady-state infusion is followed under identical conditions by ventilatory equilibration with a concentration (FI) in the gas reservoir expressed

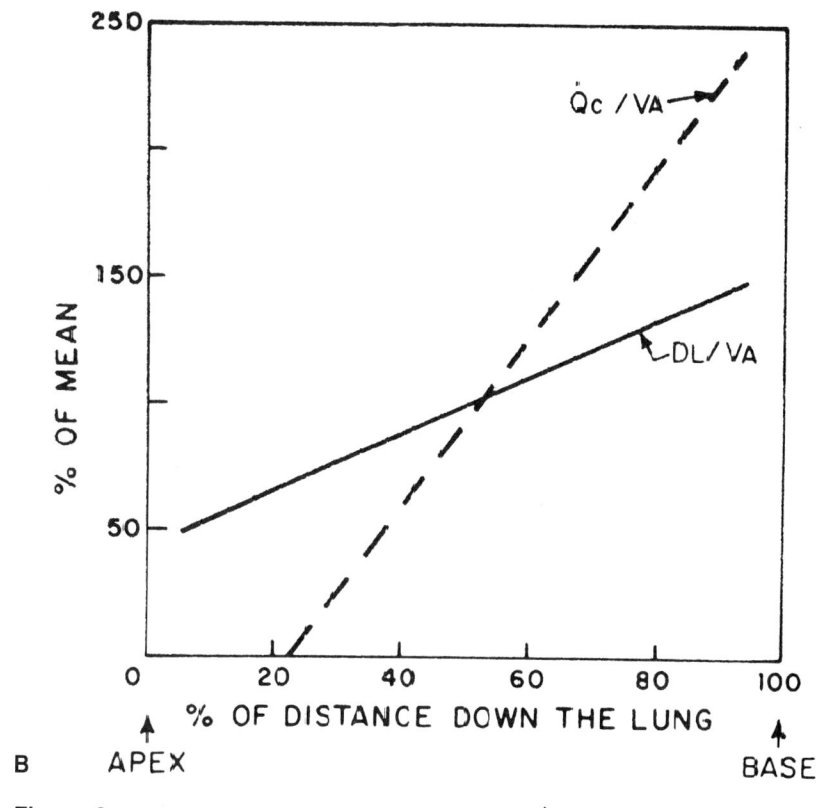

Experimental Approaches to the Study of Gas Exchange 75

Figure 9 (B) Comparative changes in blood flow $\dot{Q}$ and D$_{LCO}$ per unit lung volume measured by a bolus technique (80) similar to that of Dollfuss et al. (205).

in millicuries per liter and a constant count rate (CR$_i$). $\dot{V}_A/\dot{Q}c$ is estimated, neglecting dead space, using the following relationship:

$$\dot{V}_A/\dot{Q}c = \frac{C\bar{v} \cdot CR_i}{F_I \cdot CR_p} \tag{34}$$

Amis et al. (82,83) developed steady-state methods to measure distribution of ventilation and perfusion using a short-life radioactive isotope of krypton (^{81}Kr; half-life 13 seconds) combined with a longer-life ^{85}Kr (half-life 4.4 hours) used for volume calibration, and a gamma camera. The procedure used is to obtain regional count rates during a steady-state infusion of the relatively insoluble ^{81}Kr in saline, followed by count rates using steady-state inhalation of ^{81}Kr, followed, in turn, by regional count rates after rebreathing equilibration with a reservoir containing a known concentration of ^{85}Kr. Because ^{81}Kr has such a short half-life, alveolar delivery by either infusion or ventilation is balanced by the rate of radioactive decay as primary determinants of regional concentration of the isotope; washout rate by ventilation is a negligible component. ^{85}Kr provides a geometric factor for regional volumes seen by the counter. This technique also requires a cyclotron to provide the radioactive gases on site.

Multiple Inert Gas Elimination Technique

Radioactive inert gas techniques are useful for defining how differences in ventilation, perfusion, and $\dot{V}/\dot{Q}$ ratios are anatomically distributed in health and disease and how this pattern of distribution changes in response to changes in body position or to exercise; however, these techniques are not accurate enough to define the full extent of nonuniformity and the quantitative effects of uneven $\dot{V}/\dot{Q}$ on O_2 and CO_2 exchange. The concept of using the pulmonary elimination of multiple inert gases of different solubilities to detect nonuniformity of $\dot{V}/\dot{Q}$ ratios in the lung was introduced by Fahri (84) in a limited approach localized to a small number of $\dot{V}/\dot{Q}$ compartments, but its implementation to its full potential for approximating a continuous distribution of $\dot{V}/\dot{Q}$ ratios in the lungs at rest and exercise was performed by Wagner et al. (85–87); the test is referred to as the multiple inert gas elimination technique (MIGET). The equations describing elimination of an inert gas from the blood are essentially the same as those derived for elimination of CO_2, i.e., Eq. (11) and (13), except that the inspired concentration is zero and the CO_2 dissociation curve is replaced by a linear relationship defined by a solubility coefficient (α) so that Eq. (13) becomes:

$$\dot{V}_G(STP) = \dot{Q}\left(\alpha \cdot \frac{P\bar{v}_G}{760} - \alpha \cdot \frac{Pc'_G}{760}\right) = \frac{P_{AG}}{P_B} \cdot \dot{V}_A \cdot C_f \tag{35}$$

where $\alpha/760$ is the Bunsen solubility coefficient expressed in [milliliters gas (STP)/ milliliters blood] per millimeters mercury gas tension; $P\bar{v}_G$ and Pc'_G are mixed venous and pulmonary end-capillary inert gas tensions, respectively, in millimeters mercury. When dealing with inert gases, it is more convenient to express everything under body conditions (BTP) rather than under standard conditions (STP) and to use partition coefficients (λ) rather than the Bunsen solubility coefficient (α) where $\lambda = \alpha \cdot (273 + t/273)$; thus, dividing all terms of Eq. (35) by C_f and multiplying all terms by P_B, we obtain:

$$P_B \cdot \dot{V}_G(BTP) = \lambda \cdot \dot{Q}(P\bar{v}_G - P'_G) = P_{AG} \cdot \dot{V}_A$$

One assumption in these measurements is that regional equilibrium between alveolar air and blood is everywhere, i.e., that $Pc'_G = P_{AG}$; hence, rearranging and eliminating the subscript G for simplification, the following relationships describe inert gas elimination:

$$\frac{Pc'}{P\bar{v}} = \frac{P_A}{P\bar{v}} = \frac{\lambda}{\lambda + \dot{V}_A/\dot{Q}} \tag{36}$$

where $(Pc'/P\bar{v}) = (P_A/P\bar{v})$ represents the fractional dilution of a given mixed venous inert gas tension as it equilibrates with alveolar air; these ratios can range from zero to 1.0. Inert gases with different solubilities, i.e., different λ, are diluted differently for the same $\dot{V}_A/\dot{Q}$ ratio. If λ is small, the inert gas tension in mixed venous blood is diluted more by alveolar air during capillary transit at given $\dot{V}_A/\dot{Q}$ than if λ is large; hence, there is less retention of the gas in blood leaving the lung. If λ is large, inert gas tension in mixed venous blood is diluted less by alveolar air during capillary transit at given $\dot{V}_A/\dot{Q}$ than if λ is small; hence, if λ is large, there is greater retention of the gas in blood leaving the lung. Conversely, if λ is small, more of the gas is partitioned into alveolar air and excreted by ventilation.

In MIGET, multiple inert gases with a wide range of different solubility coefficients are dissolved in saline or 5% dextrose and infused intravenously at a constant rate until a steady state is achieved. Then mixed expired air and arterial blood are sampled simultaneously for measuring $P\bar{E}$ and Pa; these are averages from all regions of the lung weighted, respectively, for ventilation, including anatomical dead space, and blood flow. Mathematically, this mixing of an inert gas (j) partitioned into alveolar air from different regions (i) with dead space in conducting airways to yield a mixed expired gas tension ($P\bar{E}$) is described as follows:

$$P\bar{E} = \left(1 - \frac{V_D}{V_T}\right) \cdot P\bar{v} \cdot \sum^i \dot{V}_{A_i}\left(\frac{\lambda_j}{\lambda_j + \dot{V}_{A_i}/\dot{Q}_i}\right) \tag{37}$$

Mixing of an inert gas (j) retained in blood leaving different regions (i) to yield a mixed arterial tension of the gas is described in a similar equation;

$$Pa = P\bar{v} \cdot \sum^i \dot{Q}_i\left(\frac{\lambda_j}{\lambda_j + \dot{V}_{A_i}/\dot{Q}_i}\right) \tag{38}$$

In a homogeneous lung, $Pa/P\bar{v}$ should be that predicted for each inert gas based on its λ and the overall $\dot{V}_A/\dot{Q}$ ratio. Because alveolar air is diluted by the anatomical dead space, $(P\bar{E}/P\bar{v}) \neq (Pa/P\bar{v})$; rather, $(P\bar{E}/P\bar{v}) = (1 - V_D/V_T) \cdot (Pa/P\bar{v})$ for each inert gas. However, in a lung in which $\dot{V}_A/\dot{Q}$ ratios are not uniform, the predicted gas excretion and retention ratios of the different individual inert gases will not follow the pattern predicted by the mean $\dot{V}_A/\dot{Q}$ ratio for the whole lung. From the pattern of disparity between prediction and measurement for the different inert gases, the pattern of fractional distribution of perfusion and ventilation with respect to $\dot{V}_A/\dot{Q}$ ratios in an arbitrary number of assumed compartments (usually 50) can be derived (86) (Fig. 10). An initial guess as to the distribution is made, and a computer algorithm has been developed that iteratively alters the distribution to converge toward a solution that minimizes the sum of the squared differences between predicted and measured retention and excretion values for all of the inert gases used. Commonly, six gases are used, listed in order from lowest to highest solubility (sulfur hexafluoride, ethane, cyclopropane, halothane, diethyl ether, and

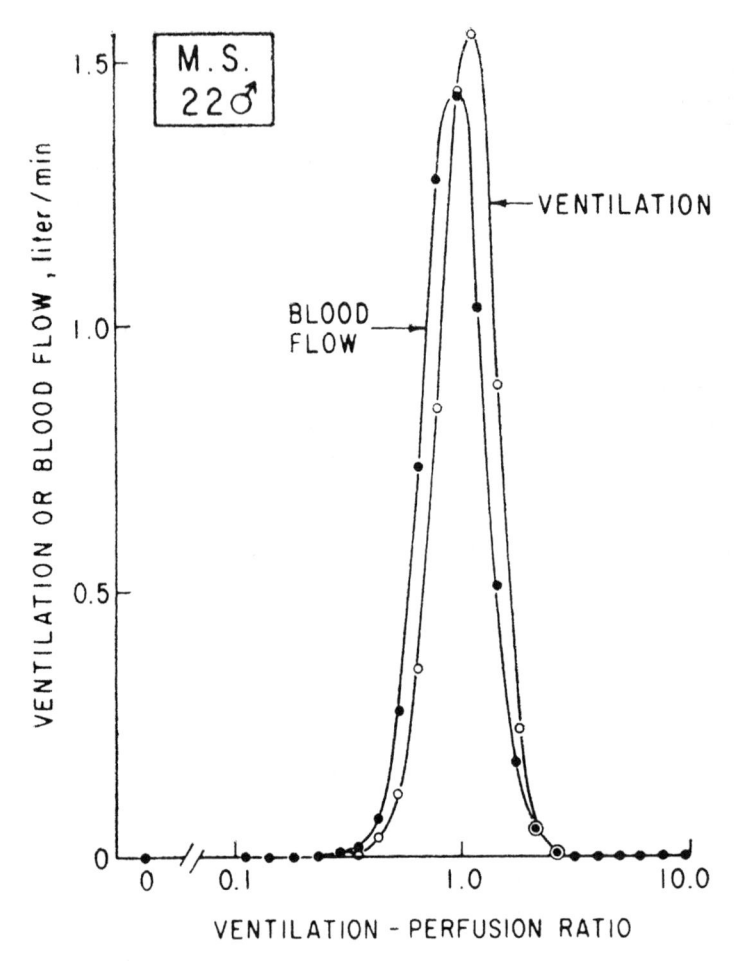

Figure 10 The distribution of ventilation and blood flow measured by MIGET in a young normal subject breathing room air. The pattern of the distribution in this normal subject is symmetrical and essentially log normal. Dispersion is measured as the SD of ventilation and of perfusion with respect to the log($\dot{V}/\dot{Q}$ ratio) and referred to as logSD$\dot{Q}$ and logSD$\dot{V}$, respectively, providing an index of the nonuniformity of distribution (86).

acetone), and are dissolved in saline or 5% dextrose and infused into a peripheral vein at a constant rate.

MIGET can be conducted at any F_{IO_2} at rest or heavy exercise. Based on the $\dot{V}_A/\dot{Q}$ compartmentation resolved by the technique, Pa_{O_2}, Pa_{CO_2}, A–aP_{O_2} and a–AP_{CO_2} can be calculated if mixed venous blood gases, pH, Hb concentration, P_{IO_2} and P_{ICO_2} are known, for comparison with measured values. Elimination of inert gases used in MIGET is not altered in the presence of severe diffusion limitation for oxygen; hence, a reliable $\dot{V}_A/\dot{Q}$ distribution can be resolved even in patients with significant alveolar capillary block. This also makes it possible to estimate the O_2 diffusing capacity (D_{LO_2}) from the difference between the measured $A-aP_{O_2}$ and that predicted on theoretical grounds based on the derived $\dot{V}_A/\dot{Q}$ distribution from MIGET (88,89). This is discussed further in the next section under Diffusive Gas Exchange for Oxygen.

MIGET has also been suggested as a means to detect the existence of gas phase limitation to inert gas exchange (90,91); this possibility is suggested when the inclusion of an inert gas with high molecular weight reduces the goodness of fit between the gas retentions measured and those predicted from the best-fitting $\dot{V}_A/\dot{Q}$ distribution (92,93). The relevance of such observations to O_2 and CO_2 exchange remains unclear.

Diffusive Gas Exchange

Background

The capacity of the lung for diffusive gas exchange determines the rapidity with which O_2 and CO_2 exchange can occur, particularly at heavy exercise; however, direct measurements of either O_2 or CO_2 diffusing capacity (D_{LO_2} and D_{LCO_2}, respectively) are difficult to obtain because uptake of both gases is primarily blood-flow–limited rather than diffusion-limited under most conditions. D_{LO_2} is defined as:

$$D_{LO_2} = \frac{\dot{V}_{O_2}}{P_{AO_2} - \overline{P}_{cO_2}} \tag{39}$$

where the numerator is O_2 uptake and the denominator is the difference between alveolar O_2 tension and the mean oxygen tension of Hb inside the red blood cell ($\overline{P}_{cO_2}$) during transit, i.e., the mean alveolar capillary O_2 tension difference driving diffusion from alveolar air into combination with intracorpuscular Hb. The $\overline{P}_{cO_2}$ is inaccessible to direct measurement.

The basic techniques for measuring diffusing capacity arose out of a controversy at the turn of the 20th century as to whether simple diffusion was sufficient to account for pulmonary O_2 uptake at rest and exercise or whether active secretion of oxygen must occur. The important investigators were Haldane, Douglas, and Bohr for the secretion hypothesis and Barcroft and the Kroghs (97,98) for passive diffusion. Both sides contributed greatly to our understanding of lung gas exchange. Bohr (94) and Haldane (95) collected data to suggest that O_2 tension in blood was higher than O_2 tension in alveolar air, suggesting active transport of O_2.

Bohr (94) was first to report a way to estimate diffusing capacity of the lung for carbon monoxide (D_{LCO}) based on measurements of CO uptake reported by Haldane (95) while breathing small concentrations of CO. He reasoned that, although O_2 was actively transported, CO, being a foreign gas would be transported by passive diffusion alone. Haldane and Smith had shown that the affinity of Hb for CO was approximately 200 times that for O_2 (96); hence, for a given carboxyhemoglobin saturation, P_{CO} is very small compared with that for O_2. Bohr used data collected by Haldane showing the slow increase in CO saturation over 15 to 20 minutes of breathing air containing 0.19% to 0.35% CO; based on an estimate of total CO capacity of the circulating blood volume and the increase in CO saturation, CO uptake was estimated ($\dot{V}_{CO}$). D_{LCO} could then be calculated from:

$$D_{LCO} = \frac{\dot{V}_{CO}}{P_{ACO} - P_{\bar{v}CO}} \tag{40}$$

$\dot{V}_{CO}$ and P_{ACO} could be easily measured and $P_{\bar{v}CO}$ was the average CO tension in venous blood during the interval of measurement. These were the first estimates of D_{LCO} by a steady-state technique. Bohr's objective in these measurements was to obtain an indirect estimate of D_{LO_2} from his estimates of D_{LCO} based on the known differences in Bunsen solubility coefficients (α) in water and molecular weights (M), i.e.,

$$D_{LO_2} = \frac{\alpha_{CO}}{\alpha_{O_2}} \cdot \frac{\sqrt{M_{O_2}}}{\sqrt{M_{CO}}} \cdot D_{LCO} \doteq 1.21 \cdot D_{LCO}$$

Bohr also derived a method for estimating how high an O_2 uptake that could be sustained by the estimated D_{LO_2} without a significant decrease in arterial oxygenation. He developed a numerical method to estimate the mean alveolar capillary O_2 tension difference ($P_{AO_2} - P_{\bar{c}O_2}$) from the O_2 dissociation curve if mixed venous and alveolar O_2 tensions are known. The method is called Bohr integration and is still used in computer algorithms for diffusive gas exchange today. Leaving off the O_2 subscripts, Bohr showed that the following relationships held:

$$P_A - P_{\bar{c}} = \frac{(S_{c'} - S_{\bar{v}})}{\int_{S_{\bar{v}}}^{S_{c'}} \frac{dS}{P_A - P_c}} \tag{41}$$

The left-hand side of the equation is the mean alveolar capillary O_2 tension difference; the numerator of the right-hand side is the oxygen saturation difference across the lung, and the denominator is the Bohr integral, which he solved numerically for any given mixed venous and end capillary saturation. Bohr wanted to know what magnitude of oxygen uptake that a given D_{LO_2} could support and could use the above equation to make that estimate:

$$\dot{V}_{O_2} = D_{LO_2} \cdot \frac{(S_{c'} - S_{\bar{v}})}{\int_{S_{\bar{v}}}^{S_{c'}} \frac{dS}{P_A - P_c}} \tag{42}$$

Based on his results, Bohr concluded from his calculations that D_{LO_2} was insufficient to explain the measured O_2 uptakes at heavy exercise, particularly at high altitude. Bohr supported Haldane's theory of active oxygen secretion by the lung, but calculations from Haldane's data were at rest.

Independently, Krogh and Krogh (97) at the same time developed a single-breath method for measuring D_{LCO} based on the same principles used by Bohr; however, because of the brief intervals over which the measurements were obtained (10 to 20 seconds) back pressures for CO in blood in most instances could be neglected. A breath of air containing approximately 0.3% CO was inspired from residual volume to TLC and then partially exhaled to collect an initial alveolar sample at time t_1; the breath was held for another 10 seconds followed by exhalation to collect a second alveolar sample at t_2. The rate of CO uptake during breath-holding is dependent on its own fractional alveolar concentration (F_A) and the D_{LCO} as follows:

$$V_A \cdot \frac{dF_{ACO}}{dt} = -F_{ACO}(P_B - P_{H_2O})D_{LCO} \tag{43}$$

This describes an exponential relationship from which D_{LCO} can be estimated:

$$D_{LCO} = \frac{V_A \cdot (P_B - P_{H_2O})}{t_2 - t_1} \cdot \ln \frac{F_{A_1}}{F_{A_2}} \tag{44}$$

V_A is volume under standard conditions (STPD). D_{LCO} by this technique significantly increased with exercise. Krogh (98) concluded that D_{LO_2} at heavy exercise was perfectly adequate to account for measured oxygen uptakes by diffusion both at sea level and high altitude without invoking oxygen secretion.

In the wake of settling this controversy, the basis for all subsequent methods for measuring diffusing capacity were in place; however, interest in diffusive gas exchange waned and was not revived until World War II stimulated an interest in high altitude.

For Oxygen

Lilienthal-Riley Method. After it became possible to routinely sample and measure arterial blood, in 1946 Lilienthal et al. (99) reported a method for separating the $A-aP_{O_2}$ into two major components, one due to $\dot{V}/\dot{Q}$ mismatching and one due to failure to reach equilibrium of P_{O_2} in alveolar air and capillary blood. Because of the shape of the O_2 dissociation curve, it was shown that, if the $A-aP_{O_2}$ breathing room air were predominantly due to diffusion impairment, the $A-aP_{O_2}$ would be exaggerated by breathing a low-oxygen mixture; however, if the $A-aP_{O_2}$ were predominantly caused by $\dot{V}/\dot{Q}$ mismatch, it would be made smaller by switching from room air to a low-oxygen mixture. Thus, by measuring the $A-aP_{O_2}$ under steady-state conditions at two different inspired O_2 tensions each measured $A-aP_{O_2}$ could be separated into a component caused by $\dot{V}/\dot{Q}$ mismatch (characterized as a relative shunt) and the remainder into a component caused by failure of the O_2 tension in capillary blood leaving the lung to reach equilibrium with that in alveolar air; this provided an estimate of end-capillary oxygen tension ($P_{c'O_2}$) and saturation ($S_{c'O_2}$). With this information, Bohr integration was used to estimate ($P_{AO_2} - P\bar{c}O_2$) and D_{LO_2} [see Eq. (41 and (42)]. The problems with the method are as follows: (1) It is a lumped parameter model that does not take into account the effects of uneven $\dot{V}/\dot{Q}$ mismatching and distribution of alveolar P_{O_2} on the efficiency of diffusive gas exchange; (2) $\dot{V}/\dot{Q}$ mismatch has been shown to change when inspired O_2 tension is changed (85); and (3) D_{LO_2} changes with inspired O_2 tension because of associated changes in resistance of red blood cells to oxygen uptake (100).

MIGET. A modification of the Lilienthal-Riley method for estimating D_{LO_2} has been provided by the MIGET technique. MIGET can provide an estimate of that component of the measured $A-aP_{O_2}$ at any given inspired oxygen concentration, which can be explained by the simultaneously measured distribution of $\dot{V}_A$ and $\dot{Q}$ with respect to $\dot{V}/\dot{Q}$ ratios in the lungs. Even in normal individuals' breathing room at heavy exercise, the measured $A-aP_{O_2}$ is significantly larger than can be explained by $\dot{V}/\dot{Q}$ mismatching (101); this can only be explained by either (1) incomplete equilibration of P_{O_2} between alveolar air and blood leaving lung capillaries or (2) postpulmonary shunts from thebesian vessels in the heart or from the bronchial circulation, which are usually a small source of discrepancy. Using iterative numerical methods, it is possible to determine the ratio of $D_L/\dot{Q}$ or $D_L/\dot{V}_A$ when uniformly distributed among regions of different $\dot{V}/\dot{Q}$, which would be necessary to explain that part of the measured $A-aP_{O_2}$ unexplained by $\dot{V}/\dot{Q}$ mismatch (88,89). The assumption has to be made that D_{LO_2} is distributed uniformly with either blood flow or ventilation; this method does take into account the effects of uneven $\dot{V}/\dot{Q}$ on diffusive gas exchange and does not require measurements at more than one inspired O_2 tension.

For CO

Steady State. The steady-state method for measuring D_{LCO} originated by Bohr was resurrected in the 1950s by Filley et al. (102) and Bates et al. (103), using modifications that were made possible by the ability to measure arterial blood gases and by rapid infrared gas analyzers. The subject breathes 0.1% CO in air until a steady state of CO uptake is reached, usually within 2 minutes. The two techniques differ primarily in the way that alveolar CO tension is estimated. Filley et al. (104) took an arterial blood sample and estimated P_{ACO} from physiological dead space calculated using Eq. (22) to obtain effective $\dot{V}_A$:

$$\text{Then} \quad \dot{V}_D/\dot{V}_E = 1 - \dot{V}_A/\dot{V}_E \tag{45}$$

$$\text{and} \quad P_{ACO} = \frac{P\bar{E}_{CO} - (\dot{V}_D/\dot{V}_E)P_{ICO}}{1 - \dot{V}_D/\dot{V}_E} \tag{46}$$

where $\dot{V}_E$ is expired ventilation, $P\bar{E}_{CO}$ is mixed expired CO tension, and P_{ICO} is inspired CO tension. Bates et al. (103) used end-tidal CO tension or an average of end-tidal and alveolar P_{CO} estimated at the end of inspiration. The CO back pressure ($P\bar{v}_{CO}$) in Eq. (40) could be estimated before and after a run using the rebreathing technique of Siosteen and Sjostrand (105); essentially, CO tension is measured while breathing 100% oxygen in a closed system with a CO_2 absorber until CO tension becomes constant. The measured CO tension is then corrected to the alveolar O_2 tension at which the measurements were made as follows:

$$P\bar{v}_{CO} = \frac{P_{CO}(\text{breathing 100\% } O_2) \cdot P_{O_2}(\text{during CO uptake measurement})}{P_{AO_2}(\text{breathing 100\% } O_2)} \tag{47}$$

Currently, $P\bar{v}_{CO_2}$ is most easily assessed by measuring CO saturation in a venous blood sample using a CO oximeter and then using the Haldane relationship to calculate $P\bar{v}_{CO}$:

$$P\bar{v}_{CO} = \frac{P_{AO_2} \cdot S\bar{v}_{CO}}{210 \cdot Sc'_{O_2}} \tag{48}$$

Single Breath. Krogh's (98) breath-holding technique for measuring D_{LCO} was modified by Ogilvie et al. (106) by the addition of an insoluble tracer gas (in this instance 10% helium) to measure the initial dilution of the inspired gas in the lung at the start of breath-holding without the necessity of obtaining an initial alveolar sample; only one alveolar sample was required at the end of breath-holding. Equation (44) was modified as follows:

$$D_{LCO} = \frac{V_A}{(P_B - P_{H_2O}) \cdot \Delta t} \cdot \ln \frac{F_{ACO}}{F_{ICO}} \cdot \frac{F_{IHe}}{F_{AHe}} = \frac{V_A}{(P_B - P_{H_2O}) \cdot \Delta t} \cdot \ln \frac{F_{ACO}}{F_{ACO_0}} \tag{49}$$

where F_{ACO_0} represents the initial fractional CO concentration in alveolar air. Typically the subject exhales to residual volume and then inspires the gas mixture, containing 0.3% CO and 10% helium in air, rapidly to near TLC, followed by approximately 10 seconds of breath-holding and rapid exhalation; after dead space is cleared during exhalation, an alveolar sample is collected. Alveolar volume (V_A) = RV (measured previously by an inert gas washout technique or by plethysmography) plus inspired volume (V_I), both expressed under standard conditions. V_A may also be estimated as $V_I \cdot (F_{IHe}/F_{AHe})$ in subjects with minimal evidence of airways obstruction. The time interval of breath-holding in the original method was taken from the beginning of inspiration to the start of sampling during exhalation. Later, Jones and Mead (207) suggested that a more appropriate measurement of time would include 0.7 of the inspiratory time to halfway through the sampling time; in people without airway obstruction, there is negligible difference in the results obtained by the different timing methods. In people with partial airway obstruction, it is often more accurate to make multiple estimates of CO disappearance using different breath-holding times and construct a linear regression curve for the relationship between $\ln \cdot (F_{ACO}/F_{ACO_0})$ and time of breath-holding; D_{LCO} is then estimated from the slope of this relationship (107). This technique is the most reliable method of eliminating errors due to timing of the effective breath-holding interval since finite intervals of time are required for inspiration and sample collection.

By adding acetylene to the inspired gas mixture, it became possible to estimate pulmonary capillary blood flow ($\dot{Q}c$) simultaneously with diffusing capacity (108). This is an important addition because D_{LCO} changes in an approximately linear relationship with cardiac output in normal subjects from rest to exercise. When acetylene is used with the breath-holding technique, it requires multiple different breath-holding intervals to construct disappearance curves for both acetylene and CO. One major advantage of the rebreathing technique is that D_{LCO} and $\dot{Q}c$ can be measured simultaneously in one maneuver. The following equations are used:

$$D_{LCO} = \frac{V_A}{P_B - H_{H_2O}} \cdot \frac{\Delta \ln(F_{ACO}/F_{ACO_0})}{\Delta t} \qquad (50)$$

$$\dot{Q}c = \frac{760}{(P_B - P_{H_2O})} \cdot \frac{(V_A + \alpha_\tau V_t)}{\alpha_b} \cdot \frac{\Delta \ln(F_{AC_2H_2}/F_{AC_2H_2o})}{\Delta t} \qquad (51)$$

where the last term in both equations is the slope of the semilog disappearance with time; α_t and α_b are Bunsen solubility coefficients for acetylene in tissue and blood, respectively; V_t is lung tissue volume in that the acetylene dissolves. Acetylene dissolves rapidly in the fine septal tissues of the lung with the first breath of the test gas mixture containing 0.6% acetylene and 10% helium; therefore, the acetylene is diluted by the tissues, whereas the He is not; this depresses the intercept of the linear plot of $\ln(F_{AC_2H_2}/F_{AC_2H_2o})$ versus time. V_t is calculated from the intercept as follows:

$$\alpha_t V_t = \frac{V_A}{\exp.\text{intercept}} - V_A \qquad (52)$$

Three-Equation Method. Originally, the single-breath method was designed to make inspiratory and expiratory time as short as possible with respect to breath-holding time. This is not always possible in patients; hence, the three-equation method was derived to take into account the pattern of CO uptake expected during intervals of slowed inspiration and/or exhalation (109,110). Errors normally introduced during inspiration and expiration are in opposite directions and tend to cancel one another out; in normal subjects and patients without significant airway obstruction, standard breath-holding analysis and application of the three-equation analysis yield identical results. Nevertheless, the three-equation model can be useful when inspiration, expiration, or both are prolonged either because of disease or purposely in an experimental protocol (111). There is not a closed solution using these equations to estimate D_{LCO}. An iterative numerical algorithm is required with the inherent assumption that D_{LCO} remains constant throughout the maneuver.

Slow Exhalation. It is also possible to estimate both D_{LCO} and $\dot{Q}c$ by following gas concentrations at the mouth during a slow constant rate of exhalation after inspiring a gas mixture containing small concentrations of CO, C_2H_2, and an inert insoluble gas such as He (112–114). Equations are as follows:

$$D_{LCO} = \frac{\dot{V}}{P_B - P_{H_2O}} \cdot \frac{\Delta \ln(F_{ACO}/F_{ACO_0})}{\Delta \ln(V_A/V_{A_0})} \tag{53}$$

$$\dot{Q}_c = \frac{760}{\alpha_b} \cdot \frac{\dot{V}}{P_B - P_{H_2O}} \cdot \frac{\Delta \ln(F_{AC_2H_2}/F_{AC_2H_2 0})}{\Delta \ln(V_A + \alpha_t V_t)/(V_{A_0} + \alpha_t V_t)} \tag{54}$$

where $\dot{V}$ is the rate of expiration in volume per unit time.

Rebreathing. The rebreathing method was developed originally by Kruhøffer (115) using a radioactive label (^{14}CO); it was modified by Lewis et al. (116), who used $C^{16}O$ with helium as an insoluble tracer, and later by Sackner et al. (117), who used as mass spectrometer with $C^{18}O$, He, and C_2H_2 for measuring D_{LCO} and cardiac output simultaneously. The basic equations for calculating D_{LCO} are Eq. (50) and (51), where system volume (V_S) replaces alveolar volume (V_A); V_S is the combined dead space, alveolar, and rebreathing bag volumes. At the end of a normal expiration, the subject inspires the test gas mixture and rebreaths the mixture in a leak-free bag, emptying the bag with each breath at approximately 30 breaths per minute for 10 to 15 seconds. Usually a mass spectrometer is used to measure the gas concentrations at the mouth; however, with a mass spectrometer, $C^{18}O$ must supplant $C^{16}O$ because $C^{16}O$ has the same mass as nitrogen. The advantages of the rebreathing technique are: (1) it can be used up to heavy levels of exercise to measure diffusing capacity, cardiac output, tissue volume, and lung volume simultaneously; (2) it requires minimal cooperation and, hence, can be used in unanesthetized animals at rest and exercise, as well as in adult humans and children; and (3) rebreathing minimizes errors resulting from uneven distribution of regional ventilation and diffusing capacity. The technique has been used to measure how diffusing capacity progressively increases from rest to heavy exercise without approaching a plateau; an upper limit remains undefined (56) (Fig. 11). The cardiac output measured by the rebreathing technique has been validated against both by dye dilution and direct Fick measurements (118,119). The major drawback of the technique is the cost of a mass spectrometer and $C^{18}O$. Compact infrared analyzers recently have become available that can simultaneously measure CO, C_2H_2, and CH_4 as the inert insoluble gas, which should make the technique more practical for general use.

Roughton-Forster Technique for Interpreting D_{LCO}. D_{LCO} is not a true diffusing capacity as defined by Krogh because it depends not only on passive diffusion of CO from alveolar air into capillary red blood cells, but also on the rate of reaction between CO and binding sites on Hb. Roughton et al. (31,120) subdivided the diffusing capacity into two components: (1) diffusing capacity of the pulmonary membrane (D_{MCO}), which includes the plasma barrier; and (2) CO uptake by red blood cells ($\Theta_{CO}V_c$), which includes both diffusion and reaction velocity. Θ_{CO} is the rate of CO uptake by a suspension of red blood cells at a normal hematocrit

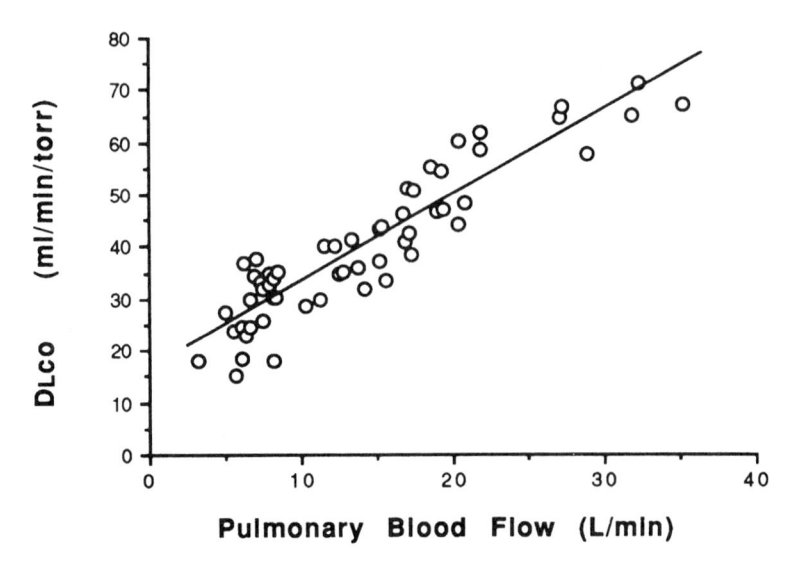

Figure 11 Diffusing capacity of the lung for CO (DLCO) plotted with respect to simultaneous measurements of cardiac output by the cardiac output measured by the acetylene technique while rebreathing a gas mixture containing 0.3% C_2H_2, 0.3% $C^{18}O$, and 10% helium in 21% to 25% O_2 in a balance of N_2. Concentrations at the mouth were measured with a mass spectrometer. (Reproduced with permission from Ref. 56)

in milliliters per minute per milliliter of blood, and Vc is the pulmonary capillary blood volume in milliliters. The reciprocals of DMCO and ΘcoVc represent the electrical analogs of conductance. The reciprocals (1/DMCO and 1/ΘcoVc, respectively) represent resistances to CO uptake by the pulmonary membrane and red blood cells, respectively; the sum of these resistances should then equal the total resistance [1/DLCO; see Eq. (4)]. This equation theoretically should hold for any gas that binds to the same heme binding site on Hb (e.g., O_2 and NO) and can be used to translate diffusing capacity with one gas to diffusing capacity for another. Because O_2 and CO compete for the same sites on Hb, the oxygen tension at which the measurement of DLCO is made has a significant effect on the measurement. Θco has been measured in vitro at different oxygen tensions by spectrophotometric measurements of the rate of carboxyhemoglobin (COHb) formation after rapid mixing with CO dissolved in saline and by a stationary thin-film technique after a sudden change of the CO tension in air. Results of the relationship between Θco and P_{O_2} have been variable, but when all existing data are plotted together, the resulting relationship is consistent with the original results of Roughton et al. in human blood (56,120):

$$\frac{1}{\Theta_{CO}} = 0.73 + 0.0058 \cdot P_{O_2} \tag{55}$$

Experimental Approaches to the Study of Gas Exchange 87

ΘCO varies with temperature in accordance with the Arrhenius equation and varies among mammalian species (121). If DLCO is measured at two or more alveolar O_2 tensions from which ΘCO can be estimated from Eq. (55), and the resulting linear relationship between 1/DLCO and 1/ΘCO is plotted based on Eq. (4), the slope and intercept of the relationship provides estimates of 1/Vc and 1/DMCO, respectively. Equation (4) is a lumped parameter model of a distributed process; the errors that may result from this oversimplification are discussed in more detail in the section Anatomical Determinants of Diffusive Gas Exchange, but the errors are probably small when the subject has a normal hematocrit.

If DMCO and Vc are known based on measurements of DLCO at different alveolar O_2 tensions, it should be possible to estimate DL for other gases using Eq. (4) if the Krogh diffusion constants are known relative to that of CO and if values of Θ are known (Table 1).

ΘO_2 estimated by Staub et al. (100) was measured with a continuous-flow reaction apparatus after rapid mixing; results of Yamaguchi et al. (122), who measured the off reaction in the presence of sodium nitrite to eliminate any unstirred layer, are probably more near to the actual value. ΘNO was measured by Carlsen and Comroe (124) is probably also too low because of an unstirred layer outside the cells; if the unstirred layer caused an error similar to that for O_2, ΘNO might be 7.2 or higher. ΘCO_2 measured by Constantine et al. (123) probably reflect the rate of hydration of CO_2 in the red blood cell; that estimated by Wagner (53) is based on the half-time for the chloride–bicarbonate shift. Thus, there is still considerable uncertainty in the values of Θ for these various gases. Furthermore, the ΘO_2 decreases progressively when O_2 saturation of Hb exceeds 80–85% in direct proportion to the reduction in O_2 binding sites; hence, DLO_2 breathing air at rest or exercise at sea level will be lower than predicted from Eq. (4) unless consideration is made for the progressive reduction in ΘO_2 when higher O_2 saturations are reached during lung capillary transit.

For CO_2

Diffusing capacity for CO_2 has been measured with $C^{18}O^{16}O$ using a mass spectrometer. A single-breath method was used with the three-equation model because the kinetics are so rapid that the maneuver had to be completed within less than 3 seconds. Average $DLCO_2$ in two normal subjects was 862 (mL/min)/mm Hg. These measurements probably represent an approximation to $DMCO_2$ and do not take into consideration the resistance imposed by CO_2 hydration in the red blood cell and the resistance imposed by the chloride shift (125).

For NO

Nitric oxide binds tenaciously to the same sites on Hb as do CO and O_2 but at a velocity of approximately 40 times that for oxygen and 200 times that for CO; hence, most of the resistance to NO uptake by blood flowing through lung capillaries is in the pulmonary membrane. DLNO tends to be four to five times that of DLCO measured simultaneously by the breath-holding technique, and it has been suggested that by measuring DLCO and DLNO simultaneously it should be possible to estimate DMCO, DMNO, and Vc using Eq. (4), without making measurements at two or more levels of PAO$_2$. The uncertainty in this technique revolves about what value to use for ΘNO. One group (208) has used the ΘNO measured by Carlsen and Comroe (124); the other group (209,210) suggests that the true ΘNO approaches infinity. Hence, the application of this technique for estimating DM and Vc is still controversial but has the potential for significantly advancing our understanding of diffusive gas exchange.

IV. Peripheral Gas Exchange

The sums of individual organ O$_2$ and CO$_2$ exchanges must equal that which can be measured at the lung. Measures of total systemic O$_2$ consumption and CO$_2$ production are the oldest and still most commonly performed assessments of gas exchange; they provide valuable information to those interested in nutrition and exercise and respiratory physiology. For the most part, however, they reveal little about the state of individual organ systems. The purpose of this section is to review briefly and critically some of the techniques used to gain knowledge of gas exchange, rather than the knowledge base itself. We discuss methods currently available to the clinician as well as those found only in the research laboratory. Each method covered here has its strengths and weaknesses, and no single test can address the adequacy of the entire O$_2$ transport system, from the lung to mitochondrial cytochrome aa$_3$. Most often, a number of methods must be combined to fully address gas exchange. It is our desire that this section will help the reader to evaluate better the data presented elsewhere in this volume.

A. Structure–Function Determinants of Gas Exchange in Microvasculature

Background

The Krogh Model of Peripheral Gas Exchange in Muscle

Because O$_2$ and CO$_2$ move in accordance with fundamental physical laws, one must define the physical environment to predict the dynamics of gas exchange. The results of such physical models or constructs provide data that can be compared with experimentally derived measurements. Such comparisons may raise questions regarding the validity of measured data, or the experimental data may force a rethinking of the assumptions underlying the model. Modeling is an another approach to investigating gas exchange, and its inception is reviewed briefly here.

The flux of a gas from point a to b is the product of its driving force (Pa−Pb) and its conductance along that path. Having first measured the diffusion constant of

Experimental Approaches to the Study of Gas Exchange

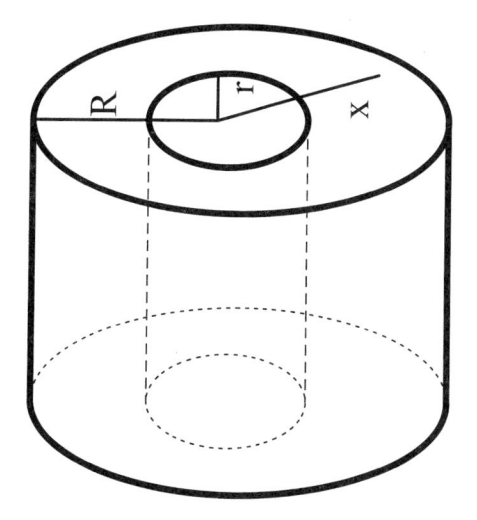

Figure 12 The Krogh tissue cylinder. (From Ref. 126.)

O_2 in animal tissues, Krogh (126) studied the vascular arrangement within various muscles of many species and concluded that "it becomes at once apparent that no serious error can be committed by supposing each capillary to supply oxygen independently of all the others to a cylinder of tissue surrounding it." Figure 12 represents a Krogh tissue cylinder with radius R surrounding a capillary of radius r. Krogh reasoned that one could calculate the difference in oxygen partial pressure between the capillary wall (Po) and at a point distance x away (Px) if one knew the O_2 consumption ($\dot{M}$), the diffusion coefficient (d), r, R, and the distance x. With the help of the mathematician Erlang, the following equation was derived:

$$P_O - P_x = \frac{\dot{M}}{d} \cdot \left(\frac{1}{2} \cdot R^2 \ln \frac{x}{r} - \frac{x^2 - r^2}{4} \right) \tag{56}$$

P is partial pressure in atmospheres; $\dot{M}$ is in minutes^{-1}; d is in centimeters squared per minute per standard atmosphere $\times 10^4$; x, r, and R are in micrometers. To find the Po_2 difference necessary to meet the oxygen needs at the periphery of the tissue cylinder, R was substituted for x, and the equation rewritten as:

$$P_O - P_R = \Delta P = \frac{\dot{M}}{d} \cdot \left(\frac{1}{2} \cdot R^2 \ln \frac{R}{r} - \frac{R^2 - r^2}{4} \right) \tag{57}$$

where ΔP is the critical pressure difference in atmospheres between the capillary and periphery of the Krogh cylinder. Putting ΔP in millimeters mercury and assuming that the ratio of $(r^2/R^2) = \emptyset$ is a good approximation to capillary blood volume/tissue volume (and index of capillary density), the equation can be put into the form:

$$\Delta P = \frac{1.9 \cdot 10^{-2} \cdot \dot{M} \cdot r^2}{d \cdot \emptyset}[\emptyset - 1 - \ln \emptyset] \qquad (58)$$

As the nondimensional term, $\emptyset$, changes between its limits of 0 and 1, the critical P_{O_2} (ΔP) changes between ∞ and 0, respectively. Krogh concluded that as long as venous P_{O_2} from a tissue is greater than this critical P_{O_2}, tissue O_2 needs should be met. Based on available data for tissue diffusion coefficients and capillary densities in different organs and species, Krogh's comparison of capillary density to resting O_2 consumption highlighted the role of capillary to cell distance as a key factor in meeting varying O_2 needs, a concept later probed by many others.

Problems with the Krogh Approximation

In an excellent review, Kreuzer (127) listed and discussed 15 different "simplifying and often unrealistic" assumptions of the Krogh model. All of these have been addressed to some degree in models subsequent to that of Krogh (for a review, see Ref. 128). Perhaps the greatest obstacle to all efforts at modeling is the accuracy of the geometry. Krogh's primary assumption was that single capillaries serve simple cylinders of tissue. Alhough Krogh was referring to muscle, which is relatively well organized, the work of investigators such as Eriksson and Myrhage (129) and Hammersen (130) contradict the concept of a terminal vascular unit, even for that tissue. Using intravital microscopy (live tissue) combined with light microscopy of stained and unstained specimens and three-dimensional microscopy of microangiograms of cat tenuissimus muscle, Eriksson and Myrhage (129) found that capillaries anastomosed to each other on average once every 200 μm; reversal of blood flow occurred frequently in capillaries, in their anastomoses, and in venules; linear flow rate in the capillaries averaged 0.5 mm/sec but was not constant, varying from 0 to 1.5 mm/sec, all of which contradicts Krogh's model assumptions. Such variability in microvascular anatomy and blood flow must be kept in mind when judging the soundness of any model of peripheral gas exchange (131,132).

Despite deficiencies of the original Krogh model, it has been of great importance conceptually by defining the major determinants of diffusive transport of oxygen between tissue capillaries and sites of oxygen use. Many subsequent refinements came about as a result of newer methods (discussed in the next two sections) that provided more accurate data for the parameters that Krogh knew to be important, namely, microvascular geometry, capillary and tissue O_2 tensions, and tissue O_2 conductance.

Newer Approaches to Structure–Function Relationships

Taylor and Weibel (133) developed a schematic approach to examine structure–function relationships, determining maximal O_2 transport at each step in the O_2

transport chain from lung to periphery. Their three hypotheses were: (1) that structural design is a rate limiting factor for O_2 flow at each level; (2) that structural design is optimized; and (3) that structural design is adaptable, i.e., can change within limits in response to changes of environmental conditions and O_2 requirements. They hypothesized that as a general principle, "no more structure is formed and maintained than what is required to satisfy functional needs," and named the principle *symmorphosis*. The principle has been examined over a wide range of mammals, requiring the development of both physiological methods for measuring maximal O_2 uptake (6) and morphometric techniques for estimating capillary blood volume, alveolar capillary surface area and mean harmonic thickness of the alveolar capillary tissue barrier for diffusive gas exchange in the lung, distribution of mitochondria and capillaries among and within skeletal muscles, inner membrane surface area of mitochondria, and length density and capillary surface area per fiber volume in skeletal muscle. The principle as stated often does not seem to hold [e.g., morphometric diffusing capacity of the lung (29)], but deviations from what is expected in a model are often more interesting and informative than confirmation.

It is not possible to present in detail all of the morphometric approaches, but it may be informative to refer some of the new techniques for defining structure back to the original Krogh cylinder model. Krogh and Erlang assumed that oxygen is used uniformly throughout the muscle cylinder; however, oxygen is used in mitochondria, and mitochondria are not distributed uniformly within the muscle fibers but tend to be more concentrated toward the fiber periphery closer to feeding capillaries (134). Gayeski and Honig (182) found a very shallow oxygen tension gradient for diffusion within highly oxidative muscle at near maximal O_2 uptake, presumably due to facilitated diffusive transport by myoglobin. They inferred that the primary O_2 diffusion gradient is in the capillary, its membrane, and adventitia. Accordingly, the major structural limitation to diffusive O_2 transport between the red blood cell and mitochondria in highly oxidative muscle would depend on the total capillary length and surface density in skeletal muscle, as well as the thickness of the capillary diffusion barrier; the morphometric technique used by Krogh did not provide that information because muscle capillaries were counted only in cross-section. The Krogh model assumed that the distribution of muscle capillaries was isotropic, i.e., straight and parallel to muscle fibers without anastomoses. Mathieu et al. (135,136) have developed quantitative morphometric techniques for estimating the degree of anisotropy in muscle capillaries to estimate their length and surface density, taking into account their tortuous and branching course with multiple anastomoses.

Newer Modeling Techniques

It was not until modern computers were developed that more complex models than that of Krogh could be studied using numerical analysis, such as finite element or finite difference modeling. These numerical methods, developed primarily by engineers for designing structurally sound and efficient buildings, chemical plants, engines, and bridges, give close approximations for solutions to physical questions with less restrictive assumptions and simplified domains required in analytical methods. Some recent examples of this approach to modeling peripheral gas exchange can be found in articles by Federspiel (33), Wang and Popel (35), or Schacterle et al. (137).

B. Physiological Measurements

Gas Exchange of Individual Organs and Tissues

Most studies of peripheral gas exchange involve the use of the Fick principle as described in detail previously. The chief considerations are the ability to obtain accurate measures of regional blood flow and O_2 contents of arterial inflow and venous outflow. Each organ system presents its own particular challenges because of variations in anatomy and ease of access. Table 2 highlights the wide variations in blood supply and O_2 uptake encountered. At rest, O_2 extraction ratio ($\dot{V}_{O_2}/\dot{Q}_{O_2}$) may be as low as 6% (skin) or as high as 66% (heart). This wide range stems from the fact that organ blood flow subserves other functions than simple gas exchange, e.g., heat exchange in skin and excretory function in kidneys.

Obviously, not all organ systems listed here have received the same attention from investigators. Heart, brain, and, more recently, bowel have been studied extensively secondary to the clinical importance of ischemic diseases affecting them. Because of its remarkable ability to vary O_2 consumption and its accessibility, skeletal muscle has also been widely studied.

Table 2 Typical Values for Regional Blood Flows, O_2 Uptakes, and Extraction Ratios in a 70-kg Man

Organ	Regional blood flow		Regional O_2 uptake		Extraction ratio (%)
	Organ weight (mL/min/kg)	Cardiac output (%)	Organ weight (mL/min/kg)	O_2 uptake (%)	
Brain	536	13	33	20	36
Heart	833	4	90	4	66
Kidney	3667	19	53	7	7
Gut	538	24	22	25	24
Skeletal muscle	39	21	2.3	30	46
Skin	139	9	1.4	2	6
Total		90		88	

Techniques to Measure Regional Blood Flow

Direct Timed Blood Volume Collection

If the anatomy permits, the most direct method is to cannulate the single large vein draining a region and redirect that blood flow to a reservoir that itself drains back to the body through another vein (138). Periodically, the blood flow can be collected into a graduated cylinder for a set time, and flow rate can be calculated. The venous circuit must be of large enough diameter to not add significantly to venous resistance and systemic anticoagulation is required.

Noncannulating Flow Probes

Alternatively, a noncannulating flow probe can be placed around either the regional vein or artery to provide a continuous estimation of flow. Earlier electromagnetic flow probes required a precise fit to the vessel and frequent in vitro calibration. These have been replaced largely by ultrasonic transit-time flow probes of remarkable accuracy ($\pm 10\%$) (139,140). Laser Doppler probes are also available that can be applied to an organ surface and give a continuous but qualitative measurement of blood flow in the underlying 1 mm^3 volume of tissue (141).

Videomicroscopy

Blood flow in microvessels lying near the transparent surface of a tissue can be estimated using videomicroscopy, as described in detail elsewhere (142,143).

Labeled Microspheres

Polystyrene spheres 15 to 25 μm diameter are injected into and mixed within the left atrium or ventricle; microspheres are distributed to peripheral tissues in proportion to regional blood flow, where they are trapped in microvessels (144). Microspheres are labeled with a radionuclide that emits gamma radiation or a colored dye (145). The animal is later killed and tissues or organs are sampled for measurement of radiation count rates or dye content per gram of tissue sampled. During the injection of the microspheres, an arterial reference sample is collected at a known flow rate over an interval of approximately 5 to 10 times the circulation time; the radioactivity or dye content in the reference sample is later measured. The reference sample acts as a surrogate organ or tissue; the gamma count rate or quantity of dye measured in the reference blood sample per unit reference blood sampling rate provides the calibration factor used to calculate regional blood flow per gram of tissue sample from the radioactivity or dye content per gram in the sample. By using multiple radionuclide labels with different energy levels or dye labels with different light absorption wavelengths, it is possible to make repeated measurements of regional blood flow under different experimental conditions. Spatial resolution of regional flow is limited only by the dissecting technique applied and by the random statistical variability in microsphere deposition, which becomes larger as the tissue sample becomes smaller; for example, Buckberg et al. (146) showed that approximately 400 microspheres per tissue sample are required to achieve 95% confidence that the flow estimates lie within ±10% of the true value. Measurement errors may also occur secondary to aggregation of microspheres, nonuniform mixing within the blood, variations in microsphere diameter, nonentrapment of microspheres, loss of microspheres from tissue during isolation, recirculation errors, and reference sampling errors (145). One must be cautious using microsphere techniques with vascular beds occurring in series. For example, Greenway and Murthy (147) showed in feline small bowel that the flow distribution of radioactive microspheres (15 ± 5 μm) between mucosa and submucosa varied with microsphere size. In addition, microspheres injected during vasoconstriction lodged in the submucosa and, with subsequent administration of vasodilators, migrated to and lodged in the mucosa, invalidating their use for estimation of blood flow to the two regions. Advantages of the microsphere technique include the ability to obtain multiple consecutive blood flow measurements in different organs, quantification of blood flow in absolute units, accuracy, reproducibility, and ease of performance (148).

Colored microspheres have certain advantages over radioactive microspheres (145). The radioactivity of radioactive microspheres decays with respect to time; therefore, in longitudinal studies, the time interval between the initial and final studies is determined by the half-life of the radionuclides used; this is not a problem with colored microspheres because leaching out of the dye is very slow. Radioactive microspheres are more costly; half-life limits the time of storage before use, and radiation hazards to personnel must be minimized. Distribution of dye-labeled microspheres within tissues also can be measured using light microscopy—not possible with radioactive microspheres. On the other hand, less manipulation of the tissues and less potential loss of microspheres during this manipulation exist for radioactive microspheres than dye labeled microspheres. When there is low tissue entrapment of microspheres, the accuracy of radioactive measurements can be enhanced by increasing the counting time, but this is not possible for colored microspheres.

Indocyanine Green

First used as an indicator for dye dilution cardiac output measurements, indocyanine green (ICG) was found to be cleared rapidly by the liver, making it useful to estimate both hepatic blood flow and provide an index of hepatic function (149). After an intravenous injection of a bolus of ICG, concentration is measured spectrophotometrically at frequent intervals in arterial and hepatic venous blood. Dye bound to plasma protein initially is distributed rapidly into the intravascular plasma volume (PV), followed by a slower exponential disappearance of the plasma concentration with time dependent entirely on a constant fractional rate of extraction of ICG across the hepatic circulation (see the semilogarithmic plot in Fig. 13). Extrapolating the linear semilog plot of arterial plasma concentration with respect to time back to time zero gives an estimate of the initial concentration of ICG (P_o) after intravascular dilution before significant extraction of ICG by the liver; from the dilution, total PV is estimated. The exponential decline of plasma concentra-

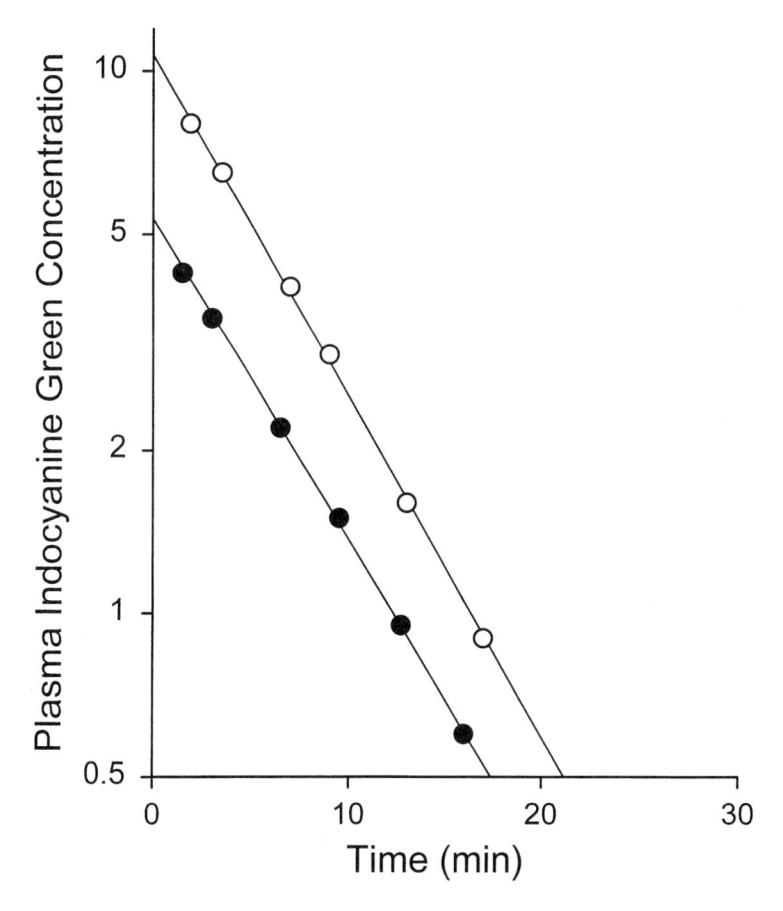

Figure 13 Peripheral arterial and hepatic venous plasma concentrations of indocyanine green (open and closed circles, respectively) at intervals after a bolus injection in a human subject. (Adapted from Ref. 149.)

tion with respect to time is given by the relationship $Pa_t = Pa_o^{-Kt}$, where Pa_t is the arterial plasma concentration of ICG at any time t. Hepatic extraction (E) is calculated as 1 minus the ratio of hepatic venous to arterial plasma concentration at the zero time intercepts $(1 - Pv_o/Pa_o)$. Hepatic plasma flow ($\dot{Q}p$) is estimated as K*PV/E. Total blood flow ($\dot{Q}_B$) is estimated as $\dot{Q}_p/(1 - Hct)$.

Thermal Dilution

One variation of the bolus thermal dilution technique for measuring cardiac output is the continuous-infusion thermal dilution method, which has been used to measure blood flow to the leg (150). Cold saline is infused into the femoral vein at a rate that is varied to achieve a stable temperature difference of 1°C at a thermocouple located a fixed distance downstream. Blood flow is calculated using thermal balance principles.

Inert Gas Techniques

Details of these techniques for peripheral-blood flow are summarized in a review by Wagner (151). These techniques can be relegated to four categories: (1) average organ blood flow by measurement of prolonged inert gas uptake; (2) instantaneous blood flow by arterial bolus injection followed by washout analysis; (3) arterial bolus injection with measurements of the height–area ratio of concentration–time curve; and (4) direct tissue injection of the tracer with washout analysis. Technique 1 is the integral approach described by Kety and Schmidt (152) for estimating cerebral blood flow but can be applied to any organ if the isolated venous blood from the organ can be sampled can be sampled to measure the inert gas concentration. A gas such as N_2O, with low solubility in blood and tissue, is breathed with frequent monitoring of arterial and organ venous partial pressure (Fig. 14). When these concentrations approach equilibrium, sampling can be stopped and organ blood flow (Q) can be estimated as follows:

$$\dot{Q} = \lambda_{ti} \cdot [G]_{eq}/A$$

where λ_{ti} is the tissue/blood partition coefficient, $[G]_{eq}$ is the gas partial pressure, and A is the area between the arterial and venous concentration curves plotted with respect to time. Measurement errors become more important when the partition coefficient is high with respect to the blood flow per gram of tissue such as fat, which has a long equilibration time. Technique 2 involves a bolus injection of ^{133}Xe into the artery leading to a tissue, followed by external radiation counting to follow the exponential decay of the count rate from the tissue. Blood flow in (milliliters per minute) per milliliter tissue is calculated as $\lambda_{ti}*0.693/t_{1/2}$, where $t_{1/2}$ is the washout half-time. This assumes homogeneous blood flow and tissue partition coefficients. Advantages are a more acute measurement assessment of tissue blood flow, the ability to repeatedly measure flow, and the fact that venous sampling is not required. However, access to the local tissue artery is required. Technique 3 differs from technique 2 only in that flow per gram of tissue is estimated as $\lambda_{ti}*(height/area)$; the whole curve is analyzed, not just the exponential count rate decay, and height refers to the maximum height of the curve. It also does not rely on the assumption of homogeneous tissue perfusion and gives a simplified value of average blood flow. Technique 4 is similar in principle to technique 2 with similar assumptions, but the arterial bolus injection is replaced by direct tissue injection of the ^{133}Xe gas in solution, followed by the decay in gamma count rates from the tissue. The additional problems encountered with this method include the possible alteration of local blood flow secondary to the volume injection. Technique 4 has been applied to the clinical setting much more than the other two methods.

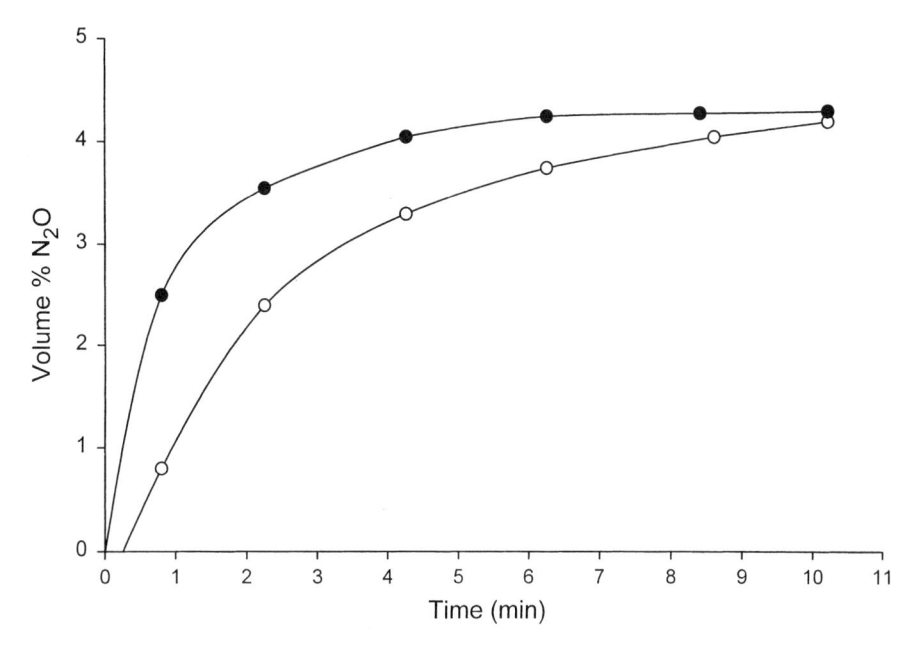

Figure 14 Arterial and jugular venous N_2O concentrations (filled and open circles, respectively) from a human subject breathing 15% N_2O in oxygen. The volume of N_2O transferred into the brain (expressed in milliliters of gas per 100 mL of tissue) is given by the area between the two curves (i.e., A in the equation). (Adapted from Ref. 152.)

Single-Photon Emission Computed Tomography/Position-Emission Tomography Imaging

In single-photon emission computed tomography (SPECT), radionuclides such as ^{99m}Tc, ^{133}Xe, or ^{123}I are injected intravascularly (153). A scintillation (gamma) counter is rotated about the subject and obtains multiple planar images from which a computer can construct two- or three-dimensional images of the organ being studied. When one of these radionuclides is complexed to a compound such as ^{99m}Tc-d,1-hexamethylpropyleneamineoxime, which after intravenous or intracarotid injection first crosses the blood brain barrier and is subsequently metabolized and thus trapped within the brain, SPECT imaging gives a quantifiable image of regional cerebral blood flow that is similar in accuracy to the Kety-Schmidt technique (152,154). Because the metabolic conversion that traps the compound in the brain is not instantaneous, computer algorithms are required to compensate for the back-diffusion and washout of the tracer from the brain during the interval of study. Coregistering the regional cerebral blood flow image with a magnetic resonance imaging or computed tomography scan can relate the distribution of flow to fairly precise anatomical locations (155). Positron-emission tomography (PET) is similar to SPECT in its use of radionuclides and type of three-dimensional information obtained; the radionuclides used with PET are positron emitters that may have short (^{11}C, ^{13}N, ^{15}O, ^{18}F) or long (^{52}Fe, ^{55}Co, ^{124}I) half-lives (156,157). Positron emission results in two gamma quanta emitted along the same line in opposite directions; this permits more precise anatomical location of the source than SPECT and gives absolute quantification of the radioactivity in becquerel per pixel. Incorporation of ^{11}C, ^{13}N, or ^{15}O into organic molecules permits the study of a wide variety of in vivo biochemical processes and also provides estimates of tissue blood flow. For example, a steady-state inhalation method using $C^{15}O_2$ has been used to noninvasively measure regional blood flow, O_2 extraction, and O_2 consumption (158). The primary disadvantage of PET techniques is the large cost, secondary to the requirement for an on-site cyclotron to generate the short half-life radionuclides.

Tissue P_{O_2}, Vascular P_{O_2}, and Hb Saturation

Tonometry

The earliest attempts to measure directly oxygen pressure within tissues was performed tonometrically (159). A gas bubble would be introduced into the tissue, allowed to equilibrate with local gas tensions, and was then removed and analyzed. Modern equivalents of this technique include balloon tonometry of the proximal bowel (160), and bladder (161), or subcutaneous tonometry (162).

Polarographic Electrodes

In the 1940s, polarographic O_2 electrodes were adapted for direct measurement in tissue in one of two ways: either incorporated into a penetrating needle for deep measurements or for application at the tissue surface (for a review of the history, see Refs. 12 and 163). By 1980, more than 90 different tissue O_2 electrodes had been developed (9). As detailed by Kreuzer and Kimmich (11), the ideal electrode would be small, have a low O_2 consumption, be sensitive only to O_2, would not damage the tissue nor alter its perfusion, have a linear response, be stable over time, and be easy to calibrate and insert. No device meets all these criteria.

Penetrating Single-Point Needle Electrodes. These electrodes are necessarily traumatic and may alter local P_{O_2}. In addition, they cannot describe the sometimes large heterogeneity of P_{O_2} present within a tissue. Still, some very interesting data have been obtained using single-point microelectrodes. For example, Duling and Berne (164) used such electrodes to examine P_{O_2} at the outside wall of arterioles on the surface of hamster cheek pouch and rat cremaster muscles, demonstrating for the first time the existence of significant precapillary O_2 diffusion.

Kessler-Lübber Multipoint Surface Electrode. Also known as the Mehrdraht, Dortmund, Oberfläche electrode) is most commonly used today. It consists of eight individual Clark-type electrodes, each 15 μm in diameter, with an Ag/AgCl reference electrode. Each wire has a predicted measuring zone of a half-sphere with a radius of 20 μm. A two-point calibration must be performed before and after use so that the data may be corrected for drift, which is generally less than 5% over 4 hours. Data can be collected continuously and presented as P_{O_2} with respect to time or as a frequency distribution histogram of P_{O_2} (Fig. 14). Typically, a Gaussian distribution is observed, with most values close to the mean. Some conditions are associated with a change in the distribution of values, with no change in the mean $Ptio_2$ (165), which can be assessed with statistics such as the Kolmogorov-Smirnov test (166). The interpretation of $Ptio_2$ measures is complex. Groebe (167) has argued that surface electrodes measure an *area* weighted average of surface P_{O_2} rather than the P_{O_2} of a tissue *volume*. Therefore, it is important that the electrode lie directly over the tissue cells of interest, without an intervening fascial layer or tissue capsule that may have a very different $Ptio_2$ profile. It need also be understood that the surface P_{O_2} represents a balance of O_2 delivery and local O_2 consumption. It says nothing regarding whether local O_2 demand is being met. Heterogeneity in $Ptio_2$ values is also a result of the relative position of each electrode to arterial and venous vessels. Use of a Mehrdraht, Dortmund, Oberfläche system requires considerable technical expertise but has yielded valuable information in studies of the gut mucosa, cerebral cortex, liver, heart, and other tissues (Fig. 15).

Transcutaneous Applications. Transcutaneous applications of polarographic O_2 and CO_2 electrodes have also been adapted for estimation of subcutaneous arterial values (168). Incorporated into the measuring device is a heating element that induces a local hyperemia that brings cutaneous capillary gas tensions close to arterial and also increases the permeability of the skin to O_2 and CO_2. Optimal "arterialization" of capillary blood occurs at 44–45°C. Because thermal trauma may occur at these temperatures, the probe must be moved frequently to other sites (12). Most often, a Clark-type electrode is used and a two-point in vitro calibration must first be performed. Transcutaneous applications work well in relatively thin-skinned neonates but give values of P_{O_2} significantly lower than arterial when perfusion is poor or in older subjects. Some investigators have used the ratio of Pa_{O_2} to Ptc_{O_2} as an index of cardiac output or to assess the viability of tissue subjected to accidental or surgical trauma. Because of the need for frequent repositioning and recalibration of transcutaneous probes, transcutaneous applications have in many situations been replaced by pulse oximeters, which give information related but not equivalent to arterial O_2 tension.

Optical Monitoring of Oxygen: Absorbance

Optical methods of measuring oxygen use either absorbance or luminescence (163). Absorbance (A) $= -\log(I/I_O) = \varepsilon \cdot C \cdot L$, where I is the intensity of the transmitted light, I_O is the intensity of the incident light, ε is the molar extinction coefficient of the indicator, C is the molar concentration of the indicator, and L is the optical path length (Beer's law). The binding of O_2 to an absorbance indicator (e.g., Hb) can change the absorbance spectrum of the indicator. Measuring absorbance at different wavelengths allows one to calculate the quantities of indicator and O_2-indicator that

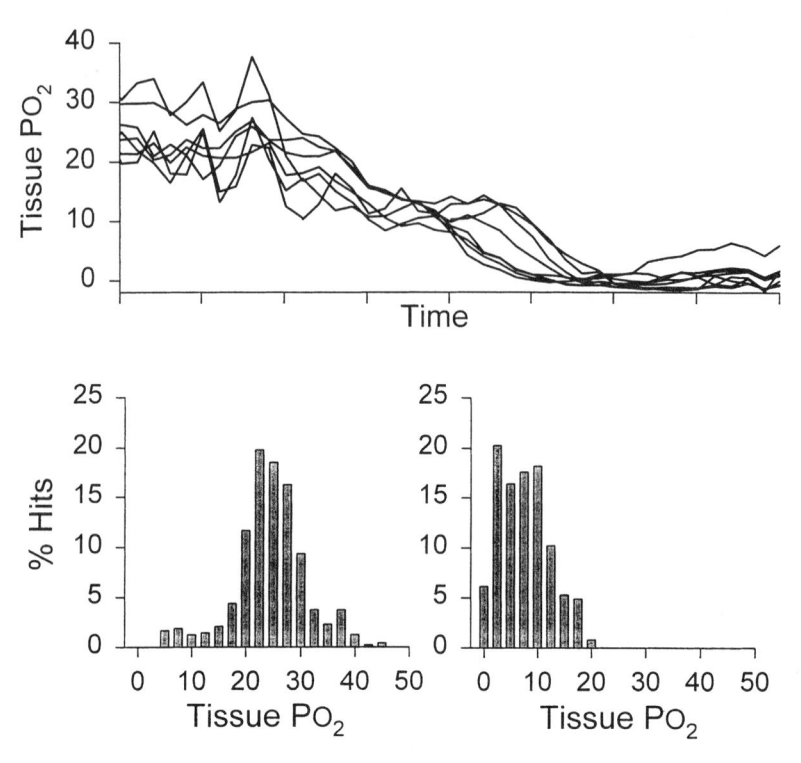

Figure 15 (Above) Continuous Mehrdraht, Dortmund, Oberfläche trace of mucosal P_{O_2} during a systemic bleed. (Below) P_{O_2} histograms before (left) and after (right) bleed.

are present. This method forms the foundation of pulse oximetry, CO oximetry, and other spectrophotometric techniques.

Pulse Oximetry. In practice, pulse oximetry involves illuminating a thin appendage, usually a digit or earlobe, and measuring the transmitted light. Generally, two wavelengths of light are used, at approximately 660 nm and 940 nm, to assess the percentage of oxyHb (%Sat) and reduced Hb (1−%Sat) present (169). With in vitro absorbance spectroscopy, one would construct a calibration curve on lysed blood plotting the ratio (R) of absorbance at the two wavelengths (y axis) versus known %Sat from a number of different samples (x axis). Because significant light scattering occurs with in vivo monitoring of intact blood, commercial monitors cannot use the aforementioned calibration curve. Instead, they are programmed with an empirically constructed plot of R versus invasively measured %Sat obtained from healthy volunteers. The amount of light transmitted depends on several relatively constant factors (tissue pigmentation, tissue thickness, venous blood) and one constantly varying (pulsating) factor—arterial blood volume. The pulse oximeter mathematically corrects for the baseline, constant light transmission so that its output reflects the absorbance spectrum of arterial blood alone. Typically, two light-emitting diodes are used as light sources. Manufacturing variability in the 660 nm light-emitting diode is often ±15 nm, which leads to inaccuracy in the calibration curve and errors in %Sat measurements when values are less than 80% (169). Other Hb species have different absorption spectra and are not adequately defined using two wavelengths. MetHb is interpreted by the pulse oximeter as a %Sat of 85% and COHb as a %Sat of 90% (170). Some other common pigments (bilirubin, fetal Hb) seem to have little effect on accuracy. Motion artifacts are significant. Advantages include continuous measurement, noninvasiveness, and insensitivity to inhaled anesthetics; in addition, calibration is not required, and it performs somewhat better than Ptco$_2$ monitors when perfusion is decreased.

In Vivo Vascular Oxyhemoglobin Spectroscopy. In the 1970s, Pittman and Duling (171) adapted a spectrophotometric method for measuring oxyHb saturation of whole blood that was able to adequately compensate for the effects of light scattering. Determining in vitro the light absorbance of whole blood at two different wavelengths isosbestic for Hb (equally absorbed by Hb and oxyHb) allows calculation of a scattering factor that can be subtracted from the absorbance measured at the nonisosbestic wavelength. They applied their new technique to make in vivo measurements of arteriolar Hb saturation in the hamster cheek pouch under conditions of normal flow at different Pao$_2$ values and during no flow (172). Their spectrophotometric results were in good agreement with Hb saturation predicted from directly measured (microelectrode) arteriolar wall Po$_2$. Subsequent use of this powerful research tool (173) has, for example, confirmed the existence of precapillary O$_2$ losses previously described (164). Combined with microvascular flow and hematocrit (Hct) measurements (142,143,174), one can estimate segmental tissue V̇o$_2$ [from arteriolar and venular saturations (Sao$_2$, Svo$_2$)] or O$_2$ extraction ratios ([Sao$_2$ − Svo$_2$]/Sao$_2$), although it is difficult to account adequately for the heterogeneity of microvascular hematocrit, flow, and saturations encountered.

Surrogate Measures of Tissue Oxygenation

To this point we have considered either direct measures of oxygen tension or the amount of oxygen bound to Hb as an indicator of tissue oxygen delivery. The following techniques are significantly less direct measures of the amount of oxygen present in tissues or its adequacy. The data they provide are thus subject to factors other than O$_2$ tension, although these can at times provide other important information. They have different goals, such as the description of intracellular Po$_2$, and different advantages, such as a noninvasive assessment of a remote tissue's oxygen sufficiency.

Optical Monitoring of Tissue Oxygenation: Luminescence

Luminescence techniques are more complicated than absorbance techniques and include fluorescence and phosphorescence reactions. When a luminescence indicator absorbs light, its electronic state changes to an excited singlet state (163). The higher energy state is not stable, and the concentration of the excited molecules decreases exponentially with time with a rate constant (K_i). The return to the ground state can occur in three ways associated with three different rate constants: (1) via strong collisions with other molecules (K_c); (2) by emission of a photon (fluorescence) (K_f); and (3) with an intermediate transition to an excited triplet state then to the ground state, also accompanied by emission of a photon (phosphorescence) (K_s). The overall rate constant K_i equals the sum of K_c, K_f, and K_s, and the mean lifetime (τ_0) of the excited indicator equals $1/(K_c + K_f + K_s)$. Oxygen can collide with the indicator, thus accelerating its energy loss (mechanism 1), shortening the mean lifetime. Less energy will be dissipated by mechanisms 2 and 3 so that fluorescence and phosphorescence intensities will be decreased (quenched). The rate constant for collisional quenching by O_2 is the product of the collisional quenching constant (K_q) and O_2 concentration. The mean lifetime with O_2 present (τ) equals $1/(K_c + K_f + K_s + K_q \cdot [O_2])$. It is important to note that K_q depends on the molecular properties of the indicator and the diffusion milieu being studied, which may be affected by pH and temperature. Lifetime can be measured after a single light pulse or by examining the phase modulation in response to a sinusoidally applied exciting light. Oxygen concentration is determined by the ratio of measured lifetimes (τ/τ_0) or luminescence intensities (F/F_0) with and without O_2 present according to the Stern Volmer equation: $\tau/\tau_0 = F/F_0 = 1/(1 + K_{sv} \cdot [O_2]) = 1/(1 + K_{sv} \cdot \alpha \cdot P_{O_2}) = 1/(1 + K_t \cdot P_{O_2})$, where α is the O_2 solubility of the milieu, $K_{sv} = K_q \cdot \tau_0$ and the overall quenching constant $K_t = K_q \cdot \tau_0 \cdot \alpha$. For in vivo measurements, τ/τ_0 or F/F_0 must first be determined for the particular indicator in vitro in a milieu that mimics the in vivo condition, some aspects of which may not be known. The indicator may simply be dissolved into the tissue topically, embedded into a polymeric membrane that is then applied to the surface of the tissue, or injected into the bloodstream either free or bound to protein (163,175,176). Protein binding adds some molecular stability to the probe and largely confines it to the intravascular space, so the technique estimates vascular P_{O_2}. With time, some of the probe does leak across vessels, which permits the measurement of extravascular P_{O_2} (177). Current research in this exciting area is focused on the development of new probes that are inexpensive, nontoxic, that absorb and emit at wavelengths different from native tissue pigments and phosphors, that are sensitive over a wide range of P_{O_2}, and that will function at various depths of tissue (178). The data are provided by quenching techniques at present is semiquantitative, but this field is barely 10 years old.

Electron Paramagnetic (Spin) Resonance

With in vivo or in vitro electron paramagnetic resonance (EPR), the area of interest is placed in a magnetic field (50 to 500 G) that fluctuates at 250 to 1200 MHz (179). A surface detector monitors the emitted spectra, which can be characterized by their peak-to-peak line width, intensity, peak height, and other features (180). The source of the spectra are paramagnetic species—atoms with unpaired electrons—that are not normally present in vivo but must first be placed into the tissue. The presence of oxygen near the paramagnetic particle affects its EPR spectrum, primarily the peak-to-peak line width. Particles may be as small as 1 to 2 μm (India ink) or as large as 0.1 × 0.1 × 0.3 mm (lithium phthalocyanine), and they have different sensitivities to O_2, which must be determined (calibrated) in vitro. The larger particles must be implanted in the tissue and give spectral data reflecting an average O_2 over a large tissue volume, but they may be stable for months (180). The limited number of in vivo studies conducted with EPR seem to give values similar to other methods of measuring extracellular tissue P_{O_2}. Further advances in this area will hinge on the development of paramagnetic species that are nontoxic with good spectra that can be placed in tissues in a minimally invasive way (181). In addition, current detectors must be placed no further than 1 cm from the site of interest, limiting the depth of study (179).

Reflectance Cryomicrospectroscopy of Myoglobin

The oxygenation state of myoglobin (Mb) in muscle tissue is related to cytosolic P_{O_2} according to its dissociation curve. If Mb saturation is known, O_2 concentration in the vicinity of the Mb can then be calculated as: $[O_2] = [MbO_2][MbP_{50}]/[Mb]$. Because of the shape of the Mb–O_2 dissociation curve ($P_{50} = 5.3$ mm Hg), small errors in saturation measurement give large errors in estimated P_{O_2} at higher levels of O_2. Mb cryomicrospectroscopy permits mapping of O_2Mb within individual cells, down to a resolution of to 1 to 2 μm (182,183). A copper block immersed in liquid N_2 is rapidly applied to a muscle surface that induces tissue freezing at a rate of approximately 10 μm/ms, which fixes Mb saturation at that point of time. Cells 100- to 500-μm deep can then be viewed on a cold-stage ($-110°$C) microscope. Four-wavelength reflectance spectroscopy is used to determine Mb saturation with O_2. Use of frozen Mb spectroscopy has increased our understanding of the role of Mb and has forced a re-evaluation of Krogh-type models, at least for muscle. In contracting skeletal muscle, Gayeski et al. (183) found that maximal $\dot{V}_{O_2}$ can be achieved with a Mb P_{O_2} down to 0.5 mm Hg. The high affinity of Mb for O_2 maintains a relatively low cellular P_{O_2}, enhancing the capillary mitochondrial O_2 gradient and unloading of O_2 from red blood cell Hb. They also found very small intracellular gradients of O_2, 1.2 mm Hg at the largest. This indicates that the cellular resistance to O_2 diffusion is small in comparison to that across the capillary, exactly opposite to Krogh's model; however, Krogh's concept of the importance of capillary density remains valid. The obvious limitations of this technique are its invasiveness and the difficulty of performing serial measurements in one subject.

Intramucosal pH

Fiddian-Green et al. (184) pioneered the technique for estimating intramucosal pH (pHi) by balloon tonometry of gastric P_{CO_2} as an indirect measure of splanchnic oxygenation. A saline-filled CO_2-permeable balloon connected to a catheter is placed into the stomach or proximal small bowel. A period of 30 to 90 minutes is allowed for the mucosal P_{CO_2} to equilibrate with the saline, which is aspirated and analyzed in a blood gas analyzer. pHi is calculated from the Henderson-Hasselbach equation with arterial HCO_3^- used as an estimate for mucosal HCO_3^-: pHi = 6.1 + log $[HCO_3^-/(P_{CO_2} \times 0.0307)]$. Reported correlation coefficients (r) between directly measured mucosal pH and tonometrically derived pHi in animals has varied from 0.69 to 0.945 (160,185). Poor correlations may be caused by inadequate equilibration of mucosal and balloon CO_2 and to the assumption that arterial HCO_3^- equals local gut HCO_3^-. Some investigators have advocated reporting balloon P_{CO_2} alone or the difference between arterial CO_2 and balloon CO_2. Mucosal P_{CO_2} (Pm_{CO_2}) is determined by the balance of local CO_2 production ($\dot{V}_{CO_2}$) and washout by venous blood. With a fixed aerobic CO_2 production, moderate decreases in gut perfusion increase Pm_{CO_2} by stagnation. Further declines in perfusion to the point where aerobic metabolism is limited will *decrease* $\dot{V}_{CO_2}$ and perhaps Pm_{CO_2}. However, the ensuing anaerobic acidosis produces CO_2 from titration of HCO_3^-, so that the net effect is usually a sharp increase in Pm_{CO_2} and decrease in pHi with critically low gut perfusion (186). Low pHi has been found in several clinical studies to be predictive of gastrointestinal hemorrhage or poor outcome (160). It is one of a very few acceptably noninvasive techniques available to clinicians to assess a regional circulation.

Lactate

Systemic blood lactate levels or lactate flux across a tissue has long been used as an indirect marker of tissue oxygenation. A little knowledge of biochemistry is needed to interpret its significance. Lactate can only be synthesized from or metabolized into pyruvate: pyruvate + NADH + H^+ ↔ lactate + NAD^+, or, [Lactate] = K[Pyruvate] ([NADH]/[NAD^+]) [H^+], so that lactate levels depend on pyruvate, pH, and cellular redox state (NADH/NAD^+) (187). In the cytosol, breakdown of glucose via glycolysis produces 85% of pyruvate, along with adenosine triphosphate (ATP) and NADH. Fifteen percent of pyruvate normally comes from protein metabolism, via alanine. In the mitochondria, pyruvate (via acetyl-CoA) enters the Kreb's cycle, yielding CO_2 and more NADH. In the electron transport chain, NADH is reconverted into NAD when its H^+ combines with oxygen to form water. With hypoxia, pyruvate and NADH levels must increase. The conversion of this pyruvate to lactate allows glycolysis and some ATP production to proceed. Normal systemic lactate levels are a balance of synthesis (25% by skin, 20% by muscle, 20% by red blood cells, 20% by brain, and 10% by gut) and uptake (60% by liver, 30% by kidneys) (187). Increased levels may be secondary to decreased uptake, increased synthesis, or both. Although a number of metabolic disturbances may affect the aforementioned pathways and increase lactate (188), by far the most common cause is global hypoxia. For such a nonspecific measurement, high lactate levels have been shown in a number of studies to be strong predictors of outcome (187,189). Still, regional hypoxia may not cause systemic lactate levels to increase, if washout is low or uptake is increased elsewhere. Conversely, a modest increase in lactate production in one region may cause large systemic changes in the presence of renal or hepatic dysfunction.

NADH Fluorescence

As previously stated, cellular hypoxia causes a buildup of NADH produced in the tricarboxylic acid (TCA) cycle (mitochondrial) and the compensatory acceleration of glycolysis increases cytosolic NADH. NAD exhibits little absorption at 365 nm, whereas NADH does and will fluoresce at a peak wavelength of approximately 470 nm (190,191). Since the introduction of the technique, numerous devices have been created to measure NADH fluorescence in vitro and in vivo in a large number of organs. Light at 365 nm penetrates tissues poorly, and any fluorescence reflects NADH in surface cells, predominantly mitochondrial NADH (190). Errors in measurement can be secondary to variations in the quantity and oxygenation status of Hb present, which absorbs both the excitation and emitted light, and with tissue motion, although various correction factors for both problems have been proposed (191). It should be emphasized that NADH fluorescence does not directly measure O_2, and other factors may affect mitochondrial NADH levels irrespective of O_2 concentration. Also, it is not possible in vivo to perform an absolute calibration of NADH fluorescence so all results are necessarily qualitative.

Near-Infrared Spectroscopy

Light in the near-infrared region (NIR; 700 to 1000 nm) has enough energy to penetrate tissues to 6- to 8-cm depth (192). Spectrophotometers have been developed that use different NIR wavelengths to quantify changes in the concentration of tissue pigments across time, although none can give absolute values of concentration (192–194). Either the amount of transmitted light or reflected light may be examined. Pigments relevant to tissue oxygenation that absorb light in the NIR range include Hb, Mb (in muscle), and mitochondrial oxidized cytochrome aa$_3$ (cyt-aa$_3$). The latter provides the most information on intracellular oxygen status of nonmuscle tissues but has the weakest signal and is most prone to measurement error. Like NADH, the redox state of cyt-aa$_3$ is linked to cellular Po$_2$. As O_2 concentration decreases, the concentration of reduced cyt-aa3 (providing substrate is available) increases accompanied by a decrease in absorbance of NIR light. In pig hind limb muscle made progressively ischemic, changes in cyt-aa$_3$ paralleled those in $\dot{V}_{O_2}$, and thus identified the same critical O_2 delivery (194). Major limitations of the technique include interference by Hb and Mb with cyt-aa$_3$ measurement, violations of Beer's law assumptions due to light scattering and unknown path lengths, susceptibility to motion artifacts, and the difficulty in performing a calibration at zero and 100% oxidation in vivo (195).

Magnetic Resonance Spectroscopy

Phosphate nuclear magnetic resonance (NMR) is based on the fact that atomic nuclei can absorb energy from a pulsating magnetic field, then release that energy as a radiofrequency signal (196). With hypoxia and continued ATP consumption (hydrolysis), ADP, H^+, and inorganic phosphate (Pi) accumulate, while phosphocreatine (PCr) stores decrease. NMR is commonly used to measure the Pi/PCr ratio and intracellular pH (which is reflected by the distance between the Pi and PCr peaks). The spectra collected are an average over both time and a significant tissue area, so localization is poor. Similar to what has been demonstrated for cyt-aa_3 (194), the Pi/PCr ratio can identify the onset of regional O_2 limitation (197). Recently, NMR has been used to assess Mb oxygenation in cardiac tissue (198). As with other techniques that measure O_2Mb, it predicts local P_{O_2} most accurately when P_{O_2} is relatively low. Disadvantages of NMR spectroscopy include cost (>$300,000) and size of the spectrometer and its narrow (and indirect) O_2 detection range. Advantages include its noninvasiveness and ability to estimate intracellular P_{O_2}.

Exercise Induced Magnetic Resonance Enhancement of Skeletal Muscle

Signal intensity in proton magnetic resonance imaging of skeletal muscle is dependent on tissue spin density and T1, T2 relaxation times, which, in turn, depend on the total water content of muscle. Water content of exercising muscle does increase in proportion to exercise load. As a consequence, there is a corresponding progressive increase in signal intensity of skeletal muscle magnetic resonance imaging as workload increases from rest to maximal load (199); hence, it becomes possible to identify the relative intensity of work by different muscle groups during limb exercise using this technique. The increase in water content is at least, in part, due to glycogenolysis and the associated increase in osmolality as lactate accumulates and draws water into the muscle; magnetic resonance imaging signal enhancement does not occur in patients with McArdle's disease (200) in which glycogenolysis and lactate production is absent. Magnetic resonance imaging complements MRS in providing high spatial resolution and less susceptibility to sampling errors.

Labeling Metabolically Active Cells in the Brain

It is possible to identify metabolically active cells in brain tissue slices obtained after an intervention performed in the living animal.

One technique is to inject radioactively labeled deoxyglucose (2-[^{14}C]deoxyglucose), which is taken up by cells in proportion to metabolic activity but cannot be metabolized. Concentration of the label after the animal is killed is measured in tissue slices by autoradiography.

A more recent technique is to measure expression of an early response gene (c-*Fos* expression) after an intervention in the living animal. The C-Fos protein is identified in the nuclei of metabolically activated neurons in tissue slices by immunocytochemical techniques (201).

Diffusive Gas Exchange Between Capillary Blood and Muscle Mitochondria

Completeness of oxygen extraction from capillaries at heavy exercise is determined partly by the uniformity with which regional blood flow is matched to local oxygen requirements and partly by diffusion limitations between capillary red blood cells and tissue mitochondria. Under a wide range of conditions of maximal induced work in isolated perfused skeletal muscle and in human limb muscles, oxygen extraction behaves as if diffusion limitation is a major determinant (202–204). Based on these observations, a minimum value for oxygen-diffusing capacity of skeletal muscle has been estimated in isolated perfused skeletal muscle in animal preparations and in limb muscles of humans at peak exercise; estimates are made from O_2 uptake by the Fick principle and mean capillary P_{O_2}:

$$D_{O_{2musc}} = \frac{\dot{V}_{O_2}}{\bar{P}c_{O_2}} \tag{59}$$

where $\bar{P}c_{O_2}$ is estimated by reverse Bohr integration between the limits of arterial and mixed venous O_2 saturation (S_{aO_2} and $\bar{P}\bar{v}_{O_2}$, respectively) as follows:

$$\bar{P}c_{O_2} = \frac{(Sc' - S\bar{v})}{\int_{Sc'}^{S\bar{v}} \frac{dS}{Pc}} \tag{60}$$

where the O_2 subscripts have been left out on the right-hand side of the equation for simplification. These estimates of $\bar{P}c_{O_2}$ and $D_{O_{2musc}}$ are based on the assumption that capillary perfusion of muscle fibers is anisotropic rather than isotropic, as assumed in the Krogh model.

V. Summary

Experimental approaches to gas exchange in the lung and periphery have similar objectives, i.e., to define (1) the structure–function relationships of each transport step in gas exchange, (2) the functional capacity of each step from rest to exercise, and (3) how uniformly adjacent steps are matched to provide efficient gas exchange. Transport steps in the lung for oxygen are alveolar ventilation ($\dot{V}_A$), diffusing capacity that includes chemical binding to Hb (D_{LO_2}), and the product of pulmonary blood flow and Hb concentration ($\dot{Q}c \times [Hb]$). Transport steps in the periphery for oxygen are $\dot{Q}c \times [Hb]$; diffusing capacity (D_{TO_2}), which includes release of bound O_2 from Hb, and O_2 use by mitochondria ($\dot{V}_{O_2}$). Study objectives currently are more easily achieved in the lung than in the periphery because of easier sampling access from the lung than from the multiple organs and wide range of locations involved in peripheral gas exchange. Furthermore, distribution of blood flow through the lung is primarily concerned with gas exchange, but distribution of blood flow to other organs may have other important functions that often overshadow gas exchange function, e.g., heat exchange in the skin, excretory function in the kidneys, and substrate absorption and transport in the gut. Furthermore, $\dot{V}_{O_2}$ and $\dot{V}_{CO_2}$ by themselves do not provide an answer to the more important question in peripheral gas exchange, i.e., whether tissue O_2 requirements are being met. Thus, other measures that indirectly reflect on adequacy of regional gas exchange must be used such as those discussed under surrogate measures of tissue oxygenation and metabolism. These difficulties, along with the practical problems of obtaining accurate regional O_2 transport and uptake in some organs drives the development of new noninvasive technologies to define efficiency with which peripheral O_2 requirements are met under different circumstances.

References

1. Weissman C. Measuring oxygen uptake in the clinical setting. In: Bryan-Brown CW, Ayres SM, eds. Oxygen Transport and Utilization. Fullerton: New Horizons, 1987; pp 25–64.
2. Ultman JS, Bursztein S. Analysis of error in the determination of respiratory gas exchange. J Appl Physiol 1981; 50:210–216.
3. Thrush DN. Spirometric versus Fick-derived oxygen consumption: which method is better? Crit Care Med 1996; 24:91–95.
4. Simonson DC, DeFrozo RA. Indirect calorimetry: methodological and interpretive problems. Am J Physiol 1990; 258 (Endocrinol Metab):E399–412.
5. Beaver WL, Lamarra N, Wasserman K. Breath-by breath measurement of true alveolar gas exchange. J Appl Physiol Respir Environ Exercise Physiol 1981; 51:1662–1665.
6. Seeherman HJ, Taylor CR, Maloiy GMO, Armstrong RB. Design of the mammalian respiratory system. II. Measuring maximum aerobic capacity. Respir Physiol 1981; 44:11–24.
7. Erickson BK, Seaman J, Kubo K, Hiraga A, Kai M, Yamaya M, Wagner PD. Mechanisms of reduction in alveolar-arterial P_{O_2} difference by helium breathing in the exercising horse. J Appl Physiol 1994; 76:2794–2801.
8. Stetz CW, Miller RG, Kelly GE, Raffin TA. Reliability of the thermal dilution method in the determination of cardiac output in clinical practice. Am Rev Respir Dis 1982; 126:1001–1004.
9. Van Slyke DD, Neil JM. The determination of gases in the blood and other solutions by vacuum extraction and manometric measurements. J Biol Chem 1924; 61:523–572.
10. Douglas AR, Jones NL, Reed JW. Calculation of whole blood CO_2 content. J Appl Physiol 1988; 65:473–477.
11. Kreuzer F, Kimmich HP, Brezina M. Polarographic determination of oxygen in biological materials. In: Koryata J, ed. Medical and Biological Applications of Electrochemical Devices. New York: John Wiley and Sons, 1981, pp 173–261.
12. Kreuzer F, Kimmich HP. Techniques using O_2 electrodes in respiratory physiology. In: Otis AB, ed. Techniques in Respiratory Physiology. New York: Elsevier, 1984, pp 1–29.
13. Weibel ER. Morphometry of the Human Lung. New York: Academic Press, 1963.
14. Rohrer F. Der Stromungswiderstand in den mensachlichens Atemwegen und Verzeigung des Bronchialsystems auf den Atmungsverlauf in verschiedenen Lungenbezwirken. Pflugers Arch 1915; 162:225–299.
15. Ross BB. Influence of bronchial tree structure on ventilation in the dog's lung as inferred from measurements of a plastic cast. J Appl Physiol 1975; 10:1–14.

16. Horsfield K, Cumming K. Functional consequences of airway morphology. J Appl Physiol 1968; 24:384–390.
17. Horsfield K, Cumming G. Morphology of the bronchial tree in man. J Appl Physiol 1968; 24:373–383.
18. Mercer RR, Crapo JD. Three dimensional reconstruction of the rat acinus. J Appl Physiol 1987; 63:785–795.
19. Fung YC. A model of the lung structure and its validation. J Appl Physiol 1988; 64:2132–2141.
20. Denny, E, Schroter RC. A mathematical model of the morphology af the pulmonary acinus. J Biomech Eng 1996; 118:210–215.
21. Horsfield K, Woldenburg MJ. Diameters and cross sectional areas in the human pulmonary arterial tree. Anat Rec 1989; 223:245–251.
22. Horsfield K. The pulmonary artery seen as a convergent tree. In: Wagner WW, Weir EK, eds. Pulmonary Circulation and Gas Exchange. Armonk, NY: Futura, 1994, pp 253–264.
23. Fung YCB. Pressure, flow, stress, and remodeling in the pulmonary vasculature. In: Wagner WW, Weir EK, eds. Pulmonary Circulation and Gas Exchange. Armonk, NY: Futura, 1994, pp 343–364.
24. Jiang ZL, Kassab GS, Fung YC. Diameter-defined Strahler system and connectivity matrix of the pulmonary arterial tree. J Appl Physiol 1994; 76:882–892.
25. Horsfield K, Cumming G. Angles of branching and diameters of branches in the human bronchial tree. Bulletin of Mathematical Biophysics 1967; 29:245–259.
26. Wilson TA. Design of the bronchial tree. Nature 1967; 18:668–669.
27. Gauthier AP, Verbank S, Estenne M, Segebarth C, Paiva M. Three dimensional reconstruction of the in vivo human diaphragm shape at different lung volumes. J Appl Physiol 1994; 76:495–506.
28. Wood SA, Zerhouni EA, Hoford JD, Hoffman EA, Mitzner W. Measurement of three-dimensional lung tree structures by using computed tomography. J Appl Physiol 1995; 79:1687–1697.
29. Weibel ER, Taylor CR, O'Neil JJ, Leith DE, Gehr P, Hoppeler H, Langman V, Baudinette RV. Maximal oxygen consumption and pulmonary diffusing capacity: a direct comparison of physiologic and morphometric measurements in canids. Respir Physiol 1983; 54:173–188.
30. Weibel ER, Gehr P, Cruz OL, Müller AE, Mwangi DK, Haussener V. Design of the mammalian respiratory system. IV Morphometric estimation of pulmonary diffusing capacity: critical evaluation of new sampling method. Respir Physiol 1981; 44:39–59.
31. Roughton FJW, Forster RE. Relative importance of diffusion and chemical reaction rates in determining the rate of exchange of gases in the human lung, with special reference to true diffusing capacity of the pulmonary membrane and volume of blood in lung capillaries. J Appl Physiol 1957; 11:290–302.
32. Hsia CCW, Chuong CJC, Johnson RL Jr. Critique of the conceptual basis of diffusing capacity estimates: a finite element analysis. J Appl Physiol 1995; 79:1039–1047.
33. Federspiel WJ, Popel AS. A theoretical analysis of the effect of the particulate nature of blood on oxygen release in capillaries. Microvasc Res 1986; 32:164–189.

34. Federspiel WJ. Pulmonary diffusing capacity: implications of two-phase blood flow in capillaries. Respir Physiol 1989; 77:119–134.
35. Wang C, Popel AS. Effect of red blood cell shape on oxygen transport in capillaries. Math Biosci 1992; 116:89–110.
36. Chuong CJ, Pean JL, Johnson RL Jr. A method of study for the passive and active deformation of the canine diaphragm. In: Spilker RL, Simon BR, eds. Computational Methods in Bioengineering. New York: The American Society of Mechanical Engineers, 1988, pp 123–134.
37. Hsia CCW, Chuong CJC, Johnson RL Jr. Red cell distortion and conceptual basis of diffusing capacity estimates: a finite element analysis. J Appl Physiol 1997; 83:1397–1404.
38. Frank AO, Chuong CJC, Johnson RL Jr. A finite element model of oxygen diffusion in the pulmonary capillaries. J Appl Physiol 1997; 82:2036–2044.
39. Cumming G, Crank J, Horsfield K, Parker I. Gaseous diffusion in the airways of the human lung. Respir Physiol 1966; 1:58–54.
40. Cumming G, Horsfield K, Preston SB. Diffusion equilibrium in the lungs examined by nodal analysis. Respir Physiol 1971; 12:329–345.
41. Scherer PW, Gobran S, Aukburg SJ, Baumgardner JE, Bartkowski R, Neufeld GR. Numerical and experimental study of steady-state CO_2 and inert gas washout. J Appl Physiol 1988; 64:1022–1029.
42. Paiva M. Gas mixing and distribution in the human lung. In: Engel LA, Paiva M, eds. Lung Biology in Health Disease. New York: Marcel Dekker, 1985, pp 221–285.
43. La Force RC, Lewis BM. Diffusional transport in the human lung. J Appl Physiol 1970; 28:291–298.
44. Wagner WW Jr. Pulmonary microcirculatory observations in vivo under physiological conditions. J Appl Physiol 1969; 26:375–377.
45. Wagner WW Jr, Latham LP. Pulmonary capillary recruitment during airway hypoxia in the dog. J Appl Physiol 1975; 39:900–905.
46. Capen RL, Latham LP, Wagner WW Jr. Diffusing capacity of the lung during hypoxia: role of capillary recruitment. J Appl Physiol Respir Environ Exercise Physiol 1981; 50:165–171.
47. Godbey PS, Graham JA, Presson RG Jr, Wagner WW Jr, Lloyd TC Jr. Effect of capillary pressure and lung distension on capillary recruitment. J Appl Physiol 1995; 79:1142–1147.
48. Lamm WJE, Kirk KR, Hanson WL, Wagner WW Jr, Albert RK. Flow through zone 1 lung utilizes alveolar corner vessels. J Appl Physiol 1991; 70:1518–1523.
49. Presson RG, Hanger CC, Godbey PS, Graham JA, Lloyd TC Jr, Wagner WW Jr. Effect of increasing flow on distribution of pulmonary transit times. J Appl Physiol 1994; 76:1701–1711.
50. Okada O, Presson RG Jr, Godbey PS, Capen RL, Wagner WW Jr. Temporal capillary perfusion patterns in single alveolar walls of intact dogs. J Appl Physiol 1994; 76:380–386.
51. Bronikowski TA, Dawson CA, Linehan JH. Model-free deconvolution techniques for estimating vascular transport function. Int J Biomed Comput 1983; 14:411–412.
52. Wagner WW, Latham LP, Capen RL. Capillary recruitment during airway hypoxia: role of pulmonary artery pressure. J Appl Physiol 1979; 47:383–387.

53. Wagner PD, West JB. Effects of diffusion impairment on O_2 and CO_2 time courses in pulmonary capillaries. J Appl Physiol 1972; 33:62–71.
54. Kelman GR. Digital computer subroutine for the conversion of oxygen tension into saturation. J Appl Physiol 1966; 21:1375–1376.
55. Kelman GR. Digital computer procedure for the conversion of P_{CO_2} into CO_2 content. Respir Physiol 1967; 3:111–115.
56. Johnson RL, Heigenhauser GJF, Hsia CCW, Jones NL, Wagner PD. Determinants of gas exchange and acid-base balance during exercise. In: Rowell LB, Shepherd JT, eds. Handbook of Physiology, Section 12, Exercise: Regulation and Integration of Multiple Systems. New York: Oxford University Press, 1996, pp 515–584.
57. Riley RL, Cournand A. 'Ideal' alveolar air and analysis of ventilation-perfusion relationships in the lungs. J Appl Physiol 1949; 1:825–847.
58. Rahn H, Otis AB. Continuous analysis of alveolar gas composition during work, hyperpnea, hypercapnia and anoxia. J Appl Physiol 1949; 1:717–724.
59. Krogh A, Lindhard J. The volume of the dead space in breathing and the mixing of gases in the lungs of man. J Physiol 1917; 51:59–90.
60. Fowler WS. Lung function studies. III. Uneven pulmonary ventilation in normal subjects and in patients with lung disease. J Appl Physiol 1949; 2:283–299.
61. Worth H, Piiper J. Diffusion of helium, carbon monoxide and sulfur hexafluoride in gas mixtures similar to alveolar gas. Respir Physiol 1978; 32:155–166.
62. Neufeld GR, Gobran S, Baumgardner JE, Aukburg SJ, Schreiner M, Scherer PW. Diffusivity, respiratory rate and tidal volume influence inert gas expirograms. Respir Physiol 1991; 84:31–47.
63. Paiva M, Verbank S, van Muylem A. Diffusion-dependent contribution to the slope of the alveolar plateau. Respir Physiol 1988; 72:257–270.
64. Anthonison NR, Danson J, Robertson PC, Ross WRD. Airway closure as a function of age. Respir Physiol 1969; 8:58–65.
65. Buist AS, Ross BB. Predicted values for closing volume using a modified single breath nitrogen test. Am Rev Respir Dis 1973; 107:744–752.
66. Burger EJ Jr, Macklem P. Airway closure: demonstration by breathing 100% O_2 at low lung volumes and by N_2 washout. J Appl Physiol 1968; 25:139–148.
67. Engel LA, Grassino A, Anthonisen NR. Demonstration of airway closure in man. J Appl Physiol 1975; 38:1117–1125.
68. Fowler WS, Cornish ER Jr, Kety SS. Lung function studies. III. Analysis of alveolar ventilation by pulmonary N_2 clearance curves. J Clin Invest 1952; 51:40–50.
69. Briscoe WA, Cournand A. Uneven ventilation of normal and diseased lungs studied by an open-circuit method. J Appl Physiol 1959; 14:284–290.
70. Ball WCJ, Steward PB, Newsham LGS, Bates DV. Regional pulmonary function studied with Xenon133. J Clin Invest 1962; 41:519–531.
71. Wagner HN Jr, Buchanan JW. Radioactive tracer studies in pulmonary disease. In: Sackner M, eds. Diagnostic Techniques in Pulmonary Disease. New York: Marcel Dekker, 1981, pp 327–349.
72. Hakim TS, Lisbona R, Dean GW. Gravity-independent inequality in pulmonary blood flow in humans. J Appl Physiol 1987; 63:1114–1121.
73. Hakim TS, Dean GW, Lisbona R. Effect of body posture on spatial distribution of pulmonary blood flow. J Appl Physiol 1988; 64:1160–1170.

74. Glenny RW, Lamm JEM, Albert RK, Robertson HT. Gravity is a minor determinant of pulmonary blood flow distribution. J Appl Physiol 1991; 71:620–629.
75. Hlastala MP, Bernard SL, Erikson HH, Fedde RM, Gaughan EM, McMurphy R, Emery NJ, Polissar N, Glenny RW. Pulmonary blood flow distribution in standing horses is not dominated by gravity. J Appl Physiol 1996; 81:1051–1061.
76. Bernard SL, Glenny RW, Erikson HH, Fedde MR, Polissar N, Basaraba RJ, Hlastala MP. Minimal redistribution of pulmonary blood flow with exercise in racehorses. J Appl Physiol 1996; 81:1062–1070.
77. Martin CJ, Cline F Jr, Marshall H. Lobar alveolar gas concentrations: effect of body position. J Clin Invest 1953; 32:617–621.
78. West JB, Dollery CT. Distribution of blood flow and ventilation-perfusion ratio in the lung measured with radioactive CO_2. J Appl Physiol 1960; 15:405–410.
79. West JB. Regional differences in gas exchange in the lung of erect man. J Appl Physiol 1962; 17:893–898.
80. Michaelson ED, Sackner MA, Johnson RL Jr. Vertical distributions of pulmonary diffusing capacity and capillary blood flow in man. J Clin Invest 1973; 52:359–369.
81. Anthonison NR, Dolovich MB, Bates DV. Steady state measurement of regional ventilation to perfusion ratios in normal man J Clin Invest 1966; 45:1349–1356.
82. Amis TC, Jones HA, Hughes JMB. Effect of posture on inter-regional distribution of pulmonary ventilation in man. Respir Physiol 1984; 56:145–167.
83. Amis TC, Jones HA, Hughes JMB. Effect of posture on inter-regional distribution of pulmonary perfusion and VA/Qc ratios in man. Respir Physiol 1984; 56:169–182.
84. Fahri LE. Elimination of inert gas by the lung. Respir Physiol 1967; 3:1–11.
85. Wagner PD, Saltzman HA, West JB. Measurements of continuous distributions of ventilation-perfusion ratios: theory. J Appl Physiol 1974; 36:588–599.
86. Wagner PD, Laravuso RB, Uhl RR, West JB. Continuous distributions of ventilation-perfusion ratios in normal subjects breathing air and 100% O_2. J Clin Invest 1974; 54:54–68.
87. Wagner PD, Nauman PF, Laravuso RB. Simultaneous measurement of eight foreign gases in the blood by gas chromatography. J Appl Physiol 1974; 36:600–605.
88. Hammond MD, Hempleman SC. Oxygen diffusing capacity estimates derived from measured V_A/Q distributions in man. Respir Physiol 1987; 69:129–147.
89. Hempleman SC, Gray AT. Estimating steady-state D_{LO_2} with nonlinear dissociation curves and V_A/Q inequality. Respir Physiol 1988; 73:279–288.
90. Hlastala MP, Scheid P, Piiper J. Interpretation of inert gas retention and excretion in the presence of stratified inhomogeneity. Respir Physiol 1981; 46:247–259.
91. Scheid P, Hlastala MP, Piiper J. Inert gas elimination from lungs with stratified inhomogeneity: theory. Respir Physiol 1981; 44:299–309.
92. Truog WE, Hlastala MP, Standaert TA, McKenna HP, Hodson WA. Oxygen-induced alteration of ventilation-perfusion relationships in rats. J Appl Physiol Respir Environ Exercise Physiol 1979; 47:1112–1117.
93. Hsia CCW, Herazo LF, Ramanathan M, Johnson RL Jr, Wagner PD. Cardiopulmonary adaptations to pneumonectomy in dogs. II. Ventilation-perfusion relationships and microvascular recruitment. J Appl Physiol 1993; 74:1299–1309.
94. Bohr C. Uber die spesifische Tatigkeit der Lungen bei der respiratorischen Gasaufnahme und ihr Verhalten zu der durch die alveolarwand stattfinden Gasdiffusion. Skand Arch Physiol 1909; 22:221–280.

95. Haldane J. The action of cabonic oxide on man. J Physiol 1895; 18:430–462.
96. Haldane J, Smith JL. The oxygen tension of arterial blood. J Physiol 1896; 20:497–518.
97. Krogh A, Krogh M. On the rate of diffusion of carbonic oxide into the lungs of man. Skand Arch Physiol 1909; 23:236–247.
98. Krogh M. The diffusion of gases through the lungs of man J Physiol 1914; 49:271–300.
99. Lilienthal JL Jr, Riley RL, Proemmel DD, Franke RE. An experimental analysis in man of the pressure gradient from alveolar air to arterial blood during rest and exercise at sea level and at high altitude. Am J Physiol 1946; 174:199–216.
100. Staub NC, Bishop JM, Forster RE. Velocity of O_2 uptake by human red cell. J Appl Physiol 1961; 17:511–516.
101. Wagner PD, Gale GE, Moon RE, Torre-Bueno JR, Stolp BW, Saltzman HA. Pulmonary gas exchange in humans exercising at sea level and simulated altitude. J Appl Physiol 1986; 61:260–270.
102. Filley GF, MacIntosh DJ, Wright GW. Carbon monoxide uptake and pulmonary diffusing capacity in normal subjects at rest and during exercise. J Clin Invest 1954; 33:530–539.
103. Bates DV, Boucot NG, Dormer AE. The pulmonary diffusing capacity in normal subjects. J Physiol (Lond) 955; 129:237–252.
104. Filley GF, MacIntosh DJ, Wright GW. Carbon monoxide uptake and pulmonary diffusing capacity in normal subjects at rest and during exercise. J Clin Invest 1954; 33:530–539.
105. Siosteen SM, Sjostrand TA. A method for the determination of low concentration of CO in the blood and the relation between the CO concentrations in the blood and that in alveolar air. Acta Physiol Scand 1951; 22:129–133.
106. Ogilvie CM, Forster RE, Blakemore WS, Morton JW. A standardized breath holding technique for the clinical measurement of the diffusing capacity of the lung for carbon monoxide. J Clin Invest 1957; 36:1–17.
107. Spicer WS Jr, Johnson RL Jr, Forster RE II. Diffusing capacity and blood flow in different regions of the lung. J Appl Physiol 1962; 17:587–595.
108. Johnson RL Jr, Spicer WS, Bishop JM, Forster RE. Pulmonary capillary blood volume, flow and diffusing capacity during exercise. J Appl Physiol 1960; 15:893–902.
109. Graham BL, Mink JT, Cotton DJ. Improved accuracy and precision of single-breath CO diffusing capacity measurements. J Appl Physiol Respir Environ Exercise Physiol 1981; 51:1306–1313.
110. Martonen TB, Wilson AF. Theoretical basis of single breath gas absorption tests. J Math Biol 1982; 14:203–220.
111. Soparkar GR, Mink JT, Graham BL, Cotton DJ. Measurement of temporal changes in DLsb/3EQ from small alveolar samples in normal subjects. J Appl Physiol 1994; 76:1494–1501.
112. Newth CJL, Cotton DJ, Nadel JA. Pulmonary diffusing capacity measured at multiple intervals during a slow exhalation in man. J Appl Physiol Respir Environ Exercise Physiol 1977; 43:617–625.

113. Huang YT, Helms NJ, MacIntyre NR. Normal values for single exhalation diffusing capacity and pulmonary capillary blood flow in sitting, supine positions and during mild exercise. Chest 1994; 105:501–508.
114. MacIntyre NR, Nadel JA. Regional diffusing capacity in normal lungs during a slow exhalation. J Appl Physiol Respir Environ Exercise Physiol 1982; 52:1487–1492.
115. Kruhøffer P. Lung diffusion coefficient for CO in human subjects by means of $C_{14}O$. Acta Physiol Scand 1954; 32:106–123.
116. Lewis BM, Lin L, Noe FE, Hayford-Welsing EJ. The measurement of pulmonary diffusing capacity for carbon monoxide by a rebreathing method. J Clin Invest 1959; 38:2073–2086.
117. Sackner MA, Greenletch D, Heiman M, Epstein S, Atkins N. Diffusing capacity, membrane diffusing capacity, capillary blood volume, pulmonary tissue volume and cardiac output by a rebreathing technique. Am Rev Respir Dis 1975; 111:157–165.
118. Hsia CCW, Herazo LF, Ramanathan M, Johnson FL Jr. Cardiac output during exercise measured by acetylene rebreathing, thermodilution and Fick techniques. J Appl Physiol 1995; 78:1612–1616.
119. Triebwasser JH, Johnson RL Jr, Burpo RP, Campbell JC, Reardon WC, Blomqvist CG. Noninvasive determination of cardiac output by a modified acetylene rebreathing procedure utilizing mass spectrometer measurements. Aviat Space Environ Med 1977; 48:203–209.
120. Roughton FJW, Forster RE, Cander L. Rate at which carbon monoxide replaces oxygen from combination with human hemoglobin in solution and in the red cell. J Appl Physiol 1957; 11:269–276.
121. Holland RAB. Rate at which CO replaces O_2 and O_2Hb in red cells of different species. Respir Physiol 969; 7:43–63.
122. Yamaguchi K, Nguyen PD, Scheid P, Piiper J. Kinetics of O_2 uptake and release by human erythrocytes studied by a stopped-flow technique. J Appl Physiol 1985; 58:1215–1224.
123. Constantine HP, Craw MR, Forster RE. Rate of reaction of carbon dioxide with human red blood cells. Am J Physiol 1965; 208:801–811.
124. Carlsen E, Comroe JH. The rate of uptake of carbon monoxide and of nitric oxide by normal human erythrocytes and experimentally produced spherocytes. J Gen Physiol 1958; 42:83–107.
125. Schuster KD. Kinetics of pulmonary CO_2 transfer studied by using labeled carbon dioxide C16O18O. Respir Physiol 1985; 60:21–37.
126. Krogh A. The number and distribution of capillaries in muscles and calculations of the oxygen pressure head necessary for supplying the tissue. J Physiol 1918; 52:409–415.
127. Kreuzer F. Oxygen supply to tissues: the Krogh model and its assumptions. Eperentia 1982; 38:1415–1426.
128. Groebe K. O_2 transport in skeletal muscle: development of concepts and current state. Adv Exp Med Biol 1994; 345:15–22.
129. Erikkson E, Myrhage R. Microvascular dimensions and blood flow in skeletal muscle. Acta Physiol Scand 1972; 86:211–222.
130. Hammersen F. The terminal vascular bed in skeletal muscle with special regard to the problem of shunts. In: Crone CC, Lassen NA, eds. Capillary Permeability. Copenhagen: Munksgard, 1970, pp 351–371.

131. Popel AS, Carny CK, Dvinsky AS. Effect of heterogeneous oxygen delivery on the oxygen distribution in skeletal muscle. Math Biosci 1986; 81:91–113.
132. Duling BR. Is red cell heterogeneity a critical variable in the regulation and limitation of oxygen transport to tissue? Adv Exp Med Biol 1994; 361:237–247.
133. Taylor CR, Weibel ER. Design of the mammalian respiratory system. I. Problem and strategy. Respir Physiol 1981; 44:1–10.
134. Hoppeler H, Mathieu O, Krauer R, Claassen H, Armstrong RB, Weibel ER. Design of the mammalian respiratory system. VI. Distribution of mitochondria and capillaries in various muscles. Respir Physiol 1981; 44:87–111.
135. Mathieu O, Cruz OL, Hoppeler H, Weibel ER. Estimating length density and quantifying anisotropy in skeletal muscle capillaries. J Microsci 1981; 131:131–146.
136. Mathieu CO, Hoppeler H, Weibel ER. Capillary tortuosity in skeletal muscles of mammals depends on muscle contraction. J Appl Physiol 1989; 66:1436–1442.
137. Schacterle RS, Adams JM, Ribando RJ. A theoretical model of gas transport between arterioles and tissue. Microvasc Res 1991; 41:210–228.
138. Vallet B, Lund N, Curtis SE, Kelly D, Cain SM. Gut and muscle P_{O_2} in endotoxemic dogs during shock and resuscitation. J Appl Physiol 1994; 76:793–800.
139. Haywood JR, Shaffer RA, Fastenow C, Fink GD, Brody MJ. Regional blood flow measurement with pulsed Doppler flowmeter in conscious rats. Am J Physiol 1981; 241 (Heart Circ Physiol 10):H273–H278.
140. Gorewit RC, Armando MC, Bristol DG. Measuring bovine mammary gland blood flow using a transit time ultrasonic flow probe. J Dairy Sci 1989; 72:1918–1928.
141. Kvietys PR, Shepherd AP, Granger DN. Laser-Doppler, H2 clearance, and microsphere estimates of mucosal blood flow. Am J Physiol 1985; 249(Gastrointest Liver Physiol 12):G221–G227.
142. Lipowsky HH, Usami S, Chien S, Pittman RN. Hematocrit determination in small bore tubes by differential specrophotometry. Microvasc Res 1982; 24:42–55.
143. Pittman RN, Ellsworth ML. Estimation of red cell flow in microvessels: consequence of the Baker-Wayland spatial averaging model. Microvasc Res 1986; 32:371–388.
144. Rudolph M, Heymann MA. The circulation of the fetus in utero: methods for studying distribution of blood flow, cardiac output amd organ blood flow. Circ Res 1967; 21:163–185.
145. Prinzen FW, Glenny RW. Developments in non-radioactive microsphere techniques for blood flow measurement. Cardiovasc Res 1994; 28:1467–1475.
146. Buckberg GD, Luck JC, Payne DB, Hoffman JIE, Archie JP, Fixler DE. Some sources of error in measuring regional blood flow with radioactive microspheres. J Appl Physiol 1971; 31:598–604.
147. Greenway CV, Murthy VS. Effect of vasopressin and isoprenaline infusions on the distribution of blood flow in the intestine: criteria for the validity of microsphere studies. Br J Pharmacol 1972; 46:177–188.
148. Von Ritter C, Hinder RA, Womack W, Bauerffeind P, Fimmel CJ, Kvietys PR, Granger DN, Blum AL. Microsphere estimates of blood flow: methodological considerations. Am J Physiol 1988; 254 (Gastrointest Liver Physiol 17):G275–G279.
149. Caeser J, Shaldon S, Guevera L, Sherlock S. The use of indocyanine green in the measurement of hepatic blood flow and as a test of hepatic function. Clin Sci 1961; 21:43–57.

150. Poole DC, Gaesser GA, Hogan MC, Knight DR, Wagner PD. Pulmonary and leg V_{O_2} during submaximal exercise: implications for muscular efficiency. J Appl Physiol 1992; 72:805–810.
151. Wagner PD. Peripheral inert gas exchange. In: Fishman AP, ed. Handbook of Physiology, Section 3: Respiratory System, Vol. IV: Gas Exchange. New York: Oxford University Press, 1987, pp 257–281.
152. Kety SS, Schmidt CF. The determination of blood flow in man by the use of nitrous oxide in low concentrations. Am J Physiol 1945; 143:53–66.
153. Early PJ. Use of diagnostic radionuclides in medicine. Health Phys 1995; 69:649–661.
154. Lassen NA, Andersen AR, Friberg L, Paulson OB. The retention of [99mTc]-d,1-HM-PAO in the human brain after intracarotid bolus injection: a kinetic analysis. J Cereb Blood Flow Metab 1988; 8:S13–S22.
155. Williamson JW, Nobrega ACL, McColl R, Mathews D, Winchester P, Friberg L, Mitchell JH. Activation of the insular cortex during dynamic exercise in humons. J Physiol 1997; 503:277–283.
156. D'Asseler YM, Koole YMM, LeMahiew I, Achten E, Boon P, De Deyn PP, Dierckx RA. Recent and future evolutions in neuroSPECT with particular emphasis on the synergistic use and fusion of imaging modalities. Acta Heurol Belg 1997; 97:154–162.
157. Paans AMJ. Position emission tomography: background, possibilities and perspectives in neuroscience. Acta Neurol Belg 1997; 97:150–153.
158. Lammertsma AA, Jones T, Frackowiak RS, Lenzi GL. A theoretical study of the steady-state model for measuring regional cerebral blood flow and oxygen utilization using oxygen-15. J Comput Assist Tomogr 1981; 5:544–550.
159. Campbell JA. Gas tension in tissues. Physiol Rev 1931; 11:1–40.
160. Fiddian-Green RG, McGough E, Pittenger G, Rothman E. Predictive value of intraluminal pH and other risk factors for massive bleeding from stress ulceration. Gastroenterology 1983; 85:613–620.
161. Bergofsky EH. Determination of O_2 tensions by hollow visceral tonometers: effect of breathing enriched O_2 mixtures. J Clin Invest 1964; 43:193–200.
162. Gys T, Van Esbroeck G, Hubens A. Assessment of the perfusion in peripheral tissue beds by subcutaneous oximetry and gastric intramucosal pH-metry in elective colorectal surgery. Intensive Care Med 1991; 7:78–82.
163. Lübbers DW. Oxygen electrodes and optodes and their application in vivo. Adv Exp Med Biol 1996; 388:13–34.
164. Duling BR, Berne RM. Longitudinal gradients in periarteriolar oxygen tension. Circ Res 1970; 28:669–678.
165. Lünd N. Ödman S, Lewis DH. Skeletal muscle oxygen pressure fields in rats: a study of the normal state and the effects of local anesthetics, local trauma and hemorrhage. Acta Anesth Scand 1980; 24:155–160.
166. Ödman S, Lünd N. Data acquisition and information processing in MDO oxygen electrode measurements of tissue oxygen pressure. Acta Anseth Scand 1980; 24:155–160.
167. Groebe K. Relating measuring signals from P_{O_2} electrodes to tissue P_{O_2}: a theoretical study. Adv Exp Med Biol 1992; 316:61–69.

168. Lübbers D. Theory and development of transcutaneous oxygen pressure measurement. Int Anesth Clin 1987; 25:31–65.
169. Pologe JA. Pulse oximetry: technical aspects of machine design. Int Anesth Clin 1987; 25:137–153.
170. Barker SJ, Tremper KK, Hyatt J. Effect of methemoglobinemia on pulse oximetry and mixed venous oximetry. Anesthesiology 1989; 70:112–117.
171. Pittman RN, Duling BR. A method for the measurement of percent oxyhemoglobin. J Appl Physiol 1975; 38:315–320.
172. Pittman RN, Duling BR. Measurement of percent oxyhemoglobin in the microvasculature. J Appl Physiol 975; 38:321–327.
173. Swain DP, Pittman RN. Oxygen exchange in the microcirculation of hamster retractor muscle. Am J Physiol 1989; 256 (Heart Circ Physiol):H245–H255.
174. Parthasarathi K, Pittman RN. Measurement of hemoglobin concentration and oxygen saturation profiles in arterioles using intravital videomicroscopy and image analysis. Adv Exp Med Biol 1994; 361:249–260.
175. Wilson DF, Vinogradov S, Lo LW, Huang L. Oxygen dependent quenching of phosphofluorescence. Adv Exp Med Biol 1996; 388:101–107.
176. Opitz N, Lübbers DW. Theory and development of fluorescence-based optochemical oxygen sensors: oxygen optodes. Int Anesth Clin 1987; 25:177–197.
177. Intaglietta M, Johnson PC, Winslow RM. Microvascular and tissue oxygen distribution. Cardiovasc Res 1996; 32:632–643.
178. Wilson DF, Vinogradov SA. Recent advances in oxygen measurements using phosphorescence quenching. Adv Exp Med Biol 1994; 36:61–66.
179. Swartz HM, Bacic B, Friedman B, Goda F, Griberg O, Hoopes PJ, Jiang J, Liu KJ, Nakashima T, O'Hara J, Walezak T. Measurement of P_{O_2} in vivo, including human subjects by electron paramagnetic resonance. Adv Exp Med Biol 1994; 361:119–128.
180. Jiang J, Nakashima T, Liu F, Goda F, Shima T, Swartz HM. Measurement of P_{O_2} in liver by using EPR oximetry. J Appl Physiol 1996; 80:552–558.
181. James PE, Grinberg OY, Goda F, Panz T, Ohara JA, Swartz HM. Gloxy: An oxygen-sensitive coal for accurate measurement of low oxygen tensions in biological systems. Magn Reson Med 1997; 38:48–58.
182. Gayeski TEJ, Honig CA. Shallow intracellular O_2 gradients and absence of perimitochondrial O_2 "wells" in heavily working red muscle. Adv Exp Med Biol 1986; 200:487–494.
183. Gayeski TEJ, Connet RJ, Honig CR. Minimum intracellular P_{O_2} for maximum cytochrome turnover in red muscle in situ. Am J Physiol 1987; 2523 (Heart Circ Physiol):H906–H915.
184. Fiddian-Green RG, Pittenger G, Whitehouse WM. Back-diffusion of CO_2 and its influence on the intramural pH in gastric mucose. J Surg Res 1982; 33:39–48.
185. Antonsson JB, Boylew III JB, Kruithoff KL, Wang H, Sacristan E, Rothschild HR, Fink MP. Validation of tonometric measurement of gut intramural pH during endotoxemia and mesenteric occlusion in pigs. Am J Physiol 1990; 259 (Gastroentest Liver Physiol 22):G519–G523.
186. Schlichtig R, Bowles SA. Distinguishing between aerobic and anaerobic appearance of dissolved CO_2 in intestine during low flow. J Appl Physiol 1994; 76:2443–2451.

187. Park R, Arieff AI. Lactic aidosis: current concepts. Clin Endocrin Metab 1983; 12:339–358.
188. Curtis SE, Cain SM. Regional and systemic oxygen delivery/uptake relations and lactate flux in hyperdynamic, endotoxemic-treated dogs. Am Rev Resp Dis 1992; 45:348–354.
189. Vincent JL. Lactate levels in critically ill patients. Acta Anesthesiol Scand 1995; 39(suppl 10):261–266.
190. Chance B, Cohen P, Jöbsis F, Schoener B. Intracellular oxidation-reduction states in vivo. Science 1962; 137:499-508.
191. Ince C, Coremans JMCC, Bruining HA. In vivo NADH fluorescence. Adv Exp Med Biol 1992; 317:277–296.
192. Edwards AD. The clinical role of near infrared spectroscopy. J Perinat Med 1994; 22:535–539.
193. Jöbsis-Vandervliet FF, Fox E, Sugioka K. Monitoring of cerebral oxygenation and cytochrome aa3 redox state. Int Anesth Clin 1987; 25:209–230.
194. Vallet B, Curtis SE, Guery B, Mangalaboyi J, Menager P, Cain SM, Chopin C, Dupuis BA. ATP sensitive K+ channel blockade impairs O_2 extraction during progressive ischemia in pig hindlimb. J Appl Physiol 1995; 79:2035–2042.
195. Hempel FG, Jöbsis FF, LaManna JL, Rosenthal MR, Saltzman HA. Oxidation of cerebral cytochrome aa3 by oxygen plus carbon dioxide at hyperbaric pressures. J Appl Physiol 1977; 43:873–879.
196. Clark BJ, Smith D, Chance B. Metabolic consequences of oxygen transport studied with phosphorus nuclear magnetic resonance spectroscopy. In: Bryan-Brown CW, Ayres SM, eds. Oxygen Transport and Utilization. Fullerton: New Horizons, 1987, pp 145–169.
197. Gutierrez G, Pohil RJ, Narayana P. Skeletal muscle O_2 consumption and energy metabolism during hypoxemia. J Appl Physiol 1989; 66:2117–2223.
198. Jue T, Kreutzer U, Chung Y. NMR approach to observed tissue oxygenation with the signals of myoglobin. Adv Exp Med Biol 1994; 361:111–118.
199. Fleckenstein JL, Archer BT, Barker BA, Vaugn T, Parkey RW, Peshock RM. Acute effects of exercise on skeletal muscle in volunteers. Am J Roentgenol 1988; 151:231–237.
200. Fleckenstein JL, Haller RG, Lewis SF, Archer BT, Barker BR, Pain J, Parkey RW, Peshock RM. Absence of exercise induced MRI enhancement of skeletal muscle in McArdles disease. J Appl Physiol 1991; 71:961–969.
201. Jianhua L, Gregory AH, Potts JT, Wilson LB, Mitchell JH. c-Fos expression in the medulla induced by static muscle contractions in cats. Am J Physiol 1997; (Heart Circ Physiol 41):H48–H56.
202. Wagner PD, Roca J, Hogan MC, Poole DC, Bebout DC, Haab P. Experimental support for the theory of diffusion limitation of maximum oxygen uptake. Adv Exp Med Biol 1990; 277:825–833.
203. Schaffartzik W, Barto ED, Poole DC, Tskimoto K, Hogan MC, Bebout DE, Wagner PD. Effect of reduced hemoglobin concentration on leg oxygen uptake during maximal exercise in humans. J Appl Physiol 1993; 75:491–498.
204. Roca J, Hogan MC, Story D, Bebout DE, Haab P, Gonzalez R, Ueno O, Wagner PD. Evidence for tissue diffusion limitation of Vo_2max in normal humans. J Appl Physiol 1989; 67:291–299.

205. Dollfuss RE, Milic-Emili J, Bates DV. Regional ventilation of the lung studied with boluses of ^{133}xenon. Respiration Physiology 1967; 2:234–246.
206. Anthonisen NR, Milic-Emili J. Distribution of pulmonary perfusion in erect man. J Appl Physiol 1966; 21:760–766.
207. Jones RS, Meade FA. A theoretical and experimental analysis of anomalies in the estimation of pulmonary diffusing capacity by the single breath method. Quarterly J of Experimental Physiology 1961; 46:131–143.
208. Borland CDR, Higenbottom TW. A simultaneous single breath measurement of pulmonary diffusing capacity with nitric oxide and carbon monoxide. Euro Respir J 1989; 2:26–63.
209. Meyer M, Schuster KD, Schulz H, Mohr M, Piiper J. Pulmonary diffusing capacities for nitric oxide and carbon monoxide determined by rebreathing in dogs. J Appl Physiol 1990; 68:2344–2357.
210. Moinard J, Guenard H. Determination of pulmonary capillary blood volume and membrane diffusing capacity in patients with COLD using the NO-CO method. Euro Respir J 1990; 3:318–322.

4

Gas Exchange in Health: Rest, Exercise, and Aging

ROBB GLENNY
Washington University
Seattle, Washington

PETER D. WAGNER
University of California, San Diego
La Jolla, California

**JOSEP ROCA and
ROBERTO RODRIGUEZ-ROISIN**
Hospital Clínic, University of Barcelona
Barcelona, Spain

The chief function of the lung is pulmonary gas exchange. The lung must match pulmonary O_2 uptake ($\dot{V}O_2$) and elimination of CO_2 ($\dot{V}CO_2$) to whole body metabolic O_2 consumption and CO_2 production, whatever the O_2 and CO_2 partial pressures in the arterial blood. The O_2 transport pathway (see Chap. 1) begins with ventilation delivering air to the alveolar surface, principally by convection. Without adequate ventilation, in relation to metabolic rate, arterial P_{O_2} will fall and arterial P_{CO_2} will rise. Oxygen crosses into pulmonary capillary blood by diffusion. Equilibration of alveolar and end-capillary P_{O_2} depends on three factors: (i) the diffusing capacity of the lungs (D_L), (ii) blood flow ($\dot{Q}$), and (iii) the capacitance of blood for O_2 (β) that is equivalent to effective solubility for O_2 (capacitance of blood for O_2 (β) is defined by the slope of the O_2Hb dissociation curve between arterial and venous P_{O_2} values). In fact, it is the ratio $D_L/\beta.\dot{Q}$ that determines the degree of equilibration and the extent that D_L is reduced and/or $\beta.\dot{Q}$ increased, arterial P_{O_2} may be less than alveolar P_{O_2}. Nonuniform distribution of inspired air and pulmonary capillary blood occurs even in normal lungs, as analyzed in this chapter. In pulmonary disease, this ventilation-perfusion ($\dot{V}_A/\dot{Q}$) inequality is usually exaggerated and may lead to significant reduction of arterial P_{O_2}. During the first half of the twentieth century (1,2), the heterogeneity of the $\dot{V}_A/\dot{Q}$ ratios within the lung was identified as a factor causing hypoxemia (Table 1). However, the importance

121

Table 1 Factors Determining Arterial Hypoxemia

Intrapulmonary	Extrapulmonary	
$\dot{V}_A/\dot{Q}$ mismatching	Primary factors:	Decreased ventilation
Shunt		Decreased cardiac output
Alveolar-end capillary		Decreased inspired P_{O_2}
O_2 diffusion limitation		Increased O_2 uptake
	Secondary factors:	Decreased P_{50}
		Decreased [Hb]
		Increased pH

$\dot{V}_A/\dot{Q}$: ventilation-perfusion; [Hb], hemoglobin concentration; P_{50}, P_{O_2} that corresponds to 50% oxyhemoglobin saturation

of $\dot{V}_A/\dot{Q}$ inequality in producing hypercapnia in patients with some forms of lung disease has been pointed out more recently (3).

Another factor that can cause severe hypoxemia in certain diseases is the presence of right-to-left shunt. Abnormalities of pulmonary gas exchange from inadequate ventilation, diffusion limitation, ventilation-perfusion inequality, or shunt have a marked impact on arterial partial pressures of respiratory gases. It is notable, however, that Pa_{O_2} and Pa_{CO_2} are finally determined by the interactions between the pulmonary factors alluded to above and by the different extrapulmonary factors indicated in Table 1.

This chapter analyzes nonuniformities of ventilation and pulmonary blood flow in health and their impact on the efficiency of the lung as O_2 and CO_2 exchanger. The role of pulmonary gas exchange and the interplay between pulmonary and extrapulmonary factors determining Pa_{O_2} and Pa_{CO_2} at rest and during exercise in healthy subjects are also examined. Finally, the effects of aging on pulmonary gas exchange are evaluated and recent data on reference values for arterial partial pressures of respiratory gases are provided.

I. Heterogeneity of Pulmonary Gas Exchange at Rest

The lung is a complex system deriving its chief function from the interaction of two very complicated networks that determine regional perfusion and ventilation, respectively. It is well accepted that normal lung is exquisitely sensitive to gravity which normally causes regional differences of blood flow, alveolar ventilation, pleural pressures, and parenchymal stress (4). It is remarkable, however, that the amount of $\dot{V}_A/\dot{Q}$ inequality due to gravity is rather small. The predicted gravitational increase in the dispersion of pulmonary blood flow distribution (Log SD_Q) is only 0.30, which accounts for a moderate rise in the AaP_{O_2} of approximately 4 mm Hg (5). The characteristic $\dot{V}_A/\dot{Q}$ distribution in seated young subjects (< 30 years) consists of narrow perfusion and ventilation curves centered around a $\dot{V}_A/\dot{Q}$ ratio of one (Figure 1). Mean values for the second moment of the distribution (Log SD_Q and Log SD_V) range between 0.35 and 0.43 (6). The upper 95% confidence limit for Log SD_Q is 0.60, and for Log SD_V is 0.65 (7–10). Nongravitational inequality, although considered separately for ventilation and perfusion, appears to result in good matching of pulmonary $\dot{V}_A/\dot{Q}$ ratios since overall Log SD_Q and Log SD_V are so small and hardly exceed values expected from gravity alone. Yet, despite the heterogeneous distribution of both blood flow and ventilation at the alveolar-capillary level, respiratory gases are exchanged efficiently in healthy man.

A. Vertical Distributions of $\dot{V}_A$, $\dot{Q}$ and $\dot{V}_A/\dot{Q}$

The most common model of pulmonary gas exchange proposes a gravitationally induced vertical distribution of perfusion and ventilation and that regional matching of ventilation and perfusion is accomplished primarily by the shared effects of

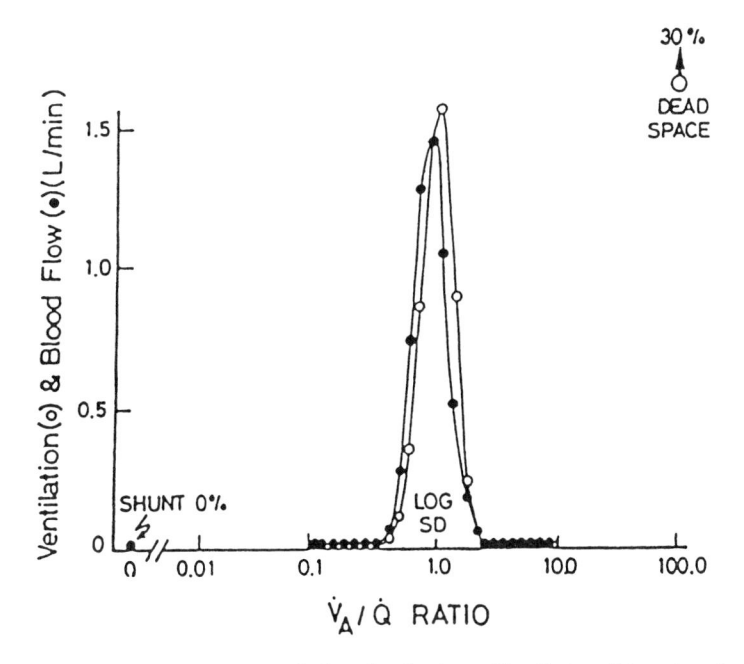

Figure 1 Ventilation-perfusion distributions. Ventilation (○) and perfusion (●) are plotted against ventilation-perfusion ($\dot{V}_A/\dot{Q}$) ratio on a logarithmic scale in a resting young healthy subject, breathing room air. Both ventilation and blood flow curves are centered (first moment) around a $\dot{V}_A/\dot{Q}$ ratio of 1 and then narrow (second moment). No perfusion to low $\dot{V}_A/\dot{Q}$ units ($\dot{V}_A/\dot{Q}$ ratios < 0.1) nor ventilation to high $\dot{V}_A/\dot{Q}$ areas ($\dot{V}_A/\dot{Q}$ ratios > 10) are observed. Note also the absence of shunt. Each individual data point represents a particular amount of blood flow (●) or alveolar ventilation (○) to the corresponding pulmonary compartment ($\dot{V}_A/\dot{Q}$ ratio). Total cardiac output corresponds to the sum of the 50 blood flow points and total alveolar ventilation is the sum of the 50 ventilation points.

gravity (4). Radioactive gases and chest-wall scintillation counters were used by a number of investigators (11–13) in the early 1960s to estimate regional ventilation and perfusion within anterior-posterior cores of lung tissue. These studies generally revealed increased ventilation and perfusion at lung bases compared to apices in upright subjects. These findings were interpreted in the context of a gravitational model where perfusion and ventilation increased down the lung due to increasing hydrostatic (14) and pleural pressures (15), respectively. West (4) integrated these observations into a model predicting the topographical distribution of regional gas exchange based on the theoretical local ventilation/perfusion ratios (Fig. 2). Local alveolar and arterial oxygen and carbon dioxide partial pressures were calculated from a hypothetical cardiac output, minute ventilation, and mixed venous gas tensions. The model produced an alveolar-arterial O_2 difference similar to that observed in man, supporting the conclusion that "most of the uneven distribution [of ventilation and perfusion] in normal upright man is accounted for by the difference in blood flow and ventilation up and down the lung" (4). West acknowledged that any perfusion or ventilation heterogeneity within isogravitational planes would not be revealed by his "relatively crude" imaging methods but stated that isogravitational heterogeneity would produce larger alveolar-arterial gas differences (4).

The vertical distribution of $\dot{V}_A/\dot{Q}$ heterogeneity and gas exchange was recently brought into question by the observation that perfusion is quite heterogeneous within isogravitational planes. Reed and Wood (16), and later Greenleaf and associates (17), observed heterogeneous blood flow within isogravitational planes

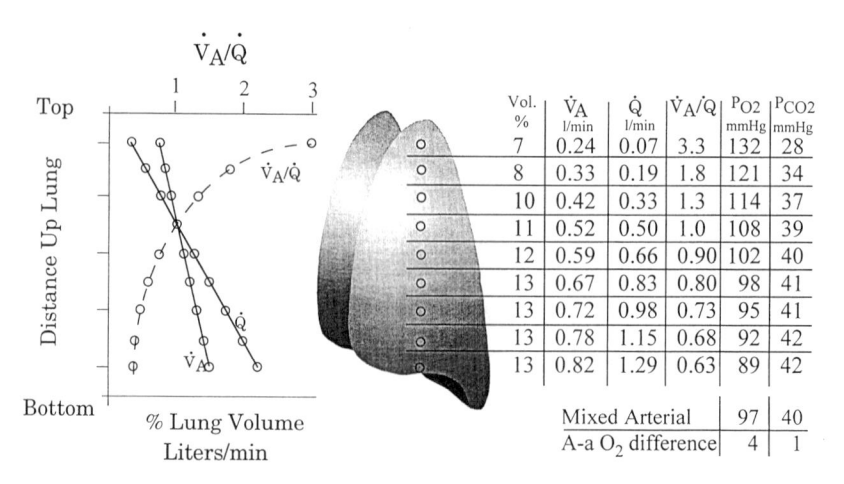

Figure 2 Gravitational model of $\dot{V}_A/\dot{Q}$ inhomogeneity in an upright lung. Both perfusion and ventilation increase down the lung but perfusion increases at a greater rate, producing variability in $\dot{V}_A/\dot{Q}$ as a function of height up the lung. The regional $\dot{V}_A/\dot{Q}$ ratios and gas tensions are theoretical predictions. (Adapted from Ref. 57.)

using high spatial resolution methods. A number of recent studies confirmed the large heterogeneity of isogravitational pulmonary blood flow with flows ranging from 0.2 to 3.5 times the mean flow within a plane (18–23). These observations were further corroborated by exhaled CO_2-concentration profiles from humans on the space shuttle that showed persistent perfusion heterogeneity under microgravity conditions (24).

Despite the heterogeneous distribution of perfusion at the alveolar-capillary level, gases are exchanged efficiently. Given the degree of isogravitational perfusion heterogeneity, matching of ventilation and perfusion cannot be governed by gravity alone. This prediction was verified recently in studies by Prisk and colleagues in Spacelabs Sciences 1 and 2 (SLS-1 and SLS-2) when they showed that ventilation/perfusion inequalities persist under conditions of microgravity (25). The authors of this study concluded that the principal determinants of ventilation/perfusion inequalities are not gravitational in origin.

B. Perfusion Heterogeneity and Fractal Models

Until recently, observed pulmonary perfusion heterogeneity has been interpreted within the context of the gravitational model as random noise. Fractal analysis, a revolutionary mathematical science, demonstrated that this "error" can be analyzed as a fundamental property of the biological system (26). Fractal analysis permits characterization of processes or structures that are not easily represented by the traditional analytical tools and provides insights and tools for constructing new models. The primary incentive for developing a fractal model of pulmonary blood flow distribution is to find a unifying mechanism that explains the heterogeneity of perfusion as well as the observation that neighboring lung regions have similar magnitudes of flow.

Fractal modeling was first used by van Beek (27) to demonstrate that perfusion heterogeneity within myocardium can be explained by a fractal branching model. In this model, the fraction of flow from parent to daughter branches is γ and $1 - \gamma$ at each bifurcation (Fig. 3). While this model does not explicitly state what determines the asymmetric distribution of flow at each branch point, heterogeneities of vascular resistance in the arterial and venous vascular trees are the key determinants. This vascular tree is extended by appending this basic element onto the ends of each daughter branch for as many generations as required to obtain the desired number of terminal branches. Flows at each terminal branch can be determined. The distribution of perfusion at the terminal branches is determined by γ and the number of generations, n, in a particular tree, and can be characterized by the coefficient of variation, CV_Q:

$$CV_Q = \frac{\sigma_Q}{\mu_Q} = \sqrt{2^n \cdot [\gamma^2 + (1-\gamma)^2]^l - 1} \tag{1}$$

where σ_Q and μ_Q are the standard deviation and mean of the perfusion distribution, respectively.

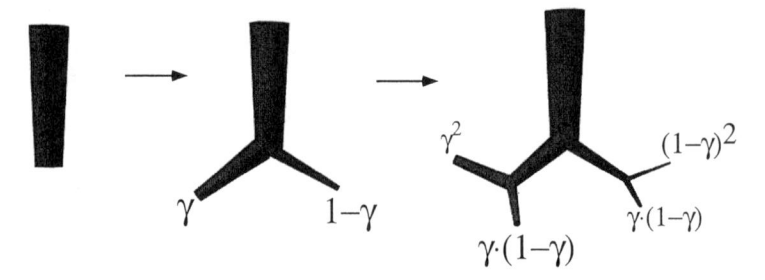

Figure 3 Dichotomously branching fractal model. *From Left:* Basic transformation is the dichotomous branching of each terminal element. The initial element is a single vessel. The asymmetric branching of the terminal branch divides flow in the vessel into two fractions, γ and $1 - \gamma$ that are distributed to daughter branches. Following a second iteration in which all terminal nodes branch again, blood flow is now distributed to four terminal branches. After a few generations, this simple recursive algorithm produces a very complex vascular tree. Flows at each terminal branch can be determined. (Adapted from Ref. 22, with permission.)

The flows generated by this network have a right-skewed distribution similar to flows obtained from experimental animals (Fig. 4). The network also demonstrates that the observed perfusion heterogeneity is dependent on the piece size. Cutting smaller organ pieces is analogous to extending the fractal network to more generations. As the organ piece size decreases, the observed heterogeneity increases (28).

An alternative, more realistic model allows the asymmetry of perfusion parameter, γ, to vary at each bifurcation (27,29). If γ is randomly selected from a normal distribution with a mean γ of 0.5, the degree of perfusion heterogeneity is dependent on the standard deviation, σ, of the distribution. The variability in perfusion at the terminal branches is uniform for $\sigma = 0$ and increases as σ deviates from zero.

Pulmonary perfusion distributions are well fitted by a fractal model. On average, a γ of 0.46 and 14 generations are needed to produce the degree of perfusion heterogeneity seen in dog lungs (29). The fractal nature of pulmonary blood flow has now been documented in a number of laboratory animals ranging in size from mice to horses (18,23,30,31).

Pulmonary blood flow is spatially correlated with neighboring regions of lung having similar magnitudes of flow, and distant pieces exhibiting negative correlation. When regional blood flow is determined to $\sim$2 cm^3 volumes of lung in dogs, high-flow regions are adjacent to other high-flow regions and low-flow regions are adjacent to other low-flow regions (32). When the spatial correlation of perfusion is determined for regional pulmonary perfusion, a strong positive correlation is noted for neighboring pieces, on average, $\rho(1.2 \text{ cm}) = 0.72$. Regions of similar flow magnitude tend to be near one another because of the shared heritage

Gas Exchange: Rest, Exercise, and Aging

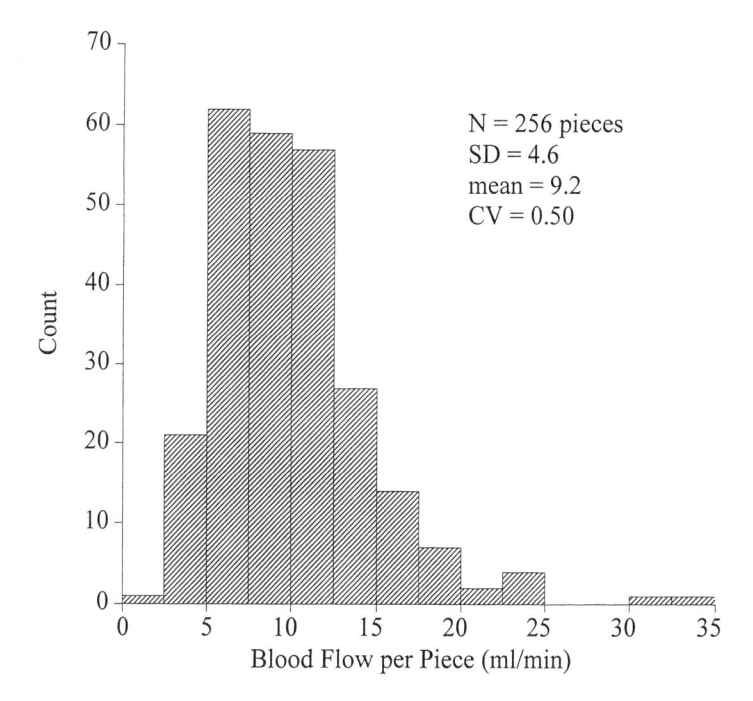

Figure 4 Perfusion distribution produced by fractal vascular model after eight generations. The simple model produces flows that are similar to those obtained from experimental animals in that they have a right skewed distribution.

of the vascular tree. The spatial correlation decreases with distance between pieces, eventually becoming negative in all cases. Because a fixed amount of blood is distributed to a limited volume, high-flow regions exist at the expense of flow to other regions. No other examples of negative spatial correlation have been reported in the natural sciences, suggesting that it may be unique to organ blood flow. Three-dimensional fractal models produce flows that are spatially correlated locally and become negatively correlated at distances (33,34).

C. Ventilation Heterogeneity and Fractal Models

In a fashion analogous to uncovering of perfusion heterogeneity, higher spatial resolution methods now show that ventilation is also heterogeneous within isogravitational planes. Amis and associates (35) were the first to note "the presence of horizontal (isogravity) gradients of lung volume or ventilation." Studies by Olson (36), Hubmayr (37), and Rodarte (38) have shown marked differences in regional lung expansion that are not related to the effects of gravity. Robertson (39) and Melsom (40) recently described new methods using fluorescent or $^{99m}T_c$ aerosols to measure the distribution of convective ventilation to lung pieces 1.9 and 1.5 cm^3 in volume. While Robertson studied anesthetized and mechanically ventilated swine and Melsom studied awake goats, both found convective ventilation to be heterogeneously distributed with average CVs of 48% and 40%, respectively. Neither investigator found a significant vertical distribution of convective ventilation and both found that isogravitational variability in ventilation was more important than a gravitational component. Recent studies performed on humans in sustained microgravity (41) confirm these findings and suggest that gravity-independent inhomogeneity of ventilation is at least as large as that induced by gravity.

Altemeier and colleagues (42) studied prone and supine pigs to determine if this marked heterogeneity of convective ventilation could be characterized by fractal analyses. They used aerosolized fluorescent microspheres to measure regional ventilation in lung pieces ∼2 cm^3 in volume, they found that ventilation distributes in a fractal pattern similar to that of perfusion, and that the fractal relationship fit the data extremely well over a broad range of piece sizes. The heterogeneity of ventilation continued to increase in the smallest pieces, suggesting that the "unit of ventilation" (the lung volume in which ventilation is uniform due to reinspired dead space and diffusion) is smaller than 2 cm^3.

Because ventilation appears to distribute in a fractal manner, regional ventilation can also be described by a fractal model similar to that used for perfusion. In such a model, the asymmetry of ventilation distribution, β, is determined by heterogeneities in local airway resistances and parenchymal compliances. The heterogeneity of ventilation can be described by Eq. (2):

$$CV_{V_A} = \frac{\sigma_{V_A}}{\mu_{V_A}} = \sqrt{2^m[\beta^2 + (1-\beta)^2]^n - 1} \qquad (2)$$

where m is the number of generations in the model. This model produces distributions of regional ventilation that are right-skewed and similar to those seen from experimental animals. Again, the model can use a varying β at each bifurcation by randomly selecting a β from a normal distribution with a mean $\beta = 0.5$ and a given σ.

D. Matching of Heterogeneous Ventilation and Perfusion

Given that both perfusion and ventilation are heterogeneously distributed, efficient exchange of gases is dependent on intimate matching of local ventilation and perfusion. In a theoretical analysis, Wilson and Beck (43) explored the impact of perfusion and ventilation heterogeneity on $\dot{V}_A/\dot{Q}$ inhomogeneity. They determined that $\dot{V}_A/\dot{Q}$ heterogeneity, expressed as the variance in the log of the $\dot{V}_A/\dot{Q}$ distribution, $\sigma^2_{\log} \dot{V}_A/\dot{Q}$, can be related to ventilation and perfusion distributions by the equation:

$$\sigma^2_{\log(V_A/Q)} = \sigma^2_{\log V_A} + \sigma^2_{\log Q} - 2\rho\sigma_{\log V_A}\sigma_{\log Q} \qquad (3)$$

where σ_{V_A} and σ_Q are the standard deviations of ventilation and perfusion distributions, respectively, and ρ is the correlation between regional ventilation and perfusion in the log domain. As the correlation between $\dot{V}_A$ and $\dot{Q}$ varies from 0 (complete independence) to 1 (tight coupling), the inhomogeneity in the $\dot{V}_A/\dot{Q}$ distribution varies from a maximum of $\sigma^2_{\log V_A} + \sigma^2_{\log Q}$ to a minimum of 0 ($\sigma_{\log V_A} = \sigma_{\log Q}$). Hence, regardless of the heterogeneities in $\dot{V}_A$ or $\dot{Q}$, tight coupling of $\dot{V}_A$ and $\dot{Q}$ results in minimal $\dot{V}_A/\dot{Q}$ inhomogeneity.

The impact of ventilation and perfusion heterogeneity and their correlation with one another on gas exchange can be further explored with the fractal ventilation and perfusion distributions presented above. For example, use $\gamma = \beta = 0.5$, $\sigma = 0.08$, and $n = m = 8$ with a total $\dot{V}_A$ and $\dot{Q}$ of 2.56 L/min. A given simulation produces 256 terminal lung pieces with a $CV_{V_A} = 0.46$ and $CV_Q = 0.46$. Correlations between $\dot{V}_A$ and $\dot{Q}$ can be produced by shuffling pairs of $\dot{V}_A$ and $\dot{Q}$ to obtain varying values of r, thus simulating different $\dot{V}_A/\dot{Q}$ distributions (Fig. 5). Flow- and ventilation-weighted $\dot{V}_A/\dot{Q}$ distributions can also be constructed so that they are directly comparable to those produced by the multiple inert gas elimination technique (MIGET). The flow-weighted σ_Q for the two simulated distributions in Fig. 5 are 0.12 and 0.35 using $\rho = 0.98$ and 0.85, respectively. The flow- and ventilation-weighted $\dot{V}_A/\dot{Q}$ information can be garnered from the ventilation vs. perfusion plots in Fig. 5. Isopleths of $\dot{V}_A/\dot{Q}$ ratios radiate from the origin in each plot. The further a lung piece lies from the origin along an isopleth indicates its relative contribution to venous admixture or wasted ventilation.

By assuming normal mixed venous O_2 and CO_2 tensions, the gas equilibration routines of Olszowka (44) can be used to determine alveolar and capillary partial pressures of O_2 and CO_2 (45) at each terminal branch in the model. Flow-weighted arterial and ventilation-weighted alveolar means of O_2 tensions can be calculated to produce an AaP_{O_2} difference for the simulated fractal ventilation and perfusion distributions depending on the given correlation coefficient, ρ. For the two simulations in Fig. 5, with $\rho = 0.98$ and 0.85, the calculated AaP_{O_2} difference are 0.5 mm Hg and 4.4, respectively.

With the advent of aerosol methods to measure regional ventilation, firm estimates of σ_{V_A}, σ_Q, and ρ at the same scale of resolution are now available. Robertson (39) and Melsom (40) both found strong correlations (mean ρ of 0.80 and 0.81, respectively) between regional ventilation and perfusion (Fig. 6). These correlations represent the coupling between $\dot{V}_A$ and $\dot{Q}$ in the linear domain and correspond to a ρ of about 0.76 in the log domain.

The correlation between regional ventilation and perfusion for all lung pieces is present in graph B. Dotted lines radiating from origin represent isopleths of $\dot{V}_A/\dot{Q}$ ratios. Histograms A and D are obtained by collapsing each point in B to the appropriate axis. Data can be reduced to a 50-compartment model by binning the $\dot{V}_A/\dot{Q}$ ratios from each lung piece and displaying them in a format familiarized by MIGET.

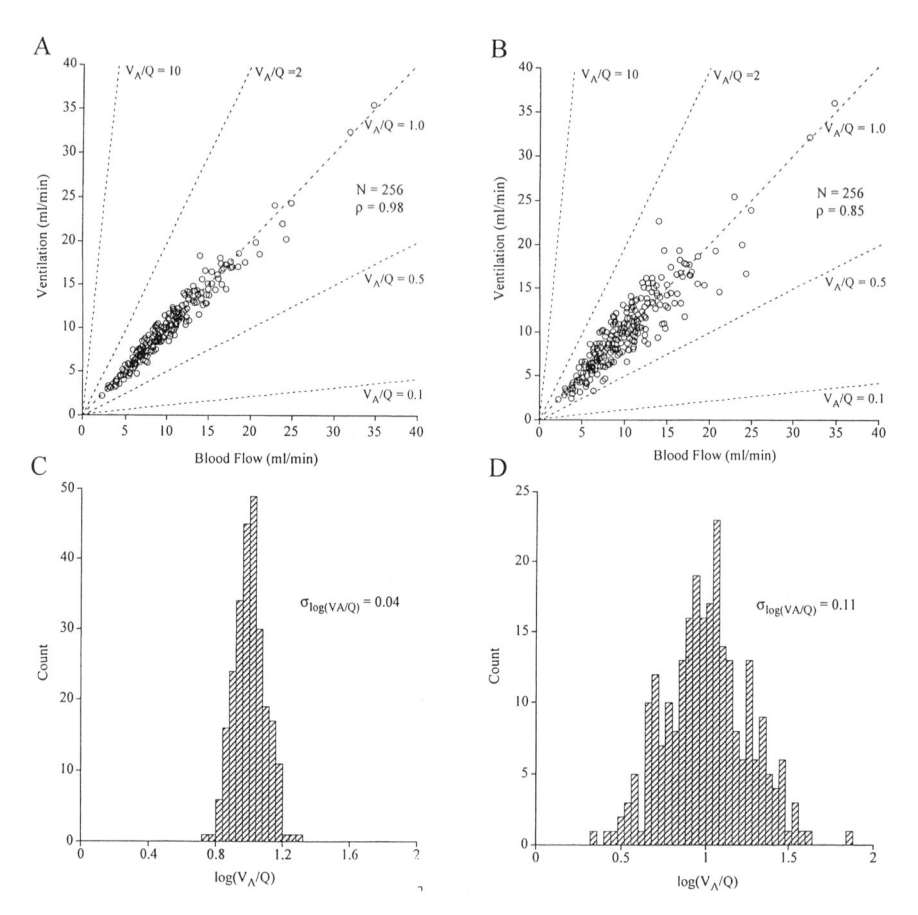

Figure 5 Simulated $\dot{V}_A$, $\dot{Q}$ and $\dot{V}_A/\dot{Q}$ distributions produced from fractal models (see text). Plots A and B present $\dot{V}_A$ and $\dot{Q}$ to 256 lung pieces with correlation coefficients of 0.98 and 0.85, respectively. The heterogeneity of perfusion and ventilation are the same in the two simulations. Plots C and D show the impact of the correlation between $\dot{V}_A$ and $\dot{Q}$ on the $\dot{V}_A/\dot{Q}$ distribution. While the heterogeneity of $\dot{V}_A$ and $\dot{Q}$ have an impact on gas exchange, the correlation between the two is equally important.

These strong correlations resulted in relatively tight $\dot{V}_A/\dot{Q}$ distributions as predicted by Wilson and Beck's model [Eq. 3)]. Melsom (40) reported a CV of the $\dot{V}_A/\dot{Q}$ distribution of 0.36 corresponding to a $\sigma_{\log(\dot{V}_A/\dot{Q})}$ of 0.16.

Altemeier and colleagues (45) explored the degree to which regional convective ventilation and perfusion predicts whole lung gas exchange. They used aerosolized and hematogenously delivered fluorescent microspheres to measure regional ventilation and perfusion to 1.9 cm^3 pieces of lung from prone pigs. Ventilation and perfusion were measured before and after vascular embolization with

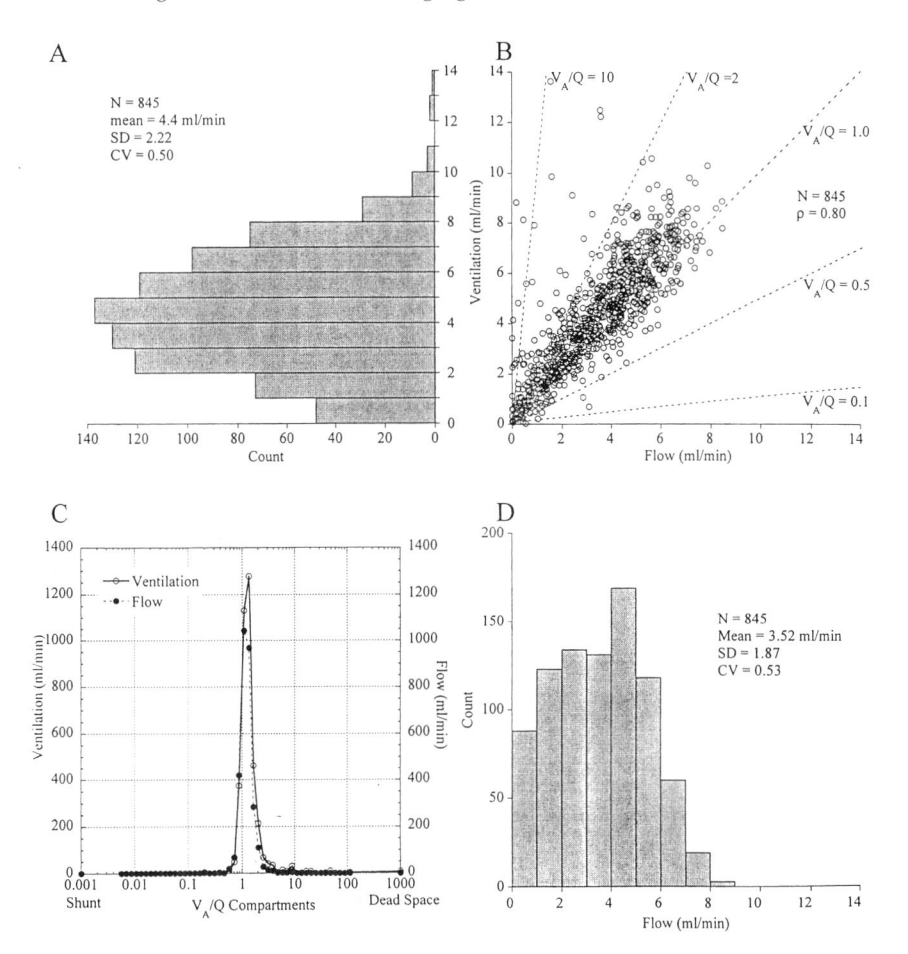

Figure 6 Ventilation and perfusion distributions measured with aerosolized and hematogenously delivered fluorescent microspheres from one animal. The ventilation and perfusion distributions to 845 lung pieces are shown in histograms A and D, respectively. The correlation between regional ventilation and perfusion for all lung pieces is present in graph B. Dotted lines radiating from origin represent isopleths of $\dot{V}_A/\dot{Q}$ ratios. Histograms A and D are obtained by collapsing each point in B to the appropriate axis. Data can be reduced to a 50-compartment model by binning the $\dot{V}_A/\dot{Q}$ ratios from each lung piece and displaying them in a format familiarized by MIGET as in C.

780 μm diameter plastic spheres. Using measured mixed venous tensions of O_2 and CO_2, they calculated the alveolar tensions of O_2 and CO_2 in each lung piece before and after embolization. Assuming complete equilibration between alveolar and capillary gases, capillary gas contents, flow-weighted averages of arterial O_2, and CO_2 tensions were calculated and compared to measured arterial gas tensions (Fig. 7).

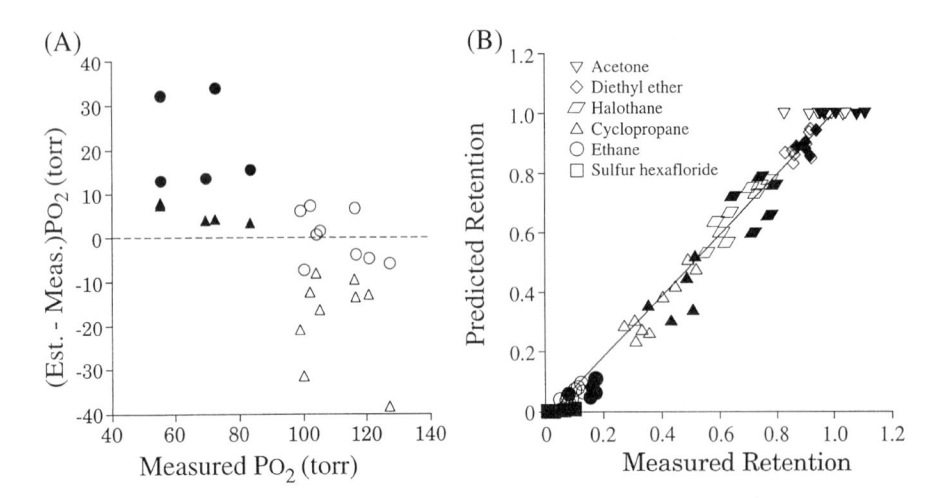

Figure 7 Gas exchange predicted from regional ventilation and perfusion estimated by aerosolized and hematogenously delivered microspheres. (A) Difference between estimated Pao₂ and measured Pao₂ in normal (open markers, repeated twice) and post embolization (closed markers) lungs of 5 animals. Circles represent Pao₂ estimated from regional ventilation and perfusion measurements and the triangles represent Pao₂ estimated from MIGET. (B) Retention of six inert gases in normal (open markers, repeated twice) and post embolization (closed markers) lungs of 5 animals. Predicted retentions are calculated from the blood:gas partition coefficients of each gas and $\dot{V}_A/\dot{Q}$ ratios in each lung piece. (Adapted from Ref. 11, with permission.)

The AaPo₂ differences calculated from regional ventilation and perfusion estimates were not statistically different from the observed AaPo₂ difference at baseline, but they underestimated the observed AaPo₂ difference following vascular embolization. The traditional six inert gases from the Multiple Inert Gas Elimination Technique (MIGET) (46) were infused intravenously and their excretions and retentions determined from exhaled and arterial gas samples. Using the blood:gas partition coefficients of each gas and measured $\dot{V}_A/\dot{Q}$ ratio in each lung piece, estimated retentions of each gas were determined for each piece and a flow-weighted average calculated for the entire lung. The retention fractions were accurately predicted for all six gases before and after vascular embolization (Fig. 7).

The estimated alveolar gas tensions of O₂ and CO₂ for each lung piece can be explored in the spatial domain for topographical patterns of distribution. Figure 8 presents the calculated partial pressure of alveolar O₂ against height up the lung in one animal. Note the large degree of variability within isogravitational planes and the slight predisposition for O₂ tensions to be higher in the superior regions. Because these animals were prone with more uniform distribution of ventilation and perfusion, a vertical gradient was not expected.

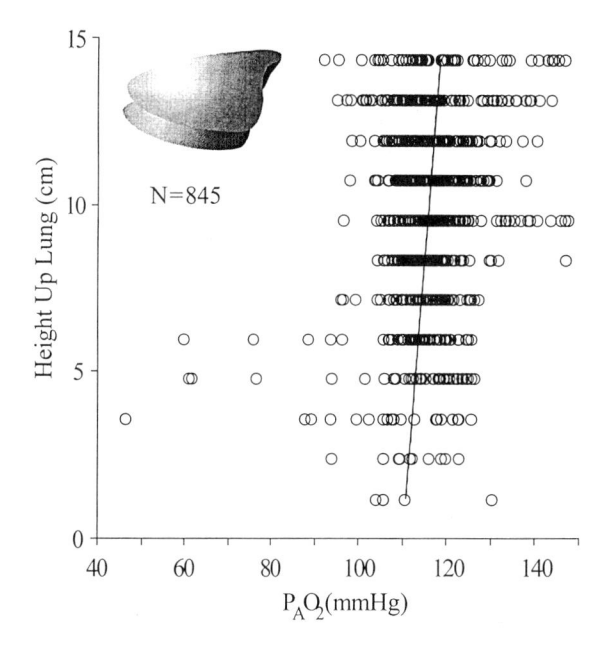

Figure 8 Vertical distribution of alveolar partial pressures of alveolar O_2 determined from the ventilation and perfusion ratios in each of 845 lung pieces from a prone pig. Note the large degree of variability within isogravitational planes and the slight predisposition for O_2 tensions to be higher in the superior regions.

The mechanisms matching heterogeneous perfusion and ventilation distributions are unknown (47). While hypoxic pulmonary vasoconstriction (HPV) has been championed as the most likely mechanism to match local perfusion to ventilation, experimental data suggest that HPV does not play an important role in the normal lung (48,49). Regional pneumoconstriction in response to local CO_2 tensions has also been proposed as a means of matching ventilation to perfusion (50–52). This effect has been shown only in experimental preparations using whole-lung pulmonary artery occlusion and can be ablated by inhalation of 3% CO_2 in air and partially blocked by inhalation of 1.5% CO_2 in air (51). Reinspiration of CO_2 from common dead space may impose a lower volume limit at which pneumonconstriction can play a significant role in redistributing ventilation.

The efficient exchange of pulmonary gases in the absence of known regulators indicates that the lung is functionally well designed. Feedback loops and local regulators are needed only for imperfect designs (53). If true, the lung is constructed so that local vascular resistances and parenchymal compliances are well matched. It is tempting to speculate that within the myriad of growth factors found in the developing lung (54), some may provide the spatial link between vascular development and parenchymal mechanics.

E. Teleological Arguments for Fractal Structures

Construction of fractal structures reveals a potential advantage in coding for growth and development of the complex gas-exchanging networks. Since a complete genetic description for every alveolus and capillary is not possible, elementary recursive rules may exist to guide their construction. Iversen and Nicolaysen (55) observed a large range of fractal dimensions across animals, but found a very strong correlation (r = 0.98) between fractal dimensions of skeletal and cardiac muscle within animals. Although these operational rules are speculative, a coding for self-similar structures is clearly the most efficient algorithm to explain both the order and complexity of ontogeny.

Efficiency of the finalized structures is also important to the organism. Lefevre (56) has shown that a self-similar branching model of the pulmonary vascular system optimizes the cost-function (energy-materials) relationship while closely approximating physiological and morphometrical data. West and colleagues (57) recently hypothesized that biological functions are limited by the transport of materials throughout the organism and demonstrated that fractal networks such as vascular and bronchial trees produce scaling relationships that follow observed allometric scaling laws.

Fractal systems provide a unifying mechanism for development and function of the vascular trees and, in particular, the pulmonary circulation and airways. By providing a geometric framework to describe these apparently irregular patterns, fractal systems capture both the richness of physiological structures and their function in a single model.

F. Reconciling Discrepancies Between Gravitational and Fractal Models

Do the above observations negate the basic principles of the gravitational model? We believe not, but that a reorientation of perspectives is necessary with a new emphasis on the geometric structure of the pulmonary vascular tree and regional parenchymal compliances. Gravity must play a role in an organ that has a large vertical dimension and a fluid filled compliant vascular system. The geometry of the pulmonary vascular tree and variability in local parenchymal compliance must also have an influence on regional perfusion and ventilation heterogeneity. It is the relative contribution of gravity and fractal structures to the heterogeneity of perfusion and ventilation that define the differences between the gravitational and fractal models.

The principle difference between the gravitational and fractal models of perfusion, ventilation, and gas exchange is the primary mechanism responsible for the observed heterogeneities. The gravitational model proposes that gravity is the primary determinant of perfusion and ventilation variability while the fractal model asserts that assymmetries in vascular branching and local compliances produce heterogeneity in perfusion and ventilation. Although not specifically stated, the gravitational model implies or predicts that perfusion and ventilation should be uniform within isogravitational planes because there are no hydrostatic or alveolar pressure gradients. A mechanism for isogravitational perfusion heterogeneity has been proposed but this variability is predicted only at the capillary level and is thought to be random (58). Hence perfusion and ventilation should be nearly uniform in saline-filled lungs (59) and under conditions of microgravity (60). In contrast, the fractal model predicts that variability in perfusion and ventilation should exist within isogravitational planes and this heterogeneity should be spatially correlated. Consequently, both perfusion and ventilation should change little with alterations in the gravity vector and should remain heterogeneous during microgravity.

The gravitational model of perfusion, ventilation, and gas exchange is largely based upon studies performed in the 1960s using chest wall scintillation counters that provided relatively crude measurements (4). Because the scintillation counters in these initial studies were unable to measure perfusion variability within isogravitational planes, only the vertical heterogeneity of perfusion and ventilation was observed. Spatial resolution of recent animal experiments can be reduced to the level of earlier experiments using chest wall scintillation counters by averaging data within isogravitational planes. When high-resolution data sets are averaged to yield a few isogravitational planes, vertical height up the lung becomes the key determinant of blood flow distribution. Thus, recent findings do not conflict with older data; higher resolution methods simply reveal other mechanisms that could not be observed previously.

The gravitational model also states that the zonal conditions within the lung are vertically stacked on top of each other. Zone 1 conditions ($P_A > P_a > P_v$) exist only above the horizontal plane of zone 2 conditions ($P_a > P_A > P_v$) which exists just above the horizontal plane of zone 3 conditions ($P_a > P_v > P_A$). With the realization that flow and driving pressures (61) are heterogeneous within isogravitational planes, it becomes apparent that multiple zonal conditions exist within a horizontal plane. Because the word ''zone'' now connotes vertical distributions, it may be less confusing to refer to these pressure relationships as occurring within ''regions.'' Each isogravitational plane has a distribution of regional pressure relationships. Gravity exerts its effects on blood flow distribution by increasing the hydrostatic pressure toward dependent lung regions. Although the mean flow per isogravitational plane increases down the lung, perfusion within isogravitational planes remains heterogeneous. Each isogravitational plane will have a distribution of ''zonal'' conditions. Gravity likely alters the statistical distribution of these regions, shifting the frequency distribution toward region 2 and 3 conditions down the lung, eventually resulting in only region 3 conditions in the most dependent regions.

Isogravitational perfusion and ventilation are not randomly distributed in space. Previous studies have revealed that perfusion and ventilation heterogeneity is spatially correlated (18,23,42,62). High-flow regions are adjacent to other high-flow regions and low-flow regions are near other low-flow regions. The spatial correlation of pulmonary perfusion may be attributed to the branching structure of the pulmonary vascular network (32) while the spatial correlation of ventilation may be due to local differences in compliance (38). Because high-flow regions are possible only at the expense of flow to other regions, flows become dissimilar and eventually correlate negatively as the distance between regions increases. A simple network, producing both heterogeneous and spatially correlated flows, can be described with a fractal model (33). Given the degree of isogravitational perfusion heterogeneity, it seems reasonable to hypothesize that gravity cannot play an important role matching ventilation and perfusion; other mechanisms must be responsible for their intimate matching.

II. Determinants of O_2 and CO_2 Exchange at Rest

It is important to note that arterial respiratory blood gases reflect not only the functional conditions of the lung as a gas exchanger, thereby their intrapulmonary determinants (i.e. ventilation-perfusion heterogeneities, intrapulmonary shunt and alveolar-end-capillary diffusion limitation for oxygen) (63–66), but also the conditions under which the lung operates, namely the composition of inspired gas and mixed venous blood (i.e. extrapulmonary factors) (63–68). Table 1 shows the intrapulmonary factors that may contribute individually, or in combination, to hypoxemia and hypercapnia as well as the extrapulmonary factors that can also influence arterial P_{O_2} and P_{CO_2}.

A. Intrapulmonary Factors

Ideally, the highest efficiency of the lung as O_2 and CO_2 exchanger should be achieved when ventilation and blood flow to each individual alveolar unit are adequately balanced ($\dot{V}_A = \dot{Q}$) and, consequently, homogeneity of $\dot{V}_A/\dot{Q}$ ratios among alveolar units is present. This so called "perfect lung," however, is not seen because mild heterogeneities of pulmonary $\dot{V}_A/\dot{Q}$ matching are present in normal subjects, as described above. The characteristic $\dot{V}_A/\dot{Q}$ distribution in normals obtained with the multiple inert gas elimination technique (MIGET) (46,69,70) is displayed in Fig. 1. It consists of narrow perfusion and ventilation distributions centered around a $\dot{V}_A/\dot{Q}$ ratio of 1.0. No ventilation to lung units with $\dot{V}_A/\dot{Q}$ ratios > 10 (high $\dot{V}_A/\dot{Q}$) is observed. Similarly, perfusion to lung units with low $\dot{V}_A/\dot{Q}$ ratio (Q_T to $\dot{V}_A/\dot{Q}$ < 0.1) is not present. *Dead space* defined as the amount of ventilation to $\dot{V}_A/\dot{Q}$ ratios > 100 (including anatomical and physiological dead space) is approximately 30% in normal subjects. *Shunt* can be due to perfusion of unventilated or extremely poorly ventilated lung regions (intrapulmonary shunt) or to direct vascular communications such as atrial septal defects with reverse (right to left) flow, or (rarely) to arterio-venous channels in the lung. As one of the standard 50 "compartments" used in the computed program of the MIGET, intrapulmonary shunt is directly estimated just as the flow to all other lung units.

The distinguishing feature of intrapulmonary shunt for the purpose of gas exchange is complete retention of all inert gases in the blood flowing through such regions. No (or virtually no) perfusion to unventilated alveolar units (shunt) is present in normal subjects (69). Physiological post-pulmonary shunt (not detectable by the MIGET) due to the Thebesian veins (71) draining blood flow from the coronary veins directly to the left atrium and the bronchial venous blood going to pulmonary veins is negligible in man ($< 1\%$ of cardiac output). *Limitation of alveolar to end capillary O_2 diffusion* is also excluded by the agreement between measured PaO_2 and estimated PO_2 by the MIGET (65).

B. Extrapulmonary Factors

Extrapulmonary factors (Table 1) can be of primary importance in modulating arterial respiratory blood gases in pulmonary diseases, as described in the following chapters. An important determinant of arterial PO_2 is the partial pressure of inspired oxygen (P_IO_2) particularly in subjects with normal lungs or a mild degree of mismatching. Patients with severe $\dot{V}_A/\dot{Q}$ inequality show a diminished response of PaO_2 as the P_IO_2 is increased. This behavior is attributed to the alveoli with very low $\dot{V}_A/\dot{Q}$ ratios, because alveolar PO_2 remains relatively low in these units, even when the inspired PO_2 is substantially increased. However, even in lungs with a very severe degrees of $\dot{V}_A/\dot{Q}$ inequality, the arterial PO_2 reaches high values during 100% O_2 breathing. By contrast, little response of arterial PO_2 to high P_IO_2 is observed when hypoxemia is caused by intrapulmonary shunt (i.e., in acute respiratory distress syndrome (ARDS)). It is important here to emphasize that while mixed venous PO_2 ($P\bar{v}O_2$) has an important role modulating arterial PO_2 in disease, changes in $P\bar{v}O_2$ have only a moderate impact on arterial oxygenation in healthy subjects. Diminished $P\bar{v}O_2$ may result from: 1) low cardiac output, 2) increased oxygen uptake, and/or 3) a decreased arterial blood oxygen content (64). As reported in Chapter 8, the impact of $P\bar{v}O_2$ on arterial PO_2 varies with the pattern and degree of severity of $\dot{V}_A/\dot{Q}$ inequality.

III. Pulmonary Gas Exchange During Exercise

It is well known that ventilation and cardiac output markedly increase during exercise to match O_2 transport with augmented cellular O_2 requirements (72). Since ventilation increases to a relatively higher extent than pulmonary blood flow, the ratio of total alveolar ventilation to blood flow (overall ratio) rises rather substantially. At moderate levels of exercise, the dispersion of the $\dot{V}_A/\dot{Q}$ distributions does not change (73–75) but the $\dot{V}_A/\dot{Q}$ ratios at the mean of both ventilation and perfusion distributions markedly increase due to the higher overall $\dot{V}_A/\dot{Q}$ ratio. Consequently, the efficiency of the lung as an O_2 and CO_2 exchanger improves at these exercise levels. Mixed venous PO_2 falls dramatically during exercise because the relative increase in $\dot{V}O_2$ is considerably greater than that of cardiac output, and mixed venous P_{CO_2} levels rise equally as remarkably. Arterial P_{O_2} levels generally remain unchanged until extremely high levels of exercise are undertaken. Arterial P_{CO_2} levels are also relatively stable until the appearance of high blood lactate levels generates acidosis, even more ventilation, and thus a fall in P_{CO_2} levels. The alveolar-arterial O_2 gradient (AaP_{O_2}), however, progressively increases with the level of exercise, reaching values of 20–30 mm Hg close to maximal exercise ($\dot{V}_{O_2}$) in average subjects, and even greater (up to 40 mm Hg or more) in some elite athletes (76). Such an increase in AaP_{O_2} indicates inefficiency of pulmonary gas exchange during heavy exercise which is even more apparent in other animal species, such as horses (77). It has been shown that the increase in the AaP_{O_2} during exercise is due, in part, to $\dot{V}_A/\dot{Q}$ mismatching (73–75) but it is mostly explained by alveolar-end capillary O_2 diffusion limitation (74,78,79). Abnormalities of pulmonary gas exchange during exercise in healthy subjects are clearly accentuated if exercise is carried out during hypoxia that is produced either breathing a low inspired O_2 fraction (79) or simulating altitude in a hypobaric chamber (73,74,78,80). The increase in the dispersion of the perfusion distribution (Log SD_Q) during heavy exercise is not associated with altered spirometry, but shows a significant correlation with the increase in mean pulmonary artery pressure. Experimental studies suggest that development of subclinical pulmonary edema (74,80) may explain the deterioration of pulmonary gas exchange during heavy exercise, but no direct evidence in man has been obtained, as yet (81). A more detailed analysis of the integrated pulmonary and systemic responses during different modalities of exercise is done in Chapter 18.

IV. Effects of Aging on Pulmonary Gas Exchange

Aging causes important changes in several physiological variables of the lung. Elastic recoil is progressively reduced (82), vital capacity and maximal expiratory flow rates fall (83), closing volume is increased (84), and arterial P_{O_2} diminishes (85). Since arterial P_{CO_2} does not rise, the fall in arterial P_{O_2} must indicate an increase in the alveolar-arterial P_{O_2} difference (AaP_{O_2}). This section examines two relevant aspects of the effects of aging on pulmonary gas exchange: 1) the underlying factors that determine the increase in AaP_{O_2} with age, and 2) the impact of age-induced fall in PaO_2 on reference values for elderly people.

The AaP_{O_2} will increase with age if any one or more of three forms of gas exchange defect develop: 1) right to left shunting of venous blood, 2) diffusion limitation of alveolar-capillary O_2 exchange, or 3) ventilation/perfusion ($\dot{V}_A/\dot{Q}$) inequality. In young healthy subjects, as described above, intrapulmonary shunts have been found to be either small or nonexistent (69), postpulmonary shunts appear to be negligible (73,74,78), and, at rest, evidence for diffusion limitation has not been found (73,74,78). For older subjects, these conclusions were only tentative, since data suggesting that $\dot{V}_A/\dot{Q}$ inequality increased significantly with age (86) had been obtained from very small numbers of subjects. However, it has been recently shown in a group of 51 healthy subjects that $\dot{V}_A/\dot{Q}$ inequality does indeed increase with age (87). Moreover, none of the other factors alluded to (intrapulmonary shunt, post-pulmonary shunt, or alveolar-end capillary O_2 diffusion limitation) seem to play a significant role decreasing the efficiency of the lung as O_2 exchanger in the elderly. It is notable, however, that the increase in $\dot{V}_A/\dot{Q}$ inequality over the span of about 50 years is physiologically very small with dispersion (ie., Log SD_Q) increasing on average by only about 0.1 from 0.36 at age 20 to 0.47 at age 70. The data fit well with Pa_{O_2} measured independently. While previously established 95% upper confidence limits for the dispersion of the perfusion and ventilation distribution (Log SD_Q and Log SD_V, respectively) in young subjects (86) were confirmed in this study, the increase in mismatch with age suggests that these limits of normalcy be raised for older subjects. Thus at age 20, the 95% upper limit on Log SD_Q is 0.60 while at age 70 it is 0.70. Those for Log SD_V are, respectively, 0.65 and 0.75, and for subjects of intermediate age, linear interpolation between these values is reasonable. These limits should be useful for interpreting $\dot{V}_A/\dot{Q}$ dispersion data in older subjects with cardiopulmonary diseases.

A. Increase of $\dot{V}_A/\dot{Q}$ Inequality with Age

The analysis of the cause(s) of the increase in $\dot{V}_A/\dot{Q}$ mismatch with age showed that only about 10% of the total variance in dispersion was attributable to age. A similar amount was due to intrasubject variability, but none was due to variation in FEV_1 (% predicted), FEV_1/FVC ratio, weight or height. Thus, a large portion of intersubject variability remained unexplained (87). It is certainly possible that age could increase $\dot{V}_A/\dot{Q}$ inequality as a result of increases in closing volume (84) such that in older subjects some airways are closed during normal tidal breathing, reducing local ventilation and producing $\dot{V}_A/\dot{Q}$ mismatch. The study (87) did not measure closing volume, but since this mechanism is highly unlikely to compromise $\dot{V}_A/\dot{Q}$ relationships in young normal subjects, and since the variance in Log SD was as great among the young as the old subjects, we would argue that closing volume was not a strong candidate for the variance in $\dot{V}_A/\dot{Q}$ matching. In a much smaller number of subjects consisting of both young and middle-aged volunteers studied for other reasons, differences in closing volume were apparent as a function of age, but there were no evident effects on $\dot{V}_A/\dot{Q}$ mismatching of increasing closing volume by water immersion to the neck (88). Both dry and immersed, the older subjects had greater $\dot{V}_A/\dot{Q}$ mismatch than the younger subjects. Taken together, these findings also do not support a role for airway closure as an explanation for age-related changes in $\dot{V}_A/\dot{Q}$ inequality. It may relate with the gradual breakdown of alveolar walls with age.

B. Influence of Errors in the Inert Gas Data (87)

One established facet of the multiple inert gas elimination technique is that there is an association between dispersion indices Log SD_Q and Log SD_V and the residual sum of squares (RSS). The RSS is the sum of squares of the differences between the measured inert gas retentions (ratio of arterial partial pressure to mixed venous partial pressure of each inert gas) (65) and those of the best fit to the measured values (which are the retentions associated with the recovered $\dot{V}_A/\dot{Q}$ distribution). If a given, initially error-free, set of retentions is perturbed with progressively increasing amounts of random error, and the data submitted to the inert gas computer analysis, the recovered values of Log SD_Q and Log SD_V will be smaller the greater the errors, and the RSS will become obviously larger (70). This, therefore, raises the question of whether experimental error that is systematically lower in older subjects is an explanation for the observed increase in Log SD_Q with age. Figure 9 shows that there is indeed a slight fall in RSS with age (bottom panel) that, at first sight, is compatible with the hypothesis that the observed increase in $\dot{V}_A/\dot{Q}$ dispersion with age is a falsely positive result due to less experimental error in

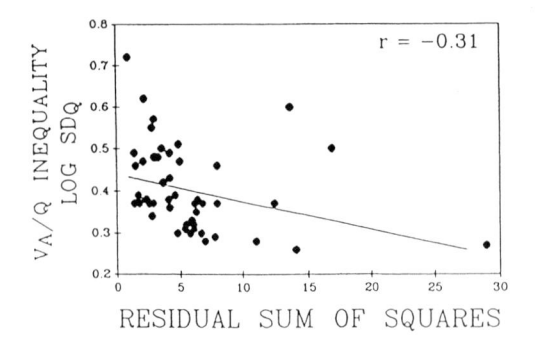

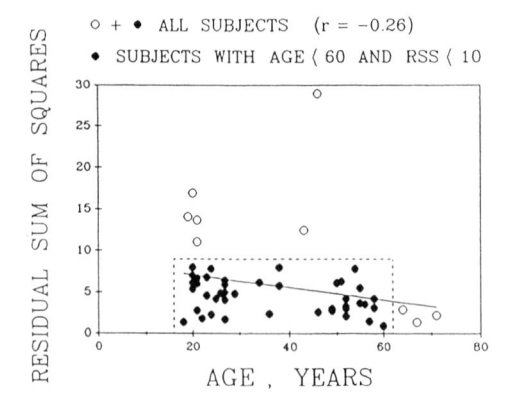

Figure 9 Relationships amongst $\dot{V}_A/\dot{Q}$ inequality (Log SD_Q), the residual sum of squares and age. See text for interpretation.

studying older subjects. Furthermore, the top panel of Fig. 9 confirms the association, weak though it is, between Log SD_Q and RSS. The situation, however, is made complicated by another reason for such an association that has nothing to do with the magnitude of random errors. For a given level of experimental error, processing a retention data set from a lung that has very little $\dot{V}_A/\dot{Q}$ mismatch will result in a larger RSS than the identical processing of a data set from a lung with more $\dot{V}_A/\dot{Q}$ mismatch (89,90). This must also lead to a negative correlation between RSS and Log SD_Q, but this is an expected and physiological result.

The question is, therefore, to choose between the two reasons for the observed association between $\dot{V}_A/\dot{Q}$ dispersion and RSS shown in Fig. 9. It is a consequence of difference in errors between young and old subjects producing an artifact, or a consequence of older subjects truly having more $\dot{V}_A/\dot{Q}$ mismatching? In Fig. 9 (bottom panel) we have divided the subjects into two sets demarcated by the dashed lines. Subjects within the lines (solid circles) show complete overlap in RSS in relation to age. Open circles show data for younger subjects with high RSS and older subjects with lower RSS. The relationship between Log SD_Q and age is the same for the entire population as for the selected group who do not show age-dependent changes in the RSS. This suggests that the small mean fall in RSS with age does not give rise to an apparent increase in Log SD_Q.

Another argument against the idea that systematic differences in error between young and old subjects cause the Log SD_Q differences comes from analysis of the duplicate data for individual subjects (a total of 120 sets obtained from the 51 subjects) (87). The agreement between duplicate sets was no better for old than young subjects, both groups (above and below 40) having a coefficient of variation of 13%.

A third point comes from multiple linear regression of Log SD_Q against both age and RSS. The regression equation was:

$$\text{Log } SD_Q = 0.362 + 0.00183 * \text{AGE} - 0.00497 * \text{RSS} \tag{4}$$

The single regression between age and Log SD_Q was:

$$\text{Log } SD_Q = 0.320 + 0.00221 * \text{AGE} \tag{5}$$

while, from Fig. 9 bottom panel, that between age and RSS for all 51 subjects was:

$$\text{RSS} = 8.62 - 0.076 * \text{AGE} \tag{6}$$

Using Eq. (2), the total increase in Log SD_Q with age over the 50 year span from age 20 to 70 is 50 * 0.00221, or 0.111. From Eq. (4), at constant RSS, the contribution from age is 50 * 0.00183, or 0.092. From Eq. (6), RSS at age 20 would average 7.1 while that at age 70 would be 3.3. These values of RSS would, via Eq. (5), reduce apparent Log SD_Q by 7.1 * 0.00497, or by 0.035, at age 20 and by 3.3 * 0.00497, or by 0.016 at age 70. The difference between 0.035 and 0.016 is then the average effect of the fall in RSS (over 50 years) in apparent Log SD_Q: 0.019. Note that this contribution (which, summed with that of age, 0.092, equals the total of 0.111) could still be based on either the artifact of potentially different error levels with age or on the physiological effect of more $\dot{V}_A/\dot{Q}$ mismatch occurring with age. But, in either case, the effects of age dominate, contributing 0.092/0.111 or 83% of the total change in Log SD_Q observed. For all of these reasons, we argue that the effects of age on Log SD_Q are real and not an artifact of experimental error.

C. Reference Values for Arterial Respiratory Blood Gases

Arterial blood gas analysis has played an important role in managing patients with cardiopulmonary diseases for approximately 30 years. Unfortunately, most reference equations still used to predict "normal" arterial blood gas values in the clinical setting are now over 20 years old (85,91–101). Respiratory blood gases are nowadays routinely analyzed on automated machines which use computer algorithms to adjust for system nonlinearities and inaccuracies. As a result, they may produce significantly different results than the manual instruments used in earlier studies. A recent study on blood gases in healthy subjects (102) reported a linear decay of Pa_{O_2} between ages 40 to 75, but no further fall in Pa_{O_2} was observed in elderly people up to 90 years old. More recently, a set of reference equations for arterial blood gas and CO-oximeter analytes based on healthy lifetime nonsmokers (ages 18 to 81) studied in different laboratories has been reported (103). The mean decline

Table 2 Regression Equations for Arterial Blood Gas Measurements Using Only Sea Level Data* (N = 96, 52 Females, 44 Males)

	Constant	Age	Gender	r^2	SEE
Pa_{O_2}	106.603	−0.2447		0.30	7.301
Pa_{CO_2}	36.837		1.256	0.41	3.059
AaP_{O_2}	−4.404	0.2610		0.38	6.478
Sa_{O_2}	97.659	−0.0296		0.32	0.847
Hb	12.32		1.717	0.45	0.952
MetHb	0.596		−0.0928	0.04	0.218

*Values under Age and Gender are regression coefficients.
Male = 1, Female = 0 (the gender coefficient is zero for females)
r^2 = coefficient of determination
SEE = standard error of estimate
Age in years
The lower limit of the reference range is calculated as: predicted value − 1.96 SEE.
No significant regressions were found for pH and COHb. Reference values are calculated using the mean and standard deviation of the measured values. Mean ± SD for pH = 7.423 ± 0.021. Mean ± SD for COHb = 1.627 ± 0.540.
Source: Ref. (103).

in Pao$_2$ with age (−0.245 mm Hg/year) (103) was consistent with other studies (92,94–96). At sea level, mean Pao$_2$ and mean AaPo$_2$ at age 20 were 100 ± 5.3 and 2.0 ± 5.7 mm Hg, respectively. The corresponding figures at age 70 and above were 88.7 ± 10.7 and 14.8 ± 8.8 mm Hg. Table 2 indicates the proposed reference equations at sea level (103).

V. Summary

It is concluded that the pulmonary system in healthy subjects is inherently heterogeneous in terms of regional perfusion and ventilation, but it has a minor impact in the efficiency of the lung as O$_2$ and CO$_2$ exchanger. The impact of gravitational and nongravitational factors on regional pulmonary heterogeneity is examined, the challenge is renewed to identify the mechanisms responsible for efficient exchange of pulmonary gases in man. The characteristics of the ventilation/perfusion distributions are summarized, as well as the interactions between intrapulmonary and extrapulmonary factors modulating arterial respiratory blood gases at rest and during exercise. The effects of aging on pulmonary gas exchange and the factors that explain the increase in alveolar-arterial Po$_2$ difference with age are examined. Finally, recent reports on reference values for arterial respiratory blood gases are provided.

References

1. Krogh A, Lindhard J. The volume of the dead space in breathing and the mixing of gases in the lungs of man. J Physiol 1917; 51:59–90.
2. Haldane JS. Respiration. New Haven, CT: Yale University Press. 1922.
3. West JB. Causes of carbon dioxide retention in lung disease. New Engl J Med 1971; 284:1232–1236.
4. West JB. Regional differences in gas exchange in the lung of erect man. J Appl Physiol 1962; 17:893–898.
5. West JB. Regional differences in the lung. New York: Academic Press. 1977.
6. Wagner PD, Laravuso RB, Uhl RR, West JB. Continuous distributions of ventilation-perfusion ratios in normal subjects breathing air and 100% O$_2$. J Clin Invest 1974; 54:54–68.
7. Gale GE, Torre-Bueno J, Moon RE, Salzman HA, Wagner PD. Ventilation-perfusion inequality in normal humans during exercise. J Appl Physiol 1985; 58:978–988.
8. Wagner PD, Gale GE, Moon RE, Torre-Bueno JE, Stolp BW, Saltzman HA. Pulmonary gas exchange in humans exercising at sea level and simulated altitude. J Appl Physiol 1986; 61:260–270.
9. Hammond MD, Gale GE, Kapitan KS, Ries A, Wagner PD. Pulmonary gas exchange in humans during exercise at sea level. J Appl Physiol 1986; 60:1590–1598.
10. Hammond MD, Gale GE, Kapitan KS, Ries A, Wagner PD. Pulmonary gas exchange in humans during normobaric hypoxic exercise. J Appl Physiol 1985; 58:978–988.

11. Ball WC, Stewart PB, Newsham LGS, Bates DV. Regional pulmonary function studied with xenon. J Clin Invest 1962; 41:519–531.
12. Dollery CT, Gillam PMS. The distribtuion of blood and gas within the lungs measured by scanning after administration of 133Xe. Thorax 1963; 18:316–325.
13. West JB, Dollery CT. Distribution of blood flow and ventilation-perfusion in the lung, measured with radioactive CO_2. J Appl Physiol 1960; 15:405–410.
14. West JB, Dollery CT, Naimark A. Distribution of blood flow in isolated lung: relation to vascular and alveolar pressures. J Appl Physiol 1964; 55:1341–1348.
15. Milic-Emili J, Henderson JAM, Dolovich MB, Trop D, Kanenko K. Regional distribution of inspired gas in the lung. J Appl Physiol 1966; 21:749–759.
16. Reed JH, Wood EH. Effect of body position on vertical distribution of pulmonary blood flow. J Appl Physiol 1970; 28:303–311.
17. Greenleaf JF, Ritman EL, Sass DJ, Wood EH. Spatial distribution of pulmonary blood flow in dogs in left decubitus position. J Appl Physiol 1974; 81:1051–1061.
18. Caruthers SD, Harris TR. Effects of pulmonary blood flow on the fractal heterogeneity in sheep lungs. J Appl Physiol 1994; 77:1474–1479.
19. Glenny RW, Lamm WJ, Albert RK, Robertson HT. Gravity is a minor determinant of pulmonary blood flow distribution. J Appl Physiol 1999; 71:620–629.
20. Hlastala MP, Bernard SL, Erickson HH, Fedde MR, Gaughan EM, McMurphy R, Emery MJ, Polissar N, Glenny RW. Pulmonary blood flow distribution in standing horses is not dominated by gravity. J Appl Physiol 1996; 81:1051–1061.
21. Melsom MN, Flatebo T, Kramer-Johansen J, Aulie A, Sjaastad OV, Iversen PO, Nicolaysen G. Both gravity and non-gravity dependent factor determine regional blood flow within the goat lung. Acta Physiol Scand 1995; 153:343–353.
22. Nicolaysen G, Shepard J, Onizuka M, Tanita T, Hattner RS, Staub NC. No gravity-independent gradient of blood flow distribution in dog lung. J Appl Physiol 1987; 57:1710–1714.
23. Parker JC, Ardell JL, Hamm CR, Barman SA, Coker PJ. Regional pulmonary blood flow during rest, tilt, and exercise in unanesthetized dogs. J Appl Physiol 1995; 78:838–846.
24. Prisk GK, Guy HJB, Elliot AR, West JB. Inhomogeneity of pulmonary perfusion during sustained microgravity on SLS-1. J Appl Physiol 1994; 76:1730–1738.
25. Prisk GK, Elliot AR, Guy HJB, Kosonen JM, West JB. Pulmonary gas exchange and its determinants during sustained microgravity on Spacelabs SLS-1 and SLS-2. J Appl Physiol 1995; 79:1290–1298.
26. Bassingthwaighte JB. Fractal nature of regional myocardial blood flow heterogeneity. Circ Res 1989; 65:578–590.
27. Van Beek JHGM, Roger SA, Bassingthwaighte JB. Regional myocardial flow heterogeneity explained with fractal networks. Am J Physiol 1989; 257:H1670–H1680.
28. Bassingthwaighte JB. Physiologic heterogeneity: fractals link determinism and randomness in structures and functions. News Physiol Sci 1988; 5–10.
29. Glenny RW, Robertson HT. Fractal modeling of pulmonary blood flow heterogeneity. J Appl Physiol 1991; 79:357–369.
30. Glenny RW, Bernard S, Barlow C, Kelly J, Robertson HT. Spatial distribution of pulmonary blood flow at a microscopic scale of resolution. American Journal of Respiratory and Critical Care Medicine 1995; 151(4):A518 (Abstract).

31. Sinclair SE, Glenny RW, Mckinney S, Bernard SL, Hlastala MP. Pulmonary blood flow distribution is fractal in resting and exercising horses. American Journal of Respiratory and Critical Care Medicine 1997; 155(4):A117 (Abstract).
32. Glenny RW. Spatial correlation of regional pulmonary perfusion. J Appl Physiol 1992; 72:2378–2386.
33. Glenny RW, Robertson HT. A computer simulation of pulmonary perfusion in three dimensions. J Appl Physiol 1995; 79:357–369.
34. Parker JC, Cave CB, Ardell JL, Hamm CR, Williams SG. Vascular tree structure affects lung blood flow heterogeneity simulated in three dimensions. J Appl Physiol 1997; 83:1370–1382.
35. Amis TC, Stewart PB, Newsham LGS, Bates JH. Effect of posture on inter-regional distribution of pulmonary ventilation in man. Respir Physiol 1984; 56:145–167.
36. Olson LE, Rodarte JR. Regional differences in expansion in excised dog lung lobes. J Appl Physiol 1984; 57:1710–1714.
37. Hubmayr, RD, Walters BJ, Chevalier PA, Rodarte JR, Olson LE. Topographical distribution of regional lung volume in anesthetized dogs. J Appl Physiol 1983; 54:1048–1056.
38. Rodarte JR, Chaniotakis M, Wilson TA. Variability of parenchymal expansion measured by computed tomography. J Appl Physiol 1989; 67:226–231.
39. Robertson HT, Glenny RW, Stanford D, Mclnnes LM, Luchtel DL, Covert D. High-resolution maps of regional ventilation utilizing inhaled fluorescent microspheres. J Appl Physiol 1997; 67:226–231.
40. Melsom MN, Kramer JJ, Flatebo T, Muller C, Nicolaysen G. Distribution of pulmonary ventilation and perfusion measured simultaneously in awake goats. Acta Physiol Scand 1997; 159:199–208.
41. Verbanck S, Linnarsson D, Prisk GK, Paiva M. Specific ventilation distribution in microgravity. J Appl Physiol 1996; 80:1458–1465.
42. Altemeier WA, Mure M, McKinney SE, Robertson HT, Glenny RW. Regional ventilation heterogeneity has fractal properties that are posture dependent. American Journal of Respiratory and Critical Care Medicine 1998; 155:A370 (Abstract).
43. Wilson TA, Beck KC. Contributions of ventilation and perfusion inhomogeneities to the VA/Q distribution. J Appl Physiol 1992; 72:2298–2304.
44. Olszowka AJ, Farhi LE. A system of digital computer subroutines for blood gas calculations. Respir Physiol 1968; 4:270–280.
45. Altemeier WA, Robertson HT, Glenny RW. Regional ventilation measured by aerosolized microspheres accurately predicts whole lung gas exchange. J Appl Physiol 1999 (In press).
46. Wagner PD, Saltzman HA, West JB. Measurement of continuous distributions of ventilation-perfusion ratios: theory. J Appl Physiol 1974; 36:588–599.
47. Marshall BE, Hanson J, Frasch F, Hanson CW. Role of hypoxic pulmonary vasoconstriction in pulmonary gas exchange and blood flow distribution: 1. Physiologic concepts. Intensive Care Med 1994; 20:291–297.
48. Hopkins SR, Johnson EC, Richardson RS, Wagner H, De RM, Wagner PD. Effects of inhaled nitric oxide on gas exchange in lungs with shunt or poorly ventilated areas. Am J Respir Crit Care Med 1997; 156:484–491.

49. Pison U, Lopez FA, Heidelmeyer CF, Rossaint R, Falke KJ. Inhaled nitric oxide reverses hypoxic pulmonary vasoconstriction without impairing gas exchange. J Appl Physiol 1995; 74:1287–1292.
50. Ingram RH. Effects of airway versus arterial CO_2 changes on lung mechanics in dogs. J Appl Physiol 1975; 38:603–607.
51. Severinghaus JW, Swenson EW, Finley TN, Lategola MT, Williams J. Unilateral hypoventilation produced in doss by occluding one pulmonary artery. J Appl Physiol 1961; 16:53–60.
52. Simon C, Tsusaki K, Venegas JC. Changes in regional lung mechanics and ventilation distribution after unilateral pulmonary artery occlusion. J Appl Physiol 1997; 82:882–891.
53. Wagner WWJ, Todoran TM, Tanabe N, Wagner TM, Glenny RW, Presson RG. Robust design of the lung: fractal patterns and capillary perfusion independence. J Appl Physiol 1999 (Submitted).
54. Stenmark KR, Mecham RP. Cellular and molecular mechanisms of pulmonary vascular remodeling. Annu Rev Physiol 1997; 59:89–144.
55. Iversen PO, Nicolaysen G. Fractals describe blood flow heterogeneity within skeletal muscle and within myocardium. Am J Physiol 1993; 265:H112–H116.
56. Lefevre J. Teleonomical optimization of a fractal model of the pulmonary arterial bed. Theor Biol 1983; 102:225–248.
57. West GB, Brown JH, Enquist BJ. A general model for the origin of allometric scaling laws in biology. Science 1997; 276:122–126.
58. West JB, Schneider AM, Mitchell MM. Recruitment in networks of pulmonary capillaries. J Appl Physiol 1975; 39:976–984.
59. West JB, Dollery CT, Matthews ME. Distribution of blood flow and ventilation in saline-filled lung. J Appl Physiol 1965; 20:1107–1117.
60. Michels DB, West JB. Distribution of pulmonary ventilation and perfusion during short periods of weightlessness. J Appl Physiol 1978; 45:987–998.
61. Kuhnle GE, Pries AR, Goetz AE. Distribution of microvascular pressure in arteriolar vessel trees of ventilated rabbit lungs. Am J Physiol 1993; 265:H1510–1515.
62. Glenny RW, Robertson HT. Fractal properties of pulmonary blood flow: characterization of spatial heterogeneity. J Appl Physiol 1990; 69:532–545.
63. West JB. Ventilation-perfusion inequality and overall gas exchange in computer models of the lung. Respir Physiol 1969; 7:88–110.
64. West JB. Ventilation-perfusion relationships. Am Rev Respir Dis 1977; 116:919–943.
65. Roca J, Wagner PD. Contribution of multiple inert gas elimination technique to pulmonary medicine, I: Principles and information content of the multiple inert gas elimination technique. Thorax 1993; 49:815–824.
66. West JB, Wagner PD. Pulmonary gas exchange. In West JB, ed., Bioengineering Aspects of the Lung. New York: Marcel Dekker, Inc. 1977, pp. 361–457.
67. Dantzker DR. The influence of cardiovascular function on gas exchange. Clin Chest Med 1983; 4:149–159.
68. Wagner PD. Ventilation-perfusion inequality in catastrophic lung disease. In Prakash O, ed. Applied Physiology in Clinical Respiratory Care. The Hague: Martinus Nijhoff, 1982, pp. 363–379.

69. Wagner PD, Laravuso RB, Uhl RR, West JB. Continuous distributions of ventilation-perfusion ratios in normal subjects breathing air and 100% O_2. J Clin Invest 1974; 54:54–68.
70. Evans JW, Wagner PD. Limits on VA\Q distributions from analysis of experimental inert gas elimination. J Appl Physiol 1977; 36:600–605.
71. West JB. Ventilation/blood flow and gas exchange. Oxford: Blackwell Scientific Publications, 1985.
72. Agustí AGN, Cotes J, Wagner PD. Responses to exercise in lung diseases. In Roca J, Whipp BJ, eds. Clinical Exercise Testing. Sheffield: ERS, 1997, pp. 32–50.
73. Gale, G. E., J. Torre-Bueno, R. E. Moon, H. A. Salzman, and P. D. Wagner. Ventilation-perfusion inequality in normal humans during exercise. J Appl Physiol 58: 978-988, 1985.
74. Wagner PD, Gale GE, Moon RE, Torre-Bueno JE, Stolp BW, Saltzman HA. Pulmonary gas exchange in humans exercising at sea level and simulated altitude. J Appl Physiol 1986; 61:260–270.
75. Hammond MD, Gale GE, Kapitan KS, Ries A, Wagner PD. Pulmonary gas exchange in humans during exercise at sea level. J Appl Physiol 1986; 60:1590–1598.
76. Dempsey JA, Hanson PG, Henderson KS. Exercise-induced arterial hypoxaemia in healthy subjects at sea level. J Physiol (London) 1984; 355:161–175.
77. Wagner PD. A comparison of man and horse during heavy exercise. In Sutton JR, Coates G, Remmers JE, eds., Hypoxia: The Adaptions. Toronto: BC Decker, Inc., 1999, pp. 142–147.
78. Torre-Bueno J, Wagner PD, Saltzman HA, Gale GE, Moon RE. Diffusion limitation in normal humans during exercise at sea level and simulated altitude. J Appl Physiol 1985; 58:989–995.
79. Hammond MD, Gale GE, Kapitan KS, Ries A, Wagner PD. Pulmonary gas exchange in humans during normobaric hypoxic exercise. J Appl.Physiol 1985; 58:978–988.
80. Wagner PD, Sutton JR, Reeves JT, Cymerman A, Groves BM, Malconian MK. Operation Everest II: pulmonary gas exchange during a simulated ascent of Mt. Everest. J Appl Physiol 1987; 63:2348–2359.
81. Wagner PD. The lungs during exercise. NIPS 1987; 2:6–10.
82. Colebatch HJH, Greaves IA, Ng CKY. Exponential analysis of elastic recoil and aging in healthy males and females. J Appl Physiol 1979; 47:683–691.
83. Knudson RJ, Clark DF, Kennedy TC, Knudson DE. Effect of aging alone on mechanical properties of the normal adult human lung. J Appl Physiol 1977; 43:1054–1062.
84. Buist AS, Ghezzo H, Anthonisen NR, et al. Relationship between the single-breath N2 test and age, sex and smoking habit in three North American cities. Am Rev Respir Dis 1979; 120:305–318.
85. Sorbini CA, Grassi V, Solinas E, et al. Arterial oxygen tension in relation to age in healthy subjects. Respiration 1968; 25:3–13.
86. Wagner PD, Hedenstierna G, Bylin G, Lagerstrand L. Reproducibility of the multiple inert gas elimination technique. J Appl Physiol 1987; 62:1740–1746.
87. Cardus J, Burgos F, Díaz O, Roca J, Barberà JA, Marrades RM, Rodriguez-Roisin R, Wagner PD. Increase in pulmonary ventilation-perfusion inequality with age in healthy individuals. Am J Respir Crit Care Med 1997; 156:648–653.

88. Derion T, Guy HJ, Tsukimoto K, Schaffartzik W, Prediletto R, Poole DC, Knight DR, Wagner PD. Ventilation-perfusion relationships in the lung during head-out water immersion. J Appl Physiol 1992; 72:64–72.
89. Kapitan KS, Wagner PD. Linear programming analysis of VA/Q distributions: limits on central moments. J Appl Physiol 1986; 60:1772–1781.
90. Kapitan KS, Wagner PD. Linear programming analysis of VA/Q distributions: average distribution. J Appl Physiol 1987; 62:1356–1362.
91. Loew PG, Die TG. Altersabhangigkeit des arteriellen Sauerstoffdruckes bei der berufstatigen Bevolkerung. Klinische Wockenschrift 1962; 40:1093–98.
92. Raine JM, Bishop JM. A-a difference in O_2 tension and physiological dead space in normal man. J Appl Physiol 1963; 18:284–288.
93. Ulmer WT, Untersuchungen RG. Uber die Altersabhangigkeit der alveolaren und arteriellen Sauerstoffund Kohlen-sauredrucke. Klinische Wochenschrift 1963; 41:1–6.
94. Conway JH, Payne WD, Tomlin PJ. Arterial oxygen tensions of patients awaiting surgery. Br J Anaesth 1965; 37:405–408.
95. Marshall BE, Millar RA. Some factors influencing post-operative hypoxaemia. Anaesthesia 1965; 20:408–428.
96. Mellemgaard K. The alveolar-arterial oxygen difference: its size and components in normal man. Acta Physiol Scand 1966; 67:10–20.
97. Weil MH, Jamieson JD, Brown DW, Grover RF. The red cell mass–arterial oxygen relationship in normal men: application to patients with chronic obstructive airways disease. J Clin Invest 1968; 47:1627–1639.
98. Kanber GJ, King FW, Eshchar YR, Sharp JT. The alveolar-arterial oxygen gradient in young and elderly men during air and oxygen breathing. Am Rev Respir Dis 1968; 97:376–81.
99. Hertle FH, Goerg R, Lange HJ. Arterial blood partial pressures as related to age and biometrical data. Respiration 1971; 28:1–30.
100. Harris J, Kenyon AM, Nisbet HD, Seelye ER, Whitlock RML. The normal alveolar-arterial oxygen-tension gradient in man. Clin Sci Mol Med 1974; 46:89–104.
101. Behn M, Renzetti Jr AD. Alveolar-arterial oxygen pressure gradient: comparison between an assumed and actual respiratory quotient in stable chronic pulmonary disease. II. Relation to aging and closing volume in normal subjects. Respir Care 1977; 22:491–500.
102. Cerveri I, Zoia MC, Fanfulla F, Spagnolatti L, Berrayah L, Grassi M, Tinelli C. Reference values of arterial oxygen tension in the middle-aged and elderly. Am J Respir Crit Care Med 1995; 152:934–941.
103. Crapo RO, Jensen RL, Hegewald M, Tashkin DP. Arterial blood gas reference values for sea level and an altitude of 1400 meters. American Journal of Respiratory and Critical Care Medicine 1999; 160:1525–1531.

5

Gas Exchange in Health: Altitude and Microgravity

JOHN B. WEST

University of California, San Diego
La Jolla, California

I. Introduction

Much important new information has been obtained on pulmonary gas exchange at high altitude and in microgravity in the last few years. It is not easy to do justice to these topics in the space allotted here. Readers who want additional information are referred to more extensive reviews (1–3).

II. High Altitude

There are many reasons why pulmonary gas exchange at high altitude is important. First, nearly 140 million people live at altitudes above 2500 m or 8000 ft (4), and many people live at altitudes that are much higher. For example, it is estimated that more than 50,000 people in Peru reside above 4000 m, and caretakers of a mine in Chile have lived at nearly 6000 m (5). Second, large numbers of people now travel to high altitudes for recreational purposes, including skiing, trekking, and mountaineering, and many become sick as a result, if only temporarily. Finally, there is a third group that is much smaller but growing rapidly, that is, people who commute to high altitudes for commercial or scientific reasons. This group provides some of the most interesting new challenges, as discussed in Section II.I.

There is a special reason why gas exchange at extreme altitude, such as near the summit of Mt. Everest, is of particular interest. Normal subjects are very near their limit of tolerance to hypoxia under these conditions, and their gas exchange responses give us unique insights into how the human organism responds to this extraordinary challenge.

A. Atmosphere

Pulmonary gas exchange is altered at high altitude because of the low partial pressure of oxygen (P_{O_2}). This results from the low barometric pressure (P_B) because the oxygen concentration of the air is constant, at least up to altitudes of interest to us. Barometric pressure decreases with distance above the earth's surface in an approximately exponential manner. Indeed, if air temperature did not decline with altitude, the relationship would be strictly exponential. In most mountainous regions of the world, the P_B is half the sea-level value of 760 mm Hg at an altitude of approximately 5800 m (19,000 ft).

The relationship between P_B and altitude frequently results in confusion. As long ago as 1878, Paul Bert, in his monumental *La Pression Barométrique* (6), correctly predicted a P_B of 248 mm Hg on the summit of Mt. Everest based on measurements reported at lower altitudes, mainly in the Andes. Subsequently, physiologists such as Zuntz et al. (7), FitzGerald (8), and Kellas (9) used the correct relationship between pressure and altitude. However, confusion arose in the 1920s and 1930s when the standard atmosphere was introduced by the aviation industry for calibrating altimeters and low-pressure chambers. The standard atmosphere was never meant to be used to predict the actual P_B at a particular location. Rather, it was developed as a model of average conditions over the surface of the world (10). In fact, the relationship between P_B and altitude depends on latitude because of the greater height of the warm air column near the equator. As a result, P_B predicted from the standard atmosphere are too low (235 vs. 253 mm Hg) for many mountainous regions, including the Himalayas and South American Andes. As an example, if the standard atmosphere is used to predict the pressure on the summit of Mt. Everest, the result is approximately 7% too low, which is highly significant in terms of the amount of work that can be performed at this extreme altitude. Nevertheless, many respiratory physiologists have based their studies on these incorrect pressures (11–14).

The relationship between P_B and altitude basically depends on the temperatures of the air in the column above the earth's surface at a particular point. It has been shown (Fig. 1) that for most of the mountainous regions of the world, including the Himalayas and South American Andes, P_B can be predicted accurately from the altitude by the model atmosphere equation:

$$P_B(\text{mm Hg}) = \exp(6.63268 - 0.1112h - 0.00149h^2) \tag{1}$$

where h is the altitude in kilometers (15).

Altitude and Microgravity 151

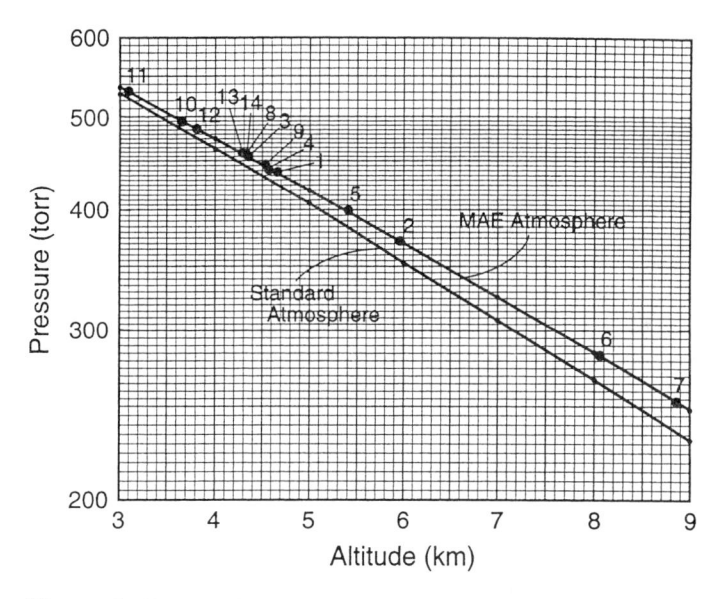

Figure 1 Barometric pressure–altitude relationships for two model atmospheres. The upper line was drawn using the model atmosphere equation given in the text. It shows how well this model atmosphere predicts the barometric pressure at 13 well-known locations where high-altitude studies have been conducted and the barometric pressures accurately measured. In numerical order, the sites are: Collahuasi mine, north Chile; Aucanquilcha mine, north Chile; Vallot Observatory, Mont Blanc; Capanna Margherita, Monte Rosa; base camp, Mt. Everest; camp 5, Mt. Everest; Summit, Mt. Everest; Cerro de Pasco, Peru; Morococha, Peru; Lhasa, Tibet; Crooked Creek, White Mountain, CA; Barcroft Laboratory, White Mountain, CA; Pikes Peak, CO; White Mountain Summit, CA. The lower line shows the standard atmosphere. (Modified from Ref. 2.)

A consequence of the dependence of P_B at altitude on temperature of the air column is that the pressure at extreme altitudes, for example, on the summit of Mt. Everest, varies considerably with season of the year and even from day to day as a result of changes of weather. As a result, the maximal oxygen consumption of a climber near the summit will certainly be affected by the season of the year and may be altered by the fluctuations caused by weather (16).

B. Ventilation

Lowlanders who travel to high altitudes undergo a series of changes known as acclimatization, which increases their tolerance to altitude. The efficiency of this process is remarkable. For example, an unacclimatized lowlander who is exposed to the P_B at the summit of Mt. Everest will lose consciousness within a few minutes. With the advantage of acclimatization, elite climbers can reach the summit without supplementary oxygen.

The most important feature of acclimatization is hyperventilation, which is brought about by hypoxic stimulation of peripheral chemoreceptors, including the carotid and aortic bodies, but chiefly the former. The ventilation increases abruptly during the first 2 hours after ascent and then increases slowly over several days (17). The slow secondary increase is a result of several factors: (1) the increased renal elimination of bicarbonate that reduces the initial respiratory alkalosis, which inhibits ventilation; (2) a loss of bicarbonate from the cerebral spinal fluid; and (3) an increased sensitivity of the carotid body as a result of the chronic hypoxia (18).

There is some evidence that the greater the hypoxic ventilatory response (HVR), the better the tolerance of climbers to extreme altitude (19,20). This is not surprising, because the climbers with the highest HVR will maintain a higher alveolar and, therefore, arterial P_{O_2}, other things being equal. However, there are certainly exceptions, and a number of elite mountain climbers have been shown to have only moderate values of HVR (21). The inverse is probably true, that is, a lowlander with a low HVR will probably have a poor tolerance for extreme altitude.

Paradoxically, some permanent residents of high altitude (highlanders) have been shown to have a low (blunted) HVR (22–24). This may reflect a difference between acclimatization (the process that occurs in lowlanders who ascend to high altitude) and true genetic adaptation (which occurs over many generations at high altitude). Presumably, native highlanders have cellular and other responses that allow them to tolerate the high altitude well despite a lower arterial P_{O_2}. The reduced HVR may have survival value in that it reduces the amount of periodic breathing during sleep (see Sec. II.H).

C. Alveolar Gas Composition

As a result of the increased ventilation at high altitude, the alveolar partial pressure of carbon dioxide (P_{CO_2}) decreases, and the alveolar P_{O_2} is maintained at a higher level than it would have been in the absence of hyperventilation. These changes are well illustrated in an oxygen–carbon dioxide diagram (Fig. 2). The two solid lines in the figure were drawn by Rahn and Otis (17) for lowlanders acutely exposed to high altitude and after acclimatization. The lower line includes data points obtained more recently, including measurements made on the American Medical Research Expedition to Everest (AMREE). The lowest open circle in the figure refers to the Everest summit (16).

Note that the bottom part of the line for acclimatized lowlanders and its extrapolation are almost vertical, indicating that above a certain altitude (approximately 7000 m, or PB of 325 mm Hg), the alveolar P_{O_2} is held essentially constant at approximately 35 mm Hg. This means that the successful climber is able to defend his alveolar P_{O_2} by extreme hyperventilation despite the decreasing P_{O_2} in the atmosphere around him as he ascends. Note that to achieve this on the summit, the alveolar P_{CO_2} has to be reduced to 7 to 8 mm Hg (16a). Only climbers with a

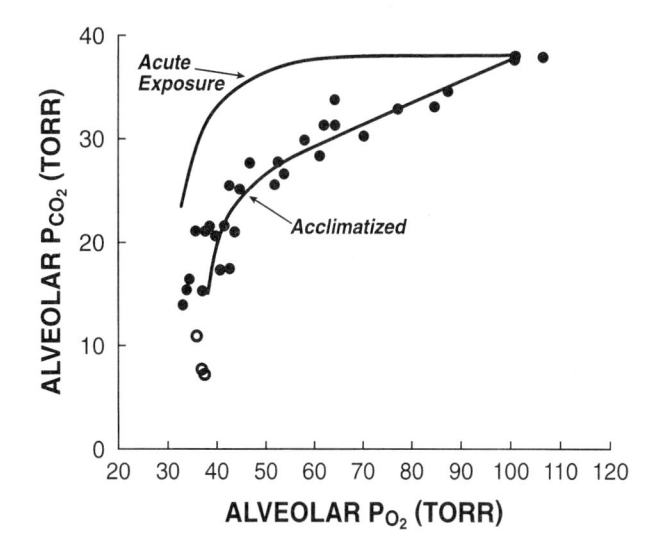

[Figure: Oxygen–carbon dioxide diagram with curves labeled "Acute Exposure" and "Acclimatized", x-axis ALVEOLAR P$_{O_2}$ (TORR) from 20 to 120, y-axis ALVEOLAR P$_{CO_2}$ (TORR) from 0 to 40.]

Figure 2 Oxygen–carbon dioxide diagram showing the two lines drawn by Rahn and Otis (17) for unacclimatized and acclimatized lowlanders at high altitude. The points show the data for acclimatized subjects, including the values obtained at extreme altitudes by the American Medical Research Expedition to Everest (open circles). (Modified from Ref. 16a.)

good HVR can generate the enormous ventilation needed for this, which is why a high HVR improves tolerance to extreme altitude.

D. Blood Gases and Acid-Base Status

The remarkable changes in alveolar P$_{O_2}$ and P$_{CO_2}$ shown in Figure 2 immediately raise the question of the values for arterial P$_{O_2}$, P$_{CO_2}$, and pH. Because of technical difficulties, these measurements have not been made in the field at very high altitudes, but valuable information was obtained in a long-term simulated ascent in a low-pressure chamber in Operation Everest II. As shown in Table 1, measurements were obtained at inspired P$_{O_2}$ values of 63, 49, and 43 mm Hg, corresponding to P$_B$ of 347, 282, and 253 mm Hg, respectively. The corresponding altitudes on Mt. Everest are also shown.

Note that both arterial P$_{O_2}$ and P$_{CO_2}$ decreased with increasing altitude and, at any given altitude, with increasing work level. The mean arterial P$_{O_2}$ on the Everest summit was only 30 mm Hg at rest, and this decreased to 28 mm Hg during exercise. The arterial P$_{CO_2}$ at rest on the summit was only 11 mm Hg, and this was associated with a marked respiratory alkalosis, giving an arterial pH of 7.56.

It is interesting to compare these data with measurements made in the field on AMREE (16a). As shown in Figure 2, the alveolar P$_{CO_2}$ was 7 to 8 mm Hg

Table 1 Arterial P_{O_2} and P_{CO_2} and pH at Extreme Altitude[a] Measured During Operation Everest II

	Work level (W)	P_{O_2} (mm Hg)	P_{CO_2} (mm Hg)	pH
P_{IO_2} = 63, 6480 m	0	41	20	7.50
	60	35	21	7.49
	120	34	19	7.48
	180-210	34	17	7.44
P_{IO_2} = 49, 8040 m	0	37	13	7.53
	60	33	13	7.51
	120	33	11	7.49
P_{IO_2} = 43, 8848 m	0	30	11	7.56
	60	28	11	7.55
	120	28	10	7.52

[a] Altitudes correspond to barometric pressures on Mt. Everest.
P_{IO_2}, partial pressure of inspired oxygen.
From Ref. 85.

on the summit, and when the arterial pH was calculated from the base excess that was measured a few hours later, the value was between 7.7 and 7.8. Part of the difference between the two studies can be ascribed to the better acclimatization that occurs in the field. Another factor is that Christopher Pizzo, who provided the data on the summit, has a high HVR. However, his alveolar P_{CO_2} values were in line with those measured on four other climbers at the slightly lower altitude of 8050 m (16a).

An interesting feature of the base excess measurements on AMREE is that the values obtained near the summit were not different from those measured in 14 subjects living for several weeks at an altitude of 6300 m. This suggests that base excess was changing extremely slowly above this altitude. This is possibly because of the chronic volume depletion found in the climbers at 6300 m. Their serum osmolality remained significantly higher than in the same subjects at sea level (25). It is known that the kidney gives a higher priority to correcting dehydration than to acid-base disturbances, and to excrete more bicarbonate to reduce the base excess, it would be necessary to lose corresponding cations, which would aggravate volume depletion. This may be the basis for the slow excretion of bicarbonate by the kidney at very high altitude.

A valuable result of the extreme respiratory alkalosis is that it greatly increases the oxygen affinity of the hemoglobin. This has the result of enhancing the loading of oxygen by the pulmonary capillaries, although it could be argued that the increased affinity also interferes with the unloading of oxygen from peripheral capillaries. However, there is abundant experimental evidence that an increased

Table 2 Strategies for Increasing Oxygen Affinity of Hemoglobin in Hypoxia

Strategy	Subject
Decrease in 2,3-DPG	Fetus of dog, horse, pig
Decrease in ATP	Trout, eel
Different type of Hb	Human fetus, Bar-headed goose, toad-fish
Mutant Hb (Andrew-Minneapolis)	Family in Minnesota
Different Hb, small Bohr effect	Tadpole
Respiratory alkalosis	Climber at extreme altitude

2,3-DPG, diphosphoglycerate; ATP, adenosine triphosphate; Hb, hemoglobin

oxygen affinity is beneficial at high altitude. Table 2 shows the variety of strategies developed by animals that live in oxygen-deprived environments. In addition, Eaton et al. (26) reported that rats whose oxygen dissociation curve had been left shifted by cyanate administration showed an increased survival when they were decompressed to a PB of 233 mm Hg. Turek et al. (27) also studied cyanate-treated rats and found that they maintained better oxygen transfer to tissues during severe hypoxia than did normal animals. Hebbel et al. (28) described a family with two members who had a hemoglobin with a very high affinity (Andrew-Minneapolis, P_{50} 17 mm Hg). These two members performed better during exercise at an altitude of 3100 m than two siblings with normal blood. It is remarkable that a climber at very high altitude uses the strategy of respiratory alkalosis to increase the oxygen affinity of his hemoglobin, as do other animals in oxygen-deprived environments (Table 2).

One of the best-known physiological responses to high altitude is the increase in red blood cell concentration of the blood. The resulting increase in hemoglobin concentration means that although the arterial PO_2 and oxygen saturation are reduced, the oxygen concentration of the arterial blood may be normal or even above normal. The polycythemia occurs in response to an increased production of erythropoietin from the kidney as a result of the tissue hypoxia.

Recently, the value of the high levels of red blood cell concentration observed at high altitude has been questioned. It is known that high hematocrit levels are associated with uneven blood flow in peripheral capillaries as a result of rouleaux formation and sludging, and that these flow phenomena may interfere with efficient oxygen unloading. Winslow and Monge (29) actually showed improvement of exercise tolerance in some high-altitude Andean natives whose very high hematocrit levels were reduced by the removal of blood over several weeks.

E. Pulmonary Diffusion

Acclimatized lowlanders have little, if any, increase in the diffusing capacity for carbon monoxide at high altitude (30–34). In one study on exercising subjects at altitudes up to 5800 m after 7 to 10 weeks of acclimatization, there was a small increase in diffusing capacity. However, the change could be accounted for by the increased rate of reaction of carbon monoxide with hemoglobin caused by the hypoxia, as well as by the increased blood hemoglobin concentration (30).

On the other hand, high-altitude natives have diffusing capacities that are approximately 20–25% higher than lowlander controls (32,33,35). These increased diffusing capacities are observed during both rest and exercise. Although there is some uncertainty about the appropriateness of the predicted values for diffusing capacity in these studies, it is likely that the higher values are a result of the development of larger lungs with a correspondingly increased alveolar surface area and capillary blood volume. Early visitors to high altitude, such as Barcroft et al. (36), commented on the remarkable chest development of Peruvian high-altitude natives. It has been shown that animals exposed to low P_{O_2} during their active growth phase develop larger lungs and greater diffusing capacities than do animals reared in a normoxic environment (37,38). The opposite is also true: animals reared in a hyperoxic environment develop small lungs (37).

A large diffusing capacity is advantageous at high altitude because oxygen transfer is likely to be diffusion-limited, especially on exercise. Barcroft et al. (36) showed that the arterial oxygen saturation decreased as a result of exercise in Cerro de Pasco (4330 m), and they correctly attributed the desaturation to failure of the P_{O_2} to equilibrate between alveolar gas and pulmonary capillary blood. This diffusion limitation of oxygen transfer at high altitude was confirmed in several subsequent studies (16a,38a,39).

To illustrate the striking change in oxygen loading in the pulmonary capillary at very high altitudes, Figure 3 compares the calculated time course for P_{O_2} in the pulmonary capillary at sea level with that for a climber at rest on the summit of Mt. Everest. Note that at sea level, the P_{O_2} increases very rapidly so that there is ample time for equilibration between alveolar gas and end-capillary blood. By contrast, at extreme altitude the P_{O_2} increases very slowly along the pulmonary capillary, reaching a value of only approximately 28 mm Hg at the end (compare with Table 1).

The reason for the slow increase of P_{O_2} along the pulmonary capillary at high altitude is the large change in arterial oxygen concentration per unit change of P_{O_2} in the blood. This, in turn, results from two factors: (1) oxygen loading is taking place very low on the oxygen dissociation curve, where it is very steep; and (2) there is substantial polycythemia. Piiper and Scheid (40) showed that whether diffusion limitation is likely depends on the factor $D/\dot{Q}\beta$, where D is the diffusing capacity, $\dot{Q}$ is the bloodflow, and β is the "effective solubility" of the gas in blood. For oxygen, this is the slope of the dissociation curve. Diffusion limitation becomes likely when this factor becomes small, and this occurs for oxygen at high altitude because of the large increase in β.

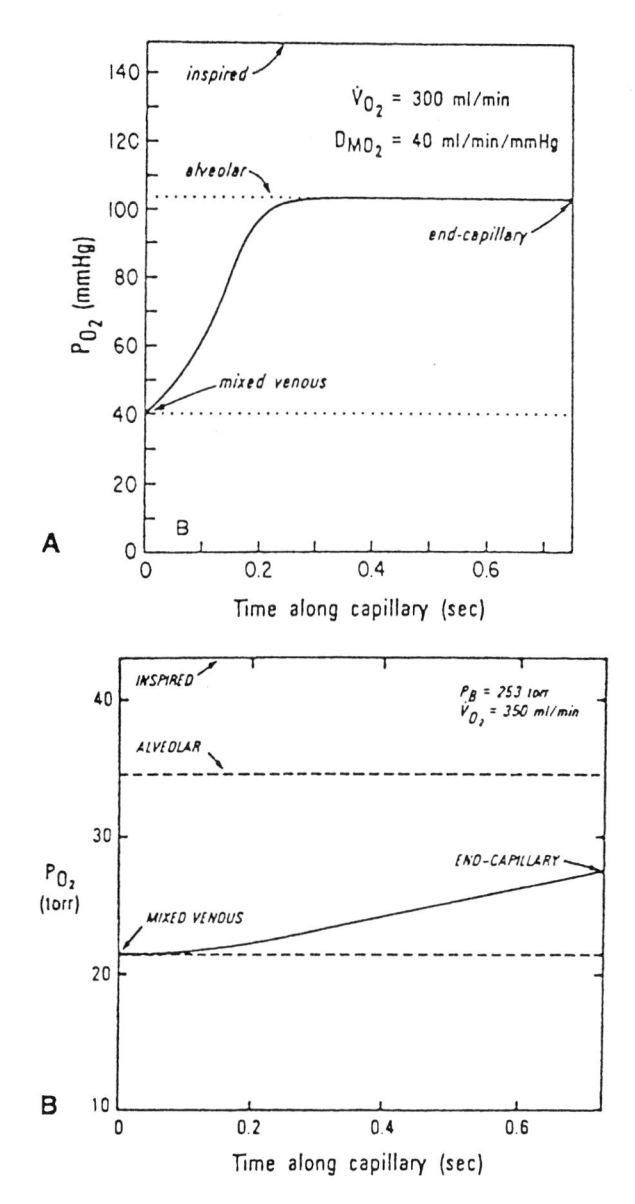

Figure 3 (A) Calculated time course for P_{O_2} in the pulmonary capillary at sea level in the resting human. Note that there is ample time for equilibration of the P_{O_2} between alveolar gas and end-capillary blood. (From Ref. 86.) (B) Similar calculations for a climber at rest on the summit of Mt. Everest. Note that there is considerable diffusion limitation of oxygen uptake with a large P_{O_2} difference between alveolar gas and end-capillary blood. (From Ref. 16a.)

F. Ventilation–Perfusion Relationships

The topographical distribution of ventilation–perfusion ratios in the lung improves at high altitude as a result of the more uniform distribution of blood flow resulting from the increased pulmonary arterial pressure (41). However, the degree of topographical inequality at sea level is such a minor factor in overall gas exchange that the effect of this change is relatively trivial.

Studies during Operation Everest II indicated that ventilation–perfusion inequality tends to become more marked at rest as altitude increases and that it further increases during exercise (39). These measurements were made using the multiple inert gas elimination technique (42) and exploited the fact that the gas exchange of inert gases is not diffusion-limited, even during maximal exercise. It was found that the log SD of blood flow (a measure of ventilation–perfusion inequality) tended to increase at rest as the simulated altitude increased from sea level to the summit of Mt. Everest (Fig. 4). In addition, an increase in exercise level at a given P_B increased the degree of ventilation–perfusion inequality, with the most severe impairment occurring at a maximal oxygen consumption of 1.75 L/min at a P_B of 347 mm Hg, equivalent to an altitude of approximately 6480 m.

In this study, it was also possible to partition the observed alveolar–arterial P_{O_2} difference caused by diffusion limitation on the one hand, and by ventilation–perfusion inequality on the other (39). The results showed that at sea level, essentially all of the alveolar–arterial P_{O_2} difference was attributable to ventilation–perfusion inequality up to an oxygen consumption of nearly 3 L/min. Above that high exercise level, some diffusion limitation apparently occurred. By contrast, at a P_B of 429 mm Hg, the measured alveolar–arterial P_{O_2} difference exceeded that predicted from the amount of ventilation–perfusion inequality when the oxygen uptake was greater than approximately 1 L/min. This was also true of a P_B of 347 mm Hg. At the highest simulated altitudes where the P_B was 282 and 240 mm Hg, almost all of the observed alveolar–arterial P_{O_2} difference during exercise could be ascribed to diffusion limitation.

G. Cardiac Output and Function

Pulmonary gas exchange in its broad sense includes the removal of oxygenated blood from the lung. Compared with normoxia, acute hypoxia results in an increase of cardiac output both at rest and for a given level of exercise (43–45). The physiological value of this response is that it increases the oxygen delivery to peripheral tissues. On the other hand, it would tend to shorten average red blood cell transit time through the lungs, which would possibly increase diffusion limitation.

However, it is remarkable that in acclimatized lowlanders at high altitude, as well as in high-altitude natives, this increase in cardiac output is not observed. Instead, the relationship between cardiac output and oxygen uptake (or work rate) returns to the sea-level value. This was shown by Pugh (46) and confirmed by

Altitude and Microgravity

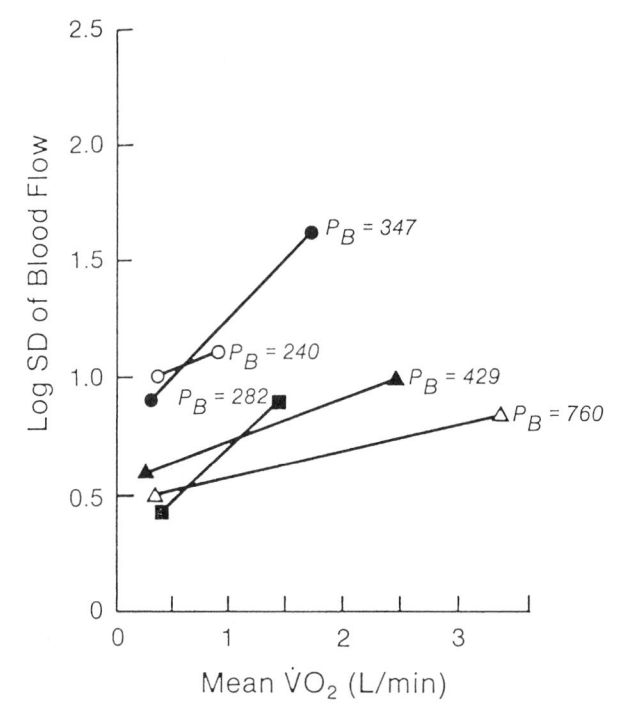

Figure 4 Relationship between the degree of ventilation–perfusion inequality in the lung and oxygen uptake in subjects during a simulated ascent of Mt. Everest in a low-pressure chamber (Operation Everest II). The vertical axis shows the log SD of blood flow, which is a measure of ventilation–perfusion inequality. Note that both a reduction of barometric pressure (P$_B$, measured in mm Hg) and increase in work rate tended to increase the degree of ventilation–perfusion inequality. (From Ref. 39.)

several subsequent studies (47–49). The regulatory mechanism for the return of the cardiac output/work rate relationship to the sea-level value is unclear. However, it is important to note that because of the polycythemia in well-acclimatized subjects, hemoglobin flow is increased. Nevertheless, it seems paradoxical that the body does not make use of the increase in oxygen delivery to the peripheral tissues that could presumably be accomplished by an increased cardiac output.

Although the cardiac output/work rate relationship is unchanged in acclimatized subjects at high altitude, heart rate is increased, and stroke volume is correspondingly reduced. Factors responsible for this may be reflex activity from the carotid body or an increase in circulating catecholamines. At one time it was suggested that the reduced stroke volume might be related to impaired myocardial contractility. However, measurements made during Operation Everest II showed that myocardial contractility was maintained up to extremely high altitudes. Indeed, there was even a suggestion that it actually improved (49,50). The measurements were made by cardiac catheterization and two-dimensional echocardiography and showed that ventricular ejection fraction, the ratio of peak systolic pressure to end-systolic volume, and mean normalized systolic volume at rest were all sustained at a P_B of 282 mm Hg, corresponding to an altitude of approximately 8040 m. These remarkable results emphasize the great difference between myocardial hypoxemia and ischemia.

H. Sleep

Pulmonary gas exchange is typically impaired during sleep at high altitude. In general, lowlanders at high altitude sleep poorly. They frequently complain that they do not feel refreshed when they wake in the morning, and an increase in the frequency of arousals from sleep occurs (51,52). However, the most important feature of sleep at high altitude from the point of view of gas exchange is the high incidence of periodic breathing. An example is shown in Figure 5. Note the waxing and waning of respiratory movements with long apneic periods. The arterial oxygen saturation (as measured by ear oximetry) fluctuated with the same frequency. Heart rate also altered in response to the periodic breathing. The administration of oxygen during periodic breathing at high altitude results in an increase in the arterial oxygen saturation and a great reduction in the strength of the periodic breathing.

Periodic breathing is extremely common in lowlanders at altitudes of 3500 m and above. The apneic periods cause a marked depression of the arterial oxygen

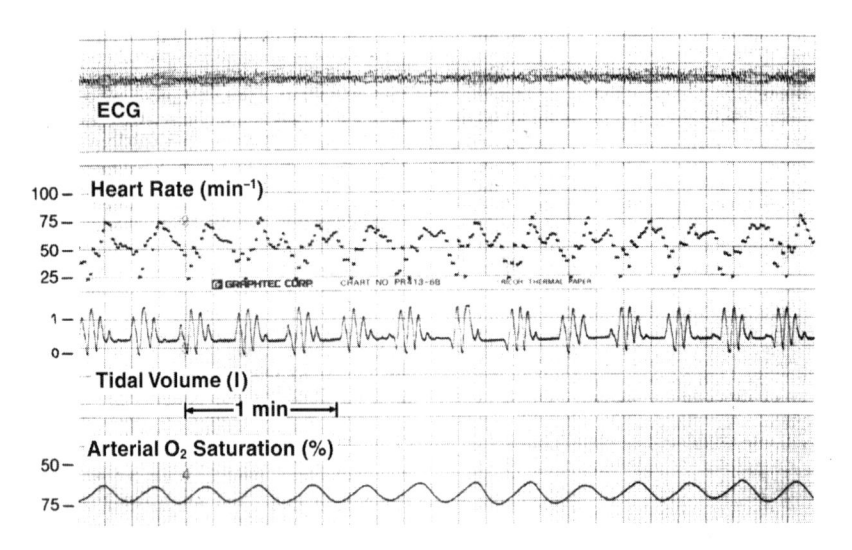

Figure 5 Example of periodic breathing at an altitude of 6300 m (P_B, 351 mm Hg). (From Ref. 87.)

saturation, and it is likely that the resulting degree of hypoxemia is the most severe of the whole 24-hour period. Interestingly, Sherpas do not generally show periodic breathing at altitudes such as 5400 m (53). It is possible that this difference in behavior is related to the blunted HVR of these native highlanders. The argument is that the periodic breathing in lowlanders is related to the very high gain of the feedback system controlling ventilation as a result of the severe hypoxia. Control systems with very high gains frequently show instability. However, because Sherpas have a reduced HVR, the gain of the system is less, and as a result the instability is avoided. Thus, the reduced HVR may have a selective advantage because of the very low values of arterial oxygen saturation that follow the apneic periods. Administration of the carbonic anhydrase inhibitor, acetazolamide, reduces the incidence and severity of periodic breathing at high altitude (54).

I. Oxygen Enrichment of Room Air for Commuters to High Altitude

An interesting recent development is the practice of commuting to work at high altitude and the consequent severe intermittent hypoxia. For example, by the turn of the century, the Collahuasi copper mine in north Chile expects to employ 2000 workers, most of whom will live on the coast and take a bus up to the mine at an altitude of 4500 to 4600 m. They will work there for 7 days, and although they will sleep at the somewhat lower altitude of approximately 3800 m, the resulting hypoxia is obviously severe. At the end of 7 days they will take a bus down to their homes on the coast for a further 7 days, and the cycle will then be repeated indefinitely. A somewhat similar problem will occur in relation to a new radiotelescope in Chile at an altitude of 5000 m. In this instance, the workers will live at approximately 2440 m and commute daily to the telescope site. One result of this pattern is that the workers will presumably never fully acclimatize to the high working altitude. The hypoxia associated with an altitude of 4500 m impairs central nervous system function, reduces the quality of sleep, and limits work capacity.

A possible way of improving the well-being of the workers, and thus the productivity of the mine, is oxygen enrichment of room air in some parts of the facility. Relatively small degrees of oxygen enrichment are very effective. It has been shown that every 1% increase in oxygen concentration (e.g., from 21% to 22%) is equivalent to a reduction of altitude of 300 m (55). Thus, increasing the oxygen concentration of the atmosphere to 26% at an altitude of 5000 m reduces the equivalent altitude to 3500 m, which is much more easily tolerated. Oxygen enrichment of relatively large areas has become feasible because of improvements in technology with oxygen concentrators and cryogenic oxygen. Places where oxygen enrichment might be valuable include dormitories, offices, conference rooms, and laboratories. It may even be possible to oxygen-enrich the air in the cabs of heavy equipment such as trucks and mechanical shovels. There is some evidence that the accident rate when these pieces of heavy equipment are being operated at high altitude is considerably greater than at sea level. Consideration must be given to the possible fire hazard of oxygen enrichment. However, studies show that if the oxygen concentration at altitudes of 4000 to 5500 m is increased so that the equivalent altitude is reduced to 3000 m, the burning rate of materials such as paper and cotton is approximately 30% less than at sea level (3).

It could be argued that oxygen enrichment represents a radical new attitude to living and working at high altitude. Until now, most people have accepted the hypoxia of high altitude as something that has to be endured. This proactive attitude of raising the oxygen concentration of the rooms could represent a major step forward.

III. Microgravity

Lay people such as journalists sometimes draw a comparison between the effects of high altitude and space flight on the body. However, there is essentially no link. Hypoxia is not a feature of the space environment because the astronaut or cosmonaut takes his atmosphere with him. Only in the event of a leak in the spacecraft or malfunction of the environmental control system is hypoxia a possibility. Indeed, the early U.S. manned space flights, including the *Apollo* flights to the moon, were characterized by hyperoxia because the astronauts breathed 100% oxygen at a reduced P_B, giving an inspired P_{O_2} of approximately 260 mm Hg.

The physiological challenges of space flight include: (1) the effects of microgravity on the body; (2) possible exposure to high levels of ionizing radiation, including exotic particles not present in the earth's environment; and (3) the consequences of living in a confined space for long periods. This last aspect of the space environment has spawned a whole area of research known as closed-environment life-support systems, where human beings and plants live symbiotically, one group taking up oxygen and giving off carbon dioxide while the other does the opposite.

The lung is exquisitely sensitive to gravity, which normally causes regional differences of blood flow, ventilation, gas exchange, alveolar size, intrapleural pressure, and parenchymal stress (56). Therefore, substantial alterations of pulmonary function are expected in microgravity. In addition, thoracic blood volume increases, at least transiently, on entering space because of the absence of pooling of blood in dependent regions of the body. The resulting increase in intrapulmonary blood volume and pressures presumably affects pulmonary function.

During the early 1990s, the successful flights of Spacelabs Life Sciences 1 and 2 (SLS-1 and SLS-2) provided the first comprehensive data on the extensive changes in pulmonary function in sustained microgravity (57–62). There were also a few previous measurements of pulmonary function in microgravity that were performed by means of parabolic flights in the high-performance aircraft (63–68). This brief review is based on the measurements made in SLS-1 and SLS-2.

A. Ventilation

Total pulmonary ventilation was measured during resting breathing on SLS-1 and SLS-2. There was a significant reduction in tidal volume of approximately 15% but an increase in respiratory frequency (9%) compared with preflight standing measurements (69). The increased frequency was chiefly caused by a reduction in expiratory time (10%) with a smaller decrease in inspiratory time (4%). Both physiological and alveolar dead space were significantly less than in preflight standing or supine measurements, consistent with the more uniform topographical distribution of blood flow. The net result was that, although total ventilation decreased, alveolar ventilation was unchanged in microgravity compared with standing in normal gravity.

B. Inhomogeneity of Ventilation

Inhomogeneity of ventilation was measured using both single-breath and multibreath nitrogen washouts. For the single-breath nitrogen washout, the subject took a vital capacity breath of oxygen, with an argon bolus at residual volume, and the nitrogen and argon concentrations in the subsequent test expiration were measured. There was a marked decrease in ventilatory inhomogeneity, as evidenced by the significant reductions in cardiogenic oscillations on the alveolar plateau, the slope of phase 3, and the height of phase 4 for both nitrogen and argon (58) (Fig. 6). This result was consistent with the known effect of gravity on the distribution of ventilation. However, considerable ventilatory inhomogeneity remained, consistent with the fact that nongravitational factors such as diffusion and convection inhomogeneity in small lung units play an important role (70,71).

The single-breath nitrogen test using a vital capacity inspiration and expiration is not a normal physiological maneuver. Therefore, we made additional measurements of the inhomogeneity of ventilation using multibreath nitrogen washouts at tidal volumes of approximately 700 mL, that is, near the normal tidal volume (61). Six indices of ventilatory inhomogeneity were derived from the data, and it was found that the degree of inhomogeneity was not significantly different in microgravity compared with that observed in normal gravity in the standing posture. This was a surprising result, indicating that the primary determinants of ventilatory inhomogeneity during tidal breathing in the upright posture are not gravitational in origin.

It might be argued that the multibreath test was not sensitive enough to pick up small differences in ventilatory inequality. However, additional measurements showed that in the supine position at normal gravity, there was a significant increase in ventilatory inhomogeneity, indicating the sensitivity of the technique to relatively minor degrees of uneven ventilation. It was therefore concluded that gravity has a negligible role on ventilatory inhomogeneity under normal breathing conditions in the upright posture.

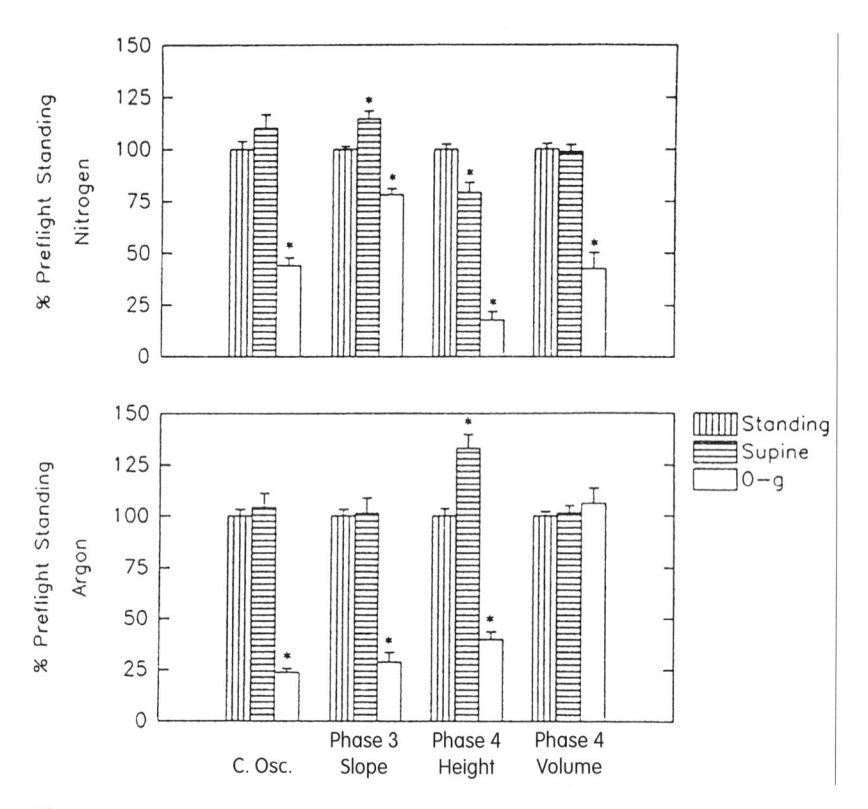

Figure 6 Effects of sustained microgravity on the single-breath nitrogen washout. An argon bolus was introduced at residual volume. Note the reduction in size of the cardiogenic oscillations (Osc) of both nitrogen and argon, indicating a more uniform distribution of ventilation; however, some inequality remained. Also note that the volume of phase 4 as measured with argon was unchanged. (From Ref. 58.)

Another unexpected finding emerged when we measured the closing volume of the lung from the onset of phase 4 using both nitrogen and argon as markers. In normal gravity, the closing volume is generally believed to be the volume of the lung at which the airways near the base of the lung close because of distortion of the lung by its weight (72). A surprising finding was that in microgravity, the closing volume measured from the argon tracing was not significantly different from that in normal gravity in the standing posture, although there was considerable variability between subjects (58). This result implies that some airways close at lung volumes above residual volume in the absence of gravity, and presumably this process is determined by the distribution of mechanical properties of the airways and parenchyma. Although this result runs counter to much contemporary thinking, it is consistent with some earlier measurements showing early airway closure in excised lungs during deflation (73). Note that although closing volume was unaltered on the average, closing capacity was reduced because of the reduction in residual volume.

The reduced inhomogeneity of ventilation in microgravity found on SLS-1 and SLS-2 is consistent with earlier results obtained during short periods of microgravity (20 to 25 seconds) on parabolic flights using high-performance aircraft (63). However, the interpretation of results obtained on parabolic flights is complicated by the fact that the period of microgravity is immediately preceded and followed by several seconds of increased gravity (g). It was therefore important to obtain measurements during the sustained microgravity of the Spacelab missions.

Measurements of maximal expiratory flow rates showed an unexpected reduction in peak flow rate on flight days 2 through 5 of up to 12.5%. However, these flow rates returned to preflight standing values by flight day 9 (62). The cause of the reduction is not clear, but it may be the lack of physical stability of the astronaut when the maneuver was performed in the absence of gravity. There was also a small reduction in flow rates at low lung volumes in some subjects, and a similar pattern had been observed previously during short exposure to microgravity in parabolic flights (65). This reduction was probably caused by the increased pulmonary blood volume, which reduces elastic recoil at low lung volumes.

C. Pulmonary Blood Flow

Total pulmonary blood flow was measured by a rebreathing technique using nitrous oxide as the soluble gas. It was found that cardiac output increased by an average of 18% compared with preflight measurements made in the standing position (57). During the week after the flight, cardiac output decreased by 9% compared with preflight measurements. The changes in stroke volume were greater because cardiac frequency decreased during the flight. Stroke volume was increased by an average of 46% inflight and decreased 14% in the first week after the flight, compared with preflight standing measurements. The increase in stroke volume was consistent with an increase of left-ventricular end-diastolic dimensions measured by echocardiography by Buckey et al. (74).

An interesting paradox emerged when the measurements of stroke volume and left-ventricular end-diastolic dimensions were compared with measurements of central venous pressure (CVP) and circulating blood volume made by Buckey et al. (74) and Udden et al. (75), respectively. When the subject entered microgravity, the CVP (measured with the catheter tip near the right atrium) decreased from an average of 15.0 to 2.5 cm H_2O in the supine position with legs elevated. In addition, the blood volume decreased by 12% in the first 24 hours of flight. The increase in stroke volume in the face of reductions in both CVP and circulating blood volume has not yet been satisfactorily explained. One possibility is that there was a decrease in the pressure outside the great vessels and heart as a result of the loss of gravity-induced compression of the lungs and mediastinal structures. This might explain how the CVP measured with a catheter might decrease but the transmural pressure of the veins increase.

D. Inhomogeneity of Blood Flow

Inhomogeneity of blood flow was measured by an indirect technique involving hyperventilation, breath holding, and measurement of the magnitude of the cardiogenic oscillations for carbon dioxide and oxygen on the alveolar plateau during a subsequent long expiration (59). It would have been valuable to study the topographical inequality of blood flow using radioactive gases, but these were not permitted in the Spacelab for safety reasons. The results showed that the distribution of pulmonary blood flow was more uniform in microgravity than in normal gravity. For example, the size of the cardiogenic oscillations in phase 3 of the test expirations was reduced to approximately 60% of the preflight standing values. In addition, the height of phase 4 (the terminal deflection after the onset of airway closure) was almost abolished. These results are consistent with the disappearance of the gravity-dependent topographical inequality of blood flow.

However, there was considerable residual inhomogeneity of pulmonary blood flow, as evidenced by the fact that the height of the cardiogenic oscillations was essentially the same in microgravity as in the supine position in normal gravity. The small height of phase 4 indicated that the differences in perfusion were probably in lung units that were not far apart. On the other hand, the inhomogeneity was probably not within the same acinus, because otherwise the cardiogenic oscillations would have been eliminated by diffusional mixing.

A number of previous studies have shown that gravity is not the only factor that causes inhomogeneity of pulmonary blood flow. Possible mechanisms include regional differences in conductance of the vessels (76), a central to peripheral gradient of blood flow within the whole lung (77), a gradient of blood flow along the acinus (78,79), and stochastic or fractal inequalities (80,81). Therefore, it is not surprising that some residual inequality of blood flow was observed. However, the measurements made in Spacelab are important because, for the first time, it was possible to see the intrinsic inhomogeneity of blood flow in the lung in the absence of the normal masking effect of gravity.

E. Diffusion

The diffusing capacity of the lung for carbon monoxide was measured with normal and high alveolar P_{O_2} values, which allowed the separation of the diffusing capacity of the alveolar membrane (D_M) and the capillary blood volume (V_c). As shown in Figure 7, the diffusing capacity was elevated by an average of 28% compared with preflight standing values and was higher than preflight supine values (57). This was a consequence of both an increase in the diffusing capacity of the alveolar membrane by 27% and an increase in capillary blood volume by 28%. The

Altitude and Microgravity

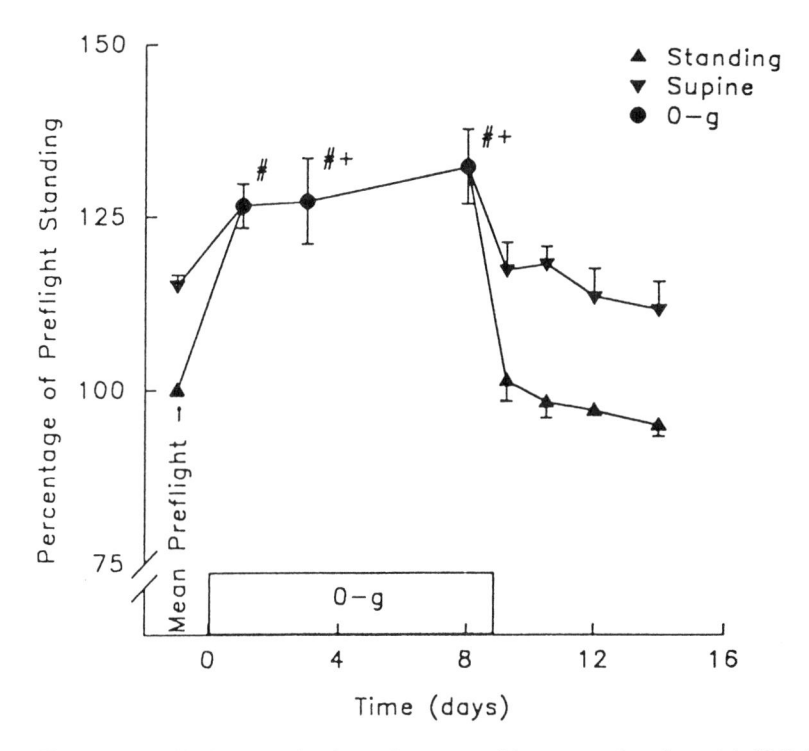

Figure 7 Diffusing capacity for carbon monoxide measured on Spacelab SLS-1. The values are shown for the mean preflight measurements, flight days 2, 4, and 9, and days 0, 1 or 2, 4, and 6 after return to $1g$. Values are means ± SE of individual DL values normalized to individual preflight standing values. Symbols denote significant differences from preflight measurements in the standing posture (see original article for details). (From Ref. 57.)

increase in diffusing capacity was expected because of the anticipated movement of blood from the dependent peripheral parts of the body to the thoracic cavity in microgravity and the resulting increased filling of the pulmonary capillaries.

However, an unexpected result became apparent when the increases in diffusing capacity of the membrane and the capillary blood volume were compared during two maneuvers: (1) the transition from the upright to the supine position in normal gravity, and (2) the transition from the upright posture in normal gravity to microgravity. It was found that the increase in capillary blood volume was comparable in the two situations (27% and 35%, respectively). However, there was a much larger increase in alveolar membrane-diffusing capacity in the transition to microgravity, the corresponding increases being 5% (not significant) and 27% ($P < 0.05$; Fig. 8). The explanation may be that, for the first time, we are seeing the effects of uniform filling of the pulmonary capillary bed because the regional

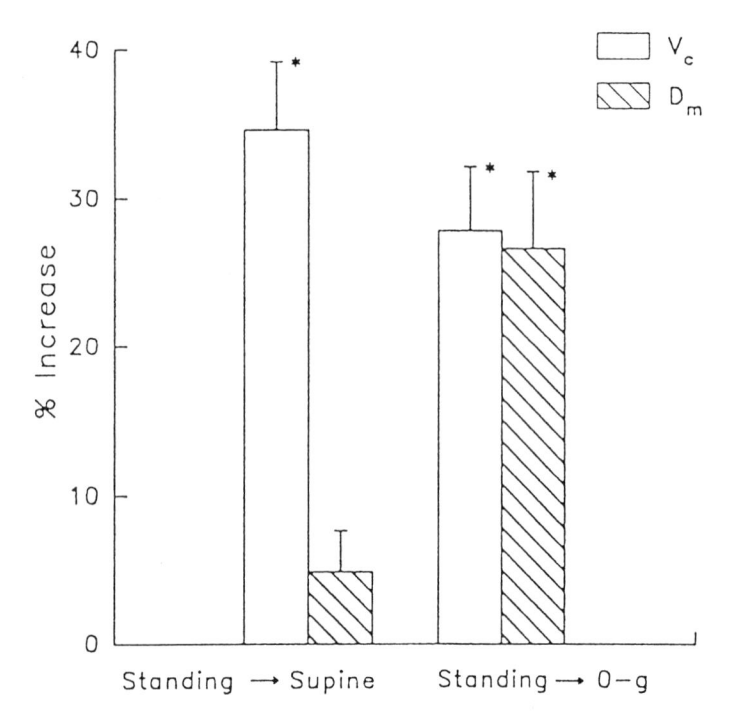

Figure 8 Percentage increase in the volume of blood in the pulmonary capillaries (V_c) and the diffusing capacity of the alveolar membrane (D_M) in the transition from standing to supine in $1g$, and standing to $0g$. Note that while the increase in V_c was comparable, there was a much larger increase in D_M in microgravity. Asterisks denote significant differences from preflight standing posture. (From Ref. 57.)

differences of capillary blood volume normally caused by gravity have been abolished. Furthermore, the surprisingly large increase in alveolar membrane-diffusing capacity may throw light on the configuration of the capillaries in microgravity. Permutt (82) noted that in the absence of gravity, all the pulmonary capillaries are either in zone 2 or zone 3, depending on whether the pulmonary venous pressure is less than or greater than alveolar pressure, respectively. The unexpectedly high value of D_M may indicate that all the capillaries are in zone 3, where the whole length of the capillary is held open, rather than in zone 2, where the downstream end of the capillary may be collapsed.

F. Pulmonary Gas Exchange

There were no significant changes in resting oxygen uptake, carbon dioxide output, or end-tidal P_{O_2} in microgravity compared with the standing posture in $1g$ (61). End-tidal P_{CO_2} was unchanged during the 9-day flight of SLS-1 but increased by 4.5

mm Hg on the 14-day flight of SLS-2, when the P_{CO_2} of the spacecraft atmosphere increased by 1 to 3 mm Hg because of the less efficient removal of the carbon dioxide by the spacecraft environmental control system.

Information about ventilation–perfusion inequality was obtained from measurements of expired P_{O_2} and P_{CO_2} during vital capacity expirations while breathing air. Cardiogenic oscillations demonstrated the presence of residual ventilation–perfusion inequality, although this was less marked than that in the standing posture with normal gravity, consistent with the aforementioned more uniform distribution of blood flow and ventilation. However, the change in respiratory exchange ratio (and, therefore, ventilation–perfusion ratio) during phase 3 of a long expiration was the same in microgravity as preflight standing values. This finding indicates that most of the ventilation–perfusion inequality in the $1g$ upright posture is not caused by gravitationally induced topographical inequality of ventilation and blood flow, which goes against some accepted thinking. On the other hand, the smaller changes in P_{O_2} and P_{CO_2} at the end of expiration after airway closure in microgravity compared with normal gravity were consistent with a more uniform topographical distribution of gas exchange. This could be expected from the earlier results showing the greater homogeneity of blood flow and ventilation.

G. Behavior of Inhaled Inert Gases of Different Molecular Weights

Some of the most provocative results emerged when the patterns of single-breath washins of helium (He) and sulfurhexafluoride (SF_6) were measured on SLS-2 (83). These two gases have very different molecular weights of 4 and 146, respectively; therefore, their diffusivities are very different. However, because diffusion rate is determined by mass, not weight, we did not expect to find any differences in the behavior of these two gases in microgravity compared with normal gravity.

Very unexpected results were obtained. As shown in Figure 9, the slope of the alveolar plateau for He was significantly less than that for SF_6 at $1g$ because of the higher diffusibility of He, which allows it to distribute itself in the peripheral regions of the lung, and also because He penetrates further into the acinus. However, when the same measurement was made in microgravity, the two slopes became the same. The mystery deepened even further when the slopes were measured during an expiration after 10 seconds of breath holding. In $1g$, both slopes became less, as would be expected because of the increased time available for mixing by diffusion and cardiogenic convection within the airways. However, in microgravity, the effect of 10 seconds of breath holding was to make the slope for SF_6 significantly smaller than that for He.

It is known that topographical inequality of ventilation has only a small effect on the slope of the alveolar plateau because the single-breath nitrogen washout is only approximately 20% flatter in microgravity (58). This means that most of the slope of the He and SF_6 plateaus is determined by the geometry of the acinus (71)

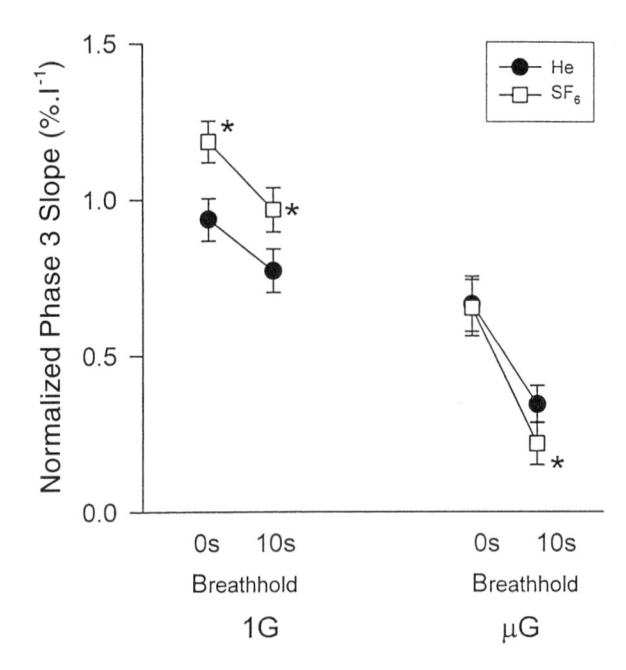

Figure 9 Normalized phase 3 slopes for helium (He) and sulfurhexafluoride (SF_6) for subjects standing in $1g$ and during microgravity (μg). Note that the data collected in $1g$ show significantly steeper phase 3 slopes for SF_6 than for He, whereas this difference is abolished in microgravity and is actually reversed after 10 seconds of breath holding. The asterisks indicate that the SF_6 slope is significantly different from that for He at the 0.05 level.

with a possible contribution from the effects of cardiogenic mixing in the airways. The inescapable conclusion seems to be that microgravity systematically affects acinar geometry in some way, conceivably because of the increase in blood volume of the lung. Very recent studies show that the equalization of the He and SF_6 slopes that were observed in sustained microgravity does not occur in brief periods of microgravity (20 to 25 seconds) during parabolic profile flight (84). Therefore, something is happening to the lung in the interval between 20 seconds and 1 or 2 days of microgravity. This totally unexpected result has thus far defied explanation.

In summary, these studies show that there are substantial changes of pulmonary function in microgravity, as would be expected from the known sensitivity of the respiratory system to gravity. However, we have not observed any changes that are likely to limit long-term space flight. It will be of considerable interest to observe pulmonary function in astronauts over longer periods of microgravity in the International Space Station.

Acknowledgments

The Spacelab studies were conducted by Harold J. B. Guy, Ann R. Elliott, G. Kim Prisk and Manuel Paiva. This work was supported by NASA contract NAS 9-16037.

References

1. West JB, Guy HJ, Elliott AR, Prisk GK. Respiratory system in microgravity. In: Fregly MJ, Blatteis CM, eds. Handbook of Physiology, Section 4: Environmental Physiology. New York: Oxford University Press, 1996, pp 675–689.
2. West JB. Physiology of extreme altitude. In: Fregly MJ, Blatteis CM, eds. Handbook of Physiology, Section 4: Environmental Physiology. New York: Oxford University Press, 1996, pp 1307–1325.
3. West JB. High Altitude. In: Crystal RG, West JB, Barnes PJ, Weibel ER, eds. The Lung: Scientific Foundations. 2nd ed. Philadelphia: Lippincott-Raven, 1997, pp 2653–2666.
4. World Health Organization. World Health Statistics Annual 1995. Geneva: WHO, 1996.
5. West JB. Highest inhabitants in the world. Nature 1986; 324:517.
6. Bert P. La Pression Barométrique. Paris: Masson, 1878.
7. Zuntz N, Loewy A, Muller F, Caspari W. Hö henklima und Bergwanderungen in ihrer Wirkung auf den Menschen. Berlin: Bong, 1906.
8. FitzGerald MP. The changes in the breathing and the blood of various altitudes. Phil Trans R Soc Lond B 1913; 203:351–371.
9. Kellas AM. A consideration of the possibility of ascending the loftier Himalaya. Geogr J 1917; 49:26–47.
10. International Civil Aviation Organization. Manual of the ICAO Standard Atmosphere. 2nd ed. Montreal, Quebec: International Civil Aviation Organization, 1964.
11. Houston CS, Riley RL. Respiratory and circulatory changes during acclimatization to high altitude. Am J Physiol 1947; 149:565–588.
12. Houston CS, Sutton JR, Cymerman A, Reeves JT. Operation Everest II: man at extreme altitude. J Appl Physiol 1987; 63:877–882.
13. Rahn H, Fenn WO. A Graphical Analysis of the Respiratory Gas Exchange. American Physiology Society, 1955.
14. Riley RL, Houston CS. Composition of alveolar air and volume of pulmonary ventilation during long exposure to high altitude. J Appl Physiol 1951; 3:526–534.
15. West JB. Prediction of barometric pressures at high altitudes using model atmospheres. J Appl Physiol 1996; 81:1850–1854.
16. West JB, Lahiri S, Maret KH, Peters RM Jr, Pizzo CJ. Barometric pressures at extreme altitudes on Mt. Everest: physiological significance. J Appl Physiol 1983; 54:1188–1194.
16a. West JB, Hackett PH, Maret KH, Milledge JS, Peters RM, Pizzo CJ, Winslow RM. Pulmonary gas exchange on the summit of Mt. Everst. J Appl Physiol 1963; 55: 678–687.

17. Rahn H, Otis AB. Man's respiratory response during and after acclimatization to high altitude. Am J Physiol 1949; 157:445–462.
18. Barnard P, Andronikou S, Pokorski M, Smatresk N, Mokashi A, Lahiri S. Time-dependent effect of hypoxia on carotid body chemosensory function. J Appl Physiol 1987; 63:685–691.
19. Schoene RB, Lahiri S, Hackett PH, Peters RM Jr, Milledge JS, Pizzo CJ, et al. Relationship of hypoxic ventilatory response to exercise performance on Mount Everest. J Appl Physiol 1984; 56:1478–1483.
20. Masuyama S, Kimura H, Sugita T, Kuriyama T, Tatsumi K, Kunitomo F, Okita S, Tojma H, Yuguchi Y, Watanabe S, Honda Y. Control of ventilation in extreme-altitude climbers. J Appl Physiol 1986; 61:500–506.
21. Oelz O, Howald H, diPrampero PE, Hoppeler H, Claassen H, Jenni R, Bühlmann A, Ferretti G, Brückner J-C, Veicstemos A, Gussoni M, Cerretelli P. Physiological profile of world-class high-altitude climbers. J Appl Physiol 1986; 60:1734–1742.
22. Severinghaus JW, Bainton CR, Carcelen A. Respiratory insensitivity to hypoxia in chronically hypoxic man. Respir Physiol 1966; 1:308–334.
23. Lahiri S, Milledge JS. Sherpa physiology. Nature 1965; 207:10–12.
24. Milledge JS, Lahiri S. Respiratory control in lowlanders and Sherpa highlanders at altitude. Respir Physiol 1967; 2:310–322.
25. Blume FD, Boyer SJ, Braverman LE, Cohen A. Impaired osmoregulation at high altitude. J Am Med Assoc 1984; 252:1580–1585.
26. Eaton JW, Skeleton TD, Berger E. Survival at extreme altitude: protective effect of increased hemoglobin–oxygen affinity. Science 1974; 183:743–744.
27. Turek Z, Kruezer F, Ringnalda BE. Blood gases at several levels of oxygenation in rats with a left shifted blood oxygen dissociation curve. Pflüger's Arch 1978; 376:7–13.
28. Hebbel RP, Eaton JW, Kronenberg RS, Zanjani ED, Moore LG, Berger EM. Human llamas: adaptation to altitude in subjects with high hemoglobin oxygen affinity. J Clin Invest 1978; 62:593–600.
29. Winslow RM, Monge CC. Hypoxia, Polycythemia, and Chronic Mountain Sickness. Baltimore: Johns Hopkins University Press, 1987.
30. West JB. Diffusing capacity of the lung for carbon monoxide at high altitude. J Appl Physiol 1962; 17:421–426.
31. Kreuzer F, Van L, Campagne P. Resting pulmonary diffusing capacity for CO and O_2 at high altitude. J Appl Physiol 1965; 20:519–524.
32. DeGraff AC, Grover RF, Johnson RL, Hammond JW, Miller JM. Diffusing capacity of the lung in Caucasians native to 3100 m. J Appl Physiol 1970; 29:71–76.
33. Dempsey JA, Reddan WG, Birnbaum ML, Forster HV, Thoden JS, Grover RF, Ronkin J. Effects of acute through life-long hypoxic exposure on exercise pulmonary gas exchange. Respir Physiol 1971; 13:62–89.
34. Guleria JS, Pande JN, Sethi PK, Roy SB. Pulmonary diffusing capacity at high altitude. J Appl Physiol 1971; 31:536–543.
35. Remmers JE, Mithoefer JC. The carbon monoxide diffusing capacity in permanent residents at high altitudes. Respir Physiol 1962; 43:357–364.
36. Barcroft J, Binger CA, Bock AV, Doggart JH, Forbes HS, Harrop G. Observations upon the effect of high altitude on the physiological processes of the human body,

carried out in the Peruvian Andes, chiefly at Cerro de Pasco. Phil Trans R Soc Lond B 1923; 211:351–480.
37. Burri PH, Weibel ER. Morphometric estimation of pulmonary diffusion capacity. II. Effect of environmental P_{O_2} on the growing lung. Respir Physiol 1971; 11:247–264.
38. Bartlett D Jr, Remmers JE. Effects of high altitude exposure on the lungs of young rats. Respir Physiol 1971; 13:116–125.
38a. West JB, Lahiri S, Gill MB, Milledge JS, Pugh LGCE, Ward MP. Arterial oxygen saturation during exercise at high altitude. J Appl Physiol 1962; 17:617–621.
39. Wagner PD, Sutton JR, Reeves JT, Cymerman A, Groves BM, Malconian MK. Operation Everest II. Pulmonary gas exchange during a simulated ascent of Mt. Everest. J Appl Physiol 1987; 63:2348–2359.
40. Piiper J, Scheid P. Blood-gas equilibration in lungs. In: West JB, ed. Pulmonary Gas Exchange, Volume 1, Ventilation, Blood Flow, and Diffusion. New York: Academic Press, 1980, pp 131–171.
41. Dawson A. Regional lung function during early acclimatization to 3100 m altitude. J Appl Physiol 1972; 33:218–223.
42. Wagner PD, Saltzman HA, West JB. Measurement of continuous distributions of ventilation-perfusion ratios: theory. J Appl Physiol 1974; 36:533–537.
43. Asmussen E, Consolazio FC. The circulation in rest and work on Mount Evans (4300 m). Am J Physiol. 1941; 32:555–563.
44. Kontos HA, Levasseur JE, Richardson DW, Mauck HP Jr, Patterson JL Jr. Comparative circulatory responses to systemic hypoxia in man and in unanesthetized dog. J Appl Physiol 1967; 23:381-386.
45. Vogel JA, Harris CW. Cardiopulmonary responses of resting man during early exposure to high altitude. J Appl Physiol 1967; 22:1124–1128.
46. Pugh LG. Cardiac output in muscular exercise at 5800 m (19,000 ft.). J Appl Physiol 1964; 19:441–447.
47. Cerretelli P. Limiting factors to oxygen transport on Mount Everest. J Appl Physiol 1976; 40:658–667.
48. Vogel JA, Hartley LH, Cruz JC. Cardiac output during exercise in altitude natives at sea level and high altitude. J Appl Physiol 1974; 36:173–176.
49. Reeves JT, Groves BM, Sutton JR, Wagner PD, Cymerman A, Malconian MK, Rock PB, Young PM, Houston CS. Operation Everest II: preservation of cardiac function at extreme altitude. J Appl Physiol 1987; 63:531–539.
50. Suarez J, Alexander JK, Houston CS. Enhanced left ventricular systolic performance at high altitude during Operation Everest II. Am J Cardiol 1987; 60:137–142.
51. Reite M, Jackson D, Cahoon RL, Weil JV. Sleep physiology at high altitude. Electroencephalogr Clin Neurophysiol 1975; 38:463–471.
52. Weil JV, Kryger MH, Scoggin CH. Sleep and breathing at high altitude. In: Guilleminault C, Dement W, eds. Sleep Apnea Syndromes. New York: Alan R. Liss, 1978, pp 119–136.
53. Lahiri S, Barnard P. Role of arterial chemoreflexes in breathing during sleep at high altitude. In: Sutton JR, Houston CS, Jones NL, eds. Hypoxia, Exercise and Altitude. New York: Alan R. Liss, 1983, pp 75–85.
54. Sutton JR, Houston CS, Mansell AL, McFadden M, Hackett P, Rigg JR, Powles AC. Effect of acetazolamide on hypoxemia during sleep at high altitude. N Engl J Med 1979; 301:1329–1331.

55. West JB. Oxygen enrichment of room air to relieve the hypoxia of high altitude. Respir Physiol 1995; 99:225–232.
56. West JB. Regional Differences in the Lung. New York: Academic Press, 1977.
57. Prisk GK, Guy HJ, Elliott AR, Deutschman RA III, West JB. Pulmonary diffusing capacity, capillary blood volume and cardiac output during sustained microgravity. J Appl Physiol 1993; 75:15–26.
58. Guy HJ, Prisk GK, Elliott AR, Deutschman RA III, West JB. Inhomogeneity of pulmonary ventilation during sustained microgravity as determined by single-breath washouts. J Appl Physiol 1994; 76:1719–1729.
59. Prisk GK, Guy HJ, Elliott AR, West JB. Inhomogeneity of pulmonary perfusion during sustained microgravity on Spacelab SLS-1. J Appl Physiol 1994; 76:1730–1738.
60. Elliott AR, Prisk GK, Guy HJ, West JB. Lung volumes during sustained microgravity on Spacelab SLS-1. J Appl Physiol 1994; 77:2005–2014.
61. Prisk GK, Guy HJ, Elliott AR, Paiva M, West JB. Ventilatory inhomogeneity determined from multiple-breath washouts during sustained microgravity on Spacelab SLS-1. J Appl Physiol 1995; 78:597–607.
62. Elliott AR, Prisk GK, Guy HJ, Kosonen J, West JB. Forced expirations and maximum expiratory flow-volume curves during sustained microgravity on Spacelab SLS-1. J Appl Physiol 1996; 81:33–43.
63. Michels DB, West JB. Distribution of pulmonary ventilation and perfusion during short periods of weightlessness. J Appl Physiol 1978; 45:987–998.
64. Michels DB, Friedman PJ, West JB. Radiographic comparison of human lung shape during normal gravity and weightlessness. J Appl Physiol 1979; 47:851–857.
65. Guy HJ, Prisk GK, Elliott AR, West JB. Maximum expiratory flow-volume curves during short periods of microgravity. J Appl Physiol 1991; 70:2587–2596.
66. Edyvean J, Estenne M, Paiva M, Engel LA. Lung and chest wall mechanics in microgravity. J Appl Physiol 1991; 71:1956–1966.
67. Paiva M, Estenne M, Engel LA. Lung volumes, chest wall configuration, and pattern of breathing in microgravity. J Appl Physiol 1989; 67:1542–1550.
68. Estenne M, Gorini M, Van Muylem A, Ninane V, Paiva M. Rib cage shape and motion in microgravity. J Appl Physiol 1992; 73:946–954.
69. Prisk GK, Elliott AR, Guy HJ, Kosonen J, West JB. Pulmonary gas exchange and its determinants during sustained microgravity on Spacelab SLS-1 and SLS-2. J Appl Physiol 1995; 79:1290–1298.
70. Crawford AB, Makowska M, Paiva M, Engel LA. Convection- and diffusion-dependent ventilation maldistribution in normal subjects. J Appl Physiol 1985; 59:838–846.
71. Paiva M, Engel LA. The anatomical basis for the sloping N_2 plateau. Respir Physiol 1981; 44:325–337.
72. Milic-Emili J, Henderson AM, Dolovich MB, Trop D, Kaneko K. Regional distribution of inspired gas in the lung. J Appl Physiol 1966; 21:749–759.
73. Glaister DH, Schroter RC, Sudlow MF, Milic-Emili J. Transpulmonary pressure gradient and ventilation distribution in excised lungs. Respir Physiol 1973; 17:365–385.
74. Buckey JC, Gaffney A, Lane LD, Levine BD, Watenpaugh DE, Wright SJ, Yancy CW, Meyer DM, Blomqvist CG. Central venous pressure in space. J Appl Physiol 1996; 81:19–25.

75. Udden MM, Driscoll TB, Pickett MH, Leach-Huntoon CS, Alfrey CP. Decreased production of red blood cells in human subjects exposed to microgravity. J Lab Clin Med 1995; 125:442–449.
76. Beck KC, Rehder K. Differences in regional vascular conductances in isolated dog lungs. J Appl Physiol 1986; 61:530–538.
77. Hakim TS, Lisbona R, Dean GW. Gravity-independent inequality in pulmonary blood flow in humans. J Appl Physiol 1987; 63:1114–1121.
78. Wagner PD, McRae J, Read J. Stratified distribution of blood flow in secondary lobule of the rat lung. J Appl Physiol 1967; 22:1115–1123.
79. West JB, Maloney JE, Castle BL. Effect of stratified inequality of bloodflow on gas exchange in liquid-filling lungs. J Appl Physiol 1972; 32:357–361.
80. Warrell DA, Evans JW, Clarke RO, Kingaby GP, West JB. Patterns of filling in the pulmonary capillary bed. J Appl Physiol 1972; 32:346–356.
81. Glenny RW, Robertson HT. Fractal properties of pulmonary blood flow: characterization of spatial heterogeneity. J Appl Physiol 1990; 69:532–545.
82. Permutt S. Pulmonary circulation and the distribution of blood and gas in the lungs. In: Anonymous Physiology in the Space Environment. Washington, DC, National Academy of Sciences National Research Council. 1485B, 1967, pp 38–56.
83. Prisk GK, Guy HJ, Elliott AR, West JB. Anomalous behavior of helium and sulfur hexafluoride in single breath washins during sustained microgravity. J Appl Physiol 1996; 80:1126–1132.
84. Lauzon AM, Prisk GK, Elliott AR, Paiva M, Verbanck S, West JB. Paradoxical helium and sulfurhexafluoride single-breath washouts in short-term versus sustained microgravity. J Appl Physiol 1997; 82:859–865.
85. Sutton JR, Reeves JT, Wagner PD, Groves BM, Cymerman A, Malconian MK, Rock PB, Young PM, Walter SD, Houston CS. Operation Everest II: oxygen transport during exercise at extreme simulated altitude. J Appl Physiol 1988; 64:1309–1321.
86. West JB, Wagner P. Predicted gas exchange on the summit of Mt. Everest. Respir Physiol 1980; 42:1–16.
87. West JB, Peters RM Jr, Aksnes G, Maret KH, Milledge JS, Schoene RB. Nocturnal periodic breathing at altitudes of 6,300 and 8,050 m. J Appl Physiol 1986; 61:280–287.

6

Anesthesia and Gas Exchange

GÖRAN HEDENSTIERNA

Uppsala University
Uppsala, Sweden

I. Introduction

Impaired oxygenation is a frequent finding in patients who undergo anesthesia for surgery (1). The impairment may be considered trivial in most patients in whom it is easily compensated for by increasing the fraction of inspired oxygen (F_{IO_2}) to 0.3 to 0.4, as is the standard today. In these cases, arterial partial pressure of oxygen (Pa_{O_2}) is "normal," and the impairment can be detected only as an increased alveolar–arterial oxygen tension difference ($P_{A-a_{O_2}}$). However, many patients develop hypoxemia for shorter or longer periods. Thus, mild to moderate hypoxemia (arterial oxygen saturation of between 85–90%) occurs in approximately half of all patients undergoing anesthesia and elective surgery, despite an F_{IO_2} of 0.3 to 0.4 (2). In 20% of patients, the saturation is less than 81% for up to 5 minutes (2). It may be argued that such hypoxemia does not cause any harm in most patients; however, it can hardly be considered a desired condition, and it is reasonable to argue that the causes of such hypoxemia should be identified and prevented if possible. Moreover, postoperative pulmonary complications occur in 1–3% of patients undergoing elective thoracic or abdominal surgery, and the complication rate may increase to 20% in emergency surgery (3,4). To what extent postoperative complications are caused by respiratory dysfunction during anesthesia is not clear. However, atelectasis that has developed during anesthesia remains in the postoperative period, and impairment in arterial oxygenation and decrease in forced spirometry correlate to the size of the atelectasis (5). Moreover, in view of the large number of anesthetics that are given in the Western world—some 30,000 to 50,000 per million inhabitants—a moderate complication rate will also have considerable social and economic consequences.

This review examines the causes of impaired oxygenation and increase in venous admixture (shunt and perfusion of regions in excess of their ventilation, so-called "low $\dot{V}_A/\dot{Q}$ regions") that is regularly observed during anesthesia. The morphological correlates (atelectasis and airway closure) to the functional impairment are then discussed. The influence of age and obstructive lung disease is also analyzed. Finally, measures that can be taken to prevent alveolar collapse and closure of airways are listed, and their advantages and disadvantages are discussed.

II. Oxygenation and Venous Admixture

Calculation of the shunt from arterial, mixed venous and alveolar P_{O_2} according to the standard shunt equation (6) has shown that it is increased from 1–2% in the awake, healthy subject to 8–10% in the anesthetized patient (1). The standard shunt equation is based on the assumption of two populations of alveoli: those that are "ideally" perfused in proportion to their ventilation and those that are perfused but not at all ventilated (the shunt). However, the lung does not contain two populations of alveoli only. There are a number of units with less ventilation than perfusion, with low ventilation–perfusion ratios (low $\dot{V}_A/\dot{Q}$ regions), as well as units that are ventilated in excess of their perfusion (high $\dot{V}_A/\dot{Q}$ regions). Perfusion of low $\dot{V}_A/\dot{Q}$ regions will also impede the oxygenation of blood and, to a varying extent, be included in the calculated shunt. The shunt, as measured by the standard oxygen technique, should therefore be called venous admixture (7) (Fig. 1). A good correspondence between venous admixture and the sum of true shunt and perfusion of low $\dot{V}_A/\dot{Q}$ regions was observed in a study of 45 anesthetized subject (8) (Fig. 1).

The magnitude of venous admixture depends on the F_{IO_2}. During room-air breathing, the influence of low $\dot{V}_A/\dot{Q}$ regions on the calculated venous admixture will be the highest. If, on the other hand, the subject is breathing or is ventilated with pure oxygen, the influence of low $\dot{V}_A/\dot{Q}$ regions will be eliminated. This is because the low $\dot{V}_A/\dot{Q}$ units will have almost as high P_{AO_2} as the better ventilated ones, and the end-capillary blood will be oxygenated to almost full extent (9). The minor difference, compared with normal lung units, is caused by the higher P_{CO_2} in the alveoli with low $\dot{V}_A/\dot{Q}$ ratios. Thus, venous admixture equals true shunt (perfusion of nonventilated alveoli) during oxygen breathing. This fact has also been used for the recording of true shunt. However, low $\dot{V}_A/\dot{Q}$ regions can be transformed to true shunt regions during oxygen breathing because of reabsorption of gas so that atelectasis is produced. Alveoli become unstable at a certain inspired

Anesthesia

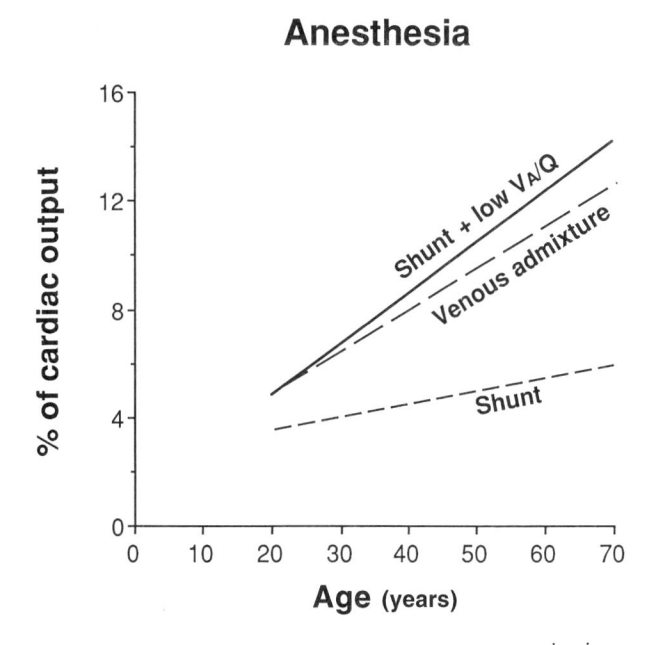

Figure 1 Plot of shunt, the sum of shunt and low $\dot{V}_A/\dot{Q}$, and venous admixture against age during anesthesia and muscle paralysis. Note the small and insignificant increase in shunt with age and the much steeper and significant increase in the sum of shunt and low $\dot{V}_A/\dot{Q}$ with increasing age. In addition, note the good agreement between venous admixture and the sum of shunt and low $\dot{V}_A/\dot{Q}$. Patients were ventilated with 40% O_2 in N_2. (From Ref. 8.)

ventilation perfusion ratio ($\dot{V}_{AI}/\dot{Q}$) that varies with the F_{IO_2}. Dantzker et al. (10) made calculations and demonstrated that during the breathing of 100% O_2, alveoli can collapse at a $\dot{V}_{AI}/\dot{Q}$ of 0.08. This means that units that are not far from the normal range of $\dot{V}_A/\dot{Q}$ ratios can collapse during oxygen breathing. Thus, true shunt can be increased by the maneuver used for measuring it. Moreover, the calculation of shunt during oxygen breathing requires that the blood gas analyzer be carefully calibrated for high Pa_{O_2}. This may be more difficult than is believed. Recording of a high Pa_{O_2} after standard calibration at normal P_{O_2} may result in underestimation of Pa_{O_2} and the calculation of an erroneously large shunt. However, other methods are available to measure shunt. This is discussed farther in the following section.

III. Distributions of Ventilation and Perfusion

The first studies on the regional distribution of ventilation during anesthesia were published in the early 1970s. Hulands et al. (11), using isotope technique in supine subjects, and Rehder et al. (12), using nitrogen washout techniques in each lung in the lateral position and isotope techniques in the supine position (13), found less-than-expected ventilation of the dependent lung regions or the dependent lung. A difference compared with the awake state was observed both in anesthetized, spontaneously breathing subjects and during muscle paralysis and mechanical ventilation. In a recent study, radioactively labeled aerosol and macroaggregated albumin were used for the assessment of ventilation and perfusion distributions by single-photo emission tomography in anesthetized patients (14). Ventilation was shown to be distributed preferentially to upper, nondependent lung regions and perfusion to lower, dependent regions, with subsequent worsening of the ventilation–perfusion matching ($\dot{V}_A/\dot{Q}$) (Fig. 2).

During anesthesia, pulmonary as well as systemic arterial pressure may be reduced. The decrease in the former will impede perfusion of the uppermost, nondependent lung regions. Institution of mechanical ventilation increases alveolar pressure, which interferes with nondependent perfusion (15). Thus, during anesthesia and/or mechanical ventilation, dependent regions become well perfused but poorly or not at all ventilated, whereas nondependent regions become well ventilated but poorly or not at all perfused. A $\dot{V}_A/\dot{Q}$ mismatch is established and interferes with pulmonary gas exchange (9). This has also been shown by means of multiple inert gas elimination technique (16). This technique is based on the infusion of a number of inert gases (usually six) in a vein and the calculations of the retention (arterial/mixed venous concentration ratio) and excretion (mixed expired/mixed venous concentration ratio) of each gas. The ratios, together with the measured solubilities of the inert gases, enable the construction of a virtually continuous distribution of ventilation and perfusion against $\dot{V}_A/\dot{Q}$ ratios.

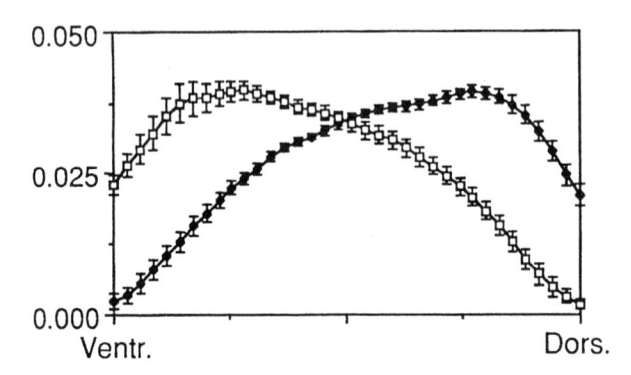

Figure 2 Vertical distributions of ventilation (□) and blood flow (♦), using single-photon emission computed tomography in supine patients (n = 10) during anesthesia and mechanical ventilation. Note the preferential distribution of ventilation to upper, nondependent lung regions and of perfusion to lower, dependent areas. The whole lung has been included for the analysis, from apex to base. This may explain why there is some ventilation at the bottom of the lung. Atelectasis is seldom near the apex. (From Ref. 14.)

Table 1 Ventilation–Perfusion Relationships During Anesthesia

	Q_{mean}	log SDQ	V_{mean}	log SDV	Shunt (% QT)	Dead space (% VT)	$Pa_{O_2}/F_{I_{O_2}}$ (kPa)
Awake	0.76	0.68	1.11	0.52	0.5	34.8	59.5
	(0.33)	(0.28)	(0.52)	(0.15)	(1.0)	(14.2)	(8.1)
Anesthesia	0.65	1.04	1.38	0.76	4.8	35.0	50.9
	(0.34)	(0.36)	(0.76)	(0.31)	(4.1)	(9.9)	(15.2)

QT = cardiac output, VT = tidal volume.
Mean (SD) ventilation–perfusion relationships in subjects with no cardiopulmonary disease (n = 45) awake and during general anesthesia and muscle paralysis. $F_{I_{O_2}}$ awake: 0.2; anesthetized: 0.42. (From Ref. 8.)

Rehder et al. (17) applied, for the first time, the multiple inert gas elimination technique to anesthesia. They studied young healthy volunteers during intravenous and inhalational anesthesia. They found that both ventilation and perfusion were distributed over wider ranges of $\dot{V}_A/\dot{Q}$ ratios after induction of anesthesia and that muscle paralysis increased dispersion of ventilation (log SDV) and blood flow (log SDQ) against $\dot{V}_A/\dot{Q}$ ratios. Increased log SDV and log SDQ were also found in another study on younger subjects during halothane anesthesia with muscle paralysis (18). In addition, a shunt was observed with a mean of 8% and a maximum of 23%.

In a study on middle-aged patients (mean age, 50 years) during halothane anesthesia and muscle paralysis before elective surgery (19), a significant increase in the mean shunt from approximately 1% to 9% was observed. There was also a doubling of the dispersion of $\dot{V}_A/\dot{Q}$ ratios. In elderly patients with impairment of lung function, halothane anesthesia with muscle paralysis caused considerable $\dot{V}_A/\dot{Q}$ mismatch (20). Shunt increased to a mean of 15% with a considerable variation between patients (Table 1).

IV. Alveolar Hypoventilation and Diffusion Limitation

There are, at least in theory, other mechanisms of hypoxia in addition to $\dot{V}_A/\dot{Q}$ mismatch and shunt. These are alveolar hypoventilation, either by reduced minute ventilation or by increased ventilation of nonperfused lung regions (increased dead space) and diffusion impairment. Alveolar hypoventilation also causes retention of CO_2.

A. Alveolar Hypoventilation

CO_2 elimination is frequently impaired during anesthesia, and it is generally held that this is caused by an increased dead space and reduced alveolar ventilation.

Single-breath washout recordings have shown anatomical dead space to be unchanged (21), indicating that the alveolar, or parallel, dead space must have been increased during anesthesia. By application of the multiple inert gas elimination technique, the increased CO_2 dead space during anesthesia was shown to be poorly perfused lung regions with high $\dot{V}_A/\dot{Q}$ ratios ($\dot{V}_A/\dot{Q}$: 10 to 100) (22). This additional high $\dot{V}_A/\dot{Q}$ can be explained by the tiny perfusion of corner vessels in interalveolar septa in upper-lung regions (where alveolar pressure may exceed pulmonary vascular pressure [Zone I]) (22). The ventilation of dead space (defined as lung regions with $\dot{V}_A/\dot{Q}$ ratios $\geq$ 100) is mostly unaffected by anesthesia (19). The impaired CO_2 elimination can be compensated for by increasing the ventilation and is seldom a problem in routine anesthesia with mechanical ventilation but may occur in the anesthetized, spontaneously breathing subject (23). Even so, hypoventilation will hardly cause any hypoxemia when the F_{IO_2} is increased to 0.3 to 0.4, as is routine during anesthesia.

B. Diffusion Limitation

In the normal lung, complete equilibration for oxygen takes place between the alveolar gas and the pulmonary end-capillary blood. Thus, there is no measurable diffusion limitation. No measurement of diffusion of gas over the alveolar–capillary membrane in the anesthetized subject has been reported. However, there seems to be no reason why diffusion should be impaired during anesthesia. For this to take place, the alveolar–capillary membrane must be thickened, the alveolar–capillary surface area must be drastically reduced, or blood flow through the capillaries must be markedly increased so that equilibration time is shortened. There are no signs of accumulation of extravascular lung water and only minor shifts in pulmonary blood volume during anesthesia that could affect the diffusion distance between the alveolar gas phase and the capillary blood (24). Cardiac output is, if anything, reduced during anesthesia so that equilibration time is at least as long as in the awake state. Finally, the increase in inspired oxygen concentration to 30–40% during anesthesia will facilitate diffusion across the alveolar–capillary membrane by increasing the driving pressure for O_2. Therefore, diffusion impairment can most likely be excluded as a cause of hypoxemia during anesthesia, unless it already existed when the patient was awake.

V. Morphologic Correlates of Shunt and Low $\dot{V}_A/\dot{Q}$

A. Reduced Functional Residual Capacity

Several studies have shown that the functional residual capacity (FRC) is reduced during anesthesia (25). In the majority of these studies, gas dilution techniques (helium equilibration, nitrogen washout) have been used. One drawback of gas distribution techniques is that the tracer gas used to assess FRC may not have been mixed with all gas in the lung because of occluded airways. This possible source of error was precluded in two studies by applying body plethysmography (26,27). This technique estimates all gas within the lung, whether located behind an occluded airway or not. Specially designed body boxes were used to allow measurements in anesthetized, supine subjects. During anesthesia, FRC was reduced both during spontaneous breathing and after muscle paralysis without difference between the two states (26,27). In the awake subject, the change from the upright to the supine position reduces FRC by 0.7 to 0.8 L. The further decrease of FRC caused by anesthesia [approximately 0.5 L, or 20% of the awake value (25)] results in a resting lung volume that is close to the awake residual volume.

There may be many mechanisms that contribute to the reduction in FRC during anesthesia: loss of tonic activity of inspiratory muscles, increased lung recoil, reduced chest wall recoil (26), development of atelectasis (28), increase in central blood volume (24), and cephalad shift of the diaphragm. However, there is some controversy over the role of the diaphragm. Froese and Bryan (29) used cineradiography and found a cranial shift of the end-expiratory position of the diaphragm during anesthesia and spontaneous breathing, without a further shift after muscle relaxation. This fits with the finding of an already reduced FRC in the anesthetized patient during spontaneous breathing, with no further decrease after muscle paralysis (26,27). Similar findings of a cranial shift of the diaphragm have been made by other groups (24,30). Other investigators have seen a caudal displacement of the dependent part of the diaphragm and a cranial shift of the nondependent part, with less overall effect of FRC (31,32). Nevertheless, it can be concluded that FRC is reduced in the anesthetized subject, along with a possible decrease in the pulmonary blood volume, further reducing thorax volume. The potential effect on the patency of airways and alveoli, and consequently pulmonary gas exchange, is the subject of the following section.

B. Airway Closure

Airways may close if pleural pressure exceeds the luminal airway pressure. This may occur during a deep expiration and begins in the dependent lung regions—an effect of the more positive pleural pressure around the lower lung regions than the upper ones (33). During the following inspiration, the airways open up again, and the subtended alveoli remain patent. Airway closure occurs at increasing lung volume with increasing age (34). In the sitting or standing position, closure of airways may take place above FRC in subjects aged 65 to 70 years. In the supine position, closure may occur at the age of 45 to 50 years because FRC is reduced by 0.7 to 1 L when lying down, whereas the lung volume at which airways begin to close during an expiration (closing capacity) is unaffected by posture (34).

Intermittent closure of airways can be expected to reduce the ventilation of dependent lung regions, which may then become low $\dot{V}_A/\dot{Q}$ units if perfusion is maintained or not reduced to the same extent as ventilation. Perfusion of low $\dot{V}_A/\dot{Q}$

regions increases with age (8), and PaO$_2$ decreases (35). It is tempting to attribute these changes to airway closure.

Because anesthesia causes a further reduction of FRC, by 0.4 to 0.5 L (25) it may be anticipated that airway closure becomes even more prominent in the anesthetized subject. A number of studies support this assumption (36,37), but there are others that do not (38,39). However, more recent studies do show a correlation between airway closure during anesthesia and $\dot{V}_A/\dot{Q}$ mismatch and shunt. Thus, a decrease of FRC during anesthesia below the awake closing capacity was accompanied by a significantly larger shunt than when FRC during anesthesia was larger than awake closing capacity (40). A correlation between airway closure, expressed as closing capacity minus FRC, and perfusion of poorly ventilated lung regions (low $\dot{V}_A/\dot{Q}$) has also been demonstrated in anesthetized patients (41). Finally, the perfusion of low $\dot{V}_A/\dot{Q}$ regions is increased during anesthesia and increases with age in a similar fashion as in awake subjects (8). All of these observations make it likely that low $\dot{V}_A/\dot{Q}$ regions during anesthesia are caused by airway closure.

C. Atelectasis

Although it has been known that shunt appears or is increased during anesthesia, its cause has remained obscure until the last 10 years. More than 30 years ago, Bendixen et al. (42) proposed "a concept of atelectasis." They had observed a successive decrease in compliance of the respiratory system and a similarly successive decrease in arterial oxygenation both in anesthetized humans and animal experiments. This was assumed to reflect progressive formation of reabsorbtion atelectasis. However, other research groups were unable to reproduce their findings but noticed a more prompt decrease in compliance and PaO$_2$ on induction of anesthesia. Moreover, atelectasis could not be demonstrated on conventional chest radiograph.

It took another 20 years to make atelectasis an attractive explanation of the shunt during anesthesia. In anesthetized small children, Damgaard-Pedersen and Qvist (43) noticed densities in dependent lung regions when the patients underwent computed tomography for diagnosis of central nervous disorders. Densities in dependent lung regions have also been observed in adult patients during anesthesia before surgery (28). They have an attenuation number of approximately zero on the Hounsfield scale, indicating airlessness. Qualitatively similar densities in anesthetized sheep (44) and horses (45) have been shown to be atelectasis with little or no interstitial edema or vascular congestion. It is therefore reasonable to conclude that the densities in anesthetized humans represent atelectasis. The atelectasis can be observed in the anesthetized subject during spontaneous breathing, and there is only a small additional increase in the size of the atelectasis with muscle paralysis and mechanical ventilation (46). The atelectasis is produced during both inhalational and intravenous anesthesia, the only exception thus far being ketamine anesthesia (47). However, when a muscle relaxant is given, atelectasis appears also with ketamine. Atelectasis is therefore common, and was observed in almost 90% of more than 100 patients (48). It is interesting to note that the atelectasis cannot be observed on conventional chest radiography, not even by an experienced radiologist who knows that a simultaneous computed tomography (CT) scan has demonstrated their existence. This may be because of the location of the atelectatis in the dorsal lung region near the spine and the transverse process of the vertebrae, which may make it difficult to distinguish the collapsed lung tissue from the bone nearby. The atelectatic area varies considerably between subjects, from zero to more than 10% of the pulmonary area at a transverse level just above the diaphragm (48). It should be remembered that the atelectasis consists of three to four times more lung tissue per unit volume than the aerated lung; therefore, the amount of collapsed tissue can be as much as one third of the lung at the level of the CT scan. The size of the atelectasis decreases from the diaphragm toward the apex of the lung in the supine subject (49). Therefore, the total lung collapse may be smaller than what can be assumed from one CT scan near the lung base. A three-dimensional reconstruction of atelectasis in an anesthetized patient, using spiral CT, is shown in Figure 3.

There is a weak correlation between the size of the atelectasis and body weight or body mass index (50,51), with obese patients showing larger atelectatic areas than lean ones. Although this was expected, it came as a surprise that the atelectasis is independent of age, with children and young people showing as much atelectasis as elderly patients (8). Another unexpected observation was that patients with chronic obstructive lung disease showed less or no atelectasis during the 45 minutes of anesthesia under which they were studied (52).

There is a good correlation between the atelectasis and the shunt as measured by multiple inert gas elimination technique. A regression equation, based on a total of 45 patients, has been calculated as: shunt $= 0.8 \times$ atelectasis $+ 1.7$ ($r = 0.8$; $P < 0.01$), with atelectasis in percent of the pulmonary area just above the diaphragm, and shunt in percent of cardiac output (modified from Ref. 8). Interestingly, shunt did not increase with age, whereas regions with poor ventilation in relation to their perfusion showed an age dependence, as previously discussed (see also Fig. 1). By combining CT scanning and single-photon emission computed tomography, the distribution of shunt and its location within the atelectatic area can be confirmed (14) (Fig. 4).

VI. Prevention of Atelectasis During Anesthesia

The procedures that can be undertaken to prevent atelectasis or to reopen collapsed alveoli are: (1) positive end-expiratory pressure (PEEP), (2) maintenance or restoration of respiratory muscle tone, (3) recruitment maneuvers, and (4) minimization of pulmonary gas resorption.

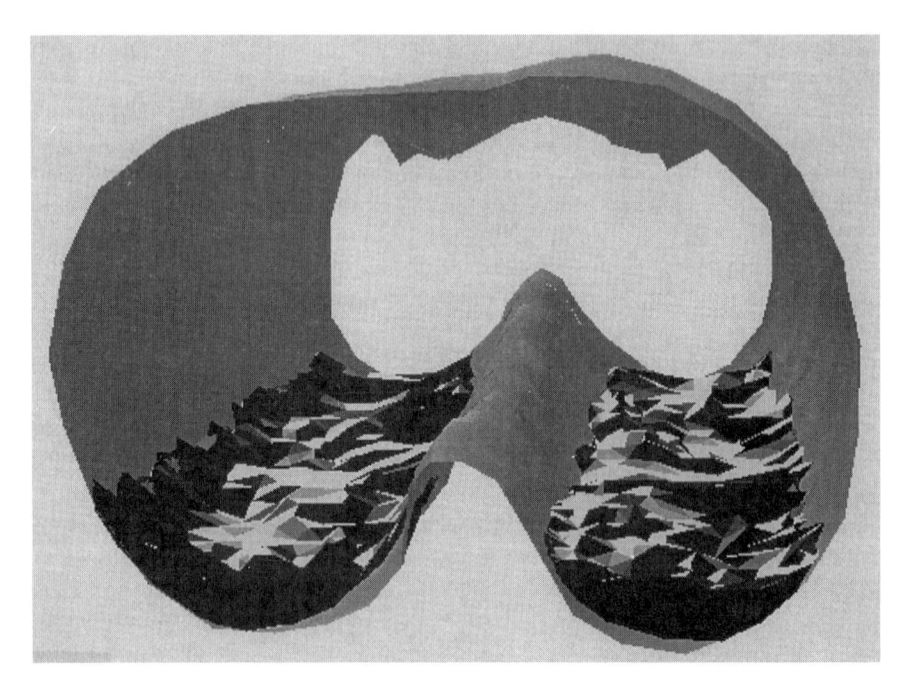

Figure 3 Three-dimensional reconstructions of the chest wall and atelectasic regions in the dependent part of the lungs in an anesthetized and paralyzed patient before commencement of surgery. The reconstruction has been performed by means of spiral computed tomography, with the patient slowly being moved through the gantry of the computed tomography scanner during continuous exposure. The chest wall is shown in grey with the anterior part up and the dorsal border down. The ridge in the dorsal part corresponds to the location of the spine. The caudal region of the chest wall is closest to the viewer who looks into the thorax as from the diaphragm. The black and white regions in the bottom of both hemithoraces correspond to the atelectasis in the dependent region of both lungs. Note the rough surface and decreasing size of the atelectasis toward the apex. (From the patient material in Ref. 49.)

A. PEEP

The application of 10 cm H_2O PEEP has been tested in several studies and consistently reopens collapsed lung tissue (28,53). However, some atelectasis persists in most patients. Further increase in the PEEP level may re-expand these areas. However, PEEP does not seem to be the ideal procedure. First, shunt is not reduced, and arterial oxygenation is therefore not improved on average. This was demonstrated in 1974 by Hewlett et al. (54), who warned against the "indiscriminate use of PEEP in routine anaesthesia." The maintenance of shunt may be explained by the redistribution of blood flow toward the most dependent parts when intrathoracic pressure

Anesthesia and Gas Exchange 187

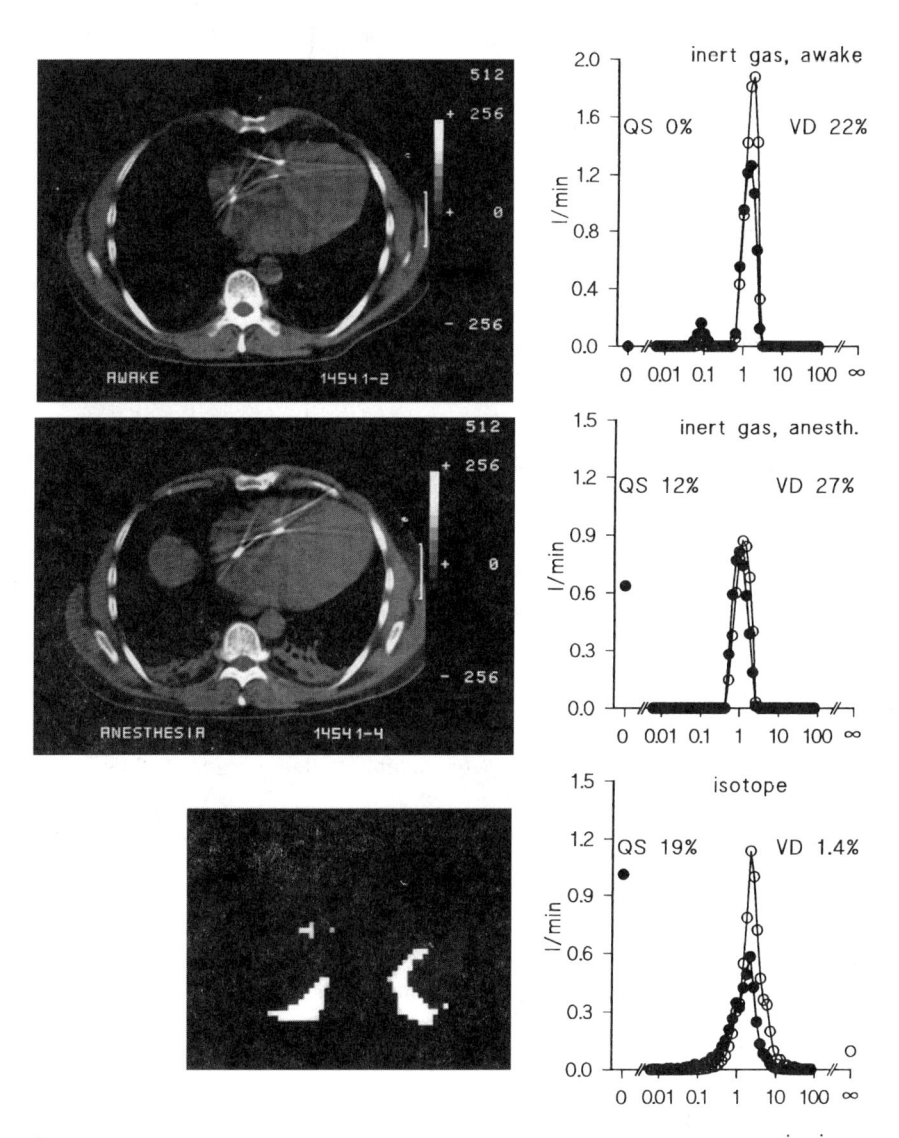

Figure 4 Computed tomography scans and inert gas ventilation–perfusion ($\dot{V}_A/\dot{Q}$) distributions in a patient when awake (uppermost panels), and when anesthetized and mechanically ventilated (midpanels). Single-photon emission computed tomography (SPECT) scan showing perfused but nonventilated regions in the lower lung (white zone) in a transverse cut similar to the computed tomography exposures (left lowermost panel). In addition, the SPECT (isotope) data have been used to reconstruct the $\dot{V}/\dot{Q}$ distribution. Note the appearance of atelectasis and shunt during anesthesia, and that the shunt blood flow is mainly in the atelectatic region. (From Ref. 14.)

is increased, so that any persisting atelectasis in the bottom of the lung receives a larger share of the pulmonary blood flow than without PEEP (55). The increased intrathoracic pressure will also impede venous return and lower cardiac output. This results in a lower venous oxygen tension for a given oxygen uptake, which will augment the desaturating effect of shunted blood and perfusion of poorly ventilated regions on the arterial oxygenation (9). Second, the lung recollapses rapidly after discontinuation of PEEP. Within 1 minute after cessation of PEEP, the collapse is as large as it was before the application of PEEP (56). This means that to bring the patient through the perioperative period without lung collapse, PEEP must be maintained without interruption, as well as during recovery and early postoperative periods. PEEP also carries the risk of overexpanding well-aerated alveoli, causing barotrauma or volotrauma (57).

B. Maintenance of Respiratory Muscle Tone

The use of the an anesthetic that allows maintenance of respiratory muscle tone will prevent atelectasis formation. As previously mentioned, ketamine does not cause atelectasis as long as it is used alone or in combination with other drugs that do not interfere with the respiratory muscle function. However, if muscle relaxation is required, atelectasis will occur as with other anaesthetics (47).

Another possibility would be to restore respiratory muscle function. This can be achieved, at least in part, by a diaphragm pacing (by applying phrenic nerve stimulation), which reduces the atelectatic area (56). However, the effect was small, and it can be argued that the technique is too complicated to become routine during anesthesia and surgery.

C. Recruitment Maneuvers

The use of a sigh maneuver, or inflation with double normal tidal volume, has been advocated to reopen any collapsed lung tissue. However, the atelectasis is not affected by an ordinary tidal volume, to an end-inspiratory airway pressure of 10 cm H_2O, nor by a deep sigh with an airway pressure to +20 cm H_2O (58). Not until an airway pressure of 30 cm H_2O was reached did the atelectasis decrease to approximately half the initial value. For a complete reopening of all collapsed lung tissue, an inflation pressure of 40 cm H_2O was required (58). Such a large inflation and subsequent expiration down to -20 cm H_2O corresponded to a vital capacity measured during spontaneous breathing with the patient awake. Although approved for lung function studies in anesthetized subjects (59), it may be argued that such a maneuver can be risky and cause baro/volotrauma (57). Therefore, another procedure was tested with repeated inflations of the lung to an airway pressure of +30 cm H_2O. However, this caused only minor further opening of lung tissue after the first maneuver (58). A full vital capacity maneuver with an inflation to +40 cm H_2O therefore seems necessary to reopen the lung completely.

D. Minimizing Gas Reabsorption

Ventilation of the lungs with pure oxygen after a vital capacity maneuver that had reopened previously collapsed lung tissue resulted in a rapid reappearance of the atelectasis (60). If, on the other hand, ventilation was made with 40% O_2 in nitrogen, atelectasis reappeared slowly, and 40 minutes after the vital capacity maneuver only 20% of the initial atelectasis had reappeared. Thus, ventilation during anesthesia should be performed with a moderate F_{IO_2} (e.g., 0.3 to 0.4), which should be increased only if arterial oxygenation is compromised.

Moreover, avoidance of the preoxygenation procedure during induction of anesthesia more or less eliminated the atelectasis formation during anesthesia (61). If the preoxygenation period was prolonged from a standard 2 to 3 minutes to 4 to 5 minutes, atelectasis increased further in size (62). Thus, avoidance of preoxygenation, or at least lowering of the F_{IO_2} during the induction phase will reduce or avoid the formation of atelectasis during the subsequent anesthesia. It is obvious that the lowering of F_{IO_2} during induction may increase the risk of hypoxemia in a difficult and prolonged intubation. However, the present findings call for a re-evaluation of current standard procedures for inducing anesthesia. It may be that induction of anesthesia with an F_{IO_2} of 50–80% is enough to ensure safe oxygenation. Moreover, the obligatory use of pulse oximeters during anesthesia in many countries makes it easy to detect dangerous hypoxemia.

A vital capacity maneuver immediately after the intubation of the airway, followed by additional vital capacity maneuvers every 30 to 40 minutes or so will keep the lung inflated during anesthesia and into the postoperative period. It is the opinion of the author that such concepts deserve attention and should be tested in larger trials.

VII. Hypoxic Pulmonary Vasoconstriction

More than 50 years ago, von Euler and Liljestrand (63) observed that hypoxia caused pulmonary vasoconstriction. It is held as a compensatory mechanism that redistributes blood flow away from hypoventilated areas and by that means counters hypoxemia. Attenuation of hypoxic pulmonary vasoconstriction (HPV) is frequently considered a mechanism of impaired gas exchange during anesthesia. Most inhalational anesthetics have been found to inhibit HPV in isolated lung preparations (64) (Fig. 5). However, no such effect has been observed with intravenous anesthetics (barbiturates (65). Results from human studies vary, reasonably explained by the complexity of the experiment, which causes several variables to change at the same time. In studies with no gross changes in cardiac output, the inhalational anesthetics isoflurane and halothane depress the HPV response by 50% at 2 minimum alveolar concentration (66). The HPV response acts efficiently both in the atelectatic lung (where HPV seems to be more important than mechanical kinking of vessels) and during ventilation with hypoxic gases (67).

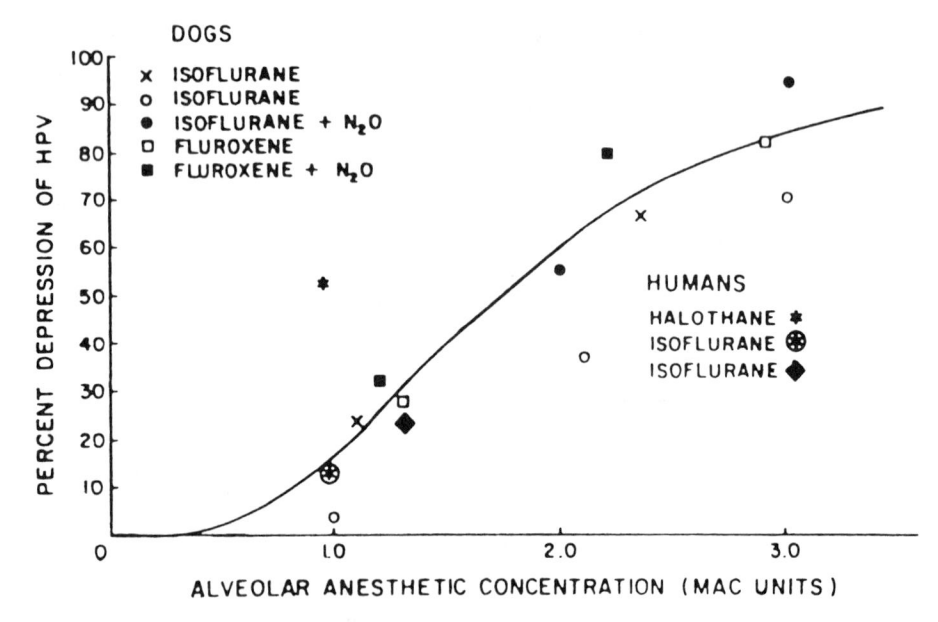

Figure 5 Inhibition of the hypoxic pulmonary vasoconstrictor response by inhalational anesthetics. Various data from humans and animals have been plotted. (From Ref. 67.)

As previously mentioned, the breathing of pure oxygen may increase the shunt by promoting alveolar collapse (10). High F_{IO_2} may also increase shunt by increasing P_{AO_2} and thus attenuating the HPV response (66). Similarly, pulmonary hypertension counters HPV, presumably by necessitating higher muscle force to constrict a vessel.

It should also be emphasized that attenuation of the HPV response cannot be the only disturbance during anesthesia to cause gas exchange impairment. If there were no corresponding ventilatory impediment, then loss of pulmonary vascular tone would not matter because adequate gas exchange would still occur. Loss of HPV can only aggravate an existing $\dot{V}_A/\dot{Q}$ mismatch.

VIII. Obstructive Lung Disease

Patients with obstructive lung disease usually suffer from more severe gas exchange impairment during anesthesia than subjects with healthy lungs (68). However, the cause and pattern of such mismatch differs from what might be anticipated. Thus, smokers with moderate airflow limitation may have less shunt during anesthesia than subjects with healthy lungs, as measured by multiple inert gas elimination. Thus, in patients with mild to moderate bronchitis who were to undergo lung surgery (69) or vascular reconstructive surgery in the leg (70), only a small shunt was noticed. However, log SDQ was increased. More recently, patients with chronic bronchitis were studied while awake and during anesthesia with both multiple inert gas elimination for assessment of $\dot{V}_A/\dot{Q}$ and CT to explore atelectasis formation (71). Interestingly, these patients developed no or very small atelectasis during anesthesia and no or only minor shunt. However, a considerable $\dot{V}_A/\dot{Q}$ mismatch was observed with large perfusion fraction to low $\dot{V}_A/\dot{Q}$ regions, as in previous studies in which the multiple inert gas elimination technique had been used. Consequently, the arterial oxygenation was more impaired than that in subjects with healthy lungs, but the cause was different to that in the normal subject. A possible reason for the absence of atelectasis and shunt may be the chronic hyperinflation, which changes the mechanical behavior of the lungs and the interaction with the chest wall, so that the tendency to collapse is reduced. Alternatively, airways may be less stable than those in subjects with healthy lungs, causing bronchioli to close before alveoli collapse. However, regions with low $\dot{V}_A/\dot{Q}$ ratios can be transferred over time to resorption atelectasis (10). Thus, the "protection" against atelectasis formation during anesthesia by the obstructive lung disease need not last for long. Regions with low $\dot{V}_A/\dot{Q}$ may be replaced at atelectasis, caused by slow resorption of gas behind occluded airways later during surgery and in the postoperative period.

IX. One-Lung Ventilation

To enable surgery of the lung and sometimes of mediastinal organs, gas exchange may have to be maintained by the ventilation of only one lung that must provide the oxygenation of blood and the elimination of CO_2. However, the nonventilated lung will receive a substantial fraction of cardiac output that is not oxygenated and thus causes a shunt. In theory, this can be countered by two different approaches. First, the persisting blood flow through the nonventilated lung can be oxygenated by a continuous small flow of oxygen to that lung, so-called "apneic oxygenation" (72). It can be executed with low levels of positive airway pressure to maintain the patency of the nonventilated alveoli. However, this may not always be enough to ensure adequate oxygenation.

Second, blood flow through the nonventilated lung can be reduced. The positioning of the patient in the lateral posture with the nonventilated lung up reduces its blood flow from 40–50% to 20–25% of cardiac output (73). By pulling a snare around the pulmonary artery or inflating a balloon in the vessel, blood flow almost can be eliminated, but the procedures are accompanied by certain risks that preclude their use in clinical routine.

Redistribution of blood flow by pharmacological means is more feasible for clinical practice and can be achieved by either constricting the vessels of the nonventilated lung (e.g., prostaglandin $F_{2\alpha}$) or dilating the vessels of the ventilated lung (e.g., prostaglandin E_1) (74,75). Recently, manipulation of the nitric oxide–guanylate cyclase system was attempted in one-lung anesthesia. Thus, blockade of the nitric oxide synthase enhances hypoxic pulmonary vasoconstriction. It also increases the pulmonary artery pressure (76). Nebulization of a nitric oxide synthase blocker into the airways of the nonventilated lung may be a way of reducing the increase in pulmonary artery pressure and producing a regional effect in the desired lung. An alternative approach is to administer nitric oxide by inhalation to the ventilated lung (77,78).

Thus, there are several means to redistribute further blood flow away from the nonventilated lung during one-lung anesthesia. Whether any of these will become clinically routine remains to be shown.

X. Postoperative Lung Function

Pulmonary function remains impaired for some days in the postoperative period (36). The extent of impairment relates to the site of surgery and the surgical technique. Procedures not involving the trunk cause minor and short-lasting reductions of ventilatory function and FRC with small effects on arterial oxygenation (36,79,80). These effects are more pronounced after lower laparotomies and are greatly magnified after upper laparotomies and thoracotomies, and they may not be restored even by the fifth postoperative day (80). Transverse abdominal incisions reduce postoperative lung function less than sagittal incisions (81). Preservation of muscle fibers in the abdominal wall by splinting them layer by layer rather than cutting them seems to preserve ventilatory capacity the most in the postoperative period (82). Laparoscopic surgery offers significant advantage regarding postoperative lung function compared with an open surgical approach (83).

Forced expiratory vital capacity and peak flows are often reduced to half and FRC to less than 70% of the preoperative value after laparotomy, mainly because of impaired diaphragmatic function (80). Although nearly normal transdiaphragmatic pressures are obtained with phrenic nerve stimulation, patients are incapable of fully activating their diaphragm in the early postoperative course despite excellent pain control by epidural analgesia (84). Thus, there seems to be a reflex inhibition of diaphragmatic function not related to pain. There is a high incidence of atelectasis in dependent lung regions detectable by CT after laparotomy and open heart surgery in patients not considered to suffer from postoperative pulmonary complications (5,85). It is possible that such atelectasis is a regular companion of abdominal and thoracic surgery, and it has been shown that the amount of venous admixture correlates to atelectasis (85). The reduction of FRC and its relation to closing volume also correlate to arterial hypoxemia (79), indicating that both airway closure and alveolar collapse contribute to the gas exchange impairment postoperatively.

The incidence of clinically significant postoperative pulmonary complications is associated with the site and length of surgery, tobacco smoking, age, obstructive lung disease, and the physical status of the patient (4,86). In an unselected group of patients, the incidence ranges from 1–2% after minor surgery to 20% after upper abdominal and thoracic surgery (4,80,86).

XI. Conclusion

Anesthesia impedes the oxygenation of blood, during both spontaneous breathing and muscle paralysis and mechanical ventilation. A likely explanation is loss of respiratory muscle tone (also during spontaneous breathing) that causes lung volume reduction, collapse of alveoli (atelectasis), and closure of airways. If muscle tone is preserved, e.g., during ketamine anesthesia, no atelectasis is produced. In addition, if the patient is breathing or is ventilated with low fractions of oxygen (FIO_2: 0.3) during the induction and the subsequent anesthesia, no atelectasis is produced. The atelectatic tissue can also be reopened by deep inflations of the lung (vital capacity maneuvers) but not by a conventional deep sigh (approximately double tidal volume). There are therefore means to prevent atelectasis formation and to improve oxygenation during anesthesia. Because atelectasis remains for a couple of days after surgery, it also may affect postoperative lung function. It is tempting to speculate that persisting atelectasis is a cause of postoperative infection, but such links need more evidence before they can be considered to be proved.

References

1. Nunn JF. Respiratory aspects of anaesthesia. In: Nunn's Applied Respiratory Physiology. 4th ed. Oxford, Heinemann, 1993, pp 407–408.
2. Moller JT, Johannessen NW, Berg H, Espersen K, Larsen LE. Hypoxaemia during anesthesia: an observer study. Br J Anaesth 1991; 66:437–444.
3. Pedersen T, Viby-Mogensen J, Ringsted C. Anaesthetic practice and postoperative pulmonary complications. Acta Anaesthesiol Scand 1992; 36:812–818.
4. Celli BR, Rodriguez KS, Snider GL. A controlled trial of intermittent positive pressure breathing, incentive spirometry, and deep breathing exercises in preventing pulmonary complications after abdominal surgery. Am Rev Respir Dis 1984; 130:12–15.
5. Lindberg P, Gunnarsson L, Tokics L, Secher E, Lundquist H, Brismar B, Hedenstierna G. Atelectasis, gas exchange and lung function in the postoperative period. Acta Anaesthesiol Scand 1992; 36:546–553.
6. Berggren SM. The oxygen deficit of arterial blood caused by nonventilating parts of the lung. Acta Physiol Scand 1942; Suppl No. 11.
7. Nunn JF. Distribution of pulmonary ventilation and perfusion. In: Nunn's Applied Respiratory Physiology. 4th ed. Oxford, Heinemann, 1993, pp 178–187.
8. Gunnarsson L, Tokics L. Gustavsson H, Hedenstierna G. Influence of age of atelectasis formation and gas exchange impairment during general anesthesia. Br J Anaesth 1991; 66:423–432.
9. West JB. State of the art: ventilation-perfusion relationships. Am Rev Resp Dis 1977; 116: 919–943.

10. Dantzker DR, Wagner PD, West JB. Instability of lung units with low V_A/Q ratios during O_2 breathing. J Appl Physiol 1975; 38:886–895.
11. Hulands GH, Greene R, Iliff LD, Nunn JF. Influence of anesthesia on the regional distribution of perfusion and ventilation in the lung. Clin Sci 1970; 38:451–460.
12. Rehder K, Hatch DJ, Sessler A, Fowler WS. The function of each lung of anesthetized and paralyzed man during mechanical ventilation. Anesthesiology 1972; 37:16–26.
13. Rehder K, Sessler AD, Rodarte JR. Regional intrapulmonary gas distribution in awake and anesthetized-paralyzed man. J Appl Physiol 1977; 42:391–402.
14. Tokics L, Hedenstierna G, Svensson L, Brismar B, Cederlund T, Lundquist H, Strandberg Å. V/Q distribution and correlation to atelectasis in anesthetized paralyzed humans. J Appl Physiol 1996; 8:1822–1833.
15. Hedenstierna G, White F, Wagner PD. Spatial distribution of pulmonary blood flow in the dog during end-expiratory pressure ventilation. J Appl Physiol 1979; 46:278–287.
16. Wagner PD, Saltzman HA, West JB. Measurement of continuous distributions of ventilation-perfusion ratios: theory. J Appl Physiol 1974; 36:588–599.
17. Rehder K, Knopp TJ, Sessler AD, Didier EP. Ventilation-perfusion relationship in young healthy awake and anesthetized-paralyzed man. J Appl Physiol 1979; 47:745–753.
18. Prutow RJ, Dueck R, Davies NJH, Clausen J. Shunt development in young adult surgical patients due to inhalation anesthesia. Anesthesiology 1982; 57:A477.
19. Bindslev L, Hedenstierna G, Santesson J, Gotlieb I, Carvallhas A. Ventilation-perfusion distribution during inhalation anesthesia: effect of spontaneous breathing, mechanical ventilation and positive end-expiratory pressure. Acta Anaesthesiol Scand 1981; 25:360–371.
20. Dueck R, Young I, Clausen J, Wagner PD. Altered distribution of pulmonary ventilation and blood flow following induction of inhalational anesthesia. Anesthesiology 1980; 52:113–125.
21. Nunn JF, Hill DW. Respiratory dead space and arterial to end-tidal CO_2 tension difference in anesthetized man. J Appl Physiol 1960; 15:383–389.
22. Hedenstierna G, White FC, Mazzone R, Wagner PD. Redistribution of pulmonary blood flow in the dog with positive end-expiratory pressure ventilation. J Appl Physiol 1979; 46:278–287.
23. Nunn JF. Effects of anaesthesia on respiration. Br J Anaesth 1990; 65:54–57.
24. Hedenstierna G, Strandberg Å, Brismar B, Lundquist H, Svensson L, Tokics L. Functional residual capacity, thoracoabdominal dimensions, and central blood volume during general anesthesia with muscle paralysis and mechanical ventilation. Anesthesiology 1985; 62:247–254.
25. Wahba RWM. Perioperative functional residual capacity. Can J Anaesth 1991; 38:384–400.
26. Westbrook PR, Stubbs SE, Sessler AD, Rehder K, Hyatt RE. Effects of anesthesia and muscle paralysis on respiratory mechanics in normal man. J Appl Physiol 1973; 34:81–86.
27. Hedenstierna G, Järnberg P-O, Gottlieb I. Thoracic gas volume measured by body plethysmography during anesthesia and muscle paralysis. Anesthesiology 1981; 55:439–443.

28. Brismar B, Hedenstierna G, Lundquist H, Strandberg Å, Svensson L, Tokics L. Pulmonary densities during anesthesia with muscular relaxation: a proposal of atelectasis. Anesthesiology 1985; 62:422–428.
29. Froese AB, Bryan C. Effects of anesthesia and paralysis on diaphragmatic mechanics in man. Anesthesiology 1974; 41:242–255.
30. Drummond GB, Allan PL, Logan MR. Changes in diaphragmatic position in association with the induction of anesthesia. Br J Anaesth 1986; 58:1246–1251.
31. Krayer S, Rehder K, Beck KC, Cameron PD, Didier EP, Hoffman EA. Quantification of thoracic volumes by three-dimensional imaging. J Appl Physiol 1987; 62:591–598.
32. Warner DO, Warner MA, Ritman EL. Human chest wall function while awake and during halothane anesthesia 1. Quiet breathing. Anesthesiology 1995; 82:6–19.
33. Milic-Emili J, Henderson JAM, Dolovich MB, Trop D, Kaneko K. Regional distribution of inspired gas in the lung. J Appl Physiol 1966; 21:749–759.
34. Leblanc P, Ruff F, Milic-Emili J. Effects of age and body position on "airway closure" in man. J Appl Physiol 1970; 28:448–451.
35. Marshall BE, Whyche MQ. Hypoxemia during and after anesthesia. Anesthesiology 1972; 37:178–209.
36. Hedenstierna G, McCarthy G, Bergstrom M. Airway closure during mechanical ventilation. Anesthesiology 1976; 44:114–123.
37. Gilmour I, Burnham M, Craig DB. Closing capacity measurement during general anesthesia. Anesthesiology 1976; 45:477–482.
38. Juno P, Marsh M, Knopp TJ, et al. Closing capacity in awake and anesthetized-paralysed man. J Appl Physiol 1978; 44:238–244.
39. Bergman NA, Tien YK. Contribution of the closure of pulmonary units to impaired oxygenation during anesthesia. Anesthesiology 1983; 59:395–401.
40. Dueck R, Prutow RJ, Davies NJH, Clausen JL, Davidson TM. The lung volume at which shunting occurs with inhalation anesthesia. Anesthesiology 1988; 69:854–861.
41. Rothen HU, Sporre B, Enhberg G, Hedenstierna G. Airway closure, atelectasis and gas exchange during general anaesthesia. Br J Anaesth 1998; 81:681–686.
42. Bendixen HH, Hedley-Whyte J, Laver MB. Impaired oxygenation in surgical patients during general anesthesia with controlled ventilation: a concept of atelectasis. N Engl J Med 1963; 269:991–996.
43. Damgaard-Pedersen K, Qvist T. Pediatric pulmonary CT-scanning. Pediatr Radiol 1980; 9:145–148.
44. Hedenstierna G, Tokics L, Lundh B, Tokics L, Strandberg Å, Brismar B, Frostell C. Pulmonary densities during anaesthesia: an experimental study on lung histology and gas exchange. Eur Respir J 1989; 2:528–535.
45. Nyman G, Funkquist B, Kvart C, Frostell C, Tokics L, Strandberg Å, Brismar B, Lundquist H, Hedenstierna G. Atelectasis causes gas exchange impairment in the anaesthetised horse. Equine Vet J 1990; 22:317–324.
46. Strandberg A, Tokics L, Brismar B, Hedenstierna G. Atelectasis during anesthesia and in the postoperative period. Acta Anaesthesiol Scand 1986; 30:145–148.
47. Tokics L, Strandberg Å, Brismar B, Lundquist H, Hedenstierna G. Computerized tomography of the chest and gas exchange measurements during ketamine anaesthesia. Acta Anaesthesiol Scand 1987; 32:684–692.

48. Lundquist H, Hedenstierna G, Strandberg Å, Tokics L, Brismar B. CT-assessment of dependent lung densities in man during general anaesthesia. Acta Radiologica 1995; 36:626–632.
49. Reber A, Engberg G, Sporre, B, Kviele L, Rothen HU, Wegenius G, Nylund U, Hedenstierna G. Volumetric analysis of aeration in the lungs during general anaesthesia. Br J Anaesth 1996; 76:760–766.
50. Strandberg Å, Tokics L, Brismar B, Lundquist H, Hedenstierna G. Constitutional factors promoting development of atelectasis during anesthesia. Acta Anaesthesiol Scand 1987; 31:21–24.
51. Rothen HU, Sporre B, Engberg G, Wegenius G, Hedenstierna G. Re-expansion of atelectasis during general anesthesia: a CT-study. Br J Anaesth 1993; 71:788–795.
52. Gunnarsson L, Tokics L, Lundquist H, Brismar B, Strandberg Å, Berg B, Hedenstierna G. Chronic obstructive pulmonary disease and anesthesia: formation of atelectasis and gas exchange impairment. Eur Respir J 1991; 4:1106-1116.
53. Tokics L, Hedenstierna G, Strandberg A, Brismar B, Lundquist H. Lung collapse and gas exchange during general anesthesia: effects of spontaneous breathing, muscle paralysis, and positive end-expiratory pressure. Anesthesiology 1987; 66:157–167.
54. Hewlett AM, Hulands GH, Nunn JF, Milledge JS. Functional residual capacity during anaesthesia III: artificial ventilation. Br J Anaesth 1974; 46:495–503.
55. West JB, Dollery CT, Naimark A. Distribution of blood flow in isolated lung: relations to vascular and alveolar pressure. J Appl Physiol 1964; 19:13–24.
56. Hedenstierna G, Tokics L, Lundquist H, Andersson T, Strandberg A, Brismar B. Phrenic nerve stimulation during halothane anesthesia: effects of atelectasis. Anesthesiology 1994; 80:751–760.
57. Dreyfuss D, Saumon G. Barotrauma is volutrauma, but which volume is the one responsible? [editorial]. Intensive Care Med 1992; 18:139–141.
58. Rothen HU, Sporre B, Engberg G, Wegenius G, Hedenstierna G. Re-expansion of atelectasis during general anaesthesia: a computed tomography study. Br J Anaesth 1993; 71:788–795.
59. Leith DE. Editorial: barotrauma in human research. Crit Care Med 1976; 4:159–161.
60. Rothen HU, Sporre B, Engberg G, Wegenius G, Hogman M, Hedenstierna G. Influence of gas composition on recurrence of atelectasis after a reexpansion maneuver during general anesthesia. Anesthesiology 1995; 82:832–842.
61. Rothen HU, Sporre B, Engberg G, Wegenius G, Reber A, Hedenstierna G. Prevention of atelectasis during general anaesthesia. Lancet 1995; 345:1387–1391.
62. Reber A, Engberg G, Wegenius G, Hedenstierna G. Lung aeration: the effect of preoxygenation and hyperoxygenation during total intravenous anaesthesia. Anaesthesia 1996; 51:733–737.
63. von Euler US, Liljestrand G. Observations on the pulmonary arterial blood pressure in cat. Acta Physiol Scand 1946; 12:310–320.
64. Sykes MK, Loh L, Seed RF, Kafer ER, Chakrabarti NK. The effects of inhalational anaesthetics on hypoxic pulmonary vasoconstriction and pulmonary vascular resistance in the perfused lungs of the dog and cat. Br J Anaesth 1972; 44:776–778.
65. Bjertnaes LJ. Hypoxia induced vasoconstriction in isolate perfused lungs exposed to injectable or inhalational anaesthetics. Acta Anaesthesiol Scand 1977; 21:133–147.

66. Marshall BE. Effects of anesthetics on pulmonary gas exchange. In: Stanley TH, Sperry RJ, eds. Anaesthesia and the Lung. London: Kluwer Academic Publishers, 1989, pp 117–125.
67. Miller FL, Chen L, Malmkvist G, Marshall C, Marshall BE. Mechanical factors do not influence blood flow distribution in atelectasis. Anesthesiology 1989; 70:481–488.
68. Nunn JF. Respiratory aspects of anaesthesia. In: Nunn's applied respiratory physiology. 4th ed. Oxford: Heinemann, 1993, pp 407–408.
69. Anjou-Lindskog E, Broman L, Broman M, Holmgren A, Settergren G, Öhqvist G. Effect of intravenous anesthesia on V_A/Q distribution. Anesthesiology 1985; 62:485–492.
70. Hedenstierna G, Lundh R, Johansson H. Alveolar stability during anesthesia for reconstructive vascular surgery in the leg. Acta Anaesthesiol Scand 1983; 27:26–34.
71. Gunnarsson L, Tokics L, Lundquist H, Brismar B, Strandberg Å, Berg B, Hedenstierna G. Chronic obstructive pulmonary disease and anesthesia: formation of atelectasis and gas exchange impairment. Eur Respir J 1991; 4:1106–1116.
72. Frumin MJ, Epstein RM, Choen G. Apneic oxygenation in man. Anesthesiology 1959; 20:789–798.
73. Benumof J. One-lung ventilation and hypoxic pulmonary vasoconstriction: implications for anesthetic management. Anesth Analg 1985; 64:821–833.
74. Scherer RW, Vigfusson G, Hultsch E, Van Aken H, Lawin P. Prostaglandin F2α improves oxygen tension and reduces venous admixture during one-lung ventilation in anesthetized, paralyzed dogs. Anesthesiology 1985; 62:23–28.
75. Chen TL, Ueng TH, Huang CH, Chen CL, Huang FY, Lin CJ. Improvement of arterial oxygenation by selective infusion of prostaglandin E1 to ventilated lung during one-lung ventilation. Acta Anaesthesiol Scand 1996; 40:7–13.
76. Sprague RS, Thiemermann C, Vane JR. Endogenous endothelium-derived relaxing factor opposes hypoxic pulmonary vasoconstriction and supports blood flow to hypoxic alveoli in anesthetized rabbits. Proc Nat Acad Sci USA 1992; 89:8711–8715.
77. Rich GF, Lowson SM, Johns RA, Daugherty MO, Uncles DR. Inhaled nitric oxide selectively decreases pulmonary vascular resistance without impairing oxygenation during one-lung ventilation in patients undergoing cardiac surgery. Anesthesiology 1994; 80:57–62.
78. Hambraeus-Jonzon K, Bindslev L, Frostell C, Hedenstierna G. Individual lung blood flow during unilateral hypoxia: effects of inhaled nitric oxide. Eur Respir J 1998; 11:565–570.
79. Alexander JI, Spencer AA, Parikh RK, Stuart B. The role of airway closure in postoperative hypoxaemia. Br J Anaesth 1973; 45:34–40.
80. Pedersen T, Viby-Mogensen J, Ringsted C. Anaesthetic practice and postoperative pulmonary complications. Acta Anaesthesiol Scand 1992; 36:812–818.
81. Halasz NA. Vertical vs horizontal laparotomies. Arch Surg 1964; 88:911–914.
82. Lindell P, Hedenstierna G. Ventilation efficiency after different incisions for cholecystectomy. Acta Chir Scand 1976; 142:561–565.
83. Putensen-Himmer G, Putensen C, Lammer H, Lingnau W, Aigner F, Benzer H. Comparison of postoperative respiratory function after laparoscopy or open laparotomy for cholecystectomy. Anesthesiology 1992; 77:675–680.

84. Simmonneau G, Vivien A, Sartene R, Kunstlinger F, Samii K, Noviant Y, Duroux P. Diaphragm dysfunction induced by upper abdominal surgery: role of postoperative pain. Am Rev Respir Dis 1983; 123:899–903.
85. Hachenberg T, Brussel T, Roos T, Lenzen N, Mollhoff T, Gockel B, Konertz W, Wendt M. Gas exchange impairment and pulmonary densities after cardiac surgery. Acta Anaesthesiol Scand 1992; 36:800–805.
86. Kroenke K, Lawrence F, Theroux JF, Tuley MR, Hilsenbeck S. Postoperative complications after thoracic and major abdominal surgery in patients with and without obstructive lung disease. Chest 1993; 104:1445–1451.

7

Asthma

IVEN H. YOUNG

Royal Prince Alfred Hospital
Sydney, Australia

A. B. HAMISH CRAWFORD

Liverpool and Westmead Hospitals
Sydney, Australia

I. Introduction

Asthma is a disease of the intrathoracic airways characterized by variable airflow limitation. A precise definition that allows a clear differentiation from other conditions causing airflow limitation is difficult. However, asthma is identified by a chronic eosinophilic inflammation of the airways, now considered to be the underlying abnormality predisposing to episodes of airway narrowing [1]. Associated with this is an increased bronchoconstrictor response to nonspecific stimuli such as aerosol histamine, methacholine, or hypertonic saline, and this reaction, labeled bronchial hyperresponsiveness, is regarded as a necessary part of the diagnosis. The episodes or attacks are usually (at least partly) reversible, either spontaneously or with treatment, and they are associated with the typical symptoms of dyspnea, chest tightness, wheeze, and cough in varying intensity and combination. It is this pattern of exacerbation and remission, regarded as responses to trigger factors interacting with the underlying inflammation and causing bronchial smooth muscle spasm and further inflammation, that clinically distinguishes asthma from other disorders of the airways. However, any exacerbation may progress to irreversible respiratory failure and death, and it is notable that more research effort into the physiology of asthma has been concentrated on the lung mechanics of the disorder rather than the progression of the gas exchange derangement, although the latter is the immediate antecedent to a fatal outcome. Nevertheless, there is a considerable body of recent literature that enhances our understanding of the mechanisms and progression of respiratory failure in asthma.

Despite advances in therapy, mortality from asthma remains disturbing. A number of factors have been implicated, including an increasing prevalence of the disease in developed and developing societies [2,3] and the possible deleterious effects of the excessive use of aerosol β-agonist bronchodilators. Certain bronchodilators have been documented as causing a transient deterioration in gas exchange, which together with an induced increase in airway hyperresponsiveness and potential cardiotoxicity, has been advanced as mechanisms contributing to mortality [4–6]. The emphasis on comprehensive asthma management plans [7] has been associated with a more recent decrease in mortality, particularly in Australia and New Zealand, where asthma prevalence is high.

Although bronchial smooth muscle spasm is an important contributor to the airway narrowing of asthma, particularly during acute attacks, postmortem studies of the lungs from patients dying of asthma have detected widespread inflammation and plugging of airways, often with complete occlusion of small- to medium-sized airways, as summarized by Hogg [8]. The advent of fiberoptic bronchoscopy has allowed easier and safer access to the asthmatic airway, and bronchial biopsy specimens from the airways of mild to moderate asthmatic patients have shown varying degrees of a chronic eosinophilic inflammatory infiltrate with edema and often smooth muscle hypertrophy [8], all of which will contribute to airway narrowing of a less transient nature. These findings provide the pathological basis for the detection of persistent gas exchange abnormality between acute attacks of asthma (discussed in Sections II.B and V.A). Interestingly, inflammatory change has also been identified in some of the pulmonary arteries accompanying these airways [9], which may have important implications for the vascular response to the airway narrowing and, hence, the matching of ventilation to perfusion. It has been recognized for a long time that this widespread, nonuniform narrowing or occlusion of airways causes a high degree of ventilation maldistribution in the lung and that this is the primary determinant of ventilation–perfusion ($\dot{V}_A/\dot{Q}$) inequality. This, in turn, results in hypoxemia and potential hypercapnia in this condition [10].

The aim of this chapter is to trace the evolution of knowledge in this field based on the development of techniques that have allowed an increasingly detailed understanding of the processes involved. The advent of blood gas electrodes, rapid gas analyzers, nuclear medicine imaging techniques, and the multiple inert gas elimination technique (MIGET) have successively contributed to a more complete picture. The contributions of the first and the last of these to the understanding of pulmonary gas exchange in asthma have been most important and are presented in more detail. The development of the concept of $\dot{V}_A/\dot{Q}$ inequality among gas exchanging units in the lung as the primary cause of impaired gas exchange, and the more recent use of digital computers to handle complex and iterative calculations [11] have been the major advances in our conceptual understanding of oxygen and carbon dioxide exchange. In conclusion, we present a summary of current knowledge of gas exchange in asthma with a final discussion of remaining questions.

II. Arterial Blood Gas Abnormalities
A. Acute Asthma

The availability of blood gas electrodes from the 1950s was the most important early advance, allowing studies of arterial blood gas tensions in asthma without the time-consuming direct measurement of gas contents. Earlier studies reported relatively mild hypoxemia, usually identified from saturation measurements, and found hypocapnia more commonly than hypercapnia during attacks of asthma; however, these studies were conducted with relatively small groups of patients under widely varying conditions. The first two studies of large patient groups presenting with acute asthma, by Tai and Read [10] and McFadden and Lyons [12], identified mild to moderate hypoxemia with a widened alveolar–arterial gradient for oxygen partial pressure (P_{AO_2}–P_{aO_2}) as the most common finding (91 of the 101 patients in the study by McFadden and Lyons). Seventy-three of these patients had hypocapnia, and these observations were similar to those of Tai and Read, who found hypoxemia in 91% and hypocapnia in 50% of their 64 patients. Importantly, both total minute and alveolar ventilation were found to increase in response to worsening airflow limitation, as measured by percent predicted forced expiratory volume in 1 second (FEV_1), until extreme reductions less than 20% predicted FEV_1 were associated with hypoventilation and hypercapnia (Fig. 1).

At modest degrees of airflow limitation, the increase in ventilation is in excess of the requirement to maintain eucapnia in the presence of $\dot{V}_A/\dot{Q}$ inequality and hence hypocapnia results, supporting the long-held hypothesis that the ventilatory drive is not from blood gas derangement in this situation. There is now evidence that hypercapnia only supervenes with task failure of the respiratory muscles [13], which may be an acute reduction in central drive "designed" to preserve essential respiratory muscle function before fatigue supervenes [14]. The central nervous system drive to ventilation is not severely chronically impaired in asthma (as would be manifest by chronic hypercapnia), unlike the depression of this drive in some patients with chronic obstructive pulmonary disease (COPD) [15]. When present, hypercapnia is a critical clinical finding in acute asthma, indicating that the need for mechanical ventilatory support may be imminent. Nevertheless, a large study of 229 episodes of acute asthma presenting over a 6-year period [16] found that only 61 episodes were associated with an arterial carbon dioxide partial pressure (P_{aCO_2}) more than 38 mm Hg (mean P_{aCO_2} of these 61 episodes was 53.6 ± 2.2 [SEM]), and only 5 required mechanical ventilation. Those with hypercapnia were generally more acutely severe and, importantly, had a history of worse chronic

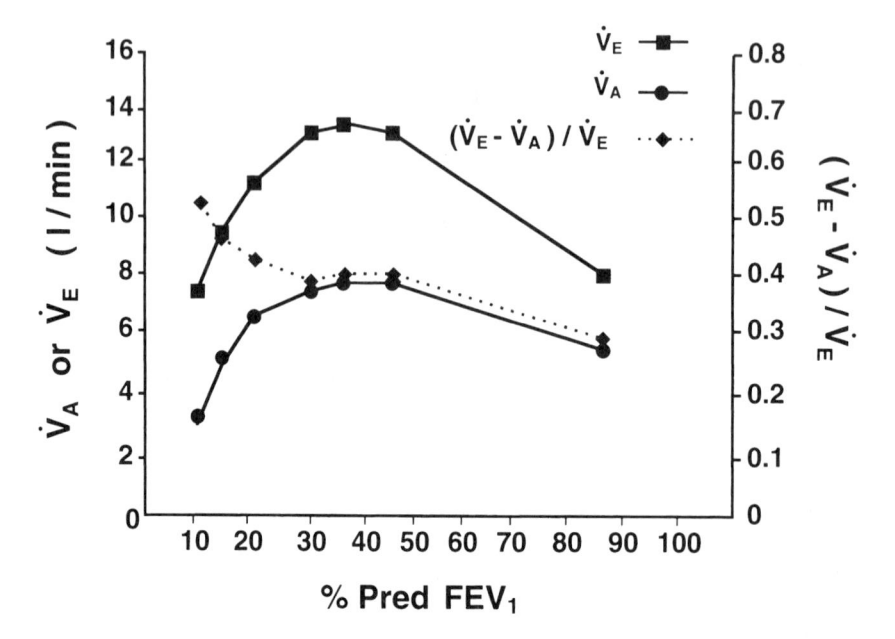

Figure 1 Minute ventilation ($\dot{V}_E$) and alveolar ventilation ($\dot{V}_A$) in relation to % predicted forced expiratory volume in 1 second (FEV_1) in a group of 30 patients presenting with acute asthma. Both $\dot{V}_E$ and $\dot{V}_A$ increase as the FEV_1 decreases, with a widening gap related to increasing ventilation–perfusion ratio ($\dot{V}_A/\dot{Q}$) inequality, causing hypocapnia until the FEV_1 decreases below 15–20% predicted. Then both ventilation measures decrease below normal, and carbon dioxide retention tends to ensue. Note the initial small increase in calculated Bohr dead space [($\dot{V}_E - \dot{V}_A$) / $\dot{V}_E$], which increases rapidly around 15–20% predicted FEV_1. (Modified from Ref. 12.)

control of their asthma. In patients who required multiple admissions, there was a correlation between the $PaCO_2$ measurements on each occasion, leading to the speculation that innate ventilatory responsiveness to CO_2 may play a role in the development of hypercapnia in acute asthma.

Although the two large studies by Tai and Read [10] and McFadden and Lyons [12] demonstrated a positive correlation between FEV_1 and PaO_2, the variance was too great for the former to be useful as a predictor of the latter in both reports. This led to the initial expression of the still-current hypothesis that obstruction or narrowing of peripheral airways may have more influence on gas exchange than the narrowing of the larger airways, which will have most influence on the reduction in FEV_1. It was also recognized then that treatment may relieve the large airway narrowing, and hence most symptoms, while leaving widespread persistent peripheral airway obstruction, and hence hypoxemia, making the patient more vulnerable to adverse effects during subsequent attacks. Age of the patient, duration of the attack, and the history of asthma severity did not relate to the gas exchange abnormality, and this has been confirmed in later studies of more severe acute asthma.

Rudolph et al. [17] reported a series of 14 patients presenting to hospital with severe attacks documented with peak expiratory flow rates (PEFR) of 4% to 22.4% of predicted normal values and followed-up with repeat arterial blood gas measurements for 1 week. On admission, all patients were hypoxemic. Nine had a Pa_{O_2} of less than 60 mm Hg, whereas only five had a Pa_{CO_2} of greater than 45 mm Hg, and only two of these were still hypercapnic at 1 hour. However, hypoxemia was persistent past 48 hours, and eight patients had a Pa_{O_2} of less than 75 mm Hg at 1 week. No clinically relevant increase in Pa_{CO_2} attributable to oxygen therapy was observed, again suggesting that, unlike some patients with exacerbations of COPD, there is no early impairment of ventilatory drive during acute exacerbations of asthma and that hypercapnia only supervenes when respiratory muscle dysfunction ensues. There is some evidence for diminished ventilatory responsiveness to hypercapnia and hypoxia in patients prone to severe asthma attacks [18], and there is also evidence for a reduced hypoxic response in children with severe persistent asthma [19]. This cannot easily be attributed to cumulative hypoxic exposure, even during sleep (see Section II.G), although the very persistent nature of hypoxemia in asthma was not recognized then (1980) as well as it is today.

B. Persistent Asthma

Hypoxemia found in these studies of acute asthma has also been found in stable asthma in clinical remission, when tests of airflow limitation are normal or near normal [17,20–22]. Therefore, there is strong evidence from studies of arterial blood gases in asthma that the distribution of $\dot{V}_A/\dot{Q}$ ratios in the lung is persistently abnormal. This has generally been attributed to a persistent maldistribution of ventilation secondary to airway narrowing in bronchi that do not make a large contribution to the standard indices of airflow limitation (PEFR and FEV_1), that is, the more peripheral airways [23].

It is generally accepted that the $\dot{V}_A/\dot{Q}$ inequality in asthma is primarily a direct consequence of maldistribution of ventilation, with changes in the distribution of perfusion being compensatory in nature (i.e., caused by hypoxic vasoconstriction) and tending to reduce the inequality. However, studies of oxygen and carbon dioxide exchange, or the steady-state exchange of any gases, cannot directly differentiate the contribution of maldistribution of ventilation from that of blood flow (per unit volume). More direct evidence for the persistent maldistribution of ventilation in asthma has come from inert gas washout methods (discussed in Section IV), whereas topographical studies using radiolabeled gases and aerosols (discussed in Section III), have provided evidence for blood flow and ventilation maldistribution.

C. Extrapulmonary Factors Influencing Gas Exchange

There is also the contribution of extrapulmonary factors such as cardiac output and mixed venous gas tensions interacting with $\dot{V}_A/\dot{Q}$ inequality, first systematically studied in computer models by West [11]. Most influences during acute asthma, such as an increase in sympathetic tone and the effects of bronchodilators, will tend to increase cardiac output and hence increase mixed venous oxygen tension if tissue oxygen consumption remains stable. This, correspondingly, will act to increase the Pa_{O_2} (and decrease the Pa_{CO_2}) as it interacts with low $\dot{V}_A/\dot{Q}$ units in the lung [24], given an unchanged distribution of $\dot{V}_A/\dot{Q}$ ratios. The increase in respiratory muscle work during an attack has the potential to decrease mixed venous oxygen content and pressure as oxygen consumption increases, but this will be more than compensated for by the increase in cardiac output. In very severe airflow limitation, cardiac output may decrease because of obstruction of venous return to the heart [25], which would be a major factor in the terminal deterioration in gas exchange in severe acute asthma. Cor pulmonale and transient pulmonary hypertension have been reported during exacerbations, one such report documenting severe hypoxemia caused by right-to-left shunting through a patent foramen ovale [26]. The shunt was not present at repeat cardiac catheterization 1 month later, and transient pulmonary hypertension associated with intense compensatory hypoxic vasoconstriction is the only plausible mechanism. The extrapulmonary influences have been clarified using MIGET and are discussed in more detail in Section V. Not surprisingly, there is sparse literature on cardiac output and mixed venous gas tension changes in asthma before the use of the MIGET technique.

D. Carbon Monoxide Transfer

The previously cited studies confirmed $\dot{V}_A/\dot{Q}$ inequality as the mechanism responsible for the changes in arterial gases by measuring increases in $Pa_{O_2}-Pa_{O_2}$ and dead space/tidal volume ratio (V_D/V_T). McFadden and Lyons [12] also measured the transfer factor for carbon monoxide by the single-breath method and found generally high normal values, implying that diffusion impairment was not a contributory cause of the hypoxemia. Although the possible mechanisms impairing oxygen diffusion through the lung, including the gas phase, are now recognized to be more complex, the constant finding of normal to high carbon monoxide diffusion (D_{CO}) in asthma is probably consistent with unimpaired oxygen diffusion across the alveolar capillary membrane, and this would be consistent with the known pathology of asthma, which does not primarily involve the lung interstitium. Later studies of D_{CO} in asthma have generally yielded normal or high results [27,28], and low values in other reports have been attributed to concomitant smoking-induced changes or very poor distribution of the test gas in patients with more severe persistent asthma.

It is now accepted that the Dco is high or normal in patients with uncomplicated acute and persistent asthma who have never smoked. The mechanism of the high Dco is most likely to be a higher capillary blood volume related to greater-than-normal perfusion of the lung apices. This is a consequence of the more negative intrapleural pressure during inspiration through narrowed airways, particularly during the test maneuver. Adding an external resistance during inspiration causes an increase in single-breath Dco in normal subjects [28], and an increase in pulmonary capillary blood volume has been demonstrated in patients who show nocturnal bronchospasm, but not in those without a nocturnal decrease in FEV_1 [29].

E. Response to Therapy

The arterial blood gas response to therapy in asthmatic patients has been of interest ever since reports from the 1960s identified a deterioration in response to certain drugs concurrent with an improvement in airflow limitation. These investigators [30–32] found that aerosol isoprenaline, systemic adrenaline, and aminophylline administration were all associated with increasing hypoxemia while these drugs were relieving airflow limitation, as indicated by an improvement in FEV_1 and symptoms. This effect was transient, and increasing P_{AO_2}–P_{aO_2} and V_D/V_T measurements indicated that it was caused by worsening $\dot{V}_A/\dot{Q}$ inequality. One hypothesis concerning the mechanism of this effect proposed that the aerosol dilators are preferentially directed to high $\dot{V}_A/\dot{Q}$ units, diverting ventilation further from low $\dot{V}_A/\dot{Q}$ units [33]. However, intravenous drugs (aminophylline) were found to cause the same effect, and attention turned to the possibility that reversal of compensatory pulmonary vasoconstriction occurs faster than the reversal of airway narrowing, which is presumably complicated by more slowly responding edema and mucus clearing.

The precise mechanism of this drug-induced reversal of pulmonary vasoconstriction remains controversial. However, it has been postulated that a drug-induced increase in cardiac output may release hypoxic vasoconstriction by increasing mixed venous oxygen pressure. The more β_2-selective dilators (e.g., salbutamol and terbutaline), which became available in the late 1960s, do not have marked cardiovascular effects and did not cause hypoxemia in other studies at that time [34–36]. Hypoxemia is clinically minor and is more likely to occur in persistent asthma than during the acute attack [32]; however, it was surmised [37] that this, together with the potential cardiotoxic effects of these drugs, may have contributed to the increasing deaths from asthma noted in the late 1960s, and this hypothesis was temporarily revived during the more recent increase in asthma deaths that occurred in the 1980s. The hypoxemia readily responds to supplemental oxygen therapy, which, in turn, will release hypoxic vasoconstriction. However, direct demonstration of this phenomenon as well as a more detailed appreciation of the interactions of cardiac output and $\dot{V}_A/\dot{Q}$ relationship changes had to await the application of MIGET.

F. Response to Challenge Testing

Starting in the 1970s, there is a large body of literature on the characteristics of the bronchoconstrictor response to challenge testing with inhaled histamine, methacholine, propranolol, and during exercise challenge. This has been recently further enlarged by reports of challenge testing with inhaled hypertonic saline and hyperventilation with dry air. Studies of the gas exchange consequences of this challenge testing were few until the application of MIGET stimulated further interest in this field (see Section V.D). Burke et al. [38] drew attention to the possibility of substantial decreases in Pa_{O_2} and increases in $P_{A_{O_2}}-Pa_{O_2}$, during histamine provocation in even mild asthmatics when they recorded a mean decrease in Pa_{O_2} of 22 mm Hg at 5-minute postchallenge, which tracked the increase in airway resistance and substantially recovered by 20 minutes. The mean baseline Pa_{O_2} was 98 mm Hg; therefore, the hypoxemia was not critical, and other investigators have reported only modest arterial oxygen saturation (Sa_{O_2}) changes during histamine challenge [39].

The Pa_{O_2} changes during exercise challenge tend to mirror the PEFR changes, with an increase in the former as the bronchodilatation occurs during the 6 to 8 minutes of exercise and then a decrease in Pa_{O_2} with the subsequent bronchoconstriction and recovery to baseline Pa_{O_2} as this recovers [40,41]. It is of interest that there seems to be no prolonged hypoxemia past the recovery in peak flow rates in these studies of exercise-induced asthma and that aerosol terbutaline blocked both the decrease in PEFR and Pa_{O_2} [42]. It seems likely that exercise challenge may only affect larger airways and not leave a persistent peripheral airway narrowing, which seems to complicate the usual exacerbations of asthma requiring hospital attendance. Subsequent MIGET studies support this conclusion.

G. Asthma During Sleep

The extensive literature on respiratory physiology during sleep over the last two decades has included a number of studies of the mechanisms and degree of nocturnal hypoxemia observed in asthmatic patients. Rarely is this hypoxemia severe, at least in relatively stable asthmatics, and the studies do not illuminate different basic mechanisms of gas exchange abnormality. There is a potential for more airway closure and loss of collateral ventilation during sleep as respiratory muscle tone decreases, thus reducing hyperinflation. Space does not allow an extensive treatment here and the interested reader is referred to a comprehensive review [43].

III. Topographical Distribution of Ventilation and Blood Flow

Radioactive ^{133}xenon (^{133}Xe) was first used in the 1960s to image the topographical distribution of ventilation and blood flow using external detectors. A study of

10 patients in the supine position with asthma in remission found that 4 had patchy areas of hypoventilation, whereas another 2 had heterogeneous ventilation in almost all regions after inhalation of this agent [44]. The lung bases were most affected. Infusion of ^{133}Xe into the peripheral venous circulation and its elimination by the lung demonstrated reduced blood flow to the regions of reduced ventilation, but the hypoventilated regions maintained low $\dot{V}_A/\dot{Q}$ ratios. This study provided one of the first direct demonstrations of ventilation inhomogeneity in asthma and the presence of low $\dot{V}_A/\dot{Q}$ regions with reduced blood flow, best understood as a result of a compensatory vasoconstriction. Before this, Woolcock et al. [45] demonstrated gross defects in perfusion lung scans obtained after injection of radioiodine (^{131}I)-labeled macroaggregated albumin in symptomatic asthma and showed that these defects tended to resolve as the symptoms did, but not always completely. Gamma camera technology has made these studies easier to analyze, and Sergysels et al. [46] measured regional residual volumes using inhaled boluses of ^{133}Xe inhaled from residual volume in 11 asymptomatic asthmatics. They found abnormally high regional residual volumes in the lower lung fields and abnormal ventilation distribution elsewhere, which suggested increased airway closure, especially in the lower zones. After inhaled fenoterol, the ventilation distribution remained abnormal, and the investigators suggested that small airway narrowing in asymptomatic asthmatics was a result of anatomical changes in addition to increased bronchomotor tone. Thus, the two studies [44,46] provide direct topographical evidence for maldistribution of ventilation and regions of low $\dot{V}_A/\dot{Q}$ ratio in persistent asthma in remission and continuing maldistribution of ventilation after aerosol bronchodilator.

Wilson et al. [47] studied 34 symptomatic asthmatics using ^{133}Xe and macroaggregated albumin ventilation–perfusion scans. They found that the severity of the ventilation maldistribution and the perfusion maldistribution each had a roughly linear relationship with the severity of symptoms, and that perfusion was less reduced to the hypoventilated regions than was ventilation, leading to low $\dot{V}_A/\dot{Q}$ regions being most prominent in the bases. The relationship to spirometric measurements of airflow limitation was not examined. Scans were performed to examine the washout of injected ^{133}Xe, which rapidly moved from the pulmonary circulation to the alveoli, and in some patients it was noted that the washout times at the lung bases were extremely prolonged. This suggested that basal airway closure was present during normal tidal breathing. There was considerable improvement, but not normalization, noted after treatment, particularly with prednisone.

A recent study (48) of airway closure in patients with variably severe asthma and in normal subjects used three-dimensional single-photon emission computed tomography to visualize regions of closure at residual volume. This technique allows a more detailed analysis without the overlap and obscuring of regions inherent in planar techniques. The study involved the inhalation of Technegas (generated from technetium 99m pertechnetate) (Tetley, Sydney, Australia) from residual volume to total lung capacity in the standing position. There was an orderly increase in the proportion of the airways closed at residual volume from the lung bases to the apices with increasing age in normal subjects. This orderly progression was lost in the asthmatic population, which showed more numerous and unevenly distributed regions of airway closure, more prevalent in the lower zones but also affecting the mid and upper zones to a greater extent than in normal subjects. The investigators concluded that the gradient of elastic recoil was the major factor determining airway closure in the normal subjects, but this was confounded by other intrinsic factors altering airway closing pressures in the asthmatic population. These factors could include airway inflammation, edema, and loss of surfactant function, as well as bronchial smooth muscle contraction.

IV. Functional Maldistribution of Ventilation

An alternative approach to studying ventilation distribution is by means of single- and multiple-breath inert gas washouts. Although ventilatory indices derived from such methods should theoretically provide a more sensitive means of quantifying ventilation maldistribution, they necessarily are more qualitative and indirect than the previously described topographical techniques. Moreover, such ventilatory indices reflect, to varying degrees, both spatial and temporal inequalities of ventilation, with the former likely to be of more direct relevance to pulmonary gas exchange [49].

Observations from both single- and multiple-breath inert gas washout studies suggest that in even mild asymptomatic disease, ventilation inequality is increased [50–52]. In relatively mild asthma, closing volume frequently occurs above functional residual capacity, that is, within the normal tidal breathing range [51]. The inhalation of a β-adrenergic aerosol typically results in a decrease in the measured closing capacity, whereas changes in the single-breath phase 3 slope may be variable [50]. Nevertheless, at least indices derived from multiple-breath washouts are relatively well correlated with the overall spirometric degree of spontaneous and drug-affected airflow obstruction [52; unpublished observations, March 1995]. This contrasts with the poor or nonexistent relationship between gas exchange impairment and spirometry, which is discussed in detail in Section V.

The predominant site and underlying mechanisms responsible for ventilation inequality in asthma are poorly defined [49]. The increase in ventilation inequality observed in asymptomatic disease with normal spirometry has been presumed to reflect persistent disease in peripheral airways [22]. The lack of any discernible differences in the relative washout characteristics of tracer gases of widely differing diffusivities suggests that such peripheral gas mixing impairment is nondiffusive in nature and hence is presumably a result of convective-dependent mechanisms [49]. Asymptomatic subjects with increased ventilation inequality are also known to display frequency dependence of dynamic compliance [22]. Thus, such increased ventilation inequality has been commonly attributed to time-constant inequality of peripheral lung units caused by inhomogeneity of their subtending airway resistances. However, whether such a mechanism significantly influences ventilation distribution during tidal breathing at rest, when breathing frequencies are low, is unknown. Both topographical [46–48] and inert gas studies [51,52] strongly suggest that, in asthma, inhomogeneous airway closure occurs during tidal breathing and is likely to be a significant determinant of ventilation distribution.

Indirect evidence that collateral ventilation also occurs in asthma is supported by the consistent absence of significant intrapulmonary shunting during MIGET studies (Section V), even when airflow obstruction is severe. Experimental simulation of inhomogeneous airway occlusion by the insufflation of ≤2-mm beads into the airways of dog lungs results in minimal gas exchange impairment [62], indicating that the subtending units of the occluded airways are at least partially ventilated via collateral channels. Interestingly, such experimentally induced peripheral airway occlusion also results in marked increases in ventilation inequality, as measured by the phase 3 slope of single-breath inert washouts [53]. Taken together, these observations suggest that collateral ventilation may result in a marked maldistribution of ventilation, which, however, may be sufficient to support adequate gas exchange of units subtended by peripherally occluded airways.

It is conventionally believed that ventilation maldistribution is the primary determinant of the ventilation–perfusion inequality occurring in asthma. Nevertheless, surprisingly, there are no published data that directly examine this relationship. We have observed in a large group of persistent asthmatics that ventilation maldistribution, as quantified by ventilatory indices derived from both single- and multiple-breath nitrogen washouts, accounted for up to 50% of the variance of ventilation–perfusion inequality as assessed by standard indices derived from MIGET (unpublished observations, March, 1995). The measured ventilation maldistribution was consistently greater than the corresponding gas exchange impairment, with the former correlating reasonably well with the spirometric degree of airflow obstruction. In contrast, and consistent with many other MIGET studies, there was no relationship between spirometric and gas exchange impairment indices. Removal of reversible hypoxic vasoconstriction by breathing 100% oxygen increased the degree of gas exchange impairment but resulted in worsening correlations between ventilatory and gas exchange impairment indices. These observations suggest that the ventilation–perfusion inhomogeneity of asthma cannot be viewed as just a simple interaction between ventilation maldistribution and compensatory reversible hypoxic vasoconstriction. It is conceivable that asthma may also produce a primary inhomogeneity of perfusion, possibly as a consequence of direct extension of airway inflammation into pulmonary vessels [9], from the mechanical effects of heterogeneous lung hyperinflation on vascular resistances [54], or from the release of chemical mediators. A study by Grant et al. [55] in open-chested vagotomized dogs provided some evidence for the latter mechanism. Challenge to the airway of one lung lobe with an *Ascaris suum* extract caused a transient decrease in the proportion of total pulmonary blood flow to that lobe, despite the administration of a hyperoxic gas mixture to eliminate hypoxic vasoconstriction.

This presumed mediator-elicited reaction did not seem to affect the local hypoxic vascular response, and it could not be attributed to pressure changes in the local airways.

V. Functional Distributions of $\dot{V}_A/\dot{Q}$ Ratios

The development of MIGET and its application to studies of patients with acute and persistent asthma has greatly increased knowledge of the mechanisms of gas exchange abnormality in this disease. Apart from allowing the description of continuous distributions of $\dot{V}_A/\dot{Q}$ ratios, the technique also provides an analysis of the influence of extrapulmonary factors such as cardiac output and mixed venous gas tensions. It also allows assessment of diffusion limitation to oxygen transfer by comparing the Pa_{O_2} calculated on the basis of the inert gas exchange data (due to $\dot{V}_A/\dot{Q}$ inequality plus shunt) with the measured Pa_{O_2}, which will be lower than the calculated Pa_{O_2} in the presence of diffusion limitation. The technical details of MIGET are discussed in Chapter 3.

A. Persistent Asthma

The first MIGET study of patients with persistent asthma was reported by Wagner et al. [56], who measured $\dot{V}_A/\dot{Q}$ distributions in a group of nine patients with widely varying FEV_1 (105% to 11% predicted) and who had not required medical attention for at least 1 month before the study. None of the patients was taking regular inhaled or oral corticosteroids, and all but one had a mild to moderate degree of hypoxemia. The $\dot{V}_A/\dot{Q}$ distributions were strikingly bimodal, with a substantial proportion (approximately 25%) of the cardiac output perfusing units with a $\dot{V}_A/\dot{Q}$ of approximately ≤ 0.1. A typical bimodal distribution is shown in Fig. 2. Other notable features were the absence of shunt and high $\dot{V}_A/\dot{Q}$ modes with no increase in dead space. A larger study of 26 stable patients with generally better-controlled asthma (mean FEV_1/forced vital capacity [FVC] 79% predicted) used a less invasive modification of MIGET that does not require arterial or mixed venous sampling [57]. These patients could be monitored with weekly measurements for 9 weeks, and bimodal distributions were only found in one third of the measurements, although 24 of the 26 patients showed bimodality at some point. The dispersion of the blood flow distribution (log SD $\dot{Q}$) averaged 0.74, exceeding the upper 95% confidence interval for the normal range, which is 0.6. Only five patients had a mean log SD less than 0.6 over the 9-week period. Importantly, this study was able to define the contribution of $\dot{V}_A/\dot{Q}$ inequality to the variance in Pa_{O_2} over time because it was measured on three occasions over the 9-week period. Sixty percent of the variance in Pa_{O_2} over time could be explained by changes in $\dot{V}_A/\dot{Q}$ distribution, with the remaining 40% presumably caused by extrapulmonary factors. The dispersion of ventilation was less abnormal, with the mean log SD $\dot{V}$ only exceeding the 95% confidence interval in four patients, confirming that regions of high $\dot{V}_A/\dot{Q}$

Asthma

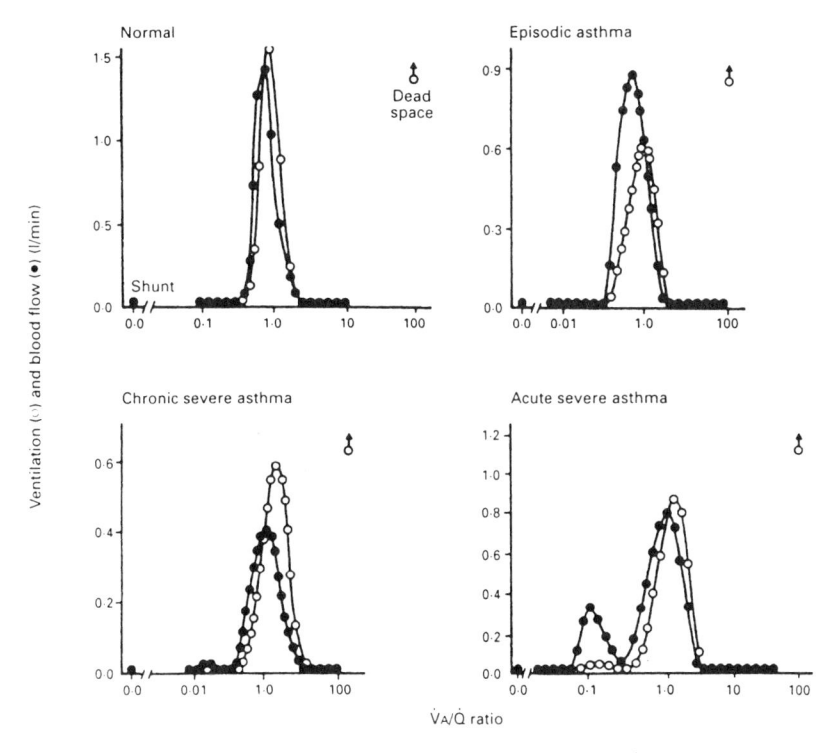

Figure 2 Typical patterns of ventilation–perfusion ratio ($\dot{V}_A/\dot{Q}$) distributions (ventilation [○] and blood flow [●]) plotted against $\dot{V}_A/\dot{Q}$ on a log scale. Healthy young adults have narrowly unimodal distributions centered around a $\dot{V}_A/\dot{Q}$ of 1. Patients with episodic or well-controlled asthma display broadly unimodal distributions, whereas more severe asthma is often characterized by a bimodal pattern. Shunt is absent and dead space (upper right, ○) is normal in each condition. (From Ref. 60.)

are not a feature of the maldistribution in asthma. This is to be expected from the underlying pathology of airway narrowing and closure unless regions of localized gas trapping and reduced capillary flow are created. High $\dot{V}_A/\dot{Q}$ regions have only been found in children during acute challenge (discussed in Section V.E; Fig. 6).

This larger study [57] emphasized the persistence of gas exchange disturbance despite better asthma control than in the earlier study [56], as measured by spirometry. The patients in the larger study were also treated with inhaled corticosteroids, which may account for the smaller frequency of bimodal distributions, as this therapy has been shown to reduce bronchial inflammation in asthma. Earlier work [58] that examined stable persistent asthma patients taking inhaled corticosteroids also found enduring $\dot{V}_A/\dot{Q}$ inequality as a wide unimodal distribution but a low prevalence of bimodal distributions. A more recent study [59] found remarkably minimal $\dot{V}_A/\dot{Q}$ inequality (mean log SD $\dot{Q}$, 0.77) in a group with severe persistent asthma with an average stable FEV_1 of 39% predicted. All of these patients were being treated with regular inhaled and oral corticosteroid drugs. These findings have been summarized and discussed by Rodriguez-Roisin and Roca [60] (Fig. 2).

The possible mechanisms underlying this rather distinctive bimodal $\dot{V}_A/\dot{Q}$ distribution, with a low mode centered around $\dot{V}_A/\dot{Q}$ 0.1, has been explored in a number of animal models, concentrating on dog lungs, which have a similar structure to human lungs. A bimodal pattern of abnormality was induced in a dog model of asthma where acute attacks were produced by nebulizing ascaris antigen and other provoking agents [61]. It was proposed that this pattern could be explained by the presence of chronically narrowed or occluded peripheral airways, creating the separate low mode of $\dot{V}_A/\dot{Q}$, which was persistent between attacks. The favored hypothesis was that complete occlusion of the major airways to these units was responsible for the appearance of a separated mode of $\dot{V}_A/\dot{Q}$, which did not become shunt because of collateral ventilation through channels such as the pores of Kohn and bronchiolar anastamoses held open by hyperinflation. This collateral ventilation is inefficient, having already undergone some gas exchange, hence its interpretation in the parallel $\dot{V}_A/\dot{Q}$ model used by MIGET as a separated low mode. Further dog experiments [62] found that the bronchoscopic instillation of 4.8-mm-diameter beads into the airways created a bimodal $\dot{V}_A/\dot{Q}$ distribution, whereas smaller beads 2.4 mm and 1.6 mm in diameter only caused widening of the distributions, placing the necessary obstruction for bimodality in somewhat larger airways than hitherto appreciated. The investigators concluded that the level of complete airway occlusion was important for the appearance of the separate mode. The potential importance of collateral channels in preventing or minimizing shunt has been supported by the clear development of shunt, without predominant low $\dot{V}_A/\dot{Q}$, when pigs are challenged with methacholine [63]. These animals have much more prominent interlobular and lobar septae minimizing these channels and making them unlike humans, at least in this respect!

To test further the hypothesis that peripheral airway edema and mucus are responsible for the airway occlusion, Lagerstrand et al. examined a rabbit model challenged with methacholine [64] and isotonic saline [65]. Rabbit lungs have a similar structure of collateral ventilation as human lungs, and methacholine challenge produced a typical bimodal pattern of $\dot{V}_A/\dot{Q}$ ratios without shunt. More specifically, the second study [65] nebulized saline droplets of 3-μm mass median diameter into peripheral airways, causing a bimodal $\dot{V}_A/\dot{Q}$ distribution without any change in measured airway resistance. Shunt steadily developed in association with decreasing lung compliance as more saline was nebulized, consistent with alveolar flooding or collapse. These findings lend strong support to the hypothesis that the bimodal distributions are related to events in peripheral airways, possibly edema and mucus and fluid accumulation.

This hypothesis, as an exclusive mechanism, has not been substantiated by subsequent work, which has found that bimodal distributions of this type can be reproduced by narrowing of large airways where collateral channels are not playing a part. Careful deposition of methacholine into central airways and, separately,

Asthma

diffusely into the periphery of the lung both caused bimodal $\dot{V}_A/\dot{Q}$ distributions in a study of eight stable human asthmatic subjects [66]. Central deposition caused a greater decrease in airway resistance than did peripheral deposition in this study, but there was a more prolonged deterioration in $\dot{V}_A/\dot{Q}$ distribution, lasting the 2 hours of the experiment, than in airway resistance, and this was independent of the pattern of deposition. Peripheral effects of neural and mediator activities were suggested after the central deposition, with more rapid clearing from the central airways accounting for the faster resolution of airflow limitation after this pattern of deposition. Again, gas exchange impairment was more prolonged than airflow limitation with both patterns of deposition, but it must be said that, whatever the mechanism, central airway challenge can result in bimodal $\dot{V}_A/\dot{Q}$ distributions. However, most evidence would suggest that persistence of bimodality with little or no airflow limitation is most consistent with persistent peripheral pathology.

B. Acute Asthma

The most comprehensive study of acute severe asthma was reported by Roca et al. [67], again using multiple MIGET measurements using the minimally invasive modification. All patients showed severe airflow limitation on admission with a mean FEV_1/FVC ratio of 34% and a mean PaO_2 of 51 mm Hg with no hypercapnia. Almost daily MIGET measurements during the hospital stay showed no correlation between the degree of $\dot{V}_A/\dot{Q}$ inequality (particularly log SD $\dot{Q}$) and spirometric indices. Such a negative correlation did develop at weeks 3 to 4 after discharge, when maximal physiological improvement had occurred. Again, the $\dot{V}_A/\dot{Q}$ pattern was a bimodal distribution at some time in 9 of the 10 patients, and shunt was small (mean, 1.1% of cardiac output). The evolution of $\dot{V}_A/\dot{Q}$ change in a representative patient is shown in Fig. 3 (see also Fig. 4 and Section V.C).

Six of eight patients with more severe asthma requiring mechanical ventilation, studied by the same group within 48 hours of admission [68], also showed typical bimodal distributions. As might be expected, the dispersion of the blood flow distribution was very high, with a mean log SD $\dot{Q}$ of 1.65, but, again, shunt was trivial or nonexistent (mean, 1.5%) and, although the dispersion of ventilation was also high (mean log SD $\dot{V}$, 1.0), there was generally no separate high mode. Administration of 100% oxygen caused the blood flow distribution to deteriorate even further and resulted in an increase in shunt, which may be interpreted as the release of compensatory hypoxic vasoconstriction that was attempting to preserve $\dot{V}_A/\dot{Q}$ matching. This response to 100% oxygen has been confirmed in persistent asthma (discussed in Section V.F).

C. Summary of Acute and Persistent Asthma Studies Using MIGET

Wagner et al. [69] published a summary analysis of the MIGET studies of acute and persistent asthma with particular emphasis on the absence of any correlation

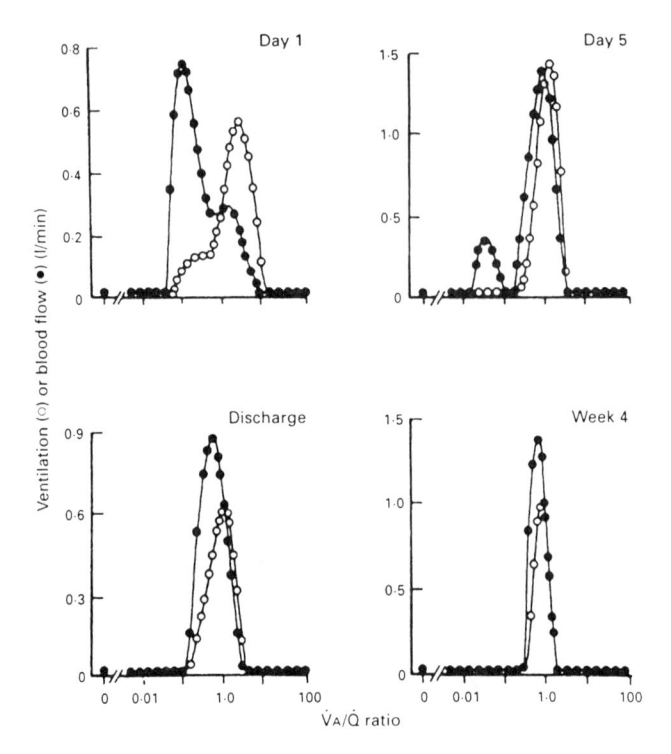

Figure 3 The evolution of ventilation–perfusion ratio ($\dot{V}_A/\dot{Q}$) inequality as acute severe asthma resolves. The axes and symbols are the same as in Fig. 2. A bimodal distribution may remain despite improvement in forced expiratory volume in 1 second (FEV_1) to approximately 60% predicted by day 5, and recovery to a normal distribution does not occur until weeks after discharge from hospital (see Fig. 4). (From Ref. 60, original figure from Ref. 67.)

between percent predicted FEV_1 and the indices of $\dot{V}_A/\dot{Q}$ inequality. They labeled the studies A to F in order of the reported severity of asthma from persistent mild disease (A and B) to acute severe hospitalized patients (E and F). Figures 4 and 5, taken from this publication, succinctly summarize a number of important points. Figure 4 summarizes the evolution in the relation between log SD $\dot{Q}$ and FEV_1 as the patients in group F [67] recovered, illustrating the stabilization of FEV_1 by day 5 but the persistence of an abnormal log SD $\dot{Q}$ past the time of discharge from hospital (see also Fig. 3). The relation between log SD $\dot{Q}$ and log SD $\dot{V}$ and FEV_1 are shown in Fig. 5. Across this spectrum of studies, there is little disturbance in the dispersion of the ventilation distribution, which is more sensitive to the presence of high $\dot{V}_A/\dot{Q}$ regions, whereas log SD $\dot{Q}$, sensitive to low $\dot{V}_A/\dot{Q}$ regions, is abnormal in mild asthma but only becomes markedly increased as the FEV_1 decreases to less than 40% predicted (see Section V.A). The more usual measures of PaO_2 and

Asthma

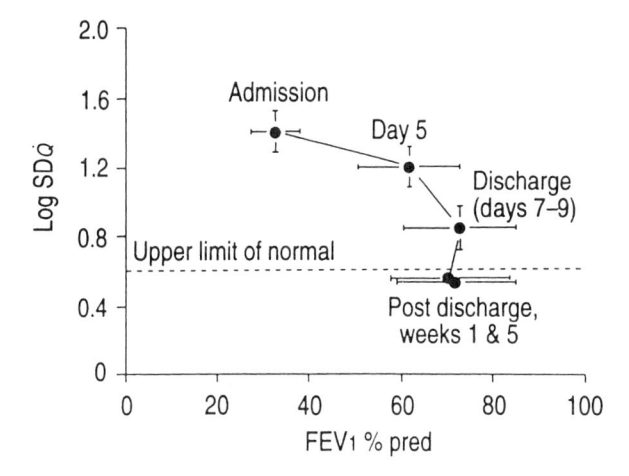

Figure 4 Relation between the dispersion of blood flow distribution (log SD $\dot{Q}$) as a measure of overall ventilation–perfusion ratio ($\dot{V}_A/\dot{Q}$) inequality, and % predicted forced expiratory volume in 1 second (FEV$_1$) as acute severe asthma resolves (data from Ref. 67, see Fig. 3). There is a faster resolution of the FEV$_1$ toward the normal range, whereas the $\dot{V}_A/\dot{Q}$ distribution remains clearly abnormal past the time of discharge from hospital. (From Ref. 69.)

P$_{AO_2}$–Pa$_{O_2}$ track the changes in these MIGET indices, although Pa$_{O_2}$ is usually in the normal range in groups A to C in the presence of a small increase in P$_{AO_2}$–Pa$_{O_2}$ and log SD $\dot{Q}$, which probably reflects the influence of extrapulmonary factors [69]. There is also no correlation between log SD $\dot{Q}$ and FEV$_1$ within each of the groups B and F [69].

D. Asthma During Provocation Challenge

Lagerstrand et al. [70] studied eight patients with a history of allergic asthma. All had normal spirometry and gas exchange at baseline (MIGET mean log SD $\dot{Q}$, 0.35) and both deteriorated immediately after the challenge with aerosol pollen or house dust mite allergens. Mean FEV$_1$ decreased from 3.9 to 2.3 L, whereas mean log SD $\dot{Q}$ increased to 0.73, mainly as a unimodal dispersion but with one definite bimodal pattern. By 2.5 hours, spirometry and $\dot{V}_A/\dot{Q}$ distributions had largely returned to normal, but there was no correlation between FEV$_1$ and log SD $\dot{Q}$ (both interindividual and intraindividual) over this period, and seven patients had a slower return of the log SD $\dot{Q}$ than the FEV$_1$ to baseline. Five patients developed a late reaction at 5 hours, but only three of them showed an increase in log SD $\dot{Q}$ at this time, suggesting that the late reaction may have been in central airways in the other patients. A similar pattern of broadening of the $\dot{V}_A/\dot{Q}$ distribution with bimodality in only 3 of 16 subjects was found after inhaled methacholine challenge

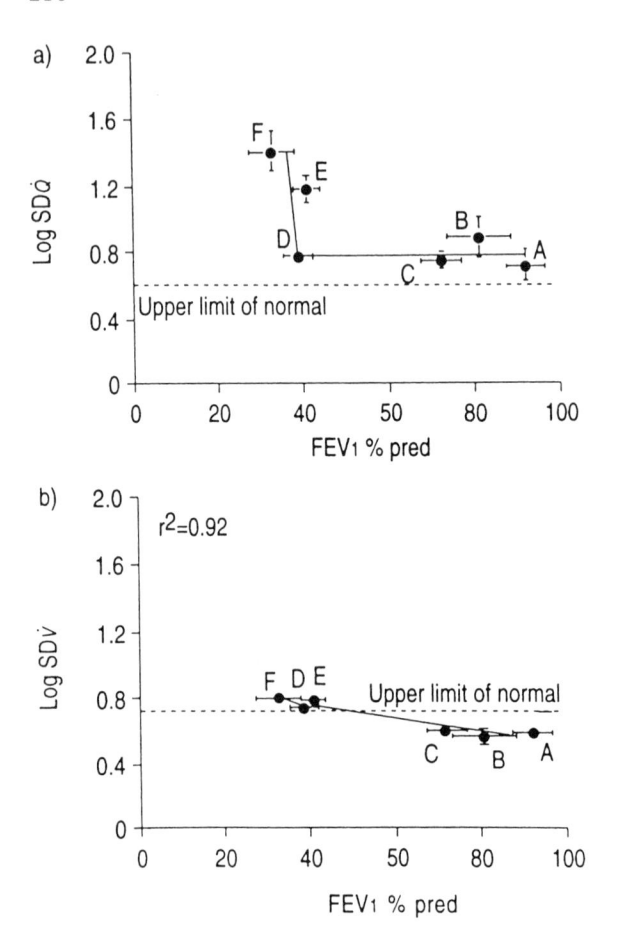

Figure 5 Relations between two measures of ventilation–perfusion ratio ($\dot{V}_A/\dot{Q}$) inequality and % predicted forced expiratory volume in 1 second (FEV_1) across the clinical spectrum of asthma. The dispersion of blood flow distribution (log SD $\dot{Q}$) (a) is abnormal in mild asthma and does not increase dramatically until the FEV_1 deteriorates to less than 40% predicted. The dispersion of ventilation distribution (log SD $\dot{V}$) (b) is only mildly abnormal, even in severe asthma (see text). (From Ref. 69.)

[71]. Again, there seemed to be no relationship between the FEV_1 as a measure of airflow limitation and indices of $\dot{V}_A/\dot{Q}$ dispersion, which included log SD V and DISP R-E*, the latter being a direct measure of overall $\dot{V}_A/\dot{Q}$ dispersion from the inert gas data excluding acetone dead space. However, other rather interesting patterns emerged from this complex study, which also incorporated the administration of aerosol salbutamol (eight patients) or placebo (eight patients) at 15 minutes after the challenge. The recovery of gas exchange indices was slower than the measures

of forced expiratory flow in the placebo group by 30 minutes after the challenge, consistent with earlier challenge studies. Nevertheless, a measure of respiratory system resistance (Rrs) obtained by an oscillation technique was slower to recover, and the improvement in this measure of airway resistance did correlate with the improvement in gas exchange indices, particularly log SD $\dot{V}$ and DISP R-E*.

The investigators [71] concluded that Rrs is likely to be more sensitive to the response of the lungs as a whole to methacholine, including the more peripheral changes that may be influencing gas exchange. The only differences between the placebo and salbutamol groups at 30–120 minutes after challenge were a lower Rrs and higher dead space in the salbutamol group. This suggests that the bronchodilator did reduce resistance to flow and increase the anatomical dead space by airway widening, although it is interesting that the FEV_1 improvement was no faster than after placebo. The other indices of gas exchange did not improve faster with salbutamol. Relatively rapid spontaneous recovery after this form of challenge, which largely just causes smooth muscle spasm, may be expected to confound the advantages of a bronchodilator. Another interesting finding was that the changes in Pa_{O_2} and P_{AO_2}–Pa_{O_2} correlated well with the changes in MIGET $\dot{V}_A/\dot{Q}$ indices with little or no changes in the extrapulmonary influences on Pa_{O_2}. This is unlike the situation in acute spontaneous asthma, before and after bronchodilators, where an increase in cardiac output is likely to partly mitigate the degree of hypoxemia.

There is little information concerning the likely mediators responsible for the typical gas exchange abnormality in acute asthma. Recent work has shown that inhaled platelet-activating factor (PAF) will induce $\dot{V}_A/\dot{Q}$ changes similar to those in patients with moderate and severe asthma when administered to subjects with mild asthma [72] and to normal subjects [73]. The inhalation of PAF causes an increase in airway resistance, the typical asthma $\dot{V}_A/\dot{Q}$ changes, and neutrophil sequestration in the lungs in both populations. Further studies [74] have indicated that pretreatment with inhaled salbutamol blocks all of these PAF-induced effects, whereas pretreatment with inhaled ipratropium only inhibits the increase in airway resistance.

Because ipratropium relaxes smooth muscle but has no vascular effects, it is reasonable to suggest that the gas exchange and neutrophil abnormalities induced by PAF are related to vascular changes in the bronchial and, perhaps, pulmonary circulations, which are inhibited by salbutamol. It seems likely that PAF will be one of a number of inflammatory mediators capable of modulating these responses (1); however, it is intriguing that inhalation of this mediator mimics many of the physiological changes of acute asthma and that pharmacological manipulation can identify a PAF-induced gas exchange effect unrelated to both bronchial smooth muscle spasm and a measurable increase in airway resistance [75].

Exercise challenge may cause a slightly different pattern of response. The only MIGET study of adult exercise-induced asthma [76] found that six subjects starting with normal $\dot{V}_A/\dot{Q}$ distributions (mean log SD $\dot{Q}$, 0.54; only one had a log SD $\dot{Q} > 0.6$) developed broad distributions to a mean log SD $\dot{Q}$ of 1.02 as the FEV$_1$ and/or PEFR decreased $\geq$ 20% in the 10- to 20-minute period after 8 minutes of treadmill exercise. Four of the $\dot{V}_A/\dot{Q}$ distributions were unimodal and two were bimodal, but all returned to baseline configuration within 1 hour, and this resolution was generally faster than the improvement in spirometric indices. This opposite finding to the recovery pattern after other challenges or spontaneous attacks may relate to the site of the major response being in large airways where drying and periciliary fluid osmotic change will be more pronounced and rapidly reversed through the influence of the bronchial circulation. These findings would suggest that exercise-induced attacks in isolation do not cause peripheral airway plugging and edema, which is slow to resolve.

E. Childhood Asthma

The only MIGET data regarding asthmatic children relate to $\dot{V}_A/\dot{Q}$ changes after challenge testing, and they show substantially different responses from adults. One study [77] of 11 children found that exercise challenge provoked an attack in 7, characterized by the development of a high $\dot{V}_A/\dot{Q}$ mode in 6 subjects. This new mode tended to center around a $\dot{V}_A/\dot{Q}$ of 10, and there was displacement of the main blood flow mode a little to the left, thus accounting for the hypoxemia that developed (Fig. 6). Another study [78], from the same center, of five children after histamine challenge found a similar pattern of response with the appearance of a slightly high $\dot{V}_A/\dot{Q}$ mode. The investigators speculated that chronically narrowed airways with the potential to produce more low $\dot{V}_A/\dot{Q}$ may not be as prevalent in children and that a check valve mechanism causing patchy hyperinflation and reduction in blood flow to these regions, because of pressure increases, may predominate in this age group.

F. Responses to Therapeutic Interventions

Response to Supplemental Oxygen

Oxygen therapy is often applied during the management of acute asthma, and the likelihood that this would result in a deterioration of $\dot{V}_A/\dot{Q}$ relationships because of release of hypoxic vasoconstriction, and possible absorption atelectasis, has been appreciated for a long time. However, before the development of MIGET, it was difficult to measure the precise changes associated with oxygen administration. Increase in the V_D/V_T ratio with oxygen in patients with COPD [79] has been interpreted as indicating release of vasoconstriction in that condition. The first MIGET study to examine the effects of 100% oxygen breathing [58] found a broadening of the $\dot{V}_A/\dot{Q}$ distribution without any shunt or change in overall cardiac output in a group of patients with acute asthma, and these findings were confirmed by a later study of a similar patient group [59]. The study by Corte and Young [58] noted little further increase in log SD $\dot{Q}$ in a few patients with a broad baseline distribution, raising the possibility that these subjects had poor compensatory hy-

Asthma 219

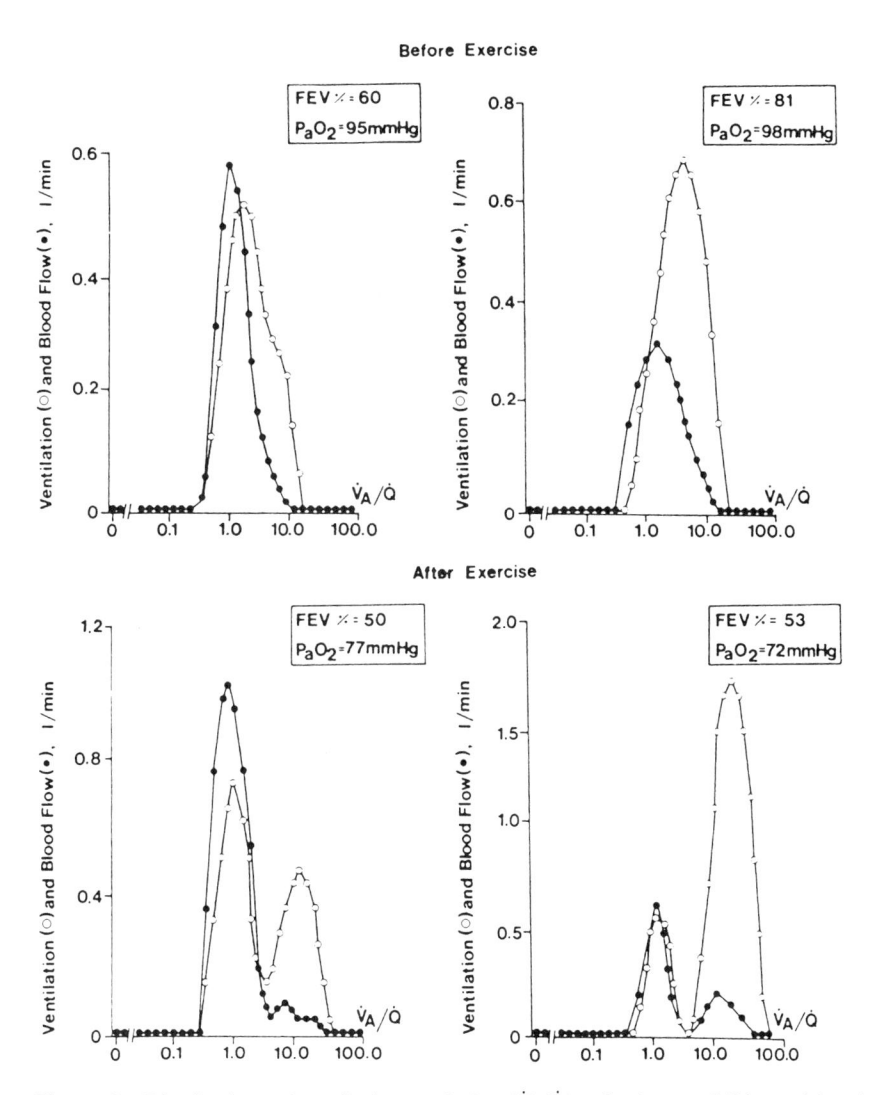

Figure 6 Distributions of ventilation–perfusion ($\dot{V}_A/\dot{Q}$) ratios in two children with asthma before and after exercise challenge. The symbols and axes are the same as in Fig. 2. A very different pattern to the adult asthma $\dot{V}_A/\dot{Q}$ abnormality developed with a mode of high $\dot{V}_A/\dot{Q}$ ratios and slight displacement of the main blood flow mode to the left causing mild hypoxemia (see text). (From Ref. 77.)

poxic vasoconstriction at baseline, perhaps because of other confounding mediator release or a poor innate hypoxic response [79]. The study by Ballester et al. [59] of subjects with severe persistent asthma (FEV_1, 39% predicted) also found that 100% oxygen caused a widening of the $\dot{V}_A/\dot{Q}$ distribution from a remarkably low baseline log SD $\dot{Q}$ of 0.77 to 1.11, with an increase in perfusion to low $\dot{V}_A/\dot{Q}$ units but no shunt and no change in cardiac output.

Presumably, all of these patient groups did not have prevalent areas of severe peripheral airway narrowing that could have led to absorption atelectasis or increase in shunt from redistribution of blood flow, as occurred in the patients on mechanical ventilation receiving supplemental oxygen [68]. The latter study detected the development of moderate amounts of shunt (mean, 8.3% of cardiac output) during the inhalation of 100% oxygen in this very severe patient group, and the two possibilities of collapse of very low $\dot{V}_A/\dot{Q}$ units through resorption atelectasis and a large increase in perfusion of small shunts was invoked by the investigators.

It is of interest that the bronchodilator effect of supplemental oxygen [80,81] measured in obstructive airway diseases does not improve $\dot{V}_A/\dot{Q}$ matching in asthma, which suggests a very important role for compensatory vasoconstriction in the matching of ventilation to blood flow in this disease.

Response to Bronchodilators

Arterial blood gas measurements during the administration of nonselective β-agonists and aminophylline [30–33] have strongly suggested that these drugs cause a deterioration in $\dot{V}_A/\dot{Q}$ relationships as a result of pulmonary vasodilatation, as previously discussed. Later MIGET studies have been less clear-cut. Aerosol isoprenaline was found to increase substantially the blood flow to the separate low mode of $\dot{V}_A/\dot{Q}$ in the small group of persistent asthmatics studied by Wagner et al. [56], although the degree of hypoxemia induced was buffered by the accompanying increase in cardiac output. Aerosol salbutamol did not cause any deterioration in $\dot{V}_A/\dot{Q}$ inequality in the group of patients with severe persistent asthma previously discussed [59] who responded to 100% oxygen, but it is of interest to note that this lack of response was in the face of a 35% increase in FEV_1. It is reasonable to presume that the aerosol salbutamol was having its major effect on large airways. However, these results are in keeping with the lack of effect on blood gases of terbutaline, another selective β_2-agonist [36,42]. On the other hand, intravenous salbutamol is associated with a deterioration in $\dot{V}_A/\dot{Q}$ relationships and an improvement in spirometric measurements in acute severe asthma [82]. Ballester et al. [82] examined 19 patients admitted to hospital with a mean FEV_1 41% predicted, and the mean log SD $\dot{Q}$ of 1.07 increased to 1.33 in a smaller subgroup given intravenous salbutamol. The subgroup given aerosol salbutamol started with a higher baseline log SD $\dot{Q}$ of 1.4 but did not change despite a similar degree of spirometric improvement. Although $\dot{V}_A/\dot{Q}$ matching deteriorated with intravenous salbutamol, the Pa_{O_2} was stable because of a concomitant increase in cardiac output.

Intravenous theophylline in usual therapeutic doses (plasma level, approximately 15 µg/mL) probably has little or no deleterious effect on gas exchange in acute severe asthma. A detailed study by Montserrat at al. [83] found no effect on the MIGET indices of $\dot{V}_A/\dot{Q}$ dispersion when compared with placebo, despite a small improvement in the FVC, with the FEV_1/FVC ratio remaining the same. There was a small increase in ventilation with a decrease in $Paco_2$ on aminophylline compared with placebo, probably because of the direct stimulation of ventilation by the drug. At first glance, this is a paradoxical finding when compared with earlier studies; however, the deleterious effect of aminophylline is probably dose-related [84], which may account for the adverse findings of the earlier studies of arterial blood gases. It is interesting to note that none of the studies of the gas exchange effects of bronchodilators actually show an immediate improvement in gas exchange to match the improvement in airflow. This is more evidence for a dissociation between peripheral pulmonary parenchymal and small airway factors affecting gas exchange on the one hand, and central larger airway factors having more influence on airflow on the other. It seems likely that an immediate deterioration in gas exchange with bronchodilators is caused by release of vasoconstriction, whereas stable $\dot{V}_A/\dot{Q}$ relations in the presence of improving airflow indicates a greater central, rather than peripheral, airway effect.

VI. Summary and Conclusions

Expired gas and topographical studies provide overwhelming evidence for an abnormally uneven distribution of ventilation per unit lung volume in asthma. There is also clear, though understandably less well documented, evidence for an uneven distribution of blood flow, and the two combined provide a physiological foundation for the gas exchange derangement on the basis of $\dot{V}_A/\dot{Q}$ inequality. That such inequality exists and is the major mechanism for the hypoxemia of asthma is now indisputable, particularly from the data accumulated through MIGET studies. These studies have also confirmed that, in asthma of widely varying severity, there is no evidence for diffusion impairment of oxygen transfer, at least across the alveolar–capillary membrane.

This $\dot{V}_A/\dot{Q}$ inequality must also impair carbon dioxide elimination; however, the vast majority of asthma patients with persistent disease, and during acute exacerbations, are able to increase ventilation sufficiently to maintain a normal or low $Paco_2$. Very severe acute attacks may be associated with hypercapnia, which is probably caused by a centrally mediated "task failure" in the face of very heavy loads rather than respiratory muscle fatigue, which is extraordinarily difficult to induce experimentally. There is evidence that patients who present on multiple occasions with hypercapnia during acute asthma do have reduced ventilatory drive to this stimulus. However, metabolic and respiratory acidosis is also likely to contribute to some respiratory muscle dysfunction in this situation, which may bring the patient to the brink of cardiac failure and reduced oxygen delivery to the muscles.

The pathological basis for abnormal airway narrowing and closure is now much better understood, and it is a complicated interaction between inflammation and edema in the airway wall causing direct narrowing and uncoupling of the elastic traction forces from the surrounding lung; bronchial smooth muscle hypertrophy and spasm; and mucus accumulation and plugging with degradation of surfactant activity. The sites in the bronchial tree where these changes are most likely to have the most effect on gas exchange is more contentious. Large volumes of lung can lack ventilation during topographical studies of asthma, suggesting that at least medium-sized airways may contribute. However, these defects can also be related to occlusion or severe narrowing of contiguous groups of smaller airways. There is strong evidence, largely from the MIGET studies, that gas exchange impairment is dissociated from measures of airflow limitation, particularly the FEV_1 and mid expiratory flow rates. This is most likely caused by a more dramatic effect of smaller airway narrowing and, in particular, closure on gas exchange than on airflow reduction, which is certainly more affected by central airway narrowing.

Relatively mild hypoxemia is commonly present in persistent asthma, with well-maintained airflow, and the hypoxemia only tends to become severe as airflow is markedly impaired [69]. The underlying $\dot{V}_A/\dot{Q}$ inequality and increase in P_{AO_2}–P_{aO_2} is often more impressive than the P_{aO_2} would suggest, and this is probably a result of the influence of extrapulmonary factors, including a small increase in cardiac output. These extrapulmonary factors also ameliorate the hypoxemic effects of some bronchodilators that can cause transiently worse $\dot{V}_A/\dot{Q}$ matching. Even severe hypoxemia seems to be rarely associated with shunt, which is somewhat surprising in view of the widespread airway plugging and closure in severe asthma. An attractive hypothesis to explain this finding is that hyperinflation opens collateral ventilation channels, converting potential shunt to populations of low $\dot{V}_A/\dot{Q}$ units, which are often seen in MIGET studies.

The most intriguing questions raised at this point of our knowledge relate to the control of the pulmonary (and bronchial) vascular responses in asthma. There is no doubt that hypoxic pulmonary vasoconstriction plays a role in reducing the $\dot{V}_A/\dot{Q}$ inequality in most degrees of severity of this condition, because oxygen administration consistently makes the inequality worse. On the other hand, there seem to be reduced pulmonary vascular responses to severe induced asthma in animal models, at least as measured by hemodynamic responses [85], and it seems likely that the inflammatory mediators released from airways will modulate the pulmonary vascular responses [55]. There is recent evidence that PAF may be an important mediator of altered bronchial vascular responses and may enhance microvascular permeability, thus contributing to airway narrowing and maldistribution of ventilation [72–75]. This mediator may also influence the pulmonary vasculature [74]. In addition, nitric oxide is released in higher-than-normal concentrations from asthmatic airways [86], and this highly diffusible vasodilator molecule may well act to inhibit compensatory vasoconstriction in associated pulmonary arterioles, hence increasing $\dot{V}_A/\dot{Q}$ inequality. However, recent work in patients with mild to moderate asthma has shown no correlation between the basal concentration of exhaled nitric oxide and the underlying distribution of ventilation–perfusion ratios. Furthermore, local inhibition of nitric oxide synthesis with nebulized NG-nitro-L-arginine methyl ester (L-NAME) did not modulate ventilation–perfusion distributions nor modify pulmonary artery pressure [87].

The interesting finding of inflammatory cells in the walls of muscular pulmonary arteries accompanying inflamed bronchioles in postmortem human specimens gives a promising lead for further research [9]. This is especially so as the inflammatory infiltrate can be found in parts of the arterial wall that are not contiguous with the bronchiole. Discrimination between pulmonary vascular and airway events and their separate effects on gas exchange will always be difficult, at least in human subjects, although the combination of expired gas measurements of ventilation distribution with MIGET estimations have the potential to yield important information. The more detailed topographical studies possible through the use of SPECT scanning may also provide useful data when combined with the other techniques. However, these techniques are demanding and difficult to apply to a disease in which the physiological processes can change over a short time period.

Finally, we do not know the prognostic significance of prolonged gas exchange impairment in the presence of near-normal airway function in asthma as measured by the standard indices, particularly the FEV_1. Is the patient with a persistently abnormal log SD $\dot{Q}$ or P_{AO_2}–P_{aO_2} (perhaps in the presence of a normal P_{aO_2}) more likely to have worse morbidity or even a fatal outcome from his or her next attack, whether it is a sudden or slow-onset exacerbation [88]? If persistent peripheral airway narrowing is responsible for the increase in log SD $\dot{Q}$ and P_{AO_2}–P_{aO_2}, will targeting these airways with smaller-particle aerosol corticosteroids improve this [89]? Is it possible or desirable to manipulate the vascular response to rematch blood flow to ventilation and hence improve gas exchange in the presence of persistent airway narrowing? Much remains to be investigated with the techniques we have, which will undoubtedly suggest new ways of learning more about the gas exchange function of the lung in this common disorder.

Acknowledgment

The authors acknowledge the support of the Institute of Respiratory Medicine, Royal Prince Alfred Hospital, Sydney, Australia.

References

1. Barnes PJ. Pathophysiology of asthma. Br J Clin Pharmacol 1996; 42:3–10.
2. Hopper J, Jenkins M, Carlin J, Giles G. Increase in self-reported prevalence of asthma and hay fever in adults over the last generation: a matched parent-offspring study. Aust J Public Health 1995; 19:120–124.

3. Lewis S, Butland B, Strachan D, Bynner J, Richards D, Butler N, Britton J. Study of the aetiology of wheezing illness at age 16 in two national British birth cohorts. Thorax 1996; 51:670–676.
4. Inman WHW, Adelstein AM. Rise and fall of asthma mortality in England and Wales in relation to use of pressurized aerosols. Lancet 1969; 2:279–285.
5. Suissa S, Ernst P, Boivin J-F, Horwitz RI, Habbick B, Cockroft D, Blais L, McNutt M, Buist AS, Spitzer WO. A cohort analysis of excess mortality in asthma and the use of inhaled β-agonists. Am J Respir Crit Care Med 1994; 149:604–610.
6. Sears MR, Taylor DR, Print CG, Lake DC, Li QQ, Flannery EM, Yates DM, Lucas MK, Herbison GP. Regular inhaled beta-agonist treatment in bronchial asthma. Lancet 1990; 336:1391–1396.
7. Comino EJ, Mitchell CA, Bauman A, Henry RL, Robertson CF, Abramson MJ, Ruffin R, Landau L. Asthma management in eastern Australia, 1990 and 1993. Med J Aust 1996; 164:403–406.
8. Hogg JC. Postgraduate course: pathology of asthma. J Allergy Clin Immunol 1993; 92:1–5.
9. Saetta M, Di Stefano A, Rosina C, Thiene G, Fabbri LM. Quantitative structural analysis of peripheral airways and arteries in sudden fatal asthma. Am Rev Respir Dis 1991; 143:138–143.
10. Tai E, Read J. Blood-gas tensions in bronchial asthma. Lancet 1967; 1:644–646.
11. West JB. Ventilation-perfusion inequality and overall gas exchange in computer models of the lung. Respir Physiol 1969; 7:88–110.
12. McFadden ER Jr, Lyons HA. Arterial blood gas tensions in asthma. N Engl J Med 1968; 278:1027–1032.
13. McKenzie DK, Allen GM, Butler JE, Gandevia SC. Task failure with lack of diaphragm fatigue during inspiratory resistive loading in human subjects. J Appl Physiol 1997; 82:2011–2019.
14. McKenzie DK, Bellemare F. Respiratory muscle fatigue. In: Gandevia SC, Enoka RM, McComas AJ, Stuart DG, Thomas CK, eds. Fatigue Neural and Muscular Mechanisms. New York: Plenum Press, 1995, pp 401–414.
15. Campbell EJM. Respiratory failure: definition, mechanisms and recent developments. Bull Eur Physiopathol Respir 1979; 15:1–12.
16. Mountain RD, Sahn SA. Clinical features and outcome in patients with acute asthma presenting with hypercapnia. Am Rev Respir Dis 1988; 138:535–539.
17. Rudolph M, Riordan JF, Grant BJB, Maberly DJ, Saunders KB. Arterial blood gas tensions in acute severe asthma. Eur J Clin Invest 1980; 10:55–62.
18. Hudgel DW, Weil JV. Depression of hypoxic and hypercapnic ventilatory drives in severe asthma. Chest 1975; 68:493–497.
19. Smith TF, Hudgel DW. Decreased ventilation response to hypoxia in children with asthma. J Pediatr 1980; 97:736–741.
20. Cade JF, Pain MCF. Pulmonary function during clinical remission of asthma: how reversible is asthma? Aust NZ J Med 1973; 3:545–551.
21. Palmer KNV, Kelman GR. Pulmonary function in asthmatic patients in remission. Br Med J 1975; 1:485–486.
22. Levine G, Housley F, MacLeod P, Macklem PT. Gas exchange abnormalities in mild bronchitis and asymptomatic asthma. New Engl J Med 1970; 282:1277–1282.

23. McFadden ER Jr, Kiser R, DeGroot WJ. Acute bronchial asthma: relationships between clinical and physiological manifestations. N Engl J Med 1973; 288:221–225.
24. West JB. State of the art: ventilation-perfusion relationships. Am Rev Respir Dis 1977; 116:919–943.
25. Tuxen DV. Detrimental effects of positive end-expiratory pressure during controlled mechanical ventilation of patients with severe airflow obstruction. Am Rev Respir Dis 1989; 140:5–9.
26. Robert R, Ferrandis J, Malin F, Herpin D, Pourrat O. Enhancement of hypoxemia by right-to-left atrial shunting in severe asthma. Intensive Care Med 1994; 20:585–587.
27. Collard P, Njinou B, Nejadnik B, Keyeux A, Frans A. Single breath diffusing capacity for carbon monoxide in stable asthma. Chest 1994; 105:1426–1429.
28. Keens TG, Mansell A, Krastins IRB, Levison H, Bryan AC, Hyland RH, Zamel N. Evaluation of the single-breath diffusing capacity in asthma and cystic fibrosis. Chest 1979; 76:41–44.
29. Desjardin JA, Sutarik JM, Suh BY, Ballard RD. Influence of sleep on pulmonary capillary blood volume in normal and asthmatic subjects. Am J Respir Crit Care Med 1995; 152:193–198.
30. Tai E, Read J. Response of blood gas tensions to aminophylline and isoprenaline in patients with asthma. Thorax 1967; 22:543–549.
31. Field GB. The effects of posture, oxygen, isoproterenol, and atropine on ventilation-perfusion relationships in the lung in asthma. Clin Sci 1967; 32:279–288.
32. Palmer KNV, Diament ML. Effect of aerosol isoprenaline on blood-gas tensions in severe bronchial asthma. Lancet 1967; 2:1232–1233.
33. Knudson RJ, Constantine HP. An effect of isoproterenol on ventilation-perfusion in asthmatic versus normal subjects. J Appl Physiol 1967; 22:402–406.
34. Palmer KNV, Legge JS, Hamilton WD, Diament ML. Effect of a selective beta-adrenergic blocker in preventing falls in arterial oxygen tension following isoprenaline in asthmatic subjects. Lancet 1969; 2:1092–1093.
35. Palmer KNV, Diament ML. Effect of salbutamol on spirometry and blood-gas tensions in bronchial asthma. Br Med J 1969; 1:31–32.
36. DaCosta J, Hedstrand U. The effect of a new beta-receptor stimulating drug (terbutaline) on arterial blood gases in bronchial asthma. Scand J Resp Dis 1970; 51:212–217.
37. Dulfano MJ. Bronchodilators, pulmonary function, and asthma (editorial). Ann Intern Med 1968; 68:955–956.
38. Burke TV, Kung MD, Burki NK. Pulmonary gas exchange during histamine-induced bronchconstriction in asthmatic subjects. Chest 1989; 96:752–756.
39. Poppius H, Stenius B. Changes in arterial oxygen saturation in patients with hyperactive airways during a histamine inhalation test. Scand J Respir Dis 1977; 58:1–4.
40. Anderson SD, Silverman M, Walker SR. Metabolic and ventilatory changes in asthmatic patients during and after exercise. Thorax 1972; 27:718–725.
41. Silverman M, Anderson SD, Walker SR. Metabolic changes preceding exercise-induced bronchoconstriction. Br Med J 1972; 1:207–209.
42. Bye PTP, Anderson SD, Daviskas E, Marty JJ, Sampson D. Plasma cyclic AMP levels in response to exercise and terbutaline sulphate aerosol in normal and asthmatic subjects. Eur J Respir Dis 1980; 61:287–297.

43. Douglas NJ, Flenley DC. State of the art: breathing during sleep in patients with obstructive lung disease. Am Rev Respir Dis 1990; 141:1055–1070.
44. Heckscher T, Bass H, Oriol A, Rose B, Anthonisen NR, Bates DV. Regional lung function in patients with bronchial asthma. J Clin Invest 1968; 47:1063–1070.
45. Woolcock AJ, McRae J, Morris JG, Read J. Abnormal pulmonary blood flow distribution in bronchial asthma. Austr Ann Med 1966; 15:196–203.
46. Sergysels R, Scano G, Vrebos J, Bracamonte M, Vandevivere J. Effect of fenoterol on small airways and regional lung function in asymptomatic asthma. Eur J Clin Pharmacol 1983; 24:429–434.
47. Wilson AF, Surprenant EL, Beall GN, Siegel SC, Simmons DH, Bennett LR. The significance of regional pulmonary function changes in bronchial asthma. Am J Med 1970; 48:416–423.
48. King GG, Eberl S, Salome CM, Young IH, Woolcock AJ. Differences in airway closure between normal and asthmatic subjects measured with single-photon emission computed tomography and Technegas. Am J Respir Crit Care Med 1998; 158:1900–1906.
49. Crawford ABH, Paiva M, Engel LA. Uneven ventilation. In: Crystal RG, West JB, eds. The Lung: Scientific Foundations. Vol. 1. New York: Raven Press, 1991, pp 1031–1041.
50. Siegler DIM, Fukuchi Y, Engel LA. Influence of bronchomotor tone on ventilation distribution and airway closure in asymptomatic asthma. Am Rev Respir Dis 1976; 114:123–130.
51. McCarthy D, Milic-Emili J. Closing volume in asymptomatic asthma. Am Rev Respir Dis 1973; 107:557–570.
52. Wall MA, Misley MC, Brown AC, Vollmer WM, Buist AS. Relationship between maldistribution of ventilation and airways obstruction in children with asthma. Respir Physiol 1987; 69:287–297.
53. Hogg W, Brunton J, Kryger M, Brown R, Macklem P. Gas diffusion across collateral channels. J Appl Physiol 1972; 33:568–578.
54. Nicholson DP, Johnson RL. Effects of isoproterenol on distribution of ventilation and perfusion in asthma. Am Rev Respir Dis 1972; 107:869–873.
55. Grant BJ, Fortune JB, West JB. Effect of local antigen inhalation and hypoxia on lobar blood flow in allergic dogs. Am Rev Respir Dis 1980; 122:39–46.
56. Wagner PD, Dantzker DR, Iacovoni VE, Tomlin WC, West JB. Ventilation-perfusion inequality in asymptomatic asthma. Am Rev Respir Dis 1978; 118:511–524.
57. Wagner PD, Hedenstierna G, Bylin G. Ventilation-perfusion inequality in chronic asthma. Am Rev Respir Dis 1987; 136:605–612.
58. Corte P, Young IH. Ventilation-perfusion relationships in symptomatic asthma: response to oxygen and clemastine. Chest 1985; 88:167–175.
59. Ballester E, Roca J, Ramis LI, Wagner PD, Rodriguez-Roisin R. Pulmonary gas exchange in chronic asthma. Response to 100% oxygen and salbutamol. Am Rev Respir Dis 1990; 141:558–562.
60. Rodriguez-Roisin R, Roca J. Contributions of multiple inert gas elimination technique to pulmonary medicine—3: Bronchial asthma. Thorax 1994; 49:1027–1033.
61. Rubinfeld AR, Wagner PD, West JB. Gas exchange during experimental canine asthma. Am Rev Respir Dis 1978; 118:525–536.

62. Lee L-N, Ueno O, Wagner PD, West JB. Pulmonary gas exchange after multiple airway occlusion by beads in the dog. Am Rev Respir Dis 1989; 140:1216–1221.
63. Kubo S, Tomioka S, Kapitan K, Wagner PD. Effect of methacholine (MCH) inflation on pulmonary gas exchange in pigs (abstr). Fed Proc 1985; 44:1383.
64. Lagerstrand L, Hedenstierna G. Gas-exchange impairment: its correlation to lung mechanics in acute airway obstruction (studies on a rabbit asthma model). Clin Physiol 1990; 10:363–380.
65. Lagerstrand L, Dahlbäck M, Hedenstierna G. Gas exchange during simulated airway secretion in the anaesthetised rabbit. Eur Respir J 1992; 5:1215–1222.
66. Schmekel B, Hedenström H, Kämpe M, Lagerstrand L, Stålenheim G, Wollmer P, Hedenstierna G. The bronchial response, but not the pulmonary response to inhaled methacholine is dependent on the aerosol deposition pattern. Chest 1994; 106:1781–1787.
67. Roca J, Ramis L, Rodriguez-Roisin R, Ballester E, Montserrat JM, Wagner PD. Serial relationships between ventilation-perfusion inequality and spirometry in acute severe asthma requiring hospitalisation. Am Rev Respir Dis 1988; 137:1055–1061.
68. Rodriguez-Roisin R, Ballester E, Roca J, Torres A, Wagner PD. Mechanisms of hypoxemia in patients with status asthmaticus requiring mechanical ventilation. Am Rev Respir Dis 1989; 139:732–739.
69. Wagner PD, Hedenstierna G, Rodriguez-Roisin R. Gas exchange, expiratory flow obstruction and the clinical spectrum of asthma. Eur Respir J 1996; 9:1278–1282.
70. Lagerstrand L, Larsson K, Ihre E, Zetterström O, Hedenstierna G. Pulmonary gas exchange response following allergen challenge in patients with allergic asthma. Eur Respir J 1992; 5:1176–1183.
71. Rodriguez-Roisin R, Ferrer A, Navajas D, Agusti AGN, Wagner PD, Roca J. Ventilation perfusion mismatch after methacholine challenge in patients with mild bronchial asthma. Am Rev Respir Dis 1991; 144:88–94.
72. Félez MA, Roca J, Barberà JA, Santos C, Rotger M, Chung KF, Rodriguez-Roisin R. Inhaled platelet-activating factor worsens gas exchange in mild asthma. Am J Respir Crit Care Med 1994; 150:369–373.
73. Rodriguez-Roisin R, Félez MA, Chung KF, Barberà JA, Wagner PD, Cobos A, Barnes PJ, Roca J. Platelet-activating factor causes ventilation-perfusion mismatch in humans. J Clin Invest 1994; 93:188–194.
74. Diaz O, Barberà JA, Marrades R, Chung KF, Roca J, Rodriguez-Roisin R. Inhibition of PAF-induced gas exchange defects by beta-adrenergic agonists in mild asthma is not due to bronchodilation. Am J Respir Crit Care Med 1997; 156:17–22.
75. Rodriguez-Roisin R. Acute severe asthma: pathophysiology and pathobiology of gas exchange abnormalities. Eur Respir J 1997; 10:1359–1371.
76. Young IH, Corte P, Schoeffel RE. Pattern and time course of ventilation-perfusion inequality in exercise-induced asthma. Am Rev Respir Dis 1982; 125:304–311.
77. Freyschuss U, Hedlin G, Hedenstierna G. Ventilation-perfusion relationships during exercise-induced asthma in children. Am Rev Respir Dis 1984; 130:888–894.
78. Hedlin G, Freyschuss U, Hedenstierna G. Histamine induced asthma in children: effects on the ventilation-perfusion relationships. Clin Physiol 1985; 5:19–34.
79. Lee J, Read J. Effect of oxygen breathing on distribution of pulmonary bloodflow in chronic obstructive lung disease. Am Rev Respir Dis 1967; 96:1173–1180.

80. Astin TW. The relationship between arterial blood oxygen saturation, carbon dioxide tension, and pH and airway resistance during 30 percent oxygen breathing in patients with chronic bronchitis with airway obstruction. Am Rev Respir Dis 1970; 102:382–387.
81. Inoue H, Inoue C, Okayama M, Sekizawa K, Hida W, Takishima Y. Breathing 30 per cent oxygen attenuates bronchial responsiveness to methacholine in asthmatic patients Eur Respir J 1989; 2:506–512.
82. Ballester E, Reyes A, Roca J, Guitart R, Wagner PD, Rodriguez-Roisin R. Ventilation-perfusion mismatching in acute severe asthma: effects of salbutamol and 100% oxygen. Thorax 1989; 44:258–267.
83. Montserrat JM, Barberà JA, Viegas C, Roca J, Rodriguez-Roisin R. Gas exchange response to intravenous aminophylline in patients with a severe exacerbation of asthma. Eur Respir J 1995; 8:28–33.
84. Lejeune P, Leeman P, Mélot C, Naeije R. Effects of theophylline and S 9795 on hyperoxic and hypoxic pulmonary vascular tone in intact dogs. Eur Respir J 1989; 2:370–376.
85. Wanner A, Friedman M, Baier H. Study of the pulmonary circulation in a canine asthma model. Am Rev Respir Dis 1977; 115:241–250.
86. Dupuy PM, Frostell CG. Bronchial effects of nitric oxide. In: Zapol WM, Bloch KD, eds. Nitric Oxide and the Lung. New York: Marcel Dekker, 1997, pp 285–311.
87. Gómez FP, Barberà JA, Roca J, Iglesia R, Ribas J, Barnes PJ, Rodriguez-Roisin R. Effect of nitric oxide synthesis inhibition with nebulized L-NAME on ventilation-perfusion distribution in bronchial asthma. Eur Respir J 1998; 12:865–871.
88. Picado C. Classification of severe asthma exacerbations: a proposal. Eur Respir J 1996; 9:1775–1778.
89. Dahl R, Ringdal N, Ward SM, Stampone P, Donnell D. Equivalence of asthma control with new CFC-free formulation HFA-134a beclomethasone dipropionate and CFC-beclomethasone dipropionate. Br J Clin Pract 1997; 51:11–15.

8

Chronic Obstructive Pulmonary Disease

JOAN ALBERT BARBERÀ

Hospital Clínic, University of Barcelona
Barcelona, Spain

I. Introduction

Chronic obstructive pulmonary disease (COPD) is defined as a disease state characterized by the presence of progressive airflow obstruction due to chronic bronchitis or emphysema [1,2]. Since the initial recognition of the disease, it has been acknowledged that abnormal gas exchange leading to hypoxemia and/or hypercapnia is one of its most characteristics features, especially in the advanced stages [3,4]. In patients with COPD, the severity of gas exchange impairment is strongly related to survival [5] and, as recently shown, to quality of life [6]. Indeed, hypoxemia correction with long-term oxygen therapy is the only treatment that has been consistently demonstrated to improve survival in patients with COPD [7,8].

That ventilation–perfusion ratio ($\dot{V}_A/\dot{Q}$) inequality may account for gas exchange abnormalities in COPD was already recognized in the early development of the concept of the disease [3]. In the mid-1960s, investigators using measurements of gas tensions in arterial blood and expired gas, as well as the slope of the nitrogen washout curve, clearly showed the presence of $\dot{V}_A/\dot{Q}$ inequality [9,10]. However, these estimates are rather insensitive in assessing the true degree of $\dot{V}_A/\dot{Q}$ inequality because they are influenced by the level of ventilation and do not take into account extrapulmonary factors, which may modify mixed venous blood gas composition.

A major advance in understanding the role of $\dot{V}_A/\dot{Q}$ inequality in gas exchange impairment in COPD has been provided by the development of the multiple inert gas elimination technique by Wagner et al. [11] and Evans and Wagner [12]. Using this technique, it has been possible to quantitate the $\dot{V}_A/\dot{Q}$ distributions in COPD and to characterize the relevance of the different factors that determine the partial pressures of O_2 and CO_2 in arterial blood under different clinical conditions.

This chapter reviews the current knowledge on pulmonary gas exchange in COPD provided by studies in which the inert gas technique has been used. First, the physiological basis of gas exchange impairment is discussed, with special emphasis on $\dot{V}_A/\dot{Q}$ distributions and the role played by extrapulmonary factors and hypoxic pulmonary vasoconstriction in the regulation of arterial oxygen partial pressure (Pa_{O_2}). Next follows a section on the correlations between lung structure and gas exchange abnormalities, followed by a discussion on the determinants of gas exchange impairment in the broad clinical spectrum of COPD, both under stable clinical conditions and during episodes of acute exacerbation. Finally, the effects of different therapeutic interventions on gas exchange in these patients is further analyzed.

II. Physiological Basis of Abnormal Gas Exchange in COPD

Despite the greater degree of gas exchange impairment seen in patients with more advanced COPD, the severity of hypoxemia or hypercapnia relates poorly to the degree of airflow obstruction. This lack of correlation is attributable to the fact that the anatomical and physiological determinants of airflow obstruction and gas exchange are of different nature. Moreover, Pa_{O_2} and arterial carbon dioxide partial pressure (Pa_{CO_2}) values are determined not only by intrapulmonary factors (i.e., $\dot{V}_A/\dot{Q}$ distributions), but also by extrapulmonary factors (i.e., minute ventilation, cardiac output, and oxygen consumption) that may be unrelated to the degree of airflow obstruction. Studies using the inert gas technique have provided the separate assessments of the intrapulmonary determinants of hypoxemia and hypercapnia in COPD and of the relevance of extrapulmonary factors in the modulation of O_2 and CO_2 levels in arterial blood. This is particularly useful in COPD, where different clinical pictures can be observed despite the same basic pathological processes.

A. Ventilation–Perfusion Inequality

In 1977, Wagner et al. [13] were the first to analyze the $\dot{V}_A/\dot{Q}$ distributions using the inert gas technique in a group of 23 patients with severe COPD. They found that all patients had some degree of $\dot{V}_A/\dot{Q}$ mismatching, as shown by increased dispersions of the distributions of both blood flow and alveolar ventilation over $\dot{V}_A/\dot{Q}$ ratios. The same group of investigators had previously shown that in healthy individuals, the second moment (or dispersion) of blood flow and ventilation distributions on a logarithmic scale (log SD $\dot{Q}$ and log SD $\dot{V}$, respectively) averaged 0.57 and 0.48, respectively [14]. By contrast, in patients with COPD, mean log SD $\dot{Q}$ was 1.12 and mean log SD $\dot{V}$ 1.27 [13] (Table 1). Furthermore, the patterns of $\dot{V}_A/\dot{Q}$ distributions were not uniform among the patients, and three different patterns were identified [13]. In some patients, $\dot{V}_A/\dot{Q}$ distributions were characterized by the presence of lung units with a very high $\dot{V}_A/\dot{Q}$ ratio that originated a distribution of ventilation with a bimodal shape ("high pattern"). In contrast, other patients showed a pattern of $\dot{V}_A/\dot{Q}$ distribution characterized by the presence of lung units with very low $\dot{V}_A/\dot{Q}$ ratios that produced a bimodally shaped distribution of blood flow ("low pattern"). A third group of patients associated features of both high and low patterns. Although the high pattern was more prevalent in patients who fulfilled the criteria of the so-called emphysematous type of COPD, according to the classification proposed by Burrows et al. [4], no other consistent associations between the pattern of $\dot{V}_A/\dot{Q}$ inequality and the clinical characteristics could be established [13]. Moreover, Wagner et al. [13] clearly demonstrated that in COPD, $\dot{V}_A/\dot{Q}$ inequality accounted for all of the observed hypoxemia and that other mechanisms of hypoxemia (i.e., intrapulmonary shunt and O_2 diffusion impairment) were generally irrelevant.

After this seminal study, a number of investigators used the inert gas approach to evaluate the $\dot{V}_A/\dot{Q}$ distributions in clinically stable COPD, covering a wide range of disease severity [15–29] (Table 1). All of these studies have consistently documented increased $\dot{V}_A/\dot{Q}$ inequality in COPD patients, as shown by greater-than-normal dispersions of both blood flow and ventilation distributions [normal upper 95% confidence limits for log SD $\dot{Q}$ and log SD $\dot{V}$, 0.60 and 0.65, respectively [30]]. As shown in Table 1, despite a wide variation in the degree of airflow obstruction among the different studies, differences in the dispersions of both blood flow and ventilation distributions seem not to be as pronounced. Although among the different studies mean forced expiratory volume in 1 second (FEV_1) ranged between 16% and 72% of predicted, log SD $\dot{Q}$ only ranged between 0.66 and 1.12, and log SD $\dot{V}$ between 0.84 and 1.43. Accordingly, the degree of $\dot{V}_A/\dot{Q}$ mismatch in clinically stable COPD patients, as assessed by the inert gas technique, usually ranges from mild to moderately severe [31], irrespective of the severity of airflow obstruction. Figure 1 shows the relationships between FEV_1 and both log SD $\dot{Q}$ and log SD $\dot{V}$ in 89 COPD patients [21,22,26–29]. Note that almost all patients have abnormally high values of log SD $\dot{Q}$ and log SD $\dot{V}$. Despite the finding that the correlations are statistically significant, there is great scatter in the relationships. Thus, patients with the same FEV_1 may show substantially different degrees of $\dot{V}_A/\dot{Q}$ inequality.

The high and low patterns of $\dot{V}_A/\dot{Q}$ distribution originally described by Wagner et al. [13] can be identified in some patients. However, accumulative experience with the inert gas technique indicates that the most frequent pattern of $\dot{V}_A/\dot{Q}$ distribution in COPD is a broad unimodal distribution of both blood flow and ventilation.

Table 1 Ventilation–Perfusion Distributions in Stable Chronic Obstructive Pulmonary Disease[a]

Reference	No. of patients	FEV$_1$ L	FEV$_1$ % Predicted	% FVC	DLCO (% predicted)	PaO$_2$ (mm Hg)	PaCO$_2$ (mm Hg)	AaPO$_2$ (mm Hg)	Mean Q̇	Log SD Q̇	Mean V̇	Log SD V̇	Shunt (%Q̇T)	Dead space (%V̇E)
Wagner et al., 1977 (13)	23	NR	40 ± 11	NR	76 ± 38	58 ± 9	45 ± 10	NR	0.6 ± 0.3	1.12 ± 0.30	2.4 ± 0.9	1.27 ± 0.35	2.1 ± 5.0	36 ± 5
Mélot et al., 1983 (15)	6	0.80 ± 0.13	NR	35 ± 4	NR	52 ± 4	46 ± 3	43 ± 2	0.6 ± 0.1	0.97 ± 0.07	2.6 ± 0.4	1.23 ± 0.20	1.7 ± 0.7	47 ± 6
Mélot et al., 1984 (16)	6	0.89 ± 0.20	NR	39 ± 8	NR	52 ± 4	44 ± 3	45 ± 2	0.5 ± 0.1	0.92 ± 0.06	1.4 ± 0.3	1.02 ± 0.11	3.5 ± 1.9	55 ± 5
Castaing et al., 1985 (17)	14	NR	NR	27 ± 8	NR	55 ± 9	51 ± 6	NR	0.7 ± 0.5	0.78 ± 0.20	1.7 ± 0.7	1.08 ± 0.41	4.2 ± 4.1	45 ± 11
Dantzker et al., 1986 (18)	7	0.56 ± 0.05	NR	36 ± 8	44 ± 15	76 ± 10	56 ± 6	NR	0.8 ± 0.2	0.73 ± 0.20	NR	NR	NR	NR
Roca et al., 1987 (19)	7	NR	NR	38 ± 4	81 ± 4	60 ± 3	48 ± 2	NR	0.5 ± 0.1	0.91 ± 0.06	1.4 ± 0.2	0.99 ± 0.10	0	46 ± 3
Ringsted et al., 1989 (20)	6	0.33 ± 0.14	16 ± 4	37 ± 15	NR	50 ± 10	48 ± 7	NR	0.5 ± 0.1	0.81 ± 0.12	2.3 ± 0.9	1.43 ± 0.25	3.3 ± 3.0	40 ± 11
Agustí et al., 1990 (21)	8	1.15 ± 0.12	36 ± 3	39 ± 3	78 ± 6	76 ± 2	39 ± 2	28 ± 2	0.8 ± 0.1	0.90 ± 0.06	2.1 ± 0.3	1.03 ± 0.11	0.6 ± 0.3	29 ± 3
Barberà et al., 1994 (23)	20	2.30 ± 0.51	72 ± 12	59 ± 10	92 ± 20	77 ± 9	37 ± 3	29 ± 9	0.7 ± 0.2	0.87 ± 0.24	1.3 ± 0.3	0.73 ± 0.25	1.0 ± 0.9	32 ± 9
Andrivet et al., 1994 (24)	8	0.85 ± 0.11	24 ± 4	42 ± 5	NR	70 ± 4	58 ± 5	30 ± 4	0.6 ± 0.1	0.66 ± 0.18	0.9 ± 0.1	0.87 ± 0.20	2.6 ± 0.8	56 ± 3
Moinard et al., 1994 (25)	14	0.89 ± 0.38	NR	49 ± 15	NR	59 ± 10	44 ± 8	NR	0.6 ± 0.2	1.20 ± 0.30	1.6 ± 0.6	1.00 ± 0.40	1.7 ± 1.3	52 ± 9
Barberà et al., 1996 (26)	13	0.90 ± 0.06	28 ± 2	36 ± 2	51 ± 5	56 ± 2	46 ± 1	35 ± 3	0.6 ± 0.1	1.11 ± 0.08	1.8 ± 0.2	0.96 ± 0.04	2.7 ± 0.9	35 ± 3
Viegas et al., 1996 (27)	24	0.93 ± 0.46	30 ± 14	42 ± 13	NR	65 ± 8	41 ± 7	37 ± 8	0.6 ± 0.2	1.11 ± 0.24	1.7 ± 0.6	0.98 ± 0.25	0.7 ± 1.3	35 ± 11
Barberà et al., 1997 (28)	13	0.91 ± 0.19	29 ± 6	35 ± 10	57 ± 23	60 ± 11	44 ± 6	NR	0.7 ± 0.3	0.96 ± 0.27	1.9 ± 0.7	1.08 ± 0.30	1.3 ± 1.7	43 ± 9
Roger et al., 1997 (29)	9	1.19 ± 0.07	39 ± 2	44 ± 4	63 ± 6	72 ± 3	41 ± 1	28 ± 4	0.7 ± 0.1	0.92 ± 0.09	1.8 ± 0.3	0.84 ± 0.08	0.5 ± 0.1	37 ± 3

[a] Dispersions are either SD or SEM.

Mean Q̇ = mean V̇A/Q̇ ratio of blood flow distribution; log SD Q̇ = dispersion of blood flow distribution; mean V̇ = mean V̇A/Q̇ ratio of ventilation distribution; log SD V̇ = dispersion of ventilation distribution; shunt = perfusion to alveolar units with V̇A/Q̇ ratios < 0.005; dead space = ventilation to units with V̇A/Q̇ ratios > 100; NR = not reported; FEV$_1$ = forced expiratory volume in 1 second; DLCO = carbon monoxide diffusing capacity; PaO$_2$ = arterial oxygen partial pressure; PaCO$_2$ = arterial carbon dioxide partial pressure; AaPO$_2$ = alveolar to arterial O$_2$ gradient.

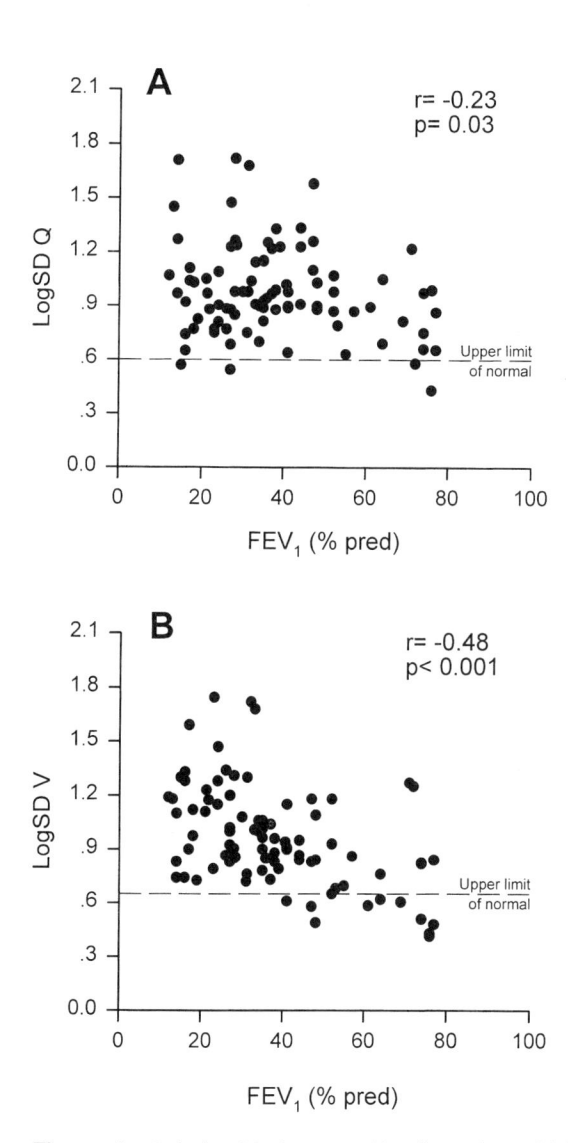

Figure 1 Relationship between (A) dispersion of blood flow distribution (log SD $\dot{Q}$) and forced expiratory volume in 1 second (FEV_1; percent predicted), and (B) dispersion of ventilation distribution (log SD $\dot{V}$) and FEV_1 in 89 patients with chronic obstructive pulmonary disease (COPD). Dashed lines indicate the normal upper 95% confidence limits of log SD $\dot{Q}$ and log SD $\dot{V}$.

In a retrospective analysis of the patterns of $\dot{V}_A/\dot{Q}$ distribution in 94 COPD patients studied under stable clinical conditions by the same laboratory [19,21,22,26–29], covering the wide clinical spectrum of COPD (FEV_1 range, 12–77% of predicted), four different patterns of $\dot{V}_A/\dot{Q}$ distribution were identified. Broad unimodal distributions of both blood flow and ventilation (Fig. 2A) were shown in 45% of patients; a bimodal distribution of blood flow, with both normal and low $\dot{V}_A/\dot{Q}$ areas (Fig. 2B), was shown in 23%; a bimodal distribution of ventilation, with normal and high $\dot{V}_A/\dot{Q}$ areas (Fig. 2C), was shown in 18%; and the remaining 14% of patients showed both bimodal blood flow and ventilation distribution patterns

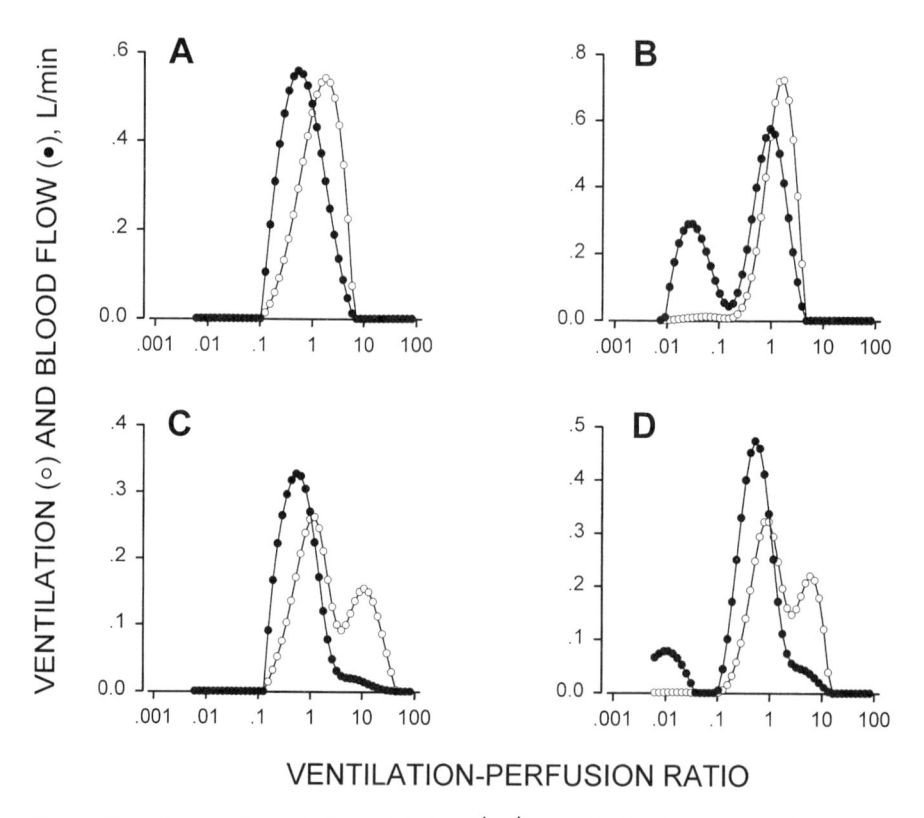

Figure 2 Patterns of ventilation–perfusion ($\dot{V}_A/\dot{Q}$) distribution in patients with chronic obstructive pulmonary disease (COPD). (A) Broad unimodal distributions of both blood flow and ventilation; (B) bimodal distribution of blood flow with a significant amount of perfusion diverted to areas with low $\dot{V}_A/\dot{Q}$ ratios; (C) bimodal distribution of ventilation with a significant amount of ventilation diverted to areas with high $\dot{V}_A/\dot{Q}$ ratios; and (D) bimodal distribution of both blood flow and ventilation. Values of shunt and dead space are not shown. The frequency of presentation of each pattern is discussed in the text.

(Fig. 2D). This diversity in the $\dot{V}A/\dot{Q}$ distribution patterns presumably reflects the heterogeneity of pathological abnormalities in the lungs of COPD patients. The association between the pattern of $\dot{V}A/\dot{Q}$ distribution and the clinical type of COPD initially reported by Wagner et al. [13] was not observed in a subsequent study by Marthan et al. [32], who studied 51 patients recovering from an acute exacerbation episode. The association between the pattern of $\dot{V}A/\dot{Q}$ mismatch and the clinical characteristics of COPD have not been addressed in other studies, presumably because of the difficulties in classifying the majority of patients into a specific group and because it has become progressively apparent that the clinical types of COPD characterized in the mid-1960s [4] are not clearly related to specific functional or pathological features [2].

B. Shunt

One of the major advantages of the inert gas technique is the ability to differentiate shunt, perfusion to nonventilated or essentially nonventilated lung units (defined as those with $\dot{V}A/\dot{Q}$ ratios < 0.005), from areas with low $\dot{V}A/\dot{Q}$ ratio caused by poor ventilation. Using the inert gas technique, it has been clearly established that shunt is of minor relevance as a mechanism of hypoxemia in COPD. As shown in Table 1, the percentage of shunt rarely exceeds 3%. From the initial work by Wagner et al. [13], who found shunt fractions greater than 5% only in 2 of 23 patients, the great majority of studies performed with the inert gas methodology have confirmed this observation, thus disregarding shunt as a mechanism of hypoxemia in COPD (15–29) (Table 1). Only Marthan et al. [32] reported shunt values greater than 5% in a significant proportion of COPD patients (11 of 51). However, this study was performed in patients recovering from an acute exacerbation episode, such that additional factors that could have potentially accounted for such an increased shunt fraction could not be excluded [32]. In our experience, in a group of 89 COPD patients studied under stable clinical conditions, only in 4 cases (4.5%) did the shunt fraction exceed 5% [19,21,22,26–29]. Accordingly, a significant amount of shunt is rarely observed in COPD, and its presence should suggest additional diagnoses [i.e., atelectasis, pneumonia, pulmonary edema, abnormal vascular or cardiac communications, or liver cirrhosis [33,34]].

C. Oxygen Diffusion Limitation

Using the estimates of the $\dot{V}A/\dot{Q}$ distribution made by the inert gas technique and measurements of total ventilation and cardiac output, it is still possible to calculate the PaO_2 value expected to result from a particular $\dot{V}A/\dot{Q}$ distribution [35]. The analysis of the differences between the calculated PaO_2 value and the measured one has been used to evaluate the presence of O_2 diffusion limitation. Measured PaO_2 values that are systematically lower than those predicted by the inert gas technique are interpreted as a reflection of alveolar end-capillary O_2 diffusion limitation, because inert gases are essentially invulnerable to this form of limitation, whereas O_2 may be diffusion-limited under certain conditions [35]. Using the inert gas technique algorithm, Wagner et al. [13] showed good agreement between predicted and measured Pa_{O_2} and that their relationship did not differ from the identity, thus indicating that in COPD, the observed $\dot{V}_A/\dot{Q}$ inequality accounts for all the measured hypoxemia. This finding ruled out limitation of O_2 diffusion between alveolar gas and capillary blood as a mechanism of hypoxemia in these patients. Subsequent studies in patients studied at rest have confirmed this observation [16,18,20,32].

D. Extrapulmonary Factors

Patients with COPD may exhibit different values of Pa_{O_2} despite similar degrees of $\dot{V}_A/\dot{Q}$ inequality. This is because extrapulmonary mechanisms, particularly total ventilation, cardiac output, and oxygen consumption, contribute to determine the final value of arterial blood gases by modulating the impact of $\dot{V}_A/\dot{Q}$ inequality [36].

Ventilation

In a condition of increased $\dot{V}_A/\dot{Q}$ inequality, where shunt is practically absent, as it is the case in COPD, changes in minute ventilation exert a significant influence over the degree of hypoxemia and hypercapnia. Because the great majority of alveolar units are ventilated to some extent, an increase in minute ventilation will increase the alveolar oxygen partial pressure (P_{AO_2}) of all units and hence the end-capillary P_{O_2}. In terms of $\dot{V}_A/\dot{Q}$ distribution, this means that the increase in alveolar ventilation shifts the distribution of blood flow toward areas with higher $\dot{V}_A/\dot{Q}$ ratios, thus increasing its mean $\dot{V}_A/\dot{Q}$ ratio. Lung units with higher $\dot{V}_A/\dot{Q}$ ratios [> 0.2 [31]] have a higher P_{AO_2} and lower alveolar carbon dioxide partial pressure (P_{ACO_2}), and the increased perfusion in these areas counterbalances the impact that perfusion in areas with lower $\dot{V}_A/\dot{Q}$ ratios has on Pa_{O_2}. The effects of ventilation on gas exchange are particularly relevant during episodes of acute exacerbation and during exercise. However, from the clinical point of view, the characteristics of the breathing pattern seem to be more important for gas exchange efficiency than the value of overall ventilation per se. As is discussed in Sec. C, changes in alveolar ventilation of approximately 1 L during exacerbation episodes had almost no effect on arterial oxygenation. By contrast, a dramatic effect of the breathing pattern on arterial blood gases was shown by Torres et al. [37] in COPD patients studied during weaning from mechanical ventilation. When patients breathed spontaneously, minute ventilation was similar to that during mechanical ventilation. However, the tidal volume decreased and the respiratory frequency increased. This pattern of rapid shallow breathing was accompanied by the shift of $\dot{V}_A/\dot{Q}$ distributions toward areas with lower $\dot{V}_A/\dot{Q}$ ratios and an increase in their dispersions, changes that yielded a decrease of Pa_{O_2} and an increase of Pa_{CO_2} [37].

Cardiac Output

In COPD, where $\dot{V}_A/\dot{Q}$ inequality is already present, cardiac output may modify gas exchange, basically through its effect on the O_2 content of mixed venous blood. A decrease in cardiac output per se will reduce mixed venous oxygen tension ($P\bar{v}_{O_2}$), and vice versa. Pa_{O_2} will then increase and decrease with the mixed venous value. Mithoefer et al. [38] were the first to identify the relevance of $P\bar{v}_{O_2}$ on arterial oxygenation in COPD. They showed that for equal abnormalities of gas exchange, estimated by the mixed venous admixture, the Pa_{O_2} level depended greatly on the patient's cardiac output, the presence of compensatory polycythemia, or both [38]. This important role of cardiac output on gas exchange has been clearly shown during acute exacerbations of COPD, where an increase in cardiac output contributed to compensate for the effect of an increased oxygen consumption by the respiratory muscles on $P\bar{v}_{O_2}$ [28].

E. Hypoxic Pulmonary Vasoconstriction

The hypoxic stimulus exerts opposite actions on systemic and pulmonary circulation. Systemic arteries relax in response to hypoxia, whereas pulmonary arteries contract. The original recognition of hypoxic pulmonary vasoconstriction was made by Von Euler and Liljestrand [39]. Hypoxic vasoconstriction is thought to be responsible for restricting blood flow through the fetal pulmonary circulation before birth and for matching perfusion to ventilation thereafter. Thus, pulmonary arteriolar constriction in response to hypoxia reduces perfusion in poorly ventilated or nonventilated lung units and diverts it to better-ventilated units, thereby partially restoring Pa_{O_2}. The mechanisms that lead to hypoxic pulmonary vasoconstriction have not been completely elucidated [40]. However, it has been shown that hypoxic vasoconstriction plays an important role in matching blood flow to ventilation in different respiratory disorders, particularly in COPD. The inhibition of hypoxic pulmonary vasoconstriction with vasodilators leads to a decrease in pulmonary artery pressure, but at the same time to a reduction in arterial oxygenation [41]. Studies using the inert gas technique have shown that this effect on Pa_{O_2} is caused by increased perfusion in poorly ventilated lung units with low $\dot{V}_A/\dot{Q}$ ratios [16,21], implying that before the administration of the vasodilator, arteriolar constriction contributed to maintain $\dot{V}_A/\dot{Q}$ matching in these units. Similar effects on $\dot{V}_A/\dot{Q}$ distributions produced by the inhibition of hypoxic vasoconstriction in COPD patients have been shown while breathing 100% oxygen [23,37] and during intravenous administration of β_2-adrenergic drugs [20].

III. Structure and Function Correlations

The relationships between the severity of pulmonary histological abnormalities, assessed morphometrically, and inert gas measurements of $\dot{V}_A/\dot{Q}$ inequality are of basic interest and have been analyzed in a group of patients with mild to moderate COPD who underwent resective lung surgery [22,23,42]. The severity of emphysema correlated with PaO_2, the alveolar to arterial O_2 gradient ($AaPO_2$), and the dispersions of blood flow and ventilation distributions [22]; all of these measurements were obtained immediately before surgery. The correlation between emphysema severity and the dispersion of blood flow distribution suggests that poorly ventilated alveolar units associated with emphysema may be one of the structural determinants of hypoxemia in COPD patients (Fig. 3). In emphysematous lungs, the number of alveolar attachments to membranous bronchioles is reduced, and hence the radial traction around bronchioles diminishes [43,44]. This causes distortion and narrowing of these small airways [45], impairing ventilation in dependent alveolar units. As a result, lung units with low $\dot{V}_A/\dot{Q}$ ratios may develop, widening the dispersion of blood flow distribution and reducing arterial oxygenation [22] (Fig. 3). This effect may be further amplified by the thickening of the airway wall secondary to the inflammatory reaction and fibrosis of membranous bronchioles [46].

Pulmonary emphysema is characterized by the destruction of alveolar walls and the enlargement of air spaces [47]. Abnormalities that are associated with the loss of pulmonary capillary network, leading to the development of lung units with greater ventilation than perfusion, i.e., with high $\dot{V}_A/\dot{Q}$ ratios, hence increasing the dispersion of ventilation distribution [22] (Fig. 3). In this case, the bimodal pattern of ventilation distribution, with a large amount of ventilation associated with high $\dot{V}_A/\dot{Q}$ ratio units, the high pattern described by Wagner et al. [13] in patients with the clinical characteristics of the emphysematous type of COPD, would be a magnification of this phenomenon, likely reflecting large areas of destroyed parenchyma in patients with advanced COPD in whom severe emphysema may be clinically apparent.

Small airway abnormalities were also associated with greater $\dot{V}_A/\dot{Q}$ inequality, as shown by a significant correlation between the severity of bronchiolar pathology and log SD $\dot{V}$ [22]. It was hypothesized that nonhomogeneous distribution of inspired air, as a result of the irregular narrowing and distortion of small airways, may account for the increased dispersion of ventilation distribution (Fig. 3). Indeed, a significant correlation between log SD $\dot{V}$ and the slope of the phase III of the nitrogen washout, which is considered an index of nonhomogeneous distribution of ventilation, was demonstrated [22]. Interestingly, in a subsequent study, the presence of small airway abnormalities did not preclude the improvement of $\dot{V}_A/\dot{Q}$ distributions during exercise in patients with mild to moderate COPD [42]. This suggests that changes in the ventilatory pattern and the increase in functional residual capacity that take place during exercise may overcome the effect of these anatomical abnormalities, leading to a more homogenous distribution of ventilation, at least in the early stage of the disease [42].

Correlations between pulmonary vascular abnormalities and indices of $\dot{V}_A/\dot{Q}$ mismatching were additionally investigated in patients with mild to moderate COPD

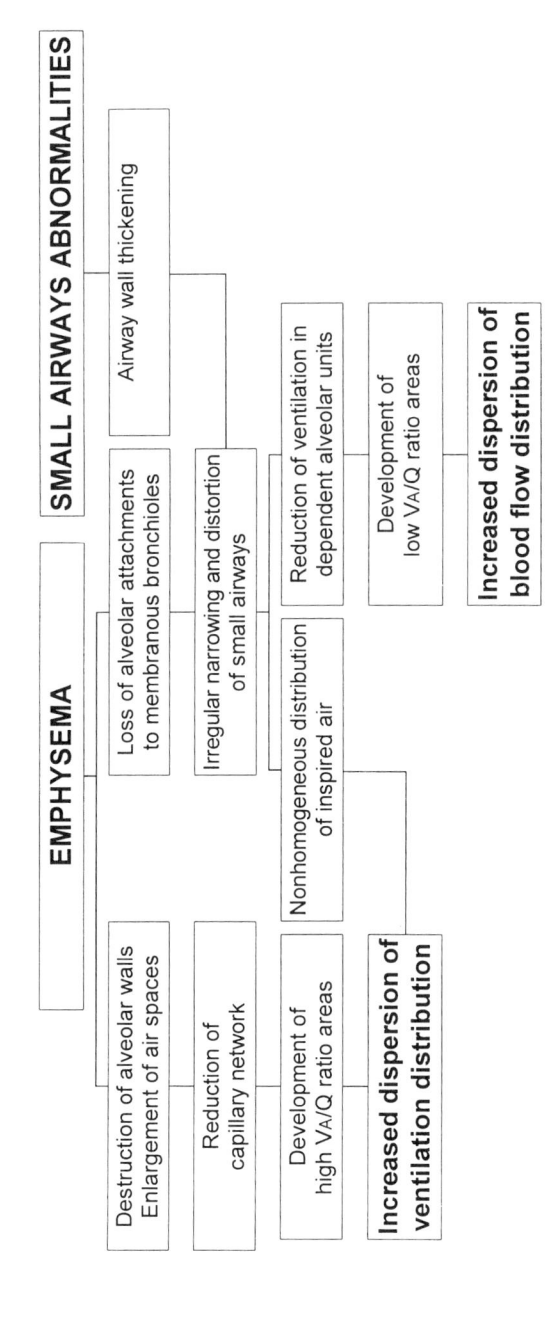

Figure 3 Schematic representation of the potential mechanisms involved in the relationships between emphysema and small airways abnormalities and the increased dispersions of ventilation–perfusion distributions in patients with chronic obstructive pulmonary disease (COPD).

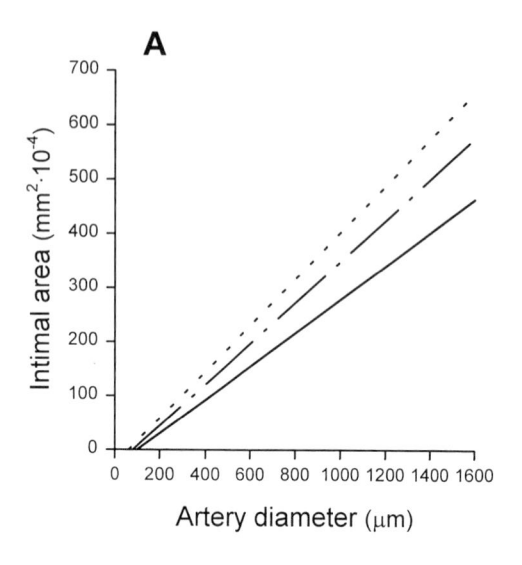

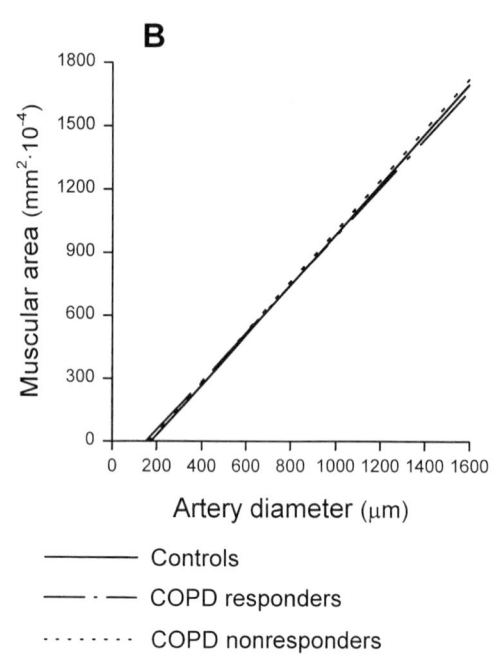

Figure 4 Regression lines of the relationship between (A) area of the intimal layer and pulmonary muscular artery diameter and (B) area of the muscular layer and pulmonary muscular artery diameter in control subjects (solid lines), chronic obstructive pulmonary disease (COPD) patient responders to oxygen breathing (dashed lines), and COPD patient nonresponders to oxygen breathing (dotted lines). The intimal layers of COPD patient nonresponders to oxygen were thickened compared with both COPD responders and controls. No differences in the thickness of the muscular layer were shown among the three groups. (From Ref. 23.)

[23]. A group of COPD patients and control subjects undergoing resective lung surgery was studied. COPD patients were further classified into two categories according to the changes in $\dot{V}_A/\dot{Q}$ distributions induced by 100% O_2 breathing. One group of patients showed a significant increase in $\dot{V}_A/\dot{Q}$ inequality (increase in log SD $\dot{Q}$ > 0.4) when breathing oxygen (COPD responders), implying that in these patients, hypoxic pulmonary vasoconstriction exerted an active role in preserving $\dot{V}_A/\dot{Q}$ matching. The other group showed a minor increase in $\dot{V}_A/\dot{Q}$ inequality (change in log SD $\dot{Q}$ < 0.4) induced by oxygen breathing (COPD nonresponders), suggesting a more modest hypoxic vascular regulation of the $\dot{V}_A/\dot{Q}$ balance. As shown in Fig. 4, morphometric measurements in pulmonary muscular arteries showed thickening of the intimal layer in COPD patients, which was more pronounced in nonresponders to oxygen, especially in arteries with small diameters [23]. This finding suggests that the damage of the intima may impair the reactivity to hypoxia and the vascular regulation of $\dot{V}_A/\dot{Q}$ matching. It is interesting to note that no differences in smooth muscle thickness were shown among arteries of the different groups [23] (Fig. 4). These observations are consistent with the prominent role that vascular endothelium has on the regulation of vessel reactivity [48]. Indeed, endothelial dysfunction of pulmonary arteries has been shown in patients with end-stage COPD undergoing lung transplantation [49], as well as in patients with moderate airflow obstruction [50]. Furthermore, the severity of endothelial dysfunction seems to be related to the degree of intimal thickening [49,50], suggesting that endothelial function may be altered in association with the remodeling process of pulmonary vessels [51]. Accordingly, in COPD, the hypoxic regulation of $\dot{V}_A/\dot{Q}$ matching may be modified by the impairment of the structure and function of pulmonary arteries.

IV. Gas Exchange in the Natural History of COPD

COPD is a progressive disease that covers a wide clinical spectrum. As discussed earlier, the degree of airflow obstruction is poorly correlated with the severity of hypoxemia and with the indices of $\dot{V}_A/\dot{Q}$ inequality (Fig. 1). However, in a particular patient, it is expected that as disease progresses and airflow rates decrease, the more severe the hypoxemia will be. Moreover, in the advanced stages of the disease, episodes of acute exacerbation, characterized by worsening gas exchange, are one of the most frequent complications. Currently available cross-sectional data obtained with the inert gas technique has allowed us to characterize the degree of $\dot{V}_A/\dot{Q}$ impairment over a wide spectrum of COPD severity and to clarify the mechanisms of gas exchange impairment during acute exacerbation episodes.

A. Stable, Mild COPD

Patients with mild to moderate COPD (FEV_1 > 50% of predicted) may show a moderate increase in $\dot{V}_A/\dot{Q}$ inequality. In a series of patients with a mean FEV_1

of 72% ± 12% of predicted, increased values of both log SD $\dot{Q}$ and log SD $\dot{V}$ were reported (0.87 ± 0.24 and 0.73 ± 0.25, respectively) [22,23]. This moderate degree of $\dot{V}_A/\dot{Q}$ inequality accounted for the increased AaPO$_2$ (29 ± 9 mm Hg) and the decrease of PaO$_2$ (77 ± 9 mm Hg). It is well known that significant impairment of peripheral structures of the lung may take place before airflow obstruction becomes apparent [52] and, as previously discussed, significant relationships between the severity of pathological abnormalities and indices of $\dot{V}_A/\dot{Q}$ inequality have been shown in these patients [22,23,42]. Accordingly, it is not surprising that gas exchange became altered by these anatomical abnormalities, despite the finding that airflow obstruction was of only moderate degree. Moreover, patients without evident airflow obstruction (FEV$_1$ > 80% of predicted) but with small airways dysfunction, as shown by reduced midexpiratory flow rates and increased slope of phase III of the nitrogen washout, may show $\dot{V}_A/\dot{Q}$ mismatching [53]. Compared with subjects with normal lung function, patients with small airways dysfunction showed increased AaPO$_2$, log SD $\dot{Q}$, and log SD $\dot{V}$ [53]. Accordingly, some degree of $\dot{V}_A/\dot{Q}$ mismatch may already be present at the very early stages of COPD, presumably as a result of the aforementioned structural impairment of peripheral lung units.

B. Stable, Severe COPD

As shown in Fig. 1 and Table 1, patients with severe airflow obstruction tend to show the greatest degree of $\dot{V}_A/\dot{Q}$ inequality. However, patients with very severe airflow obstruction may show remarkably different degrees of $\dot{V}_A/\dot{Q}$ mismatch, from log SD values almost within the normal range (≤ 0.6) to very abnormal values (> 1.5). Moreover, the rate of decline in FEV$_1$ seems not to be accompanied by a parallel increase in the severity of $\dot{V}_A/\dot{Q}$ mismatching. Indeed, some patients with severe airflow obstruction may keep $\dot{V}_A/\dot{Q}$ distributions within a moderate range of impairment (Fig. 1). In fact, in patients with stable, severe COPD, the percentage of perfusion in areas with low $\dot{V}_A/\dot{Q}$ ratio is usually moderate. This dissociation between airflow rates and indices of $\dot{V}_A/\dot{Q}$ mismatching has also been observed in patients with bronchial asthma (54), indicating that structural and functional determinants of airflow rates and gas exchange may be different.

Figure 1 shows a greater correlation of FEV$_1$ with log SD $\dot{V}$ than with log SD $\dot{Q}$, despite substantial scatter in both relationships. This may denote that log SD $\dot{V}$ may be more affected by the structural abnormalities that promote reduced airflow rates in COPD and is consistent with the correlations between log SD $\dot{V}$ and fixed structural abnormalities of the lung (emphysema and small airways pathology) alluded to previously. Patients with severe COPD show increased values of log SD $\dot{V}$ and log SD $\dot{Q}$, which do not differ significantly between them. However, no correlation between both variables was shown in a group of 89 patients ($r = -0.20$). This contrasts with observations made in patients with chronic asthma, in whom a greater correlation between both variables was shown, although log SD $\dot{V}$ was less abnormal than log SD $\dot{Q}$ [55].

C. Acute Exacerbations

Episodes of acute exacerbation of COPD are characterized by worsening hypoxemia with or without hypercapnia. Mechanisms of gas exchange worsening during acute exacerbation episodes have been recently characterized using the inert gas technique [28]. A group of patients with severe airflow obstruction (FEV$_1$, 0.91 ± 0.19 L, 29% ± 6% of predicted) were studied at the beginning of an exacerbation episode and more than 1 month later, when they were clinically stable [28]. In these patients, the decrease in PaO_2 and the increase in PaCO_2 during exacerbation were accompanied by the worsening of $\dot{V}_A/\dot{Q}$ relationships, as shown by a moderate increase in log SD $\dot{Q}$ (1.10 ± 0.29 during exacerbation, 0.96 ± 0.27 under stable conditions) (Fig. 5). This was the result of increased perfusion in poorly ventilated areas with low $\dot{V}_A/\dot{Q}$ ratios, which is consistent with airway narrowing by inflammation, bronchospasm, and mucus secretions. Interestingly, intrapulmonary shunt, which was trivial under stable conditions, did not increase during exacerbations. This gives further support to the finding that shunt is not a significant mechanism of hypoxemia in COPD, probably because these patients do not have completely occluded airways or because they possess efficient collateral ventilation. Interestingly, such a moderate increase in $\dot{V}_A/\dot{Q}$ inequality did not completely explain the worsening of arterial oxygenation, implying that other factors contributed to reduce PaO_2 [28]. The most influential factor was an increase in oxygen consumption that produced a reduction in P$\bar{v}O_2$ (Figs. 5 and 6). Such a decrease in P$\bar{v}O_2$ may decrease PaO_2 by a direct effect and, more importantly, by amplifying the impact of increased $\dot{V}_A/\dot{Q}$ inequality on end-capillary PO_2 [31]. The increase in oxygen consumption was attributed to an increased oxygen demand of the respiratory muscles as a result of the increase in airway resistance and the efforts to overcome dynamic hyperinflation. Interestingly, the effect of greater oxygen consumption on P$\bar{v}O_2$ was partially counterbalanced by an increase in cardiac output (Fig. 6). Accordingly, it was estimated that 46% of the decrease in arterial oxygenation during exacerbation was caused by increased $\dot{V}_A/\dot{Q}$ inequality, 28% to the combined changes in oxygen consumption and in cardiac output, and the remaining 26% to the amplifying effect that a decrease in P$\bar{v}O_2$ has on $\dot{V}_A/\dot{Q}$ mismatch in further decreasing end-capillary PO_2 [28] (Fig. 6).

It is interesting to note that the increase in $\dot{V}_A/\dot{Q}$ inequality during COPD exacerbations is usually moderate. Diaz et al. [56], in patients breathing spontaneously studied within the first days after hospital admission, reported a mean log SD $\dot{Q}$ of 1.08 ± 0.23. Patients requiring mechanical ventilation during exacerbations may show slightly greater dispersions of $\dot{V}_A/\dot{Q}$ distributions. In mechanically ventilated COPD patients, Castaing et al. [57] reported a mean log SD $\dot{Q}$ of 1.37 ± 0.30, and Rossi et al. [58] reported 1.33 ± 0.16. These findings contrast with the greater degree of $\dot{V}_A/\dot{Q}$ inequality that is reached during acute exacerbations of bronchial asthma. In asthmatics who breathed spontaneously, studied during an acute exacerbation episode and after hospitalization, log SD $\dot{Q}$ changed from 1.41 ± 0.12 during exacerbation to 0.53 ± 0.07 after recovery [59]. In asthmatics who

Figure 5 Change in (A) ratio of arterial oxygen tension to inspired oxygen fraction (Pa_{O_2}/F_{IO_2}), (B) ventilation–perfusion ($\dot{V}_A/\dot{Q}$) inequality (expressed as the dispersion of blood flow distribution [log SD $\dot{Q}$]), and (C) oxygen consumption ($\dot{V}_{O_2}$) from acute exacerbation (AE) to stable conditions (SC) in patients with advanced chronic obstructive pulmonary disease (COPD). Open symbols and vertical bars denote mean ± SD. (From Ref. 28.)

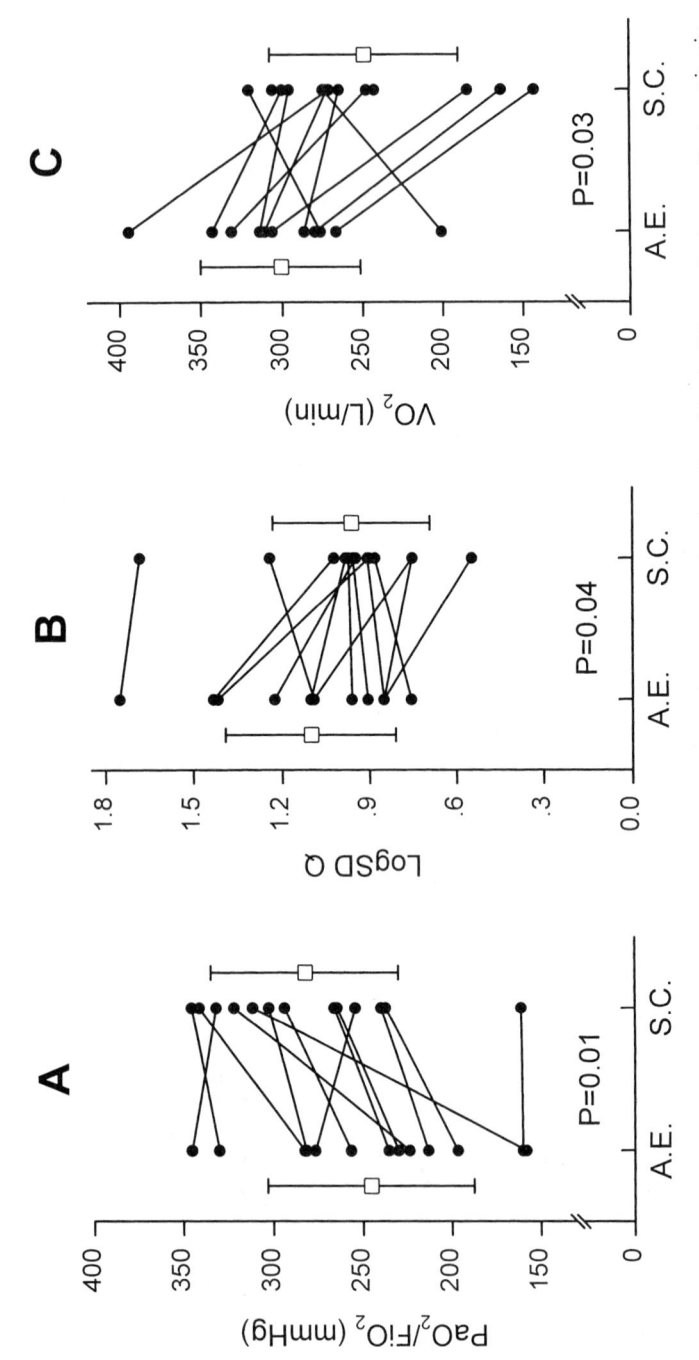

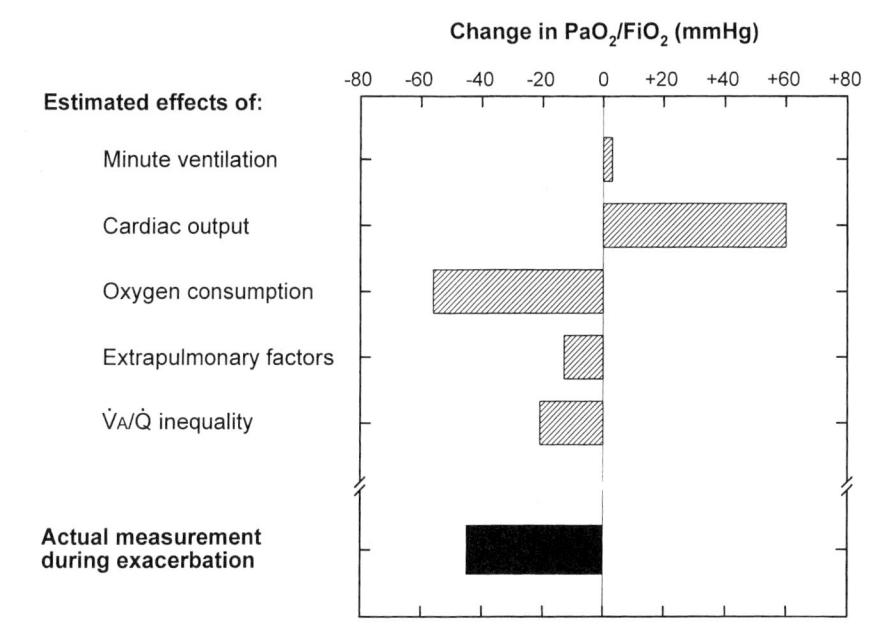

Figure 6 Theoretical analysis of the relative contributions of the factors that determined the change in the ratio of arterial oxygen tension to inspired oxygen fraction (PaO_2/FiO_2) during an acute exacerbation of chronic obstructive pulmonary disease (COPD). Dashed bars indicate the difference in PaO_2/FiO_2 measured under stable clinical conditions minus that predicted to result from a specific change, at the level corresponding to the exacerbation, in minute ventilation (V̇E), cardiac output (Q̇T), oxygen consumption (V̇O_2), all the extrapulmonary factors together (V̇E, Q̇T, and V̇O_2) and ventilation–perfusion (V̇A/Q̇) inequality. The solid bar shows the actual change in PaO_2/FiO_2 that took place during acute exacerbation. (From Ref. 28.)

required mechanical ventilation during an exacerbation episode, the mean value of log SD Q̇ was 1.65 ± 0.28 [33]. This greater degree of V̇A/Q̇ mismatch may imply that acute airway narrowing in asthma attacks is much more pronounced than in COPD exacerbations, leading to the development of a greater proportion of alveolar units with low V̇A/Q̇ ratios. This is consistent with contraction of smooth muscle in small airways acting together with thickening of airway wall by submucosal edema, which further enhances narrowing of the airway lumen [60]. In COPD exacerbations, acute changes in membranous bronchioles are less dramatic than in asthma, and hence the change in airway lumen diameter may be less pronounced. Kuwano et al. [61] have recently shown greater wall thickening in small airways of asthmatics than in COPD patients, and that such thickening especially affected the submucosa. Accordingly, thickening of the airway wall inside the smooth muscle layer acts in series with muscle shortening, amplifying the magnitude of airway narrowing [62]. These structural differences may explain the lower proportion of units with reduced $\dot{V}_A/\dot{Q}$ ratios, and thus the reduced increase in log SD $\dot{Q}$, during acute exacerbations of COPD than in asthma. In addition, the structural changes in pulmonary vessels and the reduction of the capillary network by emphysema, which are common features in COPD [22,23], may entail a limited ability to modify the distribution of pulmonary blood flow during exacerbations.

V. Gas Exchange During Exercise

In patients with COPD, Pa_{O_2} during exercise may decrease, remain unchanged, or even increase. This variable effect of exercise on Pa_{O_2} depends on the interplay between the intrapulmonary and extrapulmonary factors that govern gas exchange during exercise in human subjects. The inert gas technique has allowed a precise analysis of the role of such factors in these patients. In advanced COPD, during exercise, the degree of $\dot{V}_A/\dot{Q}$ inequality does not worsen, and it may remain the same [13,18,63] or improve slightly [21,29] (Table 2). In patients with mild COPD, a significant improvement in the degree of $\dot{V}_A/\dot{Q}$ mismatch is commonly observed during submaximal exercise [42] (Table 2). Thus, evidence accumulated to date suggests that exercise never worsens $\dot{V}_A/\dot{Q}$ inequality in COPD; on the contrary, the degree of mismatch present at rest either improves or remains unaltered, probably depending on the severity of airflow limitation. In fact, once a severe degree of $\dot{V}_A/\dot{Q}$ mismatch has been reached, a greater increase in $\dot{V}_A/\dot{Q}$ inequality exerts little effect on the relationship between Pa_{O_2} and $P\bar{v}_{O_2}$. Figure 7 shows the relationship between Pa_{O_2} and $P\bar{v}_{O_2}$ at different degrees of $\dot{V}_A/\dot{Q}$ inequality, from normal $\dot{V}_A/\dot{Q}$ distributions recovered in healthy subjects (log SD $\dot{Q} \leq 0.60$) to very abnormal $\dot{V}_A/\dot{Q}$ distributions recovered in COPD patients (log SD $\dot{Q} = 1.80$). For a given $P\bar{v}_{O_2}$, Pa_{O_2} decreased according to the degree of $\dot{V}_A/\dot{Q}$ inequality. However, $\dot{V}_A/\dot{Q}$ distributions with log SD $\dot{Q}$ values greater than 1.2 exerted little effect on further worsening Pa_{O_2} at a given $P\bar{v}_{O_2}$.

In patients in whom an amelioration of $\dot{V}_A/\dot{Q}$ distributions is shown during exercise, such an improvement is more commonly shown as a decrease in the dispersion of ventilation distribution (Table 2). This may likely be caused by the preferential diversion of ventilation to lung units with normal $\dot{V}_A/\dot{Q}$ ratios, which offer less resistance to airflow and are more susceptible to changes in ventilation and blood flow than units affected by structural abnormalities [29,42]. Moreover, the increase in functional residual capacity that takes place during exercise may stretch small airways, increasing their diameter and favoring a more homogenous distribution of ventilation [42].

Although $\dot{V}_A/\dot{Q}$ relationships do not deteriorate during exercise in COPD, some patients, particularly those with more advanced disease, often present a significant decrease in Pa_{O_2} while exercising [13,18,21,29,63] (Table 2). Such a decrease in Pa_{O_2} may have a multifactorial origin, although the most important one

Table 2 Ventilation-Perfusion Distributions During Exercise in Patients with Chronic Obstructive Pulmonary Disease[a]

					Blood flow distribution				Ventilation distribution			
			PaO2 (mm Hg)		Mean		Log SD		Mean		Log SD	
Reference	No. of patients	FEV1 (%)	Rest	Exercise	Rest	Exercise	Rest	Exercise	Rest	Exercise	Rest	Exercise
Wagner, 1977 (63)	10	43 ± 13	58 ± 11	50 ± 10	0.5 ± 0.2	0.6 ± 0.3	1.30 ± 0.31	1.48 ± 0.39	NR	NR	NR	NR
Dantzker et al., 1986 (18)	7	36 ± 8	76 ± 10	63 ± 8	0.76 ± 0.17	0.78 ± 0.18	0.73 ± 0.20	0.73 ± 0.19	NR	NR	NR	NR
Agustí et al., 1990 (21)	8	36 ± 3	76 ± 2	68 ± 4	0.79 ± 0.06	1.18 ± 0.12	0.90 ± 0.06	0.78 ± 0.07	2.14 ± 0.27	2.23 ± 0.27	1.03 ± 0.11	0.83 ± 0.09
Barberà et al., 1991 (42)	17	76 ± 4	81 ± 3	86 ± 3	0.69 ± 0.04	1.77 ± 0.08	0.75 ± 0.07	0.70 ± 0.06	1.18 ± 0.10	2.40 ± 0.08	0.66 ± 0.06	0.50 ± 0.03
Roger et al., 1977 (29)	9	39 ± 2	72 ± 3	67 ± 3	0.73 ± 0.10	1.34 ± 0.20	0.92 ± 0.09	0.84 ± 0.14	1.75 ± 0.30	2.42 ± 0.30	0.84 ± 0.08	0.66 ± 0.09

[a]Dispersions are either SD or SEM.
Mean = mean $\dot{V}_A/\dot{Q}$ ratio (first moment) of the distribution; log SD = dispersion (second moment) of the distribution on a logarithmic scale; NR = not reported; FEV1 = forced expiratory volume in 1 second; PaO2 = arterial oxygen partial pressure.

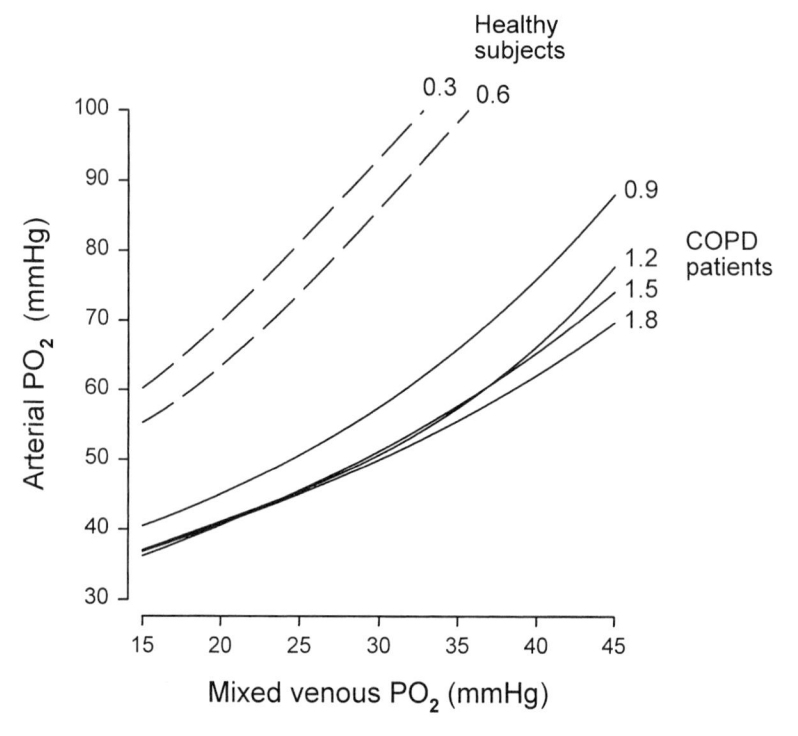

Figure 7 Relationship between oxygen tension in arterial (Pao$_2$) and mixed venous (P$\bar{v}$o$_2$) oxygen partial pressure blood calculated at different degrees of ventilation–perfusion ($\dot{V}_A/\dot{Q}$) inequality in healthy subjects (dashed lines) and in patients with chronic obstructive pulmonary disease (COPD) (solid lines). Numbers indicate the degree of $\dot{V}_A/\dot{Q}$ inequality, expressed as the dispersion of blood flow distribution (log SD $\dot{Q}$; normal, ≤ 0.6). Cardiac output (5.5 L/min) and minute ventilation (8 L/min) were kept constant in all the calculations.

is the ability to increase ventilation during exercise. Figure 8 summarizes the most relevant changes that took place during exercise in three groups of subjects. Data from healthy subjects [64], patients with mild COPD [42], and patients with severe COPD [18] are shown. Pao$_2$ decreased only in patients with severe COPD. The major difference between groups was in the change in total ventilation during exercise. During exercise, healthy subjects increased ventilation approximately 10-fold, whereas patients with severe COPD only doubled it because of their ventilatory limitation. Patients with mild COPD were in an intermediate position. The small increase in alveolar ventilation in severe COPD may be insufficient to compensate for the increase of CO$_2$ production that takes place during exercise, leading to an increase in Paco$_2$. Moreover, because differences in the ability to increase cardiac output were less pronounced than those in ventilation, the ratio between total

Chronic Obstructive Pulmonary Disease

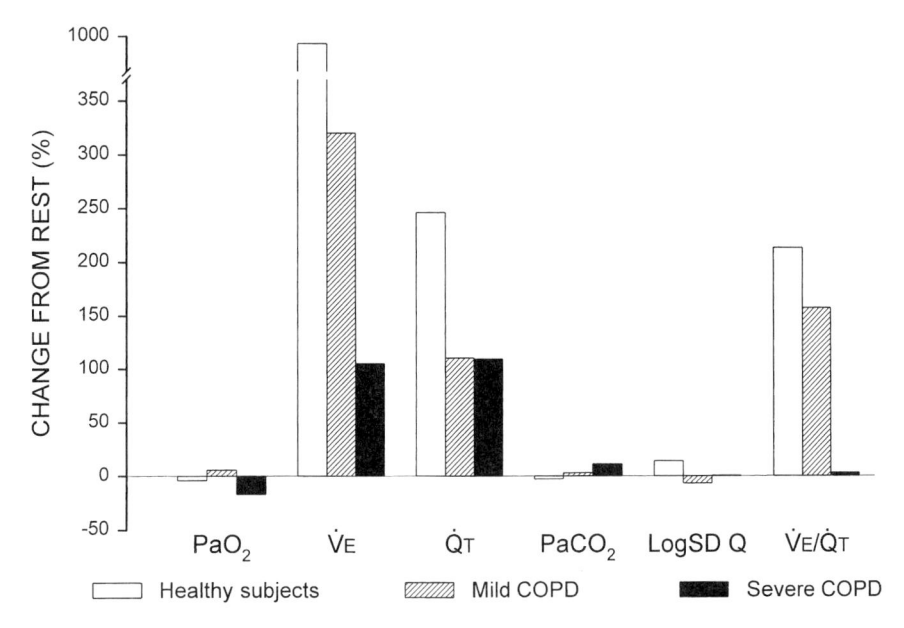

Figure 8 Percent change from rest to exercise in arterial oxygen partial pressure (Pa_{O_2}), minute ventilation (V_E), cardiac output (Q_T), arterial CO_2 partial pressure (Pa_{CO_2}), dispersion of blood flow distribution (log SD $\dot{Q}$), and the ratio between minute ventilation and cardiac output (V_E/Q_T) in healthy subjects (open bars), patients with mild chronic obstructive pulmonary disease (COPD) (dashed bars), and patients with severe COPD (solid bars). (Data from Refs. 18, 42 and 64.)

ventilation and cardiac output differed substantially among the groups. This ratio increased in healthy subjects and in patients with mild COPD, whereas it remained unaltered in patients with severe COPD (Fig. 8). As a result, patients with severe COPD could not shift the perfusion distribution toward higher $\dot{V}_A/\dot{Q}$ ratios. Such an increase in the $\dot{V}_A/\dot{Q}$ ratio of alveolar units compensates for the effect of a decreasing $P\bar{v}_{O_2}$, which normally occurs during exercise, on end-capillary P_{O_2} [31]. Such an effect was further amplified by the fact that these patients had greater $\dot{V}_A/\dot{Q}$ mismatch, i.e., lung units with more profound low $\dot{V}_A/\dot{Q}$ ratios, to begin with. Furthermore, the lowering of $P\bar{v}_{O_2}$ in COPD may be additionally promoted by the fact that these patients may develop pulmonary hypertension, particularly during exercise. A higher right ventricular afterload may result in a lower $P\bar{v}_{O_2}$ during exercise than expected if it interferes with the increase in cardiac output that normally occurs.

The potential effect of diffusion limitation to oxygen during exercise was originally investigated by Wagner et al. [13,63] using the inert gas technique algorithm. No differences between Pa_{O_2} predicted from recovered $\dot{V}_A/\dot{Q}$ distributions and that actually measured were shown. This finding indicates that in COPD, the degree of $\dot{V}_A/\dot{Q}$ inequality accounted for the measured hypoxemia during exercise. This observation demonstrates that there is no significant limitation in the diffusion of oxygen from the alveoli to the capillary blood during exercise in COPD. Other investigators have confirmed this observation [18,29].

VI. Effect of Therapeutic Interventions on Gas Exchange

A. Oxygen Breathing

The administration of high inspired O_2 fractions has two potential deleterious effects on $\dot{V}_A/\dot{Q}$ matching: (1) an increase in intrapulmonary shunt caused by the collapse of alveolar units when air is replaced by oxygen; and (2) an increase in $\dot{V}_A/\dot{Q}$ inequality caused by greater perfusion in alveolar units with low $\dot{V}_A/\dot{Q}$ ratios due to the release of hypoxic pulmonary vasoconstriction [65]. Studies using the inert gas technique in patients with COPD have shown that the increase in shunt during 100% O_2 breathing is minimal and that it rarely exceeds 5% [13,23,26,37,66]. This might be explained by the fact that in COPD, most alveolar units have $\dot{V}_A/\dot{Q}$ ratios greater than the critical value for collapse [66]. Additionally, units with $\dot{V}_A/\dot{Q}$ ratios less than such a critical value may remain open by ventilation from adjacent lung units (i.e., collateral ventilation). By contrast, 100% O_2 breathing usually worsens $\dot{V}_A/\dot{Q}$ relationships in COPD, as shown by more blood flow being diverted to units with low $\dot{V}_A/\dot{Q}$ ratios and a corresponding increase in log SD $\dot{Q}$ This is likely caused by the release of hypoxic pulmonary vasoconstriction when P_{AO_2} increases. Such worsening of $\dot{V}_A/\dot{Q}$ distributions when breathing 100% O_2 has been shown repeatedly in clinically stable COPD patients of different severity [13,23,26,66]. Furthermore, Torres et al. [37] reported significant deterioration of $\dot{V}_A/\dot{Q}$ mismatch during 100% O_2 breathing in patients with severe COPD who were in the process of being weaned from mechanical ventilation. Similar increases in $\dot{V}_A/\dot{Q}$ inequality have been shown both in patients with advanced disease recovering from an acute exacerbation [67] and in patients with mild airflow obstruction [23]. Santos et al. [66] studied the effects of increasing the inspired O_2 concentration to 100% during mechanical ventilation in patients with COPD and in patients with acute lung injury. In the latter group, 100% O_2 breathing resulted in a significant increase in the amount of intrapulmonary shunt (from 16% to 23%), whereas in COPD patients, shunt did not change, although there was a significant increase in $\dot{V}_A/\dot{Q}$ inequality (log SD $\dot{Q}$, from 1.33 to 1.80). Accordingly, it was postulated that the effect of 100% O_2 breathing on gas exchange is related to the underlying lung disorder. In patients with acute lung injury, oxygen breathing increases shunt because of the development of absorption atelectasis. By contrast, in COPD, alveolar collapse does not develop while breathing oxygen, likely because of the efficiency of collateral ventilation, and the major effect shown is worsening of $\dot{V}_A/\dot{Q}$ distributions due to the inhibition of hypoxic pulmonary vasoconstriction.

The effect of breathing supplementary oxygen at lower concentrations on $\dot{V}_A/\dot{Q}$ distributions in COPD is less clear. Castaing et al. [17] reported a significantly increased perfusion in areas with low $\dot{V}_A/\dot{Q}$ ratios while breathing 26% O_2, suggesting that low inspired O_2 concentrations may be enough for the release of hypoxic vasoconstriction. However, other studies have failed to demonstrate in COPD a significant effect on $\dot{V}_A/\dot{Q}$ distributions while breathing 28% and 40% O_2 [68]. Accordingly, in COPD patients, the potential deleterious effect on $\dot{V}_A/\dot{Q}$ distributions of low inspired O_2 fractions, which are those that are most commonly used in the clinical setting, remains controversial.

B. Mechanical Ventilation

The impact of different modalities of mechanical ventilation on $\dot{V}_A/\dot{Q}$ distributions in COPD patients has been poorly documented. In patients studied during weaning from mechanical ventilation, Torres et al. [37] showed a deterioration of the ventilatory pattern caused by the reduction of tidal volume and the increase of respiratory frequency. This breathing pattern was accompanied by a shift of $\dot{V}_A/\dot{Q}$ distributions toward areas with lower $\dot{V}_A/\dot{Q}$ ratios and an increase in their dispersions, changes that produced a decrease in Pa_{O_2} and an increase in Pa_{CO_2} [37]. Accordingly, the beneficial effect of increased cardiac output on Pa_{O_2} that resulted from the reduction of intrathoracic pressures when patients were disconnected from the ventilator was offset by the deleterious influence of the change in breathing pattern on Pa_{O_2}. Other investigators have emphasized that during weaning from mechanical ventilation, O_2 consumption may increase while breathing spontaneously, hence reducing $P\bar{v}_{O_2}$ and exerting a deleterious effect on end-capillary P_{O_2} that may result in weaning failure [69].

The use of low degrees of positive end-expiratory pressure (PEEP) in mechanically ventilated COPD patients has been recently advocated to overcome dynamic hyperinflation and intrinsic PEEP [70]. Rossi et al. [58] evaluated the effects of PEEP on $\dot{V}_A/\dot{Q}$ relationships in mechanically ventilated COPD patients. The application of a low level of external PEEP (equivalent to 50% of intrinsic PEEP) shifted $\dot{V}_A/\dot{Q}$ distributions toward units with higher $\dot{V}_A/\dot{Q}$ ratios, which have higher Pa_{O_2} and lower Pa_{CO_2}, hence improving arterial blood gases. At this low level of PEEP, no changes in respiratory mechanics or pulmonary hemodynamics were observed. By contrast, when external PEEP was increased to a value equivalent to the intrinsic PEEP level, no further improvement in gas exchange was achieved, whereas intrathoracic pressures increased significantly [58]. On the other hand, when intrinsic PEEP was reduced by modifying the ventilator settings (increase of expiratory time and decrease of both tidal volume and respiratory rate), there was a reduction in Pa_{O_2} and an increase in Pa_{CO_2}, which was caused by the worsening of gas exchange that ensued the shifting of $\dot{V}_A/\dot{Q}$ distributions toward units with low $\dot{V}_A/\dot{Q}$ ratios. However, in the latter condition, intrathoracic pressures decreased and cardiac output increased significantly; thus, the oxygen delivery to the tissues increased. A potential clinical implication of these findings is that the application of low values of PEEP, as well as the use of "controlled mechanical hypoventilation," may be adequate strategies to ventilate COPD patients during episodes of acute exacerbation [58].

Recent studies have suggested that, in acute exacerbations of COPD, noninvasive positive pressure ventilation through a facial or nasal mask can improve hypercapnia and respiratory acidosis, avoiding the need for tracheal intubation [71]. Accordingly, noninvasive ventilation is being progressively used as an alternative to conventional ventilation in patients with severe hypercapnic respiratory failure. The effect of noninvasive ventilation on $\dot{V}_A/\dot{Q}$ distributions has been recently evaluated by Diaz et al. [56]. In this study, PaO_2 increased and PaCO_2 decreased during ventilation with continuous positive airway pressure. These changes were caused by the increase in alveolar ventilation that ensued a more efficient breathing pattern, because tidal volume increased and respiratory frequency decreased. Contrasting with these effects, no changes in $\dot{V}_A/\dot{Q}$ distributions were observed during noninvasive ventilation because the indices of $\dot{V}_A/\dot{Q}$ mismatching, as well as the proportion of blood flow perfusing alveolar units with low $\dot{V}_A/\dot{Q}$ ratios, remained essentially unaltered [56]. Accordingly, it seems unlikely that recruitment of poorly ventilated or unventilated lung units took place during noninvasive ventilation. Furthermore, continuous positive airway pressure ventilation resulted in a decrease of cardiac output. Therefore, the application of high ventilatory pressures during noninvasive ventilation does not seem warranted, because the deleterious effect on cardiac output is not accompanied by an efficient recruitment of alveolar units. Interestingly, AaPO_2 increased during noninvasive ventilation, an effect that was explained by the increase in the respiratory quotient that resulted from the increased clearance of body stores of CO_2 [56].

C. Bronchodilators

Bronchodilator agents are one of the mainstays of COPD treatment. Despite their beneficial effects in reducing bronchial tone, a potential undesirable side effect is the risk of worsening $\dot{V}_A/\dot{Q}$ mismatch because of the inhibition of hypoxic pulmonary vasoconstriction. Ringsted et al. [20] showed that in COPD patients, intravenous terbutaline increased cardiac output and exerted variable effects on gas exchange, depending on disease severity. In patients who had higher PaO_2 and less airflow obstruction, terbutaline increased $\dot{V}_A/\dot{Q}$ mismatch, hence lowering PaO_2. By contrast, in patients who were more severely ill and had lower PaO_2 and FEV$_1$, terbutaline exerted no effect on $\dot{V}_A/\dot{Q}$ distributions. This different response to terbutaline was attributed to a lower hypoxic vascular response of pulmonary circulation in patients with more advanced disease and, presumably, to more severe morphologic alterations of pulmonary vessels [20].

Ballester et al. [72] pointed out that the effect of β_2-agonists on gas exchange may depend on the route of administration. In patients with bronchial asthma,

360 μg salbutamol administered intravenously worsened $\dot{V}_A/\dot{Q}$ distributions because of increased perfusion to low $\dot{V}_A/\dot{Q}$ ratio units, an effect that was ascribed to the inhibition of hypoxic vasoconstriction. By contrast, when 600 μg salbutamol was administered through a metered-dose inhaler, no effect on $\dot{V}_A/\dot{Q}$ distributions was observed [72]. Thus, contrasting with the intravenous route, the bronchodilator effect of aerosolized β_2-agonists is not accompanied by worsening of gas exchange. Viegas et al. [27] have recently shown in a group of hypoxemic patients with severe COPD that nebulized fenoterol, a less selective β_2-agonist, at doses of 1 and 5 mg, increased FEV_1 but at the same time increased significantly cardiac output and showed a trend to worsening $\dot{V}_A/\dot{Q}$ relationships. By contrast, nebulized ipratropium bromide, which lacks significant cardiovascular effects, at doses of 0.5 mg, increased FEV_1 to a similar extent but did not alter cardiac output or $\dot{V}_A/\dot{Q}$ distributions. The different effects of inhaled fenoterol and salbutamol on $\dot{V}_A/\dot{Q}$ distributions were attributed to greater cardiovascular activity of fenoterol, likely because of its lower specificity for β_2-receptors [73].

The effects of intravenous aminophylline on $\dot{V}_A/\dot{Q}$ distributions have been evaluated in a group of COPD patients recovering from an acute exacerbation [67]. Intravenous aminophylline given at a loading dose of 6 mg/kg, followed by a maintenance dose of 0.9 mg/kg/h, increased FEV_1, whereas it did not exert any significant effect on $\dot{V}_A/\dot{Q}$ distributions. This lack of effect of aminophylline on $\dot{V}_A/\dot{Q}$ relationships was not a result of diminished hypoxic vascular response of pulmonary circulation, because in this group of patients, significant $\dot{V}_A/\dot{Q}$ worsening was shown during 100% O_2 breathing. Accordingly, at doses within the therapeutic range, intravenous aminophylline seems not to impair significantly the hypoxic regulation of $\dot{V}_A/\dot{Q}$ matching.

D. Vasodilators

Because severe pulmonary hypertension may worsen the prognosis of COPD, attempts have been made to lower pulmonary hypertension in these patients by means of continuous oxygen therapy and/or pulmonary vasodilator treatment. However, a major side effect of vasodilators on the pulmonary circulation is to inhibit hypoxic pulmonary vasoconstriction, thus exerting a negative impact on $\dot{V}_A/\dot{Q}$ relationships. Mélot et al. [16] were the first to demonstrate that the decrease in pulmonary vascular resistance induced by 20 mg nifedipine, a calcium channel blocker, was accompanied by a significant decrease in PaO_2 because of the increase in perfusion of areas with low $\dot{V}_A/\dot{Q}$ ratio, suggesting that nifedipine had suppressed the beneficial effect of hypoxic vasoconstriction on $\dot{V}_A/\dot{Q}$ matching. The deleterious effect of the acute administration of systemic vasodilators on $\dot{V}_A/\dot{Q}$ distributions in COPD has been confirmed by other investigators using felodipine [74], nifedipine [21], prostaglandin E_1 [68], and atrial natriuretic factor [24]. Only in one study (performed with diltiazem) was no effect on $\dot{V}_A/\dot{Q}$ distributions shown [68].

Patients with moderate COPD may not have pulmonary hypertension at rest; however, most of them will demonstrate it during exercise. The deleterious effect of oral nifedipine on V̇A/Q̇ matching has also been shown during exercise by Agustí et al. [21]. In a group of COPD patients, 20 mg nifedipine reduced the increase in pulmonary vascular resistance induced by exercise, but at the same time worsened V̇A/Q̇ distributions and arterial oxygenation. These data illustrate that the deleterious effect of vasodilators on V̇A/Q̇ relationships is apparent also during exercise and suggest that hypoxic pulmonary vasoconstriction may be an important mechanism in enhancing V̇A/Q̇ matching also while exercising [21].

Recently, the administration of inhaled nitric oxide (NO) has been shown to exert a selective vasodilator action on pulmonary circulation [75]. The lack of systemic vasodilation when NO is given by inhalation is a result of its inactivation when combined with hemoglobin, for which it has a very high affinity. Moreover, in patients with acute respiratory distress syndrome, the administration of inhaled NO has been shown to produce a significant increase of PaO_2 because of the reduction of intrapulmonary shunt [76]. The effect of inhaled NO on COPD was first investigated by Adnot et al. [77], who performed a dose-response study of the hemodynamic and gas exchange effects of inhaled NO compared with intravenous acetylcholine. They showed that inhaled NO produced a significant decrease in pulmonary artery pressure at concentrations as low as 5 ppm (parts per million), and that higher concentrations resulted in a further decrease of pulmonary artery pressure in a dose-dependent manner. By contrast, changes in PaO_2 (from 57 ± 3 to 60 ± 3 mm Hg) were very small and were observed only at concentrations of 40 ppm (but not at lower concentrations). Moinard et al. [25] evaluated the effect of 15 ppm NO inhaled for 10 minutes in 14 COPD patients with severe airflow obstruction using the inert gas technique. Pulmonary artery pressure decreased moderately with NO inhalation, whereas PaO_2 did not change. The latter was consistent with the observed lack of changes in V̇A/Q̇ distributions. This lack of effect of NO on gas exchange could be explained by the low dose of NO that was used in that study. It is interesting to note that despite the fact that the mean value of PaO_2 increased during NO inhalation in the study by Adnot et al. [77] and did not change in the study by Moinard et al. [25], the individual responses in both studies were highly variable, some patients showing a decrease in PaO_2 during NO inhalation.

To investigate further the potential effects of inhaled NO on hypoxic pulmonary vasoconstriction, 13 patients with advanced COPD were studied while breathing NO (40 ppm) and 100% O_2 [26]. NO inhalation produced a moderate decrease of pulmonary artery pressure and also of PaO_2. The latter resulted from worsening of V̇A/Q̇ distributions, as shown by a greater dispersion of the blood flow distribution and an increased proportion of lung units with low V̇A/Q̇ ratio. Oxygen breathing reduced the mean pulmonary artery pressure to a lesser extent than NO, but caused greater V̇A/Q̇ mismatch. Intrapulmonary shunt on room air was small and did not change when breathing NO or O_2. This detrimental effect of inhaled NO on gas exchange in COPD has been confirmed in other studies [29,78] and has been attributed to the inhibition of hypoxic pulmonary vasoconstriction in units with low $\dot{V}_A/\dot{Q}$ ratios, to which the gas has access as well, exerting an effect similar to that of systemic vasodilators. Indeed, Frostell et al. [79] showed that in healthy subjects, the inhalation of 40 ppm NO abolished completely the increase in pulmonary vascular tone induced by breathing a hypoxic mixture (fraction of inspired oxygen, 12%). A potential clinical implication of these findings is that in patients in whom hypoxemia is caused essentially by $\dot{V}_A/\dot{Q}$ imbalance rather than by shunt, as it is the case in COPD, inhaled NO can worsen gas exchange because of the impairment of the hypoxic regulation of the matching between ventilation and perfusion. This may help in predicting which patients with respiratory failure should show a greater improvement of gas exchange with inhaled NO. Patients without preexisting chronic lung disease, in whom increased intrapulmonary shunt is the principal determinant of hypoxemia (i.e., acute respiratory distress syndrome, pneumonia) seem to be the most likely candidates to benefit from NO inhalation.

Additional studies on the hemodynamic and gas exchange effects of inhaled NO in COPD patients during exercise have been performed [29]. Nine patients with moderate to severe airflow obstruction were studied at rest and during steady-state submaximal exercise while breathing room air and 40 ppm NO. NO inhalation reduced pulmonary vascular resistance both at rest and during exercise. However, the effects of NO on gas exchange were different during exercise than at rest. PaO_2 decreased during exercise while breathing room air, whereas no change was shown during NO inhalation. Furthermore, at rest, NO inhalation worsened $\dot{V}_A/\dot{Q}$ distributions, whereas during exercise, $\dot{V}_A/\dot{Q}$ distributions improved while breathing both room air and NO, such that perfusion of poorly ventilated alveolar units with low $\dot{V}_A/\dot{Q}$ ratios was similar under both conditions [29]. Accordingly, from rest to exercise, the proportion of blood flow to low $\dot{V}_A/\dot{Q}$ units decreased significantly with NO, whereas it did not change while breathing room air. These findings indicate that in COPD patients, the inhalation of NO during exercise reduces pulmonary hypertension, and, contrasting with the effects shown at rest, it may prevent the development of further hypoxemia. The latter is likely explained by a preferential distribution of NO during exercise to well-ventilated lung units with faster time constants, which are more efficient in terms of gas exchange. In clinical terms, these findings may imply that if inhaled NO could be delivered specifically to alveolar units that are better ventilated and have faster time constants, possibly by adjusting the ventilator settings or delivering NO at the beginning of inspiration, the beneficial vasodilator effect of NO would not be offset by its deleterious impact on gas exchange.

E. Vasoconstrictors

Contrasting with the effect of vasodilators, an increase in pulmonary vascular resistance may enhance $\dot{V}_A/\dot{Q}$ matching. Respiratory stimulants have been used for many years for COPD treatment. One of the consequences of respiratory stimulants that act through peripheral chemoreceptor stimulation is an increase in pulmonary vascular tone [15]. Almitrine bismesylate is a peripheral chemoreceptor stimulant that may improve pulmonary gas exchange by mechanisms additional to the increase in ventilation alone [80]. Castaing et al. [81] showed that the administration of 1.5 mg/kg almitrine orally increased ventilation and PaO_2. This effect was accompanied by a significant reduction in the perfusion of areas with low $\dot{V}A/\dot{Q}$ ratios. Mélot et al. [15] confirmed this observation and showed that the diversion of blood flow from units with a low $\dot{V}A/\dot{Q}$ ratio to units with a normal ratio was associated with an increase in pulmonary vascular resistance, suggesting that the beneficial effect of almitrine on $\dot{V}A/\dot{Q}$ distributions was likely caused by the enhancement of hypoxic pulmonary vasoconstriction. These effects of almitrine were further confirmed in mechanically ventilated COPD patients [57], supporting the notion that the beneficial effects of almitrine are independent of the increase in ventilation and presumably a result of its vasoconstrictive action. However, this beneficial effect on gas exchange in patients with COPD needs to be balanced against some of the unwanted side effects of almitrine, such as peripheral neuropathy and weight loss, particularly if long-term administration of the drug is required.

VII. Conclusions

The use of the inert gas approach has provided ample information, showing that abnormal gas exchange in COPD is mainly determined by $\dot{V}A/\dot{Q}$ inequality. Such an impairment in $\dot{V}A/\dot{Q}$ matching may be already recognized in patients with mild, subclinical COPD, and its severity correlates with the degree of structural impairment in both lung parenchyma (emphysema) and small airways. During exacerbation episodes, worsening hypoxemia is explained by the combined effect of increased $\dot{V}A/\dot{Q}$ inequality and the decrease in $P\bar{v}O_2$ that results from an increased oxygen consumption by the respiratory muscles. Hypoxic pulmonary vasoconstriction is a mechanism particularly efficient for matching perfusion to ventilation in COPD patients, such that the use of pharmacological agents with vasodilator properties entail the potential for further worsening gas exchange in this condition.

References

1. American Thoracic Society. Standards for the diagnosis and care of patients with chronic obstructive pulmonary disease. Am J Respir Crit Care Med 1995; 152:S77–S120.
2. Siafakas NM, Vermeire P, Pride NB, Paoletti P, Gibson J, Howard P, Yernault JC, Decramer M, Higenbottam T, Postma DS, Rees J. Optimal assessment and management of chronic obstructive pulmonary disease (COPD). Eur Respir J 1995; 8:1398–1420.
3. Dornhorst AC. Respiratory insufficiency. Lancet 1955; 1:1185–1187.

4. Burrows B, Niden AH, Fletcher CM, Jones NL. Clinical types of chronic obstructive lung disease in London and in Chicago. Am Rev Respir Dis 1965; 90:14–27.
5. Bishop JM, Cross KW. Physiological variables and mortality in patients with various categories of chronic respiratory disease. Bull Eur Physiopathol Respir 1984; 20:495–500.
6. Okubadejo AA, Jones PW, Wedzicha JA. Quality of life in patients with chronic obstructive pulmonary disease and severe hypoxaemia. Thorax 1996; 51:44–47.
7. Nocturnal Oxygen Therapy Trial Group. Continuous or nocturnal oxygen therapy in hypoxemic chronic obstructive lung disease. Ann Intern Med 1980; 93:391–398.
8. Medical Research Council Working Party. Long term domiciliary oxygen therapy in chronic hypoxic cor pulmonale complicating chronic bronchitis and emphysema. Lancet 1981; 1:681–686.
9. Briscoe WA, Cree EM, Filler J, Houssay HEJ, Cournand A. Lung volume, alveolar ventilation and perfusion interrelationships in chronic pulmonary emphysema. J Appl Physiol 1960; 15:785–795.
10. King TKC, Briscoe WA. The distribution of ventilation, perfusion, lung volume and transfer factor (diffusing capacity) in patients with obstructive lung disease. Clin Sci 1968; 35:153–170.
11. Wagner PD, Naumann PF, Laravuso RB. Simultaneous measurement of eight foreign gases in blood by gas chromatography. J Appl Physiol 1974; 36:600–605.
12. Evans JW, Wagner PD. Limits on $\dot{V}_A/\dot{Q}$ distributions from analysis of experimental inert gas elimination. J Appl Physiol 1977; 42:889–898.
13. Wagner PD, Dantzker DR, Dueck R, Clausen JL, West JB. Ventilation-perfusion inequality in chronic obstructive pulmonary disease. J Clin Invest 1977; 59:203–216.
14. Wagner PD, Laravuso RB, Uhl RR, West JB. Continuous distributions of ventilation-perfusion ratios in normal subjects breathing air and 100% O_2. J Clin Invest 1974; 54:54–68.
15. Mélot C, Naeije R, Rothschild T, Mertens P, Mols P, Hallemans R. Improvement in ventilation-perfusion matching by almitrine in COPD. Chest 1983; 83:528–533.
16. Mélot C, Hallemans R, Naeije R, Mols P, Lejeune P. Deleterious effect of nifedipine on pulmonary gas exchange in chronic obstructive pulmonary disease. Am Rev Respir Dis 1984; 130:612–616.
17. Castaing Y, Manier G, Guénard H. Effect of 26% oxygen breathing on ventilation and perfusion distribution in patients with COLD. Bull Eur Physiopathol Respir 1985; 21:17–23.
18. Dantzker DR, D'Alonzo GE. The effect of exercise on pulmonary gas exchange in patients with severe chronic obstructive pulmonary disease. Am Rev Respir Dis 1986; 134:1135–1139.
19. Roca J, Montserrat JM, Rodriguez-Roisin R, Guitart R, Torres A, Agustí AGN, Wagner PD. Gas exchange response to naloxone in chronic obstructive pulmonary disease with hypercapnic respiratory failure. Bull Eur Physiopathol Respir 1987; 23:249–254.
20. Ringsted CV, Eliasen K, Andersen JB, Heslet L, Qvist J. Ventilation-perfusion distributions and central hemodynamics in chronic obstructive pulmonary disease: effects of terbutaline administration. Chest 1989; 96:976–983.

21. Agustí AGN, Barberà JA, Roca J, Wagner PD, Guitart R, Rodriguez-Roisin R. Hypoxic pulmonary vasoconstriction and gas exchange during exercise in chronic obstructive pulmonary disease. Chest 1990; 97:268–275.
22. Barberà JA, Ramírez J, Roca J, Wagner PD, Sánchez-Lloret J, Rodriguez-Roisin R. Lung structure and gas exchange in mild chronic obstructive pulmonary disease. Am Rev Respir Dis 1990; 141:895–901.
23. Barberà JA, Riverola A, Roca J, Ramírez J, Wagner PD, Ros D, Wiggs BR, Rodriguez-Roisin R. Pulmonary vascular abnormalities and ventilation-perfusion relationships in mild chronic obstructive pulmonary disease. Am J Respir Crit Care Med 1994; 149:423–429.
24. Andrivet P, Chabrier PE, Defouilloy C, Brun-Buisson C, Adnot S. Intravenously administered atrial natriuretic factor in patients with COPD: effects on ventilation-perfusion relationships and pulmonary hemodynamics. Chest 1994; 106:118–124.
25. Moinard J, Manier G, Pillet O, Castaing Y. Effect of inhaled nitric oxide on hemodynamics and $\dot{V}_A/\dot{Q}$ inequalities in patients with chronic obstructive pulmonary disease. Am J Respir Crit Care Med 1994; 149:1482–1487.
26. Barberà JA, Roger N, Roca J, Rovira I, Higenbottam TW, Rodriguez-Roisin R. Worsening of pulmonary gas exchange with nitric oxide inhalation in chronic obstructive pulmonary disease. Lancet 1996; 347:436–440.
27. Viegas CA, Ferrer A, Montserrat JM, Barberà JA, Roca J, Rodriguez-Roisin R. Ventilation-perfusion response after fenoterol in hypoxemic patients with stable COPD. Chest 1996; 110:71–77 (addendum 1997;111:258).
28. Barberà JA, Roca J, Ferrer A, Félez MA, Díaz O, Roger N, Rodriguez-Roisin R. Mechanisms of worsening gas exchange during acute exacerbations of chronic obstructive pulmonary disease. Eur Respir J 1997; 10:1285–1291.
29. Roger N, Barberà JA, Roca J, Rovira I, Gómez FP, Rodriguez-Roisin R. Nitric oxide inhalation during exercise in chronic obstructive pulmonary disease. Am J Respir Crit Care Med 1997; 156:800–806.
30. Cardús J, Burgos F, Diaz O, Roca J, Barberà JA, Marrades RM, Rodriguez-Roisin R, Wagner PD. Increase in pulmonary ventilation-perfusion inequality with age in healthy individuals. Am J Respir Crit Care Med 1997; 156:648–653.
31. West JB. Ventilation-perfusion relationships. Am Rev Respir Dis 1977; 116:919–943.
32. Marthan R, Castaing Y, Manier G, Guénard H. Gas exchange alterations in patients with chronic obstructive lung disease. Chest 1985; 87:470–475.
33. Rodriguez-Roisin R, Ballester E, Roca J Torres A, Wagner PD. Mechanisms of hypoxemia in patients with status asthmaticus requiring mechanical ventilation. Am Rev Respir Dis 1989; 139:732–739.
34. Rodriguez-Roisin R, Agustí AGN, Roca J. The hepatopulmonary syndrome: new name, old complexities. Thorax 1992; 47:897–902.
35. Roca J, Wagner PD. Contribution of multiple inert gas elimination technique to pulmonary medicine—1: principles and information content of the multiple inert gas elimination technique. Thorax 1994; 49:815–824.
36. West JB. Ventilation-perfusion inequality and overall gas exchange in computer models of the lung. Respir Physiol 1969; 7:88–110.

37. Torres A, Reyes A, Roca J, Wagner PD, Rodriguez-Roisin R. Ventilation-perfusion mismatching in chronic obstructive pulmonary disease during ventilator weaning. Am Rev Respir Dis 1989; 140:1246–1250.
38. Mithoefer JC, Ramirez C, Cook W. The effect of mixed venous oxygenation on arterial blood in chronic obstructive pulmonary disease: the basis for a classification. Am Rev Respir Dis 1978; 117:259–264.
39. Von Euler US, Liljestrand G. Observations on the pulmonary arterial blood pressure in the cat. Acta Physiol Scand 1946; 12:301–320.
40. Voelkel NF. Hypoxic pulmonary vasoconstriction and hypertension. In: Peacock AJ, ed. Pulmonary Circulation. London: Chapman and Hall, 1996, pp 71–85.
41. Simonneau G, Escourrou P, Duroux P, Lockhart A. Inhibition of hypoxic pulmonary vasoconstriction by nifedipine. N Engl J Med 1981; 304:1582–1585.
42. Barberà JA, Roca J, Ramírez J, Wagner PD, Ussetti P, Rodriguez-Roisin R. Gas exchange during exercise in mild chronic obstructive pulmonary disease: correlation with lung structure. Am Rev Respir Dis 1991; 144:520–525.
43. Saetta M, Ghezzo H, Kim WD, King M, Angus GE, Wang N, Cosio MG. Loss of alveolar attachments in smokers. A morphometric correlate of lung function impairment. Am Rev Respir Dis 1985; 132:894–900.
44. Petty TL, Silvers GW, Stanford RE. Radial traction and small airways disease in excised human lungs. Am Rev Respir Dis 1986; 133:132–135.
45. Nagai A, Yamawaki I, Takizawa T, Thurlbeck WM. Alveolar attachments in emphysema of human lungs. Am Rev Respir Dis 1991; 144:888–891.
46. Bosken CH, Wiggs BR, Paré PD, Hogg JC. Small airway dimensions in smokers with obstruction to airflow. Am Rev Respir Dis 1990; 142:563–570.
47. Snider GL, Kleinerman J, Thurlbeck WM, Bengali ZK. The definition of emphysema: report of a National Heart, Lung and Blood Institute, Division of Lung Diseases, Workshop. Am Rev Respir Dis 1985; 132:182–185.
48. Furchgott RF, Zawadzki JV. The obligatory role of endothelial cells in the relaxation of arterial smooth muscle by acetylcholine. Nature 1980; 288:373–376.
49. Dinh-Xuan AT, Higenbottam TW, Clelland CA, Pepke-Zaba J, Cremona G, Butt AY, Large SR, Wells FC, Wallwork J. Impairment of endothelium-dependent pulmonary artery relaxation in chronic obstructive lung disease. N Engl J Med 1991; 324:1539–1547.
50. Peinado VI, Barberà JA, Ramírez J, Gómez FP, Roca J, Jover L, Gimferrer JM, Rodriguez-Roisin R. Endothelial dysfunction in pulmonary arteries of patients with mild COPD. Am J Physiol (Lung Cell Mol Physiol) 1998; 274:L908–L913.
51. Voelkel NF, Tuder RM. Cellular and molecular mechanisms in the pathogenesis of severe pulmonary hypertension. Eur Respir J 1995; 8:2129–2138.
52. Hogg JC, Macklem PT, Thurlbeck WM. Site and nature of airway obstruction in chronic obstructive lung disease. N Engl J Med 1968; 278:1355–1360.
53. Barberà JA, Roca J, Rodriguez-Roisin R, Ussetti P, Wagner PD, Agustí-Vidal A. Gas exchange in patients with small airways dysfunction (abstract). Eur Respir J 1988; 1:27s.
54. Wagner PD, Hedenstierna G, Rodriguez-Roisin R. Gas exchange, expiratory flow obstruction and the clinical spectrum of asthma. Eur Respir J 1996; 9:1278–1282.

55. Wagner PD, Hedenstierna G, Bylin G. Ventilation-perfusion inequality in chronic asthma. Am Rev Respir Dis 1987; 136:605–612.
56. Diaz O, Iglesia R, Ferrer M, Zavala E, Santos C, Wagner PD, Roca J, Rodriguez-Roisin R. Effects of noninvasive ventilation on pulmonary gas exchange and hemodynamics during acute hypercapnic exacerbations of chronic obstructive pulmonary disease. Am J Respir Crit Care Med 1997; 156:1840–1845.
57. Castaing Y, Manier G, Guenard H. Improvement in ventilation-perfusion relationships by almitrine in patients with chronic obstructive pulmonary disease during mechanical ventilation. Am Rev Respir Dis 1986; 134:910–916.
58. Rossi A, Santos C, Roca J, Torres A, Félez MA, Rodriguez-Roisin R. Effects of PEEP on $\dot{V}_A/\dot{Q}$ mismatching in ventilated patients with chronic airflow obstruction. Am J Respir Crit Care Med 1994; 149:1077–1084
59. Roca J, Ramis L, Rodriguez-Roisin R, Ballester E, Montserrat JM, Wagner PD. Serial relationships between ventilation-perfusion inequality and spirometry in acute severe asthma requiring hospitalization. Am Rev Respir Dis 1988; 137:1055–1061.
60. Moreno RH, Hogg JC, Paré PD. Mechanics of airway narrowing. Am Rev Respir Dis 1986; 133:1171–1180.
61. Kuwano K, Bosken CH, Paré PD, Bai TR, Wiggs BR, Hogg JC. Small airways dimensions in asthma and in chronic obstructive pulmonary disease. Am Rev Respir Dis 1993; 148:1220–1225.
62. Paré PD, Wiggs BR, James A, Hogg JC, Bosken C. The comparative mechanics and morphology of airways in asthma and in chronic obstructive pulmonary disease. Am Rev Respir Dis 1991; 143:1189–1193.
63. Wagner PD. Ventilation-perfusion inequality and gas exchange during exercise in lung disease. In: Dempsey JS, Reed CS, eds. Muscular Exercise and the Lung. Madison: University of Wisconsin Press, 1977, pp 345–356.
64. Wagner PD, Gale GE, Moon RE, Torre-Bueno JR, Stolp BW, Saltzman HA. Pulmonary gas exchange in humans exercising at sea level and simulated altitude. J Appl Physiol 1986; 61:260–270.
65. Dantzker DR, Wagner PD, West JB. Instability of lung units with low $\dot{V}_A/\dot{Q}$ ratios during O_2 breathing. J Appl Physiol 1975; 38:886–895.
66. Santos C, Roca J, Torres A, Cardús J, Barberà JA, Rodriguez-Roisin R. Shunt increases during 100% O_2 breathing in patients with acute respiratory failure needing mechanical ventilation (abstract). Am Rev Respir Dis 1992; 145:A76.
67. Barberà JA, Reyes A, Montserrat JM, Roca J, Wagner PD, Rodriguez-Roisin R. Effect of intravenously administered aminophylline on ventilation/perfusion inequality during recovery from exacerbations of chronic obstructive pulmonary disease. Am Rev Respir Dis 1992; 145:1328–1333.
68. Guénard H, Castaing Y, Mélot C, Naeije R. Gas exchange during acute respiratory failure in patients with chronic obstructive pulmonary disease. In: Derenne JP, Whitelaw WA, Similowski T, eds. Acute Respiratory Failure in Chronic Obstructive Pulmonary Disease. New York: Marcel Dekker, 1996, pp 227–266.
69. Lemaire F, Teboul JL, Cinotti L, Giotto G, Abrouk F, Steg G, Macquin-Mavier I, Zapol WM. Acute left ventricular dysfunction during unsuccessful weaning from mechanical ventilation. Anesthesiology 1988; 69:171–179.

70. Ranieri VM, Giuliani R, Cinnella G, Pesce C, Brienza N, Ippolito EL, Pomo V, Fiore T, Gottfried SB, Brienza A. Physiologic effects of positive end-expiratory pressure in patients with chronic obstructive pulmonary disease during acute ventilatory failure and controlled mechanical ventilation. Am Rev Respir Dis 1993; 147:5–13.
71. Brochard L, Mancebo J, Wysocki M, Lofaso F, Conti G, Rauss A, Simonneau G, Benito S, Gasparetto A, Lemaire F, Isabey D, Harf A. Noninvasive ventilation for acute exacerbations of chronic obstructive pulmonary disease. N Engl J Med 1995; 333:817–822.
72. Ballester E, Reyes A, Roca J, Guitart R, Wagner PD, Rodriguez-Roisin R. Ventilation-perfusion mismatching in acute severe asthma: effects of salbutamol and 100% oxygen. Thorax 1989; 44:258–267.
73. Lipworth BJ, Newnham DM, Clark RA, Dhillon DP, Winter JH, McDevitt DG. Comparison of the relative airways and systemic potencies of inhaled fenoterol and salbutamol in asthmatic patients. Thorax 1995; 50:54–61.
74. Bratel T, Hedenstierna G, Nyquist O, Ripe E. The use of a vasodilator, felodipine, as an adjuvant to long-term oxygen treatment in COLD patients. Eur Respir J 1990; 3:46–54.
75. Pepke-Zaba J, Higenbottam TW, Dinh-Xuan AT, Stone D, Wallwork J. Inhaled nitric oxide as a cause of selective pulmonary vasodilation in pulmonary hypertension. Lancet 1991; 338:1173–1174.
76. Rossaint R, Falke KJ, López F, Slama K, Pison U, Zapol WM. Inhaled nitric oxide for the adult respiratory distress syndrome. N Engl J Med 1993; 328:399–405.
77. Adnot S, Kouyoumdjian C, Defouilloy C, Andrivet P, Sediame S, Herigault R, Fratacci MD. Hemodynamic and gas exchange responses to infusion of acetylcholine and inhalation of nitric oxide in patients with chronic obstructive lung disease and pulmonary hypertension. Am Rev Respir Dis 1993; 148:310–316.
78. Katayama Y, Higenbottam TW, Diaz de Atauri MJ, Cremona G, Akamine S, Barberà JA, Rodriguez-Roisin R. Inhaled nitric oxide and arterial oxygen tension in patients with chronic obstructive pulmonary disease and severe pulmonary hypertension. Thorax 1997; 52:120–124.
79. Frostell C, Blomqvist H, Hedenstierna G, Lundberg J, Zapol WM. Inhaled nitric oxide selectively reverses human hypoxic pulmonary vasoconstriction without causing systemic vasodilation. Anesthesiology 1993; 78:427–435.
80. Naeije R, Mélot C, Mols P, Hallemans R, Naeije N, Cornil A, Sergysels R. Effects of almitrine in decompensated chronic respiratory insufficiency. Bull Eur Physiopathol Respir 1981; 17:153–161.
81. Castaing Y, Manier G, Varene N, Guénard H. Effects of oral almitrine on the distribution of $\dot{V}_A/\dot{Q}$ ratio in chronic obstructive lung diseases. Bull Eur Physiopathol Respir 1981; 17:917–932.

9

Interstitial Lung Diseases

ALVAR G. N. AGUSTÍ

Hospital Universitari Son Dureta
Palma de Mallorca, Spain

I. Introduction

The term *interstitial lung disease* (ILD) includes a heterogeneous group of disorders that share common clinical, radiographic, and physiological alterations [1–6]. Among the latter, and from the gas exchange point of view, a reduced carbon monoxide diffusing capacity (D_{LCO}) and arterial hypoxemia that worsens markedly during exercise are common [7]. This chapter reviews the pathophysiological basis of these gas exchange abnormalities. For clarity of exposure, it is divided into four sections. Sections II and III present results of different studies investigating pulmonary gas exchange at rest and during exercise. Section IV attempts to integrate all of this information into a single portrait that can provide a general perspective of the mechanisms underlying the abnormal pulmonary gas exchange of ILD. Finally, Section V discusses the relationship of these mechanisms to D_{LCO}, a measurement of lung function often performed in patients with ILD for clinical purposes [8,9].

Most of the data used in this discussion has been obtained by using the multiple inert gases elimination technique (MIGET) [10,11]. MIGET is an experimental technique that allows a detailed and comprehensive analysis of all the intrapulmonary and extrapulmonary factors that govern gas exchange in humans [10,11]. Specifically, it provides a quantitative estimation of the distribution of ventilation–

perfusion ($\dot{V}_A/\dot{Q}$) ratios, as well as a quantitative evaluation of other important components of the gas transfer chain, such as the diffusion of oxygen (O_2) from the alveolar gas to the capillary blood, the presence or absence of arteriovenous shunt, and the pathophysiological role of cardiac output, minute ventilation, O_2 uptake, and mixed venous oxygen partial pressure ($P\bar{v}O_2$) [11] as determinants or modifiers of arterial oxygen partial pressure (PaO_2). Since its development in the late 1970s [10,11], MIGET has greatly facilitated the investigation of the mechanisms controlling pulmonary gas exchange in numerous disease entities, including ILD [12–16]. A detailed description of the theoretical basis and methodological peculiarities of MIGET is beyond the scope of this chapter. The interested reader is referred to some comprehensive reviews on the subject [10,11,15,17,18].

II. Resting Pulmonary Gas Exchange

A. Arterial Blood Gas Measurements

At rest, pulmonary gas exchange is relatively well preserved in ILD. When breathing room air at sea level, most patients are normoxemic or mildly hypoxemic (~70 mm Hg). Only in advanced stages of the disease does PaO_2 decrease to less than 50 mm Hg [7–9,16,19]. Hypercapnia is rare in patients with ILD. On the contrary, arterial carbon dioxide partial pressure ($PaCO_2$) at rest is typically 30 to 35 mm Hg, indicating considerable hyperventilation. This can occur even when PaO_2 is relatively high on the O_2–hemoglobin dissociation curve (i.e., $\geq$ 60 mm Hg). It is thus unlikely to be explained by hypoxic stimulation of peripheral chemoreceptors. Current speculation in ILD is that the distortion of alveolar walls caused by the fibrosis causes J-receptor activation, and thus increased ventilation [20]. The combination of mild hypoxemia and hypocapnia implies an increase in the alveolar–arterial PO_2 gradient ($AaPO_2$), that exceeds the upper limit of normal (15 to 20 mm Hg) [7]. For example, if PaO_2 is 70 mm Hg and $PaCO_2$ is 32 mm Hg, $AaPO_2$ would be approximately 40 mm Hg. This could be caused by $\dot{V}_A/\dot{Q}$ inequality, intrapulmonary shunting, or alveolar–capillary diffusion limitation, alone or in combination. Research described in Section II.B shows that all of these mechanisms may be present, although the first two are usually the most important.

B. Inert Gas Measurements

There are several published studies that used MIGET to investigate pulmonary gas exchange in ILD [16,18,21,22]. Table 1 presents the mean results of several variables of interest reported in these four studies. In general, they showed that $\dot{V}_A/\dot{Q}$ distributions at rest are generally preserved. The left column of Fig. 1 presents the $\dot{V}_A/\dot{Q}$ distribution obtained at rest in two representative subjects (patients no. 1 and 2) with idiopathic pulmonary fibrosis (IPF) breathing room air [16]. Patient no. 1 had normal PaO_2 (88.2 mm Hg) and almost normal $AaPO_2$ (22.6 mm Hg). In keeping with this, her $\dot{V}_A/\dot{Q}$ distribution was relatively well preserved: narrow and

Table 1 Mean Values of Different Clinical and Physiological Variables of Published Studies Using Multiple Inert Gas Elimination Technique in Patients with Interstitial Lung Disease

	Wagner [18]	Jernudd-Wilhelmsson et al. [21]	Eklund et al. [22]	Agustí et al. [16]
No. of patients	9	10	11	15
Type of disease	Varied	Varied	Sarcoidosis	IPF
Age (yr)	49	53	54	53
FVC (% reference)	NR	NR	67	59
TLC (% reference)	NR	64	70	69
DLCO (% reference)	45	36	73	52
KCO (% reference)	NR	NR	83	78
Pa_{O_2} rest/exercise (mm Hg)	61/50	68/46	68/64	74/59
ΔP_{O_2} rest-exercise (mm Hg)	11	22	4	15
Shunt rest/exercise (%)	5/NR	2/1	1/1	2/3
Log SD $\dot{Q}$ rest/exercise	NR	0.66/0.63	0.64/0.58	0.93/0.81
O_2 diffusion limitation rest/exercise (mm Hg)[a]	4/8	−4/13	4/10	6/21

[a]Corresponds to the difference between the predicted Pa_{O_2} (from MIGET) and the Pa_{O_2} actually measured in the patient.
NR = not reported; FVC = forced vital capacity; TLC = total lung capacity; DLCO = diffusing capacity for carbon monoxide; KCO = DLCO normalized for the measured alveolar volume; Pa_{O_2} = arterial oxygen partial pressure.
Log SD $\dot{Q}$ = dispersion of the blood flow distribution.

distributed around a $\dot{V}_A/\dot{Q}$ ratio of 1.0, with a very small amount of shunt and/or blood flow perfusing units with low $\dot{V}_A/\dot{Q}$ ratios. On the other hand, patient no. 2 had moderate hypoxemia (Pa_{O_2} 69.6 mm Hg) and increased AaP_{O_2} (41.5 mm Hg). His $\dot{V}_A/\dot{Q}$ distribution showed a higher perfusion of lung units with a $\dot{V}_A/\dot{Q}$ ratio lower than 0.1. Nonetheless, even in this patient, the $\dot{V}_A/\dot{Q}$ distribution at rest was only moderately abnormal.

III. Pulmonary Gas Exchange During Exercise

A. Arterial Blood Gas Measurements

Patients with ILD generally show typical and substantial arterial blood gas changes during exercise, even at moderate effort (Fig. 2). These are characterized by a decrease in Pa_{O_2} (which is often very profound) [7–9,16,19], whereas Pa_{CO_2} is generally unaffected [23]. Recently, it was shown that the decrease of Pa_{O_2} during exercise may be helpful to predict the deterioration of lung function over time in patients with IPF [19].

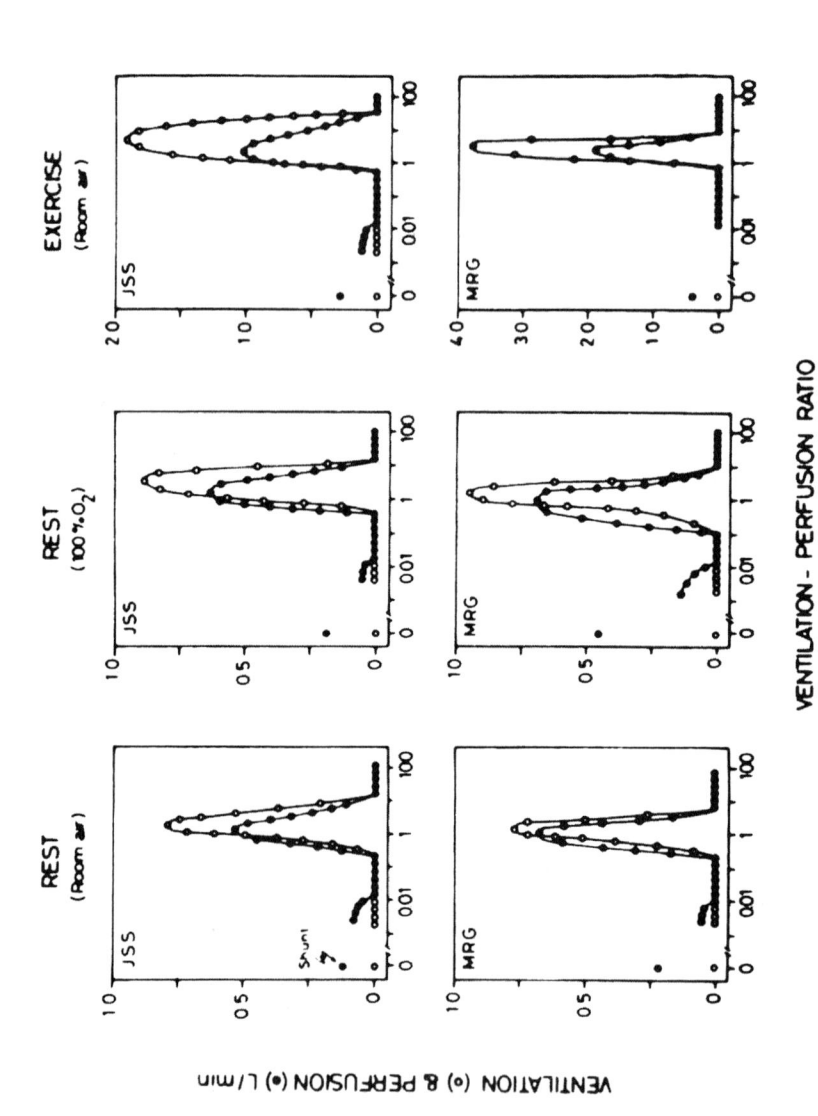

Figure 1 Ventilation–perfusion ($\dot{V}_A/\dot{Q}$) distributions obtained in two representative patients (patient no. 1, top; patient no. 2, bottom) with idiopathic pulmonary fibrosis studied at rest breathing room air (left panel), at rest breathing 100% oxygen (middle panel), and during exercise (breathing room air; right panel). See text for details. (Reprinted with permission from Ref. 16.)

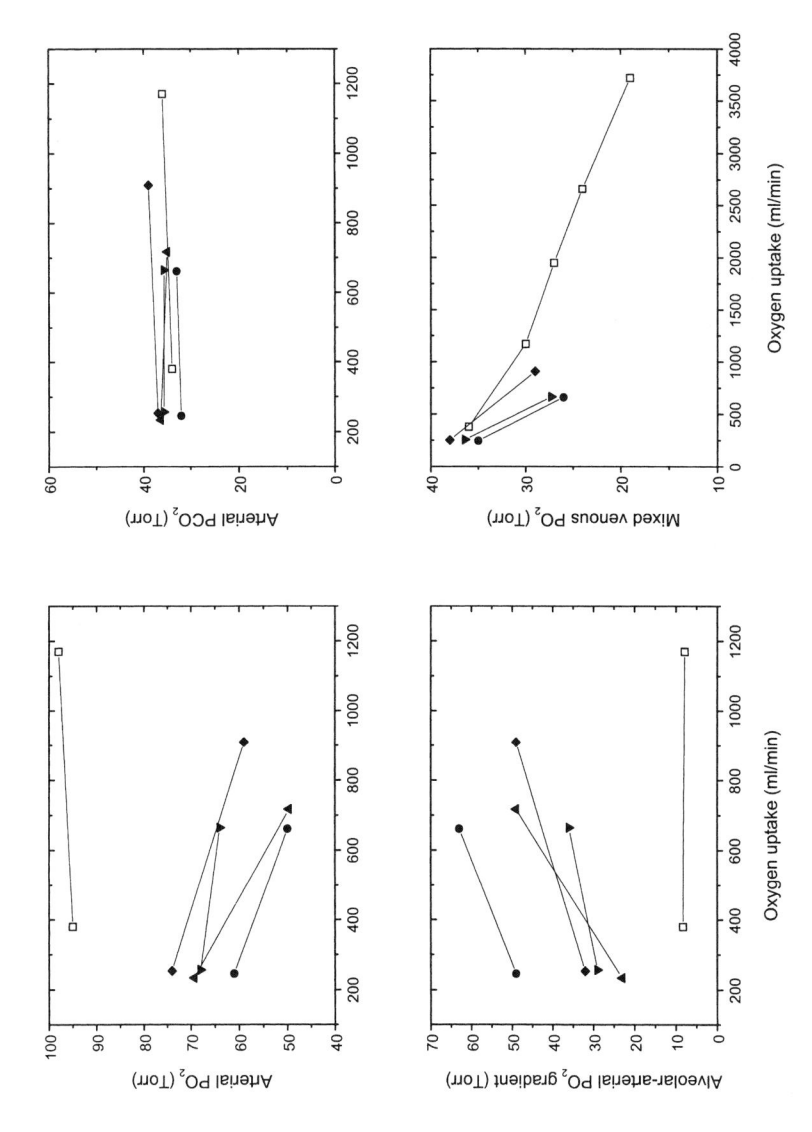

Figure 2 Mean values of arterial oxygen partial pressure (Pao$_2$), arterial carbon dioxide partial pressure (Paco$_2$), the alveolar–arterial Po$_2$ gradient (AaPo$_2$), and mixed venous Po$_2$ (P̄vo$_2$) at rest and during exercise, reported by different studies in healthy subjects (open squares) (51) and in patients with various types of ILD [circles (18) and upward triangles (21)], sarcoidosis (down triangles) (22), and IPF (diamonds) (16). See text for details.

This type of gas exchange response to exercise is very characteristic of advanced ILD. However, in early phases of the disease, Pao$_2$ may not change during exercise or may even improve slightly [16]. Also, it is important to realize that not all forms of ILD show this stereotypical response to exercise. For example, in 1988 it was shown [6] that the pattern of gas exchange during exercise was different in two groups of patients with different ILD (IPF and asbestosis), even though both groups were matched for age, sex, height, weight, smoking habits, and severity of resting ventilatory impairment [6]. In that study, patients with IPF showed a dramatic decrease in Pao$_2$ during exercise, whereas those with asbestosis did not (Fig. 3) [6]. The investigators suggested that the different structural derangement observed in asbestosis and IPF, particularly the presence of more airways disease, less pulmonary vascular involvement, and/or a lower degree of interstitial fibrotic changes in asbestosis, may play a key role in their different gas exchange response to exercise [6]. Other investigators have subsequently confirmed these findings [24].

In healthy individuals, P$\bar{v}$o$_2$ decreases during exercise [18,25,26]. As shown in Fig. 2, P$\bar{v}$o$_2$ (at a given oxygen consumption per unit time [$\dot{V}$o$_2$]) may be even lower during exercise in patients with ILD. It is known that for any given degree of pulmonary gas exchange abnormality, a low P$\bar{v}$o$_2$ results in a lower Pao$_2$ [27,28]. In addition, other factors being constant (oxygen uptake, cardiac output), a low Pao$_2$ reduces P$\bar{v}$o$_2$. The end result is that in patients with ILD, both Pao$_2$ and P$\bar{v}$o$_2$ are caught up in a vicious circle, each dragging the other down to some new steady-state level.

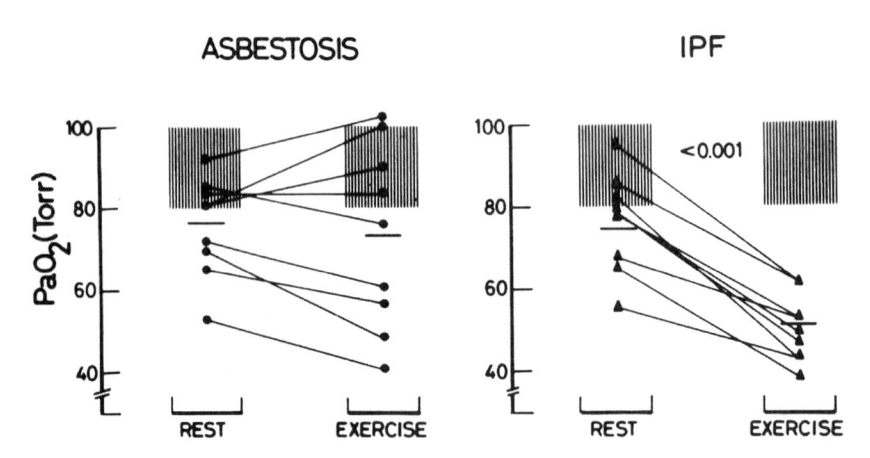

Figure 3 Arterial oxygen partial pressure (Pao$_2$) values measured at rest and during exercise in patients with asbestosis (left panel) and in patients with idiopathic pulmonary fibrosis (IPF; right panel) matched for sex, age, and degree of mechanical impairment. Patients with IPF showed an homogeneous decrease in Pao$_2$ values during exercise, whereas patients with asbestosis showed a much more heterogeneous response. See text for details. (Reprinted with permission from Ref. 8.)

B. Inert Gas Measurements

Because the alveolar interstitium is markedly thickened in patients with ILD [7,9], Austrian et al. [29] suggested that the abnormal oxygenation during exercise was caused by a limitation in the diffusion of oxygen molecules between the alveolar gas and the capillary blood ("alveolar–capillary block" syndrome). This notion was extensively incorporated into the medical literature until MIGET became available and allowed a more accurate evaluation of this hypothesis.

MIGET has the potential to discriminate between the two main mechanisms of abnormal pulmonary gas exchange proposed in patients with ILD ($\dot{V}_A/\dot{Q}$ inequality, including right-to-left shunt, vs. O_2 diffusion limitation). This is because MIGET can predict the Pa_{O_2} value (predicted Pa_{O_2}) that should result from the measured $\dot{V}_A/\dot{Q}$ distribution (plus shunt) when all of the factors that may influence gas exchange (especially fraction of inspired oxygen [F_{IO_2}], minute ventilation, and cardiac output) are taken into account on the explicit assumption that there is no oxygen diffusion limitation. This procedure uses the accepted notion that all inert gases are essentially invulnerable to alveolar–capillary diffusion limitation. Thus, the comparison of this predicted Pa_{O_2} with the actual value measured in the arterial blood (measured Pa_{O_2}) provides information on any hypothetical "alveolar–capillary block" for oxygen. Specifically, if the measured value of Pa_{O_2} is less than that predicted from MIGET, physiological factors other than shunt plus $\dot{V}_A/\dot{Q}$ inequality must be present. Basically, the only candidate mechanism is O_2 diffusion limitation.

In 1977, Wagner [18] was the first to use the MIGET to determine the relative contributions of $\dot{V}_A/\dot{Q}$ inequality and O_2 diffusion limitation to Pa_{O_2} during exercise in a group of patients with various interstitial diseases (IPF, asbestosis, sarcoidosis) [18]. Although he actually found that 17% of the total AaP_{O_2} gradient during exercise could be ascribed to failure of alveolar–capillary diffusion equilibrium, most of it (83%) was caused by the combined effects of $\dot{V}_A/\dot{Q}$ inequality and shunt [18]. In 1986, a study by Jernudd-Wilhelmsson et al. [21] reported similar results, also in patients with a wide range of interstitial lung diseases. However, as previously discussed, in 1988 it was shown that patients with different types of ILD may respond differently to exercise [6] (Fig. 3). Therefore, it was conceivable that the mechanisms leading to oxygen desaturation during exercise may also differ.

Following this line of reasoning, in 1991, MIGET was used to evaluate the mechanisms of abnormal pulmonary gas exchange in patients with only IPF (or cryptogenic fibrosing alveolitis, according to the British nomenclature) [16], which is considered the most common form of the vast group of ILD [3–5,7]. The results of this study showed that: (1) during exercise, most patients showed significant arterial desaturation, but the baseline degree of $\dot{V}_A/\dot{Q}$ inequality either did not change or improved (Fig. 1, right panels); and, (2) in contrast, the diffusion of O_2 from the alveolar gas to the capillary blood became significantly limited during exercise.

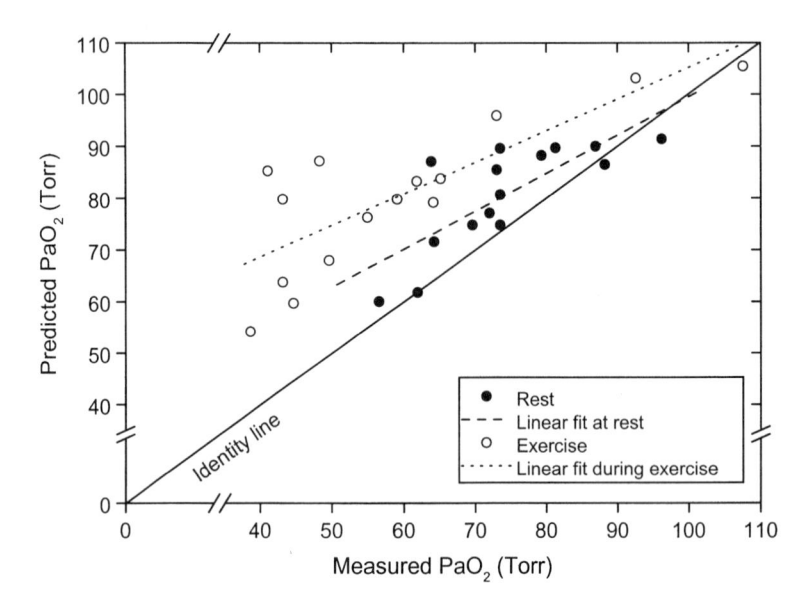

Figure 4 Plot of measured arterial oxygen partial pressure (Pao$_2$) versus the Pao$_2$ value predicted from multiple inert gas elimination technique. The line of identity and the two regression lines are also shown. See text for details. (Data from Ref. 16.)

Figure 4 shows the relationship between the Pao$_2$ value predicted from MIGET and that actually measured in that study, both at rest and during exercise. Several aspects of this figure deserve comment. First, at rest (closed symbols), most points lie to the left of the identity line, indicating that the predicted Pao$_2$ value exceeded the measured one. On average, the difference between the predicted and measured Pao$_2$ values at rest averaged 6 mm Hg, which represented 19% of the AaPo$_2$ gradient. In other words, at rest, approximately 20% of arterial hypoxemia was caused by a limitation in the diffusion of O$_2$ from the alveolar gas to the capillary blood, and 80% to $\dot{V}_A/\dot{Q}$ mismatch. Second, from Figure 4 it is also evident that the difference between the predicted and measured Pao$_2$ values at rest increases in patients with more severe hypoxemia (see the dashed line in Fig. 4, which represents the linear fit of data at rest). This indicates that the contribution of O$_2$ diffusion limitation to arterial hypoxemia at rest is higher in patients with more abnormal pulmonary gas exchange. Third, during exercise, the difference between the predicted and measured Pao$_2$ values increased from 6 to 19 mm Hg; expressed as percentage of the actual AaPo$_2$ value, this difference represented 40%. Therefore, the contribution of O$_2$ diffusion limitation to arterial hypoxemia increased during exercise. Fourth, and finally, paralleling what happened at rest, this effect was more pronounced in patients with more severe hypoxemia (see the dotted line in Figure 4, which represents the linear fit of data during exercise). In summary, oxygen diffusion is limited in patients with IPF at rest and more during exercise, particularly in patients with more severe degrees of arterial hypoxemia. These observations were subsequently substantiated in patients with stage II and III sarcoidosis [22] and by the theoretical analysis developed by Hughes [30].

IV. Integrated View: The Mechanisms of Abnormal Exercise Performance in ILD

Poor exercise tolerance and abnormal pulmonary gas exchange during exercise are very common in patients with ILD. Theoretically, exercise can be limited in these patients by a combination of factors, including an abnormal ventilatory, hemodynamic, and/or gas exchange response. This section discusses these three potential limiting factors and their interaction in ILD.

Other potential limiting factors, such as skeletal muscle dysfunction, have not been studied in patients with ILD to date. However, there is a growing body of evidence that suggests that, in other hypoxemic chronic lung diseases such as chronic obstructive pulmonary disease, they may contribute significantly to exercise intolerance [31–37]. Furthermore, these skeletal muscle abnormalities in chronic obstructive pulmonary disease (and exercise limitation) seem to persist even after the central ventilatory limitation has been removed by lung transplant [38–41]. Whether these peripheral abnormalities also occur in patients with ILD and the potential effects of lung transplant are currently not known. Accordingly, they are not discussed here. However, this is an important area that will require investigation in the near future.

A. Ventilatory Response

In normal humans, minute ventilation ($\dot{V}_E$) increases during exercise in parallel to the increase in $\dot{V}_{O_2}$. Of course, maximal exercise capacity is considerably reduced in ILD. Yet, as shown in Figure 5 (left panel), the relationship between $\dot{V}_E$ and $\dot{V}_{O_2}$ in patients with ILD generally is of the same slope as in health, despite the fact that $\dot{V}_E$ is somewhat higher than in normal subjects at the same workload. The mechanisms underlying this hyperventilatory state were discussed in Section II.A.

Normal humans initially increase $\dot{V}_E$ during exercise by increasing both tidal volume (V_T) and respiratory frequency (f) [23,42,43]. At higher work rates, V_T usually remains constant at approximately 50–60% of vital capacity (VC) [42,43]. Further increases in $\dot{V}_E$ are caused by increases in f alone [42,43]. The response of the ventilatory pattern to exercise in patients with ILD is similar to that observed in normal individuals, although V_T tends to be lower and f higher for a given level of $\dot{V}_E$ [42,43]. Differences in peak V_T are probably caused by abnormal respiratory mechanics, because there is a strong linear relationship between peak exercise V_T and VC [23].

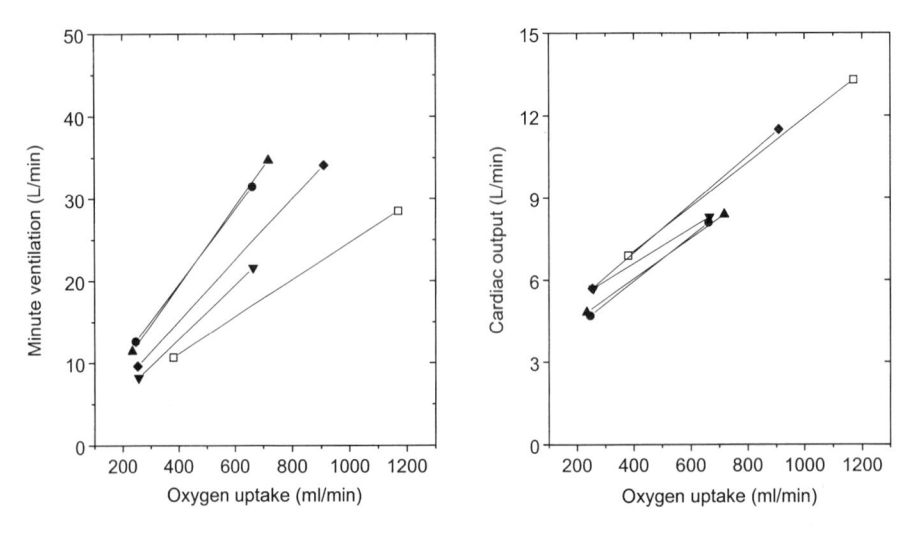

Figure 5 Mean values of minute ventilation (left panel) and cardiac output (right panel) at rest and during exercise reported by different studies in healthy subjects (open squares) (51) and in patients with various types of interstitial lung disease [circles (18) and upward triangles (21)], sarcoidosis (downward triangles) (22), and idiopathic pulmonary fibrosis (diamonds) (16). See text for details.

Normally, the ratio between dead space ventilation (V_{DS}) and V_T (V_{DS}/V_T) decreases during exercise [44]. This is mostly caused by an increased V_T, because V_{DS} does not vary greatly during exercise. In fact, the latter results from the net balance of a moderate increase in the anatomical V_{DS} (due to the augmented end-inspiratory lung volume) and some reduction in the physiological V_{DS} (due to capillary recruitment of unperfused alveoli at rest) [44]. Patients with ILD typically have increased V_{DS}/V_T values at rest (because of both lower V_T and $\dot{V}_A/\dot{Q}$ inequality) that do not show the expected decrease during exercise [8]. This abnormal response has been interpreted as evidence of abnormal pulmonary circulation in ILD [8]. However, failure to increase V_T as much as in health, as well as persistent $\dot{V}_A/\dot{Q}$ inequality during exercise, will also contribute to the high V_{DS}/V_T values.

In summary, the ventilatory response to exercise in ILD is abnormal (ventilatory pattern, V_{DS}/V_T ratio). However, it rarely limits maximal exercise in ILD [45–47]. This is supported by two different observations. First, Pa_{CO_2} does not normally increase with exercise in these patients. This is the best evidence that alveolar ventilation is matched for the metabolic load and probably does not contribute to reduced exercise capacity in ILD. Second, in 1996, Harris-Eze et al. [48] provided experimental evidence that supports this statement. These investigators studied seven patients with ILD who underwent two incremental exercise test in random order: (1) breathing room air; and (2) with added external dead space (to increase the ventilatory requirements of exercise) while breathing 60% O_2 (to avoid arterial hypoxemia). They showed that, with the added external dead space, minute ventilation was higher at a given work load, suggesting the absence of a ventilatory limitation; in addition, by preventing the development of arterial desaturation, exercise duration and oxygen uptake all increased with respect to the values measured during room air exercise [48]. These observations strongly suggest that arterial hypoxemia (not respiratory mechanics) was the main factor limiting exercise tolerance in ILD [48].

B. Hemodynamic Response

Cardiac output at peak exercise is approximately 50% lower in patients with ILD than in healthy subjects; of course, peak $\dot{V}O_2$ is also lower in ILD than in healthy subjects (Fig. 5, right panel). However, cardiac output seems to increase normally during exercise in these patients, as shown by the slope of the relationship between cardiac output and $\dot{V}O_2$ depicted in Figure 5 (right panel). It is likely that this reflects a tight control of cardiac output during exercise, such that despite capacity for a higher value, cardiac output would remain regulated to match the level of exercise and $\dot{V}O_2$ achieved. Alternatively, despite the absence of overt heart failure, the hypothesis that cardiac function may be compromised and a higher cardiac output could not be achieved should also be considered. Figure 6 shows the relationship between filling pressures and cardiac output in healthy subjects and in three different studies in patients with ILD. Although the slope of the relationship is normal, patients with ILD required a higher filling pressure to achieve a given cardiac output (Fig. 6), which may suggest some form of cardiac dysfunction in ILD. In addition, the increased right ventricular afterload that can occur in patients with ILD may limit the normal increase of cardiac output during exercise [23]. For instance, although pulmonary hypertension at rest is not frequent in ILD, at least until advanced stages of the disease (1), these patients do not show the normal decrease in pulmonary vascular resistance observed in healthy subjects during exercise (Fig. 7) [16].

The development of pulmonary hypertension in ILD has been explained classically by a reduction in capillary cross-sectional area caused by destruction of the vasculature [7]. However, some investigators have suggested that hypoxic pulmonary vasoconstriction (HPV) may also play some role [7]. To investigate the relation of the abnormal pulmonary gas exchange observed in patients with IPF and the vascular tone of the pulmonary circulation, Agustí et al. [16] gave 100% oxygen to patients with IPF (to release HPV). They observed two patterns of gas exchange response. Figure 1 (middle panels) exemplify these two types of response. The patient depicted on the top of Figure 1 (patient no. 1) did not show any noticeable change with 100% oxygen. In contrast, in the patient shown on the bottom of Figure 1 (patient no. 2), pure oxygen breathing significantly increased the amount of blood flow perfusing poorly ventilated areas.

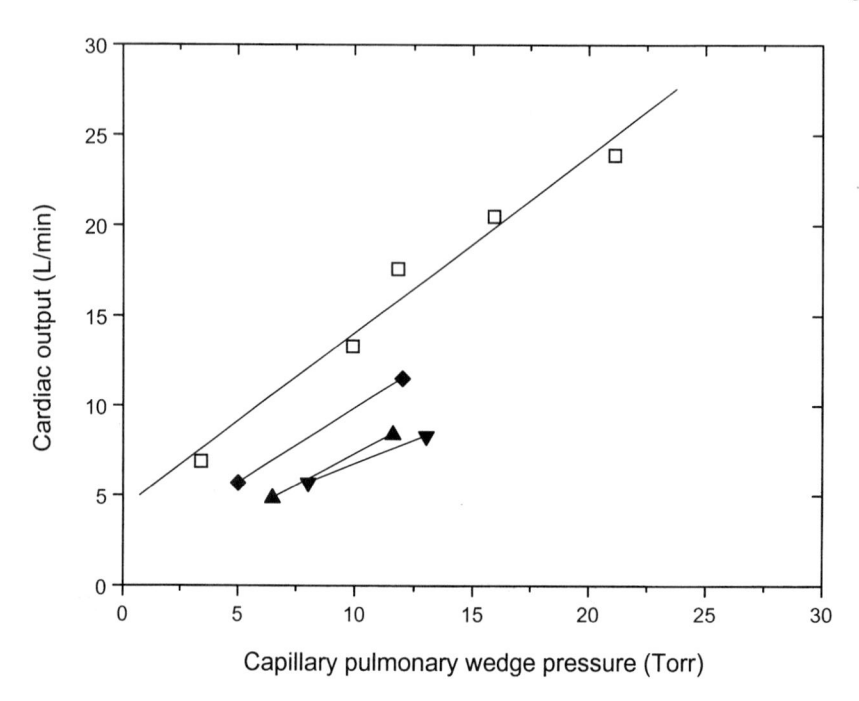

Figure 6 Relationship between cardiac output and filling pressure (capillary pulmonary wedge pressure) reported by different studies in healthy subjects (open squares) (51) and in patients with various types of interstitial lung disease [upward triangles (21)], sarcoidosis (downward triangles) (22), and idiopathic pulmonary fibrosis (diamonds) (16). See text for details.

Given that cardiac output did not change with O_2 in any of them, the observed increase in the perfusion of poorly ventilated lung units while breathing pure oxygen likely represents release of HPV [16]. Therefore, these observations suggest that the pulmonary vasculature may respond to oxygen by releasing HPV only in some patients with IPF, probably those with less anatomical vascular derangement [16]. If the increase in perfusion of low $\dot{V}_A/\dot{Q}$ units while breathing pure O_2 represents release of HPV [16], then the intensity of such response can be quantified using the change in the second moment of the blood flow distribution (log SD $\dot{Q}$). This variable is more sensitive to small changes of pulmonary vascular tone than the standard pressure-flow measurements [12]. Figure 8 shows the change in log SD $\dot{Q}$ during exercise (Δlog SD $\dot{Q}$) plotted against mean pulmonary artery pressure (left panel) and PaO_2 (right panel). It is interesting to observe that when the pulmonary vascular response to oxygen at rest is high (high Δlog SD $\dot{Q}$), the severity of the pulmonary hypertension developed during exercise is reduced and PaO_2 during exercise is preserved (Fig. 8).

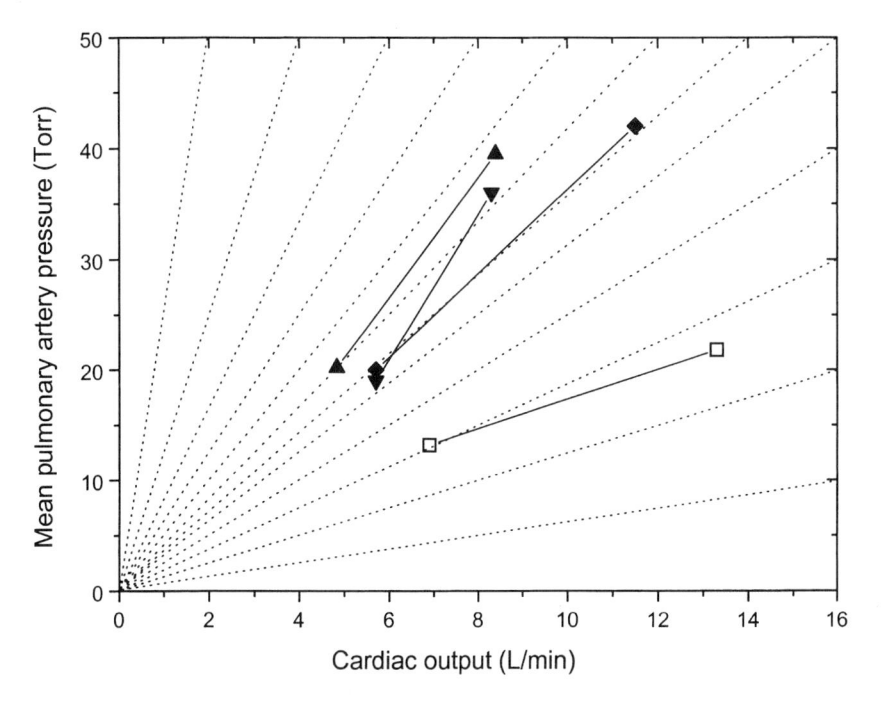

Figure 7 Mean pulmonary artery pressure/flow relationships at rest and during exercise reported by different studies in healthy subjects (open squares) (51) and in patients with various types of interstitial lung disease (upward triangles) (21), sarcoidosis (downward triangles) (22), and idiopathic pulmonary fibrosis (diamonds) (16). Dotted lines correspond to isoresistance values. Note that pulmonary vascular resistance (pressure/flow) decreases with exercise in healthy subjects, but increases in patients. See text for details.

In summary, pulmonary circulation seems to play an important regulatory role in the gas exchange response to exercise in patients with IPF [49]. The presence of reversible pulmonary vascular tone is likely associated with less disturbances in pulmonary gas exchange, both at rest and during exercise [49], as is further discussed in the following section. The basic question of whether the low peak cardiac output reflects a tight control of cardiac function, matching it to metabolic rate, or altered cardiac function in ILD remains to be answered.

C. Respiratory Gas Exchange

Several studies have now shown that: (1) patients with ILD have some (but not much) $\dot{V}_A/\dot{Q}$ inequality at rest; (2) this is not greatly modified during exercise; and (3) O_2 diffusion limitation is more important during exercise. This latter effect can be explained by the aforementioned alterations in the pulmonary vasculature, through the interplay of two different factors. On the one hand, because of the char-

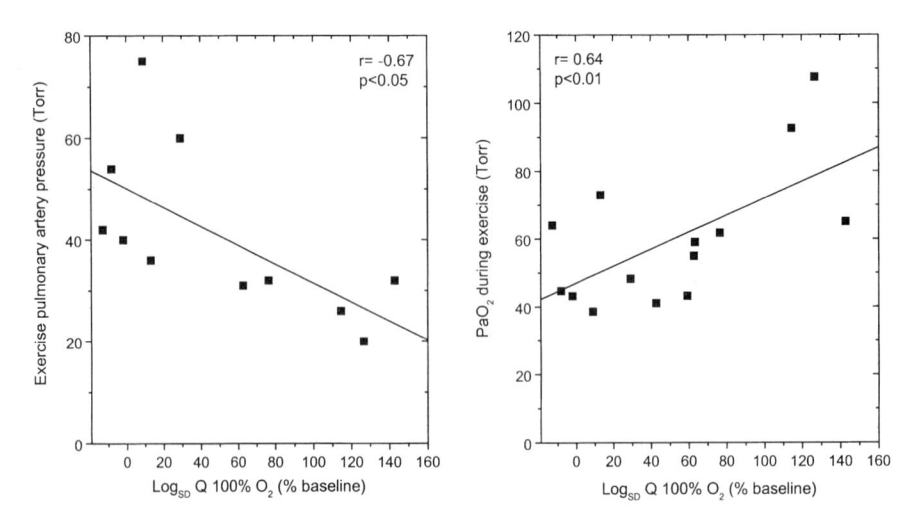

Figure 8 On the abscissa, dispersion of the perfusion distribution while breathing 100% oxygen (expressed as % change from baseline conditions, Δlog SD $\dot{Q}$). As discussed in the text, this expresses the degree of release of hypoxic pulmonary vasoconstriction. In the left panel, Δlog SD $\dot{Q}$ is plotted against the mean pulmonary artery pressure measured during exercise and, in the right panel, against arterial oxygen partial pressure also during exercise in a group of patients with idiopathic pulmonary fibrosis. See text for details. (Data from Ref. 16.)

acteristic nature of the pathological lesion of IPF, recruitment and/or distension of the pulmonary vasculature is impaired, especially in those with more advanced disease [7]. Therefore, to accommodate the higher cardiac output of exercise, these patients necessarily have to shorten capillary transit time. The end result is a significant interference with the equilibrium of oxygen between the alveolar gas and the capillary blood [18,28]. On the other hand, it is well established that, for any given amount of $\dot{V}_A/\dot{Q}$ inequality, Pao$_2$ will increase or decrease in parallel to P$\bar{v}$o$_2$ [27]. Because in patients with ILD P$\bar{v}$o$_2$ seems to decrease more than in healthy subjects (Fig. 2), this mechanism is probably relevant in the pathogenesis of arterial oxygen desaturation during exercise in these individuals. Furthermore, when there is some degree of oxygen diffusion limitation (as is the case in patients with IPF), the lower the P$\bar{v}$o$_2$, the more pronounced the defect in diffusive oxygen transfer becomes, and, consequently, the more severe is the degree of arterial hypoxemia [27].

In summary, pulmonary vasculature seems to play a key role in preventing the lung from maintaining normal arterial oxygenation during exercise in ILD. It seems now established that it is this abnormal oxygenation that mostly limits exercise in these patients [45–48].

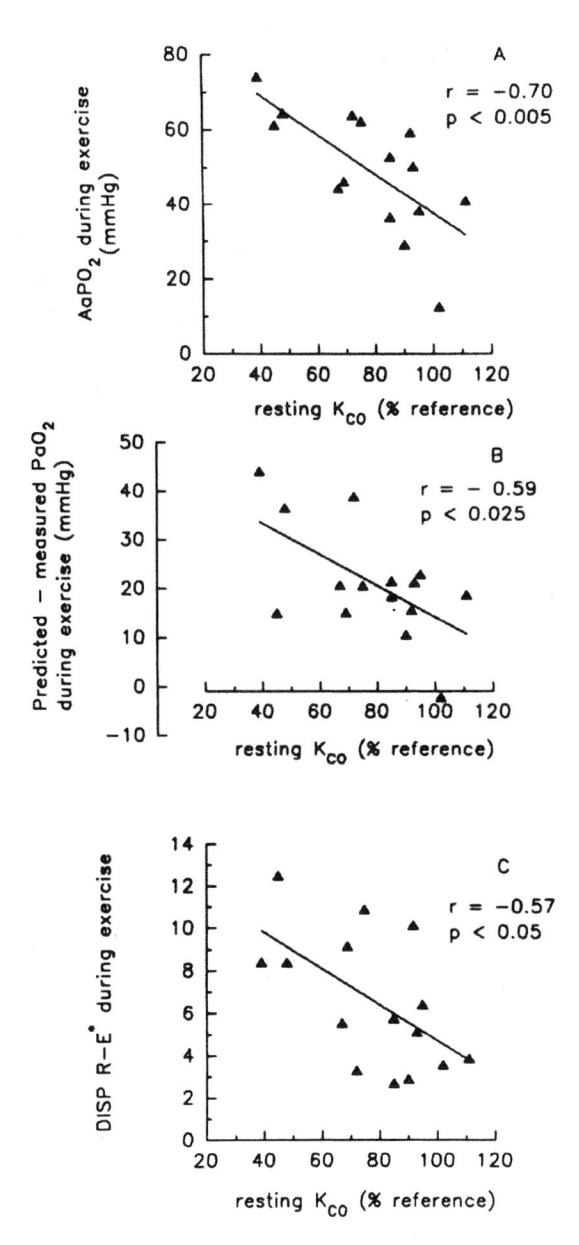

Figure 9 Relation of Kco (diffusing capacity of carbon monoxide corrected for the alveolar volume) and the alveolar–arterial oxygen partial pressure gradient (AaPo$_2$) (A), the difference between the predicted and measured arterial oxygen partial pressure (Pao$_2$) during exercise (B), and the overall degree of ventilation–perfusion ($\dot{V}_A/\dot{Q}$) inequality (DISP R-E*) (C) (51). See text for details. (Reprinted with permission from Ref. 8.)

V. Relationship Between Diffusing Capacity for Carbon Monoxide and the Mechanisms of Abnormal Pulmonary Gas Exchange in ILD

A low diffusing capacity for carbon monoxide (DLCO) is characteristic of ILD and, as such, its measurement is frequently used in the clinical management of these patients [2–5,50]. However, whether it reflects an impairment in the diffusion of oxygen (DLO$_2$) from the alveolar air to the capillary blood was a matter of debate before MIGET. In fact, it is known that DLO$_2$ must be greatly reduced before hypoxemia occurs [27,28]. This is not the case for DLCO, which can also reflect a diminished capillary surface area and capillary blood volume, as occurs in emphysema or in primary pulmonary hypertension [50].

To investigate these uncertainties, the relationship between DLCO and the different mechanisms of gas exchange impairment in IPF was specifically studied [16]. Figure 9 shows the main results of this analysis. However, because the statistical significance of all the analyzed correlations increased when KCO (which equals DLCO normalized for the measured alveolar volume) was considered [16], the latter are reported. The data presented in Figure 9 shows that, in patients with IPF, KCO is significantly related to the overall degree of pulmonary gas exchange impairment during exercise (expressed as the AaPO$_2$ gradient; panel A) and also to the two basic mechanisms of hypoxemia during exercise, i.e., a limitation in the diffusion of oxygen (expressed as the difference between the predicted and mea-

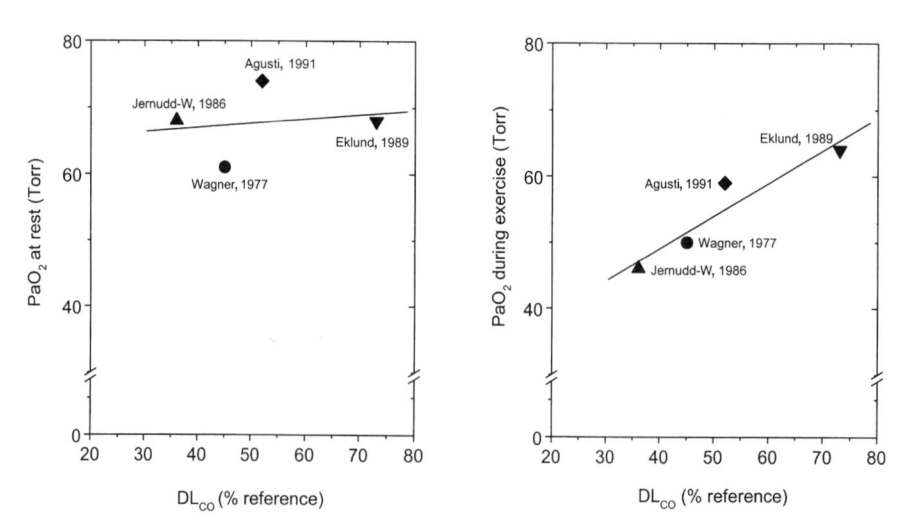

Figure 10 Relationship between diffusing capacity of carbon monoxide (DLCO; % predicted) and arterial oxygen partial pressure (PaO$_2$) at rest and during exercise. Each symbol corresponds to the mean values reported in each study (16,18,21,22).

sured Pao$_2$; panel B) and the degree of $\dot{V}_A/\dot{Q}$ inequality [expressed using an overall index of heterogeneity (DISP R-E*) as described by Wagner et al. in 1986 [51]; panel C]. It was also observed (data not shown) that the lower the Kco (expressed as percentage of reference), the greater the increase in pulmonary vascular resistance during exercise, which, as an index of pulmonary vascular compliance, is an estimate of the surface available for capillary perfusion [16]. Taken all together, these data indicate that Kco is well related to the overall degree of gas exchange impairment to be expected during exercise and also to the amount of pulmonary vascular derangement present in these patients. From the clinical standpoint, how-

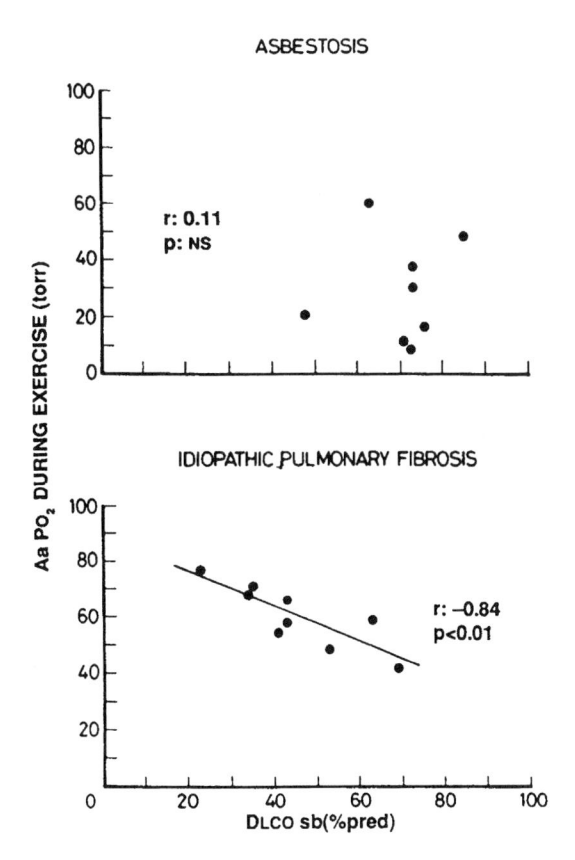

Figure 11 Relationship between diffusing capacity of carbon monoxide (Dlco; % predicted) and the alveolar–arterial O$_2$ gradient (AaPo$_2$) during exercise in patients with asbestosis (top panel) and in patients with idiopathic pulmonary fibrosis (bottom panel) matched for sex, age, and degree of mechanical impairment. Note the absence of a significant relationship in the former group and the presence of a very significant one in the latter patients. See text for details. (Reprinted with permission from Ref. 6.)

ever, it should always be kept in mind that these correlations are merely a reflection of the basic physiopathology of the disease. As such, D_{LCO} should be taken as a useful clinical descriptor of overall gas exchange dysfunction in IPF, but never as its determinant. However, with this in mind, it is interesting to see that, when the data reported by the four different studies quoted in Table 1 are plotted together (Fig. 10), the relationship previously discussed between D_{LCO} and pulmonary gas exchange during exercise (not at rest) in ILD still holds. Nonetheless, this may not be applicable to all forms of ILD, as shown in Figure 11. Apparently, in this other study [6], patients with asbestosis do not show any relationship at all between D_{LCO} and gas exchange during exercise; however, again, this relationship is very significant in patients with IPF [6]. This stresses the importance of identifying different diseases within the large group of ILD when trying to understand mechanisms of disease or effects of different therapies [19,24].

VI. Conclusions

From the discussion presented here, it follows that: (1) the relative contribution of different mechanisms of abnormal pulmonary gas exchange may vary in patients with different forms of ILD; (2) in IPF (at rest), the basic mechanism of arterial hypoxemia is $\dot{V}_A/\dot{Q}$ inequality; (3) in IPF, O_2 diffusion limitation is more in evidence during exercise because of the shorter capillary transit time and the lower $P\bar{v}_{O_2}$; (4) the presence of pulmonary vascular reactivity (as indicated by release of HPV) minimizes pulmonary gas exchange alterations in IPF, whereas when reactivity has been lost or is impaired by advancement of disease, there are greater gas exchange defects; and (5) the measurement of D_{LCO} (particularly when corrected for K_{CO}) seems to be useful in the clinical arena to predict the degree of gas exchange impairment to be expected during exercise and the amount of pulmonary vascular derangement present in these patients.

Acknowledgment

The author acknowledges the helpful comments of Dr. B. Togores (Hospital Universitori Son Dureta, Palma Mallorca, Spain).

References

1. Crystal RG, Fulmer JD, Roberts WC, Moss ML, Line BR, Reynolds HY. Idiopathic pulmonary fibrosis: clinical, histologic, radiographic, physiologic, scintigraphic, cytologic, and biochemical aspects. Ann Intern Med 1976; 85:769–788.
2. Carrington CB, Gaensler EA, Coutu RE, FitzGerald MX, Gupta RG. Natural history and treated course of usual and desquamative interstitial pneumonia. N Engl J Med 1978; 298:801–809.

3. Crystal RG, Gadek JE, Ferrans VJ, Fulmer JD, Line BR, Hunninghake GW. Interstitial lung disease: current concepts of pathogenesis, staging and therapy. Am J Med 1981; 70:542–568.
4. Crystal RG, Bitterman PB, Rennard SI, Hance AJ, Keogh BA. Interstitial lung diseases of unknown cause: disoders characterized by chronic inflamation of the lower respiratory tract (first of two parts). N Engl J Med 1984; 310:154–165.
5. Crystal RG, Bitterman PB, Rennard SI, Hance AJ, Keogh BA. Interstitial lung diseases of unknown cause: disorders characterized by chronic inflamation of the lower respiratory tract (second of two parts). N Engl J Med 1984; 310:235–244.
6. Agustí AGN, Roca J, Rodriguez-Roisín R, Xaubet A, Agustí-Vidal A. Different patterns of gas exchange response to exercise in asbestosis and idiopathic pulmonary fibrosis. Eur Respir J 1988; 1:510–516.
7. Fulmer JD, Roberts WC, Von Gal ER, Crystal RG. Morphologic-physiologic correlates of the severity of fibrosis and degree of cellularity in idiopathic pulmonary fibrosis. J Clin Invest 1979; 63:665–676.
8. Agustí AGN, Barberà JA. Chronic pulmonary diseases: chronic obstructive pulmonary disease and idiopathic pulmonary fibrosis. Thorax 1994; 49:924–932.
9. Cherniack RM, Colby TV, Flint A, Thurlbeck WM, Waldron JA, Ackerson L, Schwarz MI, King TE. Correlation of structure and function in idiopathic pulmonary fibrosis. Am J Respir Crit Care Med 1995; 151:1180–1188.
10. Wagner PD, Naumann PF, Laravuso RB, West JB. Simultaneous measurement of eight foreign gases in blood by gas chromatography. J Appl Physiol 1974; 36:600–605.
11. West JB, Wagner PD. Pulmonary gas exchange. In: West JB, ed. Bioengineering Aspects of the Lung. 1st ed. New York: Marcel Dekker, 1977, pp 361–394.
12. Wagner PD, Hedenstierna G, Rodriguez-Roisín R. Gas exchange, expiratory flow obstruction and the clinical spectrum of asthma. Eur Respir J 1996; 9:1278–1282.
13. Rodriguez-Roisín R, Roca J, Agustí AGN, Mastai R, Wagner PD, Bosch J. Gas exchange and pulmonary vascular reactivity in patients with liver cirrhosis. Am Rev Respir Dis 1987; 135:1085–1092.
14. Barberà JA, Roca J, Ferrer A, Félez MA, Díaz O, Roger N, Rodriguez-Roisín R. Mechanisms of worsening gas exchange during acute exacerbations of chronic obstructive pulmonary disease. Eur Respir J 1997; 10:1285–1291.
15. Roca J, Wagner PD. Contribution of the multiple inert gases elimination technique (MIGET) to medicine: principles and information content of the MIGET. Thorax 1994; 49:815–824.
16. Agustí AGN, Roca J, Rodriguez-Roisín R, Gea J, Xaubet A, Wagner PD. Mechanisms of gas exchange impairment in idiopathic pulmonary fibrosis. Am Rev Respir Dis 1991; 143:219–225.
17. Rodriguez-Roisín R, Roca J, Guitart R, Agustí AGN, Torres A, Wagner PD. Measurements of distributions of ventilation-perfusion ratios: multiple inert gases elimination technique. Rev Esp Fisiol 1986; 42:465–482.
18. Wagner PD. Ventilation-perfusion inequality and gas exchange during exercise in lung disease. In: Dempsey JA, Reed CE, eds. Muscular Exercise and the Lung. Madison: The University of Wisconsin Press, 1977, pp 345–356.

19. Agustí C, Xaubet A, Agustí AGN, Roca J, Ramirez J, Rodriguez-Roisín R. Clinical and functional assesment of patients with idiopathic pulmonary fibrosis: results of a 3 years follow-up. Eur Respir J 1994; 7:643–650.
20. Paintal AS. Vagal sensory receptors and their reflex effects. Physiol Rev 1973; 53:159–227.
21. Jernudd-Wilhelmsson Y, Hornblad Y, Hedenstierna G. Ventilation-perfusion relationships in interstitial lung disease. Eur J Respir Dis 1986; 68:39–49.
22. Eklund A, Broman L, Broman M, Holmgren A. V/Q and alveolar gas exchange in pulmonary sarcoidosis. Eur Respir J 1989; 2:135–144.
23. Marciniuk DD, Gallagher CG. Clinical exercise testing in interstitial lung disease. Clin Chest Med 1994; 15:287–303.
24. Agustí C, Xaubet A, Roca J, Agustí AGN, Rodriguez-Roisín R. Interstitial pulmonary fibrosis with and without associated collagen vascular disease: results of a 2 years follow-up. Thorax 1992; 47:1035–1040.
25. Wasserman K. Coupling of external to cellular respiration during exercise: the wisdom of the body revisited. Am J Physiol (Endocrinol Metab) 1994; 266:E519–E539
26. Wasserman K, Hansen JE, Sue D, Whipp BJ. Principles of Exercise Testing and Interpretation. 2nd ed. Lea & Febiger, 1994, pp 9–51.
27. Wagner PD. Influence of mixed venous P_{O_2} on diffusion of O_2 across the pulmonary blood:gas barrier. Clin Physiol 1982; 2:105–115.
28. Wagner PD. Diffusion and chemical reaction in pulmonary gas exchange. Physiol Rev 1977; 57:257–313.
29. Austrian R, McClement JH, Renzetti AD, Donald AW, Riley RL, Cournand A. Clinical and physiologic features of some types of pulmonary diseases with impairment of alveolar-capillary diffusion: the syndrome of ''alveolar-capillary block.'' Am J Med 1951; 11:667–685.
30. Hughes JMB. Diffusive gas exchange. In: Whipp BJ, Wasserman K, eds. Exercise: Pulmonary Physiology and Pathophysiology. 1st ed. New York: Marcel Dekker, 1991, pp 143–171.
31. Kutsuzawa T, Shioya S, Kurita D, Haida M, Ohta Y, Yamabayashi H. ^{31}P-NMR study of skeletal muscle metabolism in patients with chronic respiratory impairment. Am Rev Respir Dis 1992; 146:1019–1024.
32. Wuyam B, Payen JF, Levy P, Bensaidane H, Reutenauer H, Le Bas JF, Benabid AL. Metabolism and aerobic capacity of skeletal muscle in chronic respiratory failure related to chronic obstructive pulmonary disease. Eur Respir J 1992; 5:157–162.
33. Payen JF, Wuyam B, Levy P, Reutenauer H, Stieglitz P, Paramelle B, Le Bas JF. Muscular metabolism during oxygen supplementation in patients with chronic hypoxemia. Am Rev Respir Dis 1993; 147:592–598.
34. Kutsuzawa T, Shioya S, Kurita D, Haida M, Ohta Y, Yamabayashi H. Muscle energy metabolism and nutritional status in patients with chronic obstructive pulmonary disease: a ^{31}P magnetic resonance study. Am J Respir Crit Care Med 1995; 152:647–652.
35. Jakobsson P, Jorfeldt L, Henriksson J. Metabolic enzyme activity in the quadriceps femoris muscle in patients with severe chronic obstructive pulmonary disease. Am J Respir Crit Care Med 1995; 151:374–377.

36. Maltais F, Simard AA, Simard C, Jobin J, Desgagnés P, Leblanc P, Janvier R. Oxidative capacity of the skeletal muscle and lactic acid kinetics during exercise in normal subjects and in patients with COPD. Am J Respir Crit Care Med 1996; 153:288–293.
37. Sauleda J, García-Palmer FJ, Wiesner R, Tarraga S, Harting I, Tomas P, Gomez C, Saus C, Palou A, Agustí AGN. Cytochrome oxidase activity and mitochondrial gene expression in skeletal muscle of patients with chronic obstructive pulmonary disease. Am J Respir Crit Care Med 1998; 157:1413–1417.
38. Williams TJ, Patterson GA, Mcclean PA, Zamel N, Maurer JR. Maximal exercise testing in single and double lung transplant recipients. Am Rev Respir Dis 1992; 145:101–105.
39. Ambrosino N, Bruschi C, Callegari G, Baiocchi S, Felicetti G, Fracchia C, Rampulla C. Time course of exercise capacity, skeletal and respiratory muscle perfomance after heart-lung transplantation. Eur Respir J 1997; 9:1508–1514.
40. Evans AB, Al-Himyary AJ, Hrovat MI, Pappagianopoulos P, Wain JC, Ginns LC, Systrom DM. Abnormal skeletal muscle oxidative capacity after lung transplantation by ^{31}P-MRS. Am J Respir Crit Care Med 1997; 155:615–621.
41. Trulock EP. Lung transplantation. Am J Respir Crit Care Med 1997; 155:789–818.
42. Casaburi R, Petty TL. Ventilatory control in lung disease. In: Barstow TJ, Casaburi R, eds. Principles and Practice of Pulmonary Rehabilitation. Philadelphia: WB Saunders Company, 1993, pp 50–65.
43. Gallagher CG. Exercise limitation and clinical exercise testing in chronic obstructive pulmonary disease. Clin Chest Med 1994; 15:305–326.
44. Wasserman K, Hansen JE, Sue DY, Whipp BJ, Casaburi R. Principles of Exercise Testing and Interpretation. 2nd ed. Philadelphia: Lea & Febiger, 1994.
45. Marciniuk DD, Sridhar G, Clements RE, Zintel TA, Gallagher CG. Lung volumes and expiratory flow limitation during exercise in interstitial lung disease. J Appl Physiol 1994; 77:963–973.
46. Marciniuk DD, Watts RE, Gallagher CG. Dead space loading and exercise limitation in patients with interstitial lung disease. Chest 1994; 105:183–189.
47. Harris-Eze AO, Sridhar G, Clemens RE, Gallagher CG, Marciniuk DD. Oxygen improves maximal exercise performance in interstitial lung disease. Am J Respir Crit Care Med 1994; 150:1616–1622.
48. Harris-Eze AO, Sridhar G, Clemens RE, Zintel TA, Gallagher CG, Marciniuk DD. Role of hypoxemia and pulmonary mechanics in exercise limitation in interstitial lung disease. Am J Respir Crit Care Med 1996; 154:994–1001.
49. Agustí AGN. Effect of pulmonary hypertension on gas exchange. Eur Respir J 1993; 6:1371–1377.
50. Nordenfelt I, Svensson G. The transfer factor (diffusing capacity) as a predictor of hypoxaemia during exercise in restrictive and chronic obstructive pulmonary disease. Clin Physiol 1987; 7:423–430.
51. Wagner PD, Gale GE, Moon RE, Torre-Bueno JE, Stolp BW, Saltzman HA. Pulmonary gas exchange in humans exercising at sea level and simulated altitude. J Appl Physiol 1986; 61:260–270.

10

Pulmonary Vascular Diseases

CHRISTIAN MÉLOT and ROBERT NAEIJE

Erasme Hospital, Free University of Brussels
Brussels, Belgium

I. Introduction

Pulmonary vascular disease invariably leads to an abnormal increase in pulmonary vascular resistance. Pulmonary vascular disease complicates the course of many cardiac and pulmonary conditions (secondary pulmonary hypertension), but also develops either as a primary disease (primary pulmonary hypertension) or as a consequence of intraluminal thrombotic processes (acute or chronic thromboembolic pulmonary hypertension) [1]. Patients with pulmonary hypertension commonly have abnormal arterial blood gases, indicating altered pulmonary gas exchange. To answer the question how pulmonary hypertension itself affects gas exchange, it is appropriate to limit the present analysis to primary or thromboembolic pulmonary hypertension to avoid the confounding effects of the initial pulmonary parenchymal disease or of increased pulmonary capillary pressures associated with any cause of increased pulmonary venous pressure, from pulmonary veno-occlusive disease to left heart disease [2,3].

Primary and thromboembolic pulmonary hypertension are both characterized by various combinations of remodeled pulmonary arterial and arteriolar walls and intraluminal obstruction or obliteration [1]. This chapter focuses on the studies that used the multiple inert gas elimination technique (MIGET) [4,5] to understand how these pathological modifications of the pulmonary arterial tree alter the gas exchange function of the lungs. The advantage of MIGET over earlier methods based on the analysis of expired, arterial, and mixed venous Po_2 and Pco_2 has been that it makes possible the identification and quantification of all of the pulmonary and extrapulmonary determinants of abnormal blood gases. Acute pulmonary arterial obstruction, as typically occurs in pulmonary embolism, and chronic pulmonary arterial obstruction, as typically occurs in chronic thromboembolic pulmonary hypertension or in primary pulmonary hypertension, are successively reviewed.

II. Acute Pulmonary Arterial Obstruction: Pulmonary Embolism

How acute pulmonary arterial obstruction affects pulmonary gas exchange is typically illustrated by acute pulmonary embolism. These patients present with variable combinations of hypoxemia and hypocapnia. Hypoxemia is generally moderate but can be severe. Approximately one third of the patients have an arterial oxygen partial pressure (Pao_2) greater than 70 mm Hg, one third a Pao_2 between 60 and 70 mm Hg, and one third a Pao_2 less than 60 mm Hg. More than 90% of patients present with an increased alveolar–arterial oxygen partial pressure [$P(A-a)o_2$] [6]. Most patients are hypocapnic [6]. Hypocapnia results from hyperventilation, which is observed even in the presence of significant underlying lung disease [7]. Experimental animal and clinical studies using MIGET have established that acute pulmonary embolism affects approximately all of the pulmonary and extrapulmonary determinants of the composition of arterial blood gases (8–18). Accordingly, acute pulmonary embolism results in a diversity of patterns of ventilation–perfusion ($\dot{V}_A/\dot{Q}$) inequality, from unimodal distributions, only slightly wider than normal, to distributions containing either high $\dot{V}_A/\dot{Q}$ and dead space units or low $\dot{V}_A/\dot{Q}$ and shunt units (Figs. 1–3). Extrapulmonary factors, in particular total ventilation and cardiac output, with its well known effects on mixed venous Po_2 ($P\bar{v}o_2$), interact with these patterns of $\dot{V}_A/\dot{Q}$ inequality to determine the levels of Pao_2 and arterial carbon dioxide partial pressure ($Paco_2$).

A. Shunt

Shunt ($\dot{Q}s/\dot{Q}t$, ratio of shunted blood flow over total blood flow expressed in percent), or units with $\dot{V}_A/\dot{Q} = 0$, measured by the less soluble gases of MIGET in normal subjects breathing spontaneously, is 1.2% ± 0.3% (mean ± SE) with a 95% prediction interval of 0–5% [19]. In patients with acute pulmonary embolism, shunt is usually small, amounting to less than 5% in 60% of patients [8–12]. However, very large shunts, up to 39%, have occasionally been reported in patients with acute massive pulmonary embolism [8,20]. Large shunts have also be found to account for most of the abnormal gas exchange in experimental animals after microembolization with either glass or polystyrene beads [15,21,22] (Fig. 2). This has

Pulmonary Vascular Diseases 287

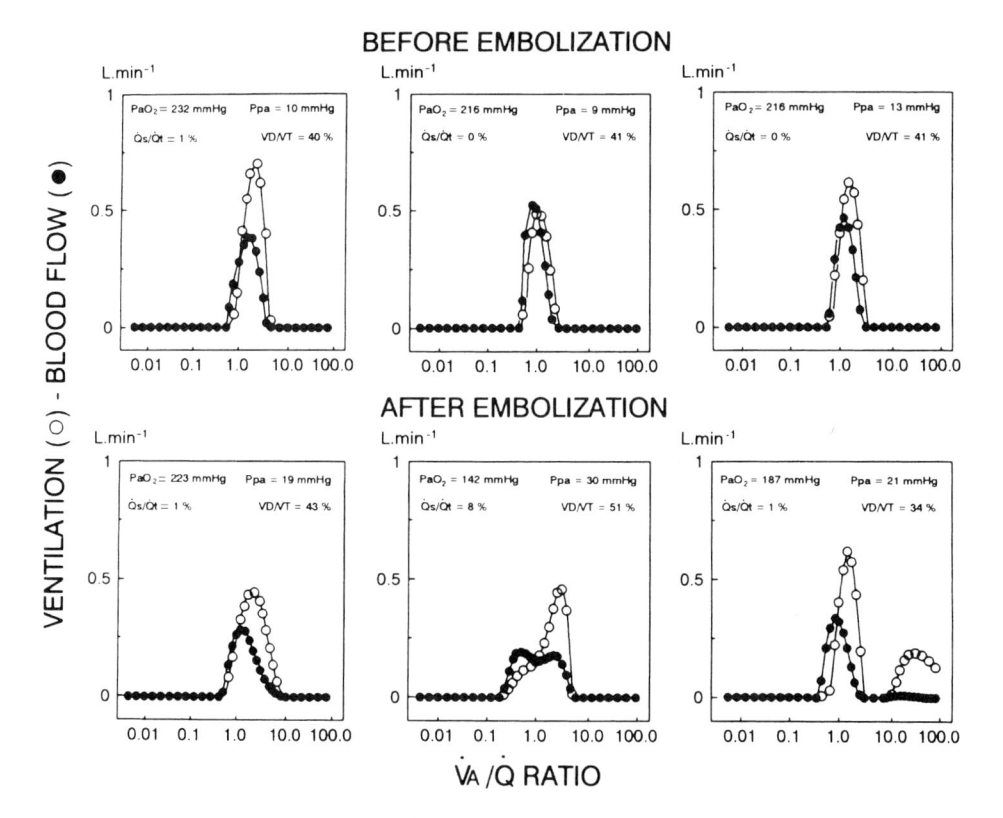

Figure 1 Ventilation–perfusion ($\dot{V}_A/\dot{Q}$) distributions before and after acute pulmonary embolization with autologous clots in dogs. Three patterns were observed: slightly broadened unimodal, hardly different from normal (left panel), broadly unimodal (middle panel), and bimodal with an additional high $\dot{V}_A/\dot{Q}$ mode (right panel). (From Ref. 14. Copyright 1990 by the American Society of Anesthesiologists, with permission.)

been shown to be caused by massive pulmonary edema, a rare finding in pulmonary embolism.

Pulmonary arterial obstruction will directly increase the $\dot{V}_A/\dot{Q}$ ratio in units by reduced perfusion. In unobstructed regions, there will be a decrease in $\dot{V}_A/\dot{Q}$ ratio because of blood flow redistribution from the obstructed vessels. Thus, the presence of shunt has to be explained by secondary events [6]. One of them is atelectasis, commonly identified on chest roentgenograms of patients with pulmonary embolism. Atelectasis has been explained by altered surfactant in embolized areas [23] and by hypocapnic hypoventilation from bronchoconstriction in units with higher than normal $\dot{V}_A/\dot{Q}$ [24]. Atelectatic lung regions would present with an increased perfusion because of pulmonary hypertension, and possibly also because

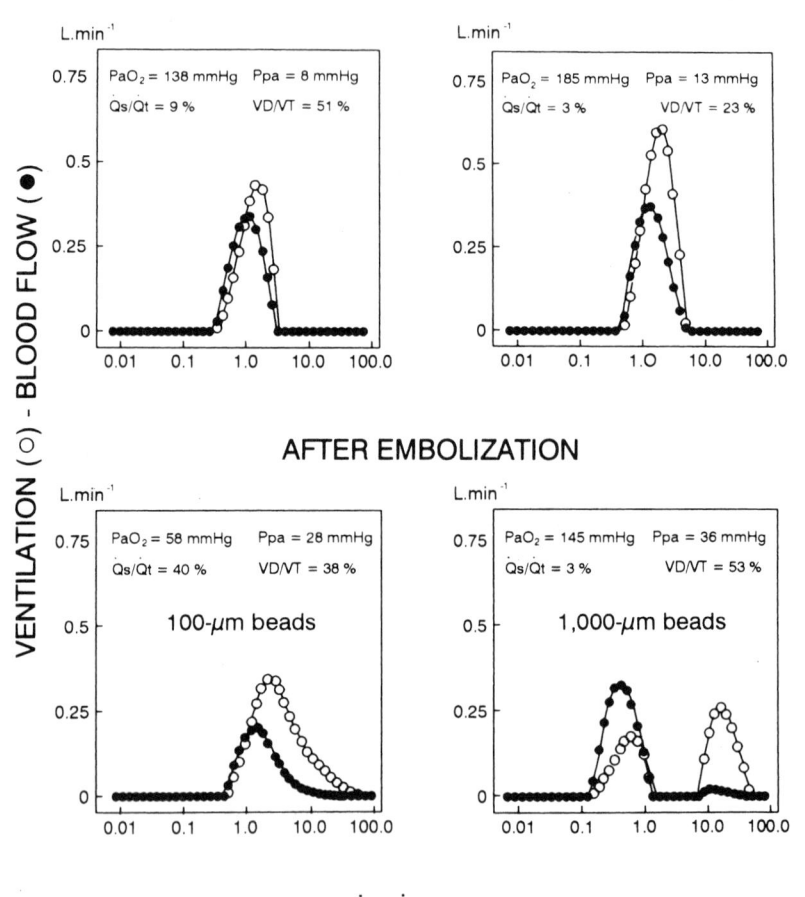

Figure 2 Ventilation–perfusion ($\dot{V}_A/\dot{Q}$) distributions before and after pulmonary embolization with 100-μm and 1000-μm diameter glass beads, respectively, in dogs. Small 100-μm bead embolization was associated with a broad unimodal pattern and an increased shunt (Qs/Qt). Large 1000-μm bead embolization was associated with a bimodal pattern, with a mode of ventilation and perfusion centered on lung units with low-normal $\dot{V}_A/\dot{Q}$, and an additional mode, mainly of ventilation, centered on units with high $\dot{V}_A/\dot{Q}$, and an increased inert gas dead space (VDS/VTIG). (From Ref. 15. Copyright 1990 by the American Physiological Society, with permission.)

ACUTE EMBOLISM BEFORE STREPTOKINASE

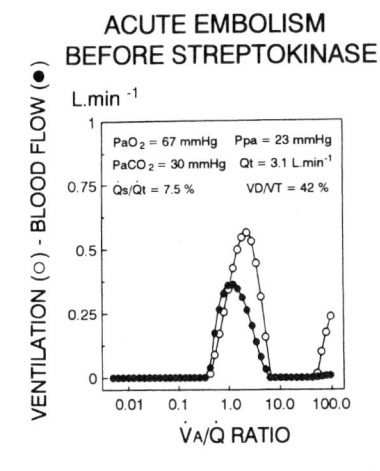

PaO$_2$ = 67 mmHg   Ppa = 23 mmHg
PaCO$_2$ = 30 mmHg   Qt = 3.1 L.min^{-1}
Qs/Qt = 7.5 %   VD/VT = 42 %

ACUTE EMBOLISM AFTER STREPTOKINASE

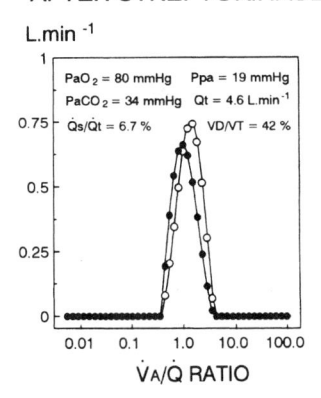

PaO$_2$ = 80 mmHg   Ppa = 19 mmHg
PaCO$_2$ = 34 mmHg   Qt = 4.6 L.min^{-1}
Qs/Qt = 6.7 %   VD/VT = 42 %

Figure 3 Ventilation–perfusion ($\dot{V}_A/\dot{Q}$) distributions in a patient with acute pulmonary embolism before and after thrombolytic therapy. Before treatment, the $\dot{V}_A/\dot{Q}$ distribution showed a bimodal pattern. Arterial hypoxemia resulted mainly from a low cardiac output and a low mixed venous oxygen partial pressure (P$\bar{v}$o$_2$). After treatment, cardiac output, arterial oxygen partial pressure (Pao$_2$), and P$\bar{v}$o$_2$ increased, and $\dot{V}_A/\dot{Q}$ distribution returned to normal except for the persistence of a slightly increased shunt.

of a relative inhibition of hypoxic pulmonary vasoconstriction [18]. A shunt may also develop as a consequence of interstitial or alveolar edema in relation to the release of vasoactive mediators from the impacted clots [6]. The importance of this mechanism seems to be related to embolus size. Acute microembolism is an experimental model of permeability lung edema [25]. We showed that embolization with 100-μm glass beads in dogs caused an increased shunt, whereas embolization with 1000-μm glass beads did not [15]. Thus, fragmentation of clots to small particles around the size of 100 μm could be a cause of increased shunt in some patients. Another cause of focal lung edema in acute pulmonary embolism could be stress failure of overperfused nonobstructed lung regions [26]. Finally, right heart failure associated with high pulmonary artery pressure may be associated with an inversion of the normal pressure gradient between the left and the right atrium, reopening a foramen ovale, which is patent in 15% of patients, and thereby creating a right-to-left cardiac shunt [20].

B. Dead Space

Inert gas dead space (VDS/VT$_{IG}$, ratio of the volume of dead space over tidal volume expressed in percent), or units with $\dot{V}_A/\dot{Q} \geq 100$, measured by the most soluble gas of MIGET in normal subjects breathing spontaneously, is 37% ± 2%

(mean ± SE) [19]. In patients with acute pulmonary embolism, $V_{DS}/V_{T_{IG}}$ is either normal (<40%) or moderately elevated (40–45%) [8–12].

The frequent absence of increase in dead space after significant embolization, also noted in experimental studies [17,27], suggests that complete occlusion of blood flow is an uncommon occurrence. Dead space may also be affected by embolus size. In dogs embolized with 1-, 5-, and 10-mm autologous clots, we found a decreased, unchanged, and increased $V_{DS}/V_{T_{IG}}$, respectively [17]. A decrease in $V_{DS}/V_{T_{IG}}$ has also been reported after experimental pulmonary embolism with 100-μm glass beads [15] and with 50- to 100-μm polystyrene beads [21]. The different effects of embolus size on dead space may be explained by (1) recruitment of poorly perfused lung units as a consequence of pulmonary hypertension; (2) common incomplete vascular obstruction; (3) variable increase in bronchial tone, redistributing ventilation from embolized lung areas, most often after small size emboli; and (4) more or less important intraregional differences in alveolar gas caused by more or less effective collateral ventilation. Collateral ventilation, especially in dogs, may be a major cause for decreased $V_{DS}/V_{T_{IG}}$ after small clots or beads, as illustrated in Fig. 4. After small clots, the most soluble inert gases and CO_2 could diffuse from perfused to unperfused alveoli through interalveolar Kohn

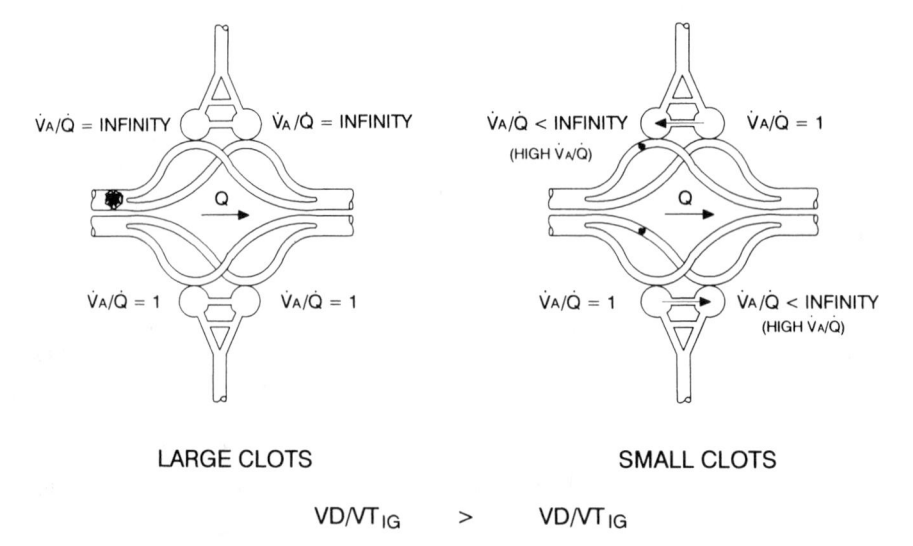

Figure 4 Explanation of differential effects of embolus size on inert gas dead space ($V_{DS}/V_{T_{IG}}$) in the presence of collateral ventilation. Diffusion of alveolar gas from perfused to unperfused alveoli through interalveolar Kohn pores and interbronchiolar Martin ducts is effective in reducing intraregional ventilation–perfusion ($\dot{V}_A/\dot{Q}$) differences only for small-size emboli. (From Ref. 17. Copyright 1990 by the American Physiological Society, with permission.)

pores and interbronchial Martin ducts, thereby making lung areas without blood flow (and thus with a $\dot{V}_A/\dot{Q}$ equal to infinity) seem to function as lung areas with a higher than normal (but not infinitely great) $\dot{V}_A/\dot{Q}$ ratio.

C. Ventilation–Perfusion Inequality

Pulmonary embolism generally impairs $\dot{V}_A/\dot{Q}$ matching, and this is the dominant mechanism of hypoxemia. After embolization, there are units that are overventilated and underperfused, with high $\dot{V}_A/\dot{Q}$ areas accounting for increased physiologic dead space (Bohr dead space), and there are units that are overperfused and underventilated, with low $\dot{V}_A/\dot{Q}$, accounting for increased physiologic shunt (or venous admixture). This heterogeneity can be explained by blood flow redistribution from embolized to nonembolized lung units [6]. Almost total occlusion of a small number of lung units will result in the development of high $\dot{V}_A/\dot{Q}$ units. However, because the total amount of blood flow diverted to the remaining uninvolved lung is, in this case, small relative to the preembolization flow, a significant number of low $\dot{V}_A/\dot{Q}$ units will not develop, and the degree of hypoxemia will be minimal. By contrast, if a large amount of the lung is embolized but the occlusion is only partial, high $\dot{V}_A/\dot{Q}$ units will not develop, and the predominant abnormality will be the creation of low $\dot{V}_A/\dot{Q}$ units caused by the diversion of blood flow to the remaining uninvolved lung. In this case, significant hypoxemia will occur. Thus, the effect on the arterial blood gases depends on the relative amount of blood flow diverted [6]. In addition, the amount of $\dot{V}_A/\dot{Q}$ inequality may be enhanced by the inhibition of hypoxic pulmonary vasoconstriction [18]. On the contrary, a well-preserved hypocapnic bronchoconstriction limits the occurrence of high $\dot{V}_A/\dot{Q}$ units and the increase in physiologic dead space [6].

D. Diffusion Impairment

Diffusion equilibrium of inert gases is complete; therefore, any diffusion abnormality causing impairment of oxygen uptake by the lung will lead to systematic overprediction of Pa_{O_2} by the mathematical lung model of MIGET and the measured $\dot{V}_A/\dot{Q}$ distribution [4]. Predicted Pa_{O_2} has been found to be either not significantly different from measured Pa_{O_2} or only slightly higher, by a maximum of 5 to 7 mm Hg, in patients with pulmonary embolism [8–12]. Predicted and measured Pa_{O_2} were not different in experimental animal pulmonary embolism [13–18]. Thus, there may be a small contribution of diffusion limitation to arterial hypoxemia in a minority of patients.

E. Extrapulmonary Factors

In the presence of altered $\dot{V}_A/\dot{Q}$ matching, Pa_{O_2} is influenced by $P\bar{v}_{O_2}$, especially in the presence of shunt and areas of low $\dot{V}_A/\dot{Q}$ ratio [6]. The hypoxemic effect of decreased $P\bar{v}O_2$ appears at $\dot{V}A/\dot{Q}$ less than and is maximal at $\dot{V}A/\dot{Q} = 0$, but decreases with increased ventilation, which is characteristic in pulmonary embolism [6]. Several studies have reported a significant contribution of low $P\bar{v}O_2$, due to decreased cardiac output, to arterial hypoxemia in patients with pulmonary embolism [9–12]. In one of these studies, correcting mixed venous hypoxemia normalized PaO_2 in 9 of 10 patients [9].

The mechanisms of increased ventilation in pulmonary embolism remain poorly understood [6]. Hypoxemic stimulation of the peripheral chemoreceptors is generally insufficient to account for the observed levels of ventilation. A possible mechanism may be a reflex increase in ventilation caused by stimulation of some pulmonary receptor sensitive to increased pulmonary artery pressures, and associated enhanced vagal afferent activity [6]. Whatever its precise cause, this increase in ventilation is the main determinant of hypocapnia in pulmonary embolism. Experimental embolism in artificially ventilated and paralyzed animals always increases $PaCO_2$ because of an increased wasted ventilation due to increased $\dot{V}A/\dot{Q}$ inequality at constant ventilation [14–16].

A recent study used MIGET to quantify the pulmonary and extrapulmonary determinants of PaO_2 in a series of 10 patients with severe pulmonary embolism [12]. The patients had a PaO_2 of 63 ± 4 mm Hg (mean $\pm$ SE), a $PaCO_2$ of 30 ± 1 mm Hg, a $P\bar{v}O_2$ of 31 ± 4 mm Hg, a ventilation of 14 ± 5 L/min, a cardiac output of 4.7 ± 1.7 L/min, and a mean pulmonary arterial pressure (Ppa) of 38 ± 17 mm Hg. As illustrated in Figure 5, most of the decrease in PaO_2 at the given level of hyperventilation could be accounted for by altered $\dot{V}A/\dot{Q}$ matching and decreased $P\bar{v}O_2$.

F. Pulmonary Vascular Tone

Embolic pulmonary hypertension is caused by a direct mechanical obstruction of the pulmonary arterial tree, but several studies have also identified a component of active pulmonary vasoconstriction [28]. The latter may be related to embolus size because it is observed experimentally after 100-μm glass-bead but not after 1000-μm glass-bead embolism [15]. The recognition of a functional component of pulmonary hypertension has been the justification for previous attempts at intravenous pharmacological pulmonary vasodilation in patients with massive pulmonary embolism and shock [29]. Such interventions would currently rather be discouraged because it is now better known that they carry a significant risk of excessive systemic hypotension, which could compromise right ventricular coronary perfusion and thereby actually aggravate right ventricular failure [30].

Intravenous pharmacological reduction of pulmonary vascular tone in pulmonary embolism could theoretically cause deterioration of arterial oxygenation, as shown in pulmonary hypertension secondary to chronic obstructive pulmonary disease [31] or to adult respiratory distress syndrome [32], and also in primary pulmonary hypertension [33]. However, this has not been reported in acute embolic

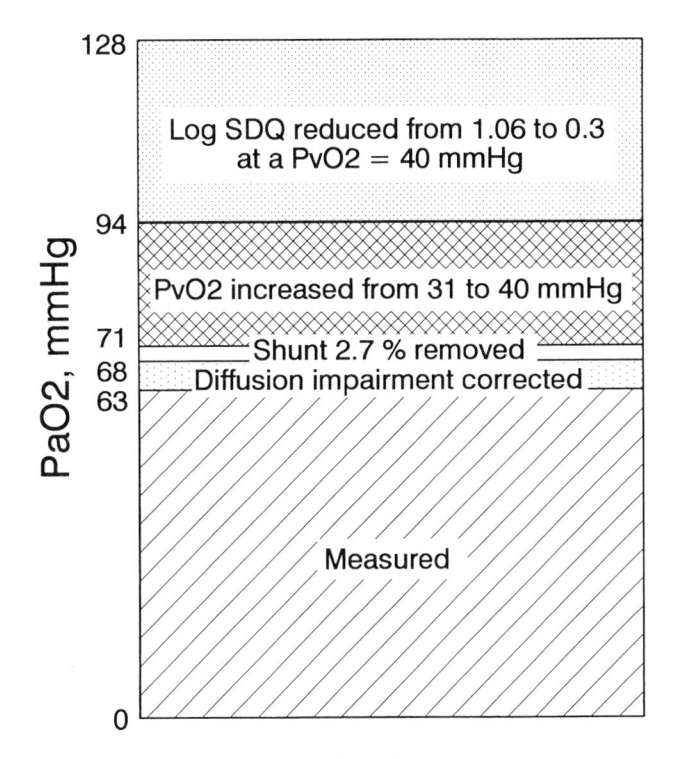

Figure 5 Quantification of the pulmonary and extrapulmonary contributors to arterial oxygen partial pressure (PaO_2) in patients with severe acute pulmonary embolism. Measured PaO_2 was 63 mm Hg. Correction of abnormal diffusion, shunt, mixed venous oxygen partial pressure (P$\bar{v}O_2$), and log SD $\dot{Q}$ successively increased PaO_2, with eventually a PaO_2 of 128 mm Hg higher than normal because of hyperventilation. (Figure drawn using the data of Ref. 12.)

pulmonary hypertension, probably because in these patients, the functional component of increased pulmonary vascular resistance is only of marginal relevance to gas exchange. Experimental acute canine autologous blood clot embolic pulmonary hypertension is slightly reversible by intravenous vasodilators such as hydralazine and nitroprusside, but without change in $\dot{V}_A/\dot{Q}$ matching when pulmonary blood flow and ventilation are kept constant [14]. We modeled pulmonary arterial pressure/flow relationships at pulmonary arterial obstructions ranging from 10–90%, using an adaptation of a viscoelastic model of the pulmonary circulation without vasoreactivity, and compared model predictions to hemodynamic measurements and pulmonary angiograms in canine autologous blood clot pulmonary embolism [34]. As shown in Figure 6, the model predicted a mean Ppa of 20 mm Hg, the upper limit of normal at a cardiac output of 3.5 L/min/m^2, at a pulmonary arterial obstruction of 50%, which is in keeping with previous findings in patients

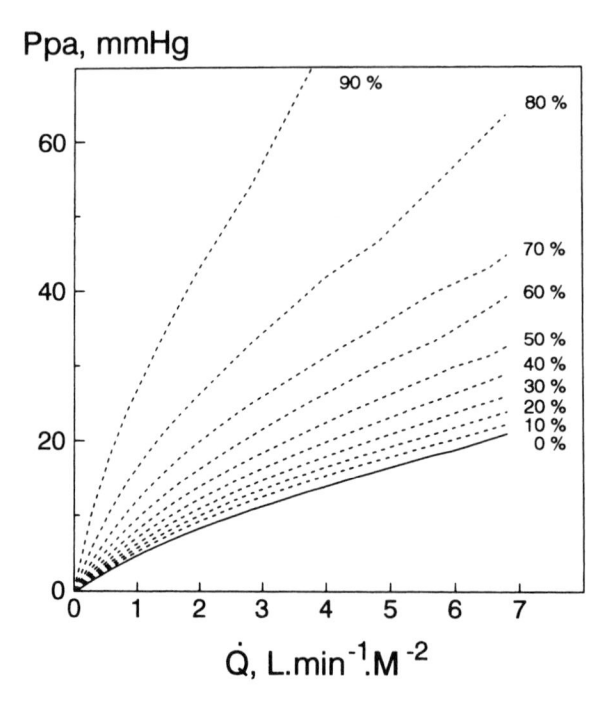

Figure 6 Relationship between mean pulmonary artery pressure (Ppa) and pulmonary blood flow ($\dot{Q}$) predicted by a viscoelastic lung model of the canine pulmonary circulation at pulmonary arterial obstruction ranging from 10–90%. At a normal pulmonary blood flow of 3.5 L/min/m², Ppa reaches the upper limit of normal of 20 mm Hg when pulmonary arterial obstruction reaches 50%. The model allowed a satisfactory prediction of Ppa/$\dot{Q}$ relationships at all levels of angiographically determined pulmonary arterial obstruction. (Figure drawn using the model of Ref. 34.)

without preexistent cardiac or pulmonary disease [28]. The model provided a satisfactory prediction of pulmonary artery pressure/flow relationships at every level of angiographic obstruction, further indicating the negligible importance of active constriction in acute embolic pulmonary hypertension.

In experimental glass-bead [35] or blood-clot [36] pulmonary embolism, cyclooxygenase inhibition has been reported to cause pulmonary vasodilation and improvement in gas exchange. In these studies, a proposed explanation was that pulmonary embolism would be associated with a release of thomboxane A_2, a pulmonary vasoconstricting and bronchoconstricting metabolite of the cyclooxygenase pathway of arachidonic acid metabolism. On the other hand, cyclooxygenase inhibition has been reported to enhance hypoxic pulmonary vasoconstriction [37]. We investigated the effects of two cyclooxygenase inhibitors, acetylsalicylic acid and indomethacin, in experimental autologous-clot pulmonary embolism [16]. Both drugs increased pulmonary vascular resistance as defined by multipoint pulmonary vascular pressure/flow relationships, and increased physiological dead space. This deterioration in pulmonary gas exchange in lung units with high $\dot{V}_A/\dot{Q}$ was accompanied by a decrease in V_DV_{TIG}, which we explained either by a bronchoconstriction caused by an inhibited production of bronchodilating prostaglandins, or by the recruitment of previously unperfused embolized areas caused by the pulmonary hypertension converting them from dead space to areas of high $\dot{V}_A/\dot{Q}$. Inhibition of cyclooxygenase had no effect on lung units with lower than normal $\dot{V}_A/\dot{Q}$, in keeping with the idea that hypoxic pulmonary vasoconstriction does not improve gas exchange in pulmonary embolism [16].

G. Effects of Treatment

The treatment of pulmonary embolism consists of the administration of anticoagulants and, in most severe cases, thrombolytics followed by anticoagulants [38]. Anticoagulant therapy reduces the early mortality of acute pulmonary embolism from 25–35% to less than 5%. Addition of thrombolytic therapy leads to a faster dissolution of clots, which is desirable in patients with massive pulmonary embolism and right heart failure, but has not been shown to further decrease the early mortality of pulmonary embolism.

The effects of 10 to 14 days of heparin therapy on pulmonary gas exchange have been recently evaluated in five patients with severe pulmonary embolism [12]. After therapy, the perfusion lung scan showed a decrease in unperfused lung segments, from 65.6% to 23.4%. Mean Ppa decreased from 35 ± 9 to 15 ± 3 mm Hg, cardiac output did not change, ventilation decreased from 13.4 ± 3 to 9 ± 0.5 L/min, $P\bar{v}O_2$ increased from 31 ± 2 to 38 ± 1 mm Hg, $PaCO_2$ increased from 32 ± 2 to 38 ± 2 mm Hg, and PaO_2 increased from 59 ± 3 to 78 ± 3 mm Hg. A bimodal $\dot{V}_A/\dot{Q}$ distribution with a high $\dot{V}_A/\dot{Q}$ mode returned to an unimodal pattern in two patients. In all five patients, both mean $\dot{V}_A/\dot{Q}$ of the ventilation distribution and mean $\dot{V}_A/\dot{Q}$ of the blood flow distribution shifted from higher than normal to normal or low-normal $\dot{V}_A/\dot{Q}$. Accordingly, physiological dead space decreased from $47\% \pm 9\%$ to $40\% \pm 6\%$ [12].

We studied the effects of thrombolytic therapy on gas exchange using the MIGET in a 69-year-old woman admitted for acute severe pulmonary embolism. A chest roentgenogram showed an area of hyperlucency at the left upper lobe. A pulmonary angiogram showed multiple emboli, with an estimated obstruction of 56% of the pulmonary arterial tree. PaO_2 was 67 mm Hg, $PaCO_2$ 30 was mm Hg, mean Ppa was 23 mm Hg, and cardiac output was 3.1 L/min. $\dot{V}_A/\dot{Q}$ distributions were measured before and after treatment by intravenous streptokinase 250,000 IU over 30 minutes followed by 100,000 IU/h during 24 hours. As shown in Fig. 3, before treatment, the patient had a bimodal pattern with a broad mode centered on $\dot{V}_A/\dot{Q}$ of 1 and an additional high $\dot{V}_A\dot{Q}$ mode. Shunt and V_D/V_{TIG} were moderately increased. After treatment, mean Ppa was 19 mm Hg, cardiac output was

4.6 L/min, and arterial blood gases improved with a PaO_2 of 80 mm Hg and a $PaCO_2$ of 34 mm Hg. The $\dot{V}A/\dot{Q}$ distributions returned to normal except for the persistence of moderately increased shunt (Fig. 3). A pulmonary angiogram performed on the second day showed a partial vascular reperfusion. Thus, treatment with anticoagulants, and more so with fibrinolytics, may rapidly reverse gas exchange abnormalities in severe pulmonary embolism.

III. Chronic Pulmonary Vascular Obstruction

A. Chronic Thromboembolic Pulmonary Hypertension

Chronic thromboembolic pulmonary hypertension is a rare complication of pulmonary embolism characterized by widespread, predominantly central, obstruction of the pulmonary arteries by organized thrombi [39]. The afflicted patient complains of progressive dyspnea and exercise intolerance and is found to be hypoxemic. The radionuclide $\dot{V}A/\dot{Q}$ scan demonstrates multiple mismatched segmental or larger defects, and the pulmonary angiogram shows widespread central obstruction of the pulmonary vascular bed in the setting of severe pulmonary hypertension. Untreated, the course is one of progressive pulmonary compromise, leading to death from right ventricular failure. Removal of the obstructing organized thrombi by surgical endarterectomy provides an effective treatment for this form of pulmonary hypertension. Thromboendarterectomy relieves pulmonary hypertension and restores right ventricular function and exercise tolerance [39]. Radionuclide perfusion scans return to near normal, and hypoxemia resolves.

The mechanisms of altered gas exchange in chronic thromboembolic pulmonary hypertension have been studied using MIGET in a series of 25 patients [40]. Mean Ppa was 45 ± 3 mm Hg, cardiac output was 1.7 ± 0.2 L/min/m², PaO_2 was 65 ± 3 mm Hg and $PaCO_2$ was 32 ± 1 mm Hg. The $\dot{V}A/\dot{Q}$ distribution was, on average, only moderately abnormal, with a characteristically widened unimodal $\dot{V}A/\dot{Q}$ centered on lung units with a normal $\dot{V}A/\dot{Q}$, no increased shunt, and no $\dot{V}A/\dot{Q}$ less than 0.1 or greater than 10. Five of the 25 patients had a bimodal distribution, with a broadened central mode plus either a small low $\dot{V}A/\dot{Q}$ mode (3 patients) or a high $\dot{V}A/\dot{Q}$ mode (2 patients). $V_D/V_{T_{IG}}$ was increased to 51% $\pm$ 1%. There was no significant difference between PaO_2 predicted from inert gas exchange and measured PaO_2, indicating that no diffusion impairment of gas exchange was present. The low cardiac output and a $P\bar{v}O_2$ decreased to 31 ± 2 mm Hg accounted for approximately 33% of the increased $P(A-a)O_2$. Gas exchange abnormalities correlated only roughly with the magnitude of pulmonary hemodynamic compromise, with correlation coefficients between the dispersion of the distribution of perfusion or $P(A-a)O_2$ and Ppa or pulmonary vascular resistance of no more than approximately 0.6 [40]. A similar pattern of abnormal $\dot{V}A/\dot{Q}$ was found in an additional patient with chronic thromboembolic pulmonary hypertension included in a study on patients with acute pulmonary embolism [12]. These investigators noted that patients with acute or chronic thromboembolic pulmonary hypertension could not be distinguished on the basis of hemodynamic, ventilatory, or gas exchange abnormalities [12].

Chronic thromboembolic pulmonary hypertension may be partially reversed by the administration of intravenous vasodilators in some patients [41]. This intervention is accompanied by an increase in cardiac output and an increase in PaO_2 as a consequence of increased $P\bar{v}O_2$.

B. Primary Pulmonary Hypertension

Primary pulmonary hypertension is primarily a disease of small muscular pulmonary arteries and arterioles, of a diameter less than 500 to 1000 μm, that presents with various combinations of medial hypertrophy, concentric or eccentric intimal fibrosis, and more complex arteritis, plexiform, or dilatation lesions, with in situ thrombosis in 30% of cases [42]. These findings contrast with predominantly proximal obstruction of the pulmonary arterial tree observed in chronic [39] or acute [43] thromboembolic pulmonary hypertension. However, patients with primary pulmonary hypertension also present with hypoxemia and hypocapnia [44]. These abnormal arterial blood gases are essentially explained, as in acute or chronic thromboembolic pulmonary hypertension, by a combination of increased ventilation, low $\dot{V}_A/\dot{Q}$ regions of the lung, and decreased $P\bar{v}O_2$ caused by a low cardiac output. Dantzker and Bower (45) reported the first MIGET study in four patients who presented with a mean Ppa of 62 ± 8 mm Hg, a cardiac output of 2.7 ± 0.5 L/min/m^2, a ventilation of 8.0 ± 0.6 L/min, a PaO_2 of 73 ± 10 mm Hg, a $PaCO_2$ of 28 ± 3 mm Hg, and a $P\bar{v}O_2$ of 33 ± 4 mm Hg. Shunt was $2.9\% \pm 1.8\%$, $V_D/V_{T_{IG}}$ was 39 ± 2, a mean of 10% of cardiac output (range, 2–19%) perfused lung units with a $\dot{V}_A/\dot{Q}$ less than 0.1, and there was no evidence for diffusion impairment as assessed by a good agreement between measured and inert gas predicted PaO_2. All of the hypoxemia was explained by the combined effects of decreased $P\bar{v}O_2$ and low $\dot{V}_A/\dot{Q}$ [45]. It is of interest that the investigators included in the same report three patients with thromboembolic pulmonary hypertension who presented very similar pulmonary hemodynamic and gas exchange abnormalities and grouped all of their patients under the global denomination "chronic obliterative pulmonary vascular disease" [45].

Exercise in patients with chronic obliterative pulmonary hypertension decreases PaO_2 and increases $P(A-a)O_2$, but does not increase $\dot{V}_A/\dot{Q}$ inequality or create a difference between measured and predicted PaO_2 [46]. Exercise-induced hypoxemia in chronic obliterative pulmonary hypertension is thus entirely explained by the effects of a decreased $P\bar{v}O_2$ in the presence of minor $\dot{V}_A/\dot{Q}$ inequality and is insufficiently mitigated by an increased ventilation [46].

Administration of vasodilators such as isoproterenol or nitroprusside in patients with chronic obliterative pulmonary hypertension decreases pulmonary vascular resistance and increases perfusion to lung units with a lower than normal $\dot{V}_A/\dot{Q}$ or shunt. However, this deterioration in $\dot{V}_A/\dot{Q}$ matching does not decrease PaO_2 because of an increase in $P\bar{v}O_2$ caused by an increase in cardiac output [33].

Administration of the calcium channel blocker diltiazem at a relatively low dose, with no effect on pulmonary vascular resistance at rest and a slight decrease in pulmonary vascular resistance at exercise, did not affect gas exchange [47].

We investigated the effects on pulmonary hemodynamics and gas exchange of two potent pulmonary vasodilators, prostaglandin E_1 (0.02 to 0.04 µg/kg/min intravenously) and nifedipine (20 mg sublingually), in five patients with primary pulmonary hypertension. Two of them have been reported previously [48]. The results are summarized in Table 1. The patients were hypoxemic because of a combination of low $P\bar{v}O_2$ and moderate $\dot{V}_A/\dot{Q}$ inequality, in keeping with previous observations. All of the patients had a bimodal pattern of $\dot{V}_A/\dot{Q}$ distributions (a major mode of normal $\dot{V}_A/\dot{Q}$ units with an additional small mode of perfusion centered on units with very low $\dot{V}_A/\dot{Q}$). Shunt ($\dot{Q}s/\dot{Q}t$) was small, except in one of the patients, who had a patent foramen ovale (Fig. 7). Prostaglandin E_1 decreased mean Ppa more than nifedipine did. Both drugs increased cardiac output, decreased pulmonary vascular resistance, and caused deterioration in $\dot{V}_A/\dot{Q}$ matching, with a shift of the blood flow distribution to lower $\dot{V}_A/\dot{Q}$ ratios. However, arterial blood gases remained unaltered, mainly because of the increase in $P\bar{v}O_2$. PaO_2 increased in the patient with a patent foramen ovale because of a decreased right-to-left cardiac shunt associated with decreased filling pressures of the right heart in response to decreased right ventricular afterload (Fig. 7).

Table 1 Blood Gases, Hemodynamic, and Gas Exchange Data in Five Patients with Primary Pulmonary Hypertension

	Baseline	Prostaglandin E_1	P[a]	Nifedipine	P[a]
PaO_2 (mm Hg)	62 ± 6	58 ± 5	NS	56 ± 6	NS
$PaCO_2$ (mm Hg)	31 ± 2	32 ± 1	NS	29 ± 2	NS
$P\bar{v}O_2$ (mm Hg)	29 ± 1	33 ± 2	NS	32 ± 2	NS
Cardiac index (L/min/m^2)	2.2 ± 0.2	3.0 ± 0.2	<.005	3.0 ± 0.1	<.001
Ppa (mm Hg)	60 ± 5	51 ± 6	<.01	58 ± 4	NS
Qva/Qt (%)	18 ± 5	24 ± 7	NS	25 ± 4	NS
Qs/Qt (%)	6.8 ± 3.6	6.3 ± 3.1	NS	6.0 ± 5.5	NS
Mean $\dot{V}_A/\dot{Q}$ blood flow	0.94 ± 0.15	0.56 ± 0.10	<.05	0.62 ± 0.06	<.05
Log SD $\dot{Q}$	1.49 ± 0.11	1.39 ± 0.17	NS	1.53 ± 0.13	NS
Mean $\dot{V}_A/\dot{Q}$ ventilation	2.01 ± 0.30	1.60 ± 0.24	NS	1.74 ± 0.09	NS
V_D/V_{TIG} (%)	46 ± 5	52 ± 8	NS	44 ± 4	NS
Log SD $\dot{V}_A$	0.50 ± 0.08	0.73 ± 0.10	<0.01	0.64 ± 0.08	NS

[a] P compared with baseline using modified t tests, after an analysis of variance.
PaO_2 = arterial oxygen partial pressure; $PaCO_2$ = arterial carbon dioxide partial pressure; $P\bar{v}O_2$ = mixed venous oxygen partial pressure; NS = not significant; Ppa = mean pulmonary artery pressure; Qva/Qt = venous admixture; $\dot{Q}s/\dot{Q}t$ = shunt; V_D/V_{TIG} = inert gas dead space; log SD $\dot{Q}$ = log standard deviation of perfusion distribution; log SD $\dot{V}_A$ = log standard deviation of ventilation distribution.

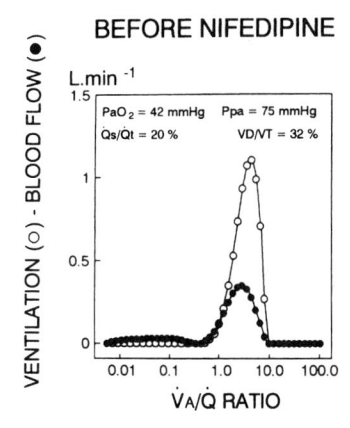

Pulmonary Vascular Diseases 299

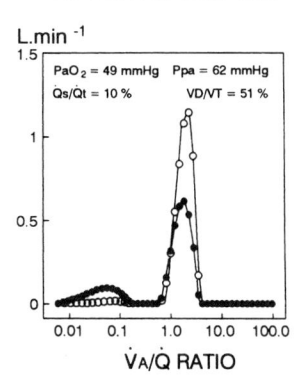

Figure 7 Ventilation–perfusion ($\dot{V}_A/\dot{Q}$) distributions before and after the administration of nifedipine in a 61-year-old woman with primary pulmonary hypertension. Before nifedipine, the $\dot{V}_A/\dot{Q}$ distribution showed a bimodal pattern with an additional low $\dot{V}_A/\dot{Q}$ mode and an increased shunt (Qs/Qt). Arterial hypoxemia resulted from an elevated shunt, partially because of a right-to-left atrial shunt demonstrated by contrast echocardiography, and a low mixed venous oxygen partial pressure ($P\bar{v}O_2$). After nifedipine, arterial oxygen partial pressure (PaO_2) increased as a result of the reduction in shunt and an increase in $P\bar{v}O_2$, in relation to increased cardiac output and decreased right ventricular afterload. Increase in inert gas dead space ($V_{DS}/V_{T_{IG}}$) was explained by a decrease in tidal volume. (From Ref. 48. Copyright 1983 by the American College of Chest Physicians, with permission.)

IV. Conclusions

Pathological processes limited to the pulmonary arterial tree such as in thromboembolic pulmonary hypertension or in primary pulmonary hypertension are associated with generally moderate alterations in pulmonary gas exchange, consisting mainly of an increased perfusion to lung units with a lower than normal $\dot{V}_A/\dot{Q}$. However, the associated hypoxemia may be severe because of the amplification effects of a reduced $P\bar{v}O_2$ related to a low cardiac output. Patients with acute thromboembolic pulmonary hypertension may present with aggravated hypoxemia caused by a secondary increase in pulmonary shunt related to the development of focal atelectasis or edema. A markedly increased shunt is sometimes observed in any patient with severe pulmonary hypertension in relation to secondary opening of a patent foramen ovale. All patients with pulmonary hypertension hyperventilate, which mitigates the hypoxemic effects of low $\dot{V}_A/\dot{Q}$ and low $P\bar{v}O_2$. The reasons for this increased ventilation, which decreases $PaCO_2$, remain unknown. Intravenous pulmonary vasodilators induce a further deterioration in $\dot{V}_A/\dot{Q}$ matching but most often do not significantly worsen arterial oxygenation because of an increased $P\bar{v}O_2$ caused by associated increases in cardiac output. Pharmacological pulmonary vasodilation may markedly improve arterial oxygenation in some patients by improvement of right heart failure, decreased right atrial pressure, and consequent decreased right-to-left cardiac shunt through patent foramen ovale.

References

1. Grossman W, Braunwald E. Pulmonary hypertension. In: Heart Disease: A Textbook of Cardiovascular Medicine, 4th ed. E Braunwald, ed. Philadelphia: Saunders, 1992, pp 790–816.
2. Manier G, Castaing Y. Gas exchange abnormalities in pulmonary vascular and cardiac disease. Thorax 1994; 49:1169–1174.
3. Dantzker DR. Ventilation-perfusion inequality in lung disease. Chest 1987; 91:749–754.
4. Wagner PD, Saltzman HA, West JB. Measurement of continuous distributions of ventilation-perfusion ratios: theory. J Appl Physiol 1974; 36:588–599.
5. Wagner PD, Nauman PF, Laravuso RB. Simultaneous measurements of eight foreign gases in blood by gas chromatography. J Appl Physiol 1974; 36:600–605.
6. D'Alonzo GE, Dantzker DR. Gas exchange alterations following pulmonary embolism. Clin Chest Med 1984; 5:411–419.
7. Lippmann M, Fein A. Pulmonary embolism in the patient with chronic obstructive pulmonary disease. Chest 1981; 79:39–42.
8. D'Alonzo GE, Bower JS, DeHart P, Dantzker DR. The mechanisms of abnormal gas exchange in acute massive pulmonary embolism. Am Rev Respir Dis 1983; 128:170–172.
9. Manier G, Castaing Y, Guénard H. Determinants of hypoxemia during the acute phase of pulmonary embolism in humans. Am Rev Respir Dis 1985; 132:332–338.
10. Huet Y, Lemaire F, Brun-Buisson C, Knaus W, Teisseire B, Payen D, Mathieu D. Hypoxemia in acute pulmonary embolism. Chest 1985; 88:829–836.
11. Manier G, Castaing Y. Influence of cardiac output on oxygen exchange in acute pulmonary embolism. Am Rev Respir Dis 1992; 145:130–136.
12. Santolicandro A, Prediletto R, Fornai E, Formichi B, Begliomini E, Gianello-Netto A, Giuntini C. Mechanisms of hypoxemia and hypocapnia in pulmonary embolism. Am J Respir Crit Care Med 1995; 152:336–347.
13. Dantzker DR, Wagner PD, Tornabene VW, Alazraki NP, West JB. Gas exchange after pulmonary thromboembolization in dogs. Circ Res 1978; 42:92–103.
14. Delcroix M, Mélot C, Lejeune P, Leeman M, Naeije R. Effects of vasodilators on gas exchange in acute canine embolic pulmonary hypertension. Anesthesiology 1990; 72:77–84.
15. Delcroix M, Mélot C, Vachiéry JL, Lejeune P, Leeman M, Vanderhoeft P, Naeije R. Effects of embolus size on hemodynamics and gas exchange in canine embolic pulmonary hypertension. J Appl Physiol 1990; 69:2254–2261.
16. Delcroix M, Mélot C, Lejeune P, Leeman M, Naeije R. Cyclooxygenase inhibition aggravates pulmonary hypertension and deteriorates gas exchange in canine pulmonary embolism. Am Rev Respir Dis 1992; 145:806–810.

17. Delcroix M, Mélot C, Vanderhoeft P, Naeije R. Embolus size affects gas exchange in canine autologous blood clot pulmonary embolism. J Appl Physiol 1993; 74:1140–1148.
18. Delcroix M, Mélot C, Vermeulen F, Naeije R. Hypoxic pulmonary vasoconstriction and gas exchange in acute canine pulmonary embolism. J Appl Physiol 1996; 80:1240–1248.
19. Mélot C. Relationships between gas exchange and the pulmonary circulation. PhD thesis, Free University of Brussels, Brussels, Belgium, 1989.
20. Hervé P, Petitpretz P, Simonneau G, Salmeron S, Laine JF, Duroux P. The mechanisms of abnormal gas exchange in acute massive pulmonary embolism (letter to the editor). Am Rev Respir Dis 1983; 128:1101.
21. Young I, Mazzone RW, Wagner PD. Identification of functional lung unit in the dog by graded vascular embolization. J Appl Physiol 1980; 49:132–141.
22. Caldini P. Pulmonary hemodynamics and arterial oxygen saturation in pulmonary embolism. J Appl Physiol 1965; 20:184–190.
23. Chernick V, Hodson WH, Greenfield LJ. Effects of chronic pulmonary artery ligation on pulmonary mechanics and surfactant. J Appl Physiol 1966; 21:1315–1320.
24. Swenson EW, Finley TN, Guzman SV. Unilateral hypoventilation in man during temporary occlusion of one pulmonary artery. J Clin Invest 1961; 40:828–835.
25. Johnson A, Malik AB. Effects of different-size microemboli on lung fluid and protein exchange. J Appl Physiol 1981; 51:461–464.
26. West JB, Mathieu-Costello O. Stress failure of pulmonary capillaries: role in lung and heart disease. Lancet 1992; 340:762–767.
27. Hlastala MP, Robertson HT, Ross BK. Gas exchange abnormalities produced by venous gas emboli. Respir Physiol 1979; 36:1–17.
28. Sharma GVRK, McIntyre KM, Sharma S, Sasahara AA. Clinical and hemodynamic correlates in pulmonary embolism. Clin Chest Med 1984; 5:421–437.
29. Bates ER, Crevey BJ, Remington Sprague F, Pitt B. Oral hydralazine therapy for acute pulmonary embolism and low output state. Arch Intern Med 1981; 141:1537–1538.
30. Tapson VF, Witty LA. Massive pulmonary embolism: diagnostic and therapeutic strategies. Clin Chest Med 1995; 16:329–340.
31. Mélot C, Hallemans R, Naeije R, Mols P, Lejeune P. Deleterious effect of nifedipine on pulmonary gas exchange in chronic obstructive pulmonary disease. Am Rev Respir Dis 1984; 130:612–616.
32. Mélot C, Lejeune P, Leeman M, Moraine JJ, Naeije R. Prostaglandin E_1 in the adult respiratory distress syndrome: benefit for pulmonary hypertension and cost for pulmonary gas exchange. Am Rev Respir Dis 1989; 139:106–110.
33. Dantzker DR, Bower JS. Pulmonary vascular tone improves $\dot{V}_A/\dot{Q}$ matching in obliterative pulmonary hypertension. J Appl Physiol 1981; 51:607–613.
34. Mélot C, Delcroix M, Closset J, Vanderhoeft P, Lejeune P, Leeman M, Naeije R. Starling resistor versus distensible vessel models for embolic pulmonary hypertension. Am J Physiol 1995; 267:H817–H827.
35. Calvin JE, Dervin G. Intravenous ibuprofen blocks the hypoxemia of pulmonary glass bead embolism in the dog. Crit Care Med 1988; 16:852–856.
36. Utsunomiya T, Krausz MM, Levine L, Shepro D, Hechtman HB. Thromboxane mediation of cardiopulmonary effects of embolism. J Clin Invest 1982; 70:361–368.

37. Leeman M, Naeije R, Lejeune P, Mélot C. Influence of cyclooxygenase inhibition and of leukotriene receptor blockade on pulmonary vascular pressure/cardiac index relationships in hyperoxic and in hypoxic dogs. Clin Sci 1987; 72:717–724.
38. Goldhaber SZ, Braunwald E. Pulmonary embolism. In: Heart Disease: A Textbook of Cardiovascular Medicine, 4th ed. E Braunwald, ed. Philadelphia: Saunders, 1992, pp 1558–1580.
39. Moser KM, Auger WR, Fedullo FF, Jamieson SW. Chronic thromboembolic pulmonary hypertension. Eur Respir J 1992; 5:334–342.
40. Kapitan KS, Buchbinder M, Wagner PD, Moser KM. Mechanisms of hypoxemia in chronic thromboembolic pulmonary hypertension. Am Rev Respir Dis 1989; 139: 1149–1154.
41. Dantzker DR, Bower JS. Partial reversibility of chronic pulmonary hypertension caused by pulmonary thromboembolic disease. Am Rev Respir Dis 1981; 124:129–131.
42. Pietra GG. The pathology of pulmonary hypertension. In: Primary Pulmonary Hypertension. Rubin LJ, Rich S, eds. New York: Marcel Dekker, 1997, pp 19–61.
43. Stein PD, Henry JW. Prevalence of acute pulmonary embolism in central and subsegmental pulmonary arteries and relation to probability interpretation of ventilation/perfusion lung scans. Chest 1997; 111:1246–1248.
44. Rich S, Dantzker DR, Ayres SM, Bergofsky EH, Brundage BH, Detre KM, Fishman AP, Goldring RM, Groves BM, Koerner SK, Levy PC, Reid LM, Vreim CE, Williams GW. Primary pulmonary hypertension: a national prospective study. Ann Intern Med 1987; 107:216–223.
45. Dantzker DR, Bower JS. Mechanisms of gas exchange abnormality in patients with chronic obliterative pulmonary vascular disease. J Clin Invest 1979; 64:1050–1055.
46. Dantzker DR, D'Alonzo GE, Bower JS, Popat K, Crevey BJ. Pulmonary gas exchange during exercise in patients with chronic obliterative pulmonary hypertension. Am Rev Respir Dis 1984; 130:412–416.
47. Crevey BJ, Dantzker DR, Bower JS, Popat KD, Walker SD. Hemodynamic and gas exchange effects of intravenous diltiazem in patients with pulmonary hypertension. Am J Cardiol 1982; 49:578–583.
48. Mélot C, Naeije R, Mols P, Vandenbossche JL, Denolin H. Effects of nifedipine on ventilation/perfusion matching in primary pulmonary hypertension. Chest 1983; 83:203–207.

11

Acute Lung Injury

CHRISTIAN PUTENSEN

University of Bonn
Bonn, Germany

I. Introduction

Acute lung injury (ALI) is associated with increased vascular permeability induced by inflammatory mediators generated outside of the lungs, resulting in interstitial pulmonary edema and alveolar collapse, or follows pulmonary consolidation caused by a direct injury to the lung parenchyma [1]. Consolidation of lung parenchyma or interstitial edema and alveolar collapse primarily in the dependent lung areas, with decrease in resting lung volume and lung compliance, result in a mismatch between ventilation and perfusion ($\dot{V}_A/\dot{Q}$). This $\dot{V}_A/\dot{Q}$ mismatch accounts entirely for the severe arterial hypoxemia observed during ALI [2,3].

Application of positive airway pressure has been commonly used to increase lung volume, recruit initially poorly ventilated or nonventilated lung units, and thereby improve ventilation distribution to well-perfused lung areas. The evolution of pathophysiological knowledge and technology has resulted in new techniques designed to improve $\dot{V}_A/\dot{Q}$ matching, and thereby oxygenation of the arterial blood in patients with ALI. This chapter attempts to clarify the principles of gas exchange abnormalities during ALI and the expected and observed effects of new strategies and techniques used in the treatment of patients with ALI on $\dot{V}_A/\dot{Q}$ matching.

II. Acute Injury of the Lungs

A. Definitions

In 1967, Ashbaugh et al. [4] first described the clinical syndrome of acute respiratory failure in adults after direct and indirect injuries to the lungs. The initial definition of the syndrome included widespread pulmonary infiltrates on chest radiograph, decreased pulmonary compliance, and severe hypoxemia refractory to an increased inspired oxygen fraction (FIO_2) in the absence of cardiac failure [4]. Minor changes of acute respiratory distress syndrome (ARDS) definitions have been proposed for at least two decades. Because of varying definitions, controversy exists not only over the frequency and outcome of ARDS, but also over the effect of various supportive therapies. All ARDS definitions tend to describe patients with severe respiratory failure and a mortality ranging from 40–70% [5]. A much larger group of patients will develop respiratory failure based on the same pathological mechanisms without the severe arterial hypoxemia and chest radiograph abnormalities observed in ARDS. The American–European Consensus Conference has defined ARDS as an ALI with diffuse radiographic infiltrates, a pulmonary artery occlusion pressure less than 18 mm Hg or no clinical evidence of cardiac failure, and an arterial oxygen partial pressure (PaO_2)/FIO_2 ratio less than 200 mm Hg [6]. The definition of ALI includes the same clinical criteria except a PaO_2/FIO_2 ratio less than 300 mm Hg [6]. Thus, ALI and ARDS represent different levels of pulmonary gas exchange disturbance caused by the same inflammatory reaction with increased vascular permeability.

B. Morphologic Findings

Although the chest radiograph typically shows diffuse alveolar infiltration [4], recent investigations suggest a heterogeneous distribution of collapsed alveoli in ARDS [7]. Computed tomography (CT) scans of patients with early ARDS have demonstrated radiographic densities corresponding to alveolar collapse localized primarily in the dependent lung regions, while the nondependent lung regions are well aerated [8,9]. It is interesting that in normal lungs, general anesthesia leads to alveolar collapse occurring immediately in dependent lung regions (see Chapter 6). Afferently, gravity plays a major role in localization of the abnormalities in both settings. The weight of the edematous lungs seem to be the main cause of alveolar collapse observed in mechanically ventilated patients with ALI [8–10]. The size and density of the lungs determine mainly the superimposed pressure on the most dependent areas of the lungs, which may vary between 4 cm H_2O in patients with mild pulmonary dysfunction and 16 cm H_2O in patients with ARDS [10]. It has been suggested that alveolar collapse should be prevented when positive end-expiratory pressure (PEEP) to a given lung region is at least equal or greater than the superimposed pressure [10]. Recruitment of dependent lung units has been shown to be a function of plateau pressure, being greater at 50 cm H_2O than at 21 cm H_2O [11]. The amount of dependent lung areas reinflated by plateau pressure that remains open at end-expiration depends on PEEP [11]. Nondependent lung areas are well aerated in early ARDS. The dimension of the aerated lung has been found to be similar to the dimensions of the lungs of a baby. Therefore, the term "baby lung" has been frequently used to characterize the ARDS lungs [9]. Because the compliance adjusted for the reduced aerated lung volume has been estimated to be normal during ARDS, the lungs have to be viewed small rather than stiff [8].

Ongoing ARDS may change the structure of the lungs. Edema may be partially resorbed, and fibrous processes may occur that prevent the persistence of compression atelectasis. In the late stage of ARDS, formation of bullae, indicating tissue lesions, has been observed mainly in the dependent previously consolidated lung areas [9].

C. Lung Mechanic Findings

Decrease in respiratory compliance is commonly observed in patients with ARDS [4,6]. Respiratory compliance correlates with the amount of normally aerated lung tissue observed in CT scans of patients with early ARDS [8]. Because the pressure/volume (P/V) relationship of the respiratory system is not linear, compliance may change with increase in lung volume. In early ARDS, lung inflation results in an inflection pressure (P_{inf}) on the static P/V curve (Fig. 1) that corresponds to a steep increase in compliance and indicates recruitment of most of the alveoli [12]. Further inflation of the lungs results in a linear increase in airway pressure until slope of the static P/V curve decreases. The corresponding deflection pressure (P_{def}) indicates overdistention of most of the alveoli [13]. In late-stage ARDS, when fibrosis is likely to have replaced edema, no P_{inf} but further decrease in slope of the static P/V curve has been observed.

Increasing PEEP in mechanically ventilated patients with early ARDS above P_{inf} corresponds to a significant increase in aerated lung tissue observed in the CT scan, decreases in venous admixture, and improvement of arterial oxygenation [12]. Therefore, a PEEP titrated above P_{inf} may recruit initially nonventilated lung units and prevent progressive loss of gas exchange area. Alveolar overdistention during inflation should be avoided by using PEEP to prevent alveolar collapse at end expiration, while minimizing the end-inspiratory lung volume below P_{def} [14,15]. Mechanical ventilation with normal lung volumes may overdistend functional lung units and contribute to $\dot{V}_A/\dot{Q}$ mismatch [2].

III. Pulmonary Gas Exchange in ARDS

A. Assessment of Pulmonary Gas Exchange

Routine assessment of pulmonary gas exchange during ARDS is based on analyses of Pa_{O_2} and arterial carbon dioxide partial pressure (Pa_{CO_2}). These variables, although sensitive to intrapulmonary factors ($\dot{V}_A/\dot{Q}$ matching and shunt in case of ARDS), are also affected by changes in extrapulmonary factors as cardiac output

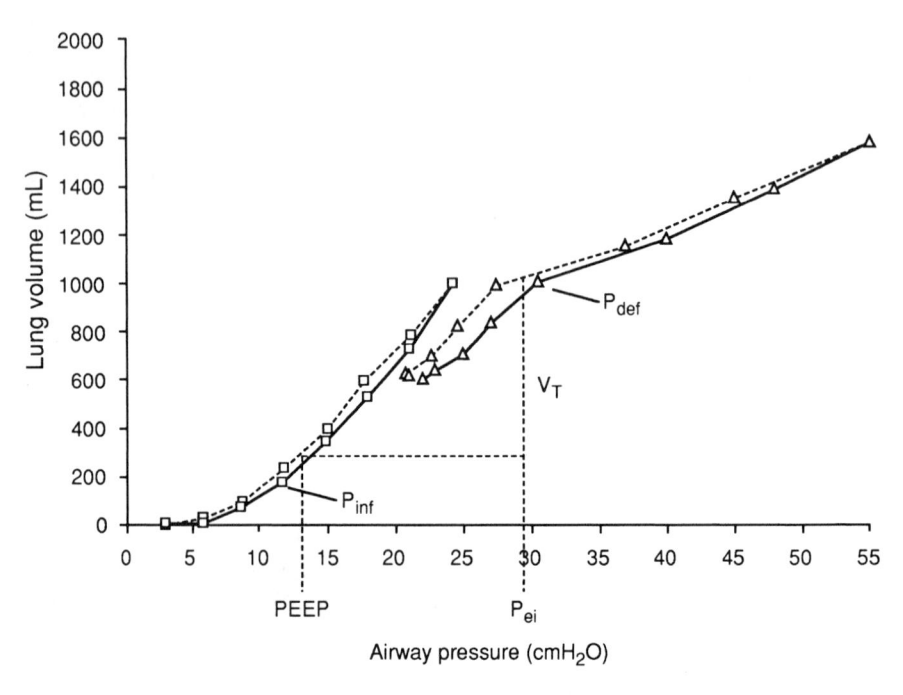

Figure 1 Pressure/volume relationships of the respiratory system in a patient with ARDS. The inflection pressure (P_{inf}) corresponds to step increase in compliance and indicates recruitment of alveoli. The deflection pressure (P_{def}) indicates a marked decrease in compliance and suggests alveolar overinflation. Titration of positive end-expiratory pressure above P_{inf} and end-inspiratory pressures below P_{def} is associated with best compliance and a decrease in venous admixture ($\dot{Q}_{VA}/\dot{Q}_T$) and volume of dead space/tidal volume (V_{DS}/V_T) (15).

(CO), oxygen consumption ($\dot{V}_{O_2}$), minute ventilation ($\dot{V}_E$), and F_{IO_2} [16]. Therefore, no index such as venous admixture ($\dot{Q}_{VA}/\dot{Q}_T$), derived from Pa_{O_2} and Pa_{CO_2}, adequately quantifies pulmonary gas exchange during ARDS. In fact, $\dot{Q}_{VA}/\dot{Q}_T$ cannot differentiate between poorly ventilated and shunt units, whereas physiological dead space (volume of dead space/tidal volume [V_{DS}/V_T]) cannot separate between poorly perfused lung units and dead space ventilation [17]. The multiple inert gas elimination technique (MIGET), using the elimination of inert gases of different solubilities (i.e., sulfur hexafluoride, ethane, cyclopropane, enflurane, diethyl ether, and acetone), allows the estimation of the continuous $\dot{V}_A/\dot{Q}$ distributions during ARDS [17,18], and thus enforces the aforementioned distinctions.

B. Shunt and Low $\dot{V}_A/\dot{Q}$ Units

Estimation of $\dot{V}_A/\dot{Q}$ distributions (using MIGET) has been performed in patients with ARDS only during ventilatory support (for clinical reasons). However, ventilatory support per se may significantly affect $\dot{V}_A/\dot{Q}$ matching [19]. In patients with ARDS, perfusion occurs in nonventilated (shunt) units ($\dot{V}_A/\dot{Q} < 0.005$) and in units with normal $\dot{V}_A/\dot{Q}$ ratios ($0.1 < \dot{V}_A/\dot{Q} < 10$) [2,3,20,21] (Fig. 2a). In some patients with early ARDS, a moderate fraction of perfusion is directed to units with a low but finite $\dot{V}_A/\dot{Q}$ ratio ($0.005 < \dot{V}_A/\dot{Q} < 0.1$; (Fig. 2b) [2,3,20,21], but it should be emphasized that the most important abnormality in most patients is shunt. Intrapulmonary shunting may occur for many reasons during ARDS: gas absorption caused by distal airway occlusion, a reduction in ventilation to below a critical $\dot{V}_A/\dot{Q}$ ratio, surfactant deficiency, or compression by the weight of the superimposed lung tissue. In early ARDS, intrapulmonary shunting has been found to correlate with the amount of nonaerated lung tissue identified as areas with Houdsfield units from -100 to 100 in the CT (Fig. 3).

Inspiratory Oxygen Fraction

Breathing high FIO_2 may cause absorption atelectasis when in the absence of the inert gas N_2, the O_2 net uptake by the blood exceeds alveolar ventilation. The effect of ventilation with high FIO_2 on intrapulmonary shunting in patients with ARDS depends largely on the presence of poorly ventilated lung units ($0.005 < \dot{V}_A/\dot{Q} < 0.1$). Dantzker et al. [22] have shown that the critical $\dot{V}_A/\dot{Q}$ level below which alveoli are vulnerable to collapse increases with FIO_2. Units with $\dot{V}_A/\dot{Q}$ less than 0.08 are likely to collapse on 100% O_2. Furthermore, an increased alveolar PO_2 (PAO_2) may release hypoxic pulmonary vasoconstriction (HPV) and increase perfusion in poorly ventilated lung units [22,23]. Because shunt accounts for most of the observed hypoxemia in patients with severe ARDS, pulmonary gas exchange may not be expected to deteriorate further during ventilation with pure oxygen [24,25]. In contrast, in ALI, poorly ventilated alveoli may contribute more to hypoxemia [23]. High airway pressures have been believed to prevent stability of theses alveoli with low $\dot{V}_A/\dot{Q}$ during mechanical ventilation with pure oxygen [25]. However, in ventilated patients with ALI, increasing FIO_2 from less than 0.4 to 1.0 for 1 hour has been observed to be associated with a 30% increase in pulmonary shunting [23]. Because blood flow to low $\dot{V}_A/\dot{Q}$ units remained essentially constant, increase in intrapulmonary shunting in these patients seems to be induced by absorption atelectasis rather than by release of HPV. Therefore, the lowest FIO_2 to assure adequate arterial oxygenation may be favorable to prevent progressive increase in nonventilated lung units from absorption atelectasis in ALI.

Cardiac Output

Alterations in CO have been shown to lead to directionally similar changes in intrapulmonary shunting in animals with induced lung injury [26] and patients with ARDS [27]. In an oleic acid–induced canine lung model, an increase in CO during dopamine infusion deteriorated, whereas reduction in CO caused by a decrease in venous return during mechanical ventilation improved intrapulmonary shunting

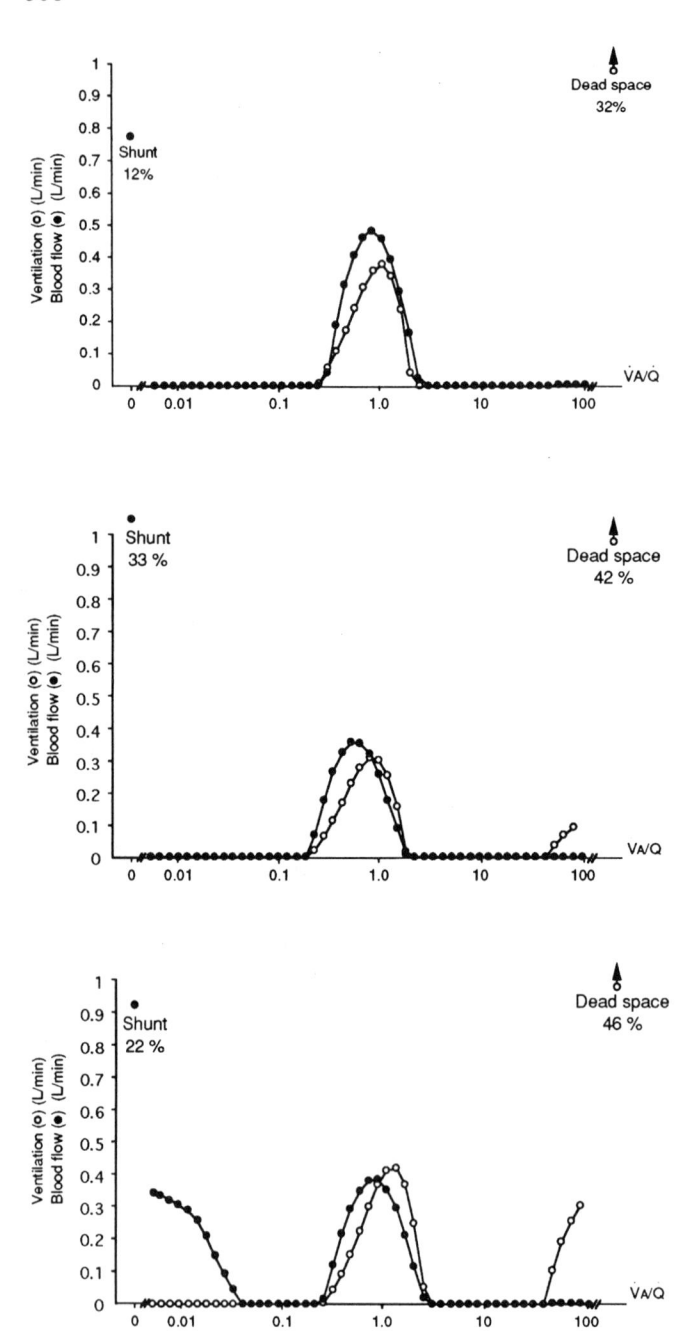

Figure 2 Representative distributions of ventilation (open circles) and perfusion (closed circles) plotted against a log scale of 50 ventilation–perfusion ($\dot{V}_A/\dot{Q}$) units in a healthy individual and two patients with acute respiratory distress syndrome.

Acute Lung Injury

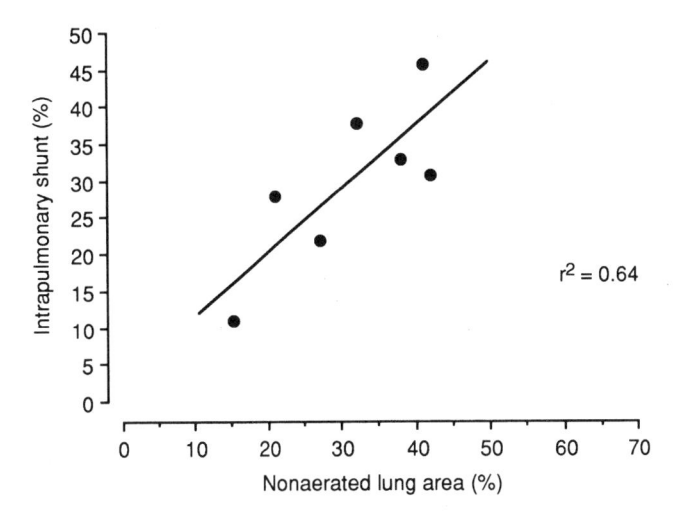

Figure 3 Relationship of the percentage of blood flow diverted to shunt units ($\dot{V}_A/\dot{Q} < 0.005$) and the percentage of essentially nonaerated lung tissue (-100 to 100 Hondsfield units) observed in the computed tomography scan in patients with acute respiratory distress syndrome.

[26]. A linear correlation between intrapulmonary shunt and CO has been observed in ARDS patients when CO was decreased by application of PEEP or of high V_T [27]. Based on these results, it was concluded that improvement in $\dot{V}_A/\dot{Q}$ matching during mechanical ventilation was at least, in part, caused by a concomitant depression in CO. In contrast, administration of dopamine in a dose from up to 12 µg/kg/min caused an increase in both CO and in intrapulmonary shunting in mechanically ventilated ARDS patients [28]. Similar results have been reported during infusion of dobutamine 5 µg/kg/min [29] and increased cardiac filling after blood volume expansion [30]. Unfortunately, in these investigations, changes in CO were produced by increase in lung volume or by infusion of inotropic drugs with pulmonary vasodilator or vasoconstrictor effects. Thus, the observed changes in $\dot{V}_A/\dot{Q}$ matching may not be entirely attributed to alterations in pulmonary blood flow. However, a linear correlation between intrapulmonary shunt and CO has also been observed in patients with ARDS when pulmonary blood flow was reduced during venoarterial lung assist while maintaining Pa_{O_2} constant [31].

The dependence of intrapulmonary shunt on CO has been explained by modulation in the vascular tone or vascular recruitment. An increase in CO has been claimed to increase perfusing pressure, resulting in vascular recruitment in nonventilated lung units [32]. However, experimental data suggest that as pulmonary blood flow is increased, the vessels supporting normal $\dot{V}_A/\dot{Q}$ units are first maximally distended and recruited, and then additional blood flow is directed to low $\dot{V}_A/\dot{Q}$ or shunt units [33]. Another factor that may change pulmonary blood flow distribution to nonventilated or poorly ventilated lung units observed with alterations in CO is the level of mixed venous O_2 tension ($P\bar{v}O_2$).

Mixed Venous P_{O_2}

Experimental data have indicated a direct relationship between intrapulmonary shunting and $P\bar{v}O_2$ during changes in FIO_2 or CO [26]. However, at constant $\dot{V}_A/\dot{Q}$ distributions, the effect of $P\bar{v}O_2$ on PaO_2 has been expected to depend mainly on the blood flow directed to shunt and low $\dot{V}_A/\dot{Q}$ units [22]. Therefore, in patients with ARDS, a decrease in $P\bar{v}O_2$ should cause a marked decrease in PaO_2. Recently, Roissant et al. [34] investigated the effect of changes in $P\bar{v}O_2$ on the $\dot{V}_A/\dot{Q}$ mismatch in patients with ARDS. Because these patients underwent extracorporal membrane oxygenation, $P\bar{v}O_2$ could be altered while maintaining FIO_2 or CO constant. Reduction in $P\bar{v}O_2$ in these patients did not affect $\dot{V}_A/\dot{Q}$ matching. However, in some patients, decrease in $P\bar{v}O_2$ was associated with a marked increase in the blood flow to shunt and low $\dot{V}_A/\dot{Q}$ units.

Hypoxic Pulmonary Vasoconstriction

The $\dot{V}_A/\dot{Q}$ mismatch during ARDS leads to alveolar hypoxia in nonventilated or poorly ventilated lung units ($\dot{V}_A/\dot{Q} < 0.1$), which, in turn, results in vasoconstriction of the perfusing arterioles [35]. The predominant stimulus for HPV is alveolar hypoxia, although lumenal pulmonary arterial hypoxemia augments this stimulus [36,37]. HPV diverts perfusion away from poorly ventilated or nonventilated lung units toward normally ventilated lung units, minimizes the effect of local hypoventilation, and promotes better $\dot{V}_A/\dot{Q}$ matching and gas exchange.

Pulmonary hypertension resulting from HPV, mediator release, and vascular obliteration complicates ARDS. Increased pulmonary vascular resistance may be associated with both structural changes in the pulmonary vasculature and right ventricular dysfunction or failure. Various vasodilator therapies are aimed at reducing pulmonary hypertension in patients with ARDS. However, intravenous vasodilators such as prostaglandin E_1 (PGE_1) [38,39] prostacyclin (PGI_2) [40], nitroprouside, ketanserine [41], calcium antagonists [42], and volatile anesthetics [43] release HPV and contribute to shunting of blood, $\dot{V}_A/\dot{Q}$ mismatch, and severe hypoxemia in ARDS. In contrast, inhalation of nitric oxide (NO) and aerosolized PGI_2 or PGE_1 in low concentrations has been shown to induce pulmonary vasodilation limited to ventilated lung areas, resulting in a redistribution of blood flow from nonventilated to ventilated lung units and an improved PaO_2 in patients with ARDS [44–46]. These findings indicate that inhalation of NO and aerosolized PGI_2 or PGE_1 apparently does not release HPV in nonventilated lung units.

Inhibition of NO synthase by L-arginine analogs has been found to enhance HPV in isolated lung preparations [47] and in animals with ALI [48]. These observations suggest that during hypoxemia secondary to ALI, NO released from endothelial cells attenuates HPV [48]. In addition, other locally released vasodilators such as PGI_2 have been shown to impair HPV [49]. Therefore, it has been suggested that endogenous release of NO and other vasodilators may contribute to impaired pulmonary gas exchange during ALI by increasing the $\dot{V}_A/\dot{Q}$ mismatch.

The contention that HPV can be enhanced has been supported by an increased pulmonary arterial pressure observed during infusion of almitrine bismesylate, a peripheral chemoreceptor stimulator with pulmonary constrictor effects, at a rate of 3 μg/kg/min in dogs while breathing 12% oxygen [50]. However, at a higher dose, almitrine has been demonstrated to inhibit HPV because of vasodilation, presumably mediated by release of endogenous PGI_2 [51]. In patients with ARDS, almitrine infusion improved PaO_2 because of a decrease in intrapulmonary shunting, whereas markers of low $\dot{V}_A/\dot{Q}$ ratios, including dispersion of pulmonary blood flow, remained essentially unchanged [52]. These results may indicate that almitrine redistributes pulmonary blood flow from nonventilated to well-ventilated lung units by a nonselective vasocontriction [50,52].

C. Dead Space Ventilation and High $\dot{V}_A/\dot{Q}$ Units

Distribution of ventilation to poorly perfused ($10 < \dot{V}_A/\dot{Q} < 100$) or nonperfused units ($\dot{V}_A/\dot{Q} > 100$) is commonly observed during ventilatory support with high V_T or PEEP levels in patients with ARDS [2,21]. Thus, ventilation distribution to high $\dot{V}_A/\dot{Q}$ or dead space units seems to correlate with the alveolar pressure and the mechanical properties of the lung units. In a canine model with oleic acid–induced lung injury, application of high inflation pressures caused compression of the intra-alveolar vessels in the nondependent lung areas, whereas the corner vessels remained perfused [53]. These histolgical findings corresponded to the appearance of high $\dot{V}_A/\dot{Q}$ units and an increased dead space ventilation [53]. Consequently, lung hyperinflation produces areas of high $\dot{V}_A/\dot{Q}$ or dead space units in ARDS. However, in animals without depression of CO, a unimodal $\dot{V}_A/\dot{Q}$ distribution was noted. Another explanation for the high $\dot{V}_A/\dot{Q}$ and dead space regions is related to microvascular obstruction, which has been reported in patients with ARDS [1].

Two mechanisms may essentially explain the occurrence of poorly perfused or nonperfused lung units in patients with ARDS during mechanical ventilation: (1) overdistension of the alveoli; and (2) redistribution of the blood flow caused by a reduction in CO. In dogs with normal and edematous lungs, increasing PEEP during mechanical ventilation with high V_T was associated with a reduction in CO and an increased ventilation of poorly perfused or nonperfused lung units [54]. In animals with normal lungs, this effect was most pronounced and caused retention of CO_2. In contrast, when, in animals with oleic acid–induced lung injury, ventilation with high airway pressures resulted in a recruitment of initially nonventilated lung units, decrease in intrapulmonary shunting was associated with no further increase in high $\dot{V}_A/\dot{Q}$ or dead space areas and a decrease in $Paco_2$. These findings may indicate that increase in high $\dot{V}_A/\dot{Q}$ or dead space areas and retention of CO_2 may mainly reflect overdistention of well-ventilated lung units during ventilatory support with high PEEP levels and large VT. In patients with ARDS, increasing PEEP up to 25 cm H_2O during mechanical ventilation with high VT of 10 to 18 mL/kg did not result consistently in an increase of high $\dot{V}_A/\dot{Q}$ units, dead space, and $Paco_2$ [2]. However, in these patients, relative hypovolemia indicated by pulmonal arterial occlusion pressures ranging between 3 and 18 mm Hg caused a marked reduction in CO that may not only explain the observed decrease in intrapulmonary shunting, but also vascular derecruitment of well-ventilated lung areas [2]. Ralph et al. [21] did not find an increase in $Paco_2$, high $\dot{V}_A/\dot{Q}$ units, and dead space while increasing PEEP from 0 to 25 cm H_2O during ventilation with VT of 10 to 12 mL/kg when CO was maintained constant. Recently, these results were confirmed in patients with severe ARDS during ventilation with moderate PEEP levels of 8 to 12 cm H_2O and VT of less than 8 mL/kg [34]. Similarly, when CO was maintained by infusion of dopamine, ventilation with high PEEP and VT did not cause high $\dot{V}_A/\dot{Q}$ units, and dead space increased only by 5% [20].

Unfortunately, the results of the inert gas measurements only quantify the high $\dot{V}_A/\dot{Q}$ mode and dead space ventilation and do not allow us to distinguish between between vascular derecruitment caused by overdistention or cardiac depression caused by increased intrathoracic pressure. Nevertheless, appearance of high $\dot{V}_A/\dot{Q}$ mode and dead space ventilation during ventilatory support may be an indicator for the risk of barotrauma in patients with ARDS.

D. Diffusion Limitation in ARDS

Intrapulmonary shunting, $\dot{V}_A/\dot{Q}$ inequality, and dead space ventilation has been observed to account entirely for the arterial hypoxemia observed during experimental induced lung injury and ARDS [1–3,20,21,26–28,38–42,45,55–61]. This concept is strongly supported by the close agreement between measured Pao_2 and the predicted Pao_2, which is derived from the excretion and retention of inert gases in patients with ARDS. Therefore, despite a histological observed interstitial thickening caused by edema, alveolar–capillary diffusion limitation does not contribute to hypoxemia in ARDS. However, $\dot{V}_A/\dot{Q}$ distributions in ARDS are determined mainly in patients in an early stage of ARDS. In contrast, in patients with fibrotic lung disease, alveolar–capillary diffusion limitation may contribute to arterial hypoxemia [62]. Based on these observations, it may be speculated that in a fibrotic stage of ARDS, alveolar–capillary diffusion limitation may also contribute to arterial hypoxemia. Unfortunately, currently there are no data available to answer the question of whether alveolar–capillary diffusion is a cause of arterial hypoxemia in late-stage ARDS.

IV. Therapeutic Concepts to Improve $\dot{V}_A/\dot{Q}$ Matching in ARDS

A. Improvement of Ventilation Distribution in ARDS

Optimized Ventilatory Support

In patients with ARDS, mechanical ventilation is commonly titrated according to arterial blood gas values. Recently, it has been suggested to set PEEP above the P_{inf} and to titrate V_T to produce an end-inspiratory lung volume below P_{def} determined from the static P/V curve of the respiratory system (Fig. 1) [14,15]. When PEEP is set above P_{inf}, initially nonventilated lung units are recruited. Reduction of end-inspiratory lung volume below P_{def} prevents alveolar overdistension. This strategy has previously been found to improve lung compliance, $\dot{Q}_{VA}/\dot{Q}_T$, and PaO_2, without causing cardiovascular impairment in patients with ARDS [14,15].

To the extent that mean intrathoracic pressure is elevated by the application of PEEP or high V_T, venous return and cardiac filling will decrease. This may lead to a reduction in CO and oxygen delivery (DO_2) if cardiac filling is not restored with fluid therapy. In addition, increased right ventricular afterload caused by compression of pulmonary microvessels and decreased left ventricular compliance caused by a leftward shift of the interventricular septum have been observed to reduce CO during positive pressure ventilation. The increase of PEEP, resulting in high end-inspiratory pressures in patients with ARDS, has been consistently shown to improve PaO_2 but to be frequently associated with a significant depression in CO and hence DO_2 [2,20,26,27,30,53]. Because appropriate fluid loading was not always effective to restore cardiac function during positive pressure ventilation, administration of inotropic drugs has been shown to improve CO without significantly affecting $\dot{V}_A/\dot{Q}$ matching and gas exchange [20]. However, the use of inotropic drugs to titrate CO above "supranormal" has not been shown to prevent multiorgan failure or improve outcome [63]. A careful titration of PEEP and V_T according to an optimal compliance may help to improve PaO_2 without affecting CO and hence DO_2 [14,15,64]. Spontaneous inspirations during sufficient partial ventilatory support cause periodic decreases in intrathoracic pressure and thus may increase venous return and cardiac filling and thereby CO [57,65,66]. In addition to an appropriate PaO_2 and CO, hemoglobin has to be kept at an adequate level to maintain DO_2. An adequate DO_2 is critical in patients with ARDS because of an abnormal relationship between DO_2 and $\dot{V}O_2$. When $\dot{V}O_2$ becomes DO_2-dependent, $P\bar{v}O_2$ may significantly affect gas exchange in patients with ARDS [16].

When cardiac function is normal, the filling of the right and left ventricle during diastole is the predominant determinant of the stroke volume and cardiac output. Spontaneous inspirations during sufficient partial ventilatory support cause periodic decreases in intrathoracic pressure, and thus increase venous return toward the right ventricle without increasing the systemic venous pressure [57,59,65]. Additionally, the outflow from the right ventricle (which depends mainly on the lung volume, the major determinant of pulmonary vascular resistance) may benefit from a decrease in intrathoracic pressure during partial ventilatory support. As a consequence, left ventricular filling can improve, and subsequently left ventricular stroke volume will increase.

Permissive Hypercapnia

In patients with ARDS, the concept of preventing end-inspiratory overinflation may result in "low" VT (< 6 mL/kg) and hypercapnia ($Paco_2$ > 60 mm Hg). This strategy of accepting a high $Paco_2$ is hypothesized to lessen barotrauma without compromizing tissue Do_2. However, acute hypercapnia and respiratory acidosis may aggravate the observed $\dot{V}_A/\dot{Q}$ mismatch in patients with ARDS [56]. Increased intrapulmonary shunting and $\dot{V}_A/\dot{Q}$ heterogeneity was observed in subjects with normal pulmonary function and ALI during hypercapnia [56], despite the known enforcement of hypoxic vasoconstriction by acidosis and hypercapnia. Increased $Paco_2$ in the presence of a low pH has been found to increase intrapulmonary shunting, which may explain the lack of sufficient improvement in Pao_2 observed in patients with ARDS ventilated with low VT to avoid alveolar overdistension [67]. Increase in intrapulmonary shunting was related to the significantly higher CO [67]. Although Pao_2 may not improve when reduction in VT is associated with a marked hypercapnia, the simultaneous decrease in intrathoracic pressure may improve systemic blood flow and oxygen supply.

Partial Ventilatory Support

Partial ventilatory support modalities provide either ventilatory assistance to every inspiratory effort and modulate the VT of the patient, such as pressure support ventilation (PSV), or modulate $\dot{V}_E$ by periodically adding mechanical insufflations to unsupported spontaneous breathing. New ventilatory support techniques such as biphasic positive airway pressure (BIPAP) [68], which is equivalent to airway pressure release ventilation (APRV) [69], provide ventilatory support by periodic switching between two levels of continuous positive airway pressure, while allowing spontaneous breathing throughout the ventilator cycle. In the absence of spontaneous breathing, APRV/BIPAP is identical with pressure-limited time-cycled mechanical ventilation.

Radiographic studies have shown a significant difference in the distribution of inspiratory gas flow between mechanical ventilation and spontaneous breathing [19]. Unsupported spontaneous ventilation is preferably directed to well-perfused, dependent lung regions, whereas a mechanically delivered VT is directed primarily to nondependent lung areas, away from regions with maximal blood flow [19]. Therefore, diaphragmatic contraction during partial ventilatory support may be expected to augment distribution of ventilation to dependent initially poorly ventilated or nonventilated, well-perfused lung areas and improve $\dot{V}_A/\dot{Q}$ matching in patients with ARDS [65].

Previous studies have corroborated findings regarding $\dot{V}_A/\dot{Q}$ matching between full and breath-to-breath synchronized partial ventilatory support. In patients with ALI, better overall $\dot{V}_A/\dot{Q}$ matching, unchanged intrapulmonary shunting, and increased dead space ventilation has been observed when comparing controlled mechanical ventilation with a combination of intermittent mandatory ventilation (IMV) and PSV [70]. Valentine et al. [71], who compared BIPAP/APRV and PSV at different pressure levels in patients recovering from open-heart surgery, found dead space to be considerably lower during BIPAP/APRV, whereas intrapulmonary shunt was not affected. However, it is difficult to evaluate the effect of the different ventilatory support modalities on $\dot{V}_A/\dot{Q}$ matching on the basis of these studies because the degree of the mechanical lung inflation was changed significantly during the investigations.

Experimental and clinical investigations have shown that minimal spontaneous breathing superimposed on mechanical ventilation during BIPAP/APRV contributes to improved $\dot{V}_A/\dot{Q}$ matching, systemic blood flow, and O_2 delivery, whereas $\dot{V}_{O_2}$ remained essentially unaffected by the work of spontaneous breathing. In an oleic acid–induced lung injury model, spontaneous breathing, accounting for 10% of $\dot{V}_E$ during BIPAP/APRV, could be attributed to a decrease in blood flow to shunt units ($\dot{V}_A/\dot{Q} < 0.005$) and an increased perfusion to normal $\dot{V}_A/\dot{Q}$ units ($0.1 < \dot{V}_A/\dot{Q} < 10$) [59]. The phenomenon that shunt units were converted directly to normal $\dot{V}_A/\dot{Q}$ units without creating regions of low $\dot{V}_A/\dot{Q}$ support the contention that initially collapsed lung areas are recruited with spontaneous breathing during APRV/BIPAP. In contrast, pulmonary blood flow distribution to shunt and normal $\dot{V}_A/\dot{Q}$ units during mechanical assistance of every breath with PSV was comparable to a pressure-controlled ventilation [57]. Consistent with these findings, in patients with ARDS, overall $\dot{V}_A/\dot{Q}$ matching, which was reflected by marked decreases in intrapulmonary shunt and dead space, improved during spontaneous breathing with BIPAP/APRV, while maintaining airway pressures limits or $\dot{V}_E$ constant (Fig. 4) [66]. In these ARDS patients, PSV did not provide any advantage in the $\dot{V}_A/\dot{Q}$ distributions when delivered with equivalent airway pressures limits or V_E [66]. These results indicate that uncoupling of spontaneous and mechanical breaths during APRV/BIPAP contributes essentially to improved $\dot{V}_A/\dot{Q}$ matching in ARDS. Apparently, the spontaneous contribution to a mechanically assisted breath is not sufficient to counteract the $\dot{V}_A/\dot{Q}$ maldistribution of positive-pressure lung insufflation during induced ALI or ARDS.

Prone Position

Because alveolar collapse is caused mainly by the adjacent pressure on dependent lung areas in ARDS patients, periodically changing the body position from supine to prone should decompress and reopen these lung units [10].

Evaluation of regional $\dot{V}_A/\dot{Q}$ distribution using the single-photon emission CT in an oleic acid–induced lung injury model indicates that during prone position, ventilation of dorsal lung units improved, whereas perfusion remained essentially

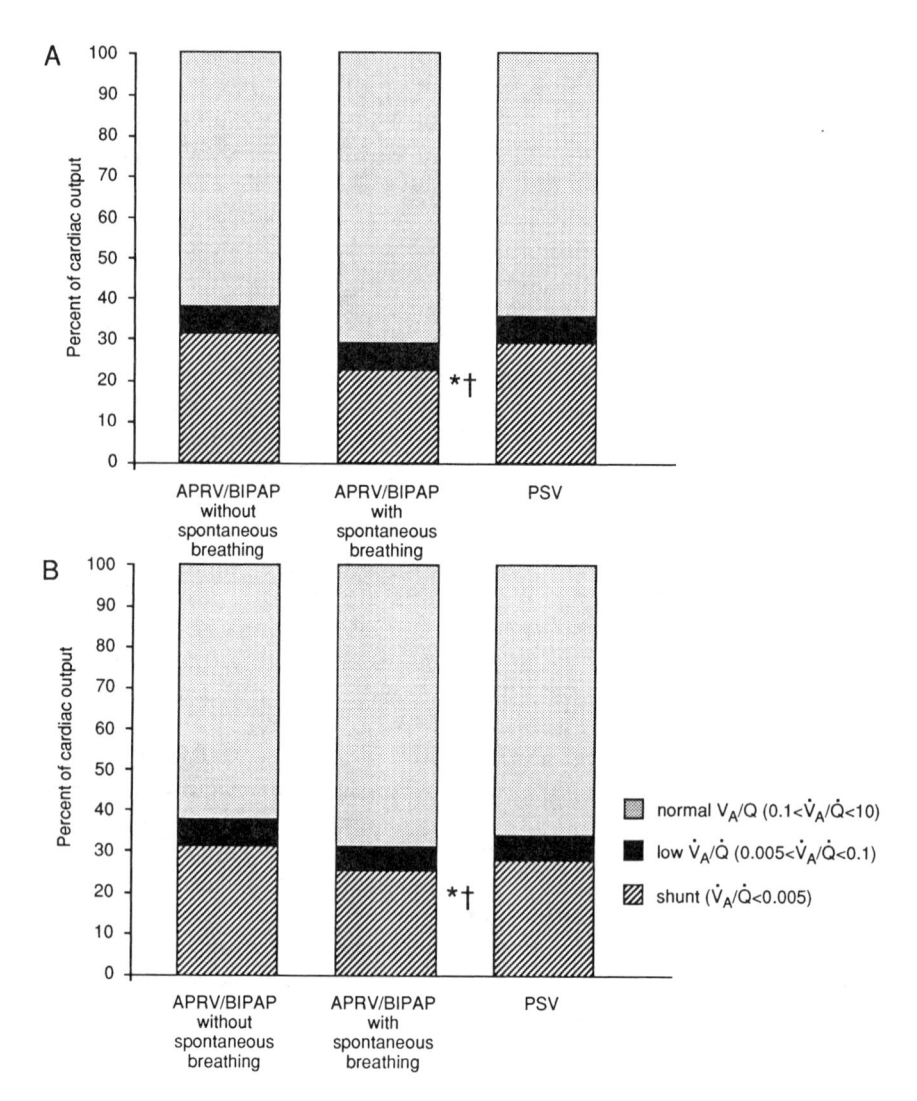

Figure 4 Distribution of pulmonary blood flow to shunt units ($\dot{V}_A/\dot{Q} < 0.005$), low $\dot{V}_A/\dot{Q}$ units ($0.005 < \dot{V}_A/\dot{Q} < 0.1$), and normal $\dot{V}_A/\dot{Q}$ units ($0.1 < \dot{V}_A/\dot{Q} < 10$) during airway pressure release ventilation (APRV)/biphasic positive airway pressure (BIPAP) with and without spontaneous breathing and pressure support ventilation delivered with equivalent airway pressure limits (A) or minute ventilation (B). * $P < .05$ vs. APRV/BIPAP without spontaneous breathing; † $P < .05$ vs. PSV.

unchanged [72]. Recruitment of dorsal lung units with decrease in intrapulmonary shunting should explain improved pulmonary oxygen transfer. In ARDS patients in the supine position, airway collapse indicated by areas of −100 to 100 Hondsfield units in the CT scan occurs in the paravertebral areas, whereas with patients in the prone position, it is more prominent in the parasternal lung regions [73]. This redistribution of density in the CT scan has been found to be associated with a decrease in $\dot{Q}_{VA}/\dot{Q}_T$ and an increase in Pa_{O_2}. Therefore, periodic prone positioning may promote recruitment of lung units while preventing excessively high PEEP levels. In 8 of 12 patients with ARDS, intrapulmonary shunting decreased and Pa_{O_2} increased during 2 hours in the prone position [74]. In the other four patients, $\dot{V}_A/\dot{Q}$ matching and Pa_{O_2} remained unchanged. Apparently, some patients with ARDS fail to improve or even show deterioration in gas exchange when turned from the supine to prone position. Currently available human data cannot explain the different response when a patient is turned several times from the supine to prone position and vice versa.

Partial Liquid Ventilation

During partial liquid ventilation (PLV), conventional gas ventilation is performed in lungs filled with perfluorocarbon to a volume equivalent to functional residual capacity (FRC; approximately 30 mL/kg) with a standard gas ventilator. The adequacy of perfluorocarbon dose is assessed during PLV by visually identifying perfluorocarbon within the tracheal tube at end expiration. Perfluorocarbons are structurally similar to hydrocarbons with the hydrogens replaced by fluorine. Perfluorocarbons are clear, odorless, relatively dense (1.7 to 1.9 mg/mL) inert fluids, immiscible in most solutions, and have excellent oxygen- and carbon dioxide–carrying capacities (50 mL O_2/dL and 180 CO_2/dL). In addition, perfluorocarbon lowers the surface tension in the alveoli. The efficacy of PLV in improving gas exchange has been investigated in various experimental models of induced lung injury but only in a small number of pediatric or adult patients with ALI.

In experimentally induced lung injury with and without surfactant deficiency, PVL has been found to increase end-expiratory lung volume, lung compliance, and to improve gas exchange, which may be suggestive for alveolar recruitment [75]. In patients with ARDS, PLV has been demonstrated to resolve the consolidations observed in the dependent lung regions [76]. Based on these data, it was claimed that perfluorocarbon, because of its density and higher hydrostatic pressure ("liquid PEEP"), which is higher in the dependent than the nondependent alveoli, may recruit collapsed lung units and improve $\dot{V}_A/\dot{Q}$ matching and gas exchange during PLV compared with gas ventilation in ARDS. In addition, the high hydrostatic pressure of perfluorocarbon may also redistribute pulmonary blood flow away from the dependent initially collapsed alveoli toward the nondependent well-aerated lung units, thereby further improving $\dot{V}_A/\dot{Q}$ matching during PVL [77]. In contrast, in animals with normal lungs, PLV caused a 50% increase in $\dot{V}_A/\dot{Q}$ heterogeneity but no significant increase in dead space ventilation [78].

In a series of adult and pedriatic patients with ARDS on extracorporal lung assist, PLV improved static lung compliance, $\dot{Q}_{VA}/\dot{Q}_T$, and arterial oxygenation over 72 hours [79]. Half of the administered perfluorocarbon evaporated from the lungs, on average, after 3.5 days in adult patients. Improved mucus clearance caused by the immiscibility of perfluorocarbon and an antiinflammatory effect during PLV has also been suggested to be beneficial in ARDS. In nine of ten patients with ARDS, responded with an marked improvement in arterial oxygenation during PLV over 96 hours [80,81]. Complications related to PLV in these patients were barotrauma and transient episodes of oxygen desaturation.

High Frequency Ventilation

Common to all high-frequency ventilation (HFV) techniques is a respiratory rate at least four times that of spontaneous breathing. The HFV techniques may not only differ in their system configuration, but also may have different effects on gas exchange. High-frequency positive pressure ventilation applies small V_T at 50 to 100 cycles/min with a conventional ventilator. During high-frequency jet ventilation, a high-pressure gas source injects small volumes of gas through a narrow catheter inserted into a common tracheal tube or integrated in the wall of specially designed high-frequency tracheal tubes. The injected gas augments the tidal gas volume. During high-frequency oscillation ventilation (HFOV), the oscillation of a piston pump or diaphragm causes an active inspiration and expiration phase of ventilation while fresh gas is supplied via a bias gas flow between the oscillator and the patient.

Because HFV delivers small gas volumes, it has been suggested that HFV may recruit lung units while avoiding alveolar ovedistention in ARDS. This would result in a better $\dot{V}_A/\dot{Q}$ matching and improved gas exchange. In animals with normal lungs, HFOV resulted in a high $\dot{V}_A/\dot{Q}$ mode [82]. The high $\dot{V}_A/\dot{Q}$ mode was caused by an enhanced transport of acetone in the conducting airways not caused by a disturbance of pulmonary blood flow distribution [82]. In a canine lung injury model characterized by large amounts of low $\dot{V}_A/\dot{Q}$ units, HFOV did not improve $\dot{V}_A/\dot{Q}$ matching and Pao_2 when compared with conventional mechanical ventilation [83]. In contrast, in other animal models of induced lung injury, an improvement in $\dot{Q}_{VA}/\dot{Q}_T$ and gas exchange was noted during HFOV [84]. Although HFOV has been shown to improve gas exchange in the neonatal respiratory distress syndrome [85], initial controlled and randomized trials failed to prove HFOV or another HFV technique as beneficial in ARDS. However, a recent pilot study observed improved arterial oxygenation with HFV in patients with ARDS that experienced failure with conventional ventilation [86].

Surfactant Replacement

Pulmonary surfactant is a complex of phospholipids, neutral lipids, and specific surfactant proteins synthesized by pneumocytes type II, which lower the surface tension of the air–liquid interface of the alveoli, thereby preventing alveolar collapse. Several mechanisms of surfactant alterations in ARDS have been proposed: (1) lack of surfactant compounds (phospholipids, apoproteins) because of a reduced synthesis/release by injured pneumocytes or increased loss in the airways during mechanical ventilation; (2) inactivation of surfactant by plasma protein leakage; and (3) inhibition of surfactant by inflammatory mediators [87]. Surfactant replacement therapy with natural or processed (bovine or porcine surfactant extracts) surfactant preparations has been tested in patients with ARDS to improve lung volume by recruiting collapsed alveoli, thereby improving $\dot{V}_A/\dot{Q}$ matching and gas exchange.

In a homogeneous lung injury model, instillation of surfactant failed to improve $\dot{V}_A/\dot{Q}$ mismatch, whereas ultrasonic nebulization efficient delivered a functionally intact surfactant to the distal bronchoalveolar space, resulting in a better $\dot{V}_A/\dot{Q}$ matching and gas exchange [88]. However, in a multicenter, randomized, placebo-controlled trial of 752 patients with sepsis-induced ARDS, administration of an artificial surfactant as an aerosol showed only little effect on lung mechanics and gas exchange and did not improve 30-day mortality [89]. In contrast, Gregory et al. [90] demonstrated in a multicenter, randomized pilot study that the bolus administration of up to 400 mg/kg natural surfactant markedly improves arterial oxygenation and reduces ventilatory requirements and mortality. These data were confirmed by Walmrath et al. [91], who observed after bronchoscopic administration of 300 mg/kg natural surfactant in 10 patients with ARDS an immediate increase in PaO_2/FIO_2 from 85 ± 7 to 200 ± 20 mm Hg mainly because of a decrease in intrapulmonary shunting from $42\% \pm 4\%$ to $20\% \pm 2\%$. In 5 of these patients, a second administration of 200 mg surfactant was necessary because PaO_2/FIO_2 deteriorated again after 18 to 24 hours.

Although the results of recent investigations are encouraging, clinical studies are warranted to provide more information on the optimal surfactant dose, dose volume, administration frequency, time of administration, and type of surfactant preparation before surfactant replacement therapy can be recommended in patients with ARDS.

B. Improvement of Perfusion Distribution in ARDS

Inhalation of Nitric Oxide

Inhalation of NO in concentrations ranging from 0.1 to 40 parts per million (ppm) has been reported to cause selective pulmonary vasodilation and to improve pulmonary gas exchange in patients with ARDS. It has been suggested that inhaled NO by its lipophilic properties diffuses at a rapid rate directly into the smooth muscle of pulmonary resistance vessels in proximity of alveoli, where it activates soluble guanylate cyclase, increases intracellular guanosine $3',5'$-cyclic monophosphate, and causes relaxation [92]. Because NO reaching the intravascular space is inactivated by rapid and avid binding to hemoglobin, systemic hypotension is avoided. Most importantly, NO inhalation results in pulmonary vasodilation limited to ventilated lung areas. This should redistribute blood away from nonventilated to well-ventilated regions, thereby improving gas exchange.

Experimental [58,92,93] and clinical [45] observations suggest that selective vasodilation in ventilated lung regions with NO inhalation improves overall $\dot{V}_A/\dot{Q}$ matching and arterial oxygenation by diversion of blood flow from essentially nonventilated to well-ventilated lung units. Roissaint et al. [45] investigated inhalation of 18 and 36 ppm NO in 10 mechanically ventilated ARDS patients. Inhalation of NO reduced pulmonary vascular resistance, while redistributing blood flow from shunt to normal $\dot{V}_A/\dot{Q}$ units and improving Pa_{O_2}. It may be of importance that in these ARDS patients, pulmonary blood flow was diverted to shunt or normal $\dot{V}_A/\dot{Q}$ units. Increasing evidence indicates that only approximately 70% of the ARDS patients respond to NO inhalation with improvement in $\dot{V}_A/\dot{Q}$ matching and Pa_{O_2} [94]. Then, recruitment of lung units may be favorable to produce a beneficial effect of NO inhalation on $\dot{V}_A/\dot{Q}$ matching and Pa_{O_2} [93]. In contrast, in patients with chronic obstructive lung disease, NO inhalation may worsen $\dot{V}_A/\dot{Q}$ mismatch and Pa_{O_2} [95]. In these patients, intrapulmonary shunt is small, whereas low $\dot{V}_A/\dot{Q}$ units are the major contributors to hypoxemia. Apparently, in poorly ventilated lung areas, inhaled NO may reach the vasculature and release regional hypoxic vasoconstriction, thereby contributing to further $\dot{V}_A/\dot{Q}$ mismatch. Consequently, increased blood flow to low $\dot{V}_A/\dot{Q}$ units may explain lack of improved $\dot{V}_A/\dot{Q}$ matching during NO inhalation in nonresponding ARDS patients.

Although several clinical trials in patients with severe ARDS demonstrated some advantageous effects on cardiopulmonary function, prolonged routine NO inhalation is controversial in ARDS patients. A mulicenter trial could not demonstrate improved outcome in patients with ARDS, although NO inhalation improved their gas exchange. Frostell [96] considered NO inhalation for more than 1 hour only appropriate in life-threatening clinical situations when previously a short NO exposure demonstrated an individual benefit. However, in patients with severe ARDS who are not responding appropriately to optimized ventilatory support, NO inhalation should be definitively considered clinically to prevent hypoxemia or before initializing extracorporal lung assist [97].

Inhalation of Prostaglandins

The arachidonic acid metabolites PGI_2 and PGE_1 are pulmonary potent vasodilators. Intravenous PGI_2 and PGE_1 cause vasodilation in ventilated and nonventilated lung units, thereby worsening intrapulmonary shunting and arterial oxygenation [38–40]. Furthermore, intravenous PGI_2 or PGE_1 administration may contribute to systemic hypotension. Inhalation of aerosolized prostanoids is expected to cause vasodilation selectively in ventilated lung areas provided that the prostanoid does not diffuse from ventilated to nonventilated lung areas and is inactivated before reaching the systemic circulation.

Some studies corroborated findings regarding the effects of aerosolized PGI_2 on $\dot{V}_A/\dot{Q}$ matching. Although PGI_2 is not inactivated within the lungs, no systemic effects were noted. In patients with ARDS, inhalation of NO or 17 to 50 ng/kg/min aerosolized PGI$_2$ has been found to improve pulmonary vascular resistance and Pa$_{O_2}$ without systemic vasodilation [60]. In patients with pneumonia-induced severe ARDS, inhalation of 6.6 ng/kg/min aerosolized PGI$_2$ was sufficient to decrease intrapulmonary shunting and increase arterial oxygenation [44]. Not surprisingly, in patients with interstitial fibrosis, increasing the dose of inhaled aerosolized PGI$_2$ to 33.6 ng/kg/min had no effect on the pulmonary vascular tone or $\dot{V}_A/\dot{Q}$ matching [44]. Similarly, inhalation of aerosolized PGE$_1$, which is deactivated rapidly within the lungs, and NO in low concentrations equivalently reduced $\dot{Q}_{VA}/\dot{T}$ and improved arterial oxygenation in patients with ARDS [46]. Although limited experimental and clinical data indicate that inhalation of aerosolized prostanoids in low concentrations improve $\dot{V}_A/\dot{Q}$ matching, further investigations are necessary to evaluate the advantage of inhaled prostanoids in critically ill patients with ARDS.

Pulmonary Vasoconstriction

Intravenous almitrine bismesylate has been suggested to enhance HPV and improve gas exchange [50]. Infusion of almitrine in a low dose to patients with ARDS increased pulmonary arterial pressure and Pa$_{O_2}$ while decreasing intrapulmonary shunt [52]. Thus, these data suggest that almitrine increases nonselectively the tone of the pulmonary vasculature, thereby redistributing the blood flow from nonventilated to well-ventilated lung areas and improving Pa$_{O_2}$.

Although the increase in the slightly elevated pulmonary arterial pressure has not been observed to be associated with a decrease in CO during almitrine infusion, an increase in pulmonary arterial pressure in ARDS patients with significant pulmonary hypertension can result in right ventricular failure and reduced systemic blood flow. In contrast to alminitrine infusion, NO inhalation, because of the selective pulmonary vasoldilation, provides a decrease of the elevated pulmonary arterial pressure and improvement in gas exchange in ARDS patients.

Combined Selective Pulmonary Vasodilation and Vasoconstriction

Endogenous NO synthesized from endogenous L-arginine by a NO synthase system causes vascular smooth muscle relaxation and vasodilation. Inhibitors of NO synthase, such as N^G-monomethyl-L-arginine (L-NMMA) or nitro^G-L-arginine-methyl-esther (L-NAME), enhance HPV in animals with induced lung injury [48]. These observations suggest that during hypoxemia secondary to ARDS, NO released from endothelial cells attenuates HPV. Therefore, endogenous NO release may contribute to impaired gas exchange during ARDS by increasing $\dot{V}_A/\dot{Q}$ mismatch.

Experimental data from an oleic acid–induced lung injury model showed that systemic L-NMMA administration alone did not affect $\dot{V}_A/\dot{Q}$ inequality and gas exchange. NO inhalation improved gas exchange by redistributing blood flow from shunt to normal $\dot{V}_A/\dot{Q}$ units [58]. Improved $\dot{V}_A/\dot{Q}$ matching and gas exchange was most pronounced when NO was inhaled in the presence of systemic L-NMMA

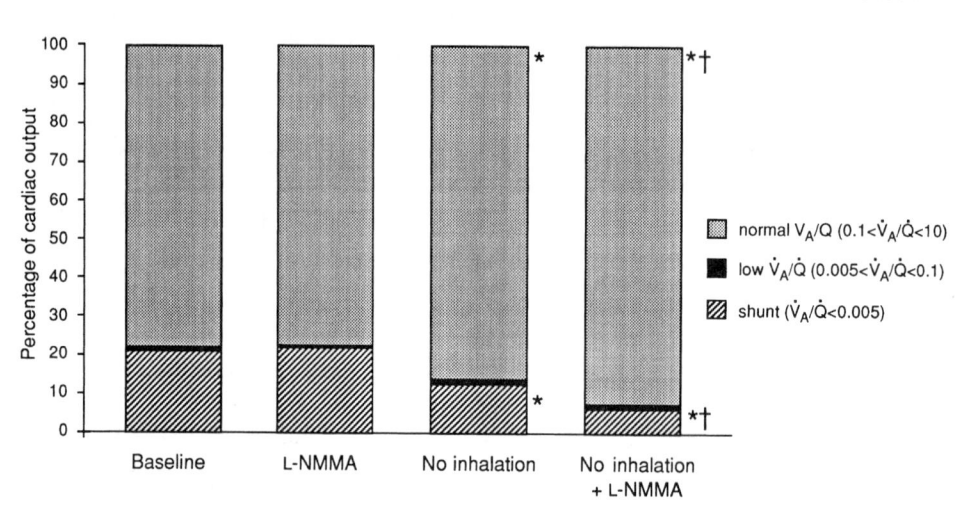

Figure 5 Distribution of pulmonary blood flow to shunt units ($\dot{V}_A/\dot{Q} < 0.005$), low $\dot{V}_A/\dot{Q}$ units ($0.005 < \dot{V}_A/\dot{Q} < 0.1$), and normal $\dot{V}_A/\dot{Q}$ units ($0.1 < \dot{V}_A/\dot{Q} < 10$) during absence of nitrous oxide (NO) inhalation or L-NMMA (control), L-NMMA infusion (5 mg/kg/h), NO inhalation (40 ppm), and L-NMMA infusion + NO (58). * $P < .05$ vs. baseline; † $P < .05$ vs. NO inhalation.

(Fig. 5). These data suggest that exogenous inhaled NO effectively reduces $\dot{V}_A/\dot{Q}$ mismatch during ALI and that this effect can be augmented by inhibiting the production of endogenous NO.

In patients with ARDS, infusion of the vasoconstrictor almitrine bismesylate improved Pa_{O_2} during NO inhalation, while pulmonary vascular resistance remained unaffected [94]. However, controlled clinical investigations are required to evaluate if enhancement of HPV during NO inhalation is advantageous in ARDS patients.

V. Conclusion

Recent developments demonstrated that in ARDS, the weight of the edematous lung causes alveolar collapse primarily in dependent lung areas, resulting in small lung volumes and a $\dot{V}_A/\dot{Q}$ mismatch that accounts entirely for the observed arterial hypoxemia. Positive airway pressures have been commonly applied to increase lung volume, recruit initially poorly ventilated or nonventilated lung units, and improve ventilation distribution to well-perfused lung areas. Minimal spontaneous breathing during BIPAP/APRV contributes to improved $\dot{V}_A/\dot{Q}$ matching, apparently by increasing ventilation of initially nonventilated or poorly ventilated lung units during diaphragmatic contraction. These data support the contention that mechanical ventilatory support techniques should allow unrestricted breathing throughout the mechanical cycle. Because alveolar collapse in ARDS patients is caused mainly by the pressure from the weight of the lung on dependent lung areas, periodically changing the body position from supine to prone should decompress and reopen these lung units, reducing intrapulmonary shunting and improving arterial oxygenation. In the future, surfactant replacement and PLV may play a role in recruiting collapsed alveoli. Although recruitment of collapsed lung units is still considered a high priority, recent developments in the treatment of ARDS have introduced techniques such as inhalation of NO or PGI_2, which causes vasodilation selectively in ventilated lung units and redistributes blood flow from nonventilated to ventilated lung areas. These mechanisms may be augmented during simultaneous infusion of nonselective vasoconstrictors such as almitrine. Thus, better $\dot{V}_A/\dot{Q}$ matching in ARDS may be achieved with techniques designed to improve ventilation or perfusion distribution.

There is no current proof that any ventilatory modality or adjunct alter the outcome of critically ill patients with mild to severe pulmonary dysfunction [98–100]. However, prevention of hypoxemia still must be the major goal in the treatment of patients with ARDS. Therefore, the search for new techniques and use of available techniques or strategies designed to improve $\dot{V}_A/\dot{Q}$ matching and gas exchange must be considered justified in patients with ARDS.

References

1. Sibbald WJ, Bone RC. The adult respiratory distress syndrome in 1987: is it a systemic disease? In: Gallagher TJ, Shoemaker WC, eds. Critical Care: State of the Art. Fullerton: Society of Critical Care Medicine, 1987, pp 279–332.
2. Dantzker DR, Brook CJ, Dehart P, Lynch JP, Weg JG. Ventilation-perfusion distributions in the adult respiratory distress syndrome. Am Rev Respir Dis 1979; 120:1039–1052.
3. Wagner PD, Laravuso RB, Uhl RR, West JB. Distributions of ventilation-perfusion ratios in acute respiratory failure. Chest 1974; 65 (suppl):32–35.
4. Ashbaugh DG, Bigelow DB, Petty TL, Levine BE. Acute respiratory disease in adults. Lancet 1967; 2:319–323.
5. Krafft P, Fridrich P, Pernerstorfer T, Fitzgerald RD, Koc D, Schneider B, Hammerle AF, Steltzer H. The acute respiratory distress syndrome: definitions, severity and clinical outcome. Intensive Care Med 1996; 22:519–529.
6. Bernard GR, Artigas A, Brigham KL, Carlet J, Falke K, Hudson L, Lamy M, Legall JR, Morris A, Spragg R. The American-European Consensus Conference on ARDS: definitions, mechanisms, relevant outcomes, and clinical trial coordination. Am J Respir Crit Care Med 1994; 149:818–824.
7. Gattinoni L, Presenti A, mm Hgesin A, Baglioni S, Rivolta M, Rossi F, Scarani F, Marcolin R, Cappelletti G. Adult respiratory distress syndrome profiles by computed tomography. J Thorac Imaging 1986; 1:25–30.

8. Gattinoni L, Pesenti A, Bombino M, Baglioni S, Rivolta M, Rossi F, Rossi G, Fumagalli R, Marcolin R, Mascheroni D. Relationships between lung computed tomographic density, gas exchange, and PEEP in acute respiratory failure. Anesthesiology 1988; 69:824–832.
9. Gattinoni L, Bombino M, Pelosi P, Lissoni A, Pesenti A, Fumagalli R, Tagliabue M. Lung structure and function in different stages of severe adult respiratory distress syndrome. JAMA 1994; 271:1772–1779.
10. Pelosi P, D'Andrea L, Vitale G, Pesenti A, Gattinoni L. Vertical gradient of regional lung inflation in adult respiratory distress syndrome. Am J Respir Crit Care Med 1994; 149:8–13.
11. Gattinoni L, Pelosi P, Crotti S, Valenza F. Effects of positive end-expiratory pressure on regional distribution of tidal volume and recruitment in adult respiratory distress syndrome. Am J Respir Crit Care Med 1995; 151:1807–1814.
12. Gattinoni L, Pesenti A, Avalli L, Rossi F, Bombino M. Pressure-volume curve of total respiratory system in acute respiratory failure: computed tomographic scan study. Am Rev Respir Dis 1987; 136:730–736.
13. Tuzzo D, Roupie E, Darmon PL, Dambrosio M, Brochard L, Lemaire F. Correlation between P-V curve and CT scan in ARDS. Am J Respir Crit Care Med 1995; 151:A72.
14. Amato MB, Barbas CS, Medeiros DM, Schettino GdP, Lorenzi-Filho G, Kairalla RA, Deheinzelin D, Morais C, Fernandes EDO, Takagaki TY, De Carvallho CR. Beneficial effects of the "open lung approach" with low distending pressures in acute respiratory distress syndrome, A prospective randomized study on mechanical ventilation. Am J Respir Crit Care Med 1995; 152:1835–1846.
15. Putensen C, Baum M, Hörmann C. Selecting ventilator settings according to variables derived from the quasi-static pressure/volume relationship in patients with acute lung injury. Anesth Analg 1993; 77:436–447.
16. Rodriguez RR, Roca J, mm Hges A. Interplay of intrapulmonary and extrapulmonary factors on pulmonary gas exchange during weaning. Intensive Care Med 1991; 17:249–251.
17. Wagner PD, Laravuso RB, Uhl RR, West JB. Continuous distributions of ventilation-perfusion ratios in normal subjects breathing air and 100 per cent O_2. J Clin Invest 1974; 54:54–68.
18. Wagner PD, Naumann PF, Laravuso RB. Simultaneous measurement of eight foreign gases in blood by gas chromatography. J Appl Physiol 1974; 36:600–605.
19. Froese AB, Bryan AC. Effects of anesthesia and paralysis on diaphragmatic mechanics in man. Anesthesiology 1974; 41:242–255.
20. Matamis D, Lemaire F, Harf A, Teisseire B, Brun BC. Redistribution of pulmonary blood flow induced by positive end-expiratory pressure and dopamine infusion in acute respiratory failure. Am Rev Respir Dis 1984; 129:39–44.
21. Ralph DD, Robertson HT, Weaver LJ, Hlastala MP, Carrico CJ, Hudson LD. Distribution of ventilation and perfusion during positive end-expiratory pressure in the adult respiratory distress syndrome. Am Rev Respir Dis 1985; 131:54–60.
22. Dantzker DR, Wagner PD, West JB. Instability of lung units with low $\dot{V}_A/\dot{Q}$ ratios during O_2 breathing. J Appl Physiol 1975; 38:886–895.

23. Santos C, Roca J, mm Hges A, Cardus J, Barbera JA, Rodriguez-Roisin R. Patients with acute respiratory failure increase shunt during 100% O_2 breathing (abstr). Eur Respir J 992; 5 (suppl 5):272.
24. Lampron N, Lemaire F, Teisseire B, Harf A, Palot M, Matamis D, Lorino AM. Mechanical ventilation with 100% oxygen does not increase intrapulmonary shunt in patients with severe bacterial pneumonia. Am Rev Respir Dis 1985; 131:409–413.
25. Lemaire F, Matamis D, Lampron N, Teisseire B, Harf A. Intrapulmonary shunt is not increased by 100% oxygen ventilation in acute respiratory failure. Bull Eur Physiopathol Respir 1985; 21:251–256.
26. Lynch JP, Mhyre JG, Dantzker DR. Influence of cardiac output on intrapulmonary shunt. J Appl Physiol 1979; 46:315–321.
27. Dantzker DR, Lynch JP, Weg JG. Depression of cardiac output is a mechanism of shunt reduction in the therapy of acute respiratory failure. Chest 1980; 77:636–642.
28. Lemaire F, Regnier B, Simonneau G, Harf A. PEEP ventilation suppresses the increase of shunting caused by dopamine infusion. Anesthesiology 1980; 52:376–377.
29. Rennotte MT, Reynaert M, Clerbaux T, Willems E, Roeseleer J, Veriter C, Rodenstein D, Frans A. Effects of two inotropic drugs, dopamine und dobutamine, on pulmonary gas exchange in artificially ventilated patients. Intensive Care Med 1989; 15:160–165.
30. Jardin F, Eveleigh MC, Gurdjian F, Delille F, Margairaz A. Venous admixture in human septic shock: cooperative effect of blood volume expansion, dopamine infusion and isoproterenol infusion or mismatch of ventilation and pulmonary blood flow in peritonitis. Circulation 1979; 60:155–159.
31. Lemaire F, Jardin F, Regnier B, Loisance D, Goudot B, Lange F. Pulmonary gas exchange during veno-arterial bypass with a membrane lung for acute respiratory failure. J Thorac Cardiovasc Surg 1978; 75:839–846.
32. Cheney FW, Colley PS. The effect of cardiac output on arterial blood oxygenation. Anesthesiology 1980; 52:496–503.
33. Wagner PD, Schaffartzik W, Prediletto R, Knight DR. Relationship among cardiac output, shunt, and inspired O_2 concentration. J Appl Physiol 1991; 71:2191–2197.
34. Rossaint R, Hahn SM, Pappert D, Falke KJ, Radermacher P. Influence of mixed venous PO_2 and inspired O_2 fraction on intrapulmonary shunt in patients with severe ARDS. J Appl Physiol 1995; 78:1531–1536.
35. Fishman AP. Vasomotor regulation of the pulmonary circulation. Ann Rev Physiol 1980; 42:211–220.
36. Domino KB, Hlastala MP, Eisenstein BL, Cheney FW. Effect of regional alveolar hypoxia on gas exchange in dogs. J Appl Physiol 1989; 67:730–735.
37. Domino KB, Cheney FW, Eisenstein BL, Hlastala MP. Effect of regional alveolar hypoxia on gas exchange in pulmonary edema. Am Rev Respir Dis 1992; 145:340–347.
38. Radermacher P, Santak B, Becker H, Falke KJ. Prostaglandin E_1 and nitroglycerin reduce pulmonary capillary pressure but worsen ventilation-perfusion distributions in patients with adult respiratory distress syndrome. Anesthesiology 1989; 70:601–606.

39. Mélot C, Lejeune P, Leeman M, Moraine JJ, Naeije R. Prostaglandin E_1 in the adult respiratory distress syndrome. Am Rev Respir Dis 1989; 139:106–110.
40. Radermacher P, Santak B, Wust HJ, Tarnow J, Falke KJ. Prostacyclin for the treatment of pulmonary hypertension in the adult respiratory distress syndrome: effects on pulmonary capillary pressure and ventilation-perfusion distributions. Anesthesiology 1990; 72:238–244.
41. Radermacher P, Huet Y, Pluskwa F, Herigault R, Mal H, Teisseire B, Lemaire F. Comparison of ketanserin and sodium nitroprusside in patients with severe ARDS. Anesthesiology 1988; 68:152–157.
42. Mélot C, Naeije R, Mols P, Hallemans R, Lejeune P, Jaspar N. Pulmonary vascular tone improves pulmonary gas exchange in the adult respiratory distress syndrome. Am Rev Respir Dis 1987; 136:1232–1236.
43. Putensen G, Putensen C, Hodges MR. Isoflurane increases ventilation-perfusion mismatch in canine acute lung injury. Crit Care Med 1994; 21:A96.
44. Walmrath D, Schneider T, Pilch J, Schermuly R, Grimminger F, Seeger W. Effects of aerosolized prostacyclin in severe pneumonia: impact of fibrosis. Am J Respir Crit Care Med 1995; 151:724–730.
45. Rossaint R, Falke KJ, Lopez F, Slama K, Pison U, Zapol WM. Inhaled nitric oxide for the adult respiratory distress syndrome. N Engl J Med 1993; 328:399–405.
46. Putensen C, Hörmann C, Kleinsasser A, Putensen-Himmer G. Cardiopulmonary effects of aerosolized prostaglandin E_1 and nitric oxide inhalation in patients with acute respiratory distress syndrome. Am J Respir Crit Care Med 1998; 157:1743–1747.
47. Archer SL, Tolins JP, Raij L, Weir EK. Hypoxic pulmonary vasoconstriction is enhanced by inhibition of the synthesis of an endothelium derived relaxing factor. Bioch Biophys Res Commun 1989; 164:1198–1205.
48. Leeman M, De BV, Gilbert E, Mélot C, Naeije R. Is nitric oxide released in oleic acid lung injury? J Appl Physiol 1993; 74:650–654.
49. Martin LD, Barnes SD, Wetzel RC. Acute hypoxia alters eicosanoid production of perfused pulmonary artery endothelial cells in culture. Prostaglandins 1992; 43:371–382.
50. Romaldini H, Rodriguez-Roisin R, Wagner PD, West JB. Enhancement of hypoxic pulmonary vasoconstriction by almitrine in the dog. Am Rev Respir Dis 1983; 128:288–293.
51. Mélot C, Dechamps P, Hallemans R, Decroly P, Mols P. Enhancement of hypoxic pulmonary vasoconstriction by low dose almitrinebismesylate in normal humans. Am Rev Respir Dis 1989; 139:111–119.
52. Reyes A, Roca J, Rodriguez RR, mm Hges A, Ussetti P, Wagner PD. Effect of almitrine on ventilation-perfusion distribution in adult respiratory distress syndrome. Am Rev Respir Dis 1988; 137:1062–1067.
53. Hedenstierna G, White FC, Mazzone R, Wagner PD. Redistribution of pulmonary blood flow in the dog with PEEP ventilation. J Appl Physiol 1979; 46:278–287.
54. Dueck R, Wagner PD, West JB. Effects of positive end-expiratory pressure on gas exchange in dogs with normal and edematous lungs. Anesthesiology 1977; 47:359–366.
55. Dantzker DR. Gas exchange in acute lung injury. Crit Care Clin 1986; 2:527–536.

56. Domino KB, Lu Y, Eisenstein BL, Hlastala MP. Hypocapnia worsens arterial blood oxygenation and increases $\dot{V}_A/\dot{Q}$ heterogeneity in canine pulmonary edema. Anesthesiology 1993; 78:91–99.
57. Putensen C, Räsänen J, Lopez FA, Downs JB. Effect of interfacing between spontaneous breathing and mechanical cycles on the ventilation-perfusion distribution in canine lung injury. Anesthesiology 1994; 81:921–930.
58. Putensen C, Räsänen J, Downs JB. Effect of endogenous and inhaled nitric oxide on the ventilation-perfusion relationships in oleic-acid lung injury. Am J Respir Crit Care Med 1994; 150:330–336.
59. Putensen C, Räsänen J, Lopez FA. Ventilation-perfusion distributions during mechanicall ventilation with superimposed spontaneous breathing in canine lung injury. Am J Respir Crit Care Med 1994; 150:101–108.
60. Walmrath D, Schneider T, Schermuly R, Olschewski H, Grimminger F, Seeger W. Direct comperison of inhaled nitric oxide and aerosolized prostacyclin in acute respiratory distress syndrome. Am J Respir Crit Care Med 1996; 153:991–996.
61. Walmrath D, Schneider T, Pilch J, Grimminger F, Seeger W. Aerosolised prostacyclin in adult respiratory distress syndrome. Lancet 1993; 342:961–962.
62. Agusti AG, Roca J, Gea J, Wagner PD, Xaubet A, Rodriguez-Roisin R. Mechanisms of gas-exchange impairment in idiopathic pulmonary fibrosis. Am Rev Respir Dis 1991; 143:219–225.
63. Gattinoni L, Brazzi, L, Pelosi P, Latini R, Tognoni G, Pesenti A, Fumagalli R. A trial of goal oriented hemodynamic therapy in critical ill patients. N Engl J Med 1995; 333:1025–1032.
64. Ranieri VM, Mascia L, Fiore T, Bruno F, Brienza A, Giuliani R. Cardiorespiratory effects of positive end-expiratory pressure during progressive tidal volume reduction (permissive hypercapnia) in patients with acute respiratoy distress syndrome. Anesthesiology 1995; 83:710–720.
65. Weisman IM, Rinaldo JE, Rogers RM, Sanders MH. Intermittent mandatory ventilation. Am Rev Respir Dis 1983; 127:641–647.
66. Putensen C, Mutz NJ, Putensen-Himmer G, Zinserling J. Spontaneous breathing during ventilatory support improves ventilation-perfusion distributions in patients with acute respiratory distress syndrome. Am J Respir Crit Care Med 1999; 159:1241–1248.
67. Langeron O, Delclaux C, Roupie E, Herigault R, Adnot S, Brochard L, Lemaire F. Hemodynamics and gas exchange alterations due to permissive hypercapnia in human ARDS: a multiple inert gas elimination technique (MIGET) study. Am Rev Respir Dis 1994; 149:A420.
68. Baum M, Benzer H, Putensen C, Koller W, Putz G. Biphasic positive airway pressure (BIPAP): a new form of augmented ventilation. Anaesthesist 1989; 38:452–458.
69. Stock MC, Downs JB, Frolicher DA. Airway pressure release ventilation. Crit Care Med 1987; 15:462–466.
70. Santak B, Radermacher P, Sandmann W, Falke KJ. Influence of SIMV plus inspiratory pressure support on $\dot{V}_A/\dot{Q}$ distributions during postoperative weaning. Intensive Care Med 1991; 17:136–140.
71. Valentine DD, Hammond MD, Downs JB, Sears NJ, Sims WR. Distribution of ventilation and perfusion with different modes of mechanical ventilation. Am Rev Respir Dis 1991; 143:1262–1266.

72. Albert RK, Leasa D, Sanderson M, Robertson HT, Hlastala MP. The prone position improves arterial oxygenation and reduces shunt in oleic-acid-induced acute lung injury. Am Rev Respir Dis 1987; 135:628–633.
73. Gattinoni L, Pelosi P, Vitale G, Pesenti A, D'Andrea L, Mascheroni D. Body position changes redistribute lung computed-tomographic density in patients with acute respiratory failure. Anesthesiology 1991; 74:15–23.
74. Pappert D, Rossaint R, Slama K, Gruning T, Falke KJ. Influence of positioning on ventilation-perfusion relationships in severe adult respiratory distress syndrome. Chest 1994; 106:1511–1516.
75. Hirschl RB, Tooley R, Parent AC, Johnson K, Bartlett RH. Perfluorocarbon-associated gas exchange in normal and acid-injured-large sheep. Chest 1995; 108:500–508.
76. Meanly JF, Kazerooni EA, Garver KA, Hirschl RB. Acute respiratory distress syndrome: CT findings during partial liquid ventilation. Radiology 1997; 202:570–573.
77. Lowe C, Schaffer T. Pulmonary vascular resiistance in the perfluorocarbon-filled lung. J Appl Physiol 1986; 60:154–159.
78. Mates EA, Hildebrandt J, Jackson JC, Tarczy-Hornoch P, Hlastala MP. Shunt and ventilation-perfusion distribution during partial liquid ventilation in healthy pigs. J Appl Physiol 1997; 82:933–942.
79. Hirschl RB, Tooley R, Parent A, Johnson K, Bartlett RH. Evaluation of gas exchange, pulmonary compliance, and lung injury during total and partial liquid ventilation in acute respiratory distress syndrome. Crit Care Med 1996; 24:1001–1008.
80. Gauger PG, Overbeck MC, Koeppe RA, Shulkin BL, Hrycko JN, Weber ED, Hirschl RB. Distribution of pulmonary blood flow and total lung water during partial liquid ventilation in acute lung injury. Surgery 1997; 122:313–323.
81. Hirschl RB, Pranikoff T, Wise C, Overbeck MC, Gauger P, Schreiner RJ, Dechert R, Bartlett RH. Initial experience with partial liquid ventilation in adult patients with the acute respiratory distress syndrome. JAMA 1996; 275:383–389.
82. Mc Evoy RD, Davies NJH, Mannino FL, Prutow RJ, Schumacker PT, Wagner PD, West JB. Pulmonary gas exchange during high-frequency ventilation. J Appl Physiol 1982; 52:1278–1287.
83. Kaiser KG, Davies NJH, Rodriguez-Roisin R, Bencowitz HZ, Wagner PD. Efficacy of high-frequency ventilation in presence of extensive ventilation-perfusion mismatch. J Appl Physiol 1985; 58:996–1004.
84. Euler US, Liljestrand G. Observations on the pulmonary aterial blood pressure. Acta Physiol Scand 1946; 12:301–320.
85. HFV Group. High-frequency oscillation ventilation compared with conventional ventilation of the respiratory failure in preterm infants. N Engl J Med 1989; 320: 88–93.
86. Fort P, Farmer C, Westerman J, Johannigman J, Beninati W, Dolan S, Derdak S. High-frequency oscillatory ventilation for adult respiratory distress syndrome: a pilot study. Crit Care Med 1997; 25:937–947.
87. Seeger W, Gunther A, Walmrath HD, Grimminger F, Lasch HG. Alveolar surfactant and adult respiratory distress syndrome: pathogenetic role and therapeutic propects. Clin Investig 1993; 71:177–190.
88. Schermuly R, Schmehl T, Gunther A, Grimminger F, Seeger W, Walmrath D. Ultrasonic nebulization for efficient delivery of surfactant in a model of acute lung injury. Am J Respir Crit Care Med 1997; 156:445–453.

89. Anzuetto A, Baugham RP, Guntupalli KK, Weg JG, Wiedemann HP, Raventos AA, Lemaire F, Long W, Zaccardelli DS, Pattishal EN. Aerosolized surfactant in adults with sepsis-induced acute respiratory distress syndrome. N Engl J Med 1996; 334:1417–1421.
90. Gregory TJ, Steinberg KP, Spragg R, Gadek JE, Hyers TM, Longmore WJ, Moxley MA, Cai GZ, Hite RD, Smith RM, Hudson LD, Crim C, Newton P, Mitchell BR, Gold AJ. Bovine surfactant therapy for patients with acute respiratory distress syndrome. Am J Respir Crit Care Med 1997; 155:1309–1315.
91. Walmrath D, Gunther A, Ghofrani HA, Schermuly R, Schneider T, Grimminger F, Seeger W. Bronchoscopic surfactant administration in patients with severe adult respiratory distress syndrome and sepsis. Am J Respir Crit Care Med 1996; 154:57–62.
92. Pison U, Lopez FA, Heidelmeyer CF, Rossaint R, Falke KJ. Inhaled nitric oxide reverses hypoxic pulmonary vasoconstriction without impairing gas exchange. J Appl Physiol 1993; 74:1287–1292.
93. Putensen C, Räsänen J, Lopez FA, Downs JB. Continuous positive airway pressure modulates effect of inhaled nitric oxide on the ventilation-perfusion distributions in canine lung injury. Chest 1994; 106:1563–1569.
94. Wysocki M, Delclaux C, Roupie E, Langeron O, Liu N, Herman B, Lemaire F, Brochard L. Additive effect on gas exchange of inhaled nitric oxide and intravenous almitrine bismesylate in the adult respiratory distress syndrome. Intensive Care Med 1994; 20:254–259.
95. Barbera J, Roger N, Roca J, Rovira I, Higenbottam TW, Rodriguez-Roisin R. Worsening of pulmonary gas exchange with nitric oxide inhalation in chronic obstructive pulmonary disease. Lancet 1996; 347:436–440.
96. Frostell CG. Nitric oxide inhalation: future drug or invitation to disaster? Paed Anaesth 1994; 4:147–150.
97. Guinard N, Beloucif S, Gatecel C, Mateo J, Payen D. Interest of therapeutic optimization in severe ARDS. Chest 1997; 111:1000–1007.
98. Amato MB, Barbas CS, Meddeiros DM, Magaldi RB, Schettino GP, Lorenzi-Fiho G, Kairalla RA, Deheinzellin D, Munzo C, Oliveira R, Takagaki TY, Carvalho CR. Effect of protective-ventilation strategy on mortality in the adult respiratory distress syndrome. N Engl J Med 1998; 338:347–354.
99. Dellinger RP, Zimmermann JL, Taylor RW, Straube RC, Hauser DL, Crine GJ, Davis K, Hyers TM, Papadakos P. Effects of inhaled nitric oxide in patients with acute respiratory distress syndrome: results of a randomized phase II trial. Crit Care Med 1998; 26:15–23.
100. Stewart TE, Meade MO, Cook DL, Granton JT, Hooder RV, Lapinsky SE, Mazer CD, McLean RF, Rogovein TS, Schouten BD, Todd TR, Slutsky AS. Evaluation of a ventilation strategy to prevent barotrauma in patients at high risk for acute respiratory distress syndrome. Pressure- and volume-limited ventilation strategy group. N Engl J Med 1998; 338:355–361.

12

Whole-Body Oxygen Transport and Use

STEPHEN M. CAIN and SCOTT E. CURTIS

University of Alabama at Birmingham
Birmingham, Alabama

I. Introduction

This chapter introduces the section devoted to gas exchange in the periphery, and its purpose is to provide an integrative approach that will act as a framework for the chapters that follow. As such, the treatment of the topic is necessarily broad rather than in-depth, and it is restricted to considerations only of oxygen (O_2) transport and use. We first consider how these two variables relate to one another in the whole body. The next step is to examine how the individual needs of the organ systems with respect to O_2 demand and O_2 supply contribute to the whole-body picture. As an example of increased O_2 demand in the healthy organism, we consider the greatly increased demands placed on the body by muscles contracting with exercise and how this calls for establishment of a priority system for the distribution of available O_2 supply. This allows us to introduce the topic of regulation of blood flow according to O_2 need and to describe in general terms how we think this operates. The scope of the chapter then broadens to include alterations in regulatory control systems with disease states and the possible consequences on tissue oxygenation. One important concept that we try to convey is that each organ system must look to its own needs with respect to O_2 supply, while at the same time it is, to a greater or lesser extent, subordinate to prioritized needs of other organ systems that are purportedly more necessary to survival of the organism.

In addition to increased O_2 demand as a stimulus to prioritize distribution of O_2 supply among the organ systems, we also explore how decreased O_2 supply evokes regulatory mechanisms to subserve both local and whole-organism requirements to maintain tissue oxygenation at adequate levels. We attempt to indicate how regulatory mechanisms achieve those ends. A major premise is developed that the general condition of a strong vasoconstrictor tone is necessary to direct blood flow and O_2 supply away from areas with lesser needs to tissues with greater demands by local modulation of that tone. Experimental evidence in whole-body and selected organs systems are cited to support that general notion. In keeping with the overall theme of the volume, the alterations in vasoregulatory controls imposed by some disease states are also considered.

II. The Interrelationship Between Oxygen Transport and Use in Health

A. Concepts of Supply-Dependent and Supply-Independent Oxygen Uptake

The Question of the Independent Variable

Oxygen transport and use are commonly considered together. A convenient way to do this is illustrated in Figure 1, in which O_2 transport ($\dot{Q}_{O_2}$) is placed on the abscissa and O_2 uptake or use ($\dot{V}_{O_2}$) on the ordinate. $\dot{Q}_{O_2}$ is defined as the product of blood flow ($\dot{Q}$) and arterial O_2 content (Ca_{O_2}):

$$\dot{Q}_{O_2} = \dot{Q} \times Ca_{O_2} \tag{1}$$

$\dot{V}_{O_2}$ is defined as the product of blood flow and the difference in O_2 content between arterial and venous blood (Cv_{O_2}):

$$\dot{V}_{O_2} = \dot{Q} \times (Ca_{O_2} - Cv_{O_2}) \tag{2}$$

In both equations, if the whole body is being considered, then $\dot{Q}$ represents the total blood flow or cardiac output. If an organ system is being considered, then $\dot{Q}$ would be the local blood flow perfusing that system. Similarly, Cv_{O_2} would either represent mixed venous blood or the venous drainage from a local area. Yet another variable can be represented on this diagram, the O_2 extraction ratio (O_2ER), which is the ratio of $\dot{V}_{O_2}$ to $\dot{Q}_{O_2}$, or the ratio of the arteriovenous O_2 content difference to the arterial O_2 content:

$$O_2ER = \dot{V}_{O_2}/\dot{Q}_{O_2} = (Ca_{O_2} - Cv_{O_2})/Ca_{O_2} \tag{3}$$

Any point on the diagram that is connected to the origin with a positive slope can represent a particular O_2ER as long as its slope is between the values of 0 and 1.

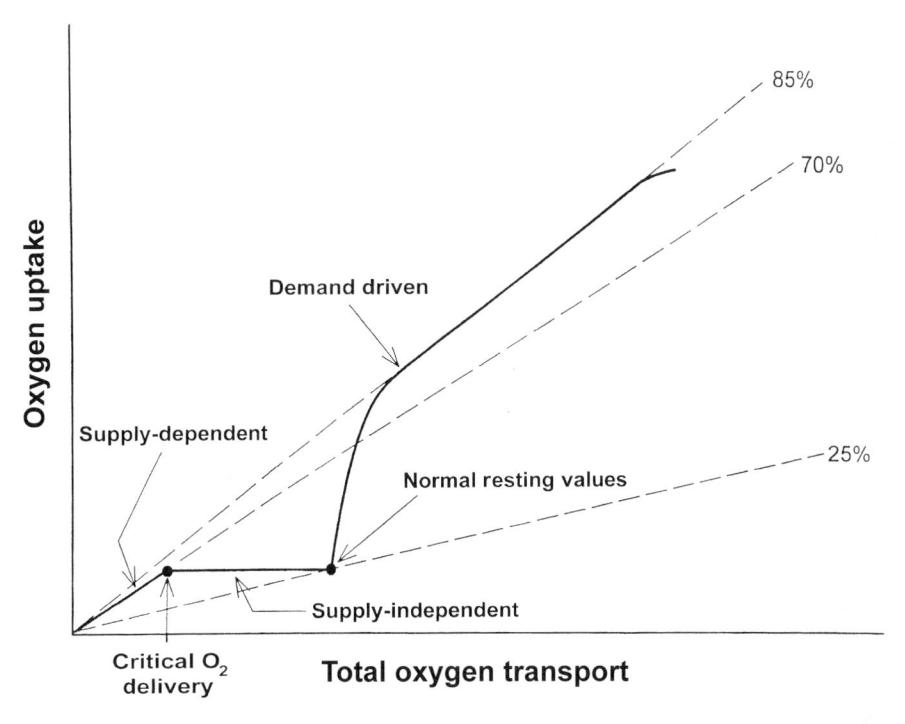

Figure 1 The solid dark line is a schematic representation of the relationship between oxygen uptake and total oxygen transport over a wide range from total deprivation of supply to maximal oxygen demand. The dashed lines represent fixed oxygen extraction ratios as a percent.

Some representative values are shown as dashed lines in Figure 1. Although actual numbers are not indicated on the ordinates, the solid line in the diagram represents this relationship between $\dot{Q}_{O_2}$ and $\dot{V}_{O_2}$ from the zero point for each to the extremes obtained by maximum effort during whole-body exercise. The shape of the relationship conforms to known facts.

However, the selection of the ordinates gives rise to the first question in that the abscissa is usually reserved for the independently manipulated variable. In that sense, either $\dot{Q}_{O_2}$ or $\dot{V}_{O_2}$ could be considered the independent factor in the relationship. If O_2 demand is being increased from the normal resting point (shown as the dashed circle) by physical exercise, for example, then it is really the manipulated variable as it drives O_2 transport. This is probably the most commonly encountered situation. On the diagram, it is represented as the "demand-driven" portion of the line in Figure 1 as the maximum O_2ER is reached, and the only way to achieve further increases in $\dot{V}_{O_2}$ is by increasing cardiac output, which, in turn, increases $\dot{Q}_{O_2}$. Conversely, if O_2 transport is being limited by any means and reduced below the normal resting level, then it is truly the independent variable. In that case, $\dot{V}_{O_2}$ is maintained by increasing O_2ER until $\dot{Q}_{O_2}$ reaches a point where O_2 uptake cannot be supported at the demand level, and tissue dysoxia ensues as uptake becomes supply-dependent [1]. In this situation, O_2 uptake will decrease with any further decrease in O_2 transport and is the dependent variable, as shown in Figure 1 as the solid line descends toward the origin of the graph. That point of descent identifies the critical level of $\dot{Q}_{O_2}$. Above the critical level of O_2 transport, increases do not affect O_2 uptake, and this is described by the plateau area of the line or the supply-independent portion of the relationship. The reason that the question of which is the independent assumes some importance is that in yet other situations, such as might be found in critically ill patients, there is still a great deal of controversy as to whether O_2 transport or O_2 demand is the independent variable and whether extensive tissue dysoxia is responsible for multiple-organ failure that often ensues in such patients [2].

Oxygen Extraction

The O_2ER is a useful quantification because it combines O_2 uptake and O_2 transport into a single quantity that provides an index of the extent to which O_2 reserves in blood are being used whenever the system is stressed. Indeed, this is a major focus of the discussion to follow because it is also an index of how well regulatory mechanisms that try to match O_2 supply with demand are functioning. In healthy individuals, whether O_2 demand is increased or O_2 supply is decreased, the first line of defense to maintain tissue oxygenation is to increase O_2ER. In Figure 1, this is represented by the fact that maintenance of resting $\dot{V}_{O_2}$, despite decreasing $\dot{Q}_{O_2}$ or increasing $\dot{V}_{O_2}$ by increasing O_2 demand, will also involve a move toward a higher O_2ER than the resting value of approximately 25%. This is accomplished by a complex regulatory system that requires an exquisite balance of constrictor and dilator forces in the microvasculature to direct convective O_2 supply to areas that need it most. Extraction is promoted by shortening the diffusion distance for O_2 from capillary to mitochondrion as much as possible.

If the periphery cannot extract most of the arterial O_2 when there is reason to believe that $\dot{Q}_{O_2}$ may be limiting $\dot{V}_{O_2}$ then, obviously, there must be a problem either in matching regional supply to demand or in the transport pathway from capillary to mitochondrion or both. As the body is pushed to the limit of O_2 uptake by physical exercise, O_2ER can reach as high as 85%. In an isolated muscle preparation stimulated to contract electrically, however, O_2ER seldom exceeds approximately 70%. The role that distribution of blood flow to and within the contracting muscles and the signals that govern it to produce this result remains part of a still-fascinating enigma [3].

B. Regional Differences in Oxygen Supply and Demand

At Rest

At rest, there is a distribution of blood flow to the organ systems that is not necessarily governed by O_2 demand. In Table 1, roughly half of total blood flow and O_2 uptake in the body are accounted for by the splanchnic and skeletal muscle systems, which extract 24% and 46%, respectively, of the O_2 transported to these regions. This compares with the 23% O_2 extraction by the body as a whole. Conversely, the kidneys receive one fifth of total blood flow, from which they extract less than 10% of the presented O_2. Because their function is to filter and adjust the composition of the blood, their high flow is understandable but does act as a functional shunt for O_2 in that renal venous blood is still nearly saturated with O_2. Skin is another area that receives far more blood flow than it needs from a nutritional standpoint, so that venous oxygen partial pressure (P_{O_2}) from that organ system is also little changed from arterial. Here again, skin's function is to dissipate heat from the core toward the surface of the body, hence the blood flow in excess of its own need.

If the relative distribution of blood flow can be regulated according to O_2 need to promote extraction when demand is increased or supply is decreased, then potentially, approximately 85% of the total amount of O_2 normally present in arterial blood can be used. This does occur by a variety of central and local control mechanisms whose interactions are still not fully understood. Furthermore, although the focus here is on O_2 transport and use, the final common pathway for the control of blood flow, the vascular smooth muscle in the resistance vessels,

Table 1 Typical Values for Regional Oxygen Uptake ($\dot{V}_{O_2}$), Blood Flow ($\dot{Q}$), Oxygen Extraction (O_2ER), and Venous P_{O_2} in a Normal Resting Subject of 70 kg

	$\dot{V}_{O_2}$ (mL/min)	Fraction of total (%)	$\dot{Q}$ (mL/min)	Fraction of total (%)	Arteriovenous O_2 (mL/dL)	O_2ER (%)	Venous P_{O_2} (mm Hg)
Splanchnic	58	25	1400	24	4.1	24	43
Renal	16	7	1100	19	1.3	7	63
Cerebral	46	20	750	13	6.3	36	34
Coronary	27	11	250	4	11.4	66	23
Skeletal muscle	70	30	1200	21	8.0	46	31
Skin	5	2	500	9	1.0	6	67
Other	12	5	600	10	3.0	17	48
Whole body	234		5800		4.0	23	

Source: Ref. 73.

can also be responding to different signals such as those related to maintenance of arterial blood pressure, exchange of other nutrients, control of blood volume, temperature control, etc. The outcome will reflect the balance achieved between vasoconstrictor and vasodilator influences.

With Increased Oxygen Demand: Whole Body

Human exercise that uses many large muscle groups provides an example of how this system is integrated (see Chapters 4 and 19 for additional information). Rowell et al. [4] postulated three types of error detection to produce a given outcome between constriction and dilation as O_2 demand is progressively increased by physical activity. Flow errors are those caused by mismatches between blood flow and metabolism, whereas pressure errors are mismatches between blood flow and vascular conductance so that blood pressure deviates from its set point. The third type of error, temperature errors, from mismatches between cutaneous blood flow and body core temperature, may also occur if body temperature increases with heavy exercise. Each error signal can alter the integrated balance of constrictor and dilator forces acting on each organ system. A detailed discussion of how this is accomplished is beyond the scope of this chapter, but more information can be found in Chapter 19. Nevertheless, some of the fundamental events that occur with exercise illustrate an important concept, namely, that there is a necessity for a strong centrally mediated increase in vasoconstrictor tone that is locally modulated so that blood flow meets the various demands placed on it.

With the onset of exercise, there is a prompt increase in blood flow to contracting muscle, as well as a redistribution of blood flow between organ systems [5]. As the muscle pump increases venous return to the heart, vagal withdrawal increases heart rate, and the baroreflex is reset to a higher level, thus insuring adequate perfusion pressure. At the same time, there is an increase in sympathetic nerve activity, the effect of which is amplified as the heart rate exceeds 100 beats/min by "spillover" of norepinephrine, which increases the circulating level as norepinephrine enters the blood, primarily from the contracting muscles. Even while cardiac output is increasing with increasing workload, both renal and splanchnic blood flows show an absolute decrease from resting levels as their vasoconstrictor tone is increased [5]. In the absence of thermoregulatory signals to the contrary, the skin is also vasoconstricted. Concurrently, venous capacitance reservoirs other than skin are also constricted to increase circulating blood volume [4]. Whether there is an actual reduction in systemic vascular compliance is still an open question, but most investigators assume this to be the case. The pattern of flow reduction and of vascular mobilization have been estimated to support an additional 500 to 600 mL of O_2 each minute for active muscles' share of the increased cardiac output. The net effect on use of O_2 stores in blood is that O_2 extraction in the whole body can attain 80–85% [6]. Furthermore, most of this increase in extraction occurs early in exercise, well before the blood flow increase has reached its maximum attainable value. This attests to the effectiveness of redistribution patterns to maximize the use of O_2 stores by matching supply to demand.

Increased Oxygen Demand: In Situ Isolated Muscle

Even in isolated in situ muscle preparations that are autoperfused and stimulated to contract electrically, there is evidence for redistribution of blood flow within the muscle. The exact reason is still not known, but neural activity may be involved. With so little of total blood flow being demanded, there is no pressure error, and the immediacy of the response would argue against a flow error. Barbee et al. [7] showed that blood flow to an in situ canine gastrocnemius muscle group stimulated to contract 4/s increased sharply within 30 seconds and continued to increase over the next 5 minutes, whereas venous O_2 concentration decreased within 30 seconds and reached a nadir within 1 minute. The stimulus that increased O_2 demand at the same time increased vascular conductance at the resistance arterioles while recruiting more of the capillary bed to increase O_2 extraction. Because less than 25% of the capillary bed is perfused in the quiescent muscle [8], further recruitment to increase capillary exchange as total flow increases allows some of that O_2 reserve in the blood to be used and thus spares additional flow requirements initially.

Both at the organ-system level and within the organ system, regulatory systems attempt to match $\dot{Q}_{O_2}$ to $\dot{V}_{O_2}$ so that more of the O_2 reserve in blood is used whenever tissue oxygenation is lowered either by increased demand or decreased supply or both. The basic mechanism to do this requires an appropriate balance of vasoconstrictor and vasodilator forces operating at vascular smooth muscle. How this is achieved remains as one of the more challenging puzzles in organ-system physiology. As an approach to unraveling the mystery, $\dot{Q}_{O_2}$ has been reduced by various means, mostly in experimental animals, both at the whole-body and organ-system levels while elements of the control system were manipulated. Although the emphasis of this chapter is on events in the whole body, much of the pertinent information has been developed on organ systems, particularly skeletal muscle and gut. Therefore, some of the information anticipates that which will be presented elsewhere, Chapters 14 and 15 in particular.

III. Matching of Oxygen Transport to Use in Health

A. Metabolic Regulation of Blood Flow

A More Detailed Look at the Control System

When O_2 supply is lowered, mechanisms are invoked that redistribute the now-limited supply on a priority basis, as previously alluded to. The priority is set by a multifactorial system that includes: (1) reflex sympathetic activation; (2) the relative richness and specificity of receptor sites for various vasoconstrictor and vasodilator substances that are either circulating or locally produced by endothelium; and (3) vasodilator action of local metabolites, as well as that of any direct effect of low P_{O_2} on vascular smooth muscle. This was described many years ago as a competition between centrally and humorally mediated vasoconstriction and local vasodilation [9]. The picture is far more complex today, with more vasoactive substances and more pathways for their actions now identified.

Figure 2 presents a summary schematic of some of these substances and pathways that does not pretend to be complete. Its main purpose is to show what seem to be redundant control systems that may work together in some hierarchical

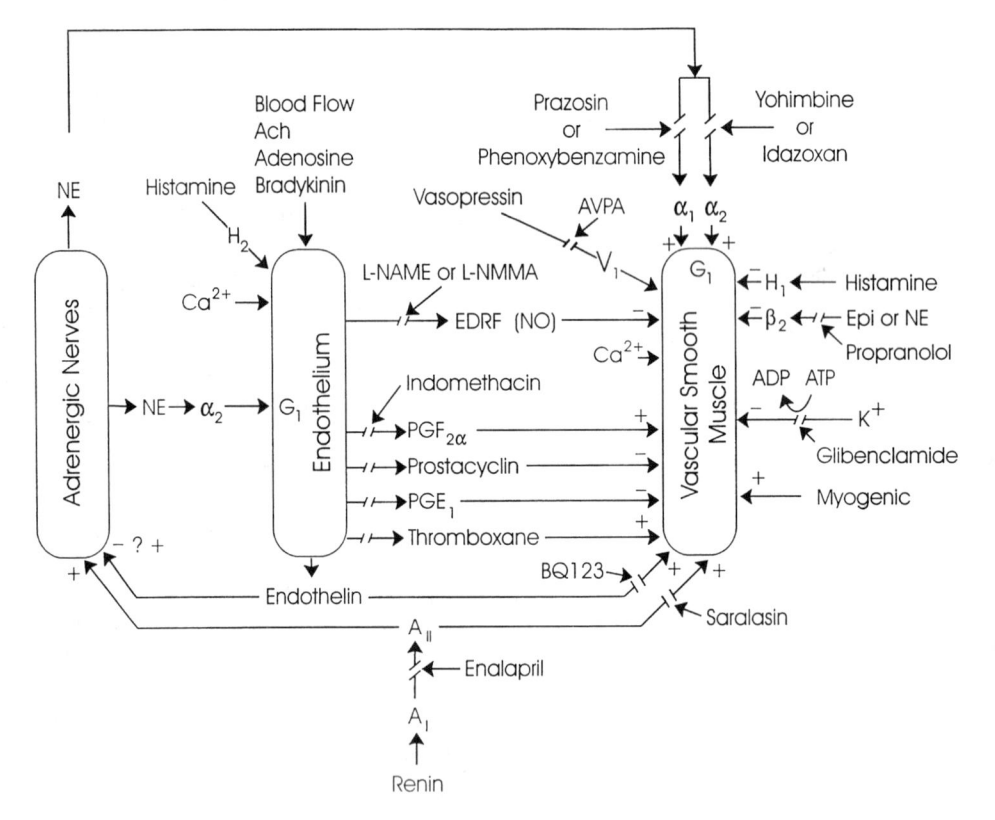

Figure 2 An attempt to illustrate the multiplicity of factors that may act on vascular smooth muscle. A plus sign represents a vasoconstrictor effect and a minus sign is a vasodilator. A break in an arrow identifies where a specific inhibitor may act. Epi = epinephrine; NE = norepinephrine; PG = prostaglandin. The authors are indebted to C. Baker and J. Price for many of the ideas incorporated here.

order or may provide backup controls when one system fails or is inactivated for any reason. Inhibitors that may allow a test of the integrative role played by these various systems are also shown, and some experimental results from their use are discussed. Rather than a competition between forces, it now seems more correct to think of this as an orchestration of effects that modulate first local distribution of $\dot{Q}_{O_2}$ within an organ system at the level of distribution controls for capillary perfusion and then the resistance vessels that control distribution between organ systems. In the latter case, the priorities are such that brain, which does not tolerate hypoxia, and constantly working muscles such as the heart and respiratory muscles (if the subject is not being ventilated) are favored. Both between and within organ systems, the assumption is that an insufficient O_2 supply will be matched as well as possible with O_2 need.

Resistance Versus Exchange Capacity

In keeping with the idea that there is an orchestration of events to accomplish the matching of O_2 supply and demand, Granger et al. [10] showed a sequence of events in response to any change that would lower tissue oxygenation. They used decreases in perfusion pressure and arterial O_2 concentration as well as increasing O_2 demand in hindlimb skeletal muscles. Effective capillary density, which was paralleled by changes in O_2ER, responded promptly to any decrease in O_2 transport before any notable change was observed in vascular resistance. They interpreted these results as showing that the metabolic sensitivity of small arterioles, which control exchange capacity, was greater than that of larger arterioles, which control resistance. These experiments were conducted in areflexic anesthetized dogs in which blood pressure and sympathetic tone were maintained by a catecholamine drip. Any signals from baroreflexes and chemoreflexes were thus avoided.

The early response of increased exchange capacity was further illustrated by a different approach in experiments in which muscle and whole-body $\dot{V}_{O_2}$ of anesthetized dogs was increased by dinitrophenol, an uncoupler of oxidative phophorylation. In an additional set of experiments, mild hypoxia was induced by ventilating the animals with 12% O_2. Although whole-body O_2 demand increased $\geq$50%, cardiac output remained unchanged or even decreased slightly. In the limb muscles, $\dot{V}_{O_2}$ was increased threefold or more, but vascular resistance did not change until O_2ER exceeded 50% [11]. The presence of mild hypoxia did not alter this result. A similar increase in $\dot{V}_{O_2}$ achieved by stimulating the muscles to contract would presumably have resulted in an immediate increase in blood flow and lowering of vascular resistance attributable to the neural component.

Autoregulatory Escape

Another observation made by Granger et al. [10] was that when neurohumoral and local mechanisms are opposed in their effects, first exchange and then resistance vessels will "escape" neurogenic vasoconstriction to maintain local tissue oxygenation. They saw resistance vessels in their areflexic preparation escape from the vasoconstrictor effect of norepipehrine only when venous P_{O_2} from the hindlimb musculature was low. This was not a necessary condition in the anesthetized dogs used by Cain and Chapter [12], who directly infused norepinephrine into the arterial supply of the hindlimb musculature. The "escape" phenomenon of exchange capacity controls was suggested by the fact that $\dot{V}_{O_2}$ was maintained by increased O_2ER even though blood flow was markedly reduced at 5 minutes of infusion. By 10 minutes, "escape" of the resistance arterioles was also evident.

The exact nature of the local vasodilator is still a matter of debate. The candidates of 20 years ago that were cited by Sparks [13] are still very much in contention. These include vessel wall P_{O_2}, interstitial K^+, tissue hyperosmolality, H^+, carbon dioxide partial pressure (P_{CO_2}), and myogenic responses. To them must be added the endothelially produced and modulated vasoactive substances that are shown in Figure 2. Notable among these substances are nitric oxide (NO; the purported endothelial-derived relaxing factor [EDRF]) and prostacyclin. Numerous references for all of these substances can be found in the report by Laughlin et al. [8]. Yet another candidate is the adenosine triphosphate–sensitive K^+ channel in vascular smooth muscle, which, when blocked by glibenclamide, prevented hypoxic vasodilation in isolated perfused guinea pig hearts [14].

Many of the pathways shown in Figure 2 are found in various vessels from large arteries to large veins, but there is considerable evidence that a metabolic imbalance is first sensed at the capillary and that a signal is then spread in a propagated fashion all the way to the larger resistance vessels [15,16]. Therefore, there seems to be a solid basis for proposing a hierarchical and coordinated control from smaller arterioles controlling exchange capacity to larger ones controlling resistance, with the greater sensitivity found in the former.

With centrally or humorally mediated vasoconstriction, therefore, a redistribution of blood flow should occur not only within but also between organ systems as the constriction is modified by local demands to restore perfusion. To the extent that this promotes better matching of O_2 transport to need, then it would remain an essential adjustment to maximize O_2ER. Conversely, if the phenomenon of autoregulatory escape in nonessential areas such as resting skeletal muscle diverts blood flow from more essential organs such as heart and brain, then it becomes part of the decompensation that is prefatory to imminent death from tissue dysoxia.

B. Responses to Reductions in Oxygen Transport

Dependence on Convective Oxygen Transport

Oxygen transport can be decreased by lowering of arterial P_{O_2} (hypoxic hypoxia), by reducing blood flow (stagnant or ischemic hypoxia), or by hemodilution (anemic or hemodilutional hypoxia). All three methods were used in anesthetized, splenectomized dogs by a single group of investigators [17]. Irrespective of the method used to produce hypoxia, they were unable to distinguish any difference in the $\dot{Q}_{O_2}$ at which either $\dot{V}_{O_2}$ began to decrease or arterial lactate levels began to increase. They concluded that $\dot{V}_{O_2}$ was primarily dependent on convective O_2 delivery. In an earlier comparison of anemic and hypoxic hypoxia, Cain [18] showed that $\dot{V}_{O_2}$ began to decrease at widely different values of mixed venous P_{O_2} (45 mm Hg vs. 17 mm Hg) for the two kinds of hypoxia but at the same value of $\dot{Q}_{O_2}$. Even in awake lambs of approximately 4 weeks of age, similar values of critical $\dot{Q}_{O_2}$ were found whether the $\dot{Q}_{O_2}$ was lowered by reducing cardiac output or by reducing arterial P_{O_2} [19,20].

The type of information gathered in such experiments is not adequate to state that diffusion limitation caused by lowered capillary driving pressure of P_{O_2} plays no role at the critical point for $\dot{V}_{O_2}$. The great similarity of critical values for $\dot{Q}_{O_2}$ on the supply side, however, does suggest that there are similar mechanisms at work in all forms of hypoxia to match supply to areas of greater O_2 need. One such mechanism is heightened vasoconstrictor tone. If the reasonable assumption is made that any local vasodilator signal will be proportional to the degree of metabolic imbalance, then those regions most in need of O_2 will escape from the increased vasoconstriction more quickly, whereas areas less in need receive less of the lowered O_2 supply.

Natural Enhancement of Vasoconstrictor Tone

Hypoxic Hypoxia

If arterial P_{O_2} is lowered for any reason, then the arterial chemoreceptors, the carotid and aortic bodies, are stimulated to increase vasoconstrictor tone [21]. This is presumably the initiating step for the O_2-conserving function of flow redistribution. That such does occur has been amply demonstrated. For example, Krasney [22] showed that blood flow in the superior vena cava increased at the expense of flow in the inferior vena cava and that this cephalad regional preference was abolished by denervation of the peripheral chemoreceptors. Wyler [23] noted in anesthetized rabbits that there was a consistent and marked decrease in renal blood flow during arterial hypoxia. More detailed information was elicted by Adachi et al. [24] with the use of labeled microspheres. In anesthetized dogs ventilated with 10% and 5% O_2, the fractions of cardiac output directed to the splanchnic bed and to the kidneys were reduced, whereas coronary and cerebral circulations were enhanced.

Another area from which blood flow is first diverted with the advent of arterial hypoxia is skeletal muscle. Cain and Chapler [25] ventilated anesthetized dogs with hypoxic gas mixtures and showed that cardiac output was elevated by severe hypoxia, whereas blood flow to the resting hindlimb muscles did not change for the first 20 minutes of hypoxia. Between 20 and 40 minutes, however, blood flow to this area also increased, an indication of autoregulatory escape from vasoconstriction. That escape was prevented in animals given the β-adrenergic inhibitor propranolol, which indicated that the vasodilator action of these receptors also participated in the final balance between dilator and constrictor forces in hypoxia.

Ischemic Hypoxia

If blood pressure is lowered by such means as hemorrhage or cardiac tamponade, then the baroreceptors initiative a strong sympathetic discharge. Schlichtig et al. [26] tested whether this was an important factor in optimizing O_2ER during hemorrhage by measuring regional values in liver, intestine, kidney, and whole body and comparing those values with the results that would have been obtained if no redistribution of blood flow had occurred. Their model predicted that O_2 supply dependency would have commenced at a higher value of $\dot{Q}O_2$ for whole body and at lower values for liver and kidney without the redistribution that actually occurred. This reaffirmed the concept that regulatory mechanisms attempt to match O_2 supply with demand at the organ-system level when supply is reduced.

In two reports from Schumacker's group [27,28], hemorrhage was used as a way to modify tone not only in the whole body of anesthetized dogs, but in two regional circulations as well: hindlimb skeletal muscle and small intestine. Blood flow was controlled by pump to the vascularly isolated but otherwise intact regions. In this manner, blood flow could be progressively lowered to establish the critical $\dot{Q}O_2$. The critical O_2ER, which is the ratio of $\dot{V}O_2$ to $\dot{Q}O_2$ at the critical $\dot{Q}O_2$ (Fig. 1), was higher in each of these regions if the animals were made hypovolemic to lower blood pressure as opposed to a normovolemic, normotensive group. This result underscored for them the significance of a strong sympathetic response to the efficient use of a reduced O_2 supply.

Hemodilutional Hypoxia

It had been a long-standing assumption since the early work of Comroe and Schmidt [29] that the peripheral chemoreceptors, the carotid and aortic bodies, responded only to decreases in arterial PO_2 and not to decreases in blood O_2 concentration. Hatcher et al. [30] then showed that, although true for the carotid body, the aortic body increased its firing markedly as hematocrit was lowered to less than 30%. Daly and Ungar [31] had shown before that although it had only weak effects on ventilation, the cardiovascular effects observed with aortic body stimulation were similar in every way to those observed with carotid body stimulation and, unlike the carotid body, were independent of lung inflation. The question of whether this might cause preferential distribution of blood flow among organ systems was answered by Fan et al. [32] in anesthetized dogs in which hematocrit was both increased and decreased below the normal value of 45%. They found that cardiac output increased with lowering of hematocrit and that the only organ system that actually decreased blood flow was the spleen. Liver, gut, and kidney maintained blood flow because these organs increased vasoconstriction, but heart and brain vasodilated and increased blood flow. The changes were modest but significant, particularly as hematocrit was decreased to less than 30%.

Skeletal muscle was not included in the organ systems studied by Fan et al. [32]. Cain and Chapler [33] measured blood flow and $\dot{V}O_2$ in whole body and in the vascularly isolated but otherwise intact hindlimb skeletal muscle of anesthetized dogs at two levels of hemodilution. Cardiac output increased at each lowering of the hematocrit, but limb blood flow increased proportionately more. At the lower level of approximately 15%, whole-body $\dot{V}O_2$ was significantly decreased, whereas that of the hindlimb was not. The limb muscles also succeeded in extracting significantly more oxygen than did the whole body, 90% versus 80% at the more severe level of anemia. This was perhaps an indication that the increased vasoconstrictor tone with anemic hypoxia was serving a useful purpose by matching O_2 supply to demand at the intraorgan level. In the case of the whole body, calculations based on reasonable assumptions showed that the kidneys were acting as a functional shunt in that their blood flow remained at a high level relative to their metabolic need so that blood close to arterial in Po_2 was being added to the venous return. This accounted for the lesser oxygen extraction measured for the whole body.

C. Experimental Alteration of Peripheral Vascular Tone

Reduced Vasoconstrictor Tone

If enhanced constrictor tone is a necessary adjunct to optimizing O_2 extraction in hypoxia, then prevention of that enhancement should have a deleterious effect. This was tested in anesthetized dogs by Cain [34], who used phenoxybenzamine to block α-adrenergic receptors. The first noticeable effect was hypotension and decreased cardiac output. An additional group of animals was given an average of 17 mL/kg dextran at this point to restore mean arterial pressure before being ventilated with an hypoxic gas mixture. The third group, which was not given phenoxybenzamine, was able to extract nearly 90% of the total $\dot{Q}O_2$ as they approached the end point of hypoxia, which was marked by a profound and rapid decrease in blood pressure, denoting decompensation. The two groups that were α-blocked, in contrast, were only able to extract 46% and 43% at that point. In that the time to reach that end point was a measure of survival time, the unblocked group survived 70 minutes of hypoxia, whereas the two treated groups survived only 35 and 40 minutes. The O_2-conserving function of enhanced vasoconstrictor tone was clearly demonstrated.

Similar results with phenoxybenzamine were obtained in another set of experiments by Cain and Chapler [35]. However, the additional goal in this study was to see if skeletal muscle contributed to the overall inability to increase O_2ER to the same level as in unblocked animals. Rather surprisingly, it did not. The O_2ER at the critical level of $\dot{Q}O_2$ was approximately 73% in the whole body of the unblocked group, as well as in the hindlimb muscles of both groups. However, at the time of that study it was generally believed that only α_1-adrenergic receptors were postjunctional so that phenoxybenzamine, an α_1-receptor inhibitor, was thought to be sufficient to the cause. Subsequently, α_2-adrenergic receptors were shown to participate in vasoconstriction in the femoral vascular bed in response to both exogenous norepinephrine and neural stimulation [36]. Kubes et al. [37] used a nerve cooler and the specific α_1- and α_2-receptor antagonists prazosin and yohimbine to show that the α_2-receptors played a substantial role in even resting sympathetic tone in skeletal muscle. Whether the combined block would affect O_2ER in hypoxic limb muscles remains to be seen.

The lack of effect of phenoxybenzamine on O_2 extraction by hypoxic seletal muscle was at odds with observations of Maginniss et al. [27] in the study cited above (35). They also used phenoxybenzamine and found similar effects on critical O_2ER in the whole body, but they found a lesser O_2 extraction ability in the hindlimb muscles as well. Indeed, the effect of α-adrenergic blockade was even more pronounced in muscle than it was in the whole body. However, the investigators pointed out that the use of hypoxic hypoxia in the earlier studies of Cain [33] and Cain and Chapler [34] differed from the ischemic hypoxia used in their studies in that the greater perfusion pressure in the former state may have helped to sustain perfusion through nutritional capillaries. Alternatively, the decreased vascular tone with decreased perfusion pressure in their study may have caused more units to shut down by altering the closing pressure as perfusion pressure decreased.

In the study by Samsel and Schumacker [28], experiments were performed similar to those described by Maginniss et al. [27], but with the small intestine as the region of interest. Again, phenoxybenzamine decreased the ability of the whole body to extract O_2 with progressive hemorrhage. They progressively reduced blood flow to the pump-perfused segment of small intestine. The critical O_2ER was significantly higher in a hypovolemic group than in a normovolemic one and was also higher in a hypovolemic group treated with phenoxybenzamine, which was slightly but significantly less than in the hypovolemic nonblocked group. The investigators suggested that this was evidence that nonadrenergic vasoconstrictors such as vasopressin and renin, which would have been elicited by hemorrhagic shock, may have acted in place of the blocked α-adrenergic receptors. An additional postulate might be that a near-maximum response was elicited by either set of mechanisms and that an additive effect was not necessary to improve critical O_2ER.

The role of enhanced vasoconstrictor tone in hemodilutional hypoxia was apparently less than in other forms of hypoxia in that regional blood flow redistribution was not as marked as in other forms of hypoxia. Skeletal muscle, for example, increased its blood flow parallel to the increase in cardiac output [33]. Arteriolar resistance vessels were observed to be not as effective when blood viscosity was lowered by hemodilution. This was emphasized in another study by Chapler and Cain [38], in which phenoxybenzamine did not lower systemic vascular resistance any further after hemodilution to a hematocrit level of approximately 15%. Vasoconstrictor tone was still important to compensate for this form of hypoxia, however, in that the loss of venous tone caused cardiac output to decrease to the point that whole-body $\dot{V}O_2$ could no longer be maintained. Volume expansion to the amount of 12 mL/kg while maintaining the hematocrit close to 15% restored cardiac output and $\dot{V}O_2$. This provided a measure of the increase in venous capacitance that occurred with α-adrenergic blockade. Chapler et al. [39] had previously shown that hemodilutional hypoxia did cause venoconstriction in the isolated hindlimb circulation of anesthetized dogs. Venoconstriction as a result of enhanced sympathetic activity thus played an essential role in compensating for a decrease in O_2-carrying capacity of blood by increasing venous return to the heart and thereby increasing cardiac output.

Enhanced Vasodilator Tone

If lessened vasoconstrictor tone detracts from the body's ability to extract O_2 from a reduced supply, then increased vasodilator tone should have a similar effect if the original hypothesis is correct that it is the balance between the two that is important for this purpose. This was demonstrated in skeletal muscles, which are vasodilated by β-adrenergic agonists at both resistance and distribution control points [40,41]. Yonekawa et al. [42] showed that tissue P_{O_2} decreased in gracilis muscles of anesthetized dogs when they infused isoproterenol, despite the fact that $\dot{Q}O_2$ to the muscle had increased more than the increase in $\dot{V}O_2$ caused by the β-agonist. They calculated the physiological tissue shunt that would account for this result and found that it increased from 41% in resting muscle to 73% in the infused muscle.

Their result was highly indicative of a mismatch between $\dot{Q}O_2$ and $\dot{V}O_2$ in the dilated skeletal muscle. An even more direct demonstration of this effect was made by Cain and Bredle [43], who used dopexamine, a moderate dopaminergic and even stronger β-adrenergic agonist, infused at 12 μg/kg/mL into anesthetized dogs while progressively lowering blood flow stepwise to the vascularly isolated but otherwise intact hindlimb muscles. The vasodilatory effect was evident in the significantly decreased vascular resistance of the limb. The critical value of $\dot{Q}O_2$ was increased from 4.0 to 6.3 mL/kg of muscle weight per minute, and the critical extraction ratio at that $\dot{Q}O_2$ was lowered from 82% to 65% in the infused animals. Whether vasoconstrictor tone is decreased or vasodilator tone is increased without a compensatory change in the other, O_2 extraction is deleteriously affected by the consequent mismatch of O_2 supply to demand within the tissue.

A practical consideration for an overbalance in vasodilator tone was shown in the study by Van der Linden et al. [44]. They examined the effect of several anesthetic agents in combination with pentobarbital on systemic critical $\dot{Q}O_2$ in dogs. These agents included isoflurane, halothane, alfentanil, and ketamine, with the latter three used at two concentrations. $\dot{Q}O_2$ was progressively lowered stepwise by hemorrhage to find the critical level. Although the agents differed in their cardiovascular effects, the unifying factor was their effect on peripheral vasodilation in that an inverse relationship was observed between critical $\dot{Q}O_2$ and systemic vascular resistance at that point. A greater vasodilator effect by the anesthetic agent was associated with a lesser ability of the body to extract O_2 from a diminishing supply.

D. Endothelial Mechanisms

Endothelial-Derived Relaxing Factor, Nitric Oxide

Figure 2 shows at least a half-dozen factors manufactured in the endothelium that modulate vasomotor tone. Notable among these is EDRF, identified by Furchgott and Zawadzki [45], which is commonly accepted to be NO. There are several effective inhibitors of the enzyme that produces EDRF-NO, NO synthase. When one of these, $N^{\prime\Omega}$-nitro-L-arginine methyl ester (L-NAME), was used in anesthetized dogs, it caused a significant increase in systemic vascular resistance and an even more dramatic increase in perfusion pressure at constant flow in the vascularly isolated hindlimb muscles [46]. The proposition that EDRF-NO was essential to hypoxic vasodilation was tested with both ischemic and hypoxic hypoxia in the intact hindlimb while the rest of the body remained normovolemic and normoxic. Although inhibition of NO synthase moved vascular resistance to a higher level both in the whole body and in the limb, hypoxic vasodilation occurred when $\dot{Q}O_2$ to the limb was lowered below the critical level. This was somewhat greater in hypoxic hypoxia than in ischemic hypoxia. Furthermore, O_2ER during hypoxia was not different between the control group and the group given L-NAME. The investigators concluded that EDRF-NO was not essential for hypoxic vasodilation or for the efficient use of a reduced O_2 supply.

Interactions Between Endothelial Mechanisms

As shown in Figure 2, in addition to EDRF-NO, there are several prostaglandins that are vasoactive and produced by endothelium. Curtis et al. [47] tested whether EDRF-NO and the prostaglandins were necessary to optimize O_2ER in the vascularly isolated hindlimb of anesthetized dogs by inhibiting their production with L-NAME and indomethacin. They went one step further and removed the endothelium itself by flushing the limb with a detergent, deoxycholate. When flow was progressively reduced in a stepwise fashion to ascertain the critical $\dot{Q}O_2$, the control group's O_2 extraction at that point was 81%. The group given L-NAME and indomethacin had a critical extraction ratio of only 66%, a significant difference. The deoxycholate group was able to extract only 42% of the transported O_2 before its $\dot{V}O_2$ became supply-limited, a very clear extraction defect presumably caused by the loss of all endothelial modulation of perfusion.

From the information presented here one can conclude that EDRF-NO is not essential to efficient use of a reduced O_2 supply. Loss of constrictor tone or any further manipulation of the multiple vasoactive controls, particularly those located in vascular endothelium, however, can lead to defective O_2 extraction in the periphery and O_2-limited metabolism at higher levels of $\dot{Q}O_2$ than when control systems are intact and operative.

IV. Matching of Oxygen Transport to Use in Disease
A. "Pathologic" Oxygen Supply Dependency
The Case For

Whether in humans or in experimental animals, it is clear that if cardiac output, for example, is lowered sufficiently to bring $\dot{Q}O_2$ below the level necessary to support the O_2 demand, then $\dot{V}O_2$ will vary directly with supply in a dependent relationship. The critical $\dot{Q}O_2$ at which this occurs also marks the limit of successful compensation by increased O_2ER. In so-called physiological supply dependency, this only occurs when two thirds or more of the CaO_2 has been extracted. The inability to increase extraction appropriately distinguishes "pathological" O_2 supply dependency. The first description of such supply-limited $\dot{V}O_2$ in the clinical setting was made by Powers et al. [48]. They examined the physiological consequences of varying positive end-expiratory pressure (PEEP) in patients ill with posttraumatic adult respiratory distress syndrome (ARDS). They observed that whichever way cardiac output went as a result of changing PEEP, $\dot{V}O_2$ went in the same direction, with O_2 extraction changing little if at all. The investigators registered their surprise at this relationship occurring at higher-than-normal cardiac outputs but were able to offer no explanation.

This observation lay dormant until 1980, when similar findings were published by Danek et al. [49], who also manipulated $\dot{Q}O_2$ with PEEP in both ARDS and non-ARDS patients. They suggested that this was a defect in O_2 extraction as a result of a failure to regulate peripheral perfusion. More importantly, they pointed out that the mixed venous PO_2 could not be relied on to indicate the state of peripheral tissue oxygenation in patients who showed supply-dependent $\dot{V}O_2$ because of functional peripheral shunting. These observations were collated with additional ones from the clinical literature and then related to parallel observations in the experimental literature by Cain [1]. He made the distinction between physiological and pathological O_2 supply dependency and went on to point out that the events that occurred in the lung microvasculature to produce the clinical state of ARDS could also affect the peripheral vasculature and thus interfere with O_2 transfer from capillary to mitochondrion. This condition was associated with or consequent to sepsis, severe trauma, and anything that caused severe tissue hypoxia. Through activated mediating systems such as the arachidonic acid cascade, complement cascade, and xanthine oxidase, further tissue events such as embolization, edema, and frank endothelial damage would set a vicious circle of events into play. In addition to these possible interferences with vasoregulation and O_2 diffusion, there also seemed to be an increased demand for O_2 in such patients that remains unexplained.

Several articles then appeared in which $\dot{Q}_{O_2}$ was manipulated in critically ill patients, usually by fluid loading, and the observation of apparent pathological O_2 supply dependency at normal and elevated cardiac outputs was repeated many times. This was the interpretation when a positive slope of $\dot{Q}_{O_2}/\dot{V}_{O_2}$ was found. These studies were cited in a report by Bihari et al. [50], who took a different approach. They hypothesized that the fact that O_2 demand was seemingly not being satisfied at normal to elevated levels of O_2 transport signified that an extensive "occult" tissue O_2 debt must therefore be present, and that this was possibly responsible for the multiple-organ-system failure that so often ensued in such cases. To detect this, they used the potent vasodilator prostacyclin infused for 30 minutes to increase $\dot{Q}_{O_2}$. The patients who responded positively to this "O_2 flux test" with an increase in $\dot{V}_{O_2}$ subsequently died, whereas those who decreased $O_2\text{ER}$ with no change in $\dot{V}_{O_2}$ survived their illness. The latter response was also observed in healthy volunteers. The investigators suggested that the results in the positive responders indicated a significant level of tissue O_2 debt and inadequate tissue oxygenation that would otherwise have been difficult to detect. The difficulties of assessing tissue oxygenation, particularly at the bedside of critically ill patients, have been the subject of several reviews [51–53] and at least one consensus conference [54].

The Case Against

Results such as those previously cited provided the impetus for many studies in which attempts were made to achieve supranormal $\dot{Q}_{O_2}$ in critically ill patients. For every study that reported improved survivability, there was another to show no improvement or even increased mortality in one instance [see Ref. 54 for specific citations]. Although such studies served a useful purpose, they also diverted attention from the root cause, which was the series of events that eroded the ability of the microvasculature to perform one of its major tasks, delivery of O_2 to the tissues. In addition, there were also some technical challenges to the validity of the measurements used to demonstrate pathological O_2 supply dependency.

Before the advent of the flow-directed pulmonary artery catheter, the measurements of cardiac output and of whole-body $\dot{V}_{O_2}$ were strictly reserved to expert teams of researchers at the bedside in critical care units and were by no means considered routine. It may be of passing interest that the first description of the flow-directed catheter was actually made by two physiologists, Lategola and Rahn [55]. With that advance in technology, and particularly the addition of the capability to measure cardiac output by thermodilution built into the same catheter, bedside measurements of cardiac output became routine in that setting. At the same time, blood gas laboratories were able to measure blood O_2 concentrations by accurate spectrophotometric instruments. This made possible frequent and convenient measurement of $\dot{Q}_{O_2}$ as the product of cardiac output and C_{aO_2} and $\dot{V}_{O_2}$ as the product of cardiac output and the O_2 concentration difference between arterial and mixed venous blood. It was the shared variable, cardiac output, that cast doubt on the hallmark of pathological O_2 supply dependency, the positive slope of the line relating $\dot{V}O_2$ to $\dot{Q}O_2$ at normal to elevated levels of $\dot{Q}O_2$.

This shared variable with its attendant measurement error makes possible mathematical coupling in which the error is multiplied on both sides of the relationship to force an apparent positive correlation that might not actually be true. Russell and Phang [56] delved into the theoretical objections extensively and cited numerous studies that showed apparent pathological supply dependency that disappeared if $\dot{Q}O_2$ and $\dot{V}O_2$ were measured independently without a shared variable. Yet another objection was raised by Dantzker et al. [57], who reminded us of the question of which was the independent variable, $\dot{Q}O_2$ or $\dot{V}O_2$. As previously noted, despite often being sedated, mechanically ventilated, and even paralyzed, many critically ill patients had elevated O_2 demands. Dantzker et al. suggested that in many cases, the positive slope of $\dot{V}O_2$ versus $\dot{Q}O_2$ was the response of the latter to an increase in the former. The increase in $\dot{V}O_2$ may represent increased activity of extramitochondrial oxidases and oxygenases such as that caused by the "respiratory burst" of activated phagocytes or to a large increase in NO synthase activity with induction of the enzyme by septic processes [52]. An intriguing possibility, if this were the case, is the fact that these extramitochondrial users of molecular O_2 have a Km that is often orders of magnitude higher than that of cytochrome oxygenase. Therefore, they would respond to any increase in tissue P_{O_2} by increasing their O_2 use even when the energy-producing $\dot{V}O_2$ was not limited by O_2 availability. This would manifest itself as apparent pathological O_2 supply dependency.

B. Pathological Oxygen Extraction Defects

Animal Studies

The true nature of pathological O_2 supply dependency as originally described in critically ill patients remains an open question as to whether it represents an artifact, an increased O_2 demand, or a relative inability to increase O_2 extraction. With respect to the last possibility, there clearly can be a disruption of normal microcirculatory control in sepsis or in an experimental animal model with infused endotoxin or live bacteria. This was shown conclusively in a series of studies conducted in Schumacker's laboratory [58–60]. Once dogs were made bacteremic or endotoxemic, they were progressively hemorrhaged while regional and whole-body blood samples and blood flows were measured. When compared with that of control animals, critical O_2ER was significantly lower for the whole body and for small intestine, whereas little effect was observed in skeletal muscle. Clearly defined supply-dependent and supply-independent portions of the $\dot{Q}O_2/\dot{V}O_2$ relationship obviated the possibility that mathematical coupling affected their conclusion in any way. Whether or not the positive slope of $\dot{Q}O_2/\dot{V}O_2$ in patients was real, the processes set in motion by endotoxin or live bacteria evidently did disturb the delicate control system in the microcirculation that is responsible for optimizing O_2 extraction from a diminishing supply. This seemed to be particularly true in the gut in that it became supply-dependent at a significantly higher systemic $\dot{Q}O_2$ than did the whole body [59].

The Gut as a Target Organ

Because the gut serves as a barrier to aid in the prevention of systemic contamination by microbes and microbial products, any incompetency in this function can have widespread and disastrous effects on the whole body. Furthermore, its structure and vascular architecture provides for a further distinction between the separate susceptibilites of the muscularis and mucosal layers of the gut wall to any lowering of $\dot{Q}O_2$ [61]. In particular, there is countercurrent blood circulation in the villus of the mucosal layer that lowers PO_2 at the tip so that it is normally less than 10 mm Hg. There are also precapillary sphincters at the villus capillaries that make possible different responses of circulation in the muscularis as opposed to the mucosal areas.

To show this, Vallet et al. [62] measured tissue PO_2 at both the muscularis (serosal) and mucosal surfaces of a segment of small intestine with multipoint electrodes of the Kessler-Lübbers type before and after infusing anesthetized dogs with endotoxin. With the shock that ensued, total blood flow to the gut decreased along with cardiac output and then was restored by volume infusion to resuscitate the animal. The tissue PO_2 value of the serosal surface decreased with cardiac output and gut blood flow and then increased again with resuscitation to near pre-endotoxin levels. The mucosal PO_2 changed only a little during the shock phase but then declined to near-zero levels during resuscitation, where it remained for the duration of the experiment. Despite a restored total blood flow to the gut and $\dot{V}O_2$ that decreased within the limits of reported normal values, the mucosal layer was practically anoxic. In many cases, this led to sloughing of the mucosal surface in these and similar experiments. A more complete discussion of the special susceptibility of the gut to practically any form of hypoxia can be found in Chapter 15. However, the disturbance in microcirculatory control with endotoxemia is not restricted to the gut. Significant tissue hypoxia and abnormal microvascular control of oxygenation were also shown even in skeletal muscle of endotoxemic rats in a recent publication [63].

C. Interventions Directed at Vascular Controls

Vasodilators

Current recommendations for the care of critically ill patients, particularly those with sepsis or a related syndrome, are aimed at correcting any hypotension with adequate volume resuscitation, inotropes, and vasoactive agents to insure adequate tissue perfusion in the periphery [64]. Dobutamine is a potent β_2-adrenergic agonist that has both positive inotropic and vasodilator effects. Its action on $\dot{Q}O_2$ and $\dot{V}O_2$ in hemodynamically stable septic patients was compared with the vasodilator, prostacyclin, in a recent study by De Backer et al. [65]. They made no attempt to use either drug as a treatment modality in that each was used in the same patient for only 20-minute infusions. This protocol was more like the one used by Bihari et al. [50] for their oxygen flux test. Both agents increased cardiac output and $\dot{Q}O_2$ and seemed to increase $\dot{V}O_2$ as well. The latter result was challengeable on the basis of mathematical coupling in that decreases in O_2ER were observed with both drugs. Unlike the earlier study, however, neither result had any prognostic value because the mortality rate was approximately 50% even though 15 of the 17 patients in the study showed a "positive" effect of the O_2 flux test.

In a study published at approximately the same time and in contrast to the result of Bihari et al. [50], Vallet et al. [66] found a much higher survival rate in patients who had a positive response to a 60-minute dobutamine infusion, i.e., both $\dot{Q}O_2$ and $\dot{V}O_2$ increased. The investigators speculated that such a positive response indicated a greater reserve capacity for supplying tissues with O_2. That this was the response observed in normal healthy volunteers was verified by Bhatt et al. [67], who avoided any question of mathematical coupling in their results by using independent measurements of $\dot{V}O_2$ and cardiac output. They also showed that dobutamine itself is a potent calorigenic agent so that the elevation of $\dot{Q}O_2$ could well have been in response to the increase in O_2 demand.

Yet another vasodilating agent was assessed in endotoxemic dogs that were resuscitated with dextran volume expansion with and without dopexamine [68]. Treatment was given only after development of endotoxic shock. $\dot{Q}O_2$ was restored to preshock values in both groups, and $\dot{V}O_2$ increased to higher than preshock values in both groups as well. Of interest was the fact that dopexamine seemed to prevent later development of tissue hypoxia in the gut, which was also studied in these experiments. Not only was its $\dot{V}O_2$ supported at slightly higher levels during the recovery period, but the positive lactate efflux from the gut observed in the dextran-resuscitated group was reversed when dopexamine was also given. The drug was also used in a randomized clinical study in which the goal was to test whether an increased $\dot{Q}O_2$ perioperatively improved mortality and morbidity in high-risk surgical patients [69]. The investigators favored this means of increasing $\dot{Q}O_2$ because it produced peripheral vasodilation and increased cardiac index without increasing O_2 demand. Although the groups were well matched with respect to initial risk factors, the treatment group in which $\dot{Q}O_2$ was significantly increased perioperatively had a 75% reduction in mortality and half the number of complications per patient. The investigators were unable to decide whether the increase in $\dot{Q}O_2$ was itself responsible for the favorable outcome or whether dopexamine had an additional and more-specific protective effect, but the result was promising.

Vasoconstrictors

The general preference among critical are practitioners is to achieve the warm hyperdynamic state in septic patients by volume resuscitation and by stimulation of the depressed myocardium by β-agonists such as dobutamine [64]. Nevertheless, there is also often concern about maintaining arterial blood pressure. Zhang et al. [70] assessed norepinephrine for this purpose in a canine model of hyperdynamic endotoxic shock, particularly with a view to its effects on peripheral-blood flow distribution and regional O_2 extraction capability. They reasoned that the observed insensitivity to adrenergic vasoconstriction observed in animal models and in septic patients might justify the early use of norepinephrine to overcome that deficit. They found that the group infused with the drug at 1 μg/kg/min maintained higher arterial pressure and cardiac index after receiving endotoxin with saline infusion than with saline alone. Furthermore, blood flow to portal, mesenteric, and renal beds was not altered. When they lowered cardiac output by cardiac tamponade, they found that the treated group was better able to extract O_2 in the whole body and in the liver. The investigators suggested that this was the result of restoring normal microvascular function with norepinephrine supplementation, a property that would not be shared by other means of increasing blood pressure such as NO synthase inhibition.

Use of NO synthase inhibitors was very inviting, however, because it was known that sepsis induced the formation of NO synthase, and at least some of the reduced reactivity to adrenergic vasoconstriction was attributed to an overabundance of NO. In a canine model of resuscitated endotoxic shock similar to that used by Zhang et al. [68], Walker et al. [71] measured blood flow, $\dot{V}O_2$, and O_2ER in whole body, hindlimb muscles, and gut. They found that in the group given the NO synthase inhibitor L-NAME at the end of a 1-hour shock period, mean arterial blood pressure was returned to the preshock level, whereas it remained depressed in the other group that was given volume but not the drug. Cardiac index was unable to reach as high a level in the L-NAME group, however, and the regional blood flows suffered a similar decrement, with the gut faring the worst. The investigators pointed out that although L-NAME successfully restored blood pressure in this model, it did so at the expense of encroaching on the O_2 transport reserve, particularly to the gut. The role of NO synthase inhibition in clinical applications was recently reviewed by Kilbourn et al. [72]. They favored a measured approach that would take into careful consideration any drug interaction with catecholamines, for example. Indeed, they viewed the use of NO synthase inhibitors as a means of restoring normal sensitivity to adrenergic controls and suggested, in addition, that effects on cardiac index might be ameliorated by other agents such as dobutamine. Their hesitancy serves as a reminder of how much more remains to be discovered before interventions such as this can be used with confidence by clinicians at the bedside.

V. Summary

In this day of molecular biology and genetic medicine, it may come as a surprise to some that there is still neither a real understanding of how the body delivers its supply of O_2 to all its tissues nor any reliable means to monitor the success with which it does so. This is nowhere more obvious than at the bedside of critically ill patients. Although systemic $\dot{Q}O_2$ and $\dot{V}O_2$ are measurable, but not always reliably, an answer to the question of whether any particular region of the body is receiving O_2 sufficient to its need remains beyond our capability. The final common pathway in the regulation of O_2 delivery to tissues resides in the vascular smooth muscle of the vessels that regulate blood flow between and within organ systems. The balance between vasodilatory and vasoconstrictor forces that accomplish this is subject to a complex array of vasoactive factors (Fig. 2), some of which yet remain to be discovered. For example, the local metabolic regulation of blood flow still cannot be described in any but the most general of terms. The extent to which the multiplicity of factors is redundant is still not known. If it is assumed that all parts of the control systems are necessary to normal function and that none are redundant, then it remains for us to discover what the hierarchy of control may be and how each factor interacts with the others. We do not know this for the healthy animal or person, and we are even more ignorant in cases in which the normal control systems are thrown into disarray by disease processes. This remains one of the more urgent problems facing those who still value the integrative approach to physiology and pathophysiology.

References

1. Cain SM. Supply dependency of oxygen uptake in ARDS: Myth or reality? Am J Med Sci 1984; 288:119–124.
2. Smithies M, Bihari DJ. Delivery dependent oxygen consumption: Asking the wrong questions and not getting any answers. Crit Care Med 1993; 21:1622–1626.
3. Cain SM. Mechanisms which control $\dot{V}O_2$ near $\dot{V}O_{max}$: An overview. Med Sci Sports Exerc 1995; 27:60–64.
4. Rowell LB, O'Leary DS, Kellogg DL Jr. Integration of cardiovascular control systems in dynamic exercise. In: Rowell LB, Shepherd JT, eds. Handbook of Physiology Section 12: Exercise: Regulation and Integration of Multiple Systems. New York: Oxford, 1996, pp 770–838.
5. Rowell LB, O'Leary DS. Reflex control of the circulation during exercise: Chemoreflexes and mechanoreflexes. J Appl Physiol 1990; 69:407–418.
6. Rowell LB. Human Circulation. New York: Oxford, 1986.
7. Barbee RW, Stainsby WN, Chirtel SJ. Dynamics of O_2, CO_2, lactate, and acid exchange during contractions and recovery. J Appl Physiol Respirat Environ Exercise Physiol 1983; 54:1687–1692.
8. Laughlin MH, Korthuis RJ, Duncker DJ, Bache RJ. Control of blood flow to cardiac and skeletal muscle during exercise. In: Rowell LB, Shepherd JT, eds. Handbook of Physiology Section 12: Exercise: Regulation and Integration of Multiple Systems. New York: Oxford, 1996, pp 705–769.
9. Costin JC, Skinner NS Jr. Competition between vasoconstrictor and vasodilator mechanisms in skeletal muscle. Am J Physiol 1971; 220:462–466.

10. Granger HJ, Goodman AH, Granger DN. Role of resistance and exchange vessels in local microvascular control of skeletal muscle oxygenation in the dog. Circ Res 1976; 38:379–385.
11. Cain SM, Chapler CK. Circulatory responses to 2,4-dinitrophenol in dog limb during normoxia and hypoxia. J Appl Physiol 1985; 59:698–705.
12. Cain SM, Chapler CK. Effects of norepinephrine and α-block on O_2 uptake and blood flow in dog hindlimb. J Appl Physiol Respirat Environ Exercise Physiol 1981; 51:1245–1250.
13. Sparks HV. Skin and muscle. In: Johnson PC, ed. Peripheral Circulation. New York: John Wiley & Sons, 1978, pp 193–230.
14. Daut J, Rudolph M, von Beckerath N, Meherke G, Gunther K, Meinen LG. Hypoxic dilation of coronary arteries is mediated by ATP-sensitive potassium channels. Science Wash DC 1990; 247:1341–1344.
15. Duling BR, Berne RM. Propagated vasodilation in the microcirculation of the hamster cheek pouch. Circ Res 1970; 26:163–170.
16. Song H, Tyml K. Evidence for sensing and integration of biological signals by the capillary network. Am J Physiol 1993; 265:H1235–H1242.
17. Cilley RE, Scharenberg AM, Bongiorno PF, Guire KE, Bartlett RH. Low oxygen delivery produced by anemia, hypoxia, and low cardiac output. J Surg Res 1991; 51:425–433.
18. Cain SM. Oxygen delivery and uptake in dogs during anemic and hypoxic hypoxia. J Appl Physiol Respirat Environ Exercise Physiol 1977; 42:228–234.
19. Fahey JT, Lister G. Postnatal changes in critical cardiac output and oxygen transport in conscious lambs. Am J Physiol 1984; 253:H100–H106.
20. Moss M, Moreau G, Lister G. Oxygen transport and metabolism in the conscious lamb: The effects of hypoxemia. Pediatr Res 1987; 22:177–183.
21. Angell JJE, Daly MDeB. Cardiovascular responses in apnoeic asphyxia: role of arterial chemoreceptors and the modification of their effects by a pulmonary vagal inflation reflex. J Physiol London 1969; 201:87–104.
22. Krasney JA. Regional circulatory responses to arterial hypoxia in the anesthetized dog. Am J Physiol 1971; 220:699–704.
23. Wyler F. Effects of hypoxia on distribution of cardiac output and organ blood flow in the rabbit. Cardiology 1975; 60:163–172.
24. Adachi H, Strauss HW, Ochi H, Wagner HN Jr. The effect of hypoxia on the regional distribution of cardiac output in the dog. Circ Res 1976; 39:314–319.
25. Cain SM, Chapler CK. Oxygen extraction by canine hindlimb during hypoxic hypoxia. J Appl Physiol Respirat Environ Exercise Physiol 1979; 46:1023–1028.
26. Schlichtig R, Kramer DJ, Pinsky MR. Flow redistribution during progressive hemorrhage is a determinant of critical O_2 delivery. J Appl Physiol 1991; 70:169–178.
27. Maginniss LA, Connolly H, Samsel RW, Schumacker PT. Adrenergic vasoconstriction augments tissue O_2 extraction during reductions in O_2 delivery. J Appl Physiol 1994; 76:1454–1461.
28. Samsel RW, Schumacker PT. Systemic hemorrhage augments local O_2 extraction in canine intestine. J Appl Physiol 1994; 77:2291–2298.
29. Comroe JH Jr, Schmidt CF. The part played by reflexes from the carotid body in the chemical regulation of respiration in the dog. Am J Physiol 1938; 121:75–97.

30. Hatcher JD, Chiu LK, Jennings DB. Anemia as a stimulus to aortic and carotid body chemoreceptors in the cat. J Appl Physiol Respirat Environ Exercise Physiol 1978; 44:696–702.
31. Daly MDeB, Ungar A. Comparison of the reflex responses elicited by stimulation of the separately perfused carotid and aortic body chemoreceptors in the dog. J Physiol London 1966; 182:379–403.
32. Fan FC, Chen RYZ, Schuessler GB, Chien S. Effects of hematocrit variations on regional hemodynamics and oxygen transport in the dog. Am J Physiol 1980; 238: H545–H552.
33. Cain SM, Chapler CK. O_2 extraction by hindlimb versus whole dog during anemic hypoxia. J Appl Physiol Respirat Environ Exercise Physiol 1978; 45:966–970.
34. Cain SM. Effects of time and vasoconstrictor tone on O_2 extraction during hypoxic hypoxia. J Appl Physiol Respirat Environ Exercise Physiol 1978; 45:219–224.
35. Cain SM, Chapler CK. O_2 extraction by canine hindlimb during α-adrenergic blockade and hypoxic hypoxia. J Appl Physiol Respirat Environ Exercise Physiol 1980; 48:630–635.
36. Chen DG, Dai X, Bache RJ. Postsynaptic adrenoceptor-mediated vasoconstriction in coronary and femoral vascular beds. Am J Physiol 1988; 254:H984–H992.
37. Kubes P, Melinyshyn M, Nesbitt K, Cain SM, Chapler CK. Participation of α_2-adrenergic receptors in neural vascular tone of canine skeletal muscle. Am J Physiol 1992; 262:H1705–H1710.
38. Chapler CK, Cain SM. Effects of α-adrenergic blockade during acute anemia. J Appl Physiol Respirat Environ Exercise Physiol 1982; 52:16–20.
39. Chapler CK, Stainsby WN, Lillie MA. Peripheral vascular responses during acute anemia. Can J Physiol Pharmacol 1981; 59:102–107.
40. Lundvall J, Järhult J. Beta adrenergic dilator component of the sympathetic vascular response in skeletal muscle. Acta Physiol Scand 1976; 96:180–192.
41. Lundvall J, Hillman J. Noradrenaline evoked beta adrenergic dilation of precapillary sphincters in skeletal muscle. Acta Physiol Scand 1978; 102:126–128.
42. Yonekawa H, Berk JL, Neuman MR, Liu CC. Tissue hypoxia and increased physiological tissue shunt caused by beta-adrenergic stimulation. Eur Surg Res 1981; 13:325–338.
43. Cain SM, Bredle DL. Actions of a dopaminergic and β_2-adrenergic agonist on O_2 extraction by canine skeletal muscle. Adv Exp Med Biol 1990; 277:569–575.
44. Van der Linden P, Gilbart E, Engelman E, Schmartz, Vincent J-L. Effects of anesthetic agents on systemic critical O_2 delivery. J Appl Physiol 1991; 71:83–93.
45. Furchgott RF, Zawadzki JV. The obligatory role of endothelial cells in the relaxation of arterial smooth muscle by acetylcholine. Nature London 1980; 288:373–376.
46. Vallet B, Curtis SE, Winn MJ, King CE, Chapler CK, Cain SM. Hypoxic vasodilation does not require nitric oxide (EDRF/NO) synthesis. J Appl Physiol 1994; 76:1256–1261.
47. Curtis SE, Vallet B, Winn MJ, Caufield JB, King CE, Chapler CK, Cain SM. Role of the vascular endothelium in O_2 extraction during progressive ischemia in canine skeletal muscle. J Appl Physiol 1995; 79:1351–1360.
48. Powers SR Jr, Mannal R, Neclerio M, English M, Marr C, Leather R, Ueda H, Williams G, Custead W, Dutton R. Physiologic consequences of positive end-expiratory (PEEP) ventilation. Ann Surg 1973; 178:265–272.

49. Danek SJ, Lynch JP, Weg JG, Dantzker DR. The dependence of oxygen uptake on oxygen delivery in the adult respiratory distress syndrome. Am Rev Respir Dis 1980; 122:387–395.
50. Bihari D, Smithies M, Gimson A, Tinker J. The effects of vasodilation with prostacyclin on oxygen delivery and uptake in critically ill patients. New Engl J Med 1987; 317:397–403.
51. Cain SM. Assessment of tissue oxygenation. Crit Care Clin 1986; 2:537–550.
52. Cain SM. Metabolic alterations with hypoxia. Réan Urg 1996; 5:174–177.
53. Soni N, Fawcett WJ, Halliday FC. Beyond the lung: Oxygen delivery and tissue oxygenation. Anaesthesia 1993; 48:704–711.
54. Consensus conference. Tissue hypoxia: How to detect, how to correct, how to prevent. Am J Respir Crit Care Med 1996; 154:1573–1578.
55. Lategola M, Rahn H. A self-guiding cathether for cardiac and pulmonary arterial catheterization and occlusion. Proc Soc Exp Biol Med 1952; 8:246–247.
56. Russell JA, Phang PT. The oxygen delivery/consumption controversy. Am J Respir Crit Care Med 1994; 149:533–537.
57. Dantzker DR. Foresman B, Gutierrez G. Oxygen supply and utilization relationships. Am Rev Respir Dis 1991; 143:675–679.
58. Nelson DP, Beyer C, Samsel RW, Wood LDH, Schumacker PT. Pathological oxygen supply dependence of O_2 uptake during bacteremia in dogs. J Appl Physiol 1987; 63:1487–1492.
59. Nelson DP, Samsel RW, Wood LDH, Schumacker PT. Pathological supply dependence of systemic and intestinal O_2 uptake during endotoxemia. J Appl Physiol 1988; 64:2410–2419.
60. Samsel RW, Nelson DP, Sanders WM, Wood LDH, Schumacker PT. Effect of endotoxin on systemic and skeletal muscle O_2 extraction. J Appl Physiol 1988; 65:1377–1382.
61. Cain SM. Gut oxygenation after reduced oxygen delivery. In: Vincent J-L, ed. Yearbook of Intensive Care and Emergency Medicine. 1996, pp 219–226.
62. Vallet B, Lund N, Curtis SE, Kelly D, Cain SM. Gut and muscle tisuse P_{O_2} in endotoxemic dogs during shock and resuscitation. J Appl Physiol 1994; 76:793–800.
63. Sair M, Etherington PJ, Curzen NP, Winlove CP, Evans TW. Tissue oxygenation and perfusion in endotoxemia. Am J Physiol 1996; 271:H1620–H1625.
64. Tuchschmidt J, Oblitas D, Fried JC. Oxygen consumption in sepsis and septic shock. Crit Care Med 1991; 19:664–671.
65. De Backer D, Berré J, Zhang H, Kahn RJ, Vincent J-L. Relationship between oxygen uptake and oxygen delivery in septic patients: Effects of prostacyclin versus dobutamine. Crit Care Med 1993; 21:1658–1664.
66. Vallet B, Chopin C, Curtis SE, Dupuis BA, Fourrier F, Mehdaoui H, LeRoy B, Rime A, Santre C, Herbecq P, Her B. Prognostic value of the dobutamine test in patients with sepsis syndrome and normal lactate values: A prospective, multicenter study. Crit Care Med 1993; 21:1868–1875.
67. Bhatt SB, Hutchinson RC, Tomlinson B, Oh TE, Mak M. Effect of dobutamine on oxygen supply and uptake in healthy volunteers. Br J Anaesth 1992; 69:298–303.
68. Cain SM, Curtis SE. Systemic and regional oxygen uptake and lactate flux in endotoxic dogs resuscitated with dextran and dopexamine or dextran alone. Circ Shock 1992; 38:173–181.

69. Boyd O, Grounds RM, Bennett ED. A randomized clinical trial of the effect of deliberate perioperative increase of oxygen delivery on mortality in high-risk surgical patients. JAMA 1993; 270:2699–2707.
70. Zhang H, Smail N, Cabral A, Rogiers P, Vincent J-L. Effects of norepinephrine on regional blood flow and oxygen extraction capabilities during endotoxic shock. Am J Respir Crit Care Med 1997; 155:1965–1971.
71. Walker TA, Curtis SE, King-VanVlack CE, Chapler CK, Ballet B, Cain SM. Effects of nitric oxide synthase inhibition on regional hemodynamics and oxygen transport in endotoxic dogs. Shock 1995; 4:415–420.
72. Kilbourn RG, Szabo C, Traber DL. Beneficial versus detrimental effects of nitric oxide synthase inhibitors in circulatory shock: Lessons learned from experimental and clinical studies. Shock 1997; 7:235–246.
73. Wade OL, Bishop JM. Cardiac Output and Regional Blood Flow. Oxford: Blackwell Scientific Publications, 1962.

13

Gas Exchange in the Heart

KEITH R. WALLEY

University of British Columbia
Vancouver, British Columbia, Canada

I. Introduction

The heart as a working muscle is uniquely dependent on its oxygen supply to continuously maintain aerobic metabolism [1]. As such, myocardial blood flow is closely regulated to match myocardial oxygen demand, which, in turn, depends on myocardial work [2]. This chapter reviews how coronary circulation accomplishes the goal of maintaining oxygen supply so that myocardial aerobic metabolism can be sustained in the face of enormous changes in oxygen demand.

The heart consumes approximately 12% of basal whole-body oxygen consumption and is almost completely dependent on adenosine triphosphate (ATP) generated by aerobic metabolism to maintain normal pump function [3]. The small amount of ATP that can be generated by the heart via anaerobic glycolysis is insufficient, so that if oxygen delivery to the heart is inadequate to meet metabolic demand, then pump function rapidly fails [1,3,4]. Oxygen consumption is thus a reasonably direct measure of energy use of the heart. Substrate metabolism by the heart generates between 19.6 (lipid) and 20.9 (carbohydrate) joules of energy per mL of oxygen consumed [5]. The main exogenous substrates of myocardial metabolism are free fatty acids, glucose, and lactate [6], which typically account for 1/2, 1/4, and 1/8 th of the oxygen consumed, respectively [7]. The remaining oxygen consumption is accounted for by metabolism of ketone bodies, pyruvate, and other minor substrates. However, the heart can adapt readily to the available substrate. For example, almost 100% of the metabolic substrate is free fatty acid after a lipid-rich meal [8]. Irrespective of the exact substrate mix, the key feature is that oxygen consumption is essential to maintain the energy supply of the heart, generating on average 20 J/mL O_2 consumed (4.8 cal/mL O_2).

The ability of the heart and other organs to extract oxygen from the arterial blood supply can be usefully illustrated using an oxygen delivery–consumption diagram (Fig. 1). In the whole body and other organs, a biphasic relationship is found between oxygen delivery and oxygen consumption [9,10]. At high oxygen deliveries sufficient to maintain aerobic metabolism, oxygen consumption is relatively constant and independent of changes in oxygen delivery. If oxygen delivery is decreased, then at some low value oxygen consumption must decrease because

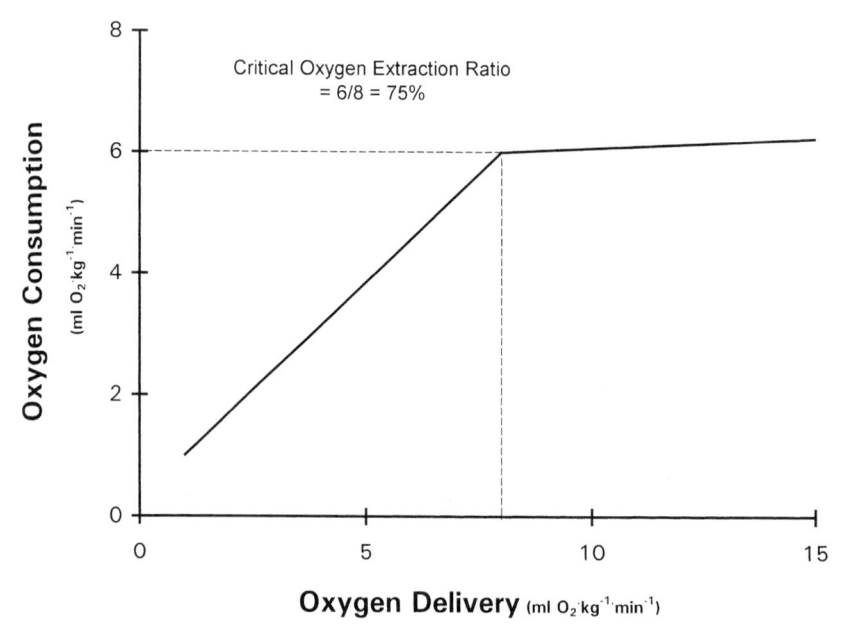

Figure 1 A typical relationship between oxygen delivery and oxygen consumption for the whole body and many noncardiac organs is shown. At high oxygen deliveries, oxygen consumption is independent of oxygen delivery and relatively constant, being set by oxygen demand. At low oxygen deliveries, oxygen consumption becomes dependent on oxygen delivery, associated with evidence of tissue hypoxia and anaerobic metabolism. The oxygen extraction ratio (oxygen consumption divided by oxygen delivery) at the transition from plateau to downslope is the critical oxygen delivery and is a measure of the ability of tissues to extract oxygen.

it is not possible to extract more oxygen than is delivered. Decreasing oxygen consumption, dependent on decreasing oxygen delivery, is associated with evidence of anaerobic metabolism, including mounting lactic acidosis [11] and decreased organ function [1]. The critical oxygen extraction ratio (oxygen consumption divided by delivery) at the transition from plateau (aerobic metabolism) to downslope (anaerobic, supply-dependent metabolism) is a key measure of oxygen extraction ability of a tissue or organ. The critical oxygen extraction ratio in health is remarkably constant at approximately 75% in many studies in various animal species and in various tissues [1,10–12].

The heart is different from the whole body and other organs in that even resting myocardial oxygen consumption is very high, typically 60–80 mL O_2/kg [1,13] (compared with 4 mL O_2/kg for the whole body and 20 mL O_2/kg for the metabolically active gut [10–12,14]), and the "aerobic plateau phase" is not a plateau [1]. Increasing myocardial oxygen demand results in increasing myocardial oxygen delivery, so that during normal aerobic metabolism there is a steeply sloped relationship (Fig. 2). The aerobic phase of the myocardial oxygen delivery–consumption relationship is approximately linear and nearly passes through the origin [1]. Thus, the myocardial oxygen extraction ratio is nearly constant at 70–80% over a wide range of cardiac work and oxygen demand states [15]. This implies that the coronary circulation very closely matches oxygen supply to demand, thereby maintaining the nearly constant oxygen extraction ratio. During extreme exercise, myocardial work and coronary blood flow can increase fivefold or more [16], yet the myocardial oxygen extraction ratio increases only slightly to 80–90% [17]. During experimentally induced severe hypoxemia, as myocardial anaerobic metabolism is approached, the myocardial oxygen extraction ratio increases to a similar level [1,16]. In this case, frank anaerobic metabolism is accompanied by a positive feedback loop of decreased ventricular function, decreased cardiac output, and decreased coronary perfusion pressure leading to cardiac arrest [1]. It is remarkable that the heart normally functions at an oxygen extraction ratio as high as the critical oxygen extraction ratio for other organs and so close to the maximum possible myocardial value consistent with life.

The close relationship between myocardial oxygen consumption and delivery is altered in a number of disease states, notably occlusive coronary artery disease [18,19] and sepsis [20,21]. The matching of myocardial oxygen supply to demand becomes an important issue when coronary artery disease limits oxygen supply at times of increased myocardial oxygen demand. Then, whole sections of the myocardium become anaerobic. In sepsis, the microvascular distribution of oxygen supply is altered, and the ability of the coronary microcirculation to match supply to demand is impaired [21]. This is associated with greatly increased heterogeneity of myocardial microcirculatory blood flow. Here, the normal myocardial oxygen extraction ratio of approximately 75% decreases to approximately 50% [7,20,21].

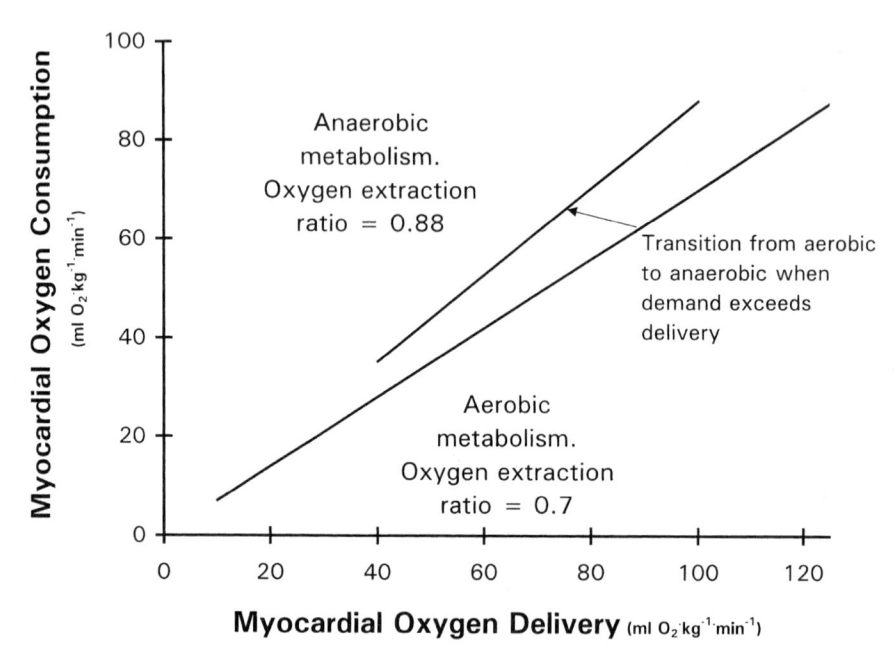

Figure 2 The relationship between oxygen delivery and oxygen consumption for the heart is shown. The downsloping delivery-dependent anaerobic phase is similar to that for the whole body and other organs. However, there is no plateau phase because the coronary circulation modulates blood flow (and thus oxygen delivery) in direct proportion to oxygen demand. Both the aerobic and anaerobic relationships are linear and nearly intersect the origin. Thus, aerobic metabolism is characterized by a fairly constant oxygen extraction ratio (slope) of approximately 70–75%, whereas anaerobic metabolism is characterized by higher oxygen extraction ratios (80–90%) when oxygen delivery is insufficient to meet demand.

II. Coronary Circulation

Coronary circulation must maintain a very high blood flow to a metabolically active myocardium to satisfy myocardial oxygen demand. Myocardial oxygen demand can change rapidly, for example, when rapidly going from rest to extreme exercise or during high catecholamine states such as "fight or flight." As a result, the coronary circulation also must adapt extremely rapidly to changing myocardial oxygen demand.

Blood flow to the heart [22] is supplied by the left and right coronary arteries that originate from the left and right sinuses of Valsalva, immediately distal to the two anterior aortic valve leaflets. The posterior leaflet of the aortic valve is not associated with a coronary artery. The left coronary artery generally is larger and supplies a greater fraction of the total coronary flow. The right coronary artery lies in the atrioventricular groove and curves to the right and posteriorly around the heart. In more than 80% of humans, the right coronary artery then supplies the posterior descending coronary artery and associated branches. Thus, the right coronary artery generally supplies blood flow to the right ventricle, the posterior wall of the left ventricle, and the posterior portion of the intraventricular septum. The left coronary artery branches within 2–10 mm of its origin into the circumflex and left anterior descending coronary arteries. The circumflex coronary artery travels laterally and posteriorly in the atrioventricular groove, supplying branches to the lateral left ventricular myocardium. In less than 20% of humans, the circumflex coronary artery supplies the posterior descending coronary artery. The left anterior descending coronary artery supplies blood flow to the anterior portion of the intraventricular septum, the anterior wall of the left ventricle, and the apex.

The main coronary arteries are very superficially located on the surface of the heart, where myocardial contraction does not mechanically cause occlusion. Branches then descend steeply into the myocardium. These vessels give rise to branched arterioles with extensive collateral connections [23] approximately 40 μm in diameter. Arterioles then give rise to capillaries that, again, form an interconnected branching pattern. For the most part, capillaries run parallel to the muscle fibers [24]. Muscle fibers of the heart are aligned in a helical pattern with changing orientation from epicardium to endocardium so that the majority of midwall fibers are circumferentially oriented [25]. Capillary length, although geometrically complex [26], is in the order of 0.5–1.5 mm. As the heart contracts, muscle fibers get shorter and wider so that capillary density decreases as predicted from geometric considerations. Coronary capillary tortuosity does not increase as much as expected, so that capillary length is less, and surface area for diffusion decreases with contraction [27].

Coronary venous drainage follows the arterial anatomy, to a large extent, for the smaller vessels. Then the posterior cardiac vein joins the great cardiac vein, which is located laterally in the atrioventricular groove and drains into the coronary sinus. The coronary sinus drains into the right atrium. The coronary sinus arises from the embryonic cardinal veins, which also give rise to the superior vena cava on the right and the hemiazgous vein on the left. The anatomy varies between different species, e.g., the left hemiazygous vein drains into the coronary sinus in the pig but not in humans. The extent of collateralization of the coronary arterial circulation is also species-specific. For example, dogs have more extensive collateralization than pigs, with humans being intermediate between the two [28].

III. Determinants of Myocardial Oxygen Demand

Over the years, different investigators have taken a number of approaches in determining the mechanical correlates of myocardial oxygen consumption. The product of heart rate and mean arterial pressure has been used by many investigators and clinicians as an easily calculated reflection of myocardial oxygen demand [29,30]. The Laplace relationship points out that wall tension is proportional to pressure multiplied by the radius of curvature of the wall. Because the contracting myocytes generate wall tension rather than generating pressure directly, a number of investigators have focused on wall tension [31] or systolic force [32] as determinants of myocardial oxygen demand. Although each approach has advantages, a number of discrepancies seem to remain [33]. Suga et al. [33–36] and other investigators [37,38] have extensively examined the relationship between mechanical variables and myocardial oxygen consumption based on the pressure–volume relationship of the left ventricle.

When the pressure–volume trajectory of a cardiac cycle is plotted, the area of the pressure–volume loop has units of work and is simply the external mechanical work that the heart performs with each beat (Fig. 3). However, when this mechanical work term is plotted against myocardial oxygen consumption per beat, these two variables are found to be poorly correlated. In particular, during experimental isovolumic contractions, no external work is performed even though the ventricle generates high systolic pressures. Thus, oxygen consumption required for the work that the myocardium does against internal elastic structures that generate pressure must also be accounted for. Suga et al. [33–36] proposed that the additional area subtended by the end systolic pressure–volume relationship be considered "potential mechanical work." Then "pressure–volume-area" (PVA) is defined as the sum of external mechanical work and potential mechanical work. The investigators found that there was a very close relationship between PVA and myocardial oxygen consumption. This unique relationship holds for a wide range of differently ejecting contractions as well as for isovolumic contractions [35]. One explanation for why this additional potential mechanical work term results in a close relationship with myocardial oxygen consumption is as follows. If the ventricle is unloaded toward the end of ejection along a trajectory that lies close to the end systolic pressure–volume relationship, then the area subtended by the end systolic pressure–volume relationship could conceivably be recovered as external work (Fig. 4).

The relationship between myocardial oxygen consumption and PVA is linear (Fig. 5). There is significant myocardial oxygen consumption at the zero PVA intercept. The intercept identifies myocardial oxygen consumption that must be maintained to keep the myocytes alive without performance of external mechanical work [33–39]. As external mechanical work increases, myocardial oxygen consumption increases. The inverse of the slope of this line is approximately 40%, demonstrating that the heart, above baseline oxygen consumption, is approximately 40% efficient in turning metabolic energy into PVA work [40].

Increased heart rate increases the slope of the myocardial oxygen consumption–PVA relationship [36]. Thus, increasing heart rate from 120 to 190 beats/min is associated with decreased efficiency of converting oxygen consumption into PVA

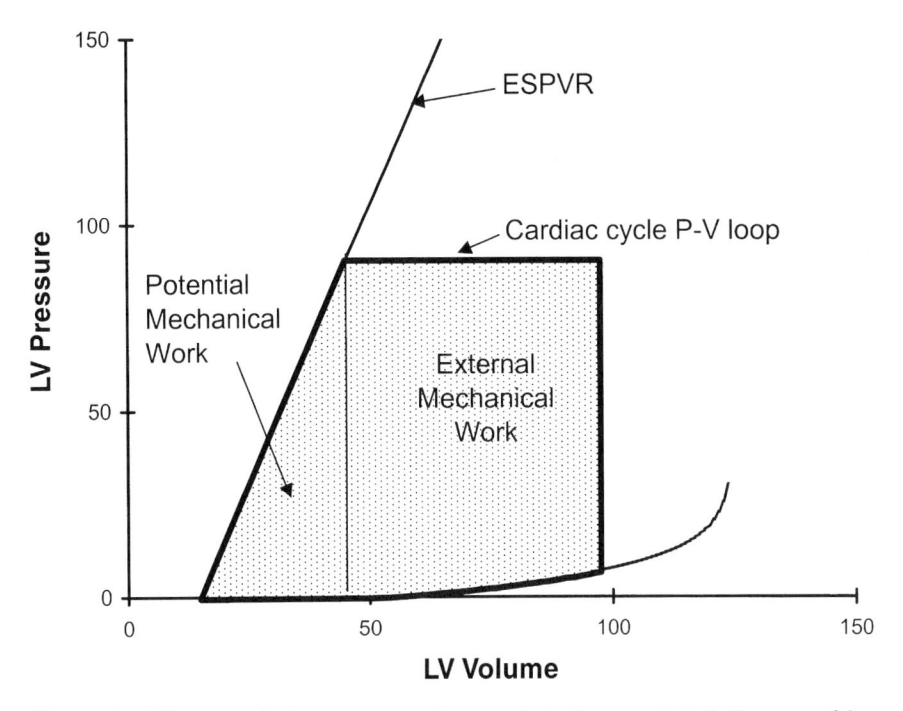

Figure 3 When ventricular pressure–volume trajectories are plotted, the area of loops has units of work. End-systolic points from many different contractions (not shown) all lie along the end-systolic pressure–volume relationship (ESPVR). The area enclosed within a cardiac cycle is external mechanical work. Potential mechanical work is the area to the left of pressure–volume loops under the ESPVR. Myocardial oxygen consumption is found to be closely correlated to pressure–volume area (shaded area), which is the sum of external mechanical work and potential mechanical work.

work. Increasing intracellular calcium concentrations directly or by the addition of catecholamines and other positive inotropic agents increases contractility. Increased contractility shifts the myocardial oxygen consumption–PVA relationship up [39] (Fig. 5B). However, the slope of the relationship does not change, demonstrating that the efficiency of the actin-myosin ATPase is approximately constant and independent of inotropic state [35,40]. When positive inotropic agents were added to a nonbeating heart, myocardial oxygen consumption did not increase [39].

Thus, Suga et al. [39] proposed that myocardial oxygen consumption can be thought of as consisting of three components (Fig. 5). The first component is directly related to PVA and supplies mechanical energy for contraction. The efficiency of conversion of consumed oxygen to PVA work is constant except that high heart

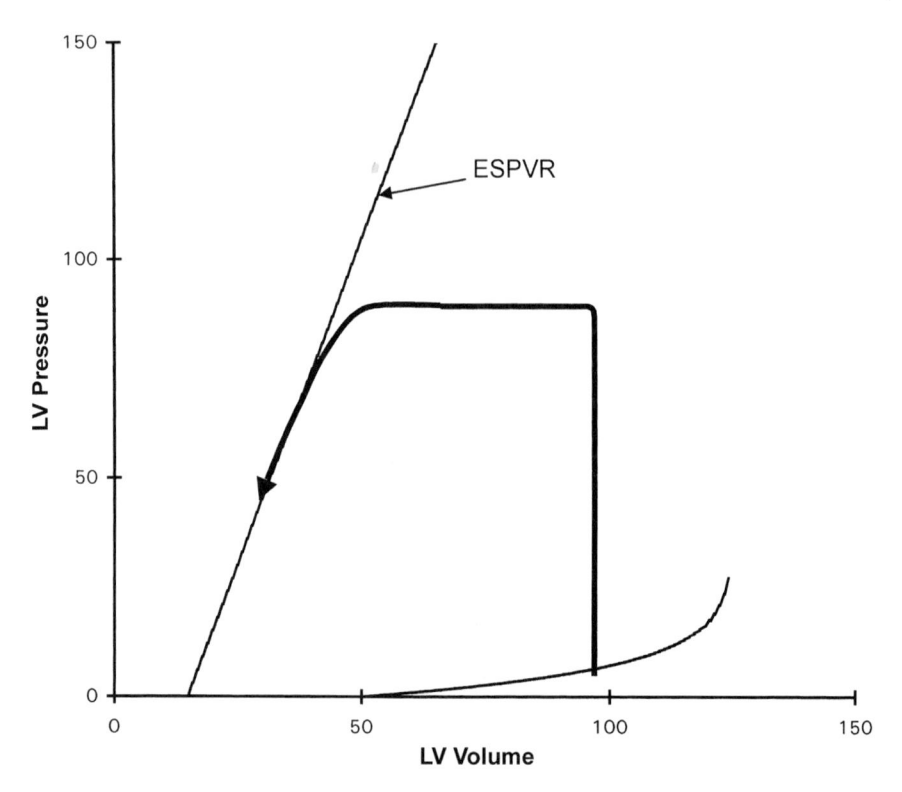

Figure 4 The area under the end-systolic pressure–volume relationship can potentially be recovered as mechanical work if the ventricle is unloaded along a trajectory similar to that illustrated here. Thus, the area under the end-systolic pressure–volume relationship is called "potential mechanical work."

rates are associated with decreased efficiency. The second component is the part of basal oxygen consumption (myocardial oxygen consumption at zero PVA) that increases with inotropic stimulation and decreases with β-adrenergic blockade. This oxygen consumption likely supplies energy for activation or excitation–contraction coupling. The third component is the part of basal oxygen consumption that is unresponsive to inotropic stimulation (as in arrested hearts). This oxygen consumption likely supports basic metabolic function and cell membrane integrity to maintain cell viability.

The PVA approach in modified form also accounts well for regional oxygen consumption [37]. Other similar analyses demonstrate that myocardial oxygen consumption can be accounted for by the sum of the oxygen consumption related to external energy expenditure plus an internal energy index of heat [41] or by preload recruitable stroke work [42].

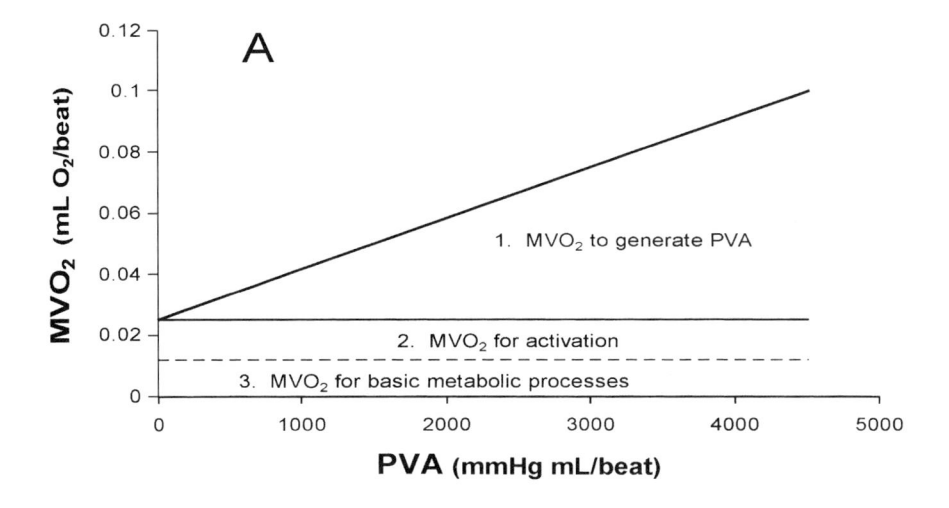

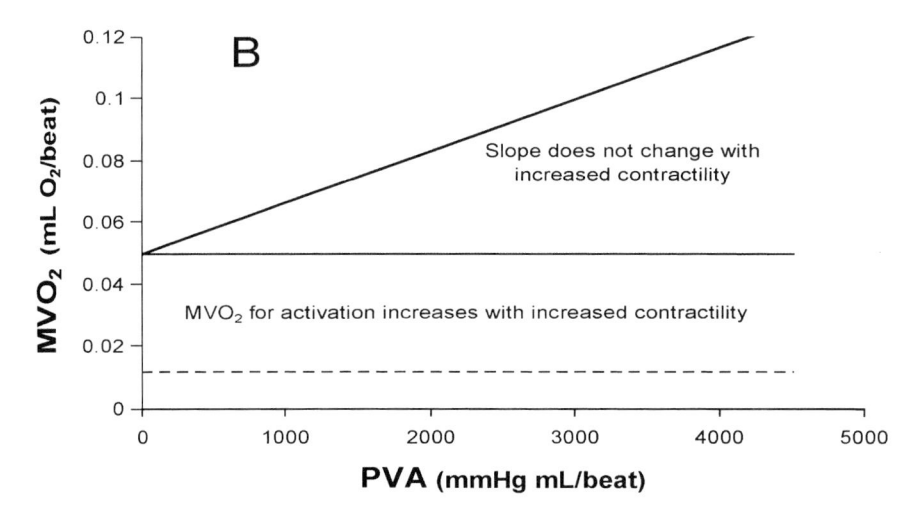

Figure 5 (A) Myocardial oxygen consumption (MVo$_2$) is linearly related to pressure–volume area (PVA) for a 100-g heart (typical of a dog or pig). Increased contractility shifts the relationship upward with no change in slope. The inverse of the slope is the efficiency of MVo$_2$/PVA conversion and is approximately 40%. (B) The increase in MVo$_2$ at zero PVA during increased contractility is postulated to be caused by increased activation, or excitation–contraction coupling, energy. Increased contractility does not change MVo$_2$ of a noncontracting heart, so that a component of basal myocardial oxygen consumption is thought to provide energy for basic metabolic processes in cell viability.

IV. Determinants of Myocardial Oxygen Supply

Normally, coronary blood flow is regulated to maintain a relatively constant myocardial oxygen extraction ratio of approximately 75%. Regulation of coronary flow depends on perfusion pressure and coronary vascular resistance. Coronary perfusion pressure changes dramatically with time through the cardiac cycle and with position across the myocardial wall. Furthermore, coronary vascular resistance changes during the cardiac cycle because coronary arteries shorten and are compressed during systolic contraction by the surrounding myocardium and by the adjacent ventricular cavity pressure.

Measurements of coronary pressure–flow relationships indicate the presence of a Starling resistor in the coronary circulation with a zero flow pressure of 20–50 mm Hg [43,44] (Fig. 6). Bellamy et al. [43] have shown that both coronary venous pressure and ventricular systole increase the zero-flow pressure of the Starling resistor by increasing surrounding myocardial tissue pressure. In addition, the epicardial coronary veins also demonstrate features of a second Starling resistor so that venous pressures less than 12 mm Hg did not influence upstream flow [45].

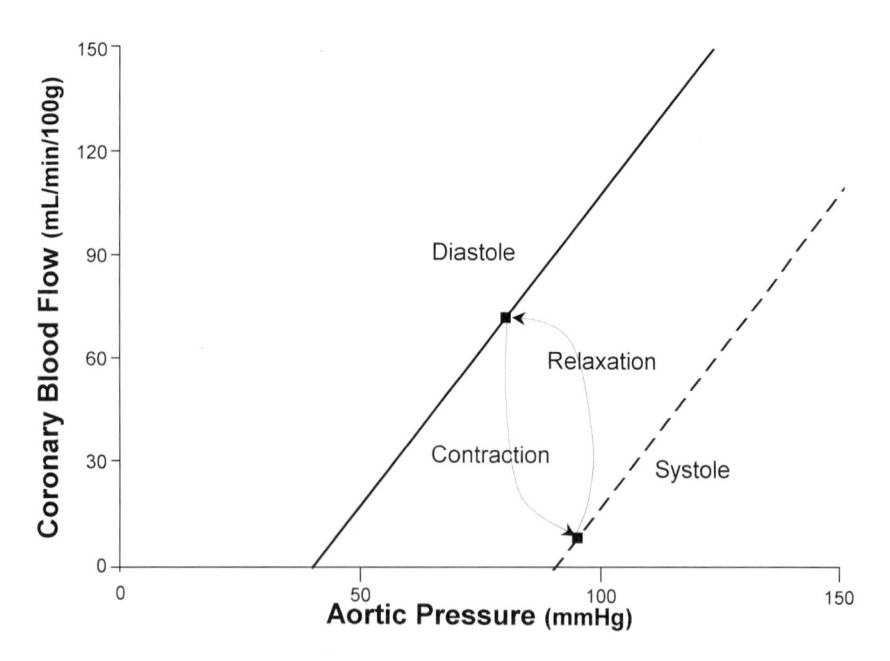

Figure 6 Representative coronary pressure–flow relationships are illustrated. The zero-flow intercept typically ranges from 30 to 50 mm Hg, indicating the presence of a Starling resistor caused by intramyocardial pressure. Systolic contraction increases intramyocardial pressure and the zero-flow intercept. To a lesser extent, an increase in coronary venous pressure also right-shifts this relationship.

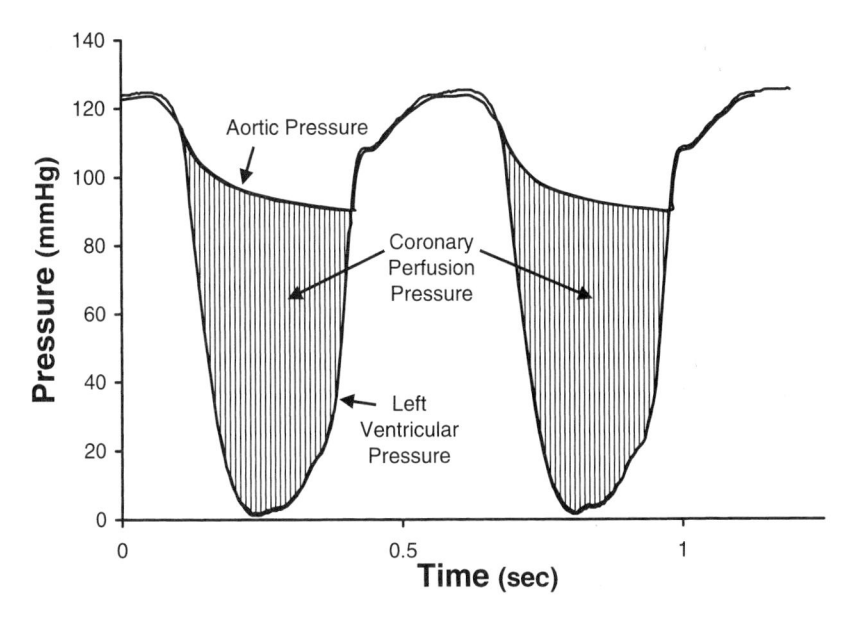

Figure 7 Coronary artery flow depends on the presence of a pressure gradient between the aorta and intramyocardial pressure. If intramyocardial pressure is approximated by ventricular intracavitary pressure, then coronary perfusion depends on diastolic perfusion pressure and the duration of diastole relative to the duration of the cardiac cycle.

Coronary perfusion pressure is complex because it is the difference between aortic pressure and pressure at the flow-limiting site (or Starling resistor) in the coronary circulation, which depends heavily on intramyocardial pressure [43]. Perfusion pressure is greatest during diastole, when the difference between aortic blood pressure and intramyocardial pressure is the greatest (Fig. 7). During diastole, the effect of vascular compression on coronary vascular resistance is also minimized. Thus, the driving pressure for coronary blood flow depends largely on the difference between diastolic aortic perfusion pressure and intraventricular pressure and the duration of diastole with respect to systole [46]. During systole, coronary blood flow decreases to almost zero because intramyocardial pressure is high. Perfusion of the outer layers of myocardium can continue because outer layers of myocardium are protected to some extent from intraventricular pressure by the inner layers of myocardium that generate that component of intraventricular pressure [47]. The difference between epicardial and endocardial coronary flow is normally small. However, this effect is important when limited oxygen delivery leads to myocardial tissue hypoxia. The endocardium becomes hypoxic before the epicardium because it exists in an environment that, on average, is at higher pressure, with a correspondingly lower perfusion pressure gradient.

There is considerable variation of flow within small regions of the heart. For example, when flow in tissue pieces less than 1% of total myocardial mass was measured, some regions had local flows as low as one third to as high as twice the average flow with a relative dispersion (SD of local flows per mean flow) of 20–30% [48,49]. Even smaller pieces demonstate greater dispersion of local blood flow. The relative dispersion of myocardial blood flow depends on the size of tissue pieces examined, in a way that can be characterized by a fractal dimension, D. That is, for relative dispersion (RD) of local regions of mass (m):

$$RD(m) = RD(m = 1g) \times (m/1g)^{1-D}$$

D for myocardial blood flow is approximately 1.2 [48]. Thus, for tissue volumes typical of capillary beds of 100 μm^3, relative dispersion increases nearly fourfold compared with that of 1-g pieces. This fractal distribution of blood flow also has the property that flows in neighboring regions are more likely to be similar than flows in distant regions. Local correlation of blood flow seems to be caused by the sharing of larger feeder vessels. Thus, while myocardial capillary flow is heterogeneous, it is not entirely random. Even at the microregional level, coronary circulation displays careful matching of flow to transport capacity [50].

Coronary vascular regulation seems to depend substantially on release of various mediators. Myocardial adenosine concentrations vary in direct proportion to myocardial oxygen consumption [51]. Furthermore, coronary vascular resistance is inversely related to myocardial adenosine concentrations [52]. Thus, adenosine seems to be a key regulator of coronary vascular tone, although other vasodilators also play important roles. Nitric oxide, released primarily from endothelial cells, is more important in regulating resistance of small arterioles (< 120 mm) than of large arterioles [53]. Increasing vagal tone mediates cholinergic vasodilation to all layers of the myocardium [54,55]. Interestingly, acetycholine itself vasodilates from the intraluminal surface but constricts from the abluminal surface [56]. Not surprisingly, tissue partial oxygen pressure (Po_2) also plays a role. Low Po_2 increases the degree and pressure range of coronary autoregulation [57].

Although a number of important mediators that regulate coronary flow have been identified, it is unclear how oxygen supply can be regulated to meet oxygen demand when the signal for inadequate supply occurs within the capillary bed yet the regulation of blood flow occurs upstream at the arteriolar level. Dietrich and Tyml [58] and Song and Tyml [59] have shown that the capillary and microvascular endothelium acts to transmit vasoactive signals upstream. A vasoconstrictive stimulus applied to capillaries can be transmitted to upstream arterioles 1000 μm away [60]. Communication from endothelial cell to endothelial cell seems to occur via gap junctions. Endothelial cells also seem to signal underlying smooth muscle using similar signal transmission via gap junctions [61]. In addition, myogenic mechanisms responding to vascular wall strain (responsive to intravascular pressure) and shear stress (responsive to intravascular flow) contribute to microvascular flow regulation [62]. These mechanisms are autoregulatory to the extent that they contribute to decreased coronary vascular resistance when aortic prefusion pressure and coronary artery flow decrease.

V. Myocardial Oxygen Extraction

During normal function, when myocardial oxygen demand increases, myocardial blood flow is extremely well regulated and increases to meet the increase in demand so that the myocardial oxygen extraction ratio is maintained constant. When myocardial oxygen demand is increased in relation to supply [16] or when supply is reduced in relation to demand [1], the myocardial oxygen extraction ratio can increase, to a small extent, to maintain aerobic metabolism. However, when the myocardial oxygen extraction ratio increases to approximately 80–90%, then evidence of anaerobic metabolism occurs with increasing lactate production, electrocardiogram changes consistent with ischemia, and decreased ventricular function [1]. Therefore, the myocardial oxygen consumption–delivery relationship is different from the oxygen delivery–consumption relationship of other organs in that there is no plateau phase. When the critical myocardial oxygen extraction ratio is exceeded, then left ventricular contractility decreases.

The observation of a critical oxygen extraction ratio suggests that the heart may be similar to the whole body and other organ systems. The presence of a critical oxygen extraction ratio indicates that not all of the delivered oxygen can be extracted at the onset of anaerobic metabolism. Therefore, there must be a percentage of arterial blood that effectively bypasses the oxygen-consuming myocardium—a physiological arteriovenous shunt fraction. When this hypothesis was tested, it was found that the myocardium was not characterized by a critical oxygen extraction ratio, but rather by a critical coronary venous P_{O_2} [63]. Left shifting the oxygen–hemoglobin dissociation curve markedly altered the critical myocardial oxygen extraction ratio but had no effect on the coronary venous P_{O_2}. This suggests that maximal oxygen uptake by the myocardium is diffusion-limited rather than limited by a physiological shunt fraction. Interestingly, working skeletal muscle is also characterized by a critical coronary venous P_{O_2} rather than by a critical oxygen extraction ratio [64]. Based on radiolabeled tracer studies, Rose and Goresky [65] also concluded that a critical capillary P_{O_2} limits myocardial aerobic metabolism. They found that the limiting step to oxygen diffusion seems to occur in oxygen transfer across the red blood cell membrane–capillary wall.

These results are consistent with the observation that cardiac myocytes demonstrate a critical P_{O_2} [66]. In a quiescent state, cardiac myocyte oxygen consumption decreases when P_{O_2} is less than 1.4 mm Hg. When P_{O_2} was decreased to less than 1 mm Hg, free adenosine diphosphate (ADP) and adenosine increased. When the cardiac myocytes were stimulated to contract, the critical myocardial P_{O_2} increased to 10 mm Hg. Oxygen consumption decreased as P_{O_2} was decreased from 10 to 5 mm Hg, but free ADP and adenosine did not change. A P_{O_2} of less than 5 mm Hg resulted in an increase of free ADP and adenosine.

Thus, the heart seems to be more dependent on the P_{O_2} of perfusing arterial blood than are other organs. Because of the importance of P_{O_2} to normal myocyte function, coronary microcirculation is well designed to maintain tissue P_{O_2}. Perfused capillary density increases by 50% as arterial P_{O_2} decreases from normal values to 30 mm Hg [67]. Normal capillary density in the heart is approximately 1,000/mm^2, although this density increases in smaller species with greater oxygen consumption per gram of myocardium. Changes in capillary density vary linearly with changes in arterial P_{O_2} and not with arterial oxygen saturation, providing further evidence that the functional design of the coronary microcirculation is focused on maintaining tissue P_{O_2}.

Once oxygen has entered the myocardium, myoglobin plays an important role in oxygen transport [68]. The oxygen dissociation curve for myoglobin is very left shifted compared with that of hemoglobin (Fig. 8). This means that oxygen saturation of myoglobin is high, and, therefore, oxygen content within the myocardium is high at low tissue P_{O_2} values. This provides a large gradient for oxygen diffusion from capillaries to tissues, thereby facilitating transport of oxygen to the cells. This

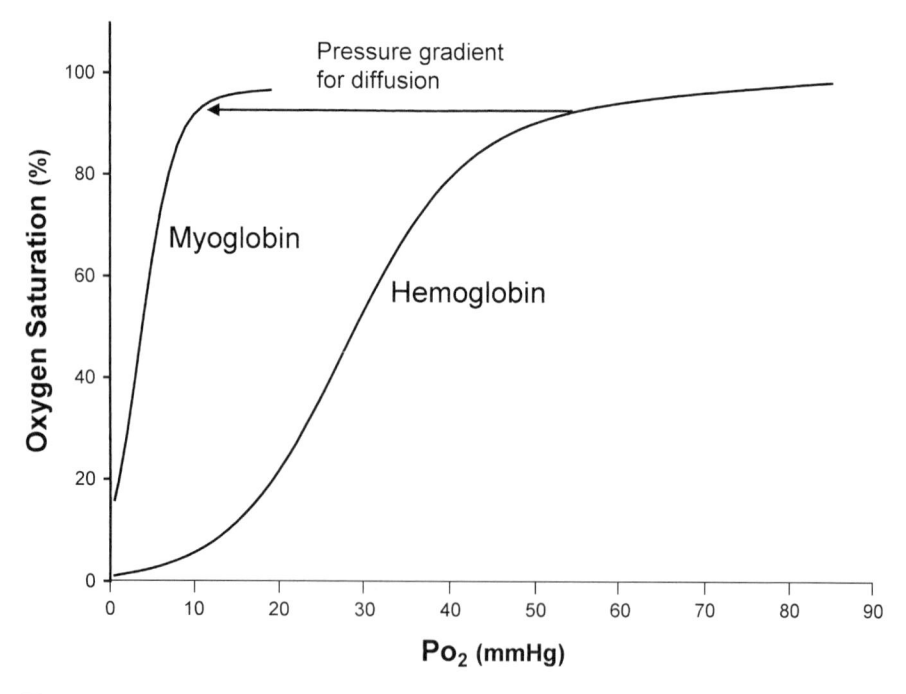

Figure 8 Hemoglobin and myoglobin oxygen dissociation curves are shown on the same set of axes to illustrate the differences. The difference between these curves provides the pressure gradient for oxygen diffusion from the capillary to the myocyte.

is important because unloading of oxygen from capillary blood is the limiting step in myocardial oxygen transport [65], in part, because of the short coronary capillary transit time of approximately 0.5 seconds [69]. The high oxygen content of the tissues also results in a remarkably uniform myocardial tissue P_{O_2} so that cells far from capillaries have a P_{O_2} that is nearly identical to that of cells near capillaries. The myocardial tissue P_{O_2} of 4–7 mm Hg [68] is easily sufficient to maintain oxygen diffusion into mitochondria that have P_{O_2} values in the range of 0.25–2 mm Hg. The distribution of tissue P_{O_2}—high within the capillaries, a sharp decrease across the capillary wall to the tissues, and uniform within myocardial tissue—is in sharp contrast to the distribution predicted from Krogh cylinder models based on oxygen diffusion alone.

VI. Relationship of Blood Flow Heterogeneity to Oxygen Extraction

In addition to diffusion limitation at a critical coronary capillary P_{O_2}, the effect on oxygen extracton of heterogeneity of microvascular oxygen supply and demand needs to be considered. Significant heterogeneity exists in microvascular blood flow distributions, and significant heterogeneity exists in distributions of coronary capillary blood flow transit times. Transit time distributions are important for gas exchange [70] and have been postulated to be closely related to the microregional ratio of oxygen supply/demand [71]. Small regions of the myocardium can be characterized by their ratios of myocardial oxygen demand to oxygen supply [72]. Regions with limited supply in relation to demand result in relatively hypoxic areas of myocardium, whereas regions with excess supply in relation to demand contribute to physiological shunting of arterial blood into the coronary venous circulation.

When the distribution of microvascular oxygen demand to supply is closely regulated with little variation at a value near the average extraction ratio, then extraction of oxygen is efficient, with few relatively hypoxic regions and little shunt of oxygenated blood past the tissues. Increasing the dispersion of the distribution of demand/supply impairs the ability of the myocardium to extract oxygen, i.e., mismatching between oxygen demand and oxygen supply impairs oxygen transport [72], much as it does in the lungs. A theoretical analysis suggests that for relative dispersions less than 20%, small changes in relative dispersion have very little effect on oxygen extraction capacity (Fig. 9) [72]. However, when relative dispersions increase beyond 30%, there is significant reason to expect a decrease in the critical myocardial oxygen extraction ratio, as observed in the coronary circulation in animal models of sepsis [7,20,21]. Normal tissues seem to decrease heterogeneity of capillary blood flow when faced with increased oxygen demand or decreased oxygen delivery [73,74].

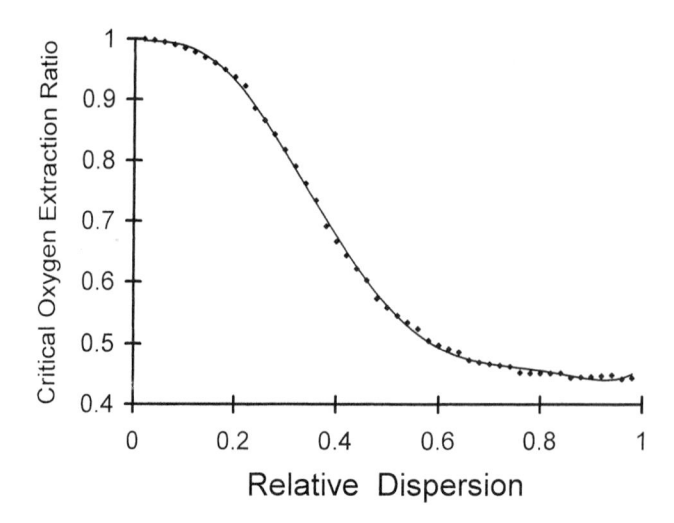

Figure 9 The effect of increasing heterogeneity of the ratio of microregional oxygen supply to demand is shown. Increased heterogeneity (relative dispersion) theoretically limits the ability of the myocardium to extract oxygen so that the critical oxygen extraction ratio decreases.

VII. Myocardial Oxygen Extraction in Sepsis

In septic patients, the myocardial oxygen extraction ratio is decreased to approximately 40–50% [7,20] compared with normal patients with a myocardial extraction ratio in the range of 75%. Coronary sinus blood flow is increased, on average, by 40% in patients with septic shock compared with that of nonseptic controls. This is related to a shift in the coronary pressure–flow relationship to the left [7]. Part of the shift seems to be caused by a decrease in coronary vascular resistance, while part may be accounted for by a decrease in the zero flow pressure of the Starling resistor of the coronary pressure–flow relationship. Metabolism of free fatty acids contributes much less to energy production in hearts of septic patients, whereas lactate extraction is maintained or increased [7]. More than half of the oxygen consumed by nonsurviving patients with sepsis cannot be accounted for by metabolism of the usual substrates of myocardial metabolism, which include free fatty acids, glucose, lactate, and ketone bodies. This suggests that endogenous substrates may be providing metabolic fuel, and this process may contribute to the impaired cardiac function that is observed in sepsis.

In animal studies of endotoxin infusion, a similar reduction in the myocardial oxygen extraction ratio is observed, decreasing from approximately 75% before endotoxin infusion to 50% after endotoxin infusion [21]. The decreased oxygen extraction ratio is accounted for by increased heterogeneity of capillary blood flow.

Impaired capillary endothelial signaling may decrease the ability of the capillaries to modulate upstream arteriolar tone to maintain a close relationship between myocardial oxygen demand and supply [75]. Hypercapnia and tissue acidosis, frequently encountered in sepsis, increase the oxygen cost of mechanical work [76], possibly because of increased energy cost of the excitation–contraction coupling due to decreased calcium sensitivity of the contractile proteins during acidosis. Leukocyte retention and plugging of coronary capillaries may also contribute to the increase in heterogeneity. After activation, neutrophils become rigid so that their 6.6 ± 0.6 μm average diameter [77] may result in occlusion of myocardial capillaries that have an average diameter of 5.6 ± 1.3 μm [78]. In animal models of sepsis, large numbers of activated leukocytes ($2 \times 10^9/100$ g myocardium) [79] are retained in the coronary capillary bed. Leukocyte retention is associated with myocyte damage, tissue edema, and decreased contractile function [80].

When inflammatory pathways involve the heart, cardiac cells are not just innocent bystanders—they actively participate. Upon activation with early pro-inflammatory mediators such as tumor necrosis factor α, nitric oxide production increases many-fold by inducible nitric oxide synthase upregulation in endothelial cells and, notably, in cardiac myocytes [81]. It is now clear that nitric oxide plays a key role in beat-to-beat modulation of rate and contractility [82]. During the inflammatory response, increased nitric oxide production decreases myocyte contractility [83] and probably oxygen consumption. Nitric oxide acts by decreasing intracellular calcium via guanylate cyclase, by formation of the peroxygnitrite free radical in the presence of oxygen free radicals, and posssibly by directly binding heme proteins involved in oxidative metabolic pathways. Upon stimulation with pro-inflammatory cytokines, cardiac myocytes produce both C-X-C and C-C chemokines that contribute to chemotaxis of neutrophils and other leukocytes [84]. Cardiac myocytes also increase espression of intercellular adhesion molecule 1, which contributes to leukocyte–myocyte interaction and to myocte damage and dysfunction [85].

VIII. Myocardial Oxygen Extraction in Coronary Occlusive Disease

The main mechanism for maintenance of aerobic myocardial metabolism and normal ventricular function in the face of increased metabolic demand is regulation of coronary flow. Thus, significant atherosclerosis that limits the ability of the coronary circulation to increase flow is an enormously important clinical issue. A number of risk factors associated with myocardial infarction contribute more than just to the genesis of atherosclerotic plaque [86–89]. For example, diabetes impairs endothelium-dependent dilation of downstream coronary vasculature. Hypercholesterolemia [88], hypertension [86], and smoking [89] also contribute to diminished downstream responsiveness to endogenous coronary vasodilators.

Ischemia reperfusion triggers an inflammatory response similar, in many respects, to the complex inflammatory signaling pathways of sepsis previously discussed. This is associated with a decrease of contractility. Normal microvascular regulatory function is impaired [90], although function of larger vessels and the response to adenosine is less affected. Leukocytes seem to play an important role in ischemia–reperfusion myocardial injury [91], as they do in sepsis. Oxygen free radicals produced by leukocytes and, importantly, by cardiac myocytes [92,93] contribute to structural and functional damage.

After ischemia–reperfusion, efficiency of conversion of consumed oxygen to mechanical work is decreased [94] because of inefficient cellular ATP use on intracellular calcium transport [95]. In the working heart, myocardial oxygen consumption is maintained despite a reduction in contractile function [94]. There is no change or a slight decrease in the slope of the myocardial oxygen consumption–PVA relationship, but the slope of the relationship between PVA-independent oxygen consumption and the slope of the end-systolic pressure-volume relationships (E_{max}) doubles [96]. After ischemia–reperfusion, fatty acid metabolism, normally the predominant metabolic substrate of the heart, is impaired [95].

IX. Summary

The heart is distinguished from other organs by its high metabolic demand that nearly exclusively requires aerobic metabolism of substrate; by its high oxygen extraction ratio and, therefore, its reliance on changes in coronary blood flow to meet changes in metabolic demand; by the multiple mechanisms that match coronary arterial flow to metabolic demand at regional and microregional levels; and by the dependence of myocardial oxygen extraction on capillary P_{O_2}. Interruption of mechanisms that result in efficient and targeted delivery of oxygen to the myocardium in sepsis or in coronary occlusive disease has dramatic effects on the ability of the heart to extract oxygen and—not surprisingly—on cardiac function.

References

1. Walley KR, Becker CJ, Hogan RA, Teplinsky K, Wood LDH. Progressive hypoxemia limits left ventricular oxygen consumption and contractility. Circ Res 1988; 63:849–859.
2. Suga H. Ventricular energetics. Physiol Rev 1990; 70:247–277.
3. Coulson RL. Energetics of isovolumic contractions of the isolated rabbit heart. J Physiol 1976; 260:45–53.
4. Neely JR, Whitmer JT, Rovetto MJ. Effect of coronary blood flow on glycolytic flux and intracellular pH in isolated rat hearts. Circ Res 1975; 37:733–741.
5. Elzinga G. Cardiac oxygen consumption and the production of heat and work. In: Drake-Holland AJ, Noble MIM, eds. Cardiac Metabolism. Chichester: John Wiley & Sons, Inc., 1983, pp 172–213.

6. Opie LH. Metabolism of the heart in health and disease. Am Heart J 1969; 77:383–410.
7. Dhainaut JF, Huyghebaert MF, Monsallier JF, Lefevre G, Dall'Ava-Santucci J, Brunet F, Villemant D, Carli A, Raichvarg D. Coronary hemodynamics and myocardial metabolism of lactate, free fatty acids, glucose, and ketones in patients with septic shock. Circulation 1987; 75:533–541.
8. Grynberg A, Demaison L. Fatty acid oxidation in the heart. J Cardiovasc Pharmacol 1996; 28 (Suppl 1):S11–S17.
9. Schumacker PT, Samsel RW. Oxygen delivery and uptake by peripheral tissues: physiology and pathophysiology. Crit Care Clin 1989; 5:255–269.
10. Nelson DP, King CE, Dodd SL, Schumacker PT, Cain SM. Systemic and intestinal limits of O_2 extraction in the dog. J Appl Physiol 1987; 63:387–394.
11. Segal JM, Phang PT, Walley KR. Low-dose dopamine hastens onset of gut ischemia in a porcine model of hemorrhagic shock. J Appl Physiol 1992; 73:1159–1164.
12. Humer MF, Phang PT, Friesen BP, Allard MF, Goddard CM, Walley KR. Heterogeneity of gut capillary transit times and impaired gut oxygen extraction in endotoxemic pigs. J Appl Physiol 1996; 81:895–904.
13. Crystal GJ, Kim SJ, Salem MM, Abdel-Latif M. Myocardial oxygen supply/demand relations during phenylephrine infusions in dogs. Anesth Analg 1991; 73:283–288.
14. Ronco JJ, Fenwick JC, Tweeddale MG, Wiggs BR, Phang PT, Cooper DJ, Cunningham KF, Russell JA, Walley KR. Identification of the critical oxygen delivery for anaerobic metabolism in critically ill septic and nonseptic humans. JAMA 1993; 270:1724–1730.
15. Knabb RM, Ely SW, Bacchus AN, Rubio R, Berne RM. Consistent parallel relationships among myocardial oxygen consumption, coronary blood flow, and pericardial infusate adenosine concentration with various interventions and beta-blockade in the dog. Circ Res 1983; 53:33–41.
16. Khouri EM, Gregg DE, Rayford CR. Effect of exercise on cardiac output, left coronary flow and myocardial metabolism in the unanesthetized dog. Circ Res 1965; 17:427–437.
17. Feinberrg H, Gerola A, Katz LN. Effect of hypoxia on cardiac oxygen consumption and coronary flow. Am J Physiol 1958; 195:593–600.
18. Vergroesen I, Kal JE, Spaan JA, Van Wezel HB. Myocardial oxygen supply:demand ratio as reference for coronary vasodilatory drug effects in humans. Heart 1997; 78:117–126.
19. Fang HK, Sturgeon C, Segil LJ, Ripper RL, Law WR. Cardiac contractile function during coronary stenosis in dogs: association of adenosine in glycolytic dependence. Am J Physiol 1997; 272:H2195–H2203.
20. Cunnion RE, Schaer GL, Parker MM, Natanson C, Parrillo JE. The coronary circulation in human septic shock. Circulation 1986; 73:637–644.
21. Herbertson MJ, Werner HA, Russell JA, Iversen K, Walley KR. Myocardial oxygen extraction ratio is decreased during endotoxemia in pigs. J Appl Physiol 1995; 79:479–486.
22. McAlpine W. Heart and Coronary Arteries. New York: Springer-Verlag, 1975.
23. Bassingthwaighte JB, Yipintsoi T, Harvey RB. Microvasculature of the dog left ventricular myocardium. Microvasc Res 1974; 7:229–249.

24. Potter RF, Groom AC. Capillary diameter and geometry in cardiac and skeletal muscle studied by means of corrosion casts. Microvasc Res 1983; 25:68–84.
25. Streeter DD Jr, Spotnitz HM, Patel DP, Ross J Jr, Sonnenblick EH. Fiber orientation in the canine left ventricle during diastole and systole. Circ Res 1969; 24:339–347.
26. Poole DC, Mathieu-Costello O. Analysis of capillary geometry in rat subepicardium and subendocardium. Am J Physiol 1990; 259:H204–H210.
27. Poole DC, Batra S, Mathieu-Costello O, Rakusan K. Capillary geometrical changes with fiber shortening in rat myocardium. Circ Res 1992; 70:697–706.
28. Schaper W. Natural defense mechanisms during ischemia. Eur Heart J 1983; 4 (Suppl D):73–78.
29. Braunwald E, Sarnoff SJ, Case RB, Stainsby WN, Welch GH. Hemodynamic determinant of coronary flow: effect of changes in aortic pressure and cardiac output on relationship between myocardial oxygen consumption and coronary flow. Am J Physiol 1958; 192:157–163.
30. Gobel FL, Norstrom LA, Nelson RR, Jorgensen CR, Wang Y. The rate-pressure product as an index of myocardial oxygen consumption during exercise in patients with angina pectoris. Circulation 1978; 57:549–556.
31. McDonald RH. Developed tension: a major determinant of myocardial oxygen consumption. Am J Physiol 1966; 210:351–356.
32. Weber KT, Janicki JS. Myocardial oxygen consumption: the role of wall force and shortening. Am J Physiol 1977; 233:H421–H430.
33. Khalafbeigui F, Suga H, Sagawa K. Left ventricular systolic pressure-volume area correlates with oxygen consumption. Am J Physiol 1979; 237:H566–H569.
34. Suga H. Total mechanical energy of a ventricle model and cardiac oxygen consumption. Am J Physiol 1979; 236:H498–H505.
35. Suga H, Yamada O, Goto Y, Igarashi Y. Oxygen consumption and pressure-volume area of abnormal contractions in canine heart. Am J Physiol 1984; 246:H154–H160.
36. Suga H, Hisano R, Hirata S, Hayashi T, Yamada O, Ninomiya I. Heart rate-independent energetics and systolic pressure-volume area in dog heart. Am J Physiol 1983; 244:H206–H214.
37. Hisano R, Cooper G IV. Correlation of force-length area with oxygen consumption in ferret papillary muscle. Circ Res 1987; 61:318–328.
38. Goto Y, Slinker BK, LeWinter MM. Similar normalized E_{max} and O_2 consumption-pressure-volume area relation in rabbit and dog. Am J Physiol 1988; 255:H366–H374.
39. Suga H, Hisano R, Goto Y, Yamada O, Igarashi Y. Effect of positive inotropic agents on the relation between oxygen consumption and systolic pressure volume area in canine left ventricle. Circ Res 1983; 53:306–318.
40. Gibbs CL, Chapman JB. Cardiac mechanics and energetics: chemomechanical transduction in cardiac muscle. Am J Physiol 1985; 249:H199–H206.
41. Elbeery JR, Lucke JC, Feneley MP, Maier GW, Owen CH, Lilly RE, Savitt MA, Hickey MS, Gall SA Jr, Davis JW. Mechanical determinants of myocardial oxygen consumption in conscious dogs. Am J Physiol 1995; 269:H609–H620.
42. Takaoka H, Suga H, Goto Y, Hata K, Takeuchi M. Cardiodynamic conditions for the linearity of preload recruitable stroke work. Heart Vessels 1995; 10:57–68.
43. Bellamy RF, Lowensohn HS, Ehrlich W, Baer RW. Effect of coronary sinus occlusion on coronary pressure-flow relations. Am J Physiol 1980; 239:H57–H64.

44. Hoffman JIE, Spaan JA. Pressure-flow relations in coronary circulation. Physiol Rev 1990; 70:331–390.
45. Uhlig PN, Baer RW, Vlahakes GJ, Hanley FL, Messina LM, Hoffman JIE. Arterial and venous coronary pressure-flow relations in anesthetized dogs: evidence for a vascular waterfall in epicardial coronary veins. Circ Res 1984; 55:238–248.
46. Rouleau J, Boerboom LE, Surjadhana A, Hoffman JI. The role of autoregulation and tissue diastolic pressures in the transmural distribution of left ventricular blood flow in anesthetized dogs. Circ Res 1979; 45:804–815.
47. Hoffman JIE. Transmural myocardial perfusion. Prog Cardiovasc Dis 1987; 29:429–464.
48. Bassingthwaighte JB, King RB, Roger SA. Fractal nature of regional mocardial blood flow heterogeneity. Circ Res 1989; 65:578–590.
49. Marcus ML, Kerber RE, Erhardt JC, Falsetti HL, Davis DM, Abboud FM. Spatial and temporal heterogeneity of left ventricular perfusion in awake dogs. Am Heart J 1977; 94:748–754.
50. Caldwell JH, Martin GV, Raymond GM, Bassingthwaighte JB. Regional myocardial flow and capillary permeability-surface area products are nearly proportional. Am J Physiol 1994; 267:H654–H666.
51. Saito D, Nixon DG, Vomacka RB, Olsson RA. Relationship of cardiac oxygen usage, adenosine content, and coronary resistance in dogs. Circ Res 1980; 47:875–882.
52. Bacchus AN, Ely SW, Knabb RM, Rubio R, Berne RM. Adenosine and coronary blood flow in conscious dogs during normal physiological stimuli. Am J Physiol 1982; 243:H628–H633.
53. Komaru T, Lamping KG, Eastham CL, Harrison DG, Marcus ML, Dellsperger KC. Effect of an arginine analogue on acetylcholine-induced coronary microvascular dilatation in dogs. Am J Physiol 1991; 261:H2001–H2007.
54. Reid JV, Ito BR, Huang AH, Buffington CW, Figl EO. Parasympathetic control of transmural coronary blood flow in dogs. Am J Physiol 1985; 249:H337–H343.
55. Clozel JP, Roberts AM, Hoffman JIE, Coleridge HM, Coleridge JCG. Vagal chemoreflex coronary vasodilation evoked by stimulating pulmonary C-fibers in dogs. Circ Res 1985; 57:450–460.
56. Ku DD, Caulfield JB, Kirklin JK. Endothelium-dependent responses in human coronary blood vessels. In: Ryan U, Rubanyi G, eds. Endothelial Regulation of Vascular Tone. New York: Marcel Dekker, 1992, pp 197–223.
57. Dole WP, Nuno DW. Myocardial oxygen tension determines the degree and pressure range of coronary autoregulation. Circ Res 1986; 59:202–215.
58. Dietrich HH, Tyml K. Capillary as a communicating medium in the microvasculature. Microvasc Res 1992; 43:87–99.
59. Song H, Tyml K. Evidence for sensing and integration of biological signals by the capillary network. Am J Physiol 1993; 265:H1235–H1242.
60. Dietrich HH, Tyml K. Microvascular flow response to localized application of norepinephrine on capillaries in rat and frog skeletal muscle. Microvasc Res 1992; 43:73–86.
61. Little TL, Xia J, Duling BR. Dye tracers define differential endothelial and smooth muscle coupling patterns within the arteriolar wall. Circ Res 1995; 76:498–504.
62. Kuo L, Davis MJ, Chilian WM. Myogenic activity in isolated subepicardial and subendocardial coronary arterioles. Am J Physiol 1988; 255:H1558–H1562.

63. Walley KR, Collins RM, Cooper DJ, Warriner CB. Myocardial anaerobic metabolism occurs at a critical coronary venous P_{O_2} in pigs. Am J Respir Crit Care Med 1997; 155:222–228.
64. King CE, Dodd SL, Cain SM. O_2 delivery to contracting muscle during hypoxic or CO hypoxia. J Appl Physiol 1987; 63:726–732.
65. Rose CP, Goresky CA. Limitations of tracer oxygen uptake in the canine coronary circulation. Circ Res 1985; 56:57–71.
66. Stumpe T, Schrader J. Phosphorylation potential, adenosine formation, and critical P_{O_2} in stimulated rat cardiomyocytes. Am J Physiol 1997; 273:H756–H766.
67. Honig CR. Modern cardiovascular physiology. Boston: Little Brown, 1988; xviii, 317.
68. Gayeski TE, Honig CR. Intracellular P_{O_2} in individual cardiac myocytes in dogs, cats, rabbits, ferrets, and rats. Am J Physiol 1991; 260:H522–H531.
69. Allard MF, Kamimura CT, English DR, Henning SL, Wiggs BR. Regional myocardial capillary erythrocyte transit time in the normal resting heart. Circ Res 1993; 72:187–193.
70. Honig CR, Odoroff CL. Calculated dispersion of capillary transit times: significance for oxygen exchange. Am J Physiol 1981; 240:H199–H208.
71. Humer MF, Phang PT, Friesen BP, Allard MF, Goddard CM, Walley KR. Heterogeneity of gut capillary transit times and impaired gut oxygen extraction in endotoxemic pigs. J Appl Physiol 1996; 81:895–904.
72. Walley KR. Heterogeneity of oxygen delivery impairs oxygen extraction by peripheral tissues: theory. J Appl Physiol 1996; 81:885–894.
73. Tyml K. Heterogeneity of microvascular flow in rat skeletal muscle is reduced by contraction and by hemodilution. Int J Microcirc Clin Exp 1991; 10:75–86.
74. Lindbom L, Tuma RF, Arfors KE. Influence of oxygen on perfused capillary density and capillary red cell velocity in rabbit skeletal muscle. Microvasc Res 1980; 19:197–208.
75. Lam C, Tyml K, Martin C, Sibbald W. Microvascular perfusion is impaired in a rat model of normotensive sepsis. J Clin Invest 1994; 94:2077–2083.
76. Hata K, Goto Y, Kawaguchi O, Takasago T, Saeki A, Nishioka T, Suga H. Hypercapnic acidosis increases oxygen cost of contractility in the dog left ventricle. Am J Physiol 1994; 266:H730–H740.
77. Doerschuk CM, Beyers N, Coxson HO, Wiggs B, Hogg JC. Comparison of neutrophil and capillary diameters and their relation to neutrophil sequestration in the lung. J Appl Physiol 1993; 74:3040–3045.
78. Grayson J, Davidson JW, Fitzgerald-Finch A, Scott C. The functional morphology of the coronary microcirculation in the dog. Microvasc Res 1974; 8:20–43.
79. Goddard CM, Allard MF, Hogg JC, Herbertson MJ, Walley KR. Prolonged leukocyte transit time in coronary microcirculation of endotoxemic pigs. Am J Physiol 1995; 269:H1389–H1397.
80. Granton JT, Goddard CM, Allard MF, van Eeden S, Walley KR. Leukocytes and decreased left-ventricular contractility during endotoxemia in rabbits. Am J Respir Crit Care Med 1997; 155:1977–1983.
81. Schulz R, Panas DL, Catena R, Moncada S, Olley PM, Lopaschuk GD. The role of nitric oxide in cardiac depression induced by interleukin-1 beta and tumour necrosis factor-alpha. Br J Pharmacol 1995; 114:27–34.

82. Kanai AJ, Mesaros S, Finkel MS, Oddis CV, Birder LA, Malinski T. Beta-adrenergic regulation of constitutive nitric oxide synthase in cardiac myocytes. Am J Physiol 1997; 273:C1371–C1377.
83. Finkel MS, Oddis CV, Jacob TD, Watkins SC, Hattler BG, Simmons RL. Negative inotropic effects of cytokines on the heart mediated by nitric oxide. Science 1992; 257:387–389.
84. Massey KD, Strieter RM, Kunkel SL, Danforth JM, Standiford TJ. Cardiac myocytes release leukocyte-stimulating factors. Am J Physiol 1995; 269:H980–H987.
85. Entman ML, Youker K, Shoji T, Kukielka G, Shappell SB, Taylor AA, Smith CW. Neutrophil induced oxidative injury of cardiac myocytes: a compartmented system requiring CD11b/CD18-ICAM-1 adherence. J Clin Invest 1992; 90:1335–1345.
86. Egashira K, Inou T, Hirooka Y, Yamada A, Maruoka Y, Kai H, Sugimachi M, Suzuki S, Takeshita A. Impaired coronary blood flow response to acetylcholine in patients with coronary risk factors and proximal atherosclerotic lesions. J Clin Invest 1993; 91:29–37.
87. Zeiher AM, Drexler H, Wollschlager H, Just H. Modulation of coronary vasomotor tone in humans: progressive endothelial dysfunction with different early stages of coronary atherosclerosis. Circulation 1991; 83:391–401.
88. Drexler H, Zeiher AM. Endothelial function in human coronary arteries in vivo: focus on hypercholesterolemia. Hypertension 1991; 18:1190–1199.
89. Quillen JE, Rossen JD, Oskarsson HJ, Minor RL Jr, Lopez AG, Winniford MD. Acute effect of cigarette smoking on the coronary circulation: constriction of epicardial and resistance vessels. J Am Coll Cardiol 1993; 22:642–647.
90. Laxson DD, Homans DS, Dai X-Z, Sublett E, Bache RJ. Oxygen consumption and coronary reactivity in postischemic myocardium. Circ Res 1989; 64:9–20.
91. Gumina RJ, Newman PJ, Kenny D, Warltier DC, Gross GJ. The leukocyte cell adhesion cascade and its role in myocardial ischemia-reperfusion injury. Basic Res Cardiol 1997; 92:201–213.
92. Vanden Hoek TL, Li C, Shao Z, Schumacker PT, Becker LB. Significant levels of oxidants are generated by isolated cardiomyocytes during ischemia prior to reperfusion. J Mol Cell Cardiol 1997; 29:2571–2583.
93. Vanden Hoek TL, Shao Z, Li C, Schumacker PT, Becker LB. Mitochondrial electron transport can become a significant source of oxidative injury in cardiomyocytes. J Mol Cell Cardiol 1997; 29:2441–2450.
94. Silverman NA. Myocardial oxygen consumption after reversible ischemia. J Cardiac Surg 1994; 9(Suppl 3):465–468.
95. Lerch R, Tamm C, Papageorgiou I, Benzi RH. Myocardial fatty acid oxidation during ischemia and reperfusion. Mol Cell Biochem 1992; 116:103–109.
96. Ohgoshi Y, Goto Y, Futaki S, Yaku H, Kawaguchi O, Suga H. Increased oxygen cost of contractility in stunned myocardium of dog. Circ Res 1991; 69:975–988.

14

Localization and Dispersion of Oxygen Demand and Supply in Skeletal Muscle

STEVEN S. SEGAL

The John B. Pierce Laboratory and Yale University School of Medicine
New Haven, Connecticut

I. Introduction

The net flux of oxygen through the body is established by the rate at which it is consumed within and delivered to respiring mitochondria. Nearly half the mass of the human body is comprised of skeletal muscle. Thus, the energy consumed in performing aerobic exercise profoundly stimulates both the demand for and the supply of oxygen to muscle fibers. Indeed, the linear relationship between exercise intensity and total body oxygen uptake (1,2) indicates that the systemic utilization and supply of oxygen are closely coupled to the energy expenditure of skeletal muscle. The strong positive correlations between muscle work, oxygen consumption ($\dot{V}O_2$), and blood flow in animals (3–5) as well as humans (6) further strengthen this conclusion. In turn, it can be argued that much of the coupling between oxygen supply and demand is mediated locally, within skeletal muscle and the peripheral vasculature (7,8).

The determinants of $\dot{V}O_2$ are expressed in general terms by the Fick principle, which states that the oxygen consumed by a tissue is the product of its delivery by convection and its removal by extraction. In turn, these processes are manifested as the flow of blood into and throughout a muscle and by the diffusion of oxygen from the blood into muscle fibers, respectively. This chapter is more specifically concerned with the nature of the physicochemical gradients that govern the flow of oxygen from arterial blood, through the microcirculation, and to the respiring mitochondria within active muscle fibers. Because the convection of oxygen throughout the body is driven by a hydrostatic pressure gradient generated by the heart and peripheral resistance vessels, blood flow and its control are considered first. I then discuss the structural and functional determinants of the gradients in the partial pressure of oxygen (Po_2) within muscle fibers and capillaries that drive the extraction (i.e., net diffusion) of oxygen from red blood cells to mitochondria. The primary emphasis of this discussion turns to consider the physiological nature of the interaction between muscle fibers and their vascular supply (Fig. 1). In the attempt to identify where and how variability may be manifested in oxygen transport to active muscle fibers, the presence of ''heterogeneity'' among these interdependent relationships is considered throughout.

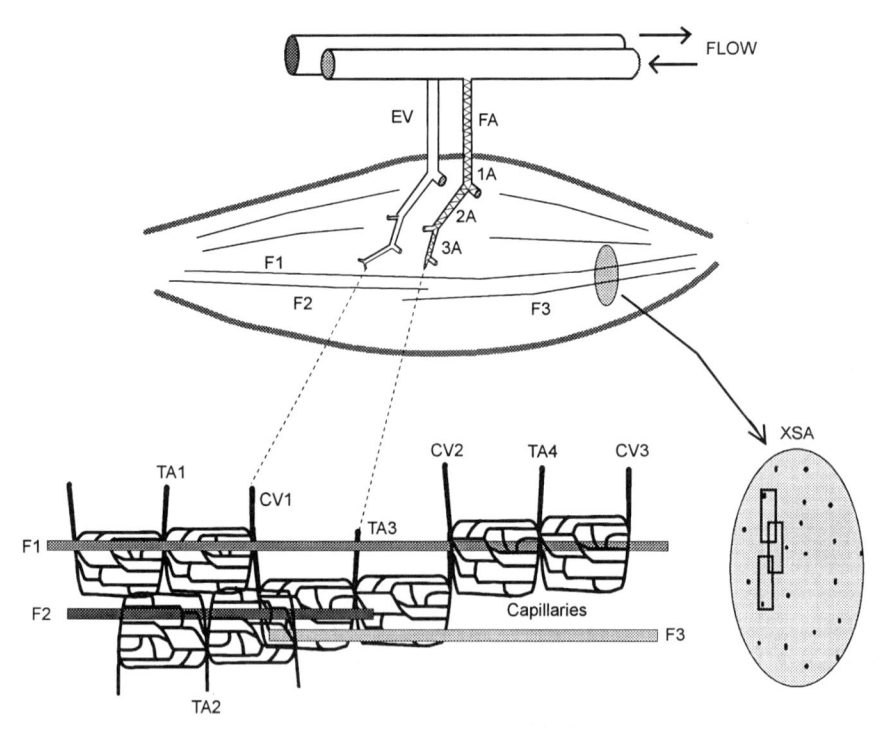

Figure 1 Schematic illustration of the physical interrelationships between skeletal muscle fibers and their microvascular supply. Blood flow is shown to enter the muscle through the feed artery (FA) and be distributed within the muscle through the first-order (1A), second-order (2A), and third-order (3A) arterioles, which are invested by sympathetic nerves (cross hatch). The terminal arterioles (TA) arise distal to the 3A branches. Each TA gives rise to a group of capillaries that supply the muscle fibers in both directions and

II. Muscle Blood Flow and Oxygen Uptake

The bulk transport of oxygen by the circulation plays a central role in the regulation of oxygen flow through the entire organism (9–11). To determine the functional capacity of human skeletal muscle for blood flow, a small fraction of the total muscle mass (e.g., the knee extensor group of one leg) was engaged in rhythmic exercise (6). Under this condition, blood flow to the active musculature approached 250 mL · min^{-1} · 100 g^{-1}; this value is slightly greater than reported for miniature swine (12) and approaches that of rats (13) obtained during maximal aerobic running. When relatively small muscle groups are exercising, muscle blood flow may be "excessive" as indicated by oxygen extraction across the leg of 12–15 vol % at $\dot{V}O_2$ max (6). This incomplete extraction (assuming ∼ 20 vol % in arterial blood) during maximal flow may be associated with extremely short transit times of red blood cells in at least some capillaries, and by the diffusion of oxygen from arterioles into capillaries and venules. These relationships are considered in detail later in the chapter.

The magnitude and the distribution of oxygen delivery to skeletal muscle are controlled through successive branches of the resistance network (Fig. 1) (14). The

---

converge into respective collecting venules (CV). Venules ultimately converge into an effluent vein (EV), which carries blood back to the heart. Each TA and the group of capillaries that it supplies are referred to as a microvascular unit (MVU); 4 MVUs are illustrated below the muscle along the fibers' axis. Note that the distance spanned by each MVU is a fraction of the length spanned by a muscle fiber (F). Within the muscle, three fibers are labeled (F1, F2, and F3); portions of these are redrawn below to illustrate corresponding MVUs. Note that F1 spans the full length of the muscle, whereas F2 and F3 originate from each end of the muscle and overlap slightly before terminating near the middle of the muscle. A portion of F1 is perfused by TA1 and by TA4, whereas TA3 is associated with F2 and F3 but not F1. (Another MVU supplies the "empty" region along F1 between CV1 and CV2 but is omitted for clarity). Note that the outflow from capillaries perfused by TA3 will converge into CV1 along with the outflow from capillaries perfused by TA1, while CV2 will carry the remaining effluent from TA3 along with a portion of the blood delivered by TA4. TA2 is derived from a different region, yet also governs perfusion of a MVU that supplies regions of F2 and F3. Diffusive interactions will occur among capillaries supplied by TA2 with those supplied by TA1 and TA3. The lower right portion of the figure shows a cross-sectional area (XSA) taken from a region within the muscle to illustrate the area of tissue contained within each MVU; the boundaries of three MVUs in cross section are shown outlined by rectangles and display some overlap. The fibers that belong to a given motor unit are indicated by the black dots. Note that the fibers within a motor unit are widely dispersed relative to the spatial domain of an individual MVU. In turn, each MVU may contain adjacent segments of 20–30 muscle fibers, with each fiber belonging to a different motor unit. In the three MVUs shown, two include fibers from the indicated motor unit; the third MVU does not.

most proximal of these vessels are the feed arteries, which are located external to the muscle and control the volume of blood flowing into the muscle. Once feed arteries enter the muscle, they give rise to the primary arterioles, which then branch into the intermediate (i.e., second and third order) arterioles that control the distribution of blood flow throughout the tissue. The distal branches of the resistance network are comprised of the terminal arterioles, which govern the entry of red blood cells into capillaries and thereby control the surface area available for capillary exchange. With exercise, vasodilation appears to be initiated in the distal arterioles and then spreads to encompass the proximal arterioles and feed arteries (15–17). In humans, such behavior is reflected by the large increase in oxygen extraction with light activity, followed by a progressive increase in blood flow as workload increases (6). In hamster skeletal muscle, vasodilation has been shown to progressively "ascend" the resistance vasculature of skeletal muscle as metabolic demand increases (18).

The flow of oxygen into a particular group of exercising muscles may be limited by vasoconstriction when another large muscle group is exercising simultaneously (19–21). Thus, during "whole body" exercise that approaches maximal cardiac output, each muscle apparently receives only a fraction of the blood flow which it would otherwise get if it were the only active muscle group in the body (20,22). Such an imposed limitation of oxygen delivery can, in turn, increase oxygen extraction (e.g., to $\sim$ 18 vol %) (21). The greater extraction when flow is restricted (21) indicates that active muscle cells are more effective in removing oxygen from the blood as flow becomes limiting (23). This improvement can be attributed to the combination of capillary recruitment and a fall in tissue Po_2 (24,25) as detailed later in this chapter. It is at the level of the feed arteries that sympathetic vasoconstriction appears to be most effective in restricting muscle blood flow during exercise (26,27). Because feed arteries are external to the muscle, their direct exposure to the products of metabolism is effectively precluded. In contrast, throughout the arteriolar network, and particularly is distal arterioles (28,29), sympathetic vasoconstriction may be antagonized by both direct and indirect actions of metabolic vasodilators (30,31) and by the conduction of vasodilation along the arteriolar wall (32). Thus, during intense aerobic activity involving large amounts of muscle mass, arterioles within the muscle can remain dilated and the capillary bed fully perfused (to promote oxygen extraction) while sympathetic vasoconstriction of feed arteries effectively constrains the total flow into active muscle.

In summary, the two primary adjustments in the delivery of oxygen to skeletal muscle fibers during exercise is an improvement in the efficacy by which oxygen is extracted by the myocytes from the circulation and an increase in the overall delivery of oxygen via an increase in blood flow. When delivery is limited, a further reduction in tissue Po_2 may explain even greater extraction of oxygen from the incoming blood. While these relationships are apparent for the whole muscle, understanding the specific processes that underlie this behavior within the muscle has remained a formidable challenge, despite over twelve decades of investigation (33). We shall now "look inside the box" with the goal of conveying an appreciation for the substantial range in the variables that are recognized as determinants of oxygen demand and supply.

III. Oxygen Flux Within Muscle Fibers

A. Mitochondria

The oxidative capacity of muscle fibers is highly correlated with their mitochondrial content (34,35). In ultrastructural studies of skeletal muscle, mitochondrial volume density provides an estimate of a cell's potential for oxidative metabolism (11,35–37). Whereas a morphological estimate is limited by uncertainty concerning the rate at which the mitochondria are actually respiring, the oxidative capacity of individual cat muscles has been shown to be directly proportional to their mitochondrial volume as determined morphometrically (35). Within myocytes, the distribution of mitochondria may reflect a balance between distances for diffusion of oxygen from capillaries to mitochondria and distances for diffusion of adenosine triphosphate (ATP) or other high-energy phosphate compounds from mitochondria to myofibrils (38–41). In muscle fiber cross-sections analyzed from a wide range of animal sizes, species, and aerobic capacities, mitochondria were found to be located predominantly near capillaries with mitochondrial density decreasing from the subsarcolemmal region towards the center of the cell (42). In hamsters and rats, this pattern of mitochondrial distribution is more prevalent in oxidative fibers when compared to glycolytic fibers (39,43) and holds as well for cardiac myocytes (38,44). Variability in mitochondrial enzymatic capacity is also apparent along the muscle fiber axis (45). It should also be remembered that capillaries contact muscle fibers at relatively discrete regions around and along the sarcolemma (37,39,46,47). Therefore, the region(s) of a muscle fiber in which oxygen is actually consumed (and P_{O_2} gradients thereby established) will vary both radially and axially throughout muscle fibers, particularly in muscle fibers suited for aerobic performance.

B. Myoglobin

During intense muscle contraction, the supply of oxygen to muscle fibers may be limited because of the compression of blood vessels (48,49). In such circumstances, myoglobin has been considered as an oxygen store, supplying it to the mitochondria during contraction and taking it from the capillary blood during relaxation (50,51). Such fluctuations in the supply and demand of oxygen are dampened with brief and moderate contractions, with the muscle operating in a steady state of oxygen flux. In this case, oxygen is presumed to flow continuously to the mitochondria from the microcirculation, and myoglobin may assume a transport function (51). In effect, deoxymyoglobin binds oxygen diffusing in from the blood and (as oxymyoglobin) facilitates its diffusion to the mitochondria.

The ability of myoglobin to effectively contribute to oxygen flux above and beyond the diffusion of free oxygen requires several conditions. These conditions include: a sufficiently high concentration of myoglobin within the cell, sufficient mobility of oxymyoglobin to permit its diffusion in the cytoplasm of the cell, and sufficiently low regions of intracellular PO_2 to allow deoxymyoglobin to exist, which provides the driving force for the diffusion of oxymyoglobin (41,52). Although myoglobin diffuses at $\sim$ 5% of the rate of free oxygen, myoglobin concentration (approaching milliMolar in highly oxidative muscle fibers) exceeds that of free oxygen in working muscle by $\sim$ 20- to 30-fold (51,52). Moreover, myoglobin molecules in concentrated solutions can slide past each other with little frictional interaction (52). Despite these biophysical properties of myoglobin, there remains substantial controversy concerning the magnitude and extent of oxygen gradients within myocytes (53–56) as well as from capillaries to myocytes (52,53).

The oxygenation of myoglobin was analyzed using cryospectrophotometry in cross-sectional and longitudinal samples of muscle obtained from dog gracilis muscle contracting in situ (53,54). Results from these studies suggested that at $\dot{V}O_2$ max, myoglobin serves to buffer intracellular PO_2 at a relatively uniform value, above that required for maintaining mitochondrial respiration but sufficiently low to promote the diffusion of oxygen from the capillary into the muscle fiber. However, a more recent and critical examination (57) has made it clear that cryospectrophotometry as originally performed (53,54) lacked sufficient spatial resolution to discern the apparent intracellular oxygen gradients (55,56) upon which such arguments were based (58). Furthermore, mitochondria were described as uniformly distributed in muscle fibers (53,54), which would minimize the likelihood of the regional heterogeneities in PO_2 ascribed to mitochondrial clustering (59). However, as discussed earlier, there is strong evidence for mitochondrial clustering within myocytes near capillaries in the heart as well as in aerobic skeletal muscle cells. Thus, calculations and assumptions based upon cryospectrophotometry in dog gracilis muscle (60–62) may require reanalysis.

In experiments performed using the rhythmically contracting dog gastrocnemius-plantaris preparation, the abolition of oxygen binding to myoglobin by its oxidation with hydrogen peroxide promptly diminished twitch tension and $\dot{V}O_2$ by more than half, and did so in an apparently specific manner (63). Nevertheless, recent experiments on mice that were homozygous null for myoglobin (myoglobin$^{-/-}$) were found to have normal exercise capacity and responded by hypoxic challenge as well as control mice (myoglobin$^{+/+}$) (64). These provocative findings directly challenge the putative role(s) of myoglobin and raise new questions regarding the intracellular transport and storage of oxygen during exercise. Whether such changes in gene expression induce compensatory responses to otherwise facilitate aerobic performance remains to be determined.

IV. Oxygen Flux from Microvessels to Muscle Fibers

A. Capillaries and Mitochondria

A basic descriptor of capillary network design is the length of capillaries per volume of muscle, as this bears on capillary blood volume, surface area, and diffusion distance (11,46). From measurements of capillary density and fiber area in muscle sections, the volume of capillary blood per unit volume of muscle tissue can be estimated as an index of capillary oxygen delivery. Capillary length density was proportional to mitochondrial volume density from muscles of mammals that spanned several orders of magnitude in body mass (42). In hindlimb muscles of the rabbit, individual fibers were surrounded by capillaries in proportion to their oxidative capacity (65). Indeed, with aerobic conditioning, both the capillarity and mitochondria of muscle fibers increase (34,43). However, from estimates of relative oxidative capacities for red and white fibers, the latter apparently had relatively more capillaries than did red fibers (65). In a cross-sectional study of muscles from five mammalian species, no correlation was found between capillarity and either muscle blood flow or oxidative capacity, suggesting that capillarity *per se* may not be the primary vascular component determining oxygen extraction and utilization by the mitochondria (47). Thus, the capillary supply of muscle fibers need not relate exclusively to their mitochondrial content or to their capacity for aerobic metabolism. Indeed, it has been noted that the functional relationship between capillaries and mitochondria is complex (37,42,66), with high capacities for oxygen flux achieved by such strategies as changing fiber size, hematocrit, and the contact area between capillaries and muscle fibers (37,43).

It will be recognized that structural indices alone cannot describe the functional properties of capillary networks, nor the diffusion of oxygen from blood to muscle fibers. In part, this is because these indices retain the assumption that the oxygen content of capillary blood is homogenous, and that the capillary is the only source of oxygen to the muscle fibers. The variability in capillary hematocrit, its potential impact on oxygen transport, and the profound diffusive interactions among arterioles, capillaries, venules and muscle fibers, and considered later in this chapter. Nevertheless, at the level of the whole muscle, there is a strong correlation between blood supply and the aerobic capacity of skeletal muscle fibers (12,13,67), apparently in the face of diffusional limitations to $\dot{V}O_2$ (60,68). The challenge we face is to integrate and explain the physiology of the intact muscle (and exercising human!) in light of the structural and functional properties of muscle fibers and their microvascular supply. Our goal is to provide insight into these fundamental relationships (Fig. 1).

B. Capillary Recruitment

In his classic studies, August Krogh (24) proposed that each capillary supplies oxygen to the region (i.e., tissue cylinder) of muscle fibers surrounding it, and did so independent of other capillaries. In collaboration with Erlang (24), it was calculated that the oxygen pressure head necessary for supplying the muscles with oxygen is so small that, even during the heaviest muscular work, the oxygen tension of the tissue will be practically equal to that of the venous blood. Thus, it was reasoned that the only way the diminished driving pressure (i.e., the P_{O_2} gradient from blood to myocyte) would be capable of maintaining adequate oxygen pressure in the tissue was if the number of perfused capillaries increased (69); i.e., through capillary recruitment during exercise (16,70).

With an increase in metabolic rate, the greater requirement for oxygen delivery can initially be met by the activity-induced fall in myocyte P_{O_2}, which steepens the gradient for oxygen diffusion from the capillary (25,69). Increasing the diffusion of oxygen in response to the fall in tissue P_{O_2} is effective only as long as the intracellular P_{O_2} remains above the value necessary to maintain mitochondrial respiration; if P_{O_2} falls below this critical level, $\dot{V}_{O_2}$ becomes flow limited (25). Such an occurrence may be forestalled in skeletal muscle by perfusing additional capillaries as metabolic rate is increased (24,25,70), which reduces the distance and increases the surface area for diffusional exchange between red blood cells and mitochondria. In addition, with reduced diffusion distances, capillary P_{O_2} can fall to lower values and still maintain tissue P_{O_2} above limiting values (25,69), as reflected by greater oxygen extraction from the blood.

The classic "tissue cylinder model" of capillary supply continues to influence thinking about oxygen transport (and its limitations) in skeletal muscle during exercise (60,68). Nevertheless, over the last few decades, substantive limitations of this model have become apparent (71–75). Of particular relevance to this discussion is that the model assumes the capillary to be a uniform source of oxygen, and that the only source of oxygen delivery to the tissue is the capillary. These relationships are considered in turn.

C. Capillary Red Blood Cell Content

Implicit in most experimental and theoretical investigations of capillary supply of oxygen to tissue is the assumption that capillary blood is homogenous with respect to the ability to deliver oxygen (6,10,24,60,68,69). However, this assumption may well be invalid. Substantive evidence indicates that there are considerable uncertainties as to the extent of uniformity of oxygen flux across various levels of the microcirculation (73–79). A fundamental observation is that the volume fraction of a capillary that is occupied by red blood cells (a key determinant of capillary oxygen content) is not a constant, but varies with the vasomotor state of resistance vessels and with the metabolic demand of the muscle fibers (74,80). Capillary or "tube" hematocrit is estimated from the number of red blood cells per unit length of capillary at a given instant, as visualized with intravital microscopy (74,76). Tube hematocrit provides an index of capillary oxygen content at that moment; the dissolved oxygen content of the plasma "gaps" between the red cells is essentially negligible in comparison to that bound to intracorpuscular hemoglobin. Capillary hematocrit is a fraction of systemic hematocrit in resting muscle, but during hyperemia it can rapidly increase by several-fold and approximate the level in the systemic circulation (74,80,81).

The oxygen delivered from capillaries is typically considered in terms of the number or volume of red blood cells traversing the capillary bed per unit time. However, it is not just the flux of red blood cells *per se* that determines oxygen delivery. Both the temporal and spatial relationships among red blood cells within the capillary may profoundly influence tissue oxygenation. At a given tissue P_{O_2}, the rate of oxygen diffusion into the tissue is determined by capillary P_{O_2} (10,24,69), which is related to capillary oxygen content by the oxygen-hemoglobin dissociation curve. The presence of red blood cells serves to "buffer" the P_{O_2} within the capillary and to thereby maintain the driving force for oxygen diffusion along the capillary (25). When capillary blood flow or oxygen content is elevated, part or all of the capillary P_{O_2} is raised, and the gradient driving oxygen diffusion is increased along the capillary (25,76,82).

The distance between successive red cells may be an important variable in determining oxygen diffusion from the capillary into muscle cells (73,82). Muscle $\dot{V}_{O_2}$ is low at rest (6), as is capillary hematocrit (74,80). During conditions of low oxygen flux from blood to tissue, P_{O_2} may be adequate along the entire capillary. However, during aerobic exercise with a low capillary hematocrit, the large plasma "gaps" between red cells may depleted of oxygen such that the P_{O_2} of plasma between red cells falls to the point where a uniform delivery of oxygen cannot be maintained at the capillary wall between two red cells. At this point, the capillary blood may no longer be homogeneous for O_2 supply, but instead assumes a "particulate" nature (51,73,82). This critical separation distance decreases as oxygen demand increases; i.e., red blood cells must be closer together in the capillary to maintain oxygen delivery as the rate of $\dot{V}_{O_2}$ increases (76,82). During hyperemia, the increase in red cell flux and the elevation in capillary hematocrit greatly reduce the plasma gaps, which would ensure that much more of the capillary surface remains functional in gas exchange (76,82).

The effect of varying the hematocrit of the blood supplying exercising muscle has been documented at several levels of investigation. Among human subjects performing under standardized conditions, blood flow to the knee extensors at constant work rate and $\dot{V}_{O_2}$ were found to differ, such that higher flows were associated with lower hemoglobin concentration (6). Analogous behavior has been shown in isolated working muscle (5). When taken with findings that blood flow was elevated in proportion to the fall in oxygen content produced by hypoxemia (20), evidence suggests that oxygen delivery may be "sensed" and regulated in the peripheral circulation by a mechanism that remains to be defined—perhaps by the red blood cell itself (83).

The presence of a plasma layer between the red cell and the capillary wall (74,79,84) would require red blood cells to be even closer together in the capillary to maintain the driving force for oxygen diffusion. This is because the red blood cell would be farther from the capillary wall, contributing to the "carrier-free layer" proposed as the principle barrier for oxygen diffusion from red cell to myocyte (53,58). However, the thickness of this layer appears to decrease as red blood cell flux and capillary hematocrit increase (74,76), thereby reducing the diffusion distance between red blood cells and muscle fibers.

The potential for these events within capillaries to limit $\dot{V}_{O_2}$ increases with the rate at which oxygen is consumed and may contribute to the diffusion limitation reported to occur within exercising skeletal muscle (60,61,68,85). Nevertheless, it is apparent that to answer the question of whether the "critical" separation distance of red blood cells really is critical to oxygen transport in tissue requires extending the analysis (51) to include a reasonable model of the surrounding tissue (38). This includes the distribution of mitochondria around the capillary, mitochondrial $\dot{V}_{O_2}$, the influence of myoglobin, and the frequency of oxygen flux variations associated with the capillary. It should also be recognized that the characteristics of red blood cell perfusion are quite variable among capillaries.

D. Capillary Transit Time and Flow Path

Capillary transit time denotes the time that red blood cells are in capillaries. It is proportional to the path length of red blood cell flow in a network and is inversely proportional to red blood cell velocity, both of which vary among capillaries (86–88). Transit time is influenced by the total volume of capillaries perfused, which can be altered acutely via capillary recruitment (70) or can be modified with training status (34). Mean capillary transit times have been calculated from measurements of organ blood flow and the estimated capillary density per unit volume of biopsied tissue (6,11). Intuitively, transit time effects the degree to which the oxygen content of the capillary blood can be lowered in the muscle; i.e. longer transit times should promote oxygen extraction. However, the idea of a mean capillary transit time is misleading as it treats the flow of red blood cells through capillaries as homogenous. This obscures the considerable variability associated with transit time indicated by anatomical measurements of flow path in conjunction with estimates of blood flow (89,90). Nevertheless, even these estimates of transit times are of limited validity as they assume that the anatomically defined capillary length correctly describes the functional flow path taken by red cells through the capillary network, and that the distribution of flow path lengths is constant. In contrast, the filling patterns for India ink in the microcirculation of rabbit leg muscles exhibited pronounced spatial heterogeneity that suggested up to a 16-fold range of flow velocities, flow path lengths, or a combination thereof (91). Such properties of microvascular perfusion underscore the importance of studying the behavior of blood cells as they course through the living microcirculation.

Intravital microscopy has revealed both temporal and spatial heterogeneity in the flow of red blood cells through capillary networks of the frog sartorius muscle (86,87). Direct measurements of capillary transit time and flow path lengths in hamster cremaster muscle revealed that the actual (functional) path lengths of labeled red blood cells were up to two-fold greater than the anatomical path length (88). This behavior was associated with broad distributions for capillary transit times, capillary red blood cell flux (cells/sec), and capillary path length (88). In the hamster tibialis muscle, variability in the distribution of red blood cells within capillary networks increased with the mean value during hyperemia, indicating that the fractional dispersion of red blood cells remained constant and was independent of blood flow or oxygen demand (92). The optimum conditions for capillary exchange appear to occur at less than maximum vasodilation (93). This may be explained by the disruption of the active regulation of red cell distribution among terminal arterioles (94), which then perturbs the distribution of perfusion among capillary networks and the exchange of substances across the capillary wall (93). Thus, a minimum level of vasomotor tone appears necessary to minimize the heterogeneity in microvascular transport, and can explain why the addition of vasodilators did not promote oxygen uptake in working muscle (68).

Because there is no correlation between (the variability in) path length and red cell velocity (86,88), both high and low red blood cell velocities occur through both short and long capillary flow paths, with a resultant dispersion of transit times. At one extreme, high velocity through a short flow path may contribute to a diffusion-limited "shunt" of oxygen from the arteriole to the venule. In a reciprocal manner, low velocities through longer flow paths may contribute to a flow-limited deficiency in local oxygen supply. Thus, based upon direct observations of the microcirculation in skeletal muscle, there are broad distributions of the multiple parameters associated with oxygen transport from the capillary (87,88,92). These data, compiled from independent laboratories, effectively preclude the assumption of the capillary as a uniform source of oxygen supply to tissue (71,75). The resulting dispersion of oxygen delivery within and among capillaries may result in "extreme" cases in which oxygen may be over-supplied or under-supplied to a particular tissue volume in relation to the local demand. As discussed below, however, diffusive interactions within and between adjacent regions within the muscle may help to offset such heterogeneity in capillary perfusion and thereby promote uniformity in oxygen delivery throughout the active muscle.

E. Functional Organization of Capillaries

The perfusion of capillaries in response to metabolic demand (i.e., muscle fiber recruitment) is discussed later. It is helpful to first consider the anatomical relationships that govern capillary perfusion (Fig. 1). With respect to the control of oxygen delivery to muscle fibers, the "functional unit" has been defined in terms of the smallest unit volume of tissue to which blood flow can be independently controlled (95). In parallel-fibered muscles, a terminal arteriole typically runs perpendicular to a bundle of several muscle fibers and gives rise to ~ 20 capillaries in each direction along the muscle fibers, which then empty into collecting venules (96–98). Because the terminal arteriole is the last branch of the arterial system that contains vascular smooth muscle, it constitutes the control element of capillary perfusion (95,97–99), with a role analogous to the "precapillary sphincter" (16). Thus, upon dilation of a terminal arteriole, the distribution of red blood cells is determined by the geometrical and rheological factors affecting the entry of red blood cells into respective capillaries (70,100) and by the distribution of resistances of respective capillary segments (88).

The capillaries governed by a terminal arteriole and the volume of tissue they encompass is referred to as a "microvascular unit" (MVU) (97,101,102). Although this volume had been estimated to approximate 1 cubic millimeter (95), measurements in the hamster indicate that each cubic millimeter of skeletal muscle may contain as many as 20 MVUs (97,102). In turn, the volume of muscle within a MVU contains segments ($\sim$ 1 mm long) of up to $\sim$ 30 muscle fibers (95,102), which may derive from as many different motor units (discussed below and refer to Fig. 1). Thus, with physiological patterns of motor unit recruitment (103), the metabolic demand within a MVU varies both spatially and temporally. As a result, a capillary within a MVU may have none, one, or all of the associated muscle fibers drawing oxygen from it at any given moment. This situation implies a distribution of Po_2 values among capillaries of any given MVU in the muscle. When taken with the gradients in mitochondrial content (and intracellular Po_2) discussed earlier, along with the heterogeneity of capillary perfusion (above), the considerable range of tissue Po_2 reported for muscles of cats (104), rabbits (105), and humans (106) may thus be accounted for. Moreover, the consistency of observations that muscle Po_2 spans a range of values (104–106) argues against tissue Po_2 as a tightly regulated variable in the local control of blood flow (107).

F. Oxygen Diffusion and Mixing Among Microvessels

Given the heterogeneity within MVUs for capillary red blood cell flux, transit times, flow path lengths, and red blood cell content (above), it seems misleading to simply consider the diffusion of oxygen from capillaries into myocytes (38,46,71). This idea carries the assumption that the oxygen content of the blood decreases progressively along the capillary path (10), which appears not to be the case. For example, countercurrent flow of red blood cells in overlapping diffusion fields from adjacent MVUs (98) may lead to mixing of capillary Po_2 rather than a progressive arterial-venous Po_2 gradient along each capillary. Recent findings demonstrate that mean Po_2 within individual capillaries, as well as arterioles and venules, can increase as well as decrease within time periods that are a fraction of a second (108). Such behavior can be explained by the gain (and loss) of oxygen from (and to) neighboring microvessels (75). In classic studies, the Po_2 of arterioles was found to decrease progressively along consecutive network branches (72). As there was no evidence for a barrier to the diffusion oxygen from the blood within the arteriole, the finding of a longitudinal gradient in P_{O_2} along the arteriolar network indicated that red cells were releasing large amounts of oxygen before even reaching the capillaries. Mathematical analyses of this behavior strongly support the contention that substantial oxygen loss occurs along the arteriolar network (78), and that the diffusion of oxygen from arterioles to capillaries is an integral component of distributing oxygen to the parenchymal cells (75,77). Moreover, the oxygen lost from arterioles may contribute a significant portion of that consumed by the tissue (109), particularly as metabolic demand increases (77). Thus, in addition to governing the convection of red blood cells into capillaries, arterioles appear to serve an important role in the diffusive delivery of oxygen to skeletal muscle fibers (72,75).

G. Venous and Tissue P_{O_2}

Early studies of the microcirculation in skeletal muscle (24,69) introduced the idea of using venous P_{O_2} as an index of end-capillary and tissue P_{O_2}. In turn, these indices were utilized to calculate the P_{O_2} gradients driving the diffusion of oxygen. From such origins, the oxygen saturation of venous blood during heavy work has widely been taken as representative of the P_{O_2} in exercising muscle. Upon considering the convection and diffusion of oxygen within the microcirculation, it becomes apparent that mixed venous P_{O_2} may well reflect what has happened to oxygen in the muscle as a whole. However, it does not provide an accurate index of the local gradients driving oxygen diffusion from blood to tissue; i.e., from red blood cells to mitochondria.

As a starting point, consider the potential variability of oxygen content with red blood cell spacing along the capillary. The effect of depleting oxygen in the plasma between red cells (73) would be masked by a time-averaged P_{O_2} measurement, even in the effluent from a single capillary. When capillaries fed by different terminal arterioles (i.e., from different MVUs) converge into a collecting venule, blood mixes from the respective MVUs (Fig. 1) (97,98,102). With differences in oxygen extraction between MVUs (which need not perfuse the same muscle fibers) (102), the mixing of blood will give an intermediate value that may not represent either MVU. The mixing and homogenizing effect is additive as venules converge into the collecting vein that carries blood from the tissue. Superimposed upon this temporal and spatial mixing of postcapillary blood is the diffusion of oxygen from capillaries and arterioles that course near the draining venules (75). Thus, the use of mixed venous P_{O_2}, or even the P_{O_2} of venous blood from a specific limb or muscle, must be questioned as an estimate of either capillary or tissue P_{O_2}. Nevertheless, for measurements based upon the Fick principle, the difference between arterial and mixed venous P_{O_2} remains a reliable measure of oxygen extraction by the muscle as a whole.

V. Intramuscular Dispersion of Metabolic Demand

Having first examined the locus and dispersion of oxygen demand within muscle fibers, the locus and dispersion of oxygen transport within the microcirculation was considered. The following discussion centers on the spatial and temporal patterns by which muscle fibers are recruited into activity, along with the effect that physiological activation of muscle fibers may have on where oxygen supply and demand occur within the muscle.

A. Functional Organization of Muscle Fibers

The functional element for the control of skeletal muscle contraction is the motor unit, which consists of a spinal motor neuron, its axon and the (often) hundreds of muscle fibers innervated by branches of the axon. A mammalian muscle is typically composed of 50 to 300 motor units that have a wide range of mechanical and metabolic properties (101,103,110). In normal, healthy muscle, the individual fibers of any given motor unit are generally not clumped together; rather, a given tissue volume is occupied by fibers interspersed from many motor units (95,101,110,111). In such manner, the functional domain of a motor unit is dispersed throughout a much larger tissue volume than occupied by the individual fibers (Fig. 1) (95,101,111). Most forms of physical activity involve only a portion of the entire motor unit population, with active units firing through a range of submaximal intensities (103). Therefore, during aerobic exercise in man, contracting skeletal muscle can be viewed as an aggregate of metabolically active and resting fibers, each with corresponding differences in local energy requirements.

A relatively simple pattern of activation occurs when muscle fibers are arranged in parallel, with each spanning the distance from tendon to tendon (Fig. 1). The force exerted by the muscle then reflects the number and size of motor units activated (110–112). This organization is well documented for unipennate muscles such as the rat soleus (113) and extensor digitorum longus (114). When complex, multipennate muscles such as the feline gastrocnemius (115) and flexor carpi radialis (116) were carefully examined, they were found to be comprised of distinct unipennate compartments that were each defined by tendonous sheaths. In turn, each compartment was spanned by individual muscle fibers arranged in parallel and innervated by a distinct, primary branch of the motor nerve (116). This type of neuromuscular organization suggests that discrete regions of a particular muscle may function independently during particular motor tasks (116,117). Such a pattern is also indicated for small, parallel-fibered and unipennate muscles of humans (118) and for distinct segments of long muscles that are separated by tendonous inscriptions, with each muscle compartment controlled by distinct primary nerves (117,119,120). It is important to note that there is a paucity of information concerning whether there is a vascular 'correlate' to this organization (121); i.e., whether (and if so, how) each compartment or subregion of a muscle may supplied by distinct feed vessels. Indeed, insight into this relationship may offer some explanation for blood flow heterogeneity at a level that has, to this point, remained unexplained (68,122).

The prevailing idea of parallel, intermingled contractile units that comprise a muscle cross-section is but one dimension of the pattern(s) by which metabolic demand may be generated within an active muscle under physiological conditions. In "long" muscles (e.g., sartorius), what may first appear as single fibers that extend from tendon to tendon, actually consists of much shorter fibers arranged in series (and in parallel) and aligned with the muscle axis (123–126). In such cases, muscle fibers typically terminate within the muscle by extensive tapering and interdigitation with other fibers. Studies of cat tenuissimus (123,125) and sartorius (124) muscles have revealed that individual fibers are activated together in series, along the entire axis of the muscle. Such a pattern for generating a stimulus for oxygen flux is in distinct contrast with the parallel organization of muscle fibers in cross section (101,110). Nevertheless, even in long muscles, a small fraction ($< 10\%$) of the fibers has been found to span the entire muscle length (118,127). Collectively, these observations support the interpretation that the metabolic demand of a motor unit (and its influence on the microcirculation) is dispersed within the muscle (101), and that any particular microvessel is influenced by muscle fibers derived from different motor units (Fig. 1).

The topological distribution of motor units within a muscle may also vary with fiber type. For example, in the unipennate feline tibialis anterior muscle, fibers in a characteristically "slow" unit spanned the full distance from tendon to tendon, with relatively constant fiber diameter (128). In contrast, the fibers of "fast" units terminated intramuscularly with extensive tapering (128). Further, there does not appear to be a 'uniform' muscle fiber length, either within or between species (118,124,126,128). In the sartorius of human infants, the longest fibers isolated from muscles 73 mm in length were 28 mm long (118), which approximates the average length (range, 20–30 mm) of fibers isolated from leg muscles of the cat (124). The range of individual fiber lengths for a given muscle can vary substantially, e.g., from < 10 to more than 50 mm in the cat tibialis anterior (128) and from 40 to nearly 200 mm in the sartorius of human adults (126).

The point to be made from the preceding discussion is that demands on the vascular supply will differ according to the pattern motor unit activation and muscle fiber dispersion. However, little is known of how blood flow may be directed to the fibers of a motor unit, all of which have similar metabolic demands but are dispersed throughout the muscle. Typically, the control of muscle blood flow has been studied by recording hemodynamic and vascular responses to electrical stimulation of whole muscle (4,61,68) or to microstimulation of a few muscle fibers (129,130). With whole muscle stimulation, the simultaneous activation of all fibers will eliminate differences in activity levels that normally exist across a population of motor units (103). Further, with graded electrical stimulation of the muscle or its motor-nerve, motor units tend to be recruited in an order that is reversed from that occurring naturally (110). Microstimulation, on the other hand, engages a small bundle of contiguous fibers, none of which may belong to the same motor unit. While these approaches have yielded valuable insights into the coupling between oxygen delivery and metabolic demand, such methods fail to emulate the complex spatial and temporal features of natural muscle activation discussed above. In turn, limitations imposed by these approaches have constrained our understanding of how oxygen transport may actually regulated in response to exercise. Indeed, a challenging area of investigation centers on how variability in the structural and functional organization of muscle fibers may determine the nature of capillary perfusion and regional blood flow (Fig. 1).

B. Interactions Between Motor Units and Microvascular Units

It is generally accepted that the flow of blood to intact skeletal muscle is matched to the intensity of muscular activity (Sec. II). However, neither the pattern nor the mechanisms by which the control elements of capillary perfusion are coordinated to meet the metabolic requirements of active fibers are well understood. As a first step in examining the complexity of interaction between motor unit recruitment and oxygen delivery to muscle fibers, we recently developed a model to simulate the perfusion of MVUs in response to the recruitment of motor units (101). Specifically, we were concerned with how differences in the spatial organization of muscle fibers into motor units could influence the pattern and magnitude of capillary perfusion throughout a muscle cross-section (101). Perfusion is considered to be distinct from blood flow in order to distinguish the following two features of vascular control. The term "perfused" indicates whether or not blood moves through a vessel. Thus, the entry of red blood cells into a capillary (or any other microvessel) is referred to as perfusion and largely determines the functional surface area for oxygen diffusion from the blood (93,131). In contrast, blood flow represents the volume of blood that traverses a blood vessel or vascular bed per unit time and reflects the total convection of oxygen into the muscle (or muscle region). In distinguishing perfusion from flow, vascular control can thus be considered as two coupled processes that reflect the Fick principle considered earlier. Because the contraction of one to several muscle fibers evokes arteriolar dilation and capillary perfusion (129,130), when any fiber(s) were active within the domain of a MVU (97,98), it was considered to be "recruited" and all of its capillaries perfused (101).

The most striking result of this model was the effectiveness with which motor unit recruitment induced MVU perfusion. Simulations of normal muscle indicated that nearly all of the MVUs would be perfused with less than 5% of the muscle fibers active. Note that robust capillary perfusion with only a modest increase in muscle (fiber) activity is consistent with actual findings in dog gracilis muscle (16) and human knee extensors (6). Because the smallest increment by which muscle fibers are activated is the motor unit, which involves many fibers scattered throughout a relatively large volume of the muscle (Sec. V.A), the recruitment of a single motor unit resulted in the perfusion of many MVUs (101). This implies that, with voluntary activation of motor units, capillary perfusion will increase dramatically with the onset of muscle activity. Moreover, the supply of blood to a single active muscle fiber requires the simultaneous perfusion of many surrounding (inactive) fibers, such that the physiological control of perfusion in skeletal muscle may well occur at an even coarser level than achieved by single MVUs. Thus, many MVUs must be perfused simultaneously to supply the fibers of a given motor unit (Fig. 1).

While the preceding argument is based primarily on a muscle cross section, it should be recognized that the millimeter distance spanned by each MVU is considerably less than the length of individual skeletal muscle fibers, which often span several centimeters. When a muscle fiber contracts, it is metabolically active along the entire length, and will require blood flow through the MVUs that supply corresponding segments of the fiber(s). The precision with which blood flow can be selectively controlled to a particular fiber or fiber group will therefore depend upon the alignment of the corresponding MVUs. As an extreme case, to increase blood flow to a single active muscle fiber without overperfusion of inactive fibers would require MVUs to be no wider than an individual fiber, (which does not occur) (97,98,102) and to be and completely aligned along a fiber's axis. We have recently examined these topological relationships in the hamster retractor muscle (102). Overall, the alignment of MVUs along muscle fibers was not significantly better than predicted for a random organization. Further, consecutive MVUs were as often derived from different parent vessels as from the same parent vessel. These findings support the conclusion that neither perfusion nor blood flow can selectively increase to a specific muscle fiber or to a particular group of fibers. Rather, perfusion must increase through a much larger region of the muscle than occupied by the active fibers. In turn, we propose that the spread ("conduction") of vasomotor responses throughout microvascular resistance networks contributes to the coordination of MVU perfusion in response to muscle fiber activation (18,81,132).

Our conclusion that perfusion cannot be exclusively directed to active muscle fibers is in direct contrast with the concept advanced from a recent study of human muscle (133). It is also argues against a reduction in the number of perfused capillaries when blood flow is limited (68) as discussed early in the chapter. Instead, we contend that the widespread dispersion of motor unit fibers promotes complete perfusion of skeletal muscle at low levels of activity. Indeed, such an arrangement could effectively constitute a "feed-forward" mechanism, with the capillaries adjacent to many *inactive* fibers also becoming perfused. In this manner, the perfusion of MVUs and the availability of oxygen may precede the activation of corresponding muscle fibers. Hence, upon the recruitment of additional motor units, much of the vascular bed would already contain red blood cells, which in turn could minimize any lag in elevating oxidative metabolism. Given the relatively low oxygen extraction of resting skeletal muscle (6), such a rapid increase in capillary surface area would facilitate oxygen extraction prior to substantial increases in total muscle blood flow (25). Based upon discussion earlier in this chapter, once the terminal arterioles dilate and MVUs are perfused, the volume of blood which then reaches the capillaries is controlled in the proximal segments of the resistance network.

Regional differences in blood flow responses to exercise are well documented between muscles and between muscle regions that are composed primarily of either oxidative or glycolytic fiber (12,13,67). When these observations are interpreted in light of the size principle of motor unit recruitment (103,110,134) and differences in the architecture and response characteristics of respective microvascular resistance networks (135,136), the apparently "selective" increase in blood flow to muscle fibers with the greatest oxidative capacity can, in fact, be readily explained (101). However, human skeletal muscles characteristically lack such regional differences in fiber type (34,137). Thus, in skeletal muscle comprised of mixed fiber type that is recruited under physiological conditions, we argue that blood flow cannot be selectively increased (or decreased) to particular muscle fibers or to particular capillaries during exercise.

VI. Conclusions

The basic determinants of oxygen transport in exercising skeletal muscle are illuminated by the Fick principle, with oxygen uptake reflecting the product of its delivery and extraction. A primary goal of this chapter has been to illustrate how and why this view constrains our thinking about the structural and functional relationships that actually determine the demand for and supply of oxygen within the exercising muscle. Attempting to bridge those relationships that are defined at the microscopic level with those that are apparent for the whole muscle or intact organism is a longstanding challenge (138). Although pronounced heterogeneity can be defined within each component, the system as a whole appears highly conducive to matching oxygen supply and demand (10). Indeed, though it is possible to design experiments and conditions that reveal diffusion as well as perfusion limitations to muscular performance, the precise determinants of these limitations remain ambiguous within the muscle. The challenge remains to integrate the determinants of oxygen transport the cellular and molecular level with the determinants of aerobic performance in the intact system.

Acknowledgment

Support for this work is awarded from the National Institutes of Health, grants RO1-HL56786 & RO1-HL41026.

References

1. Faulkner JA, Heigenhauser GF, Schork MA. The cardiac output—oxygen uptake relationship of men during graded bicycle ergometry. Med Sci Sports Exercise 1977; 9:148–154.
2. Rowell LB. Human cardiovascular adjustments to exercise and thermal stress. Physiol Rev 1974; 54:75–159.
3. Bockman EL. Blood flow and oxygen consumption in active soleus and gracilis muscles in cats. Am J Physiol 1983; 244:H546–H551.
4. Wilson BA, Stainsby WN. Relation between oxygen uptake and developed tension in dog skeletal muscle. J Appl Physiol 1978; 45:234–237.
5. Horstman DH, Gleser M, Delehunt J. Effects of altering O_2 delivery on $\dot{V}O_2$ of isolated, working muscle. Am J Physiol 1976; 230:327–334.
6. Andersen P, Saltin B. Maximal perfusion of skeletal muscle in man. J Physiol 1985; 366:233–249.
7. Shepherd JT. Circulation to skeletal muscle. In: Shepherd JT, Abboud FM (eds.). Handbook of Physiology. The Cardiovascular System. Peripheral Circulation and Organ Blood Flow, Part 1. Bethesda, MD: American Physiological Society, 1983, pp. 319–370.
8. Sparks HV. Effect of local metabolic factors on vascular smooth muscle. In: Bohr DF, Somlyo AP, Sparks HV (eds.). Handbook of Physiology. The Cardiovascular System. Vascular Smooth Muscle. Bethesda, MD: American Physiological Society, 1980, pp. 475–513.
9. Saltin B, Rowell LB. Functional adaptations to physical activity and inactivity. Fed Proc 1980; 39:1506–1513.
10. Weibel ER. The Pathway for Oxygen. Cambridge, MA: Harvard University Press, 1984, pp. 1–425.
11. Weibel ER. Scaling of structural and functional variables in the respiratory system. Ann Rev Physiol 1987; 49:147–159.
12. Armstrong RB, Delp MD, Goljan EF, Laughlin MH. Distribution of blood flow in muscles of miniature swine during exercise. J Appl Physiol 1987; 62:1285–1298.
13. Laughlin MH, Armstrong RB. Muscular blood flow distribution patterns as a function of running speed in rats. Am J Physiol 1982; 243:H296–H306.
14. Segal SS, Kurijiaka DT. Coordination of blood flow control in the resistance vasculature of skeletal muscle. Med Sci Sports Exercise 1995; 27:1–7.
15. Goodman AH, Einstein R, Granger HJ. Effect of changing metabolic rate on local blood flow control in the canine hindlimb. Circ Res 1978; 43:769–776.
16. Honig CR, Odoroff CL, Frierson JL. Capillary recruitment in exercise: rate, extent, uniformity, and relation to blood flow. Am J Physiol 1980; 238:H31–H42.
17. Granger HJ, Goodman AH, Granger DN. Role of resistance and exchange vessels in local microvascular control of skeletal muscle oxygenation in the dog. Circ Res 1976; 38:379–385.
18. Welsh DG, Segal SS. Coactivation of resistance vessels and muscle fibers with acetylcholine release from motor nerves. Am J Physiol 1997; 273:H156–H163.
19. Harms CA, Wetter TJ, McClaran SR, Pegelow DF, Nickele GA, Nelson WB, Hanson P, Dempsey JA. Effects of respiratory muscle work on cardiac output and its distribution during maximal exercise. J Appl Physiol 1998; 85:609–618.

20. Rowell LB, Saltin B, Kiens B, Christensen NJ. Is peak quadriceps blood flow in humans even higher during exercise with hypoxemia? Am J Physiol 1986; 251:H1038–H1044.
21. Secher N, Clausen JP, Noer I, Trap-Jensen J. Central and regional circulatory effects of adding arm exercise to leg exercise. Acta Physiol Scand 1977; 100:288–297.
22. Saltin B. Malleability of the system in overcoming limitations: functional elements. J Exp Biol 1985; 115:345–354.
23. Stainsby WN, Otis AB. Blood flow, blood oxygen tension, oxygen uptake, and oxygen transport in skeletal muscle. Am J Physiol 1964; 206:858–866.
24. Krogh A. The number and distribution of capillaries in muscles with calculations of the oxygen pressure head necessary for supplying the tissue. J Physiol 1918; 52:409–415.
25. Duling BR. Relationships of microvascular and tissue heterogeneities to oxygenation of skeletal muscle. In: Borer KT, Edington DW, White TP (eds.). Frontiers of Exercise Biology. Champaign: Human Kinetics, 1983, pp. 100–118.
26. Folkow B, Sonnenschein RR, Wright DL. Loci of neurogenic and metabolic effects on precapillary vessels of skeletal muscle. Acta Physiol Scand 1971; 81:459–471.
27. Lind AR, Williams CA. The control of blood flow through human forearm muscles following brief isometric contractions. J Physiol 1979; 288:529–547.
28. Kjellmer I. On the competition between metabolic vasodilatation and neurogenic vasoconstriction in skeletal muscle. Acta Physiol Scand 1965; 63:450–459.
29. McGillivray-Anderson KM, Faber JE. Effect of acidosis on contraction of microvascular smooth muscle by α_1- and α_2-adrenoreceptors. Implications for neural and metabolic regulation. Circ Res 1990; 66:1643–1657.
30. Shepherd JT, Vanhoutte PM. Local modulation of adrenergic neurotransmission. Circ Res 1981; 64:655–666.
31. Thomas GD, Victor RG. Nitric oxide mediates contraction-induced attenuation of sympathetic vasoconstriction in rat skeletal muscle. J Physiol 1998; 506:817–826.
32. Kurjiaka DT, Segal SS. Interaction between conducted vasodilation and sympathetic nerve activation in arterioles of hamster striated muscle. Circ Res 1995; 76:885–891.
33. Gaskell WH. On the changes of the blood-stream in muscles through stimulation of their nerves. J Anat Physiol 1877; 11:360–402.
34. Saltin B, Gollnick PD. Skeletal muscle adaptability: significance for metabolism and performance. In: Peachey LD, Adrian RH, Geiger SR (eds.). Handbook of Physiology. Bethesda: American Physiological Society, 1983, pp. 555–631.
35. Schwerzmann K, Hoppeler H, Kayar SR, Weibel ER. Oxidative capacity of muscle and mitochondria: Correlation of physiological, biochemical, and morphometric characteristics. Proc Natl Acad Sci 1988; 86:1583–1587.
36. Hoppeler H, Lindstedt SL. Malleability of skeletal muscle in overcoming limitations: Structural elements. J Exp Biol 1985; 115:355–364.
37. Mathieu-Costello O. Comparative aspects of muscle capillary supply. Ann Rev Physiol 1993; 55:503–525.
38. Mainwood GW, Rakusan K. A model for intracellular energy transport. Can J Physiol Pharm 1982; 60:98–102.
39. Sullivan SM, Pittman RN. Relationship between mitochondrial volume density and capillarity in hamster muscles. Am J Physiol 1987; 252:H149–H155.

40. Bessman SP, Geiger PJ. Transport of energy in muscle: the phosphorylcreatine shuttle. Science 1981; 211:448–452.
41. Meyer RA, Sweeney HL, Kushmerick MJ. A simple analysis of the "phosphocreatine shuttle." Am J Physiol 1984; 246:C365–C377.
42. Hoppeler H, Mathieu O, Weibel ER, Krauer R, Lindstedt SL, Tayler CR. Design of the mammalian respiratory system. VII. Capillaries in skeletal muscles. Resp Physiol 1981; 44:129–150.
43. Kayar SR, Claassen H, Hoppeler H, Weibel ER. Mitochondria distribution in relation to changes in muscle metabolism in rat soleus. Resp Physiol 1986; 64:1–11.
44. Kayar SR, Conley KE, Claassen H, Hoppeler H. Capillarity and mitochondrial distribution in rat myocardium following exercise training. J Exp Biol 1985; 120:189–199.
45. Hintz CS, Chi MM, Lowry OH. Heterogeneity in regard to enzymes and metabolites within individual muscle fibers. Am J Physiol 1984; 246:C288–C292.
46. Hoppeler H, Kayar SR. Capillarity and oxidative capacity of muscles. News Physiol Sci 1988; 3:113–116.
47. Maxwell LC, White TP, Faulkner JA. Oxidative capacity, blood flow, and capillarity of skeletal muscles. J Appl Physiol 1980; 49:627–633.
48. Gray SD, Staub NC. Resistance to blood flow in leg muscles of dog during tetanic isometric contraction. Am J Physiol 1967; 213:677–682.
49. Anrep GV, Von Saalfeld E. The blood flow through the skeletal muscle in relation to its contraction. J Physiol 1935; 85:375–399.
50. Folkow B, Halicka HD. A comparison between "red" and "white" muscle with respect to blood supply, capillary surface area and oxygen uptake during rest and exercise. Microvasc Res 1968; 1:1–14.
51. Popel AS. Theory of oxygen transport to tissue. Critical Views Biomed Engin 1989; 17:257–321.
52. Wittenberg BA, Wittenberg JB. Transport of oxygen in muscle. Ann Rev Physiol 1989; 51:857–878.
53. Gayeski TEJ, Honig CR. O_2 gradients from sarcolemma to cell interior in red muscle at maximal $\dot{V}O_2$. Am J Physiol 1986; 251:H789–H799.
54. Gayeski TEJ, Honig CR. Intracellular Po_2 in long axis of individual fibers in working dog gracilis muscle. Am J Physiol 1988; 254:H1179–H1186.
55. Jones DP, Kennedy FG. Analysis of intracellular oxygenation of isolated adult cardiac myocytes. J Physiol 1986; 250:C384–C390.
56. Kennedy FG, Jones DP. Oxygen dependence of mitochondrial function in isolated rat cardiac myocytes. Am J Physiol 1986; 250:C374–C383.
57. Voter WA, Gayeski TEJ. Determinants of myoglobin saturation of frozen specimens using a reflecting cryospectrophotometer. Am J Physiol 1995; 269:H1328–H1341.
58. Honig CR, Gayeski TEJ, Federspiel W, Clark A, Jr., Clark P. Muscle O_2 gradients from hemoglobin to cytochrome: new concepts, new complexities. Adv Exp Med Biol 1984; 169:23–38.
59. Jones DP. Intracellular diffusion gradients of O_2 and ATP. Am J Physiol 1986; 250:C663–C675.
60. Roca J, Hogan MC, Story D, Bebout DE, Haab P, Gonzalez R, Ueno O, Wagner PD. Evidence for tissue diffusion limitation of $VO_{2\,max}$ in normal humans. J Appl Physiol 1989; 67:291–299.

61. Hogan MC, Roca J, West JB, Wagner PD. Dissociation of maximal O_2 uptake from O_2 delivery in canine gastrocnemius in situ. J Appl Physiol 1989; 66:1219–1226.
62. Schaffartzik W, Barton ED, Poole DC, Tsukimoto K, Hogan MC, Bebout DE, Wagner PD. Effect of reduced hemoglobin concentration on leg oxygen uptake during maximal exercise in humans. J Appl Physiol 1993; 75:491–498.
63. Cole RP. Myoglobin function in exercising skeletal muscle. Science 1982; 216:523–525.
64. Garry DJ, Ordway GA, Lorenz JN, Radford NB, Chin ER, Grange RW, Bassel-Duby R, Williams RS. Mice without myoglobin. Nature 1998; 395:905–908.
65. Gray SD, Renkin EM. Microvascular supply in relation to fiber metabolic type in mixed skeletal muscles of rabbits. Microvasc Res 1978; 16:406–425.
66. Hudlicka O, Egginton S, Brown MD. Capillary diffusion distances - their importance for cardiac and skeletal muscle performance. News Physiol Sci 1988; 3:134–138.
67. Mackie BG, Terjung RL. Blood flow to different skeletal muscle fiber types during contraction. Am J Physiol 1983; 245:H265–H275.
68. Kurdak SS, Grassi B, Wagner PD, Hogan MC. Blood flow distribution in working in situ canine muscle during blood flow reduction. J Appl Physiol 1996; 80:1978–1983.
69. Krogh A. The supply of oxygen to the tissues and the regulation of the capillary circulation. J Physiol 1919; 52:457–474.
70. Klitzman B, Damon DN, Gorczynski RJ, Duling BR. Augmented tissue oxygen supply during striated muscle contraction in the hamster: Relative contributions of capillary recruitment, functional dilation, and reduced tissue P_{O_2}. Circ Res 1982; 51:711–721.
71. Kreuzer F. Oxygen supply to tissues: the Krogh model and its assumptions. Experientia 1982; 38:1415–1426.
72. Duling BR, Berne RM. Longitudinal gradients in periarteriolar oxygen tension. Circ Res 1970; 27:669–678.
73. Homer LD, Weathersby PK, Kiesow LA. Oxygen gradients between red blood cells in the microcirculation. Microvasc Res 1981; 22:308–323.
74. Klitzman B, Duling BR. Microvascular hematocrit and red cell flow in resting and contracting striated muscle. Am J Physiol 1979; 237:H481–H490.
75. Ellsworth ML, Ellis CG, Popel AS, Pittman RN. Role of microvessels in oxygen supply to tissue. News Physiol Sci 1994; 9:119–123.
76. Duling BR, Desjardins C. Capillary hematocrit—what does it mean? News Physiol Sci 1987; 2:66–69.
77. Secomb TW, Hus R. Simulation of O_2 transport in skeletal muscle: diffusive exchange between arterioles and capillaries. Am J Physiol 1994; 267:H1214–H1221.
78. Popel AS, Pittman RN, Ellsworth ML. Rate of oxygen loss from arterioles is an order of magnitude higher than expected. Am J Physiol 1989; 256:H921–H924.
79. Vink H, Duling BR. Identification of distinct luminal domains for macromolecules, erythrocytes, and leukocytes within mammalian capillaries. Circ Res 1996; 79:581–589.
80. Desjardins C, Duling BR. Microvessel hematocrit: measurement and implications for capillary oxygen transport. Am J Physiol 1987; 252:H494–H503.
81. Segal SS. Microvascular recruitment in hamster striated muscle: role for conducted vasodilation. Am J Physiol 1991; 261:H181–H189.

82. Federspiel WJ, Sarelius IH. An examination of the contribution of red cell spacing to the uniformity of oxygen flux at the capillary wall. Microvasc Res 1984; 27:273–285.
83. Ellsworth ML, Forrester T, Ellis CG, Dietrich HH. The erythrocyte as a regulator of vascular tone. Am J Physiol 1995; 269:H2155–H2161.
84. Desjardins C, Duling BR. Heparinase treatment suggests a role for the endothelial cell glycocalyx in regulation of capillary hematocrit. Am J Physiol 1990; 258:H647–H654.
85. Hogan MC, Bebout DE, Wagner PD, West JB. Maximal O_2 uptake of in situ dog muscle during acute hypoxemia with constant perfusion. J Appl Physiol 1990; 69:570–576.
86. Tyml K, Ellis CG, Safranyos RG, Fraser S, Groom AC. Temporal and spatial distributions of red cell velocity in capillaries of resting skeletal muscle, including estimates of red cell transit times. Microvasc Res 1981; 22:14–31.
87. Ellis CG, Wrigley SM, Groom AC. Heterogeneity of red blood cell perfusion in capillary networks supplied by a single arteriole in resting skeletal muscle. Circ Res 1994; 75:357–368.
88. Sarelius IH. Cell flow path influences transit time through striated muscle capillaries. Am J Physiol 1986; 250:H899–H907.
89. Honig CR, Odoroff CL. Calculated dispersion of capillary transit times: significance for oxygen exchange. Am J Physiol 1981; 240:H199–H208.
90. Honig CR, Feldstein ML, Frierson JL. Capillary lengths, anastomoses, and estimated capillary transit times in skeletal muscle. Am J Physiol 1977; 233:H122–H129.
91. Renkin EM, Gray SD, Dodd LR. Filling of microcirculation in skeletal muscles during times India ink perfusion. Am J Physiol 1981; 241:H174–H186.
92. Damon DH, Duling BR. Evidence that capillary perfusion heterogeneity is not controlled in striated muscle. Am J Physiol 1985; 249:H386–H392.
93. Renkin EM. Exchange of substances through capillary walls. In: Wolstenholm GEW, Knight J (eds.). CIBA Foundation Symposium on Circulatory and Respiratory Mass Transport. London: Churchill, 1969, pp. 50–66.
94. Sarelius IH. Cell and oxygen flow in arterioles controlling capillary perfusion. Am J Physiol 1993; 265:H1682–H1687.
95. Bloch EH, Iberall AS. Toward a concept of the functional unit of mammalian skeletal muscle. Am J Physiol 1982; 242:R411–R420.
96. Eriksson E, Lisander B. Changes in precapillary resistance in skeletal muscle vessels studied by intravital microscopy. Acta Physiol Scand 1972; 84:295–305.
97. Delashaw JB, Duling BR. A study of the functional elements regulating capillary perfusion in striated muscle. Microvasc Res 1988; 36:162–171.
98. Lund N, Damon DN, Duling BR. Capillary grouping in hamster tibialis anterior muscles: flow patterns, and physiological significance. Int J Microcirc Clin Exp 1987; 5:359–372.
99. Sweeney TE, Sarelius IH. Arteriolar control of capillary cell flow in striated muscle. Circ Res 1989; 64:112–120.
100. Honig CR, Odoroff CL, Frierson JL. Active and passive capillary control in red muscle at rest and in exercise. Am J Physiol 1982; 243:H196–H206.
101. Fuglevand AJ, Segal SS. Simulation of motor unit recruitment and microvascular unit perfusion: spatial considerations. J Appl Physiol 1997; 83:1223–1234.

102. Emerson GG, Segal SS. Alignment of microvascular units along skeletal muscle fibers of hamster retractor. J Appl Physiol 1997; 82:42–48.
103. Enoka RM. Morphological features and activation patterns of motor units. J Clin Neurophysiol 1995; 12:538–559.
104. Whalen WJ, Buerk D, Thuning CA. Blood flow-limited oxygen consumption in resting cat skeletal muscle. Am J Physiol 1973; 224:763–768.
105. Gutierrez G, Lund N, Acero AL, Marini C. Relationship of venous P_{O_2} to muscle P_{O_2} during hypoxemia. J Appl Physiol 1989; 67:1093–1099.
106. Lund N, Jorfeldt L, Lewis DH. Skeletal muscle oxygen pressure fields in healthy human volunteers: a study of the normal state and the effects of different arterial oxygen pressures. Acta Anaesth Scand 1980; 24:272–278.
107. Duling BR, Pittman RN. Oxygen tension: dependent or independent variable in local control of blood flow? Fed Proc 1975; 34:2012–2019.
108. Zheng L, Golub AS, Pittman RN. Determination of P_{O_2} and its heterogeneity in single capillaries. Am J Physiol 1996; 271:H365–H372.
109. Kuo L, Pittman RN. Influence of hemoconcentration on arteriolar oxygen transport in hamster striated muscle. Am J Physiol 1990; 259:H1694–H1702.
110. Burke R. Motor units: anatomy, physiology, and functional organization. In: Brooks VB (ed.). Handbook of Physiology. Bethesda, MD: American Physiological Society, 1981, pp. 345–422.
111. Burke RE, Tsairis P. Anatomy and innervation ratios in motor units of cat gastrocnemius. J Physiol 1973; 234:749–765.
112. Gans C. Fiber architecture and muscle function. In: Terjung RL (ed.). Exercise and Sport Sciences Reviews. Baltimore: Williams and Wilkins, 1982, pp. 160–206.
113. Segal SS, White TP, Faulkner JA. Architecture, composition, and contractile properties of rat soleus muscle grafts. Am J Physiol 1986; 250:C474–C479.
114. Balice-Gordon RJ, Thompson WJ. The organization and development of compartmentalized innervation in rat extensor digitorum longus muscle. J Physiol 1988; 398:211–231.
115. English AW, Letbetter WD. Anatomy and innervation patterns of cat lateral gastrocnemius and plantaris muscles. Am J Anat 1982; 164:67–77.
116. Galvas PE, Gonyea WJ. Motor-end-plate and nerve distribution in a histochemically compartmentalized pennate muscle in the cat. Am J Anat 1980; 159:147–156.
117. Bodine SC, Roy RR, Meadows DA, Zernicke RF, Sack RD, Fournier M, Edgerton VR. Architectural, histochemical, and contractile characteristics of a unique biarticular muscle: the cat semitendinous. J Neurophysiol 1982; 48:192–201.
118. Christensen E. Topography of terminal motor innervation in striated muscles from stillborn infants. Am J Phys Med 1959; 38:65–78.
119. Armstrong JB, Rose PK, Vanner S, Bakker GJ, Richmond FJR. Compartmentalization of motor units in the cat neck muscle, biventer cervicis. J Neurophysiol 1988; 60:30–45.
120. Richmond FJR, Armstrong JB. Fiber architecture and histochemistry in the cat neck muscle, biventer cervicis. J Neurophysiol 1988; 60:46–59.
121. Eriksson E, Myrhage R. Microvascular dimensions and blood flow in skeletal muscle. Acta Physiol Scand 1972; 86:211–222.

122. Piiper J, Pendergast DR, Marconi C, Meyer M, Heisler N, Cerretelli P. Blood flow distribution in dog gastrocnemius muscle at rest and during stimulation. J Appl Physiol 1985; 58:2068–2074.
123. Adrian ED. The spread of activity in the tenuissimus muscle of the cat and in other complex muscles. J Physiol 1925; 60:301–315.
124. Loeb GE, Pratt CA, Chanaud CM, Richmond FJR. Distribution and innervation of short, interdigitated muscle fibers in parallel-fibered muscles of the cat hindlimb. J Morphol 1987; 191:1–15.
125. Lev-Tov A, Pratt CA, Burke RE. The motor-unit population of the cat tenuissimus muscle. J Neurophysiol 1988; 59:1128–1142.
126. Heron MI, Richmond FFR. In-series fiber architecture in long human muscles. J Morphol 1993; 216:35–45.
127. Duxson MJ, Sheard PW. Formation of new myotubes occurs exclusively at the multiple innervation zones of an embryonic large muscle. Developmental Dynamics 1995; 204:391–405.
128. Ounjian M, Roy RR, Eldred E, Garfinkel A, Payne JR, Armstrong A, et al. Physiological and developmental implications of motor unit anatomy. J Neurobiol 1991; 22:547–559.
129. Gorczynski RJ, Klitzman B, Duling BR. Interrelations between contracting striated muscle and precapillary microvessels. Am J Physiol 1978; 235:H949–H504.
130. Berg BR, Sarelius IH. Functional capillary organization in striated muscle. Am J Physiol 1995;268:H1215–H1222.
131. Beer G, Yonce LR. Blood flow, oxygen uptake, and capillary filtration in resting skeletal muscle. Am J Physiol 1972; 223:492–498.
132. Kurjiaka DT, Segal SS. Interaction between conducted vasodilation and sympathetic nerve activation in arterioles of hamster striated muscle. Circ Res 1995; 76:885–891.
133. Ray CA, Dudley GA. Muscle use during dynamic knee extension: Implication for perfusion and metabolism. J Appl Physiol 1998; 85:1994–1197.
134. Henneman E, Somjen G, Carpenter DO. Functional significance of cell size in spinal motoneurons. J Neurophysiol 1965; 28:560–580.
135. Williams DA, Segal SS. Microvascular architecture in rat soleus and extensor digitorum longus muscles (published erratum in Microvasc Res 1992; 43:358). Microvasc Res 1992; 43:192–204.
136. Williams DA, Segal SS. Feed artery role in blood flow control to rat hindlimb skeletal muscles. J Physiol 1993; 463:631–646.
137. Lexell J, Henriksson-Larsen K, Sjostrom M. Distribution of different fibre types in human skeletal muscles 2. A study of cross-sections of whole m. vastus lateralis. Acta Physiol Scand 1983; 117:115–122.
138. Duling BR, Sarelius IH, Jackson WF. A comparison of microvascular estimates of capillary blood flow with direct measurements of total striated muscle flow. Int J Microcirc Clin Exp 1982; 1:409–424.

15

The Gut: Oxygen Transport and Gas Exchange Function

PAUL T. SCHUMACKER

The University of Chicago
Chicago, Illinois

I. Introduction

The primary function of the gastrointestinal system involves the controlled axial transport of ingested food, coupled with the breakdown and selective absorption of nutrients. The cellular processes required for these functions include contraction of smooth muscle, active and facilitated transport across the epithelial barrier, secretory process, neuroendocrine function, and cell growth and proliferation. Many of these processes require energy in the form of adenosine triphosphate (ATP), which is resynthesized primarily via mitochondrial oxidative phosphorylation. An important function of the gut microcirculation is to assure an adequate supply of oxygen (O_2) to all of the cells to meet these metabolic needs. Not surprisingly, the metabolic activity and gas exchange requirements of the gut vary widely depending on whether active digestion is occurring. Depending on the level of digestive activity, large variations in O_2 demand occur, accompanied by variations in splanchnic blood flow. When digestion is active, local metabolic vasodilation augments gastrointestinal blood flow to meet the increased gas exchange demands of the tissue, especially in the mucosa. Sometimes competing with local metabolic vasodilation, the powerful extrinsic neurohumoral control exerted by the autonomic nervous system over the gastrointestinal system serves to coordinate digestive processes with physical activity, stress, or other more pressing demands on the intact organism. Thus, during vigorous physical exercise, the digestive functions become inhibited, and blood flow to the gut is reduced via activation of the sympathetic nervous system. In states such as hemorrhage, reflex autonomic vasoconstriction can become maximally activated, leading to a severe restriction of blood flow and the onset of tissue hypoxia. In that case, local metabolic vasodilation begins to compete with the baroreflex-mediated vasoconstriction, restoring local tissue O_2 supply and minimizing development of ischemic tissue injury. An understanding of the regulation of gut blood flow and O_2 supply requires an understanding of the gas exchange needs of the tissue, the regional differences in those needs, and an understanding of how intrinsic and extrinsic vascular control mechanisms interact to affect diffusive and convective O_2 transport processes in the microcirculation. From that perspective, this chapter reviews the microvascular regulation of gut gas exchange function both in normal tissues and in pathophysiological states. The reader is also directed to a number of excellent reviews that have appeared in past years dealing with the regulation of gut blood flow in relation to metabolic demand [1–5] and a comprehensive chapter in the *Handbook of Physiology* dealing with the gut microcirculation [6].

II. Structure and Function of the Gut Vascular Anatomy

The splanchnic circulation receives approximately 20% of the cardiac output under resting conditions. The gut is supplied by the celiac trunk, the superior and the inferior splanchnic arteries. The celiac trunk supplies the stomach and duodenum, whereas the superior splanchnic artery supplies the small intestine and much of the colon. The inferior splanchnic artery supplies the distal region of the large bowel and the rectum. Branches of these major arteries fan out as arcades through the mesentery to supply the wall of the gut at intervals along its length. The spacing of these branches varies considerably among species, with relatively more branches per unit length of gut in porcine than canine small intestine. Obstruction of a single branch of the mesenteric artery is not catastrophic for the region of the gut it supplies, because there seems to be ample potential for collateral perfusion from adjacent regions of the gut wall. This characteristic is probably essential to prevent the development of regional ischemia as the gut changes shape under different conditions.

The wall of the gut is comprised of an inner mucosal region and an outer muscularis, separated from one another by the submucosa. The muscularis contains both longitudinal and circumferential layers of smooth muscle. The mucosa contains an outer layer composed of villi and a deeper mucosal layer of crypts where villi are formed and new epithelial cells are generated. Upon reaching the serosa of the gut, arterial vessels from a tight plexus at the mesenteric border, from which small arteries branch off radially to enter the smooth muscle wall. A minor network of conducting vessels can be observed in the smooth muscle and in the submucosal layer adjacent to the muscularis. Blood vessels supplying the mucosa arise from this network, and supply the crypts and mucosal villi [7].

Using micropipets, Gore and Bohlen [7] measured the longitudinal distribution of vascular pressures in the gut. They found large decreases in pressure in the mesenteric vessels even before they reached the gut wall. However, most of the pressure decrease occurred in arterial vessels in the gut wall upstream from the capillaries. They also estimated that capillary hydrostatic pressures were greater in muscularis than in mucosa. Unlike capillaries in the muscularis, capillaries in the mucosa seem to be fenestrated. Thus, the lower hydrostatic pressures in mucosa may help to facilitate solute exchange without excessive loss of intravascular volume. Consistent with the different metabolic requirements in mucosa and muscularis regions, density of capillaries per unit volume of mucosa is greater than capillary volume densities in muscularis [8].

Myogenic responses of the intestinal circulation have also been reported, as evidenced by an increase in vascular resistance in response to an elevation of venous pressure [9]. The arterial vessels of the intestine have also been shown to relax when arterial pressure is decreased, a response known as autoregulation [10].

III. Vascular Models of the Gut Microcirculation

The microcirculation of the gut is linked importantly to the gas exchange function of the tissue and therefore warrants careful consideration. A classical description of the gut microcirculation was proposed by Folkow [11], who described the vascular arrangement of the gastrointestinal tract as a set of parallel compartments supplying the mucosa, submucosa, and muscularis regions. According to that model, arteriolar vessels supplying these regions allowed independent adjustment of local blood flow. Because there is no evidence to suggest that capillaries are arranged in series among these regions, it is safe to assume that independent capillary–tissue exchange occurs in these three compartments. Because it is difficult to assess accurately blood flow among three layers of the gut wall experimentally, the Folkow model has received limited attention in terms of experimental verification. Nevertheless, the model is useful because O_2 demand in the submucosal region is small; therefore, blood flow to that compartment behaves much like a physiological shunt. Experimental and theoretical results suggest that such shunting may occur in the gut wall and may be regulated physiologically (see Sec. VII). Hence, that model seems to be important in understanding the gas exchange behavior of the gut under physiological and pathophysiological conditions.

A simpler model of the gut microcirculation was later proposed by Shepherd et al. [12], who described a two-compartment model comprised of mucosa and muscularis supplied by a single arterial vessel (Fig. 1). Although simplistic, this model has been useful because it attributes a large fraction of the overall

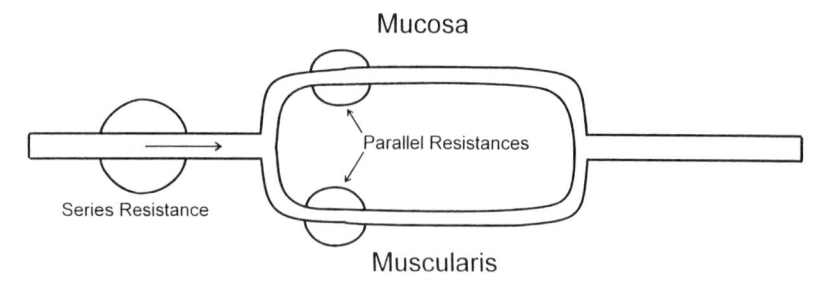

Figure 1 Two-compartment model of the gut microcirculation. Overall blood flow is controlled by an upstream resistance, whereas the distribution of blood flow between mucosa and muscularis is regulated by the relative magnitudes of the parallel resistances. Factors can affect overall blood flow without altering the intramural distribution; other factors can alter the partitioning of flow between mucosa and muscularis without an apparent effect on overall gut flow. (Redrawn with permission from Ref. 12.)

vascular resistance to the proximal upstream segment, with a relatively small fraction of the overall resistance residing in the smaller vessels immediately upstream from the capillary bed. Relative changes in the small resistances supplying the two compartments can therefore influence the intramural distribution of blood flow without necessarily changing overall mesenteric vascular resistance. As discussed in Sec. VI, this feature has important consequences for the gas exchange function of the tissue to the extent that large changes in the distribution of blood flow can occur within the microcirculation without any change in the overall vascular resistance. Conversely, large changes in overall vascular resistance can occur with little effect on the distribution of perfusion between compartments.

IV. Role of Extrinsic Autonomic Neurohumoral Control of Gut Blood Flow

Blood flow to the gut is influenced heavily by extrinsic autonomic neurohumoral control. Sympathetic vasoconstrictor fibers innervate the mesenteric vessels as well as arterial vessels within muscularis, submucosa, and mucosa. Electrical stimulation of these nerves causes constriction of resistance and capacitance vessels [11,13] and a decrease in overall blood flow. Humoral vasoconstrictors, including vasopressin and renin, can also act on the vessels supplying the small intestine. For example, McNeill et al. [14] found that the increase in gut vascular resistance during hemorrhage could only be abolished if nephrectomy and adrenalectomy were performed in addition to denervation. However, when blood flow and O_2 supply to the gut are severely reduced by increases in sympathetic vasoconstrictor activity, local metabolic vasodilation eventually competes with the vasoconstrictor activity in a phenomenon known as autoregulatory escape [15]. In this regard, the common notion that the gut is "sacrificed" during hypotensive states to preserve blood flow for "vital" organs is often overstated. As discussed in Sec. VI, a more realistic description is that hypotension both reduces the blood flow to the gut and improves its ability to extract O_2 from a limited supply. However, when O_2 supply is critically reduced, the gut has some ability to override extrinsic vasoconstriction to assure its adequate supply.

V. Metabolic Control of the Gut Microcirculation

The control of the gut microcirculation is influenced significantly by local metabolic vasodilatory mechanisms. According to the metabolic model of microcirculatory control, blood flow is distributed in accordance with local metabolic demand [3,16]. In the gut, the metabolic activity in mucosa is significantly greater than that in muscularis [17] by virtue of the active transport across the epithelial barrier, generation of secretions within epithelium and in submucosal glands, and the growth and proliferation of the cells in the mucosa. The greater metabolic activity in mucosa implies that blood flow should be distributed nonuniformly in the gut wall, assuming that regional flow remains closely matched to O_2 demand. Indeed, flow measurements in mucosa and muscularis have consistently shown that blood flow per gram of tissue is greater in the former than in the latter, for both small intestine and colon [6]. Regional differences in metabolic demand in the gut wall also are evidenced by differences in the reactive hyperemic response to transient occlusion of blood flow. In small intestine, a marked transient reactive hyperemia is observed after release of a 30–45 second arterial occlusion. Most of the increase in blood flow occurs in mucosa as opposed to muscularis, as demonstrated by Shepherd and Riedel [18,19], who found that reactive hyperemia was more vigorous in mucosa than in muscularis. Metabolic activity in the mucosa is stimulated during absorption of nutrients from the lumen, as is the reactive hyperemia response in that layer of the gut wall [9,19].

A number of studies have focused on the relationship between tissue function and blood flow in the gastrointestinal system [20]. For example, it has been noted consistently that acid secretion and O_2 consumption decrease when blood flow reaches a critically low level [4]. However, it was later recognized that this correlation is derived from the relationship between O_2 supply and consumption [1,3]. The local regulation of blood flow in the gut is importantly influenced by the balance between O_2 supply and demand. In addition, the competition between extrinsic neurohumoral vasoconstriction and local metabolic vasodilation is affected by the O_2 supply-to-demand ratio. Accordingly, an understanding of the regulation of the microcirculation requires an appreciation of the influence of O_2 on the microcirculation and the influence of the microcirculation on local regulation of O_2 supply.

VI. Oxygen Delivery–Consumption Relationships

A. Critical Oxygen Extraction

As the delivery of O_2 to the gut is reduced, increases in the O_2 extraction fraction help to maintain O_2 consumption until a cirtically low level of delivery is reached. If delivery is reduced below this point, the O_2 extraction can increase further; however, these adjustments are not sufficient to maintain oxygen consumption per unit time ($\dot{V}O_2$), which becomes O_2 supply-limited [21]. The decrease in $\dot{V}O_2$ below the critical O_2 delivery level is thought to represent O_2 starvation of some or all of the cells in the tissue. This presumption is based on the observations that (1) tissue lactate production increases [22], (2) tissue function declines [23], and (3) normal tissue function cannot be restored when O_2 supply is later increased. In cultured cells subjected to brief periods of extreme hypoxia, cellular respiration has been shown to remain independent of O_2 availability until the extracellular O_2 partial pressure (P_{O_2}) decreases to less than 3–5 mm Hg [24,25]. Extrapolation of these findings to the intact tissue suggests that supply-dependent O_2 uptake must occur because anoxic tissue regions develop. Presumably, the progressive decrease in O_2 uptake observed along the supply-dependent limb of the O_2 delivery–uptake relationship reflects a growing region of anoxic tissue, rather than a partial limitation of respiration in all of the cells simultaneously.

As the delivery of O_2 to the gut is reduced, two major mechanisms contribute to its ability to augment O_2 extraction. The first relates to the fact that tissue P_{O_2} decreases as the O_2 supply-to-demand ratio is reduced. A decrease in perivascular O_2 tension tends to augment the diffusive gradient for unloading of O_2, even in the absence of any microvascular adjustments to the distribution of blood flow. The second mechanism tending to augment O_2 extraction involves microvascular adjustments to the distribution of capillary blood flow and O_2 transport. An ability to limit O_2 delivery to capillaries with minimal O_2 demand, while augmenting blood flow in capillaries supplying metabolically active regions, tends to increase the efficiency of microvascular O_2 transport. This is manifested by an ability to achieve a greater O_2 extraction ratio at the point where $\dot{V}O_2$ begins to decrease. Experimentally, investigators have measured the critical O_2 extraction as an index of the efficiency of microvascular O_2 transport. Such studies in isolated intestine have yielded interesting insight into the factors regulating microvascular control and have served to illustrate the interactions between intrinsic microvascular regulation and extrinsic neurohumoral regulation of gut microvascular blood flow regulation [26–28].

B. Role of Resistance and Exchange Vessels in Control of Gas Exchange

In studies of skeletal muscle, Granger et al. [29] identified an important distinction between blood vessels influencing overall blood flow (resistance vessels) and those regulating the distribution of blood flow among capillary units (exchange vessels) in terms of their influence on tissue gas exchange. Evidence suggests that a similar situation exists in the intestinal circulation, with similar consequences for tissue oxygenation [3,30]. In this regard, overall blood flow to a region of the gut seems to be regulated by vasoconstrictor tone in arterial microvessels greater than approximately 30 μm in diameter. For the most part, these vessels represent the upstream series resistance element in the model of Shepherd (12) (Fig. 1). By contrast, the distribution of flow among and within the layers of the gut wall seems to be influenced by precapillary vessels located downstream from the primary site of resistance. These are analogous to the parallel resistances in the model of Shepherd et al. (12) (Fig. 1).

The distinction between resistance and exchange vessels in the gut is illustrated by studies of the effects of neurohumoral tone on critical O_2 extraction [31]. In the isolated pump-perfused gut segment, local O_2 delivery to a 30–50-g segment of ileum or jejunum was reduced by lowering the speed of the pump while the animal was kept normoxic and well perfused systemically. This yielded a low efficiency of O_2 extraction in the gut segment under study, which became O_2 supply-limited when its O_2 extraction was only 40–45%. However, when O_2 delivery was reduced simultaneously in whole body and in the gut segment, critical O_2 extraction ratios near 70% typically were found in the gut. How does systemic hypovolemia improve the O_2 extraction ability in a region of tissue whose O_2 supply is controlled by a pump? The answer relates to the role of reflex neurohumoral vasoconstrictor tone, which influences vessels both at the resistance level and at the exchange level of the microcirculation [31]. During hemorrhage, autonomic reflexes respond to the decreases in blood volume and cardiac output, and cause (1) increases in sympathetic neural activity and (2) release of vasopressin, renin, and other vasoactive compounds. These act on the upstream series resistance, tending to limit blood flow to the gut and helping to preserve systemic arterial pressure (Fig. 1). They also act on precapillary exchange vessels, tending to redistribute blood flow away from tissue regions with low O_2 demand (e.g., smooth muscle). In the intact animal, this lowers the blood flow to the gut but simultaneously improves its ability to extract sufficient O_2 from a limited supply. This effect is illustrated in Fig. 2, which shows the salutary effects of systemic hypovolemia on the gut critical O_2 extraction ratio. Moreover, when local gut O_2 uptake was reduced to create supply dependency in normovolemic animals, later hemorrhage of the whole animal caused increases in O_2 uptake at constant O_2 delivery in the isolated gut segment (Fig. 3). Interestingly, α-adrenergic blockade with phenoxybenzamine abolished the increases in gut vascular resistance but did not abolish the improvements in gut O_2 extraction observed during hypovolemia. These findings suggested that α-adrenergic vasoconstriction acted at the upstream resistance segment in the gut (Fig. 1). Other nonadrenergic vasoconstricting factors apparently acted at more distal sites, whose impact on the overall gut vascular resistance was minimal, but whose effect on gas exchange was profound. Collectively, these results indicate that overall vascular resistance in the

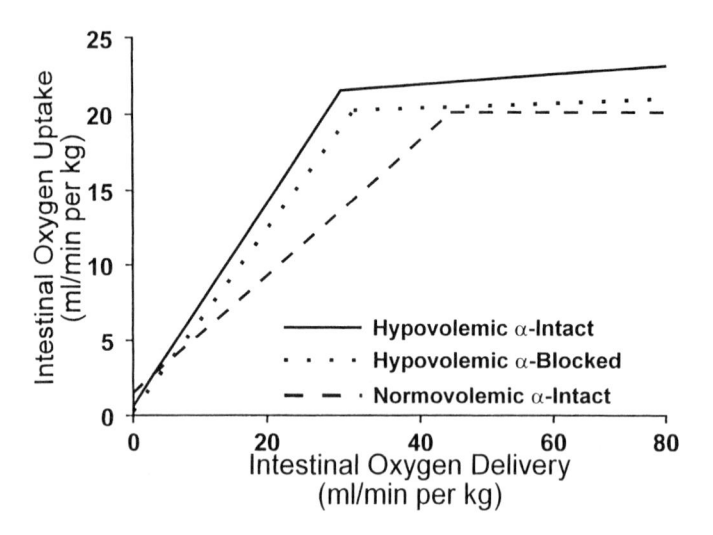

Figure 2 Effects of autonomic reflex vasoconstriction on O_2 extraction properties in an isolated, pump-perfused segment of small intestine. When local gut O_2 delivery was reduced during systemic normovolemia, the gut became O_2 supply-dependent at a higher level of O_2 delivery, indicating poor O_2 extraction efficiency. By contrast, when reflex vasoconstriction was increased by progressive hypovolemia, local gut O_2 supply dependency did not begin until significantly lower O_2 delivery was reached, indicating improved O_2 extraction efficiency. This improvement was not prevented by prior α-adrenergic blockade. (From Ref. 31, with permission.)

gut is determined by a balance between local metabolic vasodilation and extrinsic neurohumoral vasoconstriction, whereas regional control of capillary blood flow is controlled by smaller precapillary vessels. Because these vascular segments can function independently, it is not possible to infer changes in the capillary distribution or the efficiency of gas exchange from changes in overall vascular resistance.

VII. Physiological Shunting of Oxygen in the Gut Microcirculation

Gas exchange occurs between blood and tissue primarily via diffusive transport mechanisms. However, convective movement of blood through the microcirculation is required to maintain the partial pressure gradients that are necessary to maintain diffusive transport. Analogous to shunting in the lung, O_2 transport that bypasses the microcirculation does not have the opportunity to participate in gas exchange. Theoretically, functional shunting of O_2 in the microcirculation could occur by several different mechanisms, including (1) direct arteriovenous anastomoses between precapillary and postcapillary vessels; (2) diffusive shunting of O_2

The Gut: O_2 Transport and Gas Exchange

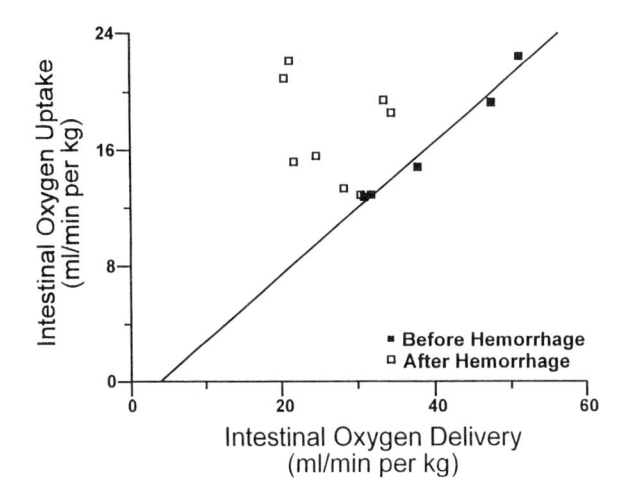

Figure 3 Effects of autonomic reflex vasoconstriction on O_2 extraction properties in an isolated pump-perfused segment of small intestine. When systemic normovolemia was maintained, local reduction in gut O_2 delivery yielded high critical O_2 delivery and low critical O_2 extraction ratios, reflecting inefficient microvascular regulation (filled symbols; solid line, indicating O_2 supply-dependent respiration). Subsequent moderate hemorrhage caused systemic O_2 extraction to increase to approximately 60%. The corresponding increase in reflex vasoconstrictor tone facilitated a local increase in O_2 extraction, causing O_2 uptake to increase at constant delivery (open symbols). (From Ref. 31, with permission.)

at sites where precapillary and postcapillary vessels come into close proximity; and (3) maldistribution of blood flow, whereby some capillaries receive far more O_2 delivery than others. All of these mechanisms have been suggested to contribute to functional shunting in the gut, and all would be expected to interfere with the efficient supply of O_2 to the cells.

Do arteriovenous shunt vessels exist in the intestinal microcirculation? Direct arteriovenous thoroughfare channels were identified in the small intestine by Vajda et al. [32], although the significance of these channels for tissue gas exchange is not known. Delaney [33] injected 20-μm microspheres into the superior mesenteric artery of the dog and recovered approximately 3% of the activity in the liver, suggesting that only a small fraction of flow passes through such large conduit channels. Likewise, Dinda et al. [34] found that all of the 15-μm spheres injected into the splanchnic artery were trapped in the gut microcirculation, but that a small percentage of 9-μm spheres reached the liver. Collectively, these and other studies [35] suggest that arteriovenous anastomotic shunt accounts for only a small fraction of the flow to the gut.

Does diffusive shunting of O_2 occur in the gut? It has been suggested that countercurrent diffusion of O_2 may occur within intestinal villi, where ascending and descending loops travel in close proximity. Anatomical studies of the villi indicate the existence of a "hairpin" arrangement of the microvessels with distances of 15–50 μm between vessels. These conditions could conceivably facilitate diffusive transport between inflowing and efferent vessels, and data from a number of studies are consistent with such an effect. However, a critical review of the literature indicates that the majority of the evidence is indirect. Using bolus arterial injections of dissolved ^{85}Krypton gas in feline intestine, Kampp et al. [36,37] measured the washout of activity from different regions of the gut wall by recording gamma emissions (which escape freely from all layers of the gut wall) and beta emissions (which escape only from the superficial 0.7-mm layer of the gut wall). Separate beta detectors were placed at the serosal surface and within the gut lumen to detect washout separately from mucosa and muscularis. When tissue washout data was analyzed, a fast initial rate of disappearance was detected, followed by a slower exponential disappearance. The investigators interpreted the fast washout component as arising from countercurrent shunting of the tracer. However, an alternative interpretation of the data is that rapid washout from a well-perfused region of tissue occurs initially, with a later washout from a larger, more poorly perfused region. Therefore, the evidence for diffusional shunting provided by these studies is rather indirect.

A more convincing demonstration of countercurrent shunting was reported by the same group using simultaneous arterial bolus injection of a mixture of oxygenated red blood cells and methemoglobin-containing cells [38]. In the absence of diffusive O_2 shunting, the oxyhemoglobin cells should appear in venous effluent at the same time as methemoglobin cells, assuming that they were well mixed and were distributed similarly in the microcirculation. As shown in Figure 4, oxygenated erythrocytes appeared at the outflow before methemoglobin cells, which suggests that diffusive loss of O_2 at some point in the vascular transit was accompanied by uptake by red blood cells farther along in their transit, allowing the O_2 to reach the venous effluent earlier than the intravascular label. Moreover, this effect seemed to disappear when blood flow was increased via pharmacological vasodilatation and was also abolished when regional sympathetic nerve fibers were stimulated. Assuming that sympathetic stimulation caused a redistribution of blood flow away from the mucosa, these results seem to be consistent with the existence of a countercurrent shunt within the mucosa.

What effect would shunting have on the relationship between O_2 delivery and uptake? Presently there are no in vivo models that are known to produce changes in the shunting of blood within the gut; therefore, it is not possible to answer this question experimentally. However, theoretical models of tissue gas exchange can be used to predict how shunting of O_2 past the capillary bed would affect the relationship between O_2 supply and uptake. In one such model based on the Krogh tissue cylinder, a biphasic relationship between O_2 delivery and uptake was predicted [39]. When a shunt was simulated by allowing a fraction of the delivered O_2 to bypass the exchange vessels, the biphasic relationship was maintained but

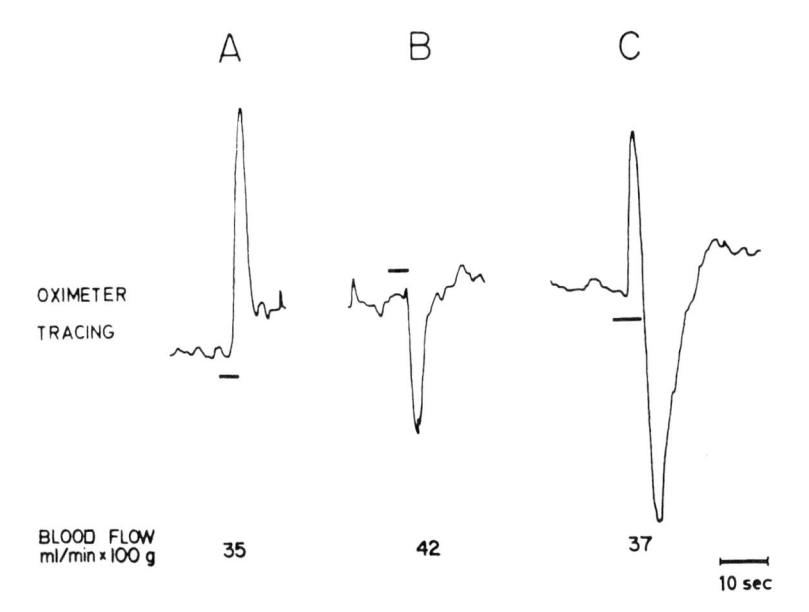

Figure 4 Evidence supporting diffusional shunting of O_2 in intestinal wall. Curves show oximeter tracings of venous blood draining a segment of small intestine after arterial injection of oxygenated red cells (A), methemoglobin-containing cells (B), or a mixture of both cell types (C). When both cells were injected simultaneously, an O_2 peak appeared at the outflow before the methemoglobin peak, suggesting that diffusional shunting allowed O_2 to reach the outflow before red blood cells could transit the circulation. (From Ref. 38, with permission.)

the critical O_2 delivery where O_2 supply dependency begins was shifted to the right (Fig. 5). Thus, the primary effect of shunt was to decrease the O_2 extraction ratio at the critical point. Interestingly, that model predicted that tissue critical O_2 extraction should be able to reach 95% in the absence of shunt, based on reasonable assumptions of microvascular geometry and tissue O_2 demand. By contrast, experimental measurements of the critical O_2 extraction ratio typically show onset of O_2 supply dependency above extractions of 65–75%. When the model was reconstructed to include a 35% shunt compartment in parallel with a Krogh "ideal tissue" compartment, it realistically predicted the O_2 extraction behavior of tissues during progressive stagnant hypoxia (reduction of blood flow with constant arterial O_2 content), hypoxic hypoxia (decreased oxyhemoglobin saturation at constant blood flow), or anemic hypoxia (decreased hemoglobin concentration with constant blood flow and saturation). Of course, this result does not prove that the tissue is comprised of ideal and shunt vessels or even that it contains any shunt at all, but it does provide insight into a possible mode of function, which needs to be tested by further experimentation.

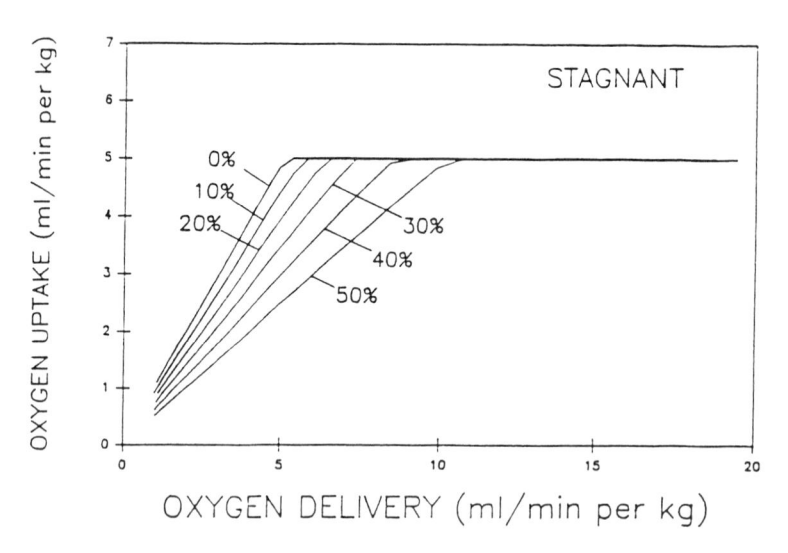

Figure 5 Theoretical effect of shunt on the relationship between O_2 delivery and uptake. Shunt effect was simulated by allowing a fraction of the blood flow to bypass the gas exchange vessels of the circulation. Increasing levels of shunt caused corresponding increases in the critical O_2 delivery, whereas the bilinear nature of the relationship was unchanged. (From Ref. 39, with permission.)

VIII. Perfusion Heterogeneity in the Gut Microcirculation

In a segment of small intestine, augmentation of sympathetic vasoconstriction could help to facilitate increases in O_2 extraction by affecting the fractional distribution of blood flow between muscularis and mucosa. Because these layers show marked differences in metabolic activity, the partitioning of blood flow and O_2 supply in accordance with O_2 demand is essential for achieving high O_2 extractions. Vasoconstriction could also influence the distribution of blood flow within each of the layers of the wall by influencing the tone in precapillary vessels, altering capillary volume, changing the percentage of perfused capillaries, or altering the geometry of individual capillaries. For a given blood flow, changes in capillary volume will cause reciprocal changes in capillary transit time, which represents the ratio of capillary volume to flow. Because the time a red blood cell spends traversing a systemic capillary influences its release of O_2, assessment of transit time is pertinent in terms of gas exchange.

An assessment of the heterogeneity of capillary transit times under known physiological conditions can provide insight into the regulation of microcirculatory gas exchange. Of course, the most useful form of heterogeneity to consider would be the distribution of transit times with respect to capillary O_2 demand. However, experimental methods are not currently available to estimate tissue O_2 demand on a capillary-by-capillary basis. It is therefore necessary to assess spatial heterogeneity, which presumes that the cellular O_2 demand is homogeneously distributed throughout the tissue. In any tissue, the experimental estimate of heterogeneity depends on the volume of tissue analyzed, with larger aliquots yielding more homogeneous estimates for the overall tissue. As smaller aliquots are examined, the estimate of heterogeneity comes closer to the true value, which would be obtained if the flow to every microvascular unit were considered. The assessment of regional heterogeneity of blood flow has been discussed extensively by Bassingthwaighte et al. [40] with respect to the heart, and the reader is referred to that literature because many of the same principles apply to other tissues, including the gut.

When assessing microvascular regulation of perfusion heterogeneity, the influence of two major factors should be considered. First, altering overall blood flow to the tissue may directly influence the distribution of perfusion by altering hemodynamic conditions. Second, changes in blood flow may affect heterogeneity by changing the O_2 supply and the distribution of Po_2 throughout the tissue. This would affect capillary flow indirectly, to the extent that local metabolic activity influences local control of capillary flow. Evidence that local changes in tissue Po_2 can affect microvascular control is supported by studies by Lindbom et al. [41] using intravital microscopy. They found significant decreases in capillary recruitment in microvascular networks superfused with solutions equilibrated to high versus low Po_2 levels. Finally, microvascular regulatory function is likely to depend on the overall O_2 supply-to-demand ratio. In this regard, microvascular control may function differently in tissues receiving ample O_2 delivery compared with hypoperfused tissues, where metabolic vasodilatation is maximal, lactate concentrations are high, and cellular hypoxia is widespread.

Several studies have assessed the role of perfusion heterogeneity in the gut for O_2 transport. In anesthetized pigs, Humer et al. [26] measured capillary transit time heterogeneity at normal levels of O_2 delivery and after whole-body delivery was reduced below the critical point. The heterogeneity of transit times in a tissue can be expressed as a histogram, where the fraction of tissue is plotted as a function of its capillary transit time. The investigators labeled the distribution of blood flow with microspheres and used radiolabeled red blood cells to measure vascular volume in the gut. The tissue was sectioned into pieces weighing 1 to 2 grams each and analyzed for radioactivity. Using morphometric analysis, they determined the ratio of capillary volume to total tissue vascular volume in representative tissue samples and used this fraction to estimate capillary volume from the measured vascular volume in the remainder of their samples. In control animals, hemorrhage of the animal caused a decrease in overall gut blood flow, yet mean capillary transit time decreased. This occurred because capillary volume decreased to a greater extent than blood flow decreased. One interpretation is that capillaries were derecruited, leading to a decrease in perfused capillary density yet a shorter transit time for a given red blood cell. Alternatively, capillary dimensions could have decreased, resulting in a shorter transit time. For that to have occurred, red blood cell spacing in the capillaries would need to have increased, as total red blood cell flow was lower. In either case, when systemic O_2 delivery was reduced by controlled hemorrhage of the animal, the heterogeneity of transit time decreased significantly. This was observed as a narrowing of the distribution of transit times (Fig. 6). Such a narrowing could represent an improvement in the regulation of capillary blood flow. However, as previously discussed, this conclusion depends on the assumption that the distribution of tissue O_2 demands is also narrow—a presumption that has not yet been verified.

In a later study of gut transit time heterogeneity, Connolly et al. [8] measured the distribution of capillary transit times in canine ileum or jejunum segments using an experimental design that permitted evaluation of the independent effects of changes in local O_2 delivery and changes in autonomic vasoconstrictor tone.

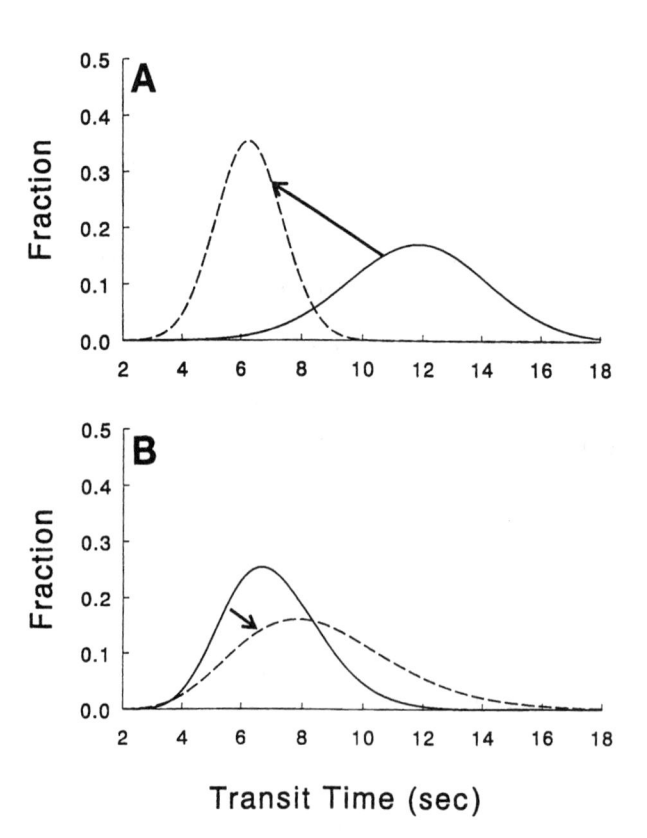

Figure 6 Effects of endotoxin on total transit time dispersions in porcine intestine. Control animals (A) showed a narrowing of the distribution when O_2 delivery was reduced from supply-independent (solid line) to supply-dependent (dashed line). During endotoxemia (B), the opposite response was noted. (From Ref. 26, with permission.)

Segments of intestine were vascularly isolated and pump perfused to permit independent control of the local O_2 supply. As in the study by Humer et al. [26], capillary blood flow was labeled with microspheres, whereas vascular volume was measured with radiolabelled red blood cells and partitioned into capillary versus conducting vessel components using morphometric point counting. During analysis of the fixed tissue, the gut wall was partitioned into approximately 120-mg pieces, which were then split into muscularis and mucosal components to permit analysis of heterogeneity in separate regions of the gut wall. In constructing the distributions of heterogeneity, data were normalized to the mean flow or transit time, which permitted the inclusion of data from multiple experiments that differed with respect to absolute flows or tissue weights. As shown in Fig. 7, significant heterogeneity was observed in both mucosal and muscularis regions of the gut wall. In this regard, some regions of smooth muscle or mucosa received four times the average tissue blood flow, whereas other regions received less than one quarter of the average flow (per gram of tissue weight). Interestingly, capillary transit time heterogeneity was similar regardless of whether the tissue was perfused under systemic normotensive or hypotensive conditions. This observation suggests that capillary volume and flow are regulated to preserve transit time control under a wide range of physiological conditions. Another interesting finding was that hemorrhage of the animal led to a significant redistribution of blood flow within the gut wall. Regardless of the flow condition, increased autonomic reflex vasoconstrictor tone caused a shift of blood flow toward mucosa at the expense of muscularis. The magnitude of this redistribution correlated with the improvement in gut O_2 consumption under O_2 supply-limited conditions when the animal was hemorrhaged. Collectively, these results and those of the study by Humer et al. (26) indicate that significant heterogeneity of capillary transit times exists within the gut wall and that extrinsic neurohumoral reflex tone plays an important role in optimizing the gas exchange function of the microcirculation in the gut.

IX. Pathophysiology of Gas Transport

The physiological mechanisms discussed previously normally contribute to the regulation of blood flow distribution among regions of the gut wall with differing metabolic demands. This promotes efficient gas exchange by limiting the wasting of excessive blood flow on tissue regions with low O_2 demands while others are starved for O_2 supply. In pathophysiological states, this regulation can become dysfunctional as a consequence of altered vasoconstrictor tone, altered responsiveness to vasoactive or neurohumoral signals, altered endothelial responsiveness, tissue edema that restricts blood flow in some tissue regions, or other factors that disrupt vasoconstrictor or vasodilator functions. This section examines known and potential mechanisms that may contribute to the disruption of normal regulatory mechanisms, along with the subsequent consequences for tissue gas exchange.

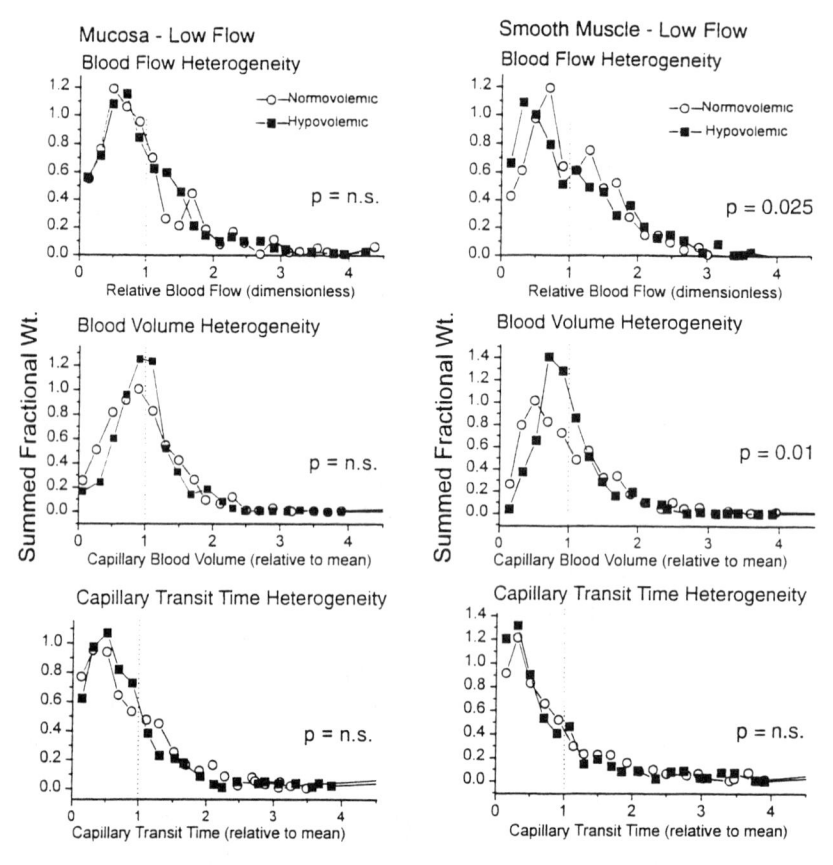

Figure 7 Perfusion heterogeneity in isolated healthy intestine perfused under O_2 supply-limited conditions. Blood flow (upper), blood volume (middle), and capillary transit time (lower) dispersions were measured mucosa (left) and muscularis (right) regions. These data show that significant heterogeneity of capillary transit times exists even in normal tissue. Open versus closed symbols indicate measurements made during systemic normovolemia and after blood removal, respectively. Interestingly, transit time dispersions were similar at the two levels of autonomic reflex activation. (From Ref. 8, with permission.)

A. Pathological Limitation of Oxygen Extraction During Sepsis

Patients with sepsis frequently develop hypotension that is refractory to vasoactive drugs, and experimental endotoxemia produces similar effects in animals [42,43] and in humans [44]. Bacterial sepsis and endotoxin have been shown to produce a significant impairment of vascular contractile responsiveness in rats [45–48] and to elicit a significant impairment of nitric oxide–mediated endothelial responsiveness to vasodilators [49]. These impairments undermine the normal vascular responsiveness to vasoconstricting and vasodilating influences, which may undermine the ability to maintain O_2 uptake in the face of a reduced O_2 supply in the gut. In anesthetized dogs, Nelson et al. studied the effects of bacteremia [50] or endotoxemia [51] on the ability to increase O_2 extraction ratio in whole body and autoperfused gut during progressive hemorrhage. Compared with nonseptic control animals, those studies showed a loss in the ability to augment O_2 extraction in whole body, which was mirrored in the behavior of the gut. As a consequence, isolated intestine segments became O_2 supply-limited at a higher critical O_2 delivery. Moreover, the gut reached that critical point at a higher level of systemic O_2 delivery, suggesting that both the regional regulation of blood flow and the microcirculatory regulation of blood flow distribution may have been affected. In one study, loss of the reactive hyperemia response to a 30-second occlusion of the gut arterial supply was observed after endotoxin administration, suggesting that microvascular dysregulation contributed to the impaired microvascular function. However, that response is not universal [52], suggesting that a complete loss of vascular responsiveness may be a specific but not a sensitive indicator of microvascular O_2 extraction failure. A number of other studies have also detected abnormal critical O_2 extraction in a variety of species and experimental protocols [26,52,53].

X. Mechanisms of Impaired Tissue Oxygen Extraction

What mechanisms contribute to a reduced ability to increase O_2 extraction in sepsis? One possible factor relates to the regulation of perfused capillary density in accordance with the local O_2 supply-to-demand ratio in the gut. Using intravital microscopy to study mucosal villi, Farquhar et al. [54] found evidence of impaired capillary recruitment in a rat model of sepsis produced using cecal ligation and perforation. In a canine model, Drazenovic et al. [55] found indirect evidence that mucosal capillaries are normally recruited when the local O_2 delivery is low and are derecruited when local blood flow is high. This response seemed to be lost after endotoxin administration, which could conceivably explain the O_2 extraction problem. However, although the adjustments in capillary density as a function of O_2 delivery apparently were impaired in that study, overall capillary recruitment was relatively high. Although some capillaries may have been better supplied than others, this observation suggests that a massive shutdown of capillaries did not occur. Technically, this issue remains unsettled because of the difficulty of assessing perfused capillary density under controlled physiological conditions.

An alternative approach to assessing capillary recruitment involves the use of multiple electrode arrays to measure surface P_{O_2} distributions in intestinal mucosa and serosa. A failure to control capillary recruitment or to regulate perfusion should be manifested by an increase in the heterogeneity of P_{O_2} values measured at the tissue surface. In a study of canine septic shock, Vallet et al. [56] used multiple electrode arrays to assess surface P_{O_2} distributions before and after resuscitation. Measurements in normal tissues showed relatively narrow distributions of mucosal P_{O_2}, suggesting that capillary flow is closely matched to local tissue O_2 requirements. During lipopolysaccharide-induced hypotension, mucosal P_{O_2}, gut $\dot{V}_{O_2}$, and tonometry-derived mucosal pH values all decreased, reflecting a marked decrease in overall blood flow. When the animals were resuscitated with dextran solution, O_2 delivery and serosal P_{O_2} returned to control levels, whereas mucosal P_{O_2} and tonometric measurements never recovered. By contrast, in nonseptic animals, global ischemia and resuscitation were associated with full recovery of gut mucosal perfusion [57]. An important conclusion from this work is that microvascular dysfunction during sepsis can disrupt adequate tissue O_2 supply in some regions such as mucosa. At the same time, other tissues, such as skeletal muscle and gut muscularis, seem to be less affected in terms of their microvascular function and tissue gas transport [58,59].

Another mechanism that may contribute to an impaired tissue O_2 extraction ability during endotoxemia involves maldistribution of capillary blood flow with respect to local O_2 demands. In the study by Humer et al. [26], endotoxemic pigs showed increases in gut capillary transit time heterogeneity, which correlated with the degree of impairment of critical O_2 extraction according to a theoretical model [60]. These findings suggest that altered microvascular regulation may be an important contributor to the tissue gas exchange dysfunction in endotoxemia. However, because that study did not examine the relative changes in perfusion to mucosa and muscularis, future studies are required to assess the importance of intramural redistribution.

A. Interstitial Edema

Another mechanism that may contribute to impaired O_2 extraction during sepsis involves the formation of tissue edema. Sepsis is associated with increases in vascular permeability [61,62], and fluid resuscitation is used to restore blood pressure in patients with septic shock. Indeed, tissue edema is often evident in septic patients with refractory hypotension during resuscitation. Conceivably, increased interstitial fluid could increase the diffusion distances for O_2 between capillary and cells, leading to the onset of an O_2 extraction defect. However, only limited data are available to address this issue. In rabbits, Ostgaard and Reed [63] showed that intestinal O_2 uptake was not impeded when portal vein occlusion and fluid administration were used to promote a modest increase in tissue edema.

Using an isolated feline intestine preparation, Crouser et al. [61] assessed endothelial permeability and examined the systemic consequences of acute lung injury. They found that increases in ileal lymph-to-plasma protein concentration ratios (suggestive of increased endothelial cell permeability) developed in an acid aspiration model of lung injury, but that this did not necessarily cause an impairment of tissue O_2 extraction. This evidence suggests that changes in endothelium do not necessarily induce an impairment of tissue gas exchange. Using the model of increased permeability, it would be interesting to study whether subsequent fluid administration induces an O_2 extraction defect related to the development of tissue edema.

B. Plasma Skimming in the Mucosa

The microcirculatory architecture of the small intestine may render the mucosa more susceptible to O_2 transport limitation during reductions in hematocrit. Vessels supplying the mucosa branch off nearly at right angles from the vascular plexus in the muscularis/submucosa. This could facilitate plasma skimming at branch points and produce different microvascular hematocrits in the layers of the gut wall. Jodal and Lundgren [65] compared hematocrits in mucosa and muscularis to the systemic hematocrit and found that the mucosal hematocrits were substantially lower than muscularis, whereas both were lower than the systemic hematocrit. In a study of porcine jejunum during progressive hemodilution, Haisjackl et al. [66] found higher surface O_2 tensions in muscularis (58 mm Hg) than in mucosa (24 mm Hg). During hemodilution, local gut flow increased while O_2 delivery decreased because of the decrease in O_2 carrying capacity. The hematocrit in muscularis vessels decreased as the systemic hematocrit decreased, and the P_{O_2} in muscularis began to decrease when systemic hematocrit reached 15%. Hematocrit in mucosa was preserved until systemic hematocrit decreased to 6.5%, and mucosal P_{O_2} was preserved until the systemic hematocrit reached 10%. These findings underscore the notion that both redistribution of blood flow within the gut wall and regional differences in hematocrit can influence O_2 transport in the intestine. The extent to which plasma skimming and regional differences in red blood cell flux may contribute to tissue gas exchange dysfunction in pathophysiological states is unknown. However, this is an interesting question because tissue edema or endothelial cell swelling may affect the distribution of red blood cell distribution in disease and thereby impact on tissue gas exchange.

XI. Pathological Oxygen Supply Dependency in Critical Illness and Sepsis

Systemic sepsis predisposes to the development of multiple organ system failure and has also been associated with increased plasma lactate levels and altered O_2 metabolism [21,43,67]. Early studies of patients with adult respiratory distress syndrome suggested that O_2 consumption is limited by O_2 supply in critically ill patients [68–72]. This is manifested by a linear relationship between O_2 delivery and uptake even at high levels of systemic O_2 transport. Although these observations are subject to varying interpretations [73], it was later realized that the calculation of O_2 uptake using measured blood O_2 contents and the measured cardiac output could create a spurious relationship between O_2 delivery and uptake [74]. Studies in which O_2 delivery and consumption were measured independently often failed to detect a significant slope in the relationship [75–78], further confirming the notion that pathological O_2 supply dependency does not exist, or at least not in the form that it was originally described. Finally, studies of terminally ill patients undergoing progressive withdrawal of life support showed that even septic patients could increase their systemic O_2 extraction ratio as cardiac output decreased [79]. Moreover these patients became O_2 supply-limited at extraction ratios near 60%, which was not dramatically impaired in comparison with those in studies with normal experimental animals. Clearly, patients in septic shock in need of resuscitation may show systemic O_2 supply dependency because their systemic O_2 delivery is inadequate to support normal tissue metabolic needs. However, the aforementioned studies suggest that, after resuscitation and stabilization, any continuing defects in tissue O_2 extraction during sepsis are not easily detected at the whole-body level. Based on these observations, it would be simple to conclude that tissue of O_2 supply and use in critically ill patients is a nonissue.

However, a substantial body of evidence suggests that a more subtle form of O_2 supply limitation may still exist in critically ill patients. This form of occult tissue hypoxia could contribute to the development of organ failure, but may not be evident at the systemic level. Moreover, it is possible that such microvascular dysregulation may develop preferentially in some tissues, creating islands of ischemic cells within otherwise well-oxygenated tissue. Evidence suggests that a situation such as this may occur in gut mucosa, and it has been suggested that the gut may thereby function as a canary for the whole body [80]. In clinical studies using gastric tonometry, abnormally increased gut mucosal carbon dioxide partial pressure and decreased interstitial pH (pHi) in some patients suggest that the gut mucosa may be underperfused despite adequate systemic O_2 supply [81–83]. Moreover, the prognosis seems to be statistically poorer for patients with poor gut mucosal perfusion who failed to respond to therapy. If gut mucosa can be selectively underperfused (and presumably hypoxic) in critically ill patients whose systemic O_2 supply is normal, it suggests that pathological O_2 supply dependency may exist at a tissue level. However, to the extent that gut mucosa is the only tissue involved, it seems unlikely that a pathological O_2 supply dependency would be evident at the systemic level because the metabolic demand of gut mucosa represents less than 5% of the whole-body O_2 uptake. To the extent that this analysis is true, one can argue that it would be folly to dismiss the importance of O_2 supply regulation in critical illness based on the failure to see a problem at the systemic level. Clearly, more studies are required to fully address this issue.

Another explanation for the apparent link between organ system failure and tissue hypoxia relates to the biochemical events that develop during sepsis [84]. Hotchkiss and Karl [85] have argued that metabolic derangements during sepsis, including defects in mitochondrial metabolism, could explain the increase in circulating lactate levels in the absence of tissue hypoxia. In porcine ileum, Vandermeer et al. [86] reported that significant mucosal acidosis developed after endotoxin without a corresponding decrease in surface PO_2 measurements or gut blood flow

[86]. They concluded that mucosal hypoxia was not responsible for the endotoxin-induced mucosal acidosis, which implies that a metabolic cause for the acidosis may have been involved. In the absence of strong evidence demonstrating tissue ischemia, derangements in metabolic control mechanisms constitute an intriguing possible explanation for the increases in lactate that have been observed. In this regard, it is possible that the increases in circulating lactate during sepsis are caused by pyruvate dehydrogenase inhibition [87] or represent a consequence of increased glycolytic flux during sepsis [84]. In those situations, both lactate and pyruvate would be increased, but their ratio would remain constant. In contrast, increases in lactate resulting from unopposed anaerobic glycolysis would involve increases in that ratio. Although this distinction has been well known for many years, very few clinical or laboratory studies of sepsis have included both lactate and pyruvate data to address this point. Future studies need to include assessment of the lactate-to-pyruvate ratio to begin to address this point.

XII. Summary

The gut is a tissue whose metabolic activity and O_2 demands vary in accordance with digestive activities. Metabolic demand for O_2 differs among the layers of the gut wall, with high metabolic activity in mucosa and relatively low metabolic rates in muscularis. These differences are reflected in the regional differences in blood flow and by the lower average tissue P_{O_2} in mucosa than in muscularis. Overall gut blood flow is regulated by a balance between metabolic activity in the tissue, which produces local vasodilation, and autonomic neurohumoral vasoconstriction, which tends to limit gut blood flow during exercise or in stressful states. Factors can influence the distribution of blood flow between mucosa and muscularis, with important consequences for the efficiency and adequacy of local O_2 supply. Interestingly, although increases in autonomic reflex-mediated vasoconstriction tend to limit overall blood flow, they also improve the microvascular distribution of flow and enhance the ability of the gut to maintain O_2 uptake in the face of reduced overall supply. Inefficiency of gut O_2 transport can occur via several distinct mechanisms. These include flow through arteriovenous shunt-like vessels, diffusive countercurrent shunting in the hairpin capillaries in mucosal villi, perfusion heterogeneity within mucosa and/or muscularis layers, and maldistribution of flow among the layers of the gut wall. In critical illness and especially sepsis, gas exchange abnormalities in the gut may contribute to local tissue hypoxia that is not evident at the systemic level. In this regard, measurements of gut mucosal perfusion may provide a window of insight into the microvascular function of the patient. This notion is supported by a growing number of clinical studies using gastric tonometry that suggest the possibility that regional defects in tissue gas exchange may occur selectively, and that show a statistical correlation with the outcome of the disease. Future studies are required to differentiate between oxygen-related and oxygen-independent causes of metabolic acidosis in sepsis, and to determine the relative contributions of these mechanisms in critical illness.

References

1. Shepherd AP. Local control of intestinal oxygenation and blood flow. Ann Rev Physiol 1982; 44:13–27.
2. Shepherd AP. Role of capillary recruitment in the regulation of intestinal oxygenation. Am J Physiol 1982; 242:G435–G441.
3. Granger HJ, Nyhof RA. Dynamics of intestinal oxygenation: interactions between oxygen supply and uptake. Am J Physiol 1982; 243:G91–G96.
4. Holm L, Perry MA. Role of blood flow in gastric acid secretion. Am J Physiol 1988; 254:G281–G293.
5. Shepherd AP. Metabolic control of intestinal oxygenation and blood flow. Fed Proc 1982; 41:2084–2089.
6. Lundgren O. Microcirculation of the gastrointestinal tract and pancreas. In: Renkin EM, Michel CC, eds. Handbook of Physiology, Sec 2, Vol 4, Part 2, The Microcirculation. Bethesda, MD: American Physiological Society, 1991, pp 799–863.
7. Gore RW, Bohlen HG. Microvascular pressures in rat intestinal muscle and mucosal villi. Am J Physiol 1977; 233:H685–H693.
8. Connolly HV, Maginniss LA, Schumacker PT. Transit time heterogeneity in canine small intestine: significance for oxygen transport. J Clin Invest 1997; 99:228–238.
9. Shepherd AP. Intestinal blood flow autoregulation during foodstuff absorption. Am J Physiol 1980; 239:H156–H162.
10. Johnson PC. Autoregulation of intestinal blood flow. Am J Physiol 1960; 199:311–318.
11. Folkow B. Regional adjustments of intestinal blood flow. Gastroeneterology 1967; 52:423–432.
12. Shepherd AP, Riedel GL, Maxwell LC, Kiel JW. Selective vasodilators redistribute intestinal blood flow and depress oxygen uptake. Am J Physiol 1984; 247:G377–G384.
13. Lautt WW, Graham SA. Effect of nerve stimulation on precapillary sphincters, oxygen extraction and hemodynamics in the intestines of cats. Circ Res 1977; 41:32–36.
14. McNeill JR, Stark RD, Greenway CV. Intestinal vasoconstriction after hemorrhage: roles of vasopressin and angiotensin. Am J Physiol 1970; 219:1442–1447.
15. Shepherd AP, Granger HJ. Autoregulatory escape in the gut: a systems analysis. Gastroenterology 1973; 65:77–91.
16. Granger HJ, Norris CP. Intrinsic regulation of intestinal oxygenation in the anesthetized dog. Am J Physiol 1980; 238:H836–H843.
17. Martin AW, Fuhrman FA. The relationship between summated tissue respiration and metabolic rate in mouse and dog. Physiol Zool 1955; 28:18–34.
18. Shepherd AP, Riedel GL. Differences in reactive hyperemia between the intestinal mucosa and muscularis. Am J Physiol 1984; 247:G617–G622.
19. Shepherd AP, Riedel GL. Laser-Doppler blood flowmetry of intestinal mucosal hyperemia induced by glucose and bile. Am J Physiol 1985; 248:G393–G397.

20. Kvietys PR, Granger DN. Relation between intestinal blood flow and oxygen uptake. Am J Physiol 1982; 242:G202–G208.
21. Schumacker PT, Cain SM. The concept of a critical oxygen delivery. Intensive Care Med 1987; 13:223–229.
22. Samsel RW, Cherqui D, Pietrabissa A, Sanders WM, Roncella M, Emond JC, Schumacker PT. Hepatic oxygen and lactate extraction during stagnant hypoxia. J Appl Physiol 1991; 17:186–193.
23. Walley KR, Becker CJ, Hogan RA, Teplinsky K, Wood LDH. Progressive hypoxemia limits left ventricular oxygen consumption and contractility. Circ Res 1988; 63:849–859.
24. Kennedy FG, Jones DP. Oxygen dependence of mitochondrial function in isolated rat cardiac myocytes. Am J Physiol 1986; 250:C374–C383.
25. Wilson DF, Erecinska M. Effect of oxygen concentration on cellular metabolism. Chest 1985; 88:229S–232S.
26. Humer MF, Phang PT, Friesen BP, Allard MF, Goddard CM, Walley KR. Heterogeneity of gut capillary transit times and impaired gut oxygen extraction in endotoxemic pigs. J Appl Physiol 1996; 81:895–904.
27. Nelson DP, King CE, Dodd SL, Schumacker PT, Cain SM. Systemic and intestinal limits of O2 extraction in the dog. J Appl Physiol 1987; 63:387–394.
28. Dodd SL, King CE, Cain SM. Gut and whole body O_2 deficit during and excess uptake after hypoxia. Adv Exp Med Biol 1986; 200:449–456.
29. Granger HJ, Goodman AH, Granger DN. Role of resistance and exchange vessels in local microvascular control of skeletal muscle oxygenation in the dog. Circ Res 1976; 38:379–385.
30. Granger HJ, Shepherd AP. Intrinsic microvascular control of tissue oxygen delivery. Microvasc Res 1973; 5:49–72.
31. Samsel RW, Schumacker PT. Systemic hemorrhage augments local O_2 extraction in canine intestine. J Appl Physiol 1994; 77:2291–2298.
32. Vajda J, Raposa T, Herpai Z. Structural bases of blood flow regulation in the small intestine. Acta Morphologica Acad Sci Hung 1968; 16:331–340.
33. Delaney JP. Arteriovenous anastomotic blood flow in the mesenteric organs. Am J Physiol 1969; 216:1556–1561.
34. Dinda PK, Buell MG, DaCosta LR, Beck IT. Simultaneous estimation of arteriolar, capillary and shunt blood flow of the gut mucosa. Am J Physiol 1983; 245:G29–G37.
35. Maxwell LC, Shepherd AP, Riedel GL. Vasodilation or altered perfusion pressure moves 15-μm spheres trapped in the gut wall. Am J Physiol 1982; 243:H123–H127.
36. Kampp M, Lundgren O, Sjostrand J. On the components of the Kr^{85} wash-out curves from the small intestine of the cat. Acta Physiol Scand 1968; 72:257–281.
37. Kampp M, Lundgren O. Blood flow and distribution in the small intestine of the cat as analysed by the Kr^{85} wash-out technique. Acta Physiol Scand 1968; 72:282–297.
38. Kampp M, Lundgren O, Nilsson NJ. Extravascular shunting of oxygen in the small intestine of the cat. Acta Physiol Scand 1968; 72:396–403.
39. Schumacker PT, Samsel RW. Analysis of oxygen delivery and uptake relationships in the Krogh tissue model. J Appl Physiol 1989; 67:1234–1244.
40. Bassingthwaighte JB, Van Beek JHGM, King RB. Fractal branchings: the basis of myocardial flow heterogeneities? Ann NY Acad Sci 1990; 591:392–401.

41. Lindbom L, Tuma RF, Arfors KE. Influence of oxygen on perfused capillary density and capillary red cell velocity in rabbit skeletal muscle. Microvasc Res 1980; 19:197–208.
42. Bigaud M, Julou-Schaeffer G, Parratt JR, Stoclet JC. Endotoxin-induced impairment of vascular smooth muscle contractions elicited by different mechanisms. Eur J Pharm 1990; 190:185–192.
43. Schumacker PT, Samsel RW. Oxygen delivery and uptake by peripheral tissues: physiology and pathophysiology. Crit Care Clin 1989; 5:255–269.
44. Suffredini AF, Fromm RE, Parker MM, Brenner M, Kovacs JA, Wesley RA, Parrillo JE. The cardiovascular response of normal humans to the administration of endotoxin. N Engl J Med 1989; 321:280–287.
45. Umans JG, Wylam ME, Samsel RW, Edwards J, Schumacker PT. Effects of endotoxin in vivo on endothelial and smooth muscle function in rabbit and rat aorta. Am Rev Respir Dis 1993; 148:1638–1645.
46. Thiemermann C, Vane J. Inhibition of nitric oxide synthesis reduces the hypotension induced by bacterial lipopolysaccharides in the rat in vivo. Eur J Pharmacol 1990; 182:591–595.
47. McKenna TM. Prolonged exposure of rat aorta to low levels of endotoxin in vitro results in impaired contractility. J Lab Clin Med 1990; 86:160–168.
48. Lam C, Tyml K, Martin C, Sibbald W. Microvascular perfusion is impaired in a rat model of normotensive sepsis. J Clin Invest 1994; 94:2077–2083.
49. Wylam ME, Samsel RW, Umans JG, Mitchell RW, Leff AR, Schumacker PT. Endotoxin impairs endothelium-dependent relaxation of canine arteries in vitro. Am Rev Respir Dis 1990; 142:1263–1267.
50. Nelson DP, Beyer C, Samsel RW, Wood LDH, Schumacker PT. Pathological supply dependence of O_2 uptake during bacteremia in dogs. J Appl Physiol 1987; 63:1487–1492.
51. Nelson DP, Samsel RW, Wood LDH, Schumacker PT. Pathological supply dependence of systemic and intestinal O_2 uptake during endotoxemia. J Appl Physiol 1988; 64:2410–2419.
52. Schumacker PT, Kazaglis J, Connolly HV, Samsel RW, O'Connor MF, Umans JG. Systemic and gut O_2 extraction during endotoxemia: role of nitric oxide synthesis. Am J Resp Crit Care Med 1995; 151:107–115.
53. Zhang H, Rogiers P, DeBacker D, Spapen H, Manikis P, Schmartz D, Vincent JL. Regional arteriovenous differences in P_{CO_2} and pH can reflect critical organ oxygen delivery during endotoxemia. Shock 1996; 5:349–359.
54. Farquhar I, Martin CM, Lam C, Potter R, Ellis CG, Sibbald WJ. Decreased capillary density in vivo in bowel mucosa of rats with normotensive sepsis. J Surg Res 1997; 61:190–196.
55. Drazenovic R, Samsel RW, Wylam ME, Doerschuk CM, Schumacker PT. Regulation of perfused capillary density in canine intestinal mucosa during endotoxemia. J Appl Physiol 1992; 72:259–265.
56. Vallet B, Lund N, Curtis SE, Kely D, Cain SM. Gut and muscle tissue P_{O_2} in endotoxemic dogs during shock and resuscitation. J Appl Pysiol 1994; 76:793–800.
57. Curtis SE, Cain SM. Systemic and regional O_2 delivery and uptake in bled dogs given hypertonic saline, whole blood, or dextran. Am J Physiol 1992; 262:778–786.

58. Samsel RW, Nelson DP, Sanders WM, Wood LDH, Schumacker PT. Effect of endotoxin on systemic and skeletal muscle O_2 extraction. J Appl Physiol 1988; 65:1377–1382.
59. Bredle DL, Samsel RW, Schumacker PT, Cain SM. Critical O_2 delivery to skeletal muscle at high and low P_{O_2} in endotoxemic dogs. J Appl Physiol 1989; 66:2553–2558.
60. Walley KR. Heterogeneity of oxygen delivery impairs oxygen extraction by peripheral tissues: theory. J Appl Physiol 1996; 81:885–894.
61. Murray JF, Matthay MA, Luce JM, Flick MR. An expanded definition of the adult respiratory distress syndrome. Am Rev Respir Dis 1988; 138:720–723.
62. Brigham KL, Meyrick B. Endotoxin and lung injury: state of the art. Am Rev Respir Dis 1986; 254:913–927.
63. Ostgaard G, Reed RK. Interstitial fluid accumulation does not influence oxygen uptake in the rabbit small intestine. Acta Anaesth Scand 1995; 39:167–173.
64. Crouser ED, Julian MW, Weisbrode SE, Dorinsky PM. Acid aspiration results in ileal injury without altering ileal $\dot{V}_{O_2}$–D_{O_2} relationships. Am J Resp Crit Care Med 1996; 153:1965–1971.
65. Jodal M, Lundgren O. Plasma skimming in the intestinal wall. Bibliotheca Anatomica 1970; 10:310–311.
66. Haisjackl M, Luz G, Sparr H, Germann R, Salak N, Friesenecker B, Deusch E, Meusburger S, Hasibeder W. The effects of progressive anemia on jejunal mucosal and serosal tissue oxygenation in pigs. Crit Care Trauma 1997; 84:538–544.
67. Schumacker PT, Samsel RW. Oxygen supply and consumption in the adult respiratory distress syndrome. Clin Chest Med 1990; 11:715–722.
68. Mohsenifar Z, Goldbach P, Tashkin DP, Campisi DJ. Relationship between O_2 delivery and O_2 consumption in the adult respiratory distress syndrome. Chest 1983; 84:267–271.
69. Powers SR, Mannal R, Neclerio M, English M, Marr C, Leather R, Ueda H, Williams G, Custead W, Dutton R. Physiological consequences of positive end-expiratory pressure. Ann Surg 1973; 3:265–271.
70. Rhodes GR, Newell JC, Shah D, Scovill W, Tauber J, Dutton RE, Powers SR. Increased oxygen consumption accompanying increased oxygen delivery with hypertonic mannitol in adult respiratory distress syndrome. Surgery 1978; 84:490–495.
71. Danek SJ, Lynch JP, Weg JG, Dantzer DR. The dependence of oxygen uptake on oxygen delivery in the adult respiratory distress syndrome. Am Rev Respir Dis 1980; 122:387–395.
72. Ronco JJ, Montaner JSG, Fenwick JC, Ruedy J, Russell JA. Pathologic dependence of oxygen consumption on oxygen delivery in acute respiratory failure secondary to AIDS-related *Pneumocystis carinii* pneumonia. Chest 1990; 98:1463–1466.
73. Dantzker DR, Foresman B, Gutierrez G. Oxygen supply and utilization relationships: a reevaluation. Am Rev Resp Dis 1991; 143:675–679.
74. Moreno LF, Stratton HH, Newell JC, Feustel PJ. Mathematical coupling of data: correction of a common error for linear calculations. J Appl Physiol 1986; 60:335–343.
75. Kruse JA, Haupt MT, Puri VK, Carlson RW. Lactate levels as predictors of the relationship between oxygen delivery and consumption in ARDS. Chest 1990; 98:959–962.

76. Manthous CA, Schumacker PT, Pohlman A, Schmidt GA, Hall JB, Samsel RW, Wood LDH. Absence of supply dependence of oxygen consumption in patients with septic shock. J Crit Care 1993; 8:203–211.
77. Phang PT, Cunningham KF, Ronco JJ, Wiggs BR, Russell JA. Mathematical coupling explains dependence of oxygen consumption on oxygen delivery in ARDS. Am J Resp Crit Care Med 1994; 150:318–323.
78. Ronco JJ, Phang PT, Walley KR, Wiggs B, Fenwick JC, Russell JA. Oxygen consumption is independent of changes in oxygen delivery in severe adult respiratory distress syndrome. Am Rev Respir Dis 1991; 143:1267–1273.
79. Ronco JJ, Fenwick JC, Tweeddale MG, Wiggs BR, Phang PT, Cooper DJ, Cunningham KF, Russell JA, Walley KR. Identification of the critical oxygen delivery for anaerobic metabolism in critically ill septic and nonseptic humans. JAMA 1993; 270:1724–1730.
80. Dantzker DR. The gastrointestinal tract: the canary of the body? JAMA 1993; 270:1247–1248.
81. Clark CH, Gutierrez G. Gastric intramucosal pH: a noninvasive method for the indirect measurement of tissue oxygenation. Am J Crit Care 1992; 1:53–60.
82. Gutierrez G, Bismar H, Dantzker DR. Gastric mucosa pH as an index of systemic oxygenation in critically ill patients (abstract). Am Rev Respir Dis 1991; 143:A86.
83. Gutierrez G, Palizas F, Doglio G, Wainsztein N, Gallesio A, Pacin J, Dubin A, Schiavi E, Jorge M, Pusajo J, Klein F, San Roman E, Dorfman B, Shottlender J, Giniger R. Gastric intramucosal pH as a therapeutic index of tissue oxygenation in critically ill patients. Lancet 1992; 339:195–199.
84. Cera FB. Hypermetabolism-organ failure syndrome: a metabolic response to injury. Crit Care Clin 1989; 5:289–302.
85. Hotchkiss RS, Karl IE. Reevaluation of the role of cellular hypoxia and bioenergetic failure in sepsis. JAMA 1992; 267:1503–1510.
86. Vandermeer TJ, Wang H, Fink MP. Endotoxemia causes ileal mucosalacidosis in the absence of mucosal hypoxia in a normodynamic porcine model of septic shock. Crit Care Med 1995; 23:1217–1226.
87. Vary TC. Sepsis-induced alterations in pyruvate dehydrogenase complex activity in rat skeletal muscle: effects on plasma lactate. Shock 1996; 6:89–94.

16

The Brain

CLAUDE A. PIANTADOSI

Duke University Medical Center
Durham, North Carolina

I. Cerebral Blood Flow and Metabolism

The brain has a very high rate of oxidative metabolism, which, in the adult human, accounts for as much as 20% of the resting oxygen consumption of the body. In addition, the brain has a respiratory quotient of approximately one, indicating that carbohydrate, in particular glucose, is the primary source of carbon for oxidative metabolism [1]. Like oxygen, the carbon reserve in the brain is minimal; consequently, maintenance of normal cerebral function depends critically on a continuous supply of oxygen and glucose from the circulation. The cerebral circulation is critical for survival of the organism, and the brain, like the heart, is a privileged organ in terms of blood flow during physiological stresses such as hypoxia, hypovolemia, and hypotension. However, equally remarkable is how the brain matches blood flow with changes in metabolism on a minute-by-minute basis. This chapter focuses on some recent conceptual progress in our understanding of how the cerebral circulation is regulated with respect to the metabolic requirements accompanying changes in brain activity.

The normal brain extracts approximately 40% of the oxygen and 10% of the glucose available from the arterial blood. This results in an arteriovenous oxygen difference of 3 μmol/mL (approximately 6 mL/dL) and an arteriovenous difference for glucose of 0.55 μmol/mL [1]. These values for the extraction of oxygen and glucose vary slightly from region to region but are relatively constant over a range of metabolic rates; under most circumstances, increased metabolic needs are met primarily by increases in the cerebral blood flow (CBF). In simplified terms, the major function of the cerebral circulation is to maintain the brain with an adequate supply of oxygen and glucose despite varying levels of neuronal activity and cellular metabolic requirements. The regulatory mechanisms by which this occurs are complex and involve a variety of potential mediators and signals. There is an ongoing debate about which of these mechanisms are responsible for the tight linkage between CBF, neuronal activity, and cellular metabolism.

The normal cerebral metabolic rate for oxygen (CMR_{O_2}) is approximately 3.5 mL O_2/min per 100 g brain cortex in the adult human [2]. More than 90% of this oxygen is reduced irreversibly to water by cytochrome c oxidase during respiration by mitochondria; this reaction is the final step in the electron transport chain that drives adenosine triphosphate (ATP) production by oxidative phosphorylation. It has been estimated that approximately half of the CMR_{O_2} is used to support synaptic transmission [3]: one quarter for maintaining resting neuronal membrane potentials, and one quarter for other, mostly unidentified homeostatic cellular functions. However, the CMR_{O_2} is virtually constant under a wide range of conditions. Exceptions occur during seizures, hypercapnia, and global hypoxia, when CMR_{O_2} is significantly increased. On the other hand, many general anesthetics and inhibitors of synaptic transmission can decrease the CMR_{O_2} significantly.

The normal cerebral metabolic rate for glucose (CMR_{gl}) is approximately 27 μmol/min/100 g in conscious humans [4]. Because the chemical reaction for the complete oxidation of glucose occurs as:

$$\text{Glucose} + 6O_2 \rightarrow 6CO_2 + 6H_2O$$

if all of the glucose taken up by the brain is oxidized and no other substrates are consumed, it follows that the ratio of the arteriovenous difference for oxygen to glucose will be 6 under steady-state conditions. In fact, this ratio has long been known to have a value of approximately 5.5. Because the nonketotic brain uses glucose almost exclusively, the measured ratio can be taken to indicate that more than 90% of the glucose is used to support aerobic metabolism, and less than 10% is used for glycolysis alone.

Normally, the rate of oxidative metabolism in the brain is determined by the cellular needs of a specific region. For the brain to maintain the CMR_{O_2} under conditions of decreased oxygen availability, it has only two options: (1) to increase the CBF; or (2) to extract more oxygen from the arterial blood. Generally, as previously mentioned, the brain relies on increasing CBF to deliver more oxygen to the tissue for increased metabolic needs or to maintain oxygen delivery during hypoxia. Increased oxygen extraction plays a relatively minor role in meeting increased metabolic needs in the brain compared with some other tissues, e.g., skeletal muscle. The same is generally true for the CMR_{gl}, although under certain conditions, such as after neuronal activation, the glucose concentration in cerebrovenous blood clearly decreases. Decreases in tissue glucose concentration of approximately 30% also have been observed by proton magnetic resonance during activation of the visual cortex [5].

II. Neurovascular Coupling: The Link Between Cerebral Blood Flow, Metabolism, and Function

The physiological relationship between cerebral blood flow, functional neuronal activity, and the metabolic rate of the brain is termed *neurovascular coupling* [6,7]. This concept is often attributed to Roy and Sherrington [8], who postulated that chemical products of metabolism could provide a link between activity and blood flow. Over the past century, many chemical mediators have been found that are released by activated neurons and that have the ability to increase or decrease local blood flow by regulating smooth muscle contraction and relaxation [9]. In addition, cerebrovascular endothelial intraluminal and neurogenic factors make important contributions to regulation of cerebral blood flow. Some of the most important of these chemical mediators and their effects are listed in Table 1. Many of these agents have been proposed to play a role in neurovascular coupling, yet the precise signaling mechanisms have not been agreed upon. Indeed, whatever the identity of the primary control mechanism(s), the result is always the prompt increase in delivery of more glucose and oxygen to an activated brain region.

It should also be pointed out as a general principle that smooth muscle function is energy dependent, i.e., ATP is required for the key phosphorylation events involved in the processes of contraction and relaxation. For instance, ATP is consumed by smooth muscle cells during phosphorylation of both the myosin light chain kinase and the myosin regulatory light chain. The molecular sites of phosphorylation determine whether ATP facilitates contraction or relaxation of the smooth muscle (Fig. 1).

Because maintenance of adequate CBF is a critical function of the circulation, it is not surprising that multiple mechanisms have been implicated in the responses of the cerebral vasculature to stimulation. Because the term *coupling* implies a link between two variables, and at least three processes must be involved, evidence for at least three regulatory mechanisms should be considered. These possibilities are vascular-metabolic, vascular-functional, and functional-metabolic coupling mechanisms. The essential features of these mechanisms are illustrated schematically in Figure 2. In this section, they are discussed individually after some comments about the general process of coupling during activation.

A. Neurovascular Coupling During Activation

The processes that trigger neuronal activation in the conscious brain obviously include various sensory afferent stimuli; however, in the case of volitional activity,

Table 1 Chemical and Physical Stimuli Known to Alter Cerebral Blood Flow

Neurogenic	Parenchyma	Neurotransmitters	Endothelium	Lumen
Extrinsic	CO_2	Serotonin	NO	O_2
Sympathetic	Adenosine	Norepinephrine	CO	ADP
Parasympathetic	H^+	Dopamine	Prostacyclin	Thrombin
Trigeminovascular	K^+	Excitatory amino acids (glutamate)	Endothelins	SNO-Hb
Intrinsic	Ca^{++}		Peptides	Peptides (substance P, CGRP, VIP)
	Lactate		Hyperpolarizing factor	Vessel stretch
	NO			Shear stress
	CO			Transmural ΔP
	Prostanoids (prostacylin, leukotrienes thromboxane)			

SNO-Hb, S-nitrosohemoglobin; CGRP, calcitonin gene-related peptide; VIP, vasoactive intestinal peptide; NO, nitric oxide; ADP, adenosine diphosphate.

The Brain 439

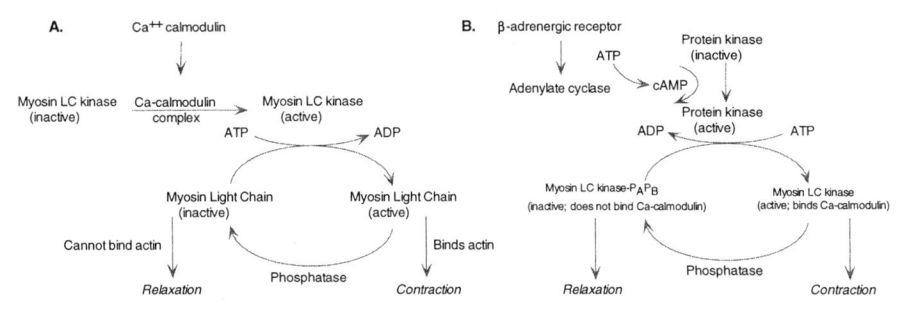

Figure 1 Two basic principles of smooth muscle contraction and relaxation in the brain. (A) Calcium–calmodulin regulation. As intracellular [Ca^{++}] increases in the cell, Ca^{++} is bound to calmodulin, and the Ca^{++}–calmodulin complex binds to and activates myosin light chain kinase. The activated kinase phosphorylates the regulatory light chain of myosin leading to actin binding and contraction. Relaxation is mediated by myosin light chain phosphatase, which dephosphorylates myosin, causing relaxation. (B) Cyclic AMP (cAMP) regulation stimulation of β-adrenergic receptors by catecholamines leads to generation of cAMP from ATP by adenylate cyclase. The cAMP-dependent protein kinase then phosphorylates myosin light chain kinase, rendering it unresponsive to Ca^{++}–calmodulin. The kinase cannot phosphorylate the regulatory light chain of myosin, allowing relaxation to occur.

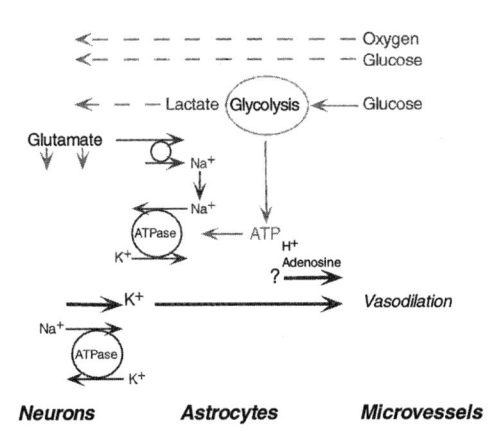

Figure 2 Schematic diagram of the potential mechanisms involved in coupling between cerebral blood flow, functional activation, and neuronal metabolism in the brain. Astrocytes are interposed between neurons and cerebral arterioles. Their foot processes make contact with and surround small arterioles in the cerebral circulation. Neuronal activation, e.g., by release of an excitatory amino acid (glutamate), leads to vasodilation and increased glucose uptake from the microcirculation. Glutamate is cotransported into astrocytes with sodium, leading to activation of the Na$^+$/K$^+$ ATPase and hydrolysis of ATP. This process could provide a metabolic signal for vasodilation. Alternatively, the increase in extracellular [K$^+$] could lead directly to hyperpolarization of cerebral vessels and vasodilation (bold arrows).

the responsible factors are largely unknown. However, whenever activation does occur, it is readily discernable with modern functional imaging techniques [6,7, 10–12]. Also problematic is the identity of the coupling mechanism, although the integrated response clearly leads to an activity-linked increase in the delivery per unit time of more substrates, i.e., oxygen and glucose, to meet the additional energy demands of the activity. Indeed, upon activation, increased glucose use can be readily detected, yet the CMR_{O_2} does not seem to increase in proportion to glucose uptake [10]. For example, visual stimulation in humans has been found to increase glucose uptake in the occipital visual centers in direct proportion to the intensity of the stimulus. Such observations have given rise to the concept that the brain relies on glucose and not oxygen uptake from the circulation as a primary response to the increased metabolic demands of activation. This interesting concept is explored further in the following section.

B. Vascular-Metabolic Coupling

The traditional view of brain metabolism has been that neuronal activity consumes energy and stimulates adenosine triphosphate (ATP) production by glycolysis and oxidative phosphorylation. The vascular response is invoked through release of metabolic products such as H^+, lactate, or carbon dioxide (CO_2) [13]. The result of such processes would be to increase the oxygen supply to match the increased energy demands of the functional activity. Such a response is logical because the energy yield for completely oxidizing a molecule of glucose to CO_2 and H_2O is far greater than for breaking it down into lactate by simple glycolysis. If coupling is intended to augment the oxygen supply to activated brain regions, however, this occurs with a large overshoot in the amount of oxygenated hemoglobin in the vasculature region serving the area of activation [12]. This overshoot phenomenon has been detected by several new techniques, including near-infrared spectroscopy and functional magnetic resonance spectroscopy. Such an increase in oxyhemoglobin content should make more oxygen available for diffusion into the tissue from the microcirculation. Whether this surplus oxygen actually is extracted by the tissue, however, would depend on whether the rate of cellular oxygen consumption increased.

Some of the aforementioned evidence suggests that a concept of coupling based on oxygen supply–demand relationships may not be correct. This tenet is strengthened by the consistent observation that increased glucose uptake occurs during functional activation. A decade ago, Fox and Raichle [10] first reported "uncoupling" between glucose uptake and CMR_{O_2} in awake humans during neuronal activation. In other words, they observed that increases in CBF and CMR_{gl} were not matched by an increase in CMR_{O_2} in the activated cortical area. This finding was subsequently confirmed in an independent study using a different method [11]. On the basis of their data, Fox and Raichle proposed that glycolysis rather than oxidative phosphorylation supplied the initial energy demand of cortical activation. Some investigators have interpreted their findings to mean that oxygen in excess is always available to the normal brain during neuronal activation, whereas the increased glucose extraction early in the activation period represents a signal that can be used to regulate the blood flow response.

Evidence from other organ systems suggests the main energy-consuming process linked to cellular activation is the turnover rate of the Na^+/K^+-ATPase. It has also been proposed that the ATP for this enzyme may be provided primarily through glycolysis and not oxidative phosphorylation [14,15]. If this is true, then the mechanism underlying the coupling between neuronal activity and glycolysis could involve the Na^+/K^+-ATPase. Other putative links between blood flow and metabolism involve the release of the excitatory amino acid glutamate and its co-transport with Na^+ [16] and the increased extracellular K^+ concentrations that accompany neuronal activity. Glutamate released from excitatory afferents is cleared within seconds by a reuptake transporter in astrocytes. Similarly, the increased K^+ released into the extracellular space is cleared into astrocytes after neuronal activation [16]. The astrocytes also surround parenchymal arterioles and capillaries that provide glucose from the circulation, and from this strategic advantage point, they may be an integral part of the mechanism for glucose uptake during activation.

In summary, current concepts of metabolic-vascular coupling make use of the idea that enhanced glucose uptake from the circulation is a primary response to neuronal activation. In addition, the neuronatomical arrangement of astrocytes and their ability to detect synaptic activity via reuptake of glutamate and K^+ may allow them to play a role in coupling neuronal activity to glucose uptake from the circulation. Although the precise control mechanisms for the accompanying blood flow response are not known, if the signal is based on glycolytic activity, then oxygen availability is not critical and plays little or no role in matching blood flow with activity under most physiological conditions.

C. Vascular-Functional Coupling

One alternative to both the conventional oxygen supply-based or more recent glucose extraction-based concepts of neurovascular coupling is that the blood flow response is linked directly to neuronal activation [7]. Stated another way, the process of activation could lead to a direct increase in the blood flow through a mediator(s) released by the activity. The efflux of K^+ from the activated neuron to the interstitial space is a case in point; K^+ is a potent dilator of cerebral vessels, and it is now generally accepted that it plays a role as an initial mediator of neurovascular coupling. Its role with respect to other mediators linked to metabolic activity, e.g., H^+, adenosine, and lactate, is not yet clear. However, it has been argued that K^+ release depends strictly on the rate of neuronal firing, whereas H^+ and adenosine accumulate when a mismatch occurs between oxygen delivery and demand. Therefore, adjustments by the metabolic signals would be expected to occur after the initial vascular response to K^+ release has been made. If the increase in oxygen supply in response to K$^+$ is adequate, then the metabolic control mechanisms would remain balanced, and no further compensation in blood flow would be necessary.

D. Functional-Metabolic Coupling

As in all living tissues, the brain shows a remarkably tight relationship between neuronal function and the provision of energy in the form of ATP. The regulation of cellular energy metabolism is a complicated process, and in many respects, our understanding of it is still overly simple. At first glance, it seems reasonable to expect that the control mechanisms regulate the ratio of ATP/adenosine diphosphate (ADP) or the phosphorylation potential of the cell to maintain constant ATP availability at the sites where it is used. In fact, this objective is met very well by the brain because the concentration of ATP in the tissue is held very close to 3 μmol/g wet weight under a wide range of conditions. Within seconds of interrupting the circulation, however, the main high-energy reserve, phosphocreatine begins to decrease, followed promptly by a decrease in the ATP/ADP ratio from its normal value of 10 to near unity. The glucose concentration decreases, and lactate increases more slowly; however, cessation of neuronal function is almost immediate. Hence, it is clear that brain function is highly dependent on oxidative phosphorylation, because glycolysis is not capable of producing enough ATP to support long-term neuronal function.

The rate of oxidative phosphorylation in mitochondria is under multiple levels of control. Oxidative phosphorylation is coupled with mitochondrial electron transport through the electrochemical proton gradient ($\Delta\Psi$), which allows energy conservation to occur. Electrons enter the system from the reactions of the citric acid cycle in the form of nicotinamide adenine dinucleotide (NADH) and flavin adenine dinucleotide (FADH$_2$) via a pair of dehydrogenases regulated, in part, by intracellular calcium concentration. Changes in the rate of electron transport are reflected by changes in the outward movement of protons across the inner mitochondrial membrane, and hence determine the proton flux required by the ATP synthase for phosphorylation of ADP to ATP.

Reductions in either glucose or oxygen supply have profound effects on the ratio of NADH/NAD$^+$ in the mitochondrion. This ratio is critical for mitochondrial electron transport and oxidative phosphorylation. Lack of carbon for the citric acid cycle can limit NADH availability, e.g., during hypoglycemia, whereas lack of oxygen relative to glucose can increase NADH levels in the mitochondria. Ultimately, however, it is the availability of ADP and inorganic phosphate for phosphorylation that drives the rate of respiration in the brain under most circumstances.

High rates of ATP turnover result in more ADP and intracellular phosphate in the cell and hence lead to a higher rate of oxidative phosphorylation and a higher rate of oxygen consumption. The net production of ATP from oxidation of one molecule of glucose is 2 from glycolysis and 24 from oxidative phosphorylation. This fact clearly illustrates the need for oxygen in the production of ATP and makes it biochemically unlikely that the increase in glucose uptake observed after activation is used entirely for glycolysis. It should not be forgotten that both products of glycolysis, pyruvate and lactate, can be used to fuel the citric acid cycle, as the lactate dehydrogenase reaction is reversible. Hence, it seems that enhanced glucose uptake during neuronal activation must be the "tip of the iceberg" insofar as the metabolic support of the activity is concerned.

III. Cerebral Hypoxia

It has been known for many years that oxygen is vasoactive. Hyperoxia causes vasoconstriction, and arterial hypoxemia causes cerebral vasodilation and an increase in the CBF. Despite intensive investigation, the detailed mechanisms by which these responses occur have not been worked out. In general, the cerebral vasculature responds to decreased oxygen availability by increasing the CBF to maintain oxygen delivery. CBF can be increased as much as fivefold during hypoxia, and it can be protected by autoregulatory mechanisms at cerebral perfusion pressures as low as 60 mm Hg. If oxygen delivery becomes limited, then cerebral oxygen extraction increases to maintain cerebral oxygen use. There are, of course, exceptions to this generalization that depend primarily on the cause of the hypoxia. Classically, the causes of hypoxia have been thought of in terms of the independent variables responsible for decreasing the oxygen concentration available to the mitochondria, e.g., hypoxic hypoxia, anemic hypoxia, CO hypoxia, ischemic hypoxia, and cytotoxic hypoxia. Most of the experimental work on the mechanisms of matching blood flow and metabolism during hypoxia has been performed under conditions of hypoxic hypoxia, and the remainder of this discussion focuses on this.

Although cerebral hypoxia of any cause produces a relatively predictable sequence of cellular dysfunction, hypoxic hypoxia is generally well tolerated provided CBF regulation is preserved. If the CBF response is inadequate, brain functions are lost incrementally. Spontaneous electrical activity is suppressed first followed by homeostatic failure and cell death. Brain hypoxia also may cause both immediate and delayed injury including programmed cell death (apoptosis) and prolonged impairment of coupling between neuronal function and blood flow.

The mechanisms of cerebral vasodilation in cerebral hypoxia are complex, and direct effects of hypoxia, neurogenic mechanisms, and release of chemical mediators and metabolic factors, e.g., adenosine, have all been implicated in the process. Metabolic control mechanisms related to either enhanced glycolysis or oxygen supply–demand imbalance are conceptually attractive but not firmly established. Roles for nitric oxide and other rapidly responding chemical mediators (Table 1) have also been put forth, but they remain incompletely characterized, and certainly no single mediator is responsible for the cerebrovascular response to all types of hypoxia.

The problem of neurovascular coupling during hypoxia can be illustrated in a number of ways. When the arterial oxygen partial pressure is reduced to ≤50 mm Hg, the CBF increases, and the cerebral concentrations of lactate increase in the interstitial and intracellular spaces. However, the increase in the intracellular lactate is offset by a decrease in CO_2 partial pressure, resulting in little or no change in pH. In fact, experimental measurements of pH in the interstitial spaces of the brain show a small shift toward alkalosis at the time the CBF response to hypoxia is maximal. Hence, regulation must be related to some other more robust signal generated during hypoxia. Nitric oxide is a potentially attractive mediator in this regard because it is produced as a result of stimulation by a wide range of endogenous vasodilators such as acetyl choline, serotonin, bradykinin, substance P, and others [17]. However, there is marked heterogeneity in the ability of endothelial cells of different cerebrovascular beds to produce nitric oxide. Furthermore, this heterogeneity does not correlate well with regional differences in the blood flow response to hypoxia. It is much better established that nitric oxide production is involved in the cerebrovascular response to CO_2, as nitric oxide synthase inhibitors nearly abolish the vasodilator response to CO_2 [18].

Another major mechanism for dilation of cerebral vessels that has been implicated in the response to hypoxia is activation of potassium channels [9]. Substances that increase the cyclic 3'-5'- adenosine monophosphate concentration inside the cell produce vasodilation by activating both K_{ATP} and BK_{Ca} channels. This process leads to hyperpolarization of cerebral vascular smooth muscle and vasodilation, but exactly how hypoxia activates these channels is not yet clear. BK_{Ca} channels but not K_{ATP} also seem to be active under basal conditions and contribute to the normal tone of the cerebral blood vessels.

IV. Summary

There has been progress recently in understanding the mechanisms responsible for regulation of CBF. A role for several vasodilator substances has been established that seem to couple CBF with neuronal activity. Other substances seem to mediate the responses to hypercapnia, hypotension, and hypoxia. Current concepts of neurovascular coupling during brain activity are centered around vascular-metabolic or vascular-functional control mechanisms. Among the early responses to increased neuronal activity seems to be an increase in glucose uptake that is out of proportion to the increase in oxygen uptake. This increase in glucose uptake may represent a signal that allows the brain to match its fuel supply with the rate of energy use. On the other hand, it is possible that blood flow is also coupled directly with neuronal function through mediators such as K^+ in the extracellular space. In any event, the biochemical mechanisms that regulate the cerebrovascular responses to activation are highly tuned to respond rapidly to changes in the metabolic demands of the brain.

References

1. Siesjo BK. Circulation and oxygen consumption in the brain. In: Energy Metabolism. New York: John Wiley & Sons, Inc. 1978, pp 56–100.
2. Kety SS, Schmidt CF. The effects of altered arterial tensions of carbon dioxide and oxygen on cerebral blood flow and cerebral oxygen consumption of normal young men. J Clin Invest 1948; 27:484–492.
3. Astrup J. Energy requiring cell functions in the ischemic brain: their critical supply and possible inhibition in protective therapy. J Neurosurg 1982; 56:482–497.
4. Cohen PJ, Alexander SC, Smith FC, Reivich M, Wellman H. Effects of hypoxia and normocarbia on cerebral blood flow and metabolism in conscious man. J Appl Physiol 1967; 23:183–189.
5. Chen W, Novotny EJ, Zhu X-H, Rothman DL, Shulman RG. Localized 1H NMR measurement of glucose consumption in the human brain during visual stimulation. Proc Natl Acad Sci USA 1994; 90:9896–9900.
6. Magistretti PJ, Pellerin L. Metabolic coupling during activation: a cellular view. In: Optical Imaging of Brain Function and Metabolism II. Advances in Experimental Medicine and Biology, vol. 413. Villringer A, Dirnagl U, eds. New York: Plenum Press, 1997; 18:161–166.
7. Kuschinsky W. Neuronal-vascular coupling. In: Optical Imaging of Brain Function and Metabolism II. 1997; 19:167–176.
8. Roy CS, Sherrington CS. On the regulation of the blood supply to the brain. J Physiol 1890; 11:85–108.
9. Brian JE, Faraci FM, Heistad DD. Recent insights into the regulation of cerebral circulation. Clin Exp Pharmacol Physiol 1996; 23:449–457.
10. Fox PT, Raichle ME. Focal physiological uncoupling of cerebral blood flow and oxidative metabolism during somatosensory stimulation in human subjects. Proc Natl Acad Sci USA 1986; 83:1140–1144.
11. Lund Madsen P, Hasselbalch SG, Hagemann LP, Olsen KS, et al. Persistent resetting of the cerebral oxygen-glucose uptake ratio by brain activation: evidence obtained with Kety-Schmidt technique. J Cereb Blood Flow Metab 1995; 15:485–491.
12. Villringer A, Planck J, Hock C, Schleinkofer L, Dirnagl U. Near infrared spectroscopy (NIRS): a new tool to study hemodynamic changes during activation of brain function in adults. Neurosci Lett 1993; 154:101–104.
13. Kuschinsky W. Role of hydrogen ions in regulation of cerebral blood flow and other regional flows. Microcirculation 1992; 11:1–19.
14. Paul RJ, Bauer M, Pease W. Vascular smooth muscle: aerobic glycolysis linked to sodium and potassium transport processes. Science 1979; 206:1414–1416.
15. Lipton P, Robacker K. Glycolysis and brain function: $[K^+]o$ stimulation of protein synthesis and K^+ uptake require glycolysis. Fed Proc 1983; 42:2875–2880.
16. Pellerin L, Magistretti PJ. Glutamate uptake into astrocytes stimulates aerobic glycolysis: a mechanism coupling neuronal activity to glucose utilization. Proc Natl Acad Sci, USA 1994; 91:10625–10629.
17. Szabo D. Physiological and pathophysiological roles of nitric oxide in the central nervous system. Brain Res Bull 1996; 41:131–141.
18. Iadecola C, Pellegrino DA, Moskowitz MA, Lassen NA. Nitric oxide synthase inhibition and cerebrovascular regulation. J Cereb Blood Flow Met 1994; 14:175–192.

17

The Kidney

SAMUEL NOAM HEYMAN and MAYER BREZIS

The Hebrew University Medical School and Hadassah University Hospital
Mount Scopus, Jersalem, Israel

I. Introduction

The kidneys receive some 20% of the cardiac output, more than any other organ of the mammalian organism. As a consequence, renal oxygen availability is remarkably high per weight of tissue—over four times the oxygen delivery to the heart, brain, or liver (Fig. 1). The high renal blood flow required for the glomerular filtration process by far exceeds the renal metabolic demands. Thus, some 80% of the delivered oxygen leaves the renal vein unconsumed [1]. In fact, high oxygen saturation has been the hallmark for proper catheter placement in the renal vein. Paradoxically, despite abundant oxygen availability, the kidney is an organ most susceptible to hypoxic damage and functional derangement after compromised systemic circulation. In this chapter we show the nature of this paradox, the consequence of the unique architecture of the renal microcirculation that leads to an uneven distribution of blood flow and tissue oxygenation. In addition, we outline the compound mechanisms known to participate in the regulation of intrarenal oxygen delivery and consumption, relate their failure to various forms of acute and chronic renal injuries, and describe the possible role of renal hypoxia in the regulation of erythropoietin production.

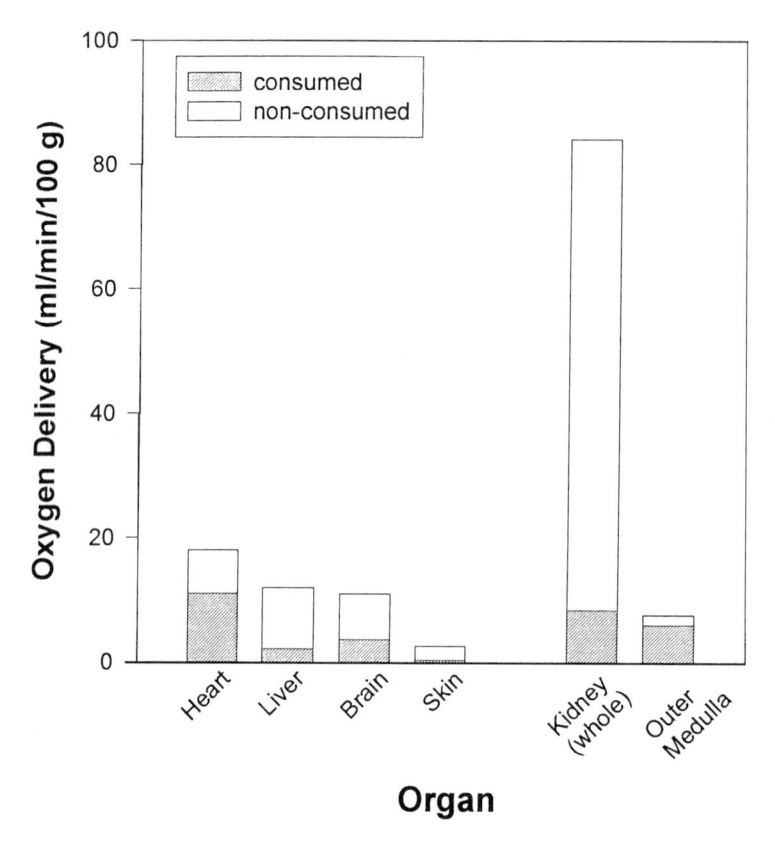

Figure 1 Oxygen delivery and consumption in various tissues. The outstandingly high renal oxygen delivery with low oxygen consumption results from the large amount of blood flow required for the filtration process. These figures mask a state of physiologic medullary oxygen insufficiency characterized by a high oxygen consumption, hardly matched by the relatively low regional oxygen delivery. The low medullary oxygen reserve renders the outer medulla susceptible to hypoxic damage. (Modified from Ref. 1.)

II. The Renal Circulation

The renal vasculature may be schematically divided into (1) the arterial system that conducts blood to the glomeruli within the cortical labyrinth; (2) the glomerular system, which consists of small afferent and efferent glomerular arteries bridged by glomerular capillaries; and (3) the postglomerular vasculature that originates from efferent glomerular arterioles, nourishes the renal tubules, and drains into the renal veins [2] (Fig. 2).

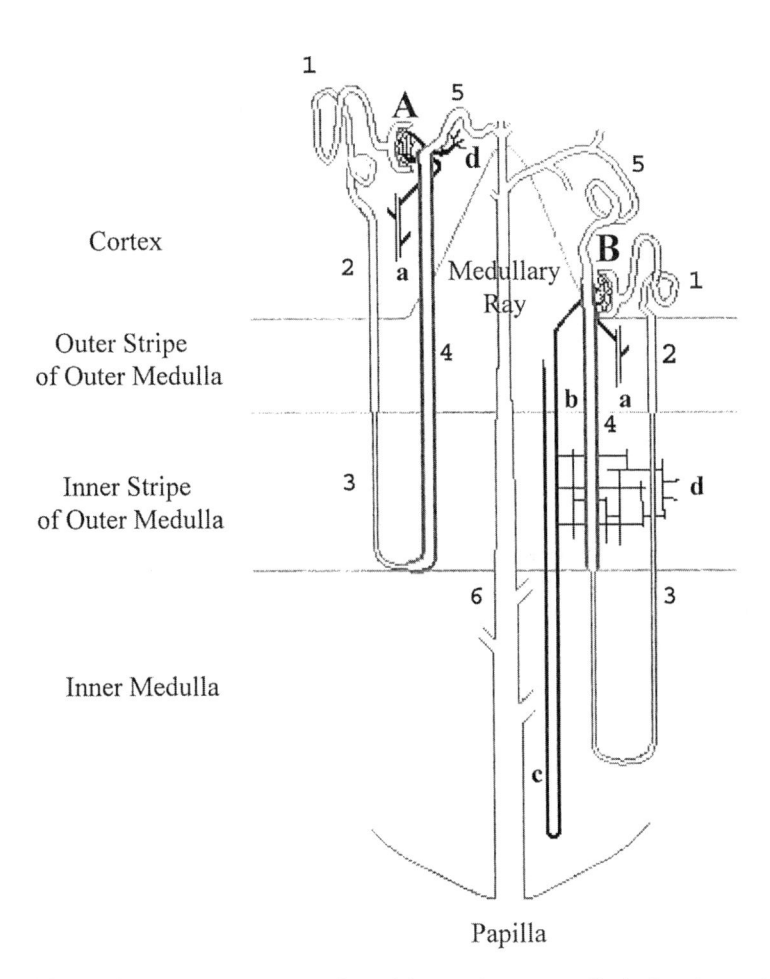

Figure 2 Schematic presentation of the renal anatomy, displaying the particular arrangement of nephron segments and blood supply. Representative nephrons are (A) a cortical nephron and (B) a juxtamedullary nephron. Nephron segments are numbered as follows: (1) proximal convoluted tubules; (2) straight portion (S_3) of proximal tubule; (3) thin limb of Henle's loop; (4) thick ascending limb of Henle's loop; (5) distal convoluted tubule, and (6) collecting duct. Microvascular segments displayed are: (a) intralobular arteries, from which emerge afferent glomerular arterioles; descending (b) and ascending (c) vasa recta, arranged in vascular bundles; and (d) a meshwork of peritubular capillaries. For simplicity, the venous system is not displayed. Please note that vasa recta originate from the efferent glomerular arterioles of juxtamedullary nephrons (B), and nourish the renal medulla, while cortical tubules are supplied by capillary meshwork that ramifies from efferent vessels of cortical nephrons (A).

The renal arterial branches penetrate the renal parenchyma as medium-size interlobar arteries that further divide into arcuate arteries at the corticomedullary junction. These, in turn, give rise to intralobular arteries that ascend toward the renal surface and ramify into small afferent glomerular arterioles.

Although the intralobular arteries may participate in the regulation of blood distribution between superficial and deep nephrons, the small glomerular arteries are the major determinants of the renal vascular resistance and intrarenal blood dispersal. Although arterial pressure is maintained close to the mean systemic pressure down to the interlobular arteries, intravascular pressure decreases from 80 to 20 mm Hg across the glomerular vasculature, markedly affecting the intrarenal blood distribution. The fine regulation of afferent and efferent arteriolar tone controls the glomerular capillary hydraulic pressure, the major determinant in the generation of glomerular filtration.

The peritubular space is supplied by a postglomerular capillary plexus. In the cortex, originating from efferent arterioles of superficial glomeruli, it nourishes the cortical tubules within the cortical labyrinth. Efferent arterioles of midcortical glomeruli also give rise to the network of capillaries, surrounding straight (S_3) proximal tubules and thick ascending limbs (TALs) of Henle's loops within medullary rays.

The medullary capillary meshwork is somewhat more compound [3–5]. Blood vessels, supplied by efferent arterioles of deep juxtamedullary glomeruli, penetrate the renal medulla from the corticomedullary junction down toward the papillary tip. Their name, vasa recta, comes from their peculiar arrangement in straight vascular bundles, surrounded by rectilinear medullary tubular segments. The vasa recta consist of descending and ascending vessels connected by a curved hairpin–like segment at their deepest end. This striking structure of closely associated vasa recta and comparably shaped Henle's loops and collecting ducts generates the countercurrent ion exchange system, the basis for the renal concentrating/diluting capabilities. A capillary plexus that originates from small side branches of the vasa recta nourishes the medullary parenchyma and drains outward into the venous system at the corticomedullary junction. At the outer stripe and extending medullary rays, this capillary plexus is sparse, in sharp contrast with a dense interbundle meshwork at the inner stripe of the outer medulla. Thus, different nephron segments are supplied by distinct capillary beds at various levels of the renal parenchyma. The heterogeneity of microcirculation is prominent even across the outer medulla, spatially separating blood perfusing different tubular segments in this region.

The cortical and medullary microcirculations also differ in their red blood cell content and blood viscosity, perhaps because of plasma skimming along the intralobular arteries (5): Glomeruli of deep nephrons are supplied by afferent arterioles exiting the intralobular artery near its origin, while cortical glomeruli receive blood that runs along its entire length. Since red blood cell density is higher in the center of the intralobular arterial cross-section, cortical nephrons (and cortical tubular segments) receive blood with a higher hematocrit level compared with juxtamedullary glomeruli (and the medullary peritubular microcirculation). Pronounced water reabsorption may also contribute to the lower medullary hematocrit. The overall effect of the regional microcirculatory hematocrit on zonal oxygenation remains speculative.

III. Intrarenal Oxygen Gradient

In the heterogeneous renal microcirculation, the finding of an uneven distribution of renal tissue oxygenation is not surprising. Using Clark-type oxygen microelectrodes for the determination of renal parenchymal oxygen partial pressure (PO_2), Aukland and Crog [6] reported in 1960 that renal medullary PO_2 was substantially lower than the arterial PO_2. This was confirmed later by Leichtweiss et al. [7] and Baumgartl et al. [8] in rats and dogs and by Leonhardt and Landes [9] in humans. More recent studies showed similar findings, with PO_2 sharply decreasing at the corticomedullary junction from 60 to 80 mm Hg in the cortex to 10 to 30 mm Hg at the outer medulla [10]. This outstanding finding is schematically illustrated in Figure 3. The prominent variability of PO_2 measurements at the deep cortex, in sharp contrast with the fairly consistent tracings at the superficial cortex and in the medulla, probably represents random sampling from the cortical labyrinth (with the higher oxygen measurements) and medullary rays (low PO_2), all placed at the same depth as determined from the renal surface. Somewhat lower PO_2 was also recorded at the very superficial, subcapsular cortical layer, a region supplied by the most remote branches of the cortical capillary meshwork [11].

IV. Outer Medullary Oxygen Balance

The measured tissue oxygen content represents the balance between local oxygen supply (determined predominantly by the regional blood flow) and the rate of tissue oxygen consumption (the reflection of local aerobic metabolism). Thus, medullary hypoxemia may result from limited oxygen supply, from high metabolic requirements, or their combination [12,13].

The medullary blood flow originating from juxtamedullary glomeruli is low, estimated as 10% of the total renal blood flow, with oxygen delivery to the deeper medullary structures appraised at 8 mL/min/100 g (Fig. 1). Low medullary blood flow is essential for the preservation of intrarenal osmotic gradient and urinary concentrating capability. Medullary oxygenation may be further compromised by an oxygen shunt. This phenomenon is believed to result from the unique arrangement of vasa recta within the vascular bundles. It is presumed that oxygen diffuses from descending to adjacent ascending vasa recta, resulting in low precapillary PO_2 in the deep medulla (Fig. 4).

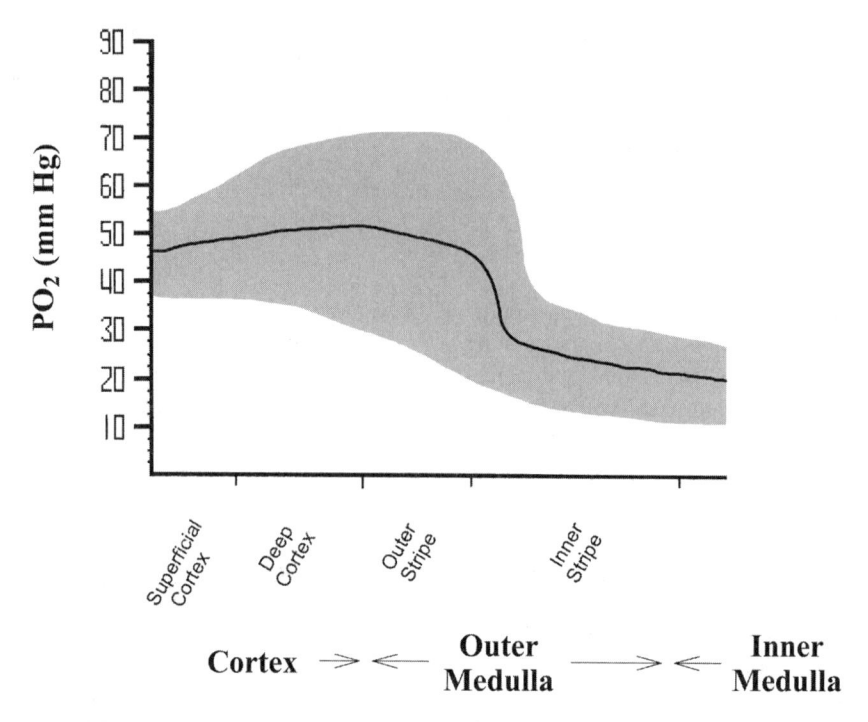

Figure 3 Schematic representation of intrarenal oxygen tension (P_{O_2}) measured at different locations in mammalian kidneys. The x-axis represents relative distance from the renal surface. The shaded area roughly represents a 95% confidence interval of measurements. While cortical P_{O_2} is close to arterial levels, a sharp decrease of tissue oxygenation is noted at the corticomedullary junction, to oxygen levels as low as 20 mm Hg. Please note the increased heterogeneity of P_{O_2} in the deep cortical region, probably reflecting determination of tissue oxygenation in both cortical tissue and medullary rays. (Modified from oxygen measurements in canine (8), rodent (7,10), and human (9) kidneys.)

The limited medullary oxygenation is hardly sufficient for the particularly high regional oxygen consumption, largely determined by tubular reabsorption. Quantitatively, medullary thick ascending limbs (mTALs), characterized histologically by numerous mitochondria, are the major participants in the regional medullary reabsorptive workload and oxygen consumption.

Thus, outer medullary physiological hypoxia results from the combined effects of low regional oxygen delivery and high local oxygen consumption (Fig. 4). The marginal oxygen reserve in the outer medulla is underscored by a very high oxygen extraction fraction, at the range of 80%, as opposed to the low total renal extraction fraction of 10% (Fig. 1). Continuous medullary oxygen deprivation can be appreciated by the substantial portion of medullary cytochrome aa$_3$, found to be in reduced state under normal circumstances [14,15].

The Kidney

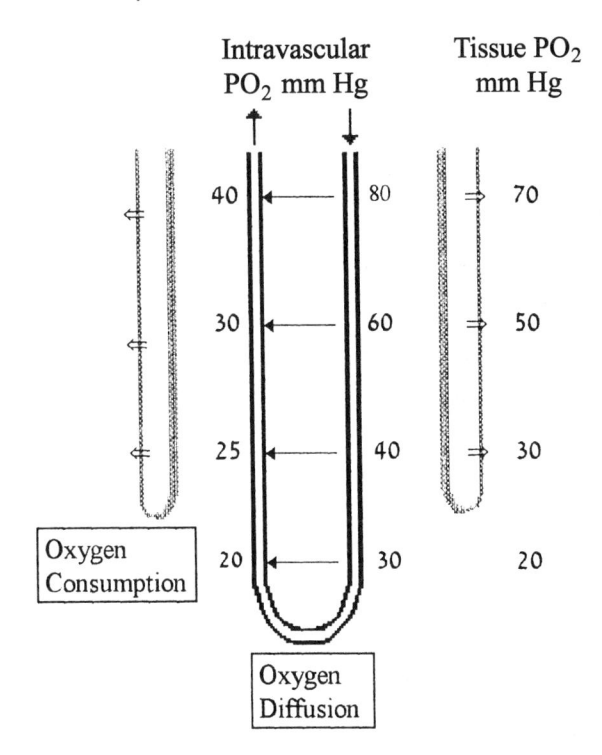

Figure 4 The postulated countercurrent oxygen shunt: medullary hypoxia results from limited oxygen supply and high oxygen consumption. Oxygen diffuses from adjacent descending-to-ascending vasa recta contribute to the reduced oxygen delivery to the renal medulla.

Thus, in reminiscence with the cardiac anginal syndrome, the limited oxygen reserve renders the outer medulla susceptible to hypoxic insult during transient or protracted oxygen imbalance after trivial daily changes in hydration state, electrolyte load, or vasomotor tone. Compound mechanisms, discussed in Sec. V, prevent hypoxic damage during trivial insults by maintaining the balance between medullary oxygen supply and consumption. Their effects, directed to preserve regional blood flow and to restrain local metabolic activity, alleviate regional oxygen insufficiency and maintain medullary tubular integrity.

V. Control of Medullary Oxygen Balance

The "corticomedullary redistribution" of blood flow, recognized for years during acute or chronic volume depletion, refers to preferential perfusion of deep juxtamedullary nephrons and diminished blood flow to superficial cortical glomeruli

[2]. As a consequence, in addition to improved salt and water preservation by the long-looped deep nephrons, the medullary perfusion is maintained despite a pronounced decrease in cortical and total renal blood flow. This brings about the clinical features of prerenal azotemia, characterized by reduced renal blood flow (RBF) and glomerular filtration rate (GFR), salt and water preservation, and intact tubular function and structural integrity. This is a fine example for the adaptive mechanisms designed to maintain medullary oxygenation [16], with locally activated vasodilating mechanisms that counteract the intense vasoconstrictive stimuli associated with hypovolemia, such as catecholamines, vasopressin, and angiotensin II.

As schematically shown in Figs. 5 and 6, two factors direct medullary oxygen balance: (1) regional oxygen supply, dictated mainly by medullary blood flow; and (2) the magnitude of distal tubular reabsorptive workload. The latter variable is governed by GFR and the intensity of proximal solute reabsorption (both affecting the solute delivery to the distal nephron), and by various neurohumoral factors that directly regulate the rate of distal tubular metabolism, in particular salt reabsorption by mTALs [12,13].

Changes in total RBF generally reflect the cortical microcirculation and may not represent alterations in outer medullary flow. Reciprocal changes were recently recorded, with medullary flow increasing while cortical flow decreases, and vice versa, indicating a different control of the various renal microvascular beds [16]. Moreover, various mediators were found to produce inverse responses at the cortical and medullary microcirculation. For instance, endothelin-1 induces profound cortical (and total renal) vasoconstriction as opposed to outer medullary vasodilation [17]. These opposing effects were found to be related to a heterogenous distribution and density of receptor subtypes, in this case endothelin-A receptors at the cortex and endothelin-B receptors in the outer medulla. These disparate responses in the medulla and cortex may preserve medullary oxygenation by the dual effect of enhanced medullary blood supply and decreased cortical blood flow and GFR (and hence reduced solute delivery to the distal nephron and diminished reabsorptive workload).

Intrarenal administration of adenosine was shown to ameliorate medullary hypoxia. Like endothelin, adenosine brings about cortical vasoconstriction (mediated by A_1 receptors), and by contrast induces medullary vasodilation (the product of A_2 stimulation) [18]. It also directly inhibits sodium-potassium ATPase (Na-K-ATPase) in mTALs. Hence, produced by the breakdown of adenosine triphosphate (ATP) during oxygen debt, adenosine seems to be an ideal candidate for the physiological maintenance of medullary oxygen sufficiency by its triple action (19). Although its local release induces vasodilation and inhibits sodium reabsorption, it may bring about cortical vasoconstriction in a paracrinic way, delivered superficially by ascending vessels. This is one of the proposed mechanisms for a tubuloglomerular feedback system generated by medullary hypoxia and decreasing GFR (Fig. 6).

Vasodilating prostaglandins, in particular prostaglandin E_2 and prostacycline, are important paracrinic outer medullary vasodilators. Inhibition of prostaglandin

The Kidney

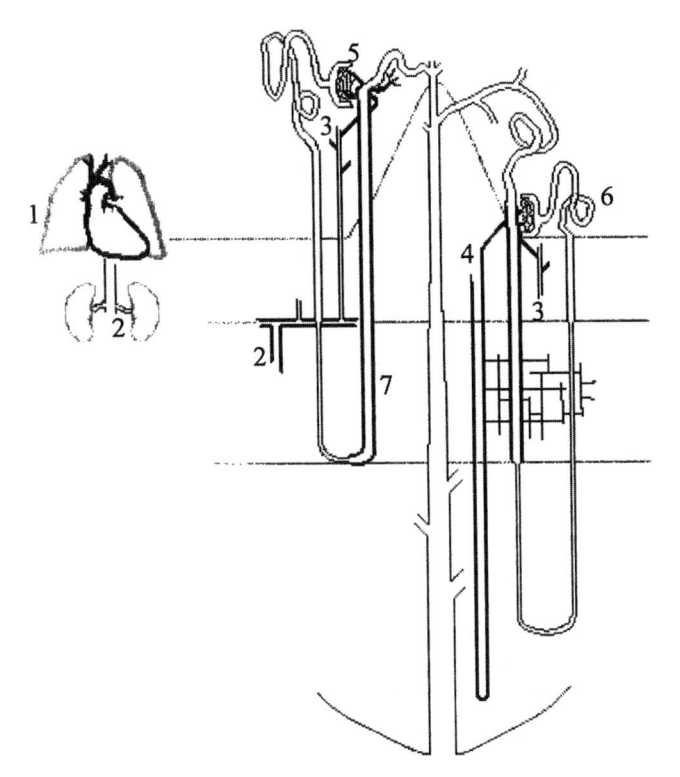

Figure 5 Schematic representation of principal determinants of medullary oxygen balance. Factors governing oxygen supply: (1) systemic factors: cardiopulmonary function, systemic hemodynamic status, blood composition and rheologic properties, status of oxygen–hemoglobin dissociation curve; (2 and 3) renal arterial vascular resistance, also determining intrarenal distribution of blood flow (preferential superficial vs. deep cortical flow, with the resulting impact on postglomerular blood distribution); (4) blood flow in vasa recta and in peritubular medullary capillary meshwork. Determinants of medullary oxygen consumption: (5) glomerular filtration rate; (6) proximal tubular reabsorption; (7) distal tubular reabsorption (see text).

synthesis selectively reduces outer medullary blood flow while cortical flow is maintained [20]. Prostaglandin E_2 also inhibits Na-K-ATPase in mTALs [21]. As a consequence, outer medullary hypoxia develops after the administration of nonsteroidal anti-inflammatory drugs (NSAIDs) [22], probably playing a central role in analgesic nephropathy. Both cyclooxygenase isoenzymes (COX-1 and COX-2) are constituent in the renal parenchyma, the latter located mainly within the renal vasculature [23], and prostaglandin E_2 receptors are located predominantly in the outer medulla [24]. Nitric oxide (NO) is another important determinant of renal hemodynamics [25]. The inhibition of its synthesis is associated with a marked

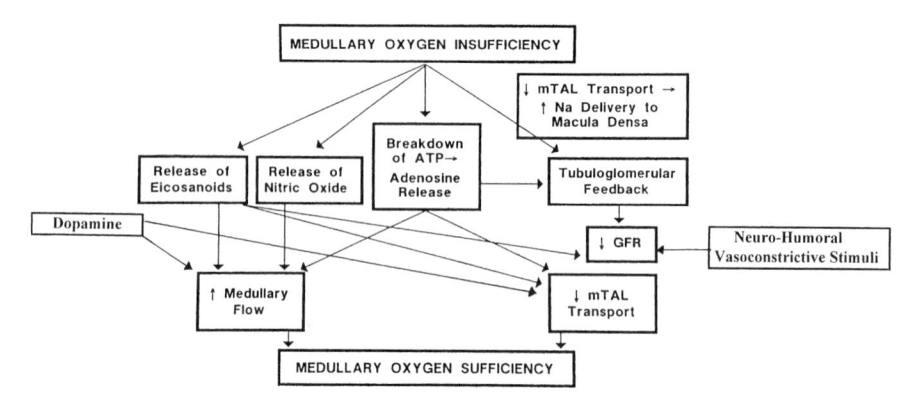

Figure 6 Mechanisms participating in the preservation of outer medullary oxygenation (see text). (Modified from Ref. 13, with permission.)

decrease of both cortical and medullary blood flow, with an intensification of the physiological medullary hypoxemia [10]. It is possible that NO bioavailability increases in the outer medulla under hypoxic conditions (because oxygen scavenges NO), ameliorating regional microcirculation [26].

Circulating or locally produced catecholamines also induce compound responses that may affect renal oxygenation, mediated by the various α-, β-, and dopamine receptors. For instance, systemic dopamine administration at low "renal dose" enhances RBF (an effect restricted to the outer medulla in volume-depleted rats) and reduces Na-K-ATPase in mTALs (through dopamine-1 receptors). However, outer medullary P_{O_2} is hardly affected [27], presumably because of enhanced GFR and reduced proximal tubular reabsorption (with increased solute delivery to the distal nephron, augmenting mTAL reabsorptive workload). At a higher dopamine infusion rate, intense β-, followed by α-receptor stimulation may predominate, with profound renal vasoconstriction and reduced GFR, with an unpredictable outcome of medullary oxygenation. On the other hand, dopamine was shown to ameliorate medullary hypoxia induced by inhibited NO and prostaglandin synthesis [27]. Medullary oxygenation was also maintained or even increased during the administration of angiotensin II (M. Brezis, unpublished data), perhaps as the result of preferential direct cortical vasoconstriction and the activation of various medullary vasodilators.

In conclusion, complex systems summarized in Fig. 6 maintain medullary oxygen balance by matching regional oxygen supply and consumption. The relative rarity of renal failure with hypoxic tubular damage in healthy subjects underscores their efficacy. The following sections outline possible links of their failure to clinical conditions that predispose to hypoxic tubular injury.

VI. Acute Tubular Necrosis and Distal Tubular Injury in Humans

Most cases of acute renal failure in the clinical practice are characterized by normal glomerular morphology despite a marked reduction in GFR. It is believed that primary tubulointerstitial damage, by virtue of intraluminal obstruction or upstream tubuloglomerular signals (tubuloglomerular feedback), reduces the GFR. Extensive cortical tubular damage is only rarely observed, almost exclusively after profound shock, as in severe puerperal hemorrhage (namely, irreversible acute cortical necrosis). In the majority of cases, cortical tubular morphology obtained by the biopsy needle is preserved, suggesting that a more distal injury takes place along the nephron. Loss of urine-concentrating capacity, the earliest clinical clue for the development of acute tubular necrosis (ATN) [28], also indicates distal tubular dysfunction.

The first morphological evidence for human distal tubular damage in the setting of acute renal failure came from autopsies performed during World War II in patients who died from acute renal failure, before the era of renal replacement therapy. A peculiar distribution of distal tubular lesion was noted, termed at that time "lower nephron nephrosis," occurring mainly in patients with crush injuries, shock, or sepsis and involving, in particular, mTALs in the outer medulla [29]. The lesions were usually focal, included tubular cell necrosis and cellular casts, and occasionally involved other nephron segments, namely, medullary collecting ducts and S_3 tubules.

It took more than four decades to confirm these findings with cytological evaluation of fragmented tubular cells obtained from kidney biopsy specimens from patients with the clinical syndrome of ATN that showed predominance of distal tubular cells, particularly mTALs [30]. Thus, the delay in the evolution of the concept of distal tubular vulnerability to hypoxic damage stems from the paucity of medullary material in kidney biopsy specimens and, as detailed in Sec. IX, from the difficulty to reproduce these lesions experimentally.

VII. Distal Tubular Injury: Experimental Evidence for Oxygen Insufficiency

Isolated kidneys perfused with erythrocyte-free oxygenated medium develop hypoxic damage restricted to the outer medulla [31]. Initially, a particular gradient of tubular injury is noted among mTALs in the inner stripe as early as 15 minutes after the beginning of the perfusion, selectively affecting tubules most remote from the vascular bundles. It progresses over the next hour to involve almost all other mTALs and spreads outward to the outer stripe of the outer medulla and into medullary rays, where S_3 segments of the proximal tubules are also affected. Morphologically, mTAL injury is first apparent as mitochondrial swelling, followed by nuclear pyknosis. Irreversible damage is finally manifested by cell membrane rupture and cell fragmentation. Programmed cell death (apoptosis) also seems to be enhanced under these conditions [32], perhaps reflecting a milder hypoxic insult to mTALs. In proximal S_3 tubules, simplification and shedding of the brush border is the hallmark of early hypoxic damage. Progressive decline in sodium reabsorption is the functional counterpart of mTAL damage, whereas mild glycosuria reflects proximal S_3 tubular injury. GFR deteriorates despite preserved glomerular structure as a secondary manifestation of tubular damage.

Alterations in oxygen availability markedly affect this injury pattern. Addition of red blood cells to the perfusate maintains tubular integrity and prevents functional impairment, whereas reduction of oxygen content in the gas mixture hastens outer medullary destruction. Manipulation of the tubular metabolic workload also affects the degree of mTAL necrosis in this model [33]. Enhancement of sodium reabsorption after polyene antibiotics, such as amphotericin B, intensifies outer medullary damage. In contrast, this injury is modified by measures that reduces mTAL oxygen requirement, such as furosemide (which prevents chloride reabsorption at the apical membrane) or ouabain (which blocks Na-K-ATPase at the basolateral membrane). Moreover, the extent of S_3 necrosis in the outer stripe and medullary rays is also attenuated by loop diuretics (which selectively act on the distal nephron), underscoring the intense competition between these two types of nephron segments on the confined regional oxygen supply [34]. In other experiments, the oncotic pressure of the perfusate was increased by the addition of albumin to a final concentration of 15 g/dL. As a result, despite ongoing renal perfusion, GFR was stopped, and solute delivery to the distal tubule was nullified. Again, outer medullary hypoxic injury was prevented [33]. In contrast, hypertrophic kidneys were found to be more vulnerable to hypoxic medullary damage during perfusion, reflecting enhanced oxygen requirement by the hypertrophic tubules [35].

Direct measurements of medullary Po_2 in the rat provided additional evidence for the impact of outer medullary oxygen balance on regional integrity. During moderate hypotension, as long as medullary blood flow was preserved, outer medullary Po_2 increased, reflecting the decline in GFR and metabolic workload at the distal nephron [16]. The injection of furosemide also markedly augmented outer medullary Po_2 despite a reduction in regional blood flow [36]. Comparable manipulations in mice induced an increase in regional cytochrome oxidation, indicating improved local oxygenation [15].

VIII. Medical Conditions Predisposing to Acute Tubular Necrosis: Implications for Medullary Oxygen Imbalance

Most threats to the renal tissue are characterized by the potential to intensify medullary hypoxia or to alter the local protective mechanisms [12,13]. Effective

The Kidney

Table 1 Factors Predisposing to Intrarenal Hypoxic Injury

Systemic causes for renal hypoperfusion
   Marked hypovolemia
   Congestive heart failure
   Decompensated hepatic cirrhosis
   Severe hypoalbuminemia
   Shock
Intrarenal causes:
   Increased medullary oxygen demand
      Compensatory hypertrophy of remnant nephrons: any chronic renal disease
      Solute diuresis: uncontrolled diabetes, hypercalcemia, mannitol, radiocontrast agents, dopamine
      Augmented glomerular filtration rate: pregnancy, early diabetes, dopamine, atrial natriuretic peptide
      Increase of medullary solute reabsorption: nonsteroidal antiinflammatory drugs, theophylline
      Miscellaneous: polyene antibiotics
   Medullary hypoperfusion
      Altered vascular architecture/external compression: chronic renal disease, obstructive uropathy, atherosclerosis, pyelonephritis, osmolar diuresis
      Rheologic alterations of the blood: endotoxemia, severe dehydration, radiological contrast agents, sickle cell anemia, falciparum malaria
      Impaired nitrovasodilation: Aging, atherosclerosis, hypertension, pigment nephropathy, radiological contrast agents
      Impaired synthesis of prostaglandins: nonsteroidal antiinflammatory drugs
      Excessive endothelin induced vasoconstriction: cyclosporine, radiological contrast agents, regional hypoxemia

Source: Ref. 13, with permission.

volume depletion (heart failure, nephrotic syndrome, cirrhosis, and hypovolemia or hypotension of any cause) may predispose to hypoxic medullary damage, providing that regulatory mechanisms designed to maintain medullary oxygenation are defective. Preexisting renal disease results in hypertrophy and increased metabolic activity and oxygen requirement of the remaining tubuli. In addition, the renal microvasculature may be altered by the evolving structural changes. Gradual reduction of the nephron population with compensatory hypertrophy of remnent nephrons may predispose the aging kidney to hypoxic damage. Early diabetes and pregnancy are characterized by renal hypertrophy, enhanced GFR, and augmented tubular reabsorptive workload. Diabetes, as well as hypertension, congestive heart failure, and aging, are all associated with defective nitrovasodilation. Obstructive uropathy predispose to medullary hypoxic injury by the increase in interstitial pressure, which leads to diminished medullary flow. Increased blood viscosity may decrease medullary oxygen availability in patients with sickle cell disease, falciparum malaria, severe dehydration, polycythemia, and other hematological disorders. Hypercalcemia, hypokalemia, and hyperglycemia may enhance solute delivery to the distal nephron, resulting in augmented reabsorptive workload.

Various endogenous and exogenous nephrotoxins exert renal damage, solely or in part, through the induction of medullary hypoxia. Administration of NSAIDs or methyl-xanthines may inactivate protective systems that act through prostaglandins and adenosine. Medullary blood flow declines and hypoxia intensifies after the administration of indomethacin [20,22]. Heme pigments such as myoglobin reduce outer medullary blood flow and Po_2 [37], perhaps through binding with NO and inactivation of nitrovasodilation. Amphothericin induces profound renal vasoconstriction and, as previously discussed, enhances outer medullary metabolic activity. As a result, medullary hypoxia increases [38]. Cyclosporine and tacrolimus (FK-506) are also potent renal vasoconstrictors. Radiological contrast agents induce cortical vasoconstriction, but medullary blood flow increases, mediated by prostaglandins, NO [39], and perhaps endothelin-B stimulation. Both cortical and medullary Po_2 decrease after radiocontrast administration, the latter decreasing to values as low as 0 to 8 mm Hg [22] despite medullary vasodilation. This probably reflects an osmotic–diuretic effect with enhancement of solute delivery and reabsorptive workload at the distal nephron, insufficiently matched by increased oxygen supply. Endotoxin alters the renal microcirculation, eliminating the medullary vasodilatory response to hypotension [40]. Marked reduction of cortical and medullary blood flow is noted after repeated exposure to endotoxin, perhaps mediated, in part, by the formation of microthrombi and endothelin.

Thus, various medical conditions and nephrotoxins may compromise medullary oxygen balance through diverse mechanisms. Nevertheless, thanks to the regulatory systems previously discussed that maintain medullary oxygen sufficiency, healthy patients do not develop hypoxic ATN after a single insult, such as acute hypovolemia. In contrast, in most cases of ATN presented in the clinical practice, a combination of predisposing factors is present [41]. For example, patients with low cardiac output and intense vasoconstrictive stimuli are particularly prone to develop renal failure after administration of NSAIDs (some reduction in GFR may result from altered glomerular hemodynamics, but ATN may develop as well). Similarly, renal failure does not develop in healthy subjects after radiocontrast administration, whereas diabetes, pre-existing renal disease, effective volume depletion, aging, or the coadministration of NSAIDs are well-known risk factors [42]. In fact, the incidence of contrast nephropathy reaches 100% in elderly patients with $\geq$ four such risk factors [43].

IX. Animal Models of Acute Renal Failure with Hypoxic Outer Medullary Necrosis

Like humans, intact animals are resistant to a single insult directed to induce renal hypoxic injury. An in vivo model for outer medullary hypoxic damage was not available for a while because of the efficient protective mechanisms that maintain medullary oxygenation. For instance, healthy animals given huge volumes of radiological contrast agents maintained tubular integrity. In contrast, in concert with the principle of predisposing factors for ATN, inactivation of nitrovasodilation and prostaglandin synthesis during radiocontrast administration were found to render the outer medulla susceptible to hypoxic damage in vivo [39] (Fig. 7). Likewise, contrast-induced renal failure developed by preconditioning of the animals with manipulations known to affect medullary oxygen balance and to predispose to clinical contrast nephropathy [13], such as salt depletion, heart failure, exogenous angiotensin II, reduction of renal mass with compensatory hypertrophy of the remnant nephrons, or obstructive uropathy. Hypoxic damage was noted in all these experiments, selectively affecting mTALs in the outer medulla and tubular segments in the medullary rays, in an identical distribution and gradient pattern noted in the isolated perfused kidney. In the same fashion, amphothericin, cyclosporine, and tacrolimus nephropathies were intensified by salt depletion, and medullary hypoxic damage was reproduced in animals subjected to ureteral obstruction or myoglobin infusion after the inactivation of nitrovasodilation and prostaglandin

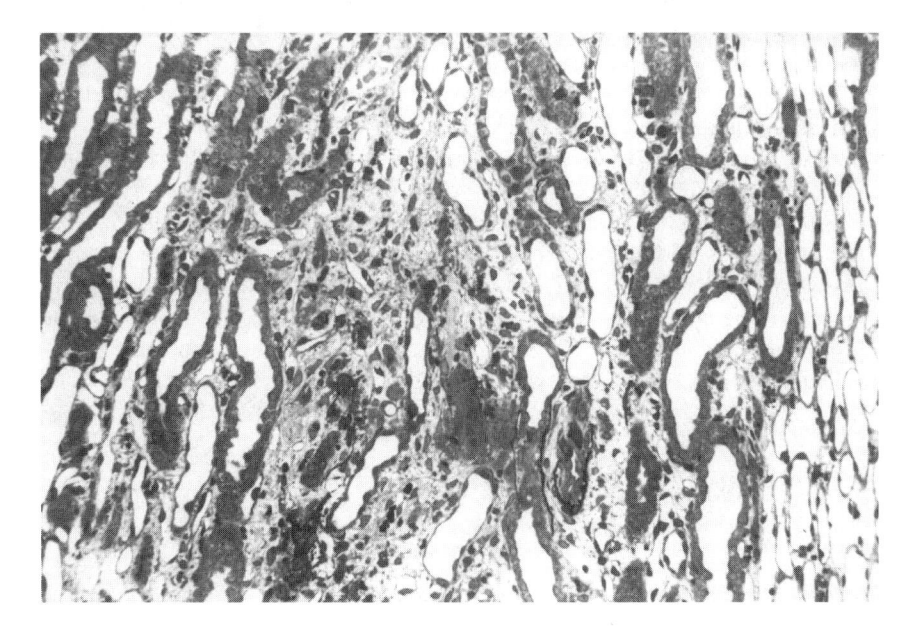

Figure 7 Outer medullary morphology in rat subjected to radiocontrast media after the administration of indomethacin and Nw-nitro-L-arginine methyl ester (L-NAME) (for the inhibition of prostaglandin and nitric oxide production). A vascular bundle is shown on the right. The midinterbundle zone is located in the center of the picture. Note a gradient of hypoxic tubular damage (with cell necrosis and cast formation), affecting mTALs in the midinterbundle zone. Tubules adjacent to the vascular bundles are spared.

synthesis [13]. Myoglobin infusion also resulted in hypoxic damage at the very superficial subcapsular cortex, another region deprived of oxygen [11].

X. Disparate Mechanisms for Hypoxic Injury in Different Nephron Segments

So far, we have discussed in depth the role of medullary hypoxia in distal ATN. Studies in the isolated perfused kidney indicate that various tubular segments differ in their response to hypoxia and metabolic inhibition. Although selective mTAL damage develops in oxygenated perfused kidneys, perfusion with hypoxic/anoxic medium results in both proximal and distal tubular injury. Metabolic inhibitors or repressors of mitochondrial respiration induce selective proximal tubular damage in the oxygenated perfused kidney, with preserved mTAL integrity [44]. Isolated proximal tubules also present a special vulnerability to hypoxic stress.

In the ischemia-reflow model of ATN in vivo, a transient clamping of the renal artery induces hypoxic damage in all animals, selectively affecting the proximal tubules, with its magnitude proportional to the length of the ischemic period [45]. The absence of distal tubular damage in this model and in isolated nonperfused kidneys seems to result from the total cessation of RBF, withholding tubular reabsorptive activity.

Thus, it seems that different sections of the nephron respond diversely to oxygen deprivation. Although proximal tubules are extremely sensitive to short-term anoxia, irrespective to metabolic workload (obligatory aerobic metabolism), mTALs resist hypoxic insult for a while, providing that reabsorptive activity ceases.

The ischemia-reflow model may mimic few clinical conditions, namely, the acute posttransplantation tubular injury and kidney failure after abdominal aortic surgery. Under such anoxic conditions, proximal tubular hypoxic damage may predominate. On the other hand, distal tubular hypoxic injury may be more common in most other clinical settings of toxic–hypoxic tubular damage, with altered renal microcirculation and hypoxia, but with ongoing reabsorptive workload in the distal nephron.

XI. Medullary Hypoxia and Chronic Tubulointerstitial Disease

Tubulointerstitial disease plays an important role in the progression of renal disease of any cause. As a matter of fact, tubulointerstitial changes were found to have a greater prognostic significance than glomerular changes even in primary glomerular diseases. Chronic or repeated hypoxic insults may induce tubular damage, either frank necrosis or enhancement of apoptosis. This results in tubular atrophy and interstitial expansion, the result of hypoxia-induced local release of various growth factors. Expanded interstitium and compensatory hypertrophy of remnant nephrons render them more susceptible to ongoing hypoxic stress [46]. In addition, glomerular pathology leads to a depletion of downstream regional microcirculation and oxygen availability.

Tubular atrophy and hypertrophy with interstitial expansion appear both in humans and in experimental models after chronic hypercalcemia or amphothericin or cyclosporine administration. Its distribution, predominantly in the corticomedullary junction and in medullary rays ("striped fibrosis"), suggests chronic hypoxic damage as the principal pathophysiological factor [12,13]. It is also conceivable that medullary hypoxia induces sickling and microvascular stagnation that leads to progressive medullary damage in sickle cell anemia. Outer medullary injury has also been suggested to precede papillary necrosis in obstructive and analgesic nephropathy [47], perhaps resulting from compromised vasa recta transversing the injured outer medulla [48].

Thus, hypoxic medullary damage seems to participate in various forms of chronic hypoxic and toxic nephropathies and to perpetuate tissue destruction once irreversible structural changes have taken place.

XII. Medullary Oxygen Balance and the Prevention/Treatment of Acute Tubular Necrosis

Because the reduction of GFR is a protective mechanism designed to refine medullary oxygenation, pharmacological interventions that enhance GFR may be potentially hazardous. This may explain why, despite preliminary reports, the attempts to augment GFR have consistently failed to improve the outcome of ATN in large-scale, well-controlled studies. This has occurred with dopamine and theophylline and now seems to occur with atrial natriuretic peptide and its analogs. From the medullary point of view, the decline in GFR is, in fact, a renal success in the restoration of medullary oxygenation that may not be intervened as long as it is required.

Diuretics have also been used to enhance urine production and to prevent tubular obstruction by inspissated debri. However, their use has generally failed to improve renal function and to reduce morbidity or mortality. Moreover, mannitol was shown to decrease medullary oxygenation [36], probably as the result of the osmotic effects that enhance solute delivery and reabsorptive workload at the distal nephron. In fact, mannitol in large doses was reported to reproduce ATN. Its only beneficial effect, shown in patients with crush syndrome, may be related to a reduction of muscle damage. On the other hand, furosemide improves medullary oxygenation [36] and cytochrome oxidation in the inner stripe of the outer medulla [15] by the inhibition of tubular reabsorption and oxygen requirement, and in the isolated perfused kidneys it prevents hypoxic damage [33,34]. In a rat model of contrast nephropathy, mTAL necrosis was abolished by furosemide [49]. However, thus far in clinical practice, loop diuretics failed to prevent radiocontrast-induced renal failure, and their use was associated with a significant decline in renal function [50], perhaps reflecting incomplete volume replacement with the addition of a prerenal component of azotemia [51]. Further studies are required to address the protective properties of loop diuretics supplemented with appropriate hydration.

Thus, currently, the only measures considered effective in the prevention of hypoxic ATN is the identification of patients at risk, correction of treatable risk factors such as volume depletion or the unnecessary use of NSAIDs, and avoidance of needless exposure to conditions that may endanger medullary oxygen availability.

XIII. Control of Erythropoietin Production: A Role for Renal Parenchymal Oxygen Insufficiency

The kidney is the major source of erythropoietin (Epo), the circulating hormone that regulates the rate of red blood cell production. It is an ideal candidate to govern the degree of oxygen-carrying capacity of the blood, given the peculiar intrarenal heterogeneity of oxygen availability. In situ hybridization studies have recently demonstrated that in the kidney, the *Epo* gene is expressed predominantly in cortical and outer medullary fibroblasts. The mechanisms by which *Epo* gene expression are regulated within these cells have been the subject of intensive research, recently reviewed in the February 1997 issue of *Kidney International* [52]. Renal anatomical integrity is required for the synthesis of Epo by these interstitial cells. By yet-undetermined mechanisms, they lose their capability to produce Epo after acute and chronic renal injury or when cultured ex vivo. Hypoxia and anemia stimulate renal Epo production, as shown experimentally in vivo during hypobaric hypoxia or after maneuvers that reduce red blood cell mass. These factors may counteract: for instance, in transfused animals, Epo response to hypoxia is blunted. Possibly, a minor change in oxygen availability as the consequence of changing hematocrit is sensed by the regulatory mechanisms that control Epo production. Alternatively, this could be related to a direct stimulatory effect of Epo on *Epo* gene expression. In addition, a cross-talk between Epo-sensitive cells in hematopoietic tissue and Epo-producing cells may also exist, modulating *Epo* expression. For instance, acute inhibition of hematopoiesis enhances Epo response to hypoxia, even at the absence of anemia.

The cellular oxygen sensing pathway is mediated, in part, by the induction of hypoxia-inducible factor-1, a protein complex that serves as an enhancer element, controlling a broad range of genes in response to hypoxia. Intracellular H_2O_2 and other reactive oxygen species could be the ultimate key signals for down-regulation of *Epo* gene expression.

In summary, despite high RBF and oxygen supply, physiological hypoxia exists at the outer medulla, the result of limited regional blood flow and high oxygen demand for solute reabsorption by mTALs. This is the price the mammalian kidney pays for the urinary-concentrating capability. Medullary hypoxia plays a pivotal role in the pathophysiology of acute and chronic renal failure, the consequence of failure of compound systems designed to maintain medullary oxygen sufficiency. From that perspective, the marked gradient of renal tissue oxygenation makes the renal interstitium a most appropriate sensor of oxygen availability for the control of red blood cell production.

References

1. Brezis M, Rosen S, Silva P, Epstein FH. Renal ischemia: a new perspective. Kidney Int 1984; 26:375–383.
2. Dwarkin LD, Brenner BM. The renal circulation. In: Brenner BM, Rector FC, eds. The Kidney, 4th edition. Philadelphia: WB Saunders Co. 1991, pp 164–204.
3. Bankir L, Bouby N, Trinh-Trang-Tan MM. Heterogeneity of nephron anatomy. Kidney Int 1987; 31(Suppl 20):S25–S39.
4. Jamison RL, Kritz W. Structure of the medulla as a whole. In: Urinary Concentration Mechanism: Structure and Function. New York: Oxford University Press, 1982, pp 55–76.
5. Pallone TL, Robertson CR, Jamison RL: Renal medullary microcirculation. Physiol Rev 1990; 70:885–920.
6. Aukland K, Crog J. Renal oxygen tension. Nature 1960; 188:671.
7. Leichtweiss HP, Lubbers DW, Weiss CH, Baumgartl H, Reschke W. The oxygen supply of the rat kidney: measurements of intrarenal P_{O_2}. Pflugers Arch 1969; 309:328–349.
8. Baumgartl H, Leichtweiss HP, Lubbers DW, Weiss CH, Huland H. The oxygen supply of the dog kidney: measurements of intrarenal P_{O_2}. Microvasc Res 1972; 4:247–257.
9. Leonhardt KO, Landes RR. Oxygen tension of the urine and renal structures: preliminary report of clinical findings. N Engl J Med 1963; 269:115–121.
10. Brezis M, Heyman SN, Dinur D, Epstein FH, Rosen S. Role of nitric oxide in renal medullary oxygen balance: studies in isolated and intact rat kidneys. J Clin Invest 1991; 88:390–395.
11. Schurek HJ, Jost U, Baumgartl H, Bertram H, Heckmann U. Evidence for a preglomerular oxygen diffusion shunt in the renal cortex. Am J Physiol 1990; 259:F910–F915.
12. Brezis M, Rosen S. Hypoxia of the renal medulla: its implications for disease. N Engl J Med 1995; 332:647–655.
13. Heyman SN, Fuchs S, Brezis M. The role of medullary ischemia in acute renal failure. New Horizons 1995; 3:597–607.
14. Epstein FH, Balaban RS, Ross BD. Redox state of cytochrome a,a3 in isolated perfused rat kidney. Am J Physiol 1982; 243:F356–F363.
15. Atkins JL, Lankford SP. Changes in cytochrome oxidation in outer stripe and inner stripe of the outer medulla. Am J Physiol 1991; 261:F849–F857.
16. Brezis M, Heyman SN, Epstein F. Determinants of intrarenal oxygenation: II: hemodynamic effects. Am J Physiol 1994; 267:F1063–F1062.

17. Gurbanov K, Rubinstein I, Hoffman A, Abassi Z, Better O, Winaver J. Differential regulation of renal regional blood flow by endothelin-1. Am J Physiol 1996; 271:F1166–F1172.
18. Agmon Y, Dinour D, Brezis M. Disparate effects of adenosine A1 and A2 receptor agonists on intrarenal blood flow. Am J Physiol 1993; 265:802–806.
19. Dinour D, Agmon Y, Brezis M. Adenosine: an emerging role in the control of renal medullary oxygenation. Exp Nephrol 1993; 1:152–157.
20. Agmon Y, Brezis M. Effects of nonsteroidal anti-inflamatory drugs upon intrarenal blood flow: selective medullary hypoperfusion. Exp Nephrol 1993; 1:357–363.
21. Lear S, Silva P, Kelley VE, Epstein FH. Prostaglandin E_2 inhibits oxygen consumption in rabbit medullary thick ascending limb. Am J Physiol 1990; 258:F1372–F1378.
22. Heyman SN, Brezis M, Epstein FH, Spokes K, Silva P, Rosen S. Early renal medullary hypoxic injury from radiocontrast and indomethacin. Kidney Int 1991; 40:632–642.
23. Komhoff M, Grone HJ, Klein T, Seyberth HW, Nusing RM. Localization of cyclooxygenase-1 and -2 in adult and fetal human kidney: implication for renal function. Am J Physiol 1997; 272:F460–F468.
24. Eriksen EF, Richelsen B, Gesser BP, Jacobsen NO, Stengraad-Pedersen K. Prostaglandin-E_2 receptors in the rat kidney: biochemical characterization and location. Kidney Int 1987; 32:181–186.
25. Kone BC, Baylis C. Biosynthesis and homeostatic roles of nitric oxide in the normal kidney. Am J Physiol 1997; 272:F561–F578.
26. Heyman SN, Karmeli F, Rachmilewitz D, Haj Yehia A, Brezis M. Intrarenal nitric oxide monitoring with a clark-type electrode: potential pitfalls. Kidney Int 1997; 51:1619–1623.
27. Heyman SN, Kaminski N, Brezis M. Dopamine increases medullary blood flow without improving regional hypoxia. Exp Nephrol 1995; 3:331–337.
28. Landes RG, Lillehei RC, Lindsay WG, Nocoloff DM. Free water clearence and the early recognition of acute renal insufficiency after cardiopulmonary bypass. Ann Thorac Surg 1976; 22:41–43.
29. Lucke B. Lower nephron nephrosis. Milit Surg 1946; 99:371–396.
30. Olsen TS, Hansen HE. Ultrastructure of medullary tubules in ischemic acute tubular necrosis and acute interstitial nephritis in man. APMIS 1990; 98:1139–1148.
31. Brezis M, Rosen S, Silva P, Epstein FH. Selective vulnerability of the medullary thick ascending limb to anoxia in isolated perfused rat kidney. J Clin Invest 1984; 73:182–190.
32. Beeri R, Symon Z, Brezis M, Ben Sasson SA, Baehr PH, Rosen S, Zager RA. Rapid DNA fragmentation from hypoxia along the thick ascending limb of rat kidneys. Kidney Int 1995; 47:1806–1810.
33. Brezis M, Rosen S, Silva P, Epstein FH. Transport activity modifies thick ascending limb damage in the isolated perfused kidney. Kidney Int 1984; 25:65–72.
34. Heyman SN, Rosen S, Epstein FH, Spokes K, Brezis M. Loop diuretics reduce hypoxic damage to proximal tubules of the isolated perfused rat kidney. Kidney Int 1994; 45:981–985.
35. Epstein FH, Silva P, Spokes K, Brezis M, Rosen S. Renal medullary Na-K-ATPase and hypoxic injury in perfused rat kidneys. Kidney Int 1989; 36:768–772.
36. Brezis M, Agmon Y, Epstein FH. Determinants of intrarenal oxygenation I: effects of diuretics. Am J Physiol 1994; 267:F1059–F1062.

37. Heyman SN, Rosen S, Fuchs S, Epstein FH, Brezis M. Myoglobinuric acute renal failure in the rat: a role for medullary hypoperfusion, hypoxia and tubular obstruction. J Am Soc Nephrol 1996; 7:1066–1074.
38. Brezis M, Heyman SN, Sugar AM. Reduced amphotericin toxicity in albumin vehicle. J Drug Targeting 1993; 1:185–189.
39. Agmon Y, Peleg H, Greenfeld Z, Rosen S, Brezis M. Nitric oxide and prostanoids protect the renal outer medulla from radiocontrast toxicity in the rat. J Clin Invest 1994; 94:1069–1075.
40. Heyman SN, Darmon D, Goldfarb M, Bitz H, Shima A, Rosen S, Brezis M. Endotoxin-induced renal failure. I. A role for altered renal microcirculation. Exp Nephrol 2000, in press.
41. Rasmussen HH, Ibels LS. Acute renal failure: multivariate analysis of causes and risk factors. Am J Med 1982; 73:211–218.
42. Brezis M, Epstein FH. A closer look at radiocontrast-induced nephropathy. New Engl J Med 1989; 320:179–181.
43. Rich MW, Crecelius CA. Incidence, risk factors and clinical course of acute renal insufficiency after cardiac catheterization in patients 70 years of age or older. Arch Intern Med 1990; 150:1237–1242.
44. Brezis M, Shanley P, Silva P, Spokes K, Epstein FH, Rosen S. Disparate mechanisms for hypoxic cell injury in different nephron segments: studies in isolated perfused rat kidney. J Clin Invest 1985; 76:1796–1806.
45. Glaubermann B, Trump BF. Studies on the pathogenesis of ischemic cell injury: III: morphological changes of the proximal pars recta tubule (P3) of the rat kidney made ischemic in vivo. Virchows Arch B 1975; 19:303–323.
46. Schrier RW, Shapiro JI, Chan L, Harris DC. Increased nephron oxygen consumption: potential role in progression of chronic renal failure. Am J Kidney Dis 1994; 23:176–182.
47. Eknoyan G, Qunibi WY, Grissom RT, Tuma SN, Ayus J. Renal papillary necrosis: an update. Medicine 1982; 61:55–73.
48. Heyman SN, Fuchs S, Yafe R, Beeri R, Elazarian L, Brezis M, Rosen S. Renal microcirculation and tissue damage during acute ureteral obstruction: the effect of saline infusion, indomethacin and radiocontrast. Kidney Int 1997; 51:653–663.
49. Heyman SN, Brezis M, Greenfeld Z, Rosen S. Protective role of furosemide and saline in radiocontrast-induced acute renal failure in the rat. Am J Kidney Dis 1989; 14:377–385.
50. Solomon R, Werner C, Mann D, D'Elia J, Silva P. Effects of saline, mannitol and furosemide on acute decreases in renal function induced by radiocontrast agents. N Engl J Med 1994; 331:1416–1420.
51. Weinstein JM, Heyman SN, Brezis M. Potential deleterious effect of furosemide in radiocontrast nephropathy. Nephron 1992; 62:413–415.
52. Bauer C, Kurtz A (eds). Forefronts in nephrology: oxygen sensing on the cellular and molecular levels. Kidney Int 1997; 51:371–590.

18

Pulmonary and Peripheral Gas Exchange During Exercise

DAVID C. POOLE and TIMOTHY I. MUSCH

Kansas State University
Manhattan, Kansas

I. Introduction

Dynamic physical exercise that engages a large muscle mass presents the most potent physiological challenge to the cardiopulmonary, vascular, and muscle oxygen (O_2) delivery/use systems. Pulmonary gas exchange is considered to represent the ultimate global manifestation of metabolic events in the periphery as transduced through a series of intervening structural and functional barriers. In this regard, the lung may be viewed as the servant of these peripheral metabolic requirements, but under some circumstances, it may govern them. Such circumstances include altitude (in health) and several forms of lung disease. This chapter synthesizes current knowledge regarding the coordinated functional response to exercise of systems that are key to the uptake, transport, and exchange of O_2. To illustrate the behavior of these systems, three exercise scenarios are considered: (1) The transient after an increase in metabolic demand; (2) constant-load exercise; and (3) incremental or ramp exercise. Traditionally, pulmonary gas exchange measurements have provided insights into muscle function with the tacit acknowledgment that intervening gas stores and transit delays likely distort the true underlying muscle response. Recent technological advances have permitted simultaneous measurement of pulmonary and muscle gas exchange and, therefore, show the true nature of the muscle metabolic response and the relationship between gas exchange events in the muscle and the lungs. Section II examines the temporal and quantitative relationships between gas exchange events across the lungs and exercising muscles. Section III briefly evaluates the bulk cardiovascular responses that provide the essential link between lung and muscle. In addition, the effect of exercise on blood flow redistribution from different organs to active skeletal muscle and within active skeletal muscle is considered. Section IV focuses on the role of structural and functional elements that impact the efficacy of O_2 exchange within the muscle capillary bed. Finally, Section V presents maximum O_2 uptake per unit time ($\dot{V}O_{2max}$) as the culmination of multiple convective and diffusive steps in the pathway for O_2 from the lungs to mitochondria. Within this context, the mechanistic bases for the reduced $\dot{V}O_{2max}$ found in chronic disease states is evaluated.

The purpose of this chapter is to present key features of the pulmonary/peripheral gas exchange responses to exercise and to examine potential sites of control and/or limitation. Emphasis is placed on recent experimental advances and how these extend or alter conventional standpoints. The reader is referred to excellent pertinent reviews and texts [1–19].

II. Pulmonary and Muscle Gas Exchange

A. Facets of the Pulmonary and Muscle Oxygen Uptake Response

Exercise Transient

At exercise onset or across the transition to a higher work rate, the rate of muscle adenosine triphosphate (ATP) splitting increases instantaneously. In contrast, it has long been established that pulmonary $\dot{V}O_2$ increases with finite kinetics [20]. Specifically, three phases of the $\dot{V}O_2$ response can be discriminated (Fig. 1). Phase 1 consists of an immediate, although quantitatively modest, increase in pulmonary $\dot{V}O_2$ primarily in response to an augmented pulmonary blood flow [21], with secondary contributions from a lowered mixed venous O_2 content [22] and altered lung gas stores [4]. The duration of phase 1 corresponds to the transit delay of venous blood from the exercising muscle to the lung (approximately 10–20 seconds). Upon arrival of this lowered O_2 content blood at the lung, phase 2 is initiated and $\dot{V}O_2$ increases monoexponentially with a time constant, τ_1, of 30–45 seconds to achieve a steady state, phase 3, within 3 minutes. Thus, for all moderate work rates, $\dot{V}O_2$ increases according to:

$$\dot{V}O_{2(t)} = \dot{V}O_{2(b)} + A_1(1 - e^{-(t-TD_1)/\tau 1}) \tag{1}$$

where $\dot{V}O_{2(t)}$ denotes $\dot{V}O_2$ at time t above the baseline, $\dot{V}O_{2(b)}$. A_1 is the increase of $\dot{V}O_2$ above $\dot{V}O_{2(b)}$ at steady state, and TD_1 represents the early delay-like feature that incorporates phase 1. For a given subject, τ_1 is invariant with work rate in the domain of moderate intensity exercise (i.e., below the lactate threshold, T_{lac},

Pulmonary/Peripheral Gas Exchange During Exercise 471

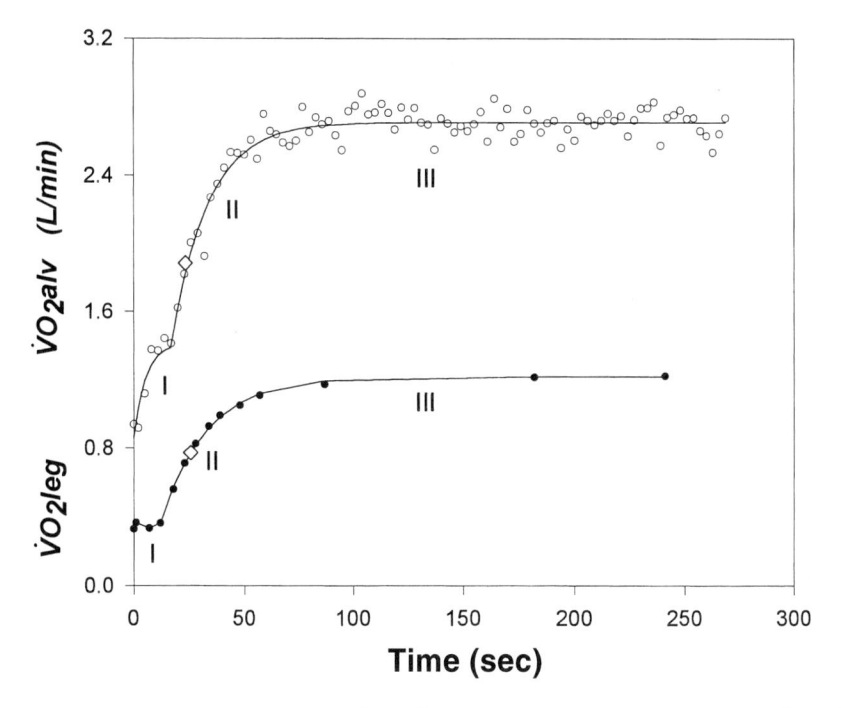

Figure 1 Response of muscle $\dot{V}O_2$ ($\dot{V}O_{2leg}$, solid symbols) and alveolar $\dot{V}O_2$ ($\dot{V}O_{2alv}$, hollow symbols) across the transition to moderate cycle exercise. Monoexponential functions are fitted to data points during phase 2. Open diamond denotes time necessary to reach 50% of difference between baseline and steady-state values. Note the close temporal correspondence between the two phase 2 profiles and also that $\dot{V}O_{2leg}$ does not increase appreciably for several seconds after exercise onset (phase 1) despite the augmented $\dot{V}O_{2alv}$. See text for further details. (From Ref. 26.)

[1,23]) but can be speeded by exercise training or alternatively markedly slowed by cardiopulmonary disease or inactivity [11]. Interestingly, these basic responses are not unique to humans. It has recently been demonstrated that the horse shows very similar $\dot{V}O_2$ transient responses at exercise onset, except that they are much faster [τ = approximately 10 seconds (24)]. Faster $\dot{V}O_2$ kinetics confer the distinct advantage of reducing the O_2 deficit (calculated as τ in minutes $\times$ A_1) incurred at exercise onset and constraining the degree of intracellular metabolic perturbation. This tighter metabolic control is thought to be important in reducing the reliance on expendable muscle glycogen stores while promoting fat metabolism during the course of the entire exercise bout [13].

Until very recently, insights into the control of skeletal muscle $\dot{V}O_2$ during the transient had relied principally on two indirect approaches: (1) mathematical models or extrapolations based on pulmonary or alveolar $\dot{V}O_2$ profiles; and (2) analysis of phosphocreatine breakdown at exercise onset using ^{31}P-nuclear magnetic resonance spectroscopy of mammalian muscle or biochemically in frog muscle during the recovery from exercise [1,25]. In 1996, Grassi et al. [26] measured the $\dot{V}O_2$ of the exercising leg (i.e., muscle $\dot{V}O_2$) simultaneously with pulmonary $\dot{V}O_2$ across the on-transient to moderate exercise. As seen in Figure 1, despite the interposition of transit delays and O_2 stores, the temporal correspondence between pulmonary and muscle $\dot{V}O_2$ is compelling. Although the muscle $\dot{V}O_2$ increase observed in phase 1 was either less pronounced than that for pulmonary $\dot{V}O_2$ or absent, the $\dot{V}O_2$ half times for all six subjects were remarkably similar (i.e., 25.5 seconds and 27.9 seconds for pulmonary and muscle $\dot{V}O_2$, respectively). These experiments substantiated findings in dog muscle and earlier claims in humans that the kinetic profile of muscle $\dot{V}O_2$ was reproduced faithfully at the mouth [1,26]. Moreover, because the exercising muscle is the predominant site of the augmented exercise $\dot{V}O_2$, both muscle and pulmonary $\dot{V}O_2$ increase with a gain of 9–11 mL/W/min, which gives a calculated delta work efficiency of approximately 30% and approximates closely that estimated based on cellular energetics considerations [1,27,28].

The mechanisms that limit $\dot{V}O_2$ kinetics at the transition to higher metabolic rates have not been unequivocally resolved. Some investigators have considered bulk muscle blood flow and O_2 delivery to constitute the limiting step [29]. Among the strongest evidence for this notion is the observation that supine exercise slows both cardiovascular and $\dot{V}O_2$ kinetics. In these same studies, lower-body negative pressure that should increase muscle blood flow speeded the kinetics toward normal [29]. What has not been adequately explained is how muscle $\dot{V}O_2$ kinetics can be limited by blood flow kinetics when the increase in cardiac output [30] and muscle blood flow precedes that of $\dot{V}O_2$ in most instances [26].

Furthermore, proponents of the blood flow limitation hypothesis have never demonstrated that speeding muscle blood flow improves $\dot{V}O_2$ kinetics in healthy individuals performing upright cycle ergometry. An opposing viewpoint considers that the site of the kinetic limitation for $\dot{V}O_2$ resides in the intracellular compartment, specifically, that inertia of muscle oxidative enzymes limits $\dot{V}O_2$ kinetics [1,6,7,26]. Some of the strongest evidence for an intramuscular limitation to $\dot{V}O_2$ kinetics comes from the measurements of leg blood flow and muscle O_2 extraction across the exercise transition [26]. As shown in Figure 2, after an increase in work rate, increased leg (predominantly muscle) O_2 delivery clearly precedes that of muscle $\dot{V}O_2$ such that the fractional O_2 extraction (arterial minus venous O_2 difference) actually decreases for the first 10–15 seconds. Although this evidence places the kinetic limitation to $\dot{V}O_2$ within the exercising muscle, as discussed by Grassi et al. [26], these studies cannot resolve definitively whether the ultimate mechanism for this limitation resides with some extracellular (microvascular blood flow distribution, red blood cell, [RBC]-O_2 offloading, capillary–myocyte O_2 exchange) or intracellular (mitochondrial) process. However, preliminary investigations using pump perfusion in the electrically stimulated dog gastrocnemius under control and adenosine vasodilated conditions suggest that the microvascular flow distribution

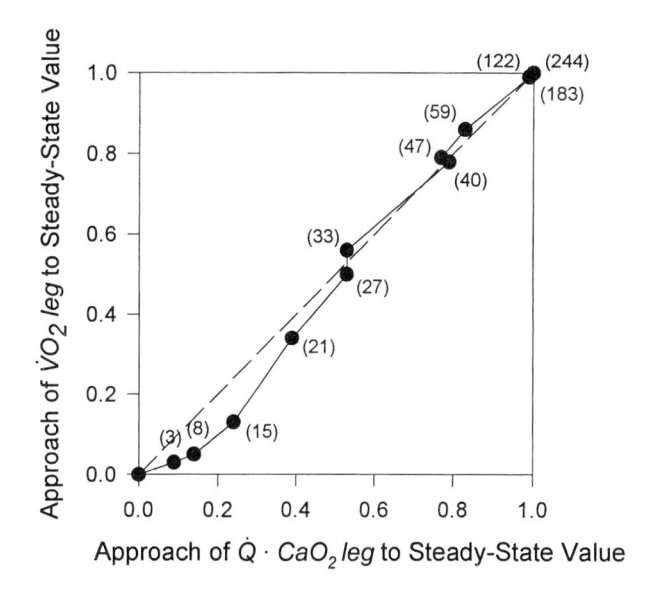

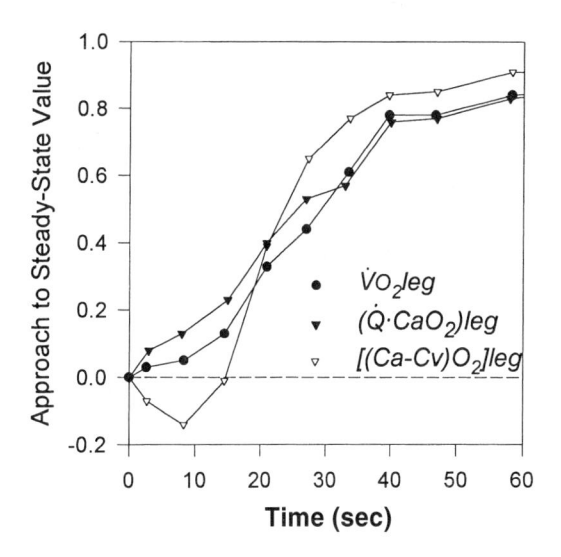

Figure 2 (Top) Group mean (n = 6) values for muscle $\dot{V}O_2$ ($\dot{V}O_{2leg}$) versus muscle O_2 delivery ($\dot{Q} \cdot CaO_{2leg}$). Data are normalized such that 0 = baseline and 1 = steady-state response. Numbers in parentheses correspond to elapsed time (in seconds) from exercise onset. Dashed line is line of identity. (Bottom) Mean (n = 6) temporal responses of $\dot{V}O_2$, O_2 delivery ($\dot{Q} \cdot CaO_{2leg}$), and O_2 extraction (Ca-CvO_{2leg}) across the exercising muscles during the transition to moderate exercise. Note that O_2 extraction actually decreases for 10–15 seconds after exercise onset. See text for further details. (From Ref. 26.)

might not limit $\dot{V}O_2$ kinetics at the onset of exercise [31]. Specifically, neither speeding the blood flow kinetics nor vasodilating the muscle significantly altered $\dot{V}O_2$ kinetics, thereby implicating an intracellular site for the limitation to $\dot{V}O_2$ kinetics.

As for $\dot{V}O_2$, carbon dioxide output ($\dot{V}CO_2$) kinetics in the moderate intensity domain can be well described by a delay function followed by a monoexponential increase to the steady state [analogous to Eq. (1)]. However, τ is appreciably longer (60–70 seconds), reflecting an increased CO_2 storage primarily in the muscle and venous blood compartments. In addition, the steady-state gain during moderate exercise will not simply be a function of the prevailing work rate (as for $\dot{V}O_2$), but also the respiratory exchange ratio (R). Typically, R becomes elevated at higher work rates and may increase further with the proportion of carbohydrate calories consumed before exercise [9].

Constant-Load Exercise

Three discrete domains of exercise intensity can be characterized with respect to their attendant $\dot{V}O_2$ and blood lactate responses (Fig. 3). As previously mentioned, the domain of moderate exercise incorporates the range of work rates that can be achieved without a sustained elevation of blood lactate (i.e., below the lactate threshold [T_{lac}]) and for which $\dot{V}O_2$ kinetics are well described by a monoexponential function [1,4,32]. The heavy exercise domain emerges at the lowest pulmonary $\dot{V}O_2$ at which blood lactate becomes elevated for the duration of the exercise bout. The upper limit to this domain is the highest $\dot{V}O_2$ at which blood lactate (and $\dot{V}O_2$) can be stabilized, reflecting a reestablishment of the equilibrium between lactate production and removal rates, albeit at an elevated level. Within the heavy exercise domain, the temporal profiles of blood lactate and $\dot{V}O_2$ are closely matched, and there are only very rare instances in which this coherence has been absent (4). Within the heavy exercise domain, $\dot{V}O_2$ kinetics become more complex, and 80–110 seconds after exercise onset, a secondary "slow component" of the $\dot{V}O_2$ response becomes superimposed on the rapid initial increase (or "fast component") associated with exercise onset [1,4,24,33]. Thus, in the heavy domain:

$$\dot{V}O_{2(t)} = \dot{V}O_{2(b)} + A_1(1 - e^{-(t-TD_1)/\tau 1}) + A_2(1 - e^{-(t-TD_2)/\tau 2}) \tag{2}$$

where A_2, TD_2, and τ_2 represent the asymptote, time delay, and time constant for the slow component, respectively. It should be mentioned that, in some individuals, τ_2 is impossibly long, suggesting a linear rather than exponential process. In most instances, τ for the fast component (τ_1) is slowed in the heavy exercise domain, and emergence of the slow component further delays achievement of the steady state [4,24]. It is crucial to appreciate that this slow component constitutes an additional or excess $\dot{V}O_2$ above that predicted from the sub-T_{lac} $\dot{V}O_2$–work rate relationship, resulting in an elevated $\dot{V}O_2$ per watt and a reduced work efficiency in this domain

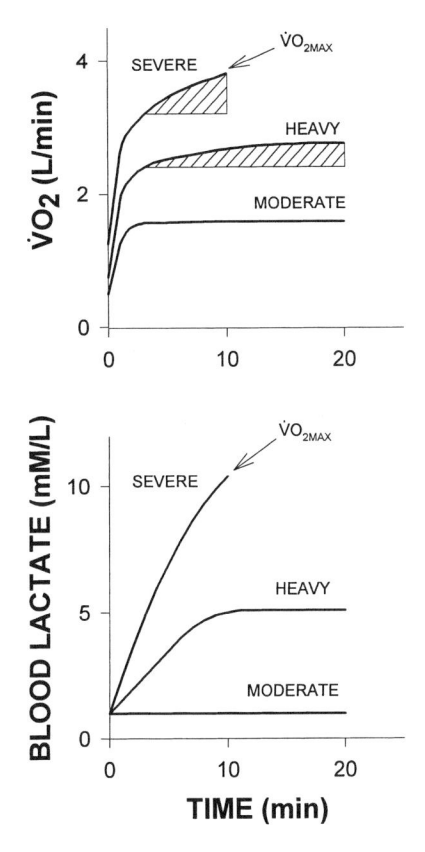

Figure 3 Schematic illustrating the response profiles of $\dot{V}O_2$ (top) and blood lactate (bottom) to constant-load exercise in the moderate, heavy, and severe domains. Hatched area corresponds to the $\dot{V}O_2$ slow component. Note that in the severe domain, $\dot{V}O_2$ slow component drives $\dot{V}O_2$ to its maximum ($\dot{V}O_{2max}$) at fatigue.

[1,33]. One surprising consequence of this behavior is that at a given absolute work rate, a fitter individual may show a lower $\dot{V}O_2$ than a less fit counterpart who invokes a large slow component [4,11].

All higher work rates (i.e., > heavy exercise) fall within the severe exercise domain, where both blood lactate and $\dot{V}O_2$ increase inevitably until the point of fatigue. At fatigue in the severe domain, the $\dot{V}O_2$ slow component drives pulmonary $\dot{V}O_2$ to its maximum (i.e., $\dot{V}O_{2max}$ [1,34,35]). It is remarkable that a disappearingly small difference in work rate (i.e., 5–10 W) can exert such drastic metabolic and performance consequences when it moves the individual from the heavy to the severe exercise domain. For instance, heavy exercise can be sustained for an extended period of time (e.g., up to 1–2 hours), and fatigue ensues when muscle glycogen reserves are ostensibly depleted [9]. In marked contrast, severe exercise fatigue occurs within a much more limited time frame (e.g., < 20 minutes) and is accompanied by a marked lactic acidosis and creatine phosphate depletion but with substantial glycogen reserves remaining in all but the type IIb fibers [4]. Within the severe exercise domain, the $\dot{V}O_2$ slow component may account for up to 1.5 L O_2/min and is immutably linked with the fatigue process. Despite the magnitude of this slow component and its association with the fatigue process, its precise etiology remains obscure. What is known is that it originates principally from within the exercising muscles (Fig. 4) [35], is facilitated approximately equally by augmented blood flow and O_2 extraction, and does not seem to be driven by the potentially calorigenic effects of either elevated catecholamines or blood lactate (4). There is solid evidence that quadriceps fiber-type composition correlates with features of both fast and slow components of the $\dot{V}O_2$ kinetics during cycle exercise [14]. Furthermore, the recruitment pattern of metabolically less-efficient type II fibers constitutes the most tenable explanation for slow component behavior. Unfortunately, direct evidence in the latter regard has yet to be forthcoming [4,14].

As previously mentioned, for exercise that engages a large muscle mass, the $\dot{V}O_2$ increase arising from within the exercising muscles overwhelms that from support processes such as increased cardiac and respiratory muscle work, hormonal perturbations (e.g., catecholamines), and augmented body temperature (Q_{10} effect) at sites removed from the exercising muscles. For example, although higher ventilations, do demand some additional $\dot{V}O_2$ cost [4], the effect of this is proportionally modest, and muscle $\dot{V}O_2$ increases as a percentage of pulmonary $\dot{V}O_2$ from approximately 70% for moderate to $\geq$80% in the heavy and severe intensity domains [35]. Furthermore, as exercise is continued at a given work rate in the severe exercise domain, the $\dot{V}O_2$ slow component becomes increasingly larger, reflecting a proportionally greater contribution of muscle energetic demands to the pulmonary $\dot{V}O_2$.

Incremental Exercise

The incremental exercise test, popularized most notably by Wasserman et al. [33], has provided a powerful physiological investigative tool for the understanding of human physiology and pathophysiology. For example, this test permits determination of work efficiency, lactate and ventilatory thresholds (T_{lac} and T_{vent}), $\dot{V}O_{2max}$, and the maximum exercising ventilation. As shown in Figure 5, when the work rate is increased in equal increments of 25–50 W/min to the limit of the subject's tolerance, after a brief lag the duration of which is determined by $\tau\dot{V}O_2$ (not shown), $\dot{V}O_2$ increases in a closely linear fashion up to $\dot{V}O_{2max}$ with a slope of 9–11 mL/W/min [1,3,28,33]. During tests with either smaller (< 25 W) or more prolonged (> 1 minute) work rate increments, $\dot{V}O_2$ loses its linear characteristic and becomes steeper at the supra-T_{lac} work rates as the slow component becomes

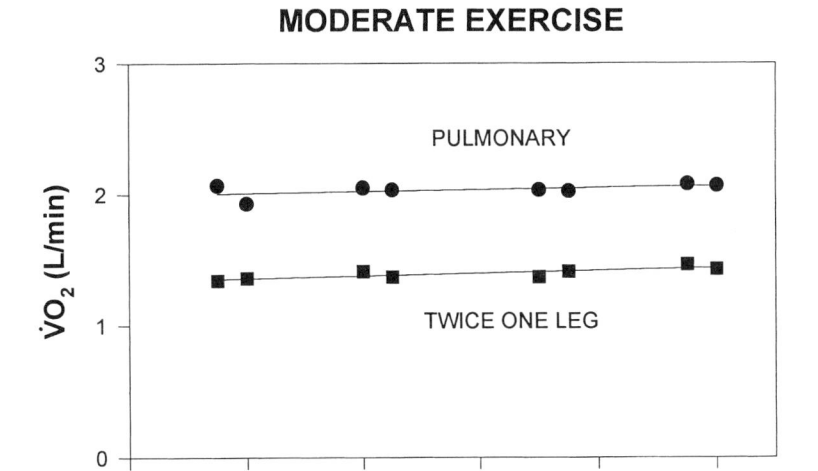

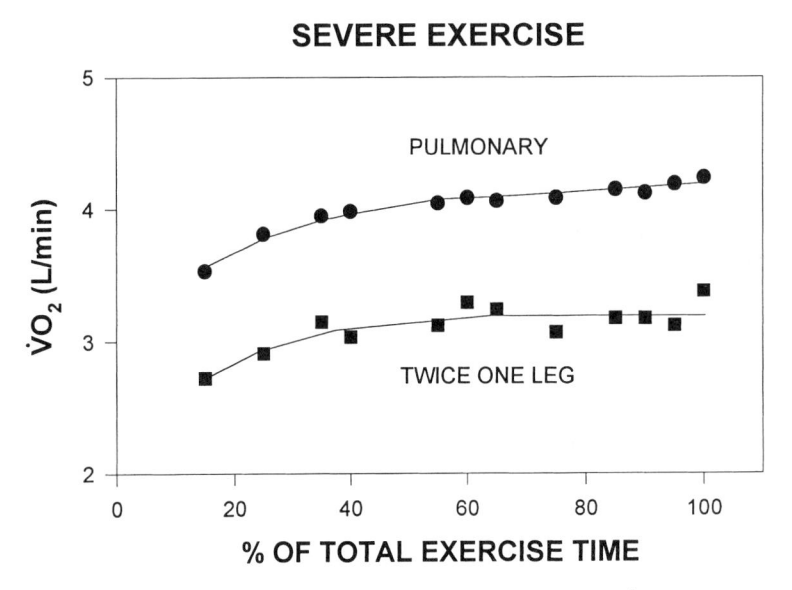

Figure 4 Mean response (n = 6) of pulmonary and muscle $\dot{V}O_2$ (twice one leg) to moderate (top) and severe (bottom) constant-load exercise. One hundred percent of exercise time represents 24 and 20.8 (fatigue) minutes for moderate and severe exercise, respectively. For severe exercise, exponential fits are plotted. Increase of muscle $\dot{V}O_2$ accounted for 86% of pulmonary $\dot{V}O_2$ increase beyond 15% exercise time (i.e., slow component). (From Ref. 35.)

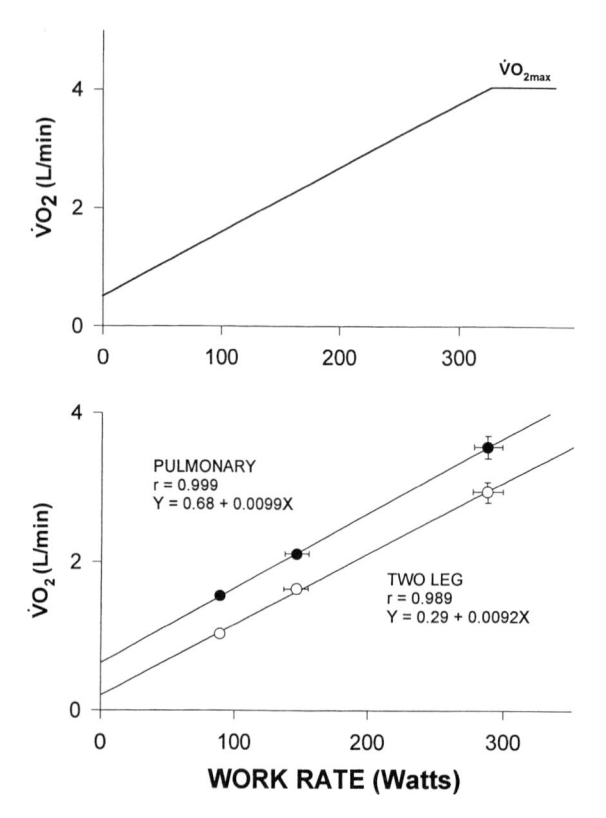

Figure 5 (Top) Schematic showing increase of pulmonary $\dot{V}O_2$ to $\dot{V}O_{2max}$ during rapidly incremented exercise testing protocol. (Bottom) Pulmonary and muscle (twice, one leg) $\dot{V}O_2$ during incremental exercise. Note close correspondence between the two slopes. (From Ref. 28.)

manifest [33]. When the testing protocol is designed to preclude development of the slow component, the linear pulmonary $\dot{V}O_2$ response reflects closely that occurring in the exercising muscles such that the slopes of these responses are not different (Fig. 5). Furthermore, for subjects in whom pulmonary $\dot{V}O_2$ "plateaus" at $\dot{V}O_{2max}$, this is associated with a leveling of muscle $\dot{V}O_2$ [36].

B. Pulmonary Ventilation

From rest to maximal exercise, expired ventilation ($\dot{V}E$) may increase more than 20-fold to achieve levels in excess of 100–140 L/min in healthy individuals. This is accomplished by an approximately sixfold increase in tidal volume (VT) to approximately 60% of vital capacity and a threefold increase in breathing frequency to 50–60 breaths/min (Fig. 6 [6,7,37]). The manner in which $\dot{V}E$ increases attempts

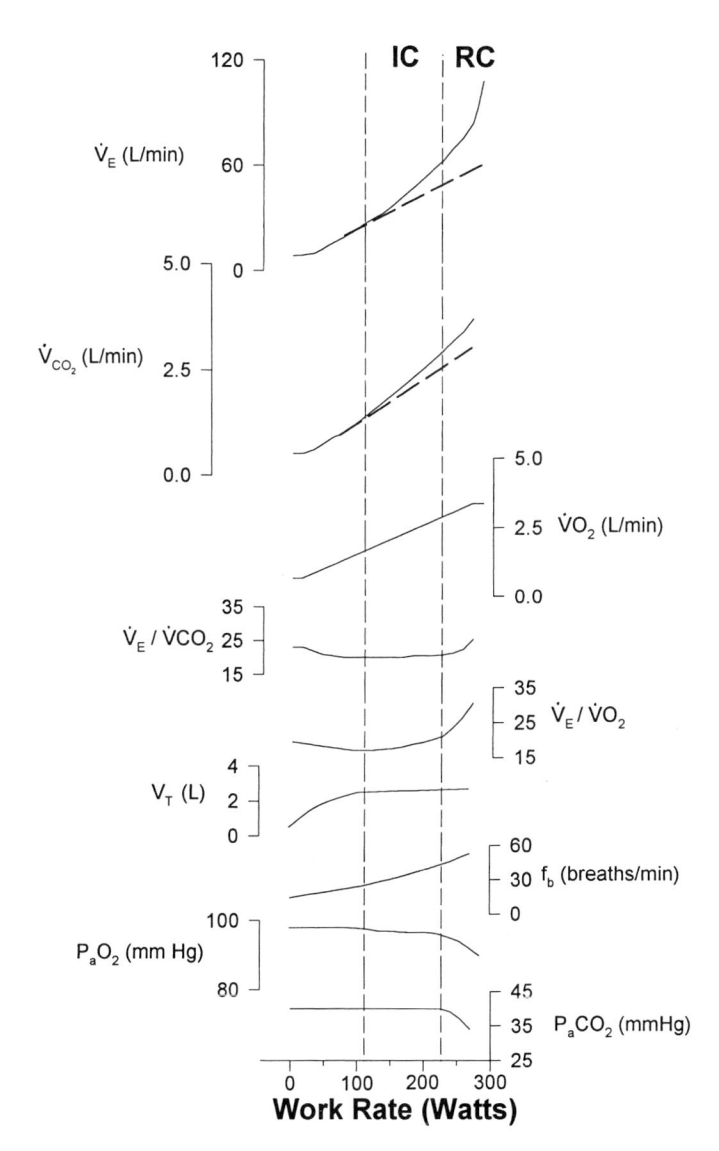

Figure 6 Ensemble responses of expired ventilation ($\dot{V}_E$), CO_2 output ($\dot{V}_{CO_2}$), $\dot{V}_{O_2}$, ventilatory equivalents for O_2 and CO_2 ($\dot{V}_E/\dot{V}_{O_2}$, $\dot{V}_E/\dot{V}_{CO_2}$), tidal volume (V_T), breathing frequency (f_b), and arterial P_{O_2} and P_{CO_2} (Pa_{O_2}, Pa_{CO_2}) to a rapidly incremented testing protocol. Left-most dashed vertical line is the ventilation threshold, and that to the right is the respiratory compensation (RC) threshold. Interposed region (IC) denotes isocapnic buffering.

to minimize dead space ventilation ($\dot{V}_D$) and work expended inflating and deflating the lung. Thus, at moderate work rates, $\dot{V}_E$ increases predominantly via augmented V_T, which reduces the proportion of each breath that is wasted in the non–gas exchanging regions of the lung (V_D/V_T). Above 40–60% $\dot{V}_{O_2max}$, further increases in V_T are limited, and $\dot{V}_E$ continues to increase almost entirely via breathing frequency [37]. This strategy limits the work performed on the lung by avoiding upper, less-steep regions of the pulmonary compliance curve where volume excursions are energetically more expensive.

The primary role of the exercise hyperpnea is to facilitate CO_2 removal rates of from approximately 0.2 L/min at rest up to 4–6 L/min during maximal exercise so as to maintain arterial blood gas and acid-base status. Across the range of achievable work rates, $\dot{V}_E$ increases according to the following relation [38]:

$$\dot{V}_E = 863 \ \dot{V}_{CO_2}/[P_aCO_2(1 - V_D/V_T)] \tag{3}$$

where 863 is the product of barometric pressure, temperature, and water vapor corrections needed to express $\dot{V}_E$ at BTPS (body temperature and pressure, saturated), $\dot{V}_{CO_2}$ at standard temperature and pressure, dry (STPD), and arterial CO_2 as a partial pressure (P_aCO_2). From this equation, the $\dot{V}_E$ requirement at any given level of exercise is defined by three factors: (1) $\dot{V}_{CO_2}$; (2) the level or ''set point'' at which P_aCO_2 is regulated; and (3) V_D/V_T.

At maximal exercise, $\dot{V}_E$ is only 50–60% of that achieved on a (typically) 15-second maximum voluntary ventilation test and uses only 50–60% of the maximum flow–volume loop. Such ventilations have been considered to be sustainable indefinitely [39]. That observation, coupled with the maintenance of arterial O_2 content and hypocapnia at maximal exercise, has strengthened the opinion that the respiratory sytem is unlikely to limit exercise tolerance in healthy humans. In marked contrast, recent evidence demonstrates that the diaphragm shows significant fatigue at high work rates [40], and that limb muscle blood flow (and thereby O_2 delivery) may be altered by varying the energetic demands placed on the inspiratory muscles [41]. Specifically, this very recent evidence indicates the highly oxidative respiratory muscles may subvert or ''steal'' blood flow that otherwise would support the nutritive requirements of the limb muscles during intense exercise. In addition, in highly trained athletes and certain females, arterial O_2 partial pressure (P_aO_2) and arterial O_2 saturation (S_aO_2) may decrease markedly during heavy exercise. The mechanisms for this decrease in P_aO_2 include mechanical limitation to $\dot{V}_E$ that constrains the increase in alveolar P_{O_2}, altered chemoresponsiveness, RBC transit time limitation in the pulmonary capillary [10,12,42], and possibly ventilation/perfusion mismatch [53].

Exercise Transient

Similar to that observed for $\dot{V}_{O_2}$, in the moderate intensity domain, the ventilatory response at exercise onset may be partitioned into three discrete phases. Phase 1 is initiated within the first breath after exercise onset (Fig. 7) and is associated with

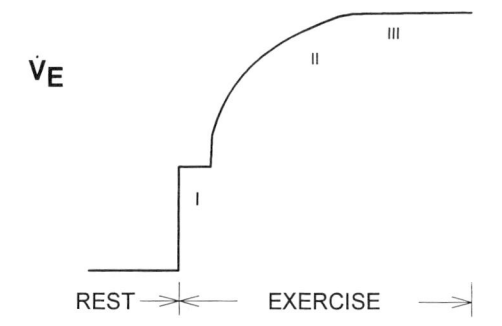

Figure 7 Response of pulmonary ventilation across the transition to moderate exercise. Phases 1, 2, and 3 are designated. See text for further details.

a decrease in functional residual capacity. At very low work rates, phase 1 may constitute the entire ventilatory response. However, at higher (although still sub-T_{lac}) work rates, a distinct phase 2 begins some 10–20 seconds after exercise onset, and $\dot{V}_E$ increases monoexponentially with $\tau = 60$–70 seconds to achieve the steady state, phase 3, within 4–5 minutes for moderate exercise. Consistent with the notion of feedforward "cardiodynamic hyperpnea" (i.e., the precise matching of $\dot{V}_E$ to pulmonary blood flow [21]) in phase 1, increases in $\dot{V}_{O_2}$ and $\dot{V}_{CO_2}$ are proportional to those of $\dot{V}_E$ such that R ($\dot{V}_{CO_2}/\dot{V}_{O_2}$) and the end-tidal P_{O_2} and P_{CO_2} ($P_{ET O_2}$ and $P_{ET CO_2}$) remain unaltered [2,5,21,33,38]. The more sluggish phase 2 $\dot{V}_{CO_2}$ kinetics (compared with $\dot{V}_{O_2}$) results from the greater solubility and thus storage of CO_2 in the tissues. One consequence of this is that R will decrease transiently in phase 2 before increasing to its steady-state level. As pulmonary blood flow and mixed venous P_{CO_2} increase, there is an augmented slope of the alveolar P_{CO_2} such that $P_{ET CO_2}$ increases in the face of a constant Pa_{CO_2} [2]. In phase 2, increases in $\dot{V}_{CO_2}$ precede those of $\dot{V}_E$ by a very few seconds [5,23], which may implicate some form of error signal in Pa_{CO_2} profile in the control of the exercise hyperpnea [2,5].

Constant-Load Exercise

In the moderate domain, $\dot{V}_E$ increases in proportion to $\dot{V}_{CO_2}$ to achieve a well-defined phase 3, and arterial CO_2 remains at resting levels [see Eq. (3)]. In contrast, for exercise in the heavy or severe domains, $\dot{V}_E$ continues to increase beyond the initial transient such that there is no clear phase 3. This occurs principally by means of an increased breathing frequency in accordance with the Hey relationship [37], and $P_{ET CO_2}$ decreases and $P_{ET O_2}$ increases [5,33]. Akin to the $\dot{V}_{O_2}$ response, there is a pronounced difference in the $\dot{V}_E$ behavior in response to heavy versus severe exercise. Thus, a "ventilatory threshold for long-term exercise" has been described [43]. Specifically, at heavy work rates given sufficient time, $\dot{V}_E$ seems to approach stable levels in contrast to severe exercise, where $\dot{V}_E$ continues to increase (and

Paco$_2$ to decrease) until fatigue ensues [4,5,43]. The precise control mechanisms for the ventilatory response to moderate, heavy, and severe exercise remain the topic of heated debate. What is clear is that in humans, Paco$_2$ and arterial pH are regulated at or very close to resting levels for moderate exercise, whereas in the heavy and severe domains, a marked lactic acidosis and compensatory hypocapnia become evident. The peripheral chemoreceptors or carotid bodies are thought to be important in determining the speed of the $\dot{V}$E kinetics during moderate exercise, and there is convincing evidence that these organs do play a major role in the ventilatory response to heavy and severe exercise, where they stimulate ventilation as a means of constraining the decrease in arterial pH [2,5]. In addition to their hypoxic sensitivity (which is probably not of great importance during exercise in healthy humans), the carotid bodies respond to alterations in arterial H$^+$, catecholamines, blood temperature, K$^+$, and blood osmolarity [2]. With the exception of K$^+$, each of these variables changes in a time-dependent fashion during heavy and severe exercise and, therefore, may contribute to the marked hypocapnia (Paco$_2$ as low as 25–30 mm Hg) found in these intensity domains [2,5].

Incremental Exercise

A progressive incremental increase in work rate to the maximum elicits a coordinated ensemble of ventilatory and gas exchange responses (Fig. 6 [1,3,5,38]). Within the moderate domain, $\dot{V}$E increases as a function of $\dot{V}$co$_2$ in a close-to-linear fashion with a slope of some 25–30 L/L (exact value dependent on work efficiency, R, Paco$_2$, and VD/VT ratio) as described in Eq. (3). As VT increases in the moderate domain, VD/VT decreases, which drives the ventilatory equivalents for O$_2$ and CO$_2$ ($\dot{V}$E/$\dot{V}$O$_2$, $\dot{V}$E/$\dot{V}$co$_2$) downward with increased work rate. In proximity to T$_{lac}$, there is an acceleration of $\dot{V}$E (T$_{vent}$, denoted by the left-most vertical dashed line in Fig. 6) consequent to the augmented $\dot{V}$co$_2$ derived from the bicarbonate buffering of H$^+$ originating from lactic acid. Because this CO$_2$ source is in addition to that produced by mitochondrial respiration, the rate of increase for $\dot{V}$co$_2$ accelerates, whereas that of $\dot{V}$o$_2$ remains constant. Thus, the ventilatory equivalent for O$_2$ ($\dot{V}$E/$\dot{V}$O$_2$) begins to increase as a hyperventilatory response is observed with respect to $\dot{V}$o$_2$. As $\dot{V}$E and $\dot{V}$co$_2$ increase proportionally in this region, Paco$_2$ remains constant, and VD/VT stabilizes [reflecting the switch to an increased breathing frequency rather than VT as a means to increase $\dot{V}$E (3,5,33,37)] with $\dot{V}$E/$\dot{V}$co$_2$ leveling off. This phenomenon has been termed *isocapnic buffering* (IC in Fig. 6) and is absent from more prolonged tests where the work rate increments are of ≥ 4 minutes. However, in tests with shorter work rate intervals, isocapnic buffering may last for up to several minutes. It has not been resolved why the carotid bodies do not respond to the reduced pH by driving down Paco$_2$ in this region. After the isocapnic buffering period, a clear respiratory compensation (RC in Fig. 6) occurs, with $\dot{V}$E increasing out of proportion to $\dot{V}$co$_2$ (start of the increased $\dot{V}$E/$\dot{V}$co$_2$), and, consequently, Paco$_2$ decreases to below its resting value.

Following their description of the gas exchange and metabolic responses to increased work rate [44], Wasserman et al. coined the term *anaerobic threshold*, which attempted to link the respiratory events at the mouth with those occurring in the active muscle. Subsequently, the principal tenets of this relationship have been challenged. In brief, although it is well accepted that any perturbation that either reduces muscle O_2 delivery or Pa_{O_2} increases the accumulation of blood lactate, it has yet to be convincingly demonstrated that exercising muscle becomes hypoxic or operates "anaerobically" at $\geq T_{vent}$. Indeed, Brooks [45] argued that an augmented intracellular lactate results simply from an accelerated rate of glycolysis and the high activity of lactate dehydrogenase coupled with an imbalance in the rates of lactate production and removal. Thus, a state of intracellular anaerobiosis is unnecessary. Moreover, Connett et al. [46] have been unable to demonstrate limiting intracellular P_{O_2} values even in muscle at $\dot{V}_{O_2max}$. Indeed, these investigators have proposed that lactate production in wholly aerobic muscle subserves an essential metabolic regulatory role and, therefore, should not be taken as an indication of obligatory lack of O_2. In this regard, the observations of Wilson et al. [47] may be insightful. Using a suspension of hepatocyte mitochondria, these investigators demonstrated that at given $\dot{V}_{O_2}$, there was an inverse relationship between P_{O_2} and adenosine diphosphate (ADP)/ATP ratio. Thus, in vivo it may be that the ADP/ATP ratio must increase to defend a given mitochondrial ATP flux in the face of a reduced intracellular P_{O_2}. An increased ADP/ATP ratio will stimulate glycolysis, and thereby lactate production, by disinhibition of the enzyme phosphofructokinase, which is a primary site for control of the glycolytic pathway. Accordingly, the term *anaerobic threshold* is considered by many to be a complete misnomer.

The linkage between elevated blood lactate levels and the ventilatory responses to incremental exercise has been challenged. There is no doubt that in humans and animals, the carotid bodies are stimulated by increased arterial H^+ and that this is a powerful ventilatory stimulus [2,5,38]. However, several groups have dissociated T_{vent} and T_{lac} by means of experimental interventions such as exercise training [48] or glycogen depletion [45,48]. In addition, the observation of a T_{vent} and consequent respiratory alkalosis in McArdle's patients who lack glycogen phosphorylase, and thus cannot produce lactate or the associated H^+ [49], has been used to discredit the ability to gain useful metabolic information from noninvasive respiratory measurements. However, it has been argued pointedly that severe muscle pain is pathognomonic to McArdle's patients on exercise and that this induces the hyperventilatory response in these individuals. The fact that normal subjects do not become hypocapnic after T_{vent} suggests that very different respiratory control mechanisms are operative in this particular pathology. How might the training and glycogen depletion–induced alteration/dissociation in T_{vent}–T_{lac} be explained? Traditional methods for detecting T_{vent} have relied ultimately on the ventilatory response (e.g., $\dot{V}_E$, $\dot{V}_E/\dot{V}_{O_2}$, $\dot{V}_E/\dot{V}_{CO_2}$), which itself is subject to much biological and measurement imprecision. To evoke any ventilatory nonlinearity, the rate (not absolute quantity) of arterial lactate, and thus H^+ accumulation and bicarbonate buffering, must be adequate to produce an increase in CO_2 evolution sufficient to stimulate (by some as-yet unresolved mechanism) a detectable ventilatory response, the magnitude and clarity of which is likely dependent on the sensitivity of the ventilatory control mechanisms and which may be obscured by breath-to-breath variability in ventilation. To circumvent these problems, Beaver et al. [50] developed the V-slope method for threshold detection. The V-slope relies solely on the relationship between $\dot{V}_{CO_2}$ and $\dot{V}_{O_2}$ and thus avoids problems associated with ventilatory sensitivity by detecting directly the extra CO_2 evolved from the bicarbonate buffering of H^+. During exercise, there is a plethora of potential humoral sources of carotid body stimulation during exercise [2,5]. Nevertheless, before any definitive conclusions can be reached regarding the fidelity of the T_{lac}–T_{vent} relationship, a reexamination of the training and glycogen-depletion studies using the V-slope method would be appropriate.

C. Pulmonary Gas Exchange

In a population of young, healthy individuals at rest, Pa_{O_2} typically varies between 90 and 100 mm Hg and Pa_{CO_2} between 35 and 40 mm Hg (Fig. 6 [6,51]). During exercise, Pa_{O_2} remains largely unchanged up to the heavy and severe exercise domains, at which point it may decrease slightly, although it usually remains greater than 90 mm Hg (Fig. 6). As depicted in Figure 6, Pa_{CO_2} decreases to below resting levels as the respiratory system hyperventilates to constrain the decreasing arterial pH consequent to the exercise-induced lactic acidosis. During constant-load exercise, this occurs for all work rates in the heavy and severe domains. However, the isocapnic buffering (IC) that follows T_{vent} during incremental exercise temporally delays the respiratory compensation (RC) for several minutes such that Pa_{CO_2} does not decrease until a work rate and $\dot{V}_{O_2}$ considerably greater than T_{vent}. In the extreme conditions present at maximal exercise, Pa_{CO_2} may decrease to ≤ 30 mm Hg.

At Pa_{O_2} values greater than 90 mm Hg, the slope of the O_2 dissociation curve is close to zero and thus, regardless of the rightward shift induced by increased blood temperature and H^+, no appreciable O_2 desaturation occurs. In contrast, as mentioned previously, this is not the case for some human or animal (horse, dog) athletes who develop arterial hypoxemia and a reduced respiratory compensation for the lactic acidosis at high work rates or running speeds [42]. This behavior has been attributed primarily to diffusion limitation secondary to extremely short mean pulmonary capillary RBC transit times. These individuals may also be mechanically limited in their ability to develop airway pressure and flow [52].

As demonstrated in Figure 8, alveolar–arterial P_{O_2} difference (A-aP_{O_2}), averages 5–11 mm Hg at rest and increases in a fairly systematic fashion above 30–40% $\dot{V}_{O_{2max}}$ to approximately 25 mm Hg in normal healthy males and even higher in athletes [6,7,42,51]. In the absence of hypoventilation, this exercise-induced A-aP_{O_2} increase may be attributed to some combination of ventilation/

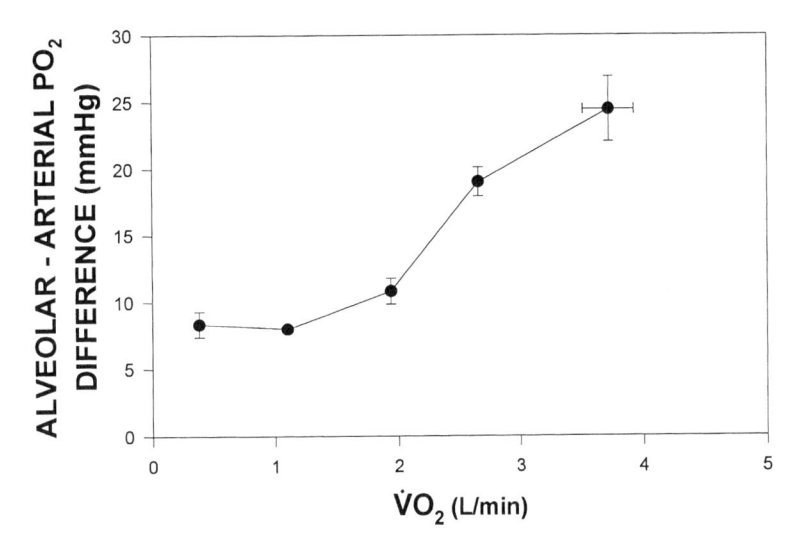

Figure 8 Alveolar–arterial P_{O_2} difference as a function of pulmonary $\dot{V}_{O_2}$. (From Ref. 51.)

perfusion ($\dot{V}_A/\dot{Q}$) mismatch, diffusion limitation, and postpulmonary shunt [6,7,42, 51,52]. Although not measurable directly, less than 1% of the cardiac output is considered to undergo postpulmonary shunting. This would reduce Pa_{O_2} by 3–7 mm Hg and increase A-aP_{O_2} by the same amount. Consistent with this small postpulmonary shunt, the multiple inert gas elimination technique has demonstrated that $\dot{V}_A/\dot{Q}$ mismatch and/or diffusion limitation are responsible for almost all of the A-aP_{O_2}. Approximately 50% of males examined do develop $\dot{V}_A/\dot{Q}$ mismatch, which becomes manifest in individuals with the most severe lactic acidosis and highest cardiac outputs [53]. Animal studies suggest that heavy/severe exercise can evoke subclinical pulmonary edema with peribronchial fluid accumulation and perivascular cuffing, which may lead to $\dot{V}_A/\dot{Q}$ mismatch [53]. Technical limitations preclude confirmation of this mechanistic basis for $\dot{V}_A/\dot{Q}$ mismatch in humans, whereas it is estimated to account for 5–10 mm Hg of the increased A-aP_{O_2} found in males at $\dot{V}_{O_2\text{max}}$ [51,53].

Under normoxic conditions, diffusion limitation is only apparent above a $\dot{V}_{O_2}$ of approximately 3 L/min. As discussed by Piiper and Scheid [54], the extent of diffusional disequilibration is governed by the ratio of diffusional (across the blood gas barrier [D_L]) to perfusional (pulmonary vasculature [$\beta\dot{Q}c$]) O_2 conductance. Thus:

$$(P_A - P_{c'})/(P_A - P\bar{v}) = e^{-D_L/\beta\dot{Q}c} \qquad (4)$$

where P_A, $P_{c'}$, and $P\bar{v}$ denote alveolar, end capillary, and mixed venous P_{O_2}, respectively. β is the slope of the O_2 dissociation curve in the physiologically relevant range. As exercise intensity increases, the ratio $D_L/\beta\dot{Q}c$ decreases primarily because from rest to $\dot{V}O_{2max}$, the proportional increase in D_L is only 30–50% that of the associated increase in $\dot{Q}c$ (Fig. 9). β also increases almost threefold since $CaO_2 - C\bar{v}O_2$ increases more than $PaO_2 - P\bar{v}O_2$. Thus, at $\dot{V}O_{2max}$, $D_L/\beta\dot{Q}$ decreases to approximately one sixth of its value at rest. Factors governing the increase in cardiac output, and thus $\dot{Q}c$ as a function of $\dot{V}O_2$, are described in Section III. D_L increases during exercise as a consequence of an augmented effective gas–blood contact surface, which results from a pressure-induced dilation of open and recruitment of additional, pulmonary capillaries. In addition, the exercise-induced increase of pulmonary artery pressure produces a more homogeneous vertical distribution of blood perfusion [6,7]. Also, in his recent review, Wagner [8] points out an often overlooked phenomenon related to capillary RBC transit time that probably contributes substantially to the increased D_L during exercise. Specifically, as at rest, RBCs become essentially fully O_2 saturated within the first third of their capillary transit and, thus, the remaining two thirds of available capillary length merely subsumes a conduit function. However, as $\dot{Q}c$ increases and RBC transit time decreases, an increasing proportion of the capillary length and surface area becomes recruited for gas exchange. This mechanism of increasing the gas-exchanging area does not depend on either vessel recruitment or distension per se.

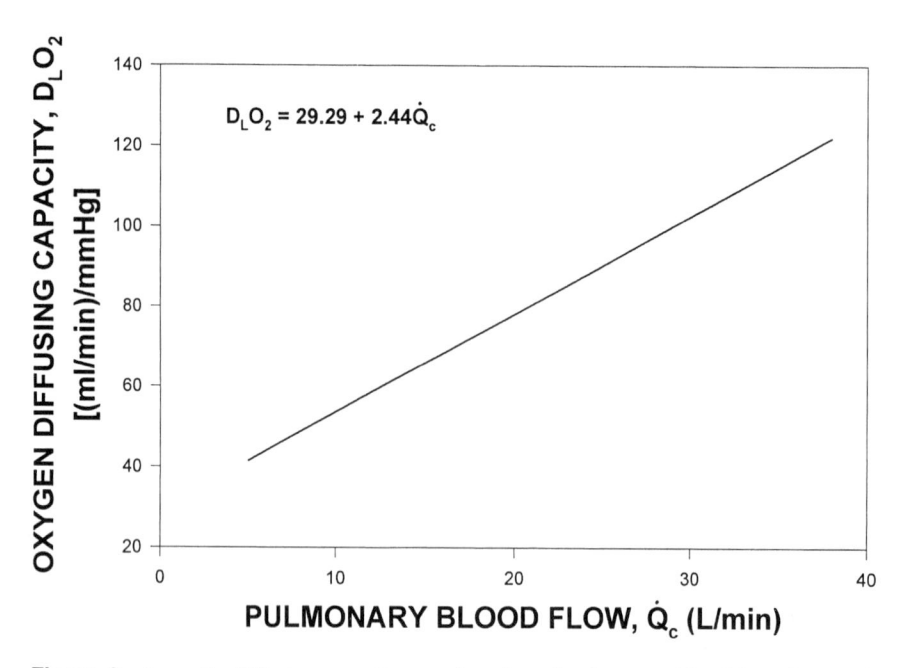

Figure 9 Lung O_2 diffusing capacity as a function of pulmonary blood flow. Regression line drawn from data compiled by Johnson et al. (51).

Compilation of the data from several different studies in Figure 9 indicates that there is an eightfold increase in $\dot{Q}c$ from rest to maximal $\dot{V}O_2$ compared with a threefold to fourfold elevation of D_L [51]. As a consequence of this behavior, pulmonary RBC capillary transit time becomes insufficient to permit equilibration between alveolar and end-capillary PO_2. Strong experimental evidence in humans and animals supports the notion that events within the capillary are important determinants of muscle diffusing capacity (DO_{2m}) as well. Specifically, increased systemic (and by assumption, capillary) hematocrit increases DO_{2m} [55,56], most likely via a combination of enhanced hemoglobin–O_2 offloading kinetics and increased effective capillary surface area (see Section IV). Thus, by extrapolation, gas exchange studies in muscles of exercising humans and dogs support the concept that pulmonary capillary hematocrit is likely to be of major importance in determining lung diffusing capacity (D_L) [57].

D. Blood Oxygen-Carrying Capacity

Plasma volume may decrease up to 20% during bouts of severe exercise [6,7,9,10] as the muscle concentration of osmotically active solutes increases and water is drawn from the vascular space. This effect is further exacerbated by elevated capillary luminal pressure and surface area. In addition, during prolonged bouts of moderate or heavy exercise, thermoregulatory requirements will lower circulating plasma volume. As shown in Figure 10, this effect increases the arterial O_2-carrying capacity, which effectively counteracts the slight decrease in percentage O_2 saturation that results from the rightward temperature- and H^+-induced shift in the O_2 dissociation curve and modest reduction in PaO_2 (see Fig. 6). The rightward-shifted O_2 dissociation curve is thought to be critical for enhancing O_2 offloading in the exercising muscle in the presence of a finite DO_{2m} [58], and as previously stated, does not effect any major deficit in O_2 loading in the lung in normal humans at sea level. However, in athletes or normal individuals at altitude in whom arterial O_2 desaturation occurs, and thus O_2 loading is confined to the steep portion of the dissociation curve, the exercise-induced rightward shift potentially is a double-edged sword. Namely, it facilitates O_2 off-loading in the muscle but acts to impair O_2 loading in the lung (see Sec. V).

Given the hemoconcentration and elevated plasma osmolarity that accompany severe exercise, it might be expected that RBC volume and, therefore, geometry might be affected. If so, this could have a major effect on the microrheological properties of blood and impact muscle capillary O_2 exchange. However, this is not the case, at least in humans. One remarkable feature of human blood is that after severe exercise in the face of an approximately 7% increase in osmolarity, mean corpuscular (RBC) volume, hemoglobin content, and water content are unchanged [59]. The implication of these findings is that during exercise, the human erythrocyte can increase its osmolarity equivalent to that of the plasma without permitting an alteration of volume.

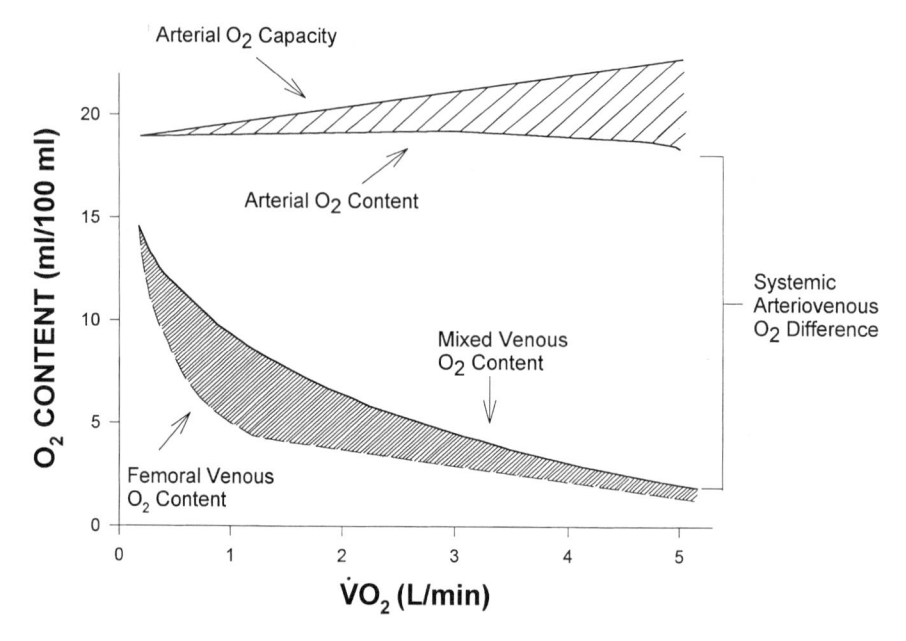

Figure 10 Schematic demonstrating profiles of arterial O_2 capacity and content and also mixed venous and femoral vein O_2 content as a function of pulmonary $\dot{V}O_2$. (From Ref. 10.)

III. Cardiovascular System

The cardiovascular system forms an integral conduit for O_2 and CO_2 between the lungs and peripheral tissues. The blood flow capacity of all skeletal muscles combined greatly exceeds the maximal cardiac output (maximum $\dot{Q}_{tot}$). Consequently, this $\dot{Q}_{tot}$ ceiling limits mass specific O_2 delivery when a large muscle mass is recruited during cycling or running exercise. Indeed, at maximal exercise levels, it is essential to maintain sufficient arteriolar vasoconstrictor tone in the active (as well as the inactive) muscles to prevent a catastrophic decrease in arterial blood pressure. To date, maximal muscle vasodilation, and thus maximal muscle vascular conductance has only been demonstrated in humans while performing single-leg knee extensor exercise that recruits approximately 2 kg of muscle [60]. This places the limitation to muscle O_2 delivery during cycling or running with the left ventricular pumping capacity rather than the muscles' capacity to accept the available blood flow. At exercise onset, $\dot{Q}_{tot}$ increases rapidly via an almost instantaneous heart rate response (latency < 0.5 seconds [61]) driven by parasympathetic withdrawal [10,62]. This heart rate increase is combined with an elevated stroke volume, resulting, in part, from mechanical compression of muscle veins ("muscle pump" [15]), which augments venous return and left ventricular end diastolic volume and recruits the Frank-Starling mechanism. Increased contractility, as evidenced by the increase in ejection fraction, also contributes to the elevated stroke volume. These feedforward cardiovascular responses precede those of muscle $\dot{V}O_2$ [10,26,63] such that in the first few seconds after exercise onset, increased $\dot{Q}_{tot}$ and pulmonary $\dot{V}O_2$ occur in the absence of altered muscle $\dot{V}O_2$ (Fig. 1) [26].

This section reviews briefly: (1) The relationship among $\dot{V}O_2$, $\dot{Q}_{tot}$, and O_2 extraction (a-$\bar{v}O_2$ difference), i.e., Fick equation; (2) the distribution of $\dot{Q}_{tot}$ among different organs during exercise; and (3) factors controlling blood flow and thus O_2 distribution within exercising skeletal muscle. Where pertinent, the effect of exercise training is used to illustrate the underlying control features.

A. Relationship Among Oxygen Uptake, Cardiac Output, and Oxygen Extraction

In all exercise intensity domains, $\dot{Q}_{tot}$ is coupled to pulmonary and muscle $\dot{V}O_2$ ($\dot{V}O_{2m}$) via the Fick equation:

$$\dot{V}O_2 = \dot{Q}_{tot}(\text{a-}\bar{v}O_2 \text{ difference}) \tag{5}$$

where $\dot{V}O_2$ and $\dot{Q}_{tot}$ are expressed in liters per minute and both a and $\bar{v}$ are expressed in liters O_2 per liter of blood flow, Q. During exercise, $\dot{Q}_{tot}$ increases from 5 to 6 L/min at rest to its maximal value of 15–25 L/min in healthy individuals (or possibly as high as 40 L/min in highly trained athletes) in a linear fashion with a slope of between 5 and 6 L/min $\dot{Q}$ per L/min pulmonary $\dot{V}O_2$, ($\dot{V}O_{2pul}$ [6,7,10,64]; Fig. 11). According to Eq. (5) and the proportionality between $\dot{Q}_{tot}$ and $\dot{V}O_{2pul}$, a-$\bar{v}O_2$ difference will increase (because of venous O_2 content decreasing) as a hyperbolic function of $\dot{V}O_2$ (Fig. 10) such that [64]:

$$\text{a-}\bar{v}O_2 \text{ difference} = 20\dot{V}O_{2pul} \cdot (1 + \dot{V}O_{2pul})^{-1} \tag{6}$$

where a-$\bar{v}O_2$ difference is expressed in milliliters O_2 per 100 ml blood and $\dot{V}O_{2pul}$ is expressed in liters per minute. The above proportionality is governed, in part, by the 5–6 L/min positive intercept for $\dot{Q}_{tot}$ (Fig. 11). When this relationship is determined empirically across the exercising muscles [11], the $\dot{Q}$ intercept is far lower (2.8 L/min) because it denotes leg $\dot{Q}$ rather than $\dot{Q}_{tot}$. In addition, the slope of $\dot{Q}$ becomes 5.3 L/min $\dot{Q}$ per L/min $\dot{V}O_{2m}$, and Eq. (6) becomes:

$$\text{a-v}O_2 \text{ difference} = 22\dot{V}O_{2m} \cdot (1 + \dot{V}O_{2m})^{-1} \tag{7}$$

with the a-vO_2 difference reflecting the O_2 content of the muscle effluent venous blood (which can decrease as low as 1–2 mL O_2/100 mL blood) rather than that of the so-called mixed venous blood returning to the lung from all body compartments as considered in Eq. (6) (Fig. 10).

Because $\dot{Q}_{tot}$ is the product of stroke volume and heart rate, and because maximum heart rate is primarily a function of age (i.e., 220-age), differences in maximum $\dot{Q}_{tot}$ among individuals derive from the variability in stroke volume

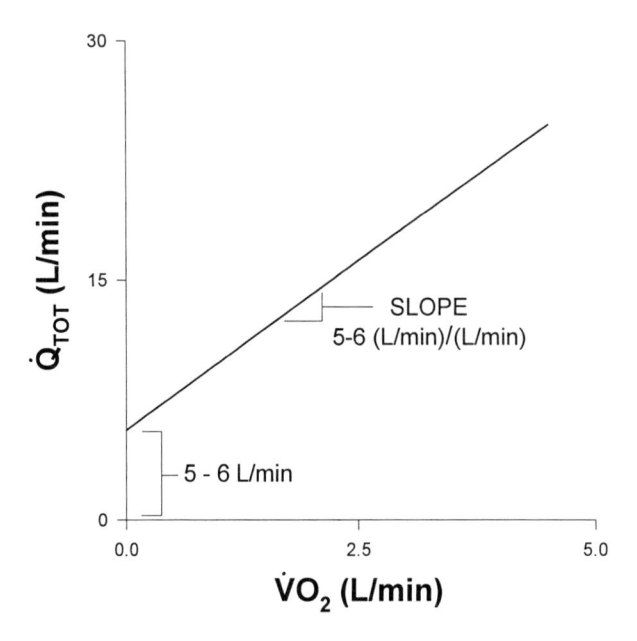

Figure 11 Schematic illustrating the relationship between pulmonary $\dot{V}O_2$ and cardiac output ($\dot{Q}_{tot}$).

found during maximum exercise. In addition, highly trained athletes achieve their impressive values of $\dot{Q}_{tot}$ via inordinately high stroke volumes (> 180 mL/beat). Whereas the aforementioned slope of $\dot{Q}_{tot}$ to $\dot{V}O_2$ is invariant among individuals, at any given work rate the size of the stroke volume will determine the heart rate response to submaximal exercise. Thus, individuals with a smaller stroke volume can only achieve a given $\dot{Q}_{tot}$ and, therefore, $\dot{V}O_2$ by elevating heart rate above that found in their fitter counterparts, who are endowed with a larger stroke volume.

B. Effect of Exercise on Cardiac Output Distribution Among Organs

Exercise induces a massive redistribution of $\dot{Q}_{tot}$, which ensures preferential perfusion of active skeletal muscle (up to 90% of $\dot{Q}_{tot}$ at $\dot{V}O_{2max}$) while preserving $\dot{Q}$ and O_2 delivery to essential organs such as the brain [10] (Table 1). This is effected largely via sympathetic vasoconstriction and is most pronounced in the splanchnic and renal vascular beds, where absolute $\dot{Q}$ is reduced 70–80% from rest to maximum exercise. In relative terms, this means that the %$\dot{Q}_{tot}$ that perfuses these organs is reduced from approximately 50% at rest to less than 3% during maximal exercise. Coronary $\dot{Q}$ is increased approximately fourfold to support the elevated energetic requirements associated with pumping the threefold to fivefold

Table 1 Blood Flow Expressed in Absolute Terms and as a Percentage of Cardiac Output ($\dot{Q}_{tot}$), and Oxygen Uptake ($\dot{V}_{O_2}$) for Each Organ at Rest and During Maximum Exercise

Region	Blood flow (mL/min) Rest	Blood flow (mL/min) Exercise	Cardiac output (%) Rest	Cardiac output (%) Exercise	Oxygen uptake (mL/min) Rest	Oxygen uptake (mL/min) Exercise
Splanchnic	1,500	350	27	1.4	60	60
Kidneys	1,200	360	22	1.4	14	10
Muscle						
Active	NA	21,840	NA	87.4	NA	3,931
Inactive	1,000	200	18	0.8	60	30
Brain	750	850	14	3.4	60	68
Skin	500	300	9	1.2	10	10
Coronary	250	1,000	5	4.0	35	140
Other	300	100	5	0.4	11	11
Total	5,500	25,000	100	100	250	4,260

NA, not available.
Source: Adapted from Ref. 10.

increase of $\dot{Q}_{tot}$. In addition, brain blood flow increases modestly, whereas that to the skin and other tissues is reduced. In absolute terms, however, organs that experience a reduced $\dot{Q}$ (i.e., splanchnic, kidneys, resting muscle, skin) increase their %O_2 extraction such that their $\dot{V}_{O_2}$ is unaffected. Not only is this vasoconstriction important for redirecting the elevated $\dot{Q}_{tot}$ to the exercising muscles, it also redistributes substantial blood volume away from the extremely compliant vascular beds of the skin and splanchnic organs [10].

C. Distribution of Blood Flow Within Exercising Skeletal Muscle

From Table 1, it is evident that a substantial heterogeneity of $\dot{Q}$ exists among different muscles and muscle groups depending on whether they are recruited during exercise. In the past two decades, microsphere measurements of muscle $\dot{Q}$ ($\dot{Q}_m$) at rest and during exercise in the rat and dog have shown considerable spatial and temporal $\dot{Q}$ heterogeneity within a given muscle [15,16,65]. In many instances, this $\dot{Q}$ heterogeneity has been considered synonymous with the inability of skeletal muscle to match effectively regional tissue metabolic requirements ($\dot{V}_{O_2req}$) with muscle O_2 delivery ($\dot{Q}_{O_2m}$). However, given the inhomogeneity of muscle structure (stratification/mozaic of fiber types and mitochondrial volumes, regional capillary-to-fiber geometrical variations) and function (fiber recruitment patterns, mechanical effects of muscle contractions and length excursions, vascular control mechanisms) within a given muscle, it would be both surprising and counterproductive to supply all muscle fibers and regions with the same $\dot{Q}O_2$. Despite directing more than 85% of $\dot{Q}_{tot}$ to active skeletal muscle at maximum exercise, the relationship between $\dot{Q}_{tot}$ and $\dot{V}O_2$ is maintained (Fig. 11), and muscle extraction peaks at 80–90% [36]. Under these conditions, it is inconceivable that substantial $\dot{V}O_{2req}/\dot{Q}O_{2m}$ heterogeneity persists. Therefore, the implication is that the regional differences in blood flow detected by microspheres are, in fact, a manifestation of local blood flow control to match $\dot{V}O_2$ to $\dot{Q}O_2$ within different areas of the muscle.

One situation in which there is the potential for $\dot{V}O_{2req}/\dot{Q}O_{2m}$ mismatch is at exercise onset. As mentioned in Section II, muscle O_2 extraction actually decreases for 10–15 seconds after the initiation of exercise [26]. One potential mechanism for this response is that at exercise onset, the muscle pump or other "feed forward" mechanisms rapidly increase whole-muscle $\dot{Q}_m$, whereas mechanisms responsible for $\dot{V}O_{2req}/\dot{Q}O_{2m}$ matching depend on some type of metabolic feedback from the recruited muscle fibers, which has a finite delay. Thus, early-on nonrecruited fibers may be overperfused and extract little of the available O_2, causing venous effluent PO_2 and O_2 content to increase. As exercise progresses, metabolic feedback processes fine tune $\dot{V}O_{2req}/\dot{Q}O_{2m}$ matching, and O_2 extraction increases (see Figs. 1 and 2).

There exists a plethora of mechanical, neural, and humoral mechanisms that function to augment and distribute muscle $\dot{Q}_m$ during exercise. These operate at multiple levels ranging from the level of the whole muscle (muscle pump [15,16,66]) down to that of a single-capillary module and its associated muscle fibers [67]. In addition, the rapidity of onset varies greatly from instantaneous with muscle contraction (muscle pump, neurotransmitter release) to that observed after creation and diffusion of vasoactive metabolites from contracting muscle fibers. The remainder of this section considers the potential role of each mechanism to effect $\dot{V}O_{2req}/\dot{Q}O_{2m}$ matching during exercise based on its potency and spatial (extent of vascular bed affected) and temporal (rapidity of response) characteristics.

Muscle Pump

The muscle pump mechanism refers to the mechanical interaction between the relaxing muscle mass and the venous vasculature. Specifically, during rhythmic exercise, muscle contraction partially collapses the venular vessels and impedes flow. On muscle relaxation, the vessel lumen is expanded, forcing intraluminal pressure to plummet. This mechanism increases the arteriovenous pressure differential and, thus, $\dot{Q}_m$ is augmented in the absence of large increases in mean arterial pressure. The majority of the instantaneous increase in $\dot{Q}_m$ at exercise onset (< 5 seconds) is thought to be attributable to this pumping action [15,16,66], the magnitude of which is determined by the degree of muscle activation, as expected [66]. Because the muscle pump effect occurs on a whole-muscle basis and is relatively independent of arterial vascular tone [15,16], there is great potential to create or exacerbate

$\dot{V}_{O_2req}/\dot{Q}_{O_2m}$ mismatch. This is especially true because the $\dot{V}_{O_2req}$ is likely to be extremely heterogeneous throughout the muscle [15,16,19].

Thus, the muscle pump provides a mechanism for rapidly and uniformly increasing $\dot{Q}_m$ (and $\dot{Q}_{O_2m}$) accepting that in some regions where $\dot{V}_{O_2req}$ is low, this will lead to an overabundance of $\dot{Q}_{O_2m}$, causing O_2 extraction to decrease. This mechanism may well account for the reduced O_2 extraction found across human muscle at exercise onset [26] (Fig. 2). Subsequently, neural and/or metabolic feedback systems engage and help resolve the $\dot{V}_{O_2req}/\dot{Q}_{O_2m}$ mismatch, thereby allowing whole-muscle O_2 extraction to increase rapidly.

Skeletal Muscle and Vascular Coactivation

Release of the neurotransmitter acetylcholine at the neuromuscular junction may induce both muscle contraction and a vasodilation of the feed arteries and arterioles [68]. This "feed forward" mechanism has the potential to augment regional $\dot{Q}_m$ within approximately 5 seconds in proportion to the degree of muscle contraction, and thereby presents an attractive mechanism for rapidly matching $\dot{Q}_{O_2m}$ to $\dot{V}_{O_2req}$. Welsh and Segal [68] demonstrated that this mechanism was sufficiently potent to account for up to 60% of the total hyperemic response. What remains uncertain, however, is how coactivation of muscle contraction with the vascular tree vasodilation might be integrated with the muscle pump at the whole-muscle level. One current challenge to help answer this question is to develop an intravital microscopy preparation that facilitates direct microvascular observation under contractile conditions necessary to recruit the muscle pump.

Endothelial Factors

The role of endothelial-derived relaxing factors in the exercise hyperemic response has not been unequivocally resolved. It is known that increases in shear stress acting on the arteriolar endothelium will result in the release of endothelial-derived nitric oxide and prostaglandins, which ultimately induces smooth muscle relaxation and vasodilation [69]. Accordingly, increases in shear stress produced by the rapid increases in $\dot{Q}_m$ by either the muscle pump and/or acetylcholine-mediated vasodilation at exercise onset could potentiate the increase of $\dot{Q}_m$. However, it is important to recognize that this mechanism is secondary in nature. Furthermore, if it potentiates the $\dot{Q}_m$ increase resulting from the muscle pump (and therefore perfuses both active and nonrecruited muscle fibers irrespective of their $\dot{V}_{O_2req}$), such vasodilation will further augment $\dot{V}_{O_2req}/\dot{Q}_{O_2m}$ mismatch. In contrast, the acetylcholine-mediated vasodilation would induce a secondary increase in $\dot{Q}_m$ spatially synchronous with $\dot{V}_{O_2req}$. The latter scenario would be expected to enhance $\dot{V}_{O_2req}/\dot{Q}_{O_2m}$ matching and reverse the earlier reduction in O_2 extraction found close to exercise onset. The initial lag followed by the rapid increase in O_2 extraction at exercise onset demonstrated in Figures 1 and 2 is consistent with an early $\dot{Q}_m$ increase with poor $\dot{V}_{O_2req}/\dot{Q}_{O_2m}$ matching preceding further increases in

$\dot{Q}_m$ and subsequently improved $\dot{V}O_{2req}/\dot{Q}O_{2m}$ matching that facilitates the observed augmentation of O_2 extraction after approximately 15 seconds of exercise.

Metabolic Control

The tight association between $\dot{Q}O_{2m}$ and $\dot{V}O_{2m}$ presents a compelling case for muscle metabolism ultimately controlling $\dot{Q}O_{2m}$ [10,15,19,28,36,70] (Fig. 11). Moreover, the notion that exercise-induced metabolites can provide a negative feedback vasodilatory stimulus that is graded both spatially and in intensity is attractive. However, this requires that the signal somehow travel upstream to the resistance arterioles, whereas the vasoactive substances themselves are flushed downstream via the capillaries and venular network. To this end, Kurjiaka and Segal [71] demonstrated that a cell-to-cell propagated vasodilation can occur along the arteriolar wall for several millimeters, encompassing multiple vessel branch orders (see also Duling and Dora [19]. Furthermore, this propagated vasodilation can originate from within the capillaries of a single "capillary module" in response to stimulation of the adjacent muscle fibers in an "exercise-intensity"–dependent fashion [67,72].

In addition to this upstream propagation, there are responses that may arise from the venous circulation per se. For example, this may occur via the outward diffusion of vasoactive metabolites from the venules to adjacent upstream arterioles [73,74]. The potential efficacy of this mechanism is facilitated by the anatomical proximity of the resistance arterioles to the effluent venules. Moreover, on the issue of venous control, Groebe [75] has proposed a well-defined servo-control of upstream arteriolar vascular control that is initiated by venular dilation and that does not depend on the spatial relationship between the arteriole and venule. Thus, the reduction of postcapillary resistance will decrease capillary hydrostatic pressure and increase $\dot{Q}_m$ in upstream arterioles, thereby initiating shear stress-induced vasodilation, which potentiates the initial response. Both of these mechanisms can potentially reduce $\dot{V}O_{2req}/\dot{Q}O_{2m}$ mismatch after the onset of exercise.

Whether metabolic rate and metabolic feedback mechanisms possibly related to the release of metabolites or other vasoactive substances (e.g., CO_2, H^+, K^+) constitute the primary determinants of $\dot{Q}_m$ in exercising whole muscle at pulmonary $\dot{V}O_{2max}$ can be challenged using the following rationale. Previous studies have shown that maximal $\dot{Q}_m$ to the functionally isolated leg extensors approaches 400 mL/min/100 g [60,70]. For this exercise paradigm, the recruited muscle mass is so small (approximately 2.3 kg) that $\dot{Q}_{tot}$ cannot be the limiting factor to $\dot{Q}_m$, and thus local features (i.e., vascular structure, muscle pump, neural, metabolic) constitute the primary determinants of the hyperemic response. In contrast, if a sufficiently large muscle mass (approximately 15 kg) is engaged (e.g., during conventional cycle ergometry), the vasodilatory capacity of the recruited muscle by far outstrips maximal $\dot{Q}_{tot}$. Under these conditions, neural reflexes and sympathetic activation constrain the whole-muscle hyperemic response to prevent a catastrophic decrease in arterial blood pressure. Under these circumstances, one could argue that the sympathetic nervous system represents the primary determinant of $\dot{Q}_m$ in exercising skeletal muscle because it provides a governor that overides any locally released vasodilatory stimuli. There is also the question as to whether metabolic feedback mechanisms are sufficiently fast to account for the rapid increase in $\dot{Q}_m$ at exercise onset [10,15,16,66]. In this regard, proposed metabolic feedback mechanisms are relatively slow, requiring at least 20 seconds to take effect. This supports the notion that the role of metabolic feedback processes is one of fine regional tuning rather than that of primary control of flow to the muscle as a whole.

One worthy challenge that faces physiologists today is defining the the quantitative importance of each vasodilatory mechanism previously addressed within the context of unhindered physiological function.

IV. Muscle Microcirculation

As previously discussed, the transport of O_2 from the atmosphere to the electron transport chain located on the mitochondrial inner membranes depends on the integrated function of convective (ventilation, circulation) and diffusive (lung, muscle tissue) O_2 transport. Ultimately, the number of respiratory complexes and the sum of their combined turnover rates will determine the rate of O_2 use. At submaximal exercise levels, beyond the initial transient at exercise onset, $\dot{V}_{O_2pul}$ and $\dot{V}_{O_2m}$ are set primarily by the work rate (see Sec. II). Specifically, if arterial blood O_2 content (CaO_2) is either reduced (e.g., by inspiratory hypoxia or reduced hematocrit) or increased (e.g., by inspiratory hyperoxia or increased hematocrit), muscle blood flow is adjusted so as to maintain O_2 delivery ($\dot{Q}_{O_2m}$) and $\dot{V}_{O_2}$ constant. In contrast, at maximal exercise levels, $\dot{V}_{O_2pul}$ and $\dot{V}_{O_2m}$ are exquisitely sensitive to alterations in CaO_2 and $\dot{Q}_{O_2m}$. Thus, $\dot{V}_{O_2max}$ is increased or decreased by increasing or decreasing CaO_2 and, therefore, $\dot{Q}_{O_2m}$ [12,76,77]. There is compelling evidence that during maximal cycling exercise which recruits a large muscle mass, the increase of $\dot{Q}_m$ is constrained by the $\dot{Q}_{tot}$ (and resultant $\dot{Q}_m$) ceiling. This becomes obvious when comparing mass-specific $\dot{Q}_m$ and $\dot{V}_{O_2}$ during maximal cycle ergometry [36], which recruits approximately 15 kg of muscle with values achieved during leg extensor exercise, which recruits only approximately 2.3 kg of muscle (see Section III [70,78]). The observation that muscle $\dot{V}_{O_2max}$ varies in proportion to $\dot{Q}_{O_2m}$ in animals and humans has for many years diverted attention away from the actual processes of O_2 exchange within the muscle microcirculation. However, it is intuitively and empirically obvious that muscle O_2 diffusing capacity (D_{O_2m}) cannot be infinite and, thus, effluent venous P_{O_2} will not decrease to zero [12,77]. According to the Fick equation, $\dot{V}_{O_2m}$ is the product of $\dot{Q}_m$ and arterial minus venous O_2 content:

$$\dot{V}_{O_2m} = \dot{Q}_m(CaO_2 - C\bar{v}O_2) \tag{8}$$

Because the transfer of O_2 from the RBC to muscle mitochondria is a diffusional process, it is more instructive to consider $\dot{V}O_{2m}$ as a function of DO_{2m} and the PO_2 differential between the RBC (mean capillary PO_2 [$P_{cap}O_2$]) and the mitochondrial sink ($P_{mit}O_2$):

$$\dot{V}O_{2m} = DO_{2m}(P_{cap}O_2 - P_{mit}O_2) \tag{9}$$

$P_{cap}O_2$ may be obtained from measurements of arterial and effluent venous blood gases and $\dot{Q}_m$ using a stepwise Bohr integration procedure [79]. During maximal exercise, $P_{mit}O_2$ may be considered as zero with little error [17,77]. From the above relationship, it is apparent that DO_{2m} is a major determinant of muscle O_2 extraction and, thus, $\dot{V}O_{2m}$. However, it is important to recognize that DO_{2m} and $\dot{Q}_m$ are interdependent variables such that [12,77,79]:

$$\dot{V}O_{2m} = \dot{Q}O_{2m}(1 - e^{-DO_{2m}/\beta \dot{Q}_m}) \tag{10}$$

where β is the slope of the O_2 dissociation curve in the physiological range. Thus, O_2 extraction will be dependent on the ratio of $DO_{2m}/\dot{Q}_m$ rather than their individual levels:

$$\dot{V}O_{2m}/\dot{Q}O_{2m} = \text{fractional } O_2 \text{ extraction} = 1 - e^{-DO_{2m}/\beta \dot{Q}_m} \tag{11}$$

Consequently, extraction cannot be considered simply as a "peripheral parameter" because of its dependence on $\beta \dot{Q}$ as well as DO_{2m}, i.e., both central and peripheral components.

DO_{2m} may be considered to represent an apparent muscle O_2 diffusing capacity, which is a composite of up to four discrete processes [77]: (1) the total O_2 diffusional conductance between hemoglobin and mitochondria; (2) functional (rather than structural) shunting of arterial blood into the venous effluent; (3) diffusional shunting of O_2 from arterioles and capillaries to venules; and (4) O_2 requirement to O_2 delivery ($\dot{V}O_{2req}/\dot{Q}O_{2m}$) inequality.

There is little or no experimental evidence to suggest that significant functional or diffusional O_2 shunting (no. 2 and 3 above) occurs in exercising muscle. By elimination, therefore, muscle O_2 diffusional conductance (no. 1) and $\dot{V}O_{2req}/\dot{Q}O_{2m}$ inequality (no. 4) determine DO_{2m} and, thus, O_2 extraction at any given $\dot{Q}_m$. The overall importance of $\dot{V}O_{2req}/\dot{Q}O_{2m}$ inequality remains uncertain because of technical limitations in measuring both $\dot{V}O_{2req}$ and $\dot{Q}O_{2m}$ simultaneously with the required temporal and spatial resolution (i.e., seconds and individual capillary/capillary module and motor unit). If techniques such as phosphorescence quenching, cryomicrospectroscopy, and magnetic reasonance spectroscopy can be refined sufficiently, they may permit elucidation of the contribution of $\dot{V}O_{2req}/\dot{Q}O_{2m}$ mismatch to DO_{2m}. Using microspheres (rest and exercising muscle) and intravital (resting muscle) observations of the muscle microcirculation, it is apparent that substantial heterogeneity of $\dot{Q}O_2$ does exist among individual capillaries, capillary modules, and discrete tissue regions. However, this may reflect different metabolic demands (i.e., $\dot{V}O_{2req}$) among regions sampled. Notwithstanding the inability to quantify the magnitude of any $\dot{V}_{O_{2req}}/\dot{Q}_{O_{2m}}$ inequality, the presence of myoglobin within oxidative muscle fibers likely minimizes intercellular and intracellular P_{O_2} gradients [17], and local vasoregulatory processes redistribute $\dot{Q}_{O_{2m}}$ according to the local $\dot{V}_{O_{2req}}$. An elegant series of experiments by Hogan et al. [55] and Wagner et al. [12,77] have demonstrated that $D_{O_{2m}}$ is extremely sensitive to intracapillary manipulations such as altered hemoglobin–O_2 binding properties and also hemoglobin concentration. For example, altering blood hemoglobin–O_2 affinity in the electrically stimulated dog gastrocnemius muscle changes $\dot{V}_{O_{2max}}$ in accordance with predictions based on a diffusion-limited system [77]. These findings limit the potential importance of $\dot{V}_{O_{2req}}/\dot{Q}_{O_{2m}}$ inequality in setting muscle O_2 diffusional properties, i.e., $D_{O_{2m}}$ at least beyond the transient at exercise onset.

From rest to maximal exercise, $D_{O_{2m}}$ and $\dot{Q}_m$ increase 50- to 100-fold. Section III dealt with the increase of $\dot{Q}_m$ and its intramuscular distribution. The bulk of Section IV is devoted to consideration of the structural and functional determinants of $D_{O_{2m}}$ and the mechanistic basis for its increase during exercise and after training.

A. Determinants of Muscle Oxygen Diffusing Capacity

The pathway for O_2 from the RBC in the capillary to the mitochondrial cytochromes is comprised of the following sequential steps (Fig. 12): (1) chemical dissociation of O_2 from hemoglobin; (2) diffusion from the RBC across the plasma to the capillary endothelium; (3) diffusion across the capillary endothelium, extravascular space, and sarcolemma (steps 2 and 3 constitute the "carrier-free region" described by Honig et al. [17]); (4) intramyocyte diffusion from sarcolemma to mitochondria; and (5) transmitochondrial membrane diffusion. At $\dot{V}_{O_{2max}}$, the P_{O_2} decrease between hemoglobin and plasma is considered to be small (< 4 mm Hg [80]) compared with the precipitous decrease (up to 80 mm Hg depending on RBC distance traveled down capillary and $\dot{V}_{O_{2req}}/\dot{Q}_{O_{2m}}$ ratio) across that short distance (2–3 μm) between hemoglobin in the RBC and the immediately subsarcolemmal cytoplasmic space. As a consequence, intramyocyte P_{O_2} is low (1–3 mm Hg) and also extremely uniform throughout the transverse and longitudinal expanse of the myocyte, with any P_{O_2} gradients being extremely modest (< 3 mm Hg) despite the potentially long diffusion distances (Figs. 12 and 13) [17]. These low intracellular P_{O_2} values are not thought to limit mitochondrial oxidative function because of the very small (approximately 0.2 mm Hg) cytosol-to-cytochrome P_{O_2} decrease and the ability of the cytochromes to operate maximally at P_{O_2} values less than 1 mm Hg [81]. The potential importance of myoglobin for facilitating intracellular O_2 transport is well recognized, and one component of this might be the inherent mobility of myoglobin among intracellular sites [77]. An additional consideration is that, particularly at high mitochondrial volume densities, the mitochondrial system itself forms a catenated network that may enhance intracellular O_2 and high-energy phosphate transport [77].

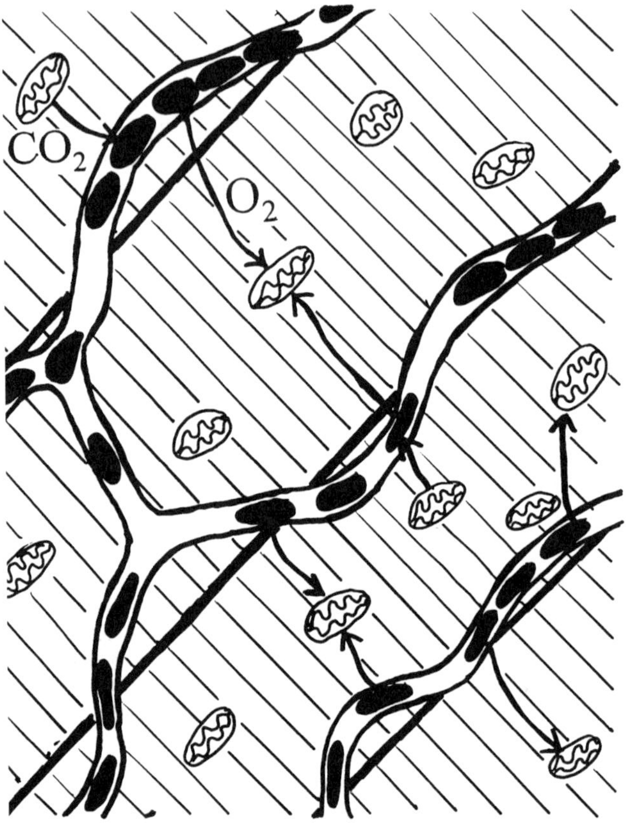

Figure 12 Schematic representation of muscle fibers and associated capillaries illustrating the pathway for O_2 and CO_2 between the red blood cells (RBCs) and mitochondria in skeletal muscle. Note that capillaries show tortuosity and branching, and there is great variability in capillary diameter and RBC spacing within and among capillaries. In addition, the physical distance for O_2 movement from RBC to myocyte sarcolemma is often far less than the intramyocyte distance from the sarcolemma to the mitochondrial matrix. As discussed in the text, the principal resistance to O_2 diffusion seems to reside in that very short physical distance between the RBC and the intracellular matrix.

The measurements of Honig et al. [17], which demonstrate very low intramyocyte P_{O_2} values, are supported by theoretical estimations [82] and nuclear magnetic spectroscopy measurements of similarly low myoglobin saturations in the human quadriceps at $\dot{V}_{O_2 max}$ [83]. All of these approaches lead to the inescapable conclusion that the vast majority of the muscle O_2 diffusional resistance resides within very few microns of the RBC, and myocyte P_{O_2} is independent of intramyocyte diffusion distance, i.e., fiber cross-sectional area and mitochondrial distribution.

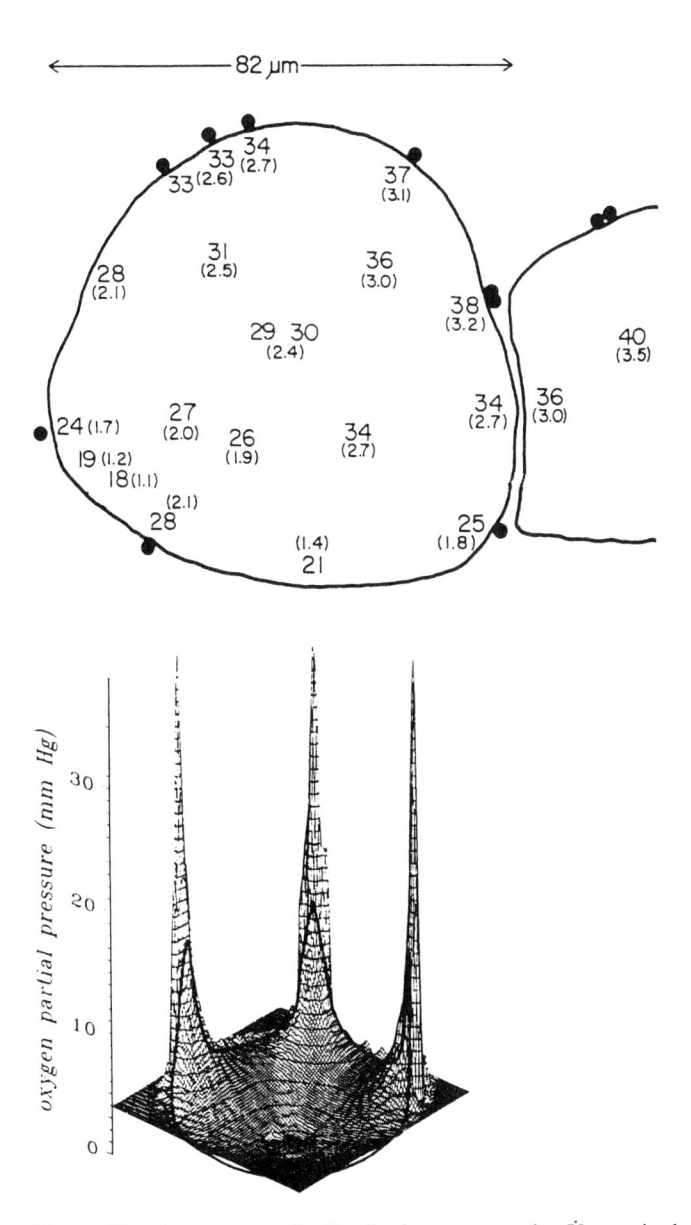

Figure 13 Intramyocyte O_2 distributions measured at $\dot{V}_{O_2max}$ in dog gracilis. (Top) Solid circles indicate RBC-containing capillaries. Numbers indicate myoglobin saturation with (parentheses) myoglobin P_{O_2}. (Bottom) P_{O_2} contours at intervals of 1 mm Hg. (From Ref. 17.)

This realization has forced a marked rethinking of what structural and functional attributes of skeletal muscle are most important for facilitating blood–tissue O_2 exchange. In addition, the concept of O_2 flux density developed by Honig et al. [17] is instructive because it enables a quantitative partitioning of the aforementioned diffusive steps in the O_2 pathway from hemoglobin to cytochrome oxidase. Specifically, because the net O_2 flux across the capillary and mitochondrial membranes is the same, but the aggregate surface area of the external mitochondrial membranes is two to three orders of magnitude greater than that capillary surface area available for O_2 exchange, the O_2 flux density and, thus, the transcapillary Po_2 decrease must be correspondingly larger. Thus, all evidence suggests that the pericapillary region is of paramount importance in setting Do_{2m}.

Structure: Muscle Capillary and Fiber Geometry

The capillary bed represents the principal location for blood–tissue O_2 exchange and, as previously discussed, is the site of the greatest intramuscular O_2 flux density. Thus, alterations in capillary geometry and surface area available for O_2 exchange have great potential to alter Do_{2m}. Within the last 10 to 15 years, the work of Mathieu-Costello et al. [84,85] and other investigators [86] has demonstrated that capillaries cannot be considered simply as straight, unbranched structures running parallel to the muscle fibers (Figs. 12 and 14). Rather, capillaries have a range of different luminal diameters (i.e., 2–8 μm; mean, 4–6 μm) and show a complex geometry with tortuosity and branching components that add substantially to capillary length and surface area and which may affect flow patterns and transit times within the capillary bed. Traditional descriptors of capillarity, such as capillary density (capillary number per fiber area) and capillary-to-fiber ratio (capillary number per fiber number), cannot account for these important geometrical features of the capillary bed. Central to the description and quantification of muscle capillarity is the realization that skeletal muscle operates over a discrete range of sarcomere lengths. Because alterations of sarcomere length within and among muscles can profoundly change measured muscle cross-sectional area and capillary density, tortuosity, length, and luminal diameter, it is essential that these variables be normalized with respect to sarcomere length [85].

If the primary purpose of the capillary bed is to facilitate O_2 (and CO_2) exchange, it is intuitively reasonable that its size be matched to the size of the mitochondrial O_2 sink. Accordingly, in humans, quadriceps capillary-to-fiber ratio is highly correlated with pulmonary $\dot{V}o_{2max}$ [13], and in perfusion-fixed animal muscles, capillary length per fiber volume is correlated with the oxidative capacity of that muscle [87]. However, given the plethora of capillary bed descriptors, there has been some confusion regarding which is the best or most appropriate descriptor to quantify the O_2 exchange potential of the capillary bed. To this end, Mathieu-Costello et al. [85] pioneered the concept of capillary surface per fiber surface as a structural measurement of capillary exchange potential. Irrespective of muscle fiber

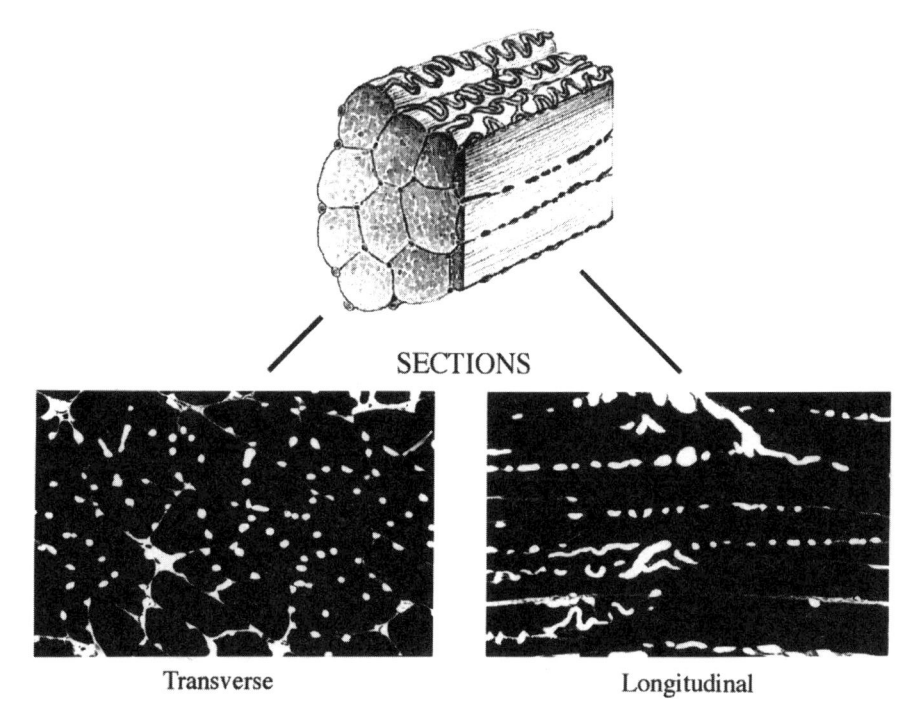

Figure 14 Schematic illustrating three-dimensional geometry of skeletal muscle capillary bed and the appearance of this structure in transverse and longitudinal sections as observed by light microscopy. Quantification of capillary length and surface area requires an appreciation of this geometry. (From Ref. 89.)

type or oxidative capacity, capillary surface per fiber surface seems to be regulated as a unique function of fiber mitochondrial volume (or maximal O_2 demand) in rat soleus and plantaris muscles across training states (Figure 15) [88]. Whether this relationship holds for other muscles, species, and conditions remains to be elucidated.

Function: Capillary Hemodynamics and Oxygen Exchange

The understanding of intracapillary events and transcapillary O_2 exchange processes within exercising muscle has been hindered by the technical challenges of making quantitative microscopic observations in moving tissue. This is unfortunate, because it is becoming clear that chronic pathological conditions such as heart failure, emphysema [89], renal failure, and possibly diabetes are associated with compromised muscle O_2 exchange.

Quantification of capillary structure alone does not permit determination of that capillary surface actually available for O_2 exchange at any instant in time,

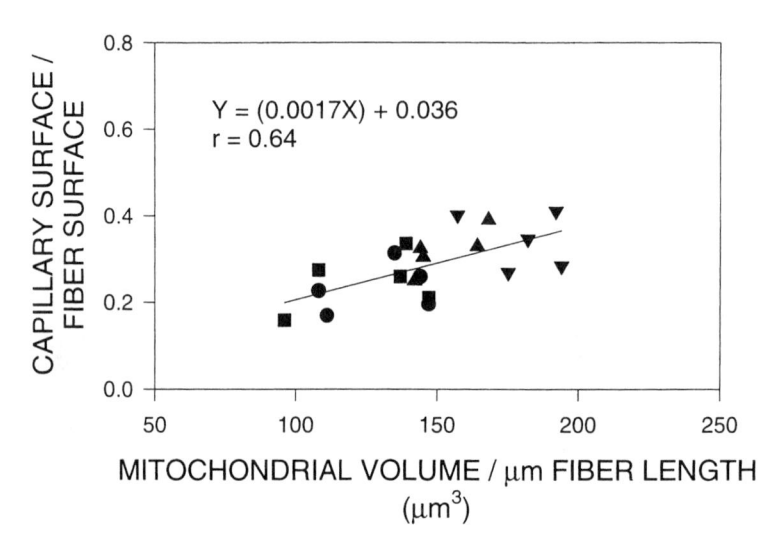

Figure 15 Relationship between capillary surface per fiber surface and mitochondrial volume per fiber length in soleus and plantaris muscles from untrained and trained rats. (From Ref. 88.)

i.e., effective capillary surface area. Rather, the effective capillary surface area will be dependent on several functional variables, including: (1) proportion of flowing capillaries; (2) capillary tube hematocrit (which may differ considerably from and is usually much less than systemic values); (3) RBC orientation; (4) RBC pathlength; and (5) RBC capillary transit time. In addition, the efficacy of O_2 offloading will be influenced by the presiding physicochemical conditions (pH, temperature, P_{CO_2}) because they affect hemoglobin–O_2 binding affinity and also the intracellular P_{O_2} and resultant myoglobin saturation.

Proportion of Flowing Capillaries

Unlike the situation in the lung, it is doubtful whether capillary recruitment and distension play a major role in increasing muscle capillary surface area during exercise. There is good evidence that the majority of capillaries (> 80%) contain RBCs and support flow at rest [90], and it is almost certain that close to 100% do so during rhythmic muscle contractions. In skeletal muscle, tissue extravascular pressures and the presence of collagenous capillary-to-myocyte struts likely limit any capillary distension during exercise. However, this issue remains to be systematically addressed. It should be mentioned that there are a few very narrow capillaries approximately 2 μm in diameter that may support plasma but not RBC flow. These diminutive capillaries may be important for equalizing intracapillary pressures within the network as opposed to facilitating blood–tissue O_2 exchange per se.

Capillary "Tube" Hematocrit

In resting muscle, capillary "tube" hematocrit averages only 25–50% of systemic values. However, the discharge hematocrit (i.e., that of the capillary effluent blood) is no different from systemic. The most cogent hypothesis invoked to explain this phenomenon is that the endothelial glycocalyx that projects into the capillary lumen acts to retard plasma flow in the proximity of the endothelium such that RBC velocity is twofold to fourfold that of the plasma. Removal of this glycocalyx using heparinase perfusion elevates capillary tube hematocrit to systemic values [91]. In addition, hyperemic states such as vasodilation and muscle contractions increase capillary tube hematocrit [92]. Capillary tube hematocrit is thought to be a critically important component of Do_{2m}, and alteration of systemic hematocrit undoubtedly changes capillary tube hematocrit in the same direction [93]. This effect likely underlies the increased Do_{2m} and contributes to the increased $\dot{V}o_{2max}$ found during exercise in dog [55] and human [56] muscle with elevated systemic hematocrit. At present, it is not known what proportion of this increased Do_{2m} results from augmented O_2 offloading kinetics versus increased effective capillary surface area.

The modelling studies by Federspiel and Popel [94,95] and Groebe and Thews [82] suggest that the number of RBCs along the fiber surface (i.e., within a capillary directly apposed to the fiber) at any instant constitutes the principal determinant of Do_{2m}. Thus, capillary length (and volume) combined with capillary tube hematocrit are extremely important components of Do_{2m}. Malvin and Wood [96] provided direct experimental support for this notion by demonstrating that O_2 exchange in frog skin capillaries was correlated with RBC density over a range of hematocrit levels achieved by hemodilution. In contrast, Hogan et al. [97] were unable to increase Do_{2m} in the electrically stimulated dog gastrocnemius muscle by increasing O_2 solubility with a perfluorocarbon emulsion. $\dot{V}o_{2max}$ was elevated; however, the expected increase of Do_{2m} predicted by recruiting additional capillary endothelial surface area for O_2 exchange was not found. Obviously, more investigative work is necessary to clarify this issue.

Red Blood Cell Orientation

In the absence of an O_2 carrier, plasma within the capillary has been considered to represent a high resistance region for O_2 diffusion [17,77,94]. Accordingly, that portion of the RBC membrane most closely apposed to the capillary endothelium will represent the preferential pathway for O_2 offloading. To a large extent, the capillary diameter dictates RBC orientation, and narrower capillaries will tend to

CAPILLARY DIAMETER (μm)

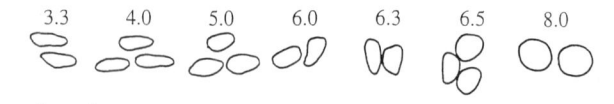

Figure 16 Schematic representation of RBC profiles in capillaries of different diameters in rat spinotrapezius muscle. Bar = 10 μm. (From Ref. 90.)

increase the RBC surface apposed to the capillary endothelium (Figs. 12 and 16). This consideration might help explain why muscle capillary luminal diameters are smaller than RBCs. As previously mentioned, if plasma does indeed represent a significant barrier to O_2 diffusion, increasing plasma solubility should increase Do_{2m} and $\dot{V}o_{2max}$ substantially. That Do_{2m} does not increase experimentally under these conditions [97] is an important problem to resolve because it will help define what sets Do_2 in the capillary and will further improve our understanding of the mechanistic basis for the peripheral O_2 exchange deficits found in heart failure and diabetic patients.

Red Blood Cell Pathlength

Historically, recruitment of additional capillaries or capillary modules has been invoked to explain the greater Do_{2m} during exercise. However, as detailed previously, more than 80% of capillaries are perfused in resting muscle, which leaves room for only a modest increase on exercise. Another mechanism that recruits capillary endothelium but does not depend on perfusing additional capillaries relies on the exercise-induced increase in capillary RBC velocity. This concept was considered previously for the pulmonary capillaries [8] and is based on the premise that at low RBC velocities, the bulk or entirety of O_2 exchange occurs close to the arteriolar end of the capillary. Thus, capillary length and surface area further downstream do not contribute to O_2 exchange. Because RBC velocity increases during exercise, progressively more of each capillary can be used for O_2 exchange. This notion remains to be tested empirically. However, if O_2 exchange is rapid and thus biased toward the early capillary segments at rest, this effect may be substantial and be further compounded by the fact that the actual RBC capillary pathlength may be somewhat longer than that determined anatomically [98].

Red Blood Cell Capillary Transit Time

The slope of the O_2–hemoglobin dissociation curve favors fast loading of O_2 in the lung but slow unloading of O_2 in the muscle. This raises the possibility that muscle capillary O_2 offloading might be transit time–limited. Within a given capillary, RBC transit time denotes the ratio of RBC pathlength to velocity. Most conveniently, however, mean capillary RBC transit time can be calculated as perfused capillary volume divided by $\dot{Q}_m$, acknowledging that there may be a considerable spread about the mean value. At intramyocyte P_{O_2} values less than 5 mm Hg, O_2 offloading has been considered to be 90% complete within 0.3 seconds [17]. In contrast, there is excellent evidence in humans that mean RBC transit times can decrease to below this without compromising O_2 offloading, i.e., O_2 extraction. Specifically, the highest blood flows yet measured in humans average 385 mL/100 g/min in the quadriceps performing maximal single leg–knee extensor exercise [78]. Assuming a reasonable value for capillary volume (1.2%) in the muscles of these trained cyclists [13], this blood flow will force mean capillary RBC transit time to less than 0.2 seconds [78]. Interestingly, even at these extraordinary $\dot{Q}_m$ values, O_2 extraction achieved approximately 85%, which is not appreciably different from that measured at much lower mass specific blood flows during maximal cycle ergometry (150 mL/100 g/min) [36]. This implies that short RBC capillary transit times may not limit O_2 offloading.

Intramyocyte Diffusion

Within the fiber, myoglobin-facilitated diffusion substantially increases O_2 conductivity. Because of the left-shifted myoglobin–O_2 dissociation curve (P_{50} (i.e., that P_{O_2} at which myoglobin is 50% saturated) = approximately 3 mm Hg), myoglobin facilitation of O_2 transport becomes pronounced only at very low intramyocyte P_{O_2} values, which are necessary to (partly) desaturate myoglobin. Thus, in resting muscle, the $\dot{V}_{O_2req}$ is low, and intramyocyte P_{O_2} is sufficiently high that most myoglobin–O_2 binding sites are saturated. Under these conditions, myoglobin-facilitated O_2 transport is poor, and such fibers or regions where this occurs may be considered as functionally carrier-depleted regions, (FCDR) (Fig. 17) [17]. This situation is comparable to a Los Angeles freeway at rush hour, where there is a high density of cars, all going nowhere. However, as fiber $\dot{V}_{O_2req}$ increases, intramyocyte P_{O_2} decreases, causing the thickness of the FCDR to be reduced. More myoglobin–O_2 binding sites become emptied, and myoglobin can function to markedly enhance O_2 conductivity. Continuing the freeway analogy, increased $\dot{V}_{O_2req}$ is akin to more off-ramps opening up, allowing a greater velocity and flux of vehicles, albeit with greater intercar spacing and, thus, a lower density.

B. Mechanistic Basis for Increased Muscle Oxygen Diffusing Capacity During Exercise

Extracellular events undoubtedly contribute to the augmented muscle oxygen diffusing capacity (D_{O_2m}) found during exercise. However, it is difficult to account for the up to 100-fold increase actually observed. Specifically, recruitment of additional capillaries and distension of the capillary lumen is probably far less important in skeletal muscle than in the lung because most capillaries are already perfused at rest, and the muscle capillaries likely have only a very limited distensibility. Capillary tube hematocrit may increase by twofold to threefold, thereby increasing the effective capillary surface area by a similar amount. Heterogeneity of $\dot{Q}_m$ and

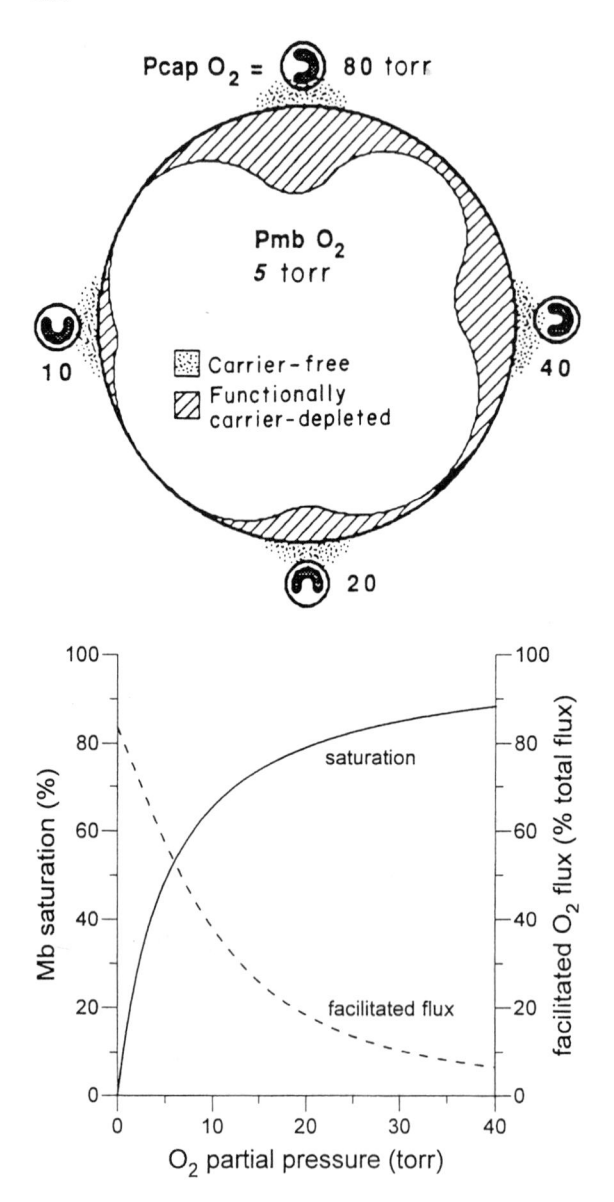

Figure 17 (Top) Effect of decreasing capillary P_{O_2} on penetration of functionally carrier-depleted region (FCDR, hatched regions) into myocyte. Note that the distance over which diffusion (slow) rather than myoglobin-facilitated transport (fast) is the predominant mechanism for O_2 movement, increases markedly as a function of the FCDR thickness. Alteration of FCDR permits rapid modulation of intramyocyte and intermyocyte diffusion properties and, thus, O_2 flux. (Bottom) Solid curve is the myoglobin dissociation curve. Dashed curve illustrates the increased facilitation of O_2 flux as myoglobin saturation decreases. (From Ref. 17.)

$\dot{V}_{O_{2}req}/\dot{Q}_{O_{2}m}$ are not thought to play major roles in limiting $D_{O_{2}m}$ and, thus, whatever improvements in $\dot{V}_{O_{2}req}/\dot{Q}_{O_{2}m}$ matching that occur are likely to be modest. The altered physicochemical environment with elevated H^{+}, temperature, and $P_{CO_{2}}$ will undoubtedly augment offloading [58], but, again, this effect will be relatively small and alters capillary $P_{O_{2}}$ or O_{2} content rather than $D_{O_{2}m}$. The notion has become popular that capillary RBC transit time might be sufficiently short so as to limit O_{2} offloading. However, as previously discussed, the shortest calculated transit times achieved in human muscle do not seem to constitute any sizeable impediment to O_{2} offloading [70,78]. The observation that O_{2} offloading in vivo is sufficiently fast that mean RBC capillary transit times of less than 0.3 seconds permit excellent O_{2} extraction suggests that increased capillary RBC velocities greater than those found at rest would permit recruitment of additional capillary length and surface area. Thus, provided RBC transit time is never so short that O_{2} offloading becomes compromised, any increase in $\dot{Q}_{m}$ would be matched by increased $D_{O_{2}m}$ via recruitment of additional capillary length and surface area mostly within already-perfused capillaries. This mechanism is, at present, speculative. However, none of the other exercise-induced extracellular changes previously listed can account for the major portion of the exercise-induced increase in $D_{O_{2}m}$.

Notwithstanding the importance of the previously mentioned extracellular events, it is likely that intracellular mechanisms quantitatively overshadow those occuring at the capillary level with respect to their potential to increase $D_{O_{2}m}$ during exercise. Initial claims that cryospectroscopy could measure myoglobin $P_{O_{2}}$ within very few microns below the sarcolemma, and the findings of very low $P_{O_{2}}$ values in this region, may have obscured the presence and, thus, importance of the FCDR and its modulation with fiber $\dot{V}_{O_{2}}$. However, such modulation of intracellular O_{2} conductivity as a function of the thickness of the FCDR represents one potentially powerful mechanism for increasing $D_{O_{2}m}$ in proportion to fiber $\dot{V}_{O_{2}req}$ (Fig. 17). In addition, longitudinal alterations in the FCDR thickness offer the potential to substantially alter local $D_{O_{2}}$ along the capillary to distribute blood–tissue O_{2} flux more evenly throughout the fiber.

C. Effect of Training on Muscle Oxygen Exchange

Endurance exercise training increases pulmonary and muscle $\dot{V}_{O_{2}}$ during maximal exercise ($\dot{V}_{O_{2}max}$) by as much as 40–60% and also speeds $\dot{V}_{O_{2}}$ kinetics at exercise onset [11]. $\dot{V}_{O_{2}max}$ increases as a function of increased cardiac output ($\dot{Q}_{tot}$) and $\dot{Q}_{m}$ coupled with a modest increase in O_{2} extraction (Fig. 18). Muscles recruited during training undergo profound structural and functional adaptations that include capillary and mitochondrial proliferation and a reduced intracellular perturbation at any given submaximal work rate, which, in turn, reduces lactate production and glycogen depletion. In humans, as opposed to laboratory animals, training does not increase muscle myoglobin concentration [11]. One feature that often escapes notice is that even modest training-induced elevations in O_{2} extraction

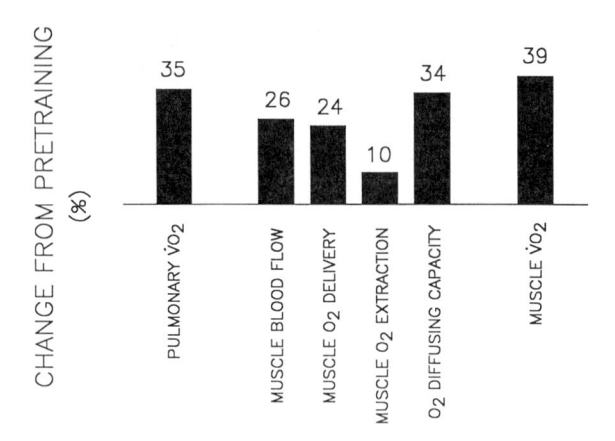

Figure 18 Nine weeks of training enhances muscle O_2 delivery and extraction, thereby increasing muscle $\dot{V}O_{2max}$. Note the large increase in muscle O_2 diffusing capacity. (Data from Ref. 79.)

demand proportionally large increases in DO_{2m} because of the interdependence of DO_{2m} and $\dot{Q}_m$ [see Eqs. (10) and (11)]. Thus, Roca et al. [79] demonstrated that, after 8 weeks of training which increased pulmonary and muscle $\dot{V}O_{2max}$ by 35–39%, a 34% increase in DO_{2m} was required to increase O_2 extraction by just 10% (Fig. 18). Had the 26% increase in $\dot{Q}_m$ not been accompanied by this sizeable increase in DO_{2m}, O_2 extraction would be expected to decrease [Eqs. (10) and (11)]. Indeed, across the muscles of patients in chronic heart failure when $\dot{Q}_m$ is acutely increased by vasodilator treatment, O_2 extraction decreases [99] because of the inability of their muscles to attain a sufficiently high DO_{2m}. What is the mechanism for the increased DO_{2m} found after training? Training does not alter systemic hematocrit and, therefore, would not be expected to change capillary tube hematocrit or O_2 offloading kinetics. Depending on the proportionality between the increased capillary volume and $\dot{Q}_m$ (capillary-to-fiber number increases, but individual capillary length remains constant), mean transit time may increase by a small amount. However, the major extracellular consequence of training will be to increase effective capillary surface area by providing more capillary length per fiber volume, which would augment DO_{2m}. Intracellularly, a higher mitochondrial O_2 flux might reduce the FCDR to a greater extent, thereby also contributing to the increased DO_{2m}.

D. Effects of Muscle Tension and Length on Microcirculatory Structure–Function

As detailed in Section III, during isotonic exercise, $\dot{Q}_m$ is controlled at a level commensurate with the external work and muscle $\dot{V}O_{2req}$ by a complex array of neural, humoral, and mechanical influences. It has long been recognized that muscle blood flow is reduced by mechanical compression of microvessels during contraction, and akin to the myocardium, blood flow oscillates, with the highest flows occurring during muscle relaxation. During heavy or even severe ($\dot{V}_{O_2max}$) cycle ergometry, $\dot{Q}_m$ never seems to be completely impeded, and this effect produces only approximately 20% oscillation about the mean [28,35].

Muscle blood flow is reduced by stretch over the physiological range of sarcomere lengths. For many years, the assumption has been that this results from mechanical compression of microvessels. However, recent experiments have shown a very different scenario. As muscle sarcomere length is increased from 1.6 to 3.2 μm, vessels aligned principally with the fiber longitudinal axis (i.e., arterioles and capillaries) progressively become less tortuous, and above 2.3 to 2.7 μm are stretched [84,100]. This stretch reduces their luminal diameter and markedly increases their flow resistance. This is associated with up to 50% reduction in $\dot{Q}_m$ and the proportion of capillaries that sustain flow [90]. Within those flowing capillaries, RBC velocity is also compromised (Fig. 19). In the hamster retractor muscle, approximately two thirds of this stretch response may be blocked by tetrodotoxin, prazosin, or phentolamine, and thus is attributed to active vasoconstriction [101]. Presumably, the remaining one third involves passive mechanical effects at the microvascular level. It remains to be demonstrated whether this active vasoconstrictor response is sufficiently fast to operate in a muscle-performing rhythmic exercise. What is certain is that many skeletal muscles, including those of the limbs and diaphragm, operate over a range of sarcomere lengths, where microvessels are cyclically stretched, and understanding the mechanistic basis for poor flow at longer muscle lengths is of great physiological importance. Moreover, these studies provide insights into the impaired muscle performance and possibly discomfort in muscles placed in chronically extended positions.

V. Maximum Oxygen Consumption in Health and Disease

The peak energetic demands of skeletal muscle myosin ATPase greatly surpass the capacity of the respiratory system to replenish high-energy phosphates by means of mitochondrial oxidative phosphorylation. Consequently, there exists a broad range of exercise scenarios in which the ATP requirement exceeds that which can be supported by O_2 delivery and use. Under these conditions, given sufficient time, pulmonary $\dot{V}_{O_2}$ increases to its maximum ($\dot{V}_{O_2max}$), and an obligatory anaerobiosis is incurred. Pulmonary $\dot{V}_{O_2max}$ is elicited by exercise modalities such as cycling, running, or swimming, which recruit a substantial muscle mass. One crucial conceptual appreciation in understanding the determinants of $\dot{V}_{O_2max}$ is that the full oxidative potential of skeletal muscle mitochondria cannot be exploited during large-muscle-mass exercise, at least in trained subjects. A dramatic demonstration of this is the twofold to threefold higher mass-specific $\dot{V}_{O_2}$ achieved during

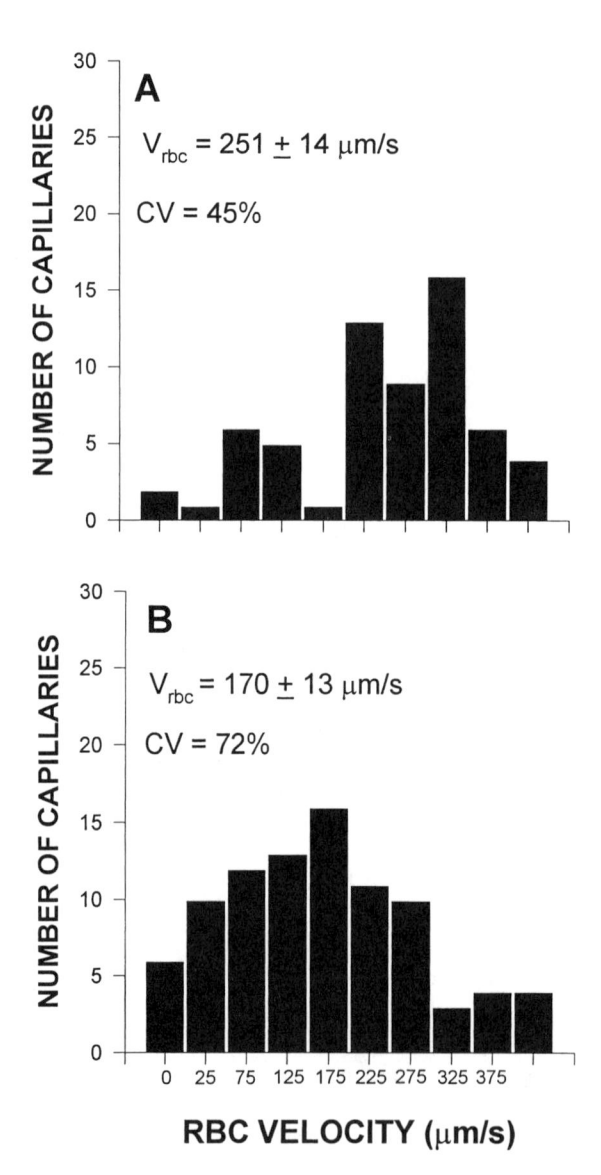

Figure 19 Frequency histograms demonstrating the reduction in capillary RBC velocities (V_{rbc}) when the spinotrapezius muscle is stretched from short (top) to extended (bottom) sarcomere lengths within the physiological range. (From Ref. 90.)

maximal knee extensor exercise (approximately 600 mL/kg/min) [60,70], which recruits only 2–3 kg of muscle compared with conventional cycling (approximately 250 mL/kg/min) [36] that recruits approximately 15 kg of muscle. This effect is caused by the finite limit to cardiac output, which places a restrictive ceiling on the mass-specific muscle blood flow, O_2 delivery, and $\dot{V}_{O_2max}$ during exercise that recruits a muscle mass more than 4–5 kg. Further support for this notion comes from experimental conditions in which muscle O_2 delivery is elevated in humans and animals and that invariably results in an increased $\dot{V}_{O_2max}$ [102]. Examples of this include inspiratory hyperoxia [76], elevated hemoglobin concentration via blood reinfusion [103], and pericardectomy experiments in foxhounds [104]. These experiments further substantiate the findings of Richardson et al. [60,70], that muscle $\dot{V}_{O_2}$ at pulmonary $\dot{V}_{O_2max}$ is limited by O_2 delivery to the mitochondria and not by oxidative enzyme capacity.

Within a given individual running, cycling, or swimming at an intensity sufficient to yield $\dot{V}_{O_2max}$, that $\dot{V}_{O_2max}$ represents the interactive culmination of multiple steps in the O_2 pathway [12,102]. Some of these steps, such as cardiovascular O_2 transport, may be more influential than others. However, each single step contributes to setting $\dot{V}_{O_2max}$ in that any change in its capacity will alter $\dot{V}_{O_2max}$ predictably. This concept has been developed by Wagner et al. [12,102] and forms an insightful construct within which to understand the determinants of $\dot{V}_{O_2max}$ and its plasticity in health (exercise training, altitude) and disease. Briefly, the integrative analysis presented in Figure 20 combines the Fick principle for convective O_2 transport ($\dot{V}_{O_2} = \dot{Q}(CaO_2 - C\bar{v}O_2)$; see Eq. (8) and the curved line in Fig. 20A) and Fick's law for diffusive O_2 transport ($\dot{V}_{O_2} = D_{O_2}[P_{cap}O_2 - P_{mito}O_2]$; see Eq. (9) and the straight line in Fig. 20A). As detailed in Section IV, $\dot{Q}_m$ denotes muscle blood flow, and D_{O_2} is muscle diffusing capacity. CaO_2 and $C\bar{v}O_2$ are the concentrations of O_2 in the arterial and venous effluent blood, and $P_{cap}O_2$ and $P_{mito}O_2$ are mean capillary and mitochondrial P_{O_2}, respectively. For a simple diffusion-limited system in which P_{O_2} decreases exponentially along the capillary from the arteriolar to venular end, $P_{cap}O_2$ and $P\bar{v}O_2$ will change in proportion to each other, and $P_{mito}O_2$ is close to zero (see Section IV), the diffusive O_2 transport equation reduces to:

$$\dot{V}_{O_2} = D_{O_2} * K * P\bar{v}O_2 \tag{12}$$

where K is a constant that relates $P\bar{v}O_2$ to $P_{cap}O_2$. As is evident from Figure 20, $\dot{V}_{O_2max}$ is dictated by the laws of mass balance and can only occur at the intersection of the conductive and diffusive relationships. The characteristics and position of the curved line in Figure 20 will be altered by any change in O_2 delivery [i.e., $\dot{Q}$ or CaO_2; Eq. (8)]. If D_{O_2} remains unchanged, the resultant perturbation of $P\bar{v}O_2$ and $\dot{V}_{O_2max}$ is readily apparent from Figure 20. By the same token, any alteration in D_{O_2} independent of O_2 delivery will alter $\dot{V}_{O_2max}$ by either decreasing or increasing $P\bar{v}O_2$ and, thus, the point of intersection in Figure 20 in a predictable fashion. This behavior has been demonstrated for healthy muscle in humans [79] and across each animal species examined to date (e.g., rat [105], dog [106], and horse [107]).

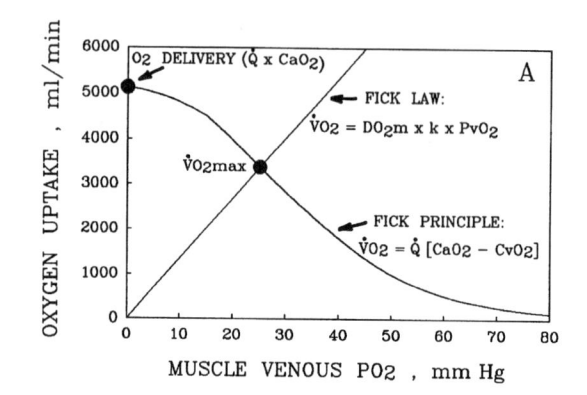

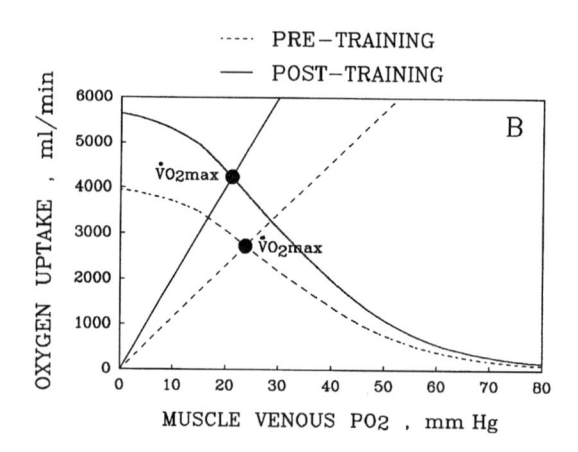

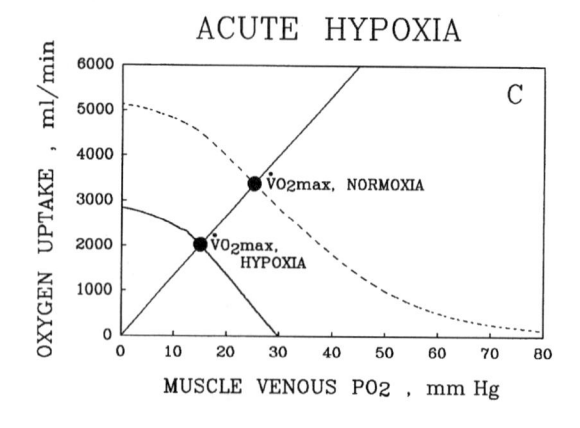

Within the aforementioned model, the relative potency of each physiological variable to alter $\dot{V}_{O_2max}$ is shown in Figure 21. This analysis is particularly valuable for understanding the mechanistic bases for physiological function and pathophysiological dysfunction because it forces consideration of convective and diffusive elements within the O_2 pathway and their interaction.

A. Exercise Training

Endurance exercise training increases pulmonary $\dot{V}_{O_2max}$ up to 60% depending on the training parameters and initial fitness levels [11]. In part, because of the strong linear correlation between $\dot{V}_{O_2}$ and convective O_2 delivery (i.e., $\dot{Q}_m$ × arterial O_2 content) from rest to maximum exercise, the training-induced augmentation of $\dot{V}_{O_2max}$ has often been attributed almost exclusively to cardiovascular adaptations (increased stroke volume) that elevate O_2 delivery. However, as is obvious from Figure 21, increased blood flow ($\dot{Q}_m$) represents a potent means of increasing $\dot{V}_{O_2max}$, but because of the interactive nature of $\dot{Q}_m$ and muscle diffusing capacity [D_{O_2m}; Eqs. 10 and 11] in determining O_2 extraction, if $\dot{Q}_m$ increased after training but D_{O_2m} did not, O_2 extraction would be expected to decrease. Direct measurement of D_{O_2m} by Roca et al. [79] demonstrated that several weeks of training increased O_2 extraction by a modest 10% via an impressive 34% increase of D_{O_2m}. In comparison, $\dot{Q}_m$ increased 26%. Thus, after training, $\dot{V}_{O_2max}$ in Figure 20B is elevated by an upward shift in the conductive O_2 delivery curve combined with an increased slope of the diffusive O_2 transport relationship. Although the precise determinants of D_{O_2m} have not been resolved (see Sec. IV), the size of the capillary bed and, more specifically, that of the capillary-to-fiber interface, is thought to be an important component of D_{O_2m} [85,88]. This is consistent with the established observation that exercise training induces capillary neogenesis [13,88] and that the capillary-to-myocyte surface maintains a constant relationship to the mitochondrial volume subserved across training states and fiber types [88]. It is notable that arterial O_2 content ([Hb] in Fig. 21) is not elevated after training.

B. Altitude/Inspired Hypoxia

The sigmoid shape of the hemoglobin–O_2 dissociation curve defends arterial O_2 content and $\dot{V}_{O_2max}$ in response to modest acute reductions of inspired P_{O_2} (or F_{IO_2}

Figure 20 Integrative analysis of convective and diffusive components of O_2 transport to muscle. The curved line denotes mass balance according to the Fick principle. The straight line passing through the origin represents Fick's law of diffusion and relates $\dot{V}_{O_2}$ to O_2 partial pressure gradient. The point of intersection gives $\dot{V}_{O_2max}$. (A) The underlying relationship. (B) Endurance exercise training elevates $\dot{V}_{O_2max}$ by increasing muscle O_2 delivery and D_{O_2m}. (C) Acute hypoxia lowers $\dot{V}_{O_2max}$ by reducing O_2 delivery in the face of unchanged D_{O_2}. See text for further details.

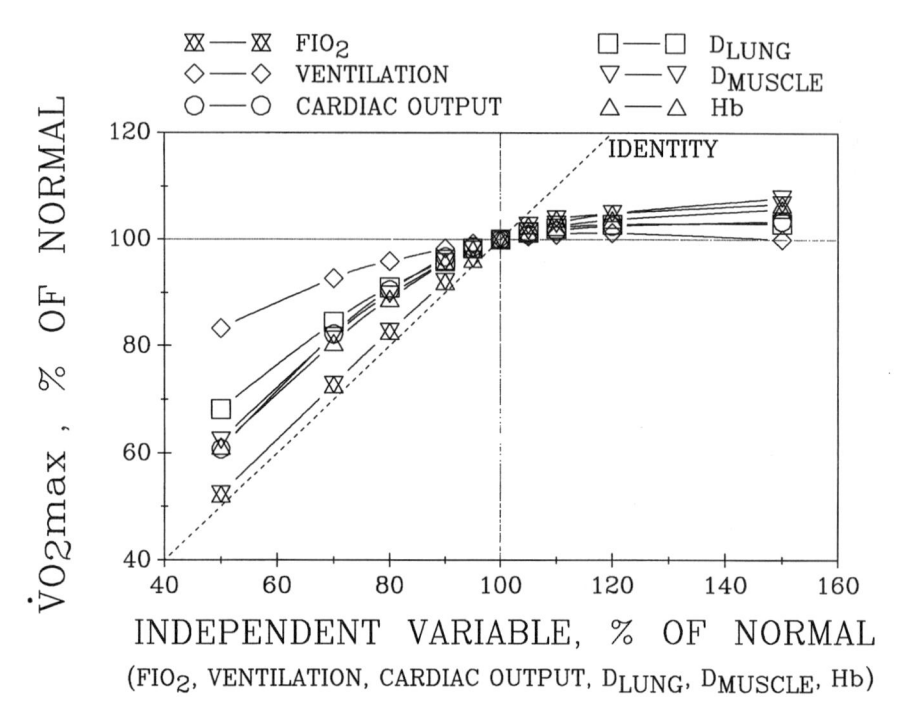

Figure 21 Relative potency of O_2 transport components to elicit changes in $\dot{V}O_{2max}$. D_{LUNG}, lung diffusive capacity; D_{MUSCLE}, muscle diffusing capacity; F_{IO_2}, % of implied O_2; Hb, arterial hemoglobin concentration.

down to approximately 120 mm Hg; Fig. 21). However, further reductions decrease arterial O_2 content, and $\dot{V}O_{2max}$ decreases systematically. For example, $\dot{V}O_{2max}$ is reduced to approximately 70% of its sea level value at an inspired P_{O_2} of 90 mm Hg. At an inspired P_{O_2} equivalent to that found at the summit of Mt. Everest (approximately 43 mm Hg), $\dot{V}O_{2max}$ plummets to 25% of sea level values [12]. This dramatic reduction of $\dot{V}O_{2max}$ occurs largely because of the lowered alveolar P_{O_2} and is exacerbated by pulmonary O_2 uptake being restricted to the steep region of the O_2 dissociation curve and the reduced pulmonary capillary RBC transit time. Thus, at altitude, pulmonary O_2 uptake becomes diffusion-limited and a substantial A-aP_{O_2} difference is manifest.

Not only does reduced inspired P_{O_2} lower arterial O_2 content, O_2 delivery is further constrained by a poorly understood reduction in maximum heart rate, which limits maximum cardiac output [108]. Consequently, inspired hypoxia reduces $\dot{V}O_{2max}$ in proportion to the decreased O_2 delivery in the face of unchanged $D_{O_{2m}}$ (Fig. 20C) [79,106]. Reductions in P_{aO_2} below approximately 60 mm Hg stimulate the carotid chemoreceptors and induce a hyperventilation that lowers alveolar and arterial P_{CO_2}. The resultant increase of arterial pH drives the O_2 dissociation curve to the left as O_2 becomes more tightly bound to hemoglobin. This will act to enhance O_2 loading in the lung but impair off-loading at the tissue. However, notwithstanding this, modeling studies suggest that substantial perturbations (left or right shifts) in the position of the O_2 dissociation curve (P_{50} 15–47 mm Hg) exert only a very minimal effect on $\dot{V}O_{2max}$ [109]. As opposed to acute hypoxia, chronic hypoxia stimulates erythropoiesis, and the resulting polycythemia improves arterial O_2 content. The improved O_2-carrying capacity of the blood facilitates a reduced cardiac output that elevates RBC transit time in the pulmonary capillaries and reduces the A-aP_{O_2} difference [110].

C. Chronic Diseases

Accepting that in trained healthy humans, $\dot{V}O_{2max}$ is O_2 supply–dependent and $D_{O_{2m}}$ is an integral determinant of this supply, if we seek to understand the mechanistic basis for the reduced $\dot{V}O_{2max}$ in disease, it would seem derelict to ignore the effects of that disease on $D_{O_{2m}}$. Furthermore, it is possible that correction of the primary myopathy, for example, in chronic heart failure, renal failure, or type I diabetes, does not resolve the muscle D_{O_2} problem, and, consequently, $\dot{V}O_{2max}$ remains lower than expected. Examples of this include the inability of acute increases in muscle O_2 delivery to elevate $\dot{V}O_{2max}$ [111] in chronic heart failure or the lower-than-expected improvements in exercise performance after heart or lung transplantation [112,113] or erythropoietin therapy [114] despite substantial recovery of $\dot{Q}$ and/or C_{aO_2}. Wagner [77] demonstrated empirically that much of this effect can potentially be attributable to an inability to correct the underlying O_2 conductance deficit.

It is clear that a greater understanding of the muscle adaptations that attend these chronic conditions is warranted. In Section IV, evidence was presented that the capillary-to-myocyte contact surface represents an important component of $D_{O_{2m}}$, with the bulk of the resistance to blood–tissue O_2 transfer residing in that short physical space between the RBC and the immediately subsarcolemmal cytoplasmic space. In at least three of the aforementioned chronic disease states—chronic heart failure [115], renal failure [116], and type I diabetes [117]—there is emerging evidence that the capillary bed undergoes substantial remodeling. In addition, there may be arteriolar dysfunction that contributes to elevated peripheral resistance and interferes with the distribution of O_2 delivery within the muscle. Furthermore, intravital microscopy observations in resting muscles of animals with chronic heart failure or type I diabetes show marked microvascular flow perturbations, suggesting that the ability of the capillary bed to support and distribute O_2 flux is compromised [118,119]. It is anticipated that future scientific investigation and the design of therapeutic interventions will aim to understand and ameliorate the muscle microvascular structural and functional consequences of these chronic disease states.

VI. Summary and Conclusions

The coupling of pulmonary O_2 uptake with muscle O_2 requirements during exercise requires the precise coordination of ventilatory, cardiovascular, and muscle microcirculatory responses. The fidelity of these responses is such that, beyond the initial transient at exercise onset, there exists a broad range of metabolic rates (i.e., moderate and heavy exercise domains) in which the rate of muscle O_2 exchange is equal to the requirement. It is only in the obligatory non–steady state of severe exercise that so-called anaerobic energy sources are continually used to supplement the ATP turnover. Contrasting exercise scenarios and, to a certain extent, individuals reveals different limitations in the systems for muscle O_2 delivery and exchange, specifically: (1) At exercise onset, muscle O_2 delivery is so rapid that $\dot{V}O_2$ kinetics seem not to be limited by bulk O_2 delivery, but rather by some intramuscular process. Inefficient O_2 delivery to O_2 requirement matching and inertia of the oxidative machinery remain prime candidates in this regard. (2) At pulmonary $\dot{V}O_{2max}$, blood flow to the active muscles (and mass-specific muscle $\dot{V}O_2$) is constrained by the cardiac output ceiling (by means of a powerful sympathetic vasoconstriction that defends arterial blood pressure) in combination with a finite muscle O_2 diffusing capacity that sets an upper limit for O_2 extraction at any given blood flow. There is also the opportunity for the respiratory muscles to subvert blood flow that otherwise would have benefitted the limb muscles. (3) When exercise is limited to a small muscle mass (approximately 2–3 kg), muscle maximum blood flow is not under central control and is limited simply by the geometry and size of the vascular bed, the efficacy of the muscle pump, and the arteriovenous pressure differential. Under these conditions, muscle $\dot{V}O_2$ is determined by the O_2 delivery and muscle O_2 diffusing capacity and the activity of the mitochondrial oxidative enzymes. (4) In some highly fit athletes, their superb cardiac output exceeds that of the pulmonary system to oxygenate the blood, and SaO_2 decreases. Some of the most compelling questions facing physiologists today relate to elucidating the mechanisms responsible for the rapid increases in muscle blood flow at exercise onset and how O_2 delivery is spatially matched to O_2 requirements within exercising muscle. Central to this issue is understanding the determinants of muscle O_2 conductance, its extraordinary increase during exercise, and the impairment of this increase in chronic disease states.

Acknowledgments

The authors thank Dr. Robert L. Johnson, Jr., for providing the regression equation for Figure 9, Dr. Peter D. Wagner for generating Figures 20 and 21, and Drs. Thomas J. Barstow, Craig A. Harms, and Richard M. McAllister, and Mr. Casey A. Kindig for their review of the manuscript. During preparation of the manuscript, D.C.P. and T.I.M. were supported by grants no. HL-50306, HL-17731, and AG-11535 from the National Institutes of Health (Bethesda, MD).

References

1. Whipp BJ, Mahler M. Dynamics of pulmonary gas exchange during exercise. In: West JB, ed. Pulmonary Gas Exchange, volume II. New York: Academic, 1980, pp 33–96.
2. Whipp BJ. The control of exercise hyperpnea. In: Hornbein T, ed. Regulation of Breathing. New York: Marcel Dekker, 1981, pp 1069–1139.
3. Whipp BJ. Dynamics of pulmonary gas exchange. Circulation 1987; 76(Suppl VI): V1–18.
4. Gaesser GA, Poole DC. The slow component of oxygen uptake kinetics in humans. In: Holloszy JO, ed. Exercise and Sports Science Reviews, volume 25. Baltimore: Williams and Wilkins, 1996, pp 35–70.
5. Wasserman K, Whipp BJ, Casaburi R. Respiratory control during exercise. In: Fishman AP, Chemisek NS, Liddicombe JE, eds. Handbook of Physiology: The Respiratory System. Bethesda: American Physiological Society, 1986, pp 595–619.
6. Cerretelli P, DiPrampero PE. Gas exchange in exercise. In: Handbook of Physiology: The Respiratory System. Bethesda: American Physiological Society, 1986, pp 297–339.
7. Cerretelli P, DiPrampero PE. Pulmonary gas exchange during exercise. In: Crystal RG, West JB, Weibel ER, Barnes PJ, eds. The Lung: Scientific Foundations. 2nd Edition. Philadelphia: Lippincott-Raven, 1997, pp 2011–2020.
8. Wagner WW. Recruitment of gas exchange vessels. In: Crystal RG, West JB, Weibel ER, Barnes PJ, eds. The Lung: Scientific Foundations. 2nd Edition. Philadelphia: Lippincott-Raven, 1997, pp 1537–1547.
9. Astrand PO, Rodahl K. Textbook of Work Physiology. 3rd Edition. New York: McGraw-Hill, 1986.
10. Rowell LB. Human Cardiovascular Control. New York: Oxford University Press, 1993.
11. Poole DC. Influence of exercise training on skeletal muscle oxygen delivery and utilization. In: Crystal RG, West JB, Weibel ER, Barnes PJ, eds. The Lung: Scientific Foundations. 2nd Edition. Philadelphia: Lippincott-Raven, 1997, pp 1957–1967.
12. Wagner PD, Hoppeler H, Saltin B. Determinants of maximal oxygen uptake. In: Crystal RG, West JB, Weibel ER, Barnes PJ, eds. The Lung: Scientific Foundations. 2nd Edition. Philadelphia: Lippincott-Raven, 1997, pp 2033–2041.
13. Saltin B, Gollnick PD. Skeletal muscle adaptability: significance for metabolism and performance. In: Peachey LD, Adrian RH, eds. Handbook of Physiology. Section 10. Bethesda: American Physiological Society, 1983, pp 555–631.
14. Barstow TJ, Jones AM, Nguyen PH, Casaburi R. Influence of muscle fiber type and pedal frequency on oxygen uptake kinetics of heavy exercise. J Appl Physiol 1996; 81:1642–1650.
15. Laughlin MH, Korthuis RJ, Duncker DJ, Bache RJ. Control of blood flow to cardiac and skeletal muscle during exercise. In: Rowell LB, Shepherd JT, eds. Handbook of Physiology. New York: Oxford University Press, 1996, pp 705–769.
16. Laughlin MH, McAllister RM, Delp MD. Heterogeneity of blood flow in striated muscle. In: Crystal RG, West JB, Weibel ER, Barnes PJ, eds. The Lung: Scientific Foundations. 2nd Edition. Philadelphia: Lippincott-Raven, 1997, pp 1945–1955.

17. Honig CR, Gayeski TEJ, Groebe K. Myoglobin and oxygen gradients. In: Crystal RG, West JB, Weibel ER, Barnes PJ, eds. The Lung: Scientific Foundations. 2nd Edition. Philadelphia: Lippincott-Raven, 1997, pp 1925–1933.
18. Hoofd L, Kreuzer F. Oxygen transfer from blood to mitochondria. In: Crystal RG, West JB, Weibel ER, Barnes PJ, eds. The Lung: Scientific Foundations. 2nd Edition. Philadelphia: Lippincott-Raven, 1997, pp 1913–1923.
19. Duling BR, Dora K. Control of striated muscle blood flow. In: Crystal RG, West JB, Weibel ER, Barnes PJ, eds. The Lung: Scientific Foundations. 2nd Edition. Philadelphia: Lippincott-Raven, 1997, pp 1935–1943.
20. Hill AV, Lupton H. Muscular exercise, lactic acid, and the supply and utilization of oxygen. Q J Med 1923; 16:135–171.
21. Wasserman K, Whipp BJ, Castagna J. Cardiodynamic hyperpnea: hyperpnea secondary to cardiac output increase. J Appl Physiol 1974; 36:457–464.
22. Casaburi R, Daly J, Hansen JE, Effros RM. Abrupt changes in mixed venous blood gas composition after the onset of exercise. J Appl Physiol 1989; 67:1106–1112.
23. Linnarsson D. Dynamics of pulmonary gas exchange and heart rate changes at start and end of exercise. Acta Physiol Scand Suppl 1974; 415:1–68.
24. Langsetmo I, Weigle GE, Fedde MR, Erickson HH, Poole DC. $\dot{V}O_2$ kinetics in the horse at moderate and heavy exercise. J Appl Physiol 1997; 83:1235–1241.
25. Mahler M. First-order kinetics of muscle oxygen consumption, and equivalent proportionality between $\dot{Q}O_2$ and phosphorylcreatine level: implications for the control of respiration. J Gen Physiol 1985; 86:135–165.
26. Grassi B, Poole DC, Richardson RS, Knight DR, Erickson BK, Wagner PD. Muscle O_2 kinetics in humans: implications for metabolic control. J Appl Physiol 1996; 80:988–998.
27. Gaesser GA, Brooks GA. Muscular efficiency during steady-rate exercise: effects of speed and work rate. J Appl Physiol 1975; 38:1132–1139.
28. Poole DC, Gaesser GA, Hogan MC, Knight DR, Wagner PD. Pulmonary and leg $\dot{V}O_2$ during submaximal exercise: implications for muscular efficiency. J Appl Physiol 1992; 72:805–810.
29. Hughson RL, Cochrane JE, Butler GC. Faster O_2 uptake kinetics at onset of supine exercise with than without lower body negative pressure. J Appl Physiol 1993; 75:1962–1967.
30. Sheriff DD, Rowell LB, Scher AM. Is rapid rise in vascular conductance at onset of dynamic exercise due to muscle pump? Am J Physiol 1993; 265:H1227–1234.
31. Grassi B, Gladden LB, Samaja N, Stary CM, Hogan MC. Faster adjustment of O_2 delivery does not affect $\dot{V}O_2$ on kinetics in isolated in situ canine muscle. J Appl Physiol 1998; 85:1394–1403.
32. Whipp BJ, Wasserman K. Oxygen uptake kinetics for various intensities of constant-load work. J Appl Physiol 1972; 33:351–356.
33. Wasserman K, Hansen JE, Sue DY, Whipp BJ, Casaburi R, eds. Principles of Exercise Testing and Interpretation. Philadelphia: Lea and Febiger, 1994.
34. Sloniger MA, Cureton KA, Carrasco DI. Effect of the slow-component rise in oxygen uptake on $\dot{V}O_{2max}$. Med Sci Sports Exerc 1996; 28:72–78.
35. Poole DC, Schaffartzik W, Knight DR, Derion T, Kennedy B, Guy HJB, Prediletto R, Wagner PD. Contribution of exercising legs to the slow component of oxygen uptake kinetics in man. J Appl Physiol 1991; 71:1245–1253.

36. Knight DR, Poole DC, Schaffartzik W, Guy HJ, Prediletto R, Hogan MC, Wagner PD. Relationship between body and leg $\dot{V}O_2$ during maximal cycle ergometry. J Appl Physiol 1992; 73:1114–1121.
37. Hey EN, Lloyd BB, Cunningham DJC, Jukes MGM, Bolton DPG. Effects of various respiratory stimuli on the depth and frequency of breathing in man. Respir Physiol 1966; 1:193–205.
38. Whipp BJ, Ward SA. Ventilatory control dynamics during muscular exercise in man. Int J Sports Med 1980; 1:146–159.
39. Tenney SM, Reese RE. The ability to sustain great breathing efforts. Respir Physiol 1968; 5:187–201.
40. Johnson BD, Babcock MA, Suman OE, Dempsey JA. Exercise-induced diaphragmatic fatigue in healthy humans. J Physiol (Lond) 1993; 460:385–405.
41. Harms CA, Babcock MA, McClaran SR, Pegelow DF, Nickele GA, Nelson WB, Dempsey JA. Respiratory muscle work compromises leg blood flow during maximal exercise. J Appl Physiol 1997; 82:1573–1583.
42. Powers SK, Lawler J, Dempsey JA, Dodd S, Landry G. Effects of incomplete pulmonary gas exchange on $\dot{V}O_{2max}$. J Appl Physiol 1989; 66:2491–2495.
43. Reybrouk T, Ghesquire J, Cattaert A, Fagard R, Amery A. Ventilatory thresholds during short- and long-term exercise. J Appl Physiol 1983; 55:1694–1700.
44. Wasserman K, McIlroy MB. Detecting the threshold of anaerobic metabolism. Am J Cardiol 1964; 14:844–852.
45. Brooks GA. Anaerobic threshold: review of the concept and directions for future research. Med Sci Sports Exerc 1985; 17:22–31.
46. Connett RJ, Gayeski TEJ, Honig CR. Lactate efflux is unrelated to intracellular Po_2 in a working red muscle in situ. J Appl Physiol 1986; 61:402–408.
47. Wilson DF, Erecinska M, Drown C, Silver IA. Effect of oxygen tension on cellular energetics. Am J Physiol 1977; 233:C135–140.
48. Gaesser GA, Poole DC. Lactate and ventilatory thresholds: disparity in time course of adaptations to training. J Appl Physiol 1986; 61:999–1004.
49. Hagberg J, Coyle EM, Carroll JE, Miller JM, Martin WH, Brooke MH. Exercise hyperventilation in patients with McArdle's disease. J Appl Physiol 1982; 52:991–994.
50. Beaver WL, Wasserman K, Whipp BJ. A new method for detecting anaerobic threshold by gas exchange. J Appl Physiol 1986; 60:2020–2027.
51. Johnson RL, Heigenhauser GJF, Hsia CCW, Jones NL, Wagner PD. Determinants of gas exchange and acid-base balance during exercise. In: Rowell LB, Shepherd JT, eds. Handbook of Physiology. New York: Oxford University Press, 1996, pp 515–584.
52. Johnson BD, Saupe KW, Dempsey JA. Mechanical constraints on exercise hyperpnea in endurance athletes. J Appl Physiol 1992; 73:874–886.
53. Schaffartzik W, Poole DC, Derion T, Tsukimoto K, Hogan MC, Arcos J, Bebout E, Wagner PD. $\dot{V}_A/\dot{Q}$ distribution during heavy exercise and recovery in humans: implications for pulmonary edema. J Appl Physiol 1992; 72:1657–1667.
54. Piiper J, Scheid P. Models for a comparative functional analysis of gas exchange organs in vertebrates. J Appl Physiol 1982; 53:1321–1329.
55. Hogan MC, Bebout DE, Wagner PD. Effect of hemoglobin concentration on maximal O_2 uptake in canine gastrocnemius muscle in situ. J Appl Physiol 1991; 70:1105–1112.

56. Schaffartzik W, Barton ED, Poole DC, Hogan MC, Tsukimoto K, Bebout DE, Wagner PD. The effect of altered hemoglobin concentration on O_2 diffusion from blood to muscle at maximal exercise. J Appl Physiol 1993; 75:491–498.
57. Wu EY, Ramanathan M, Hsia CCW. Role of hematocrit in the recruitment of pulmonary diffusing capacity: comparison of human and dog. J Appl Physiol 1996; 80:1014–1020.
58. Stringer W, Wasserman K, Casaburi R, Porszasz J, Maehara K, French W. Lactic acidosis as a facilitator of oxyhemoglobin dissociation during exercise. J Appl Physiol 1994; 76:1462–1467.
59. Buono MJ, Faucher PE. Intraerythrocyte and plasma osmolarity during graded exercise in humans. J Appl Physiol 1985; 58:1069–1072.
60. Richardson RS, Knight DR, Poole DC, Kurdak S, Hogan MC, Grassi B, Wagner PD. Determinants of $\dot{V}o_{2max}$ during single leg knee extensor exercise in man. Am J Physiol 1995; 268:H1453–1461.
61. Petro JK, Hollander AP, Bouman LN. Instantaneous cardiac acceleration in man induced by a voluntary muscle contraction. J Appl Physiol 1970; 29:794–798.
62. Robinson BF, Epstein SE, Beiser GD, Braunwald E. Control of heart rate by the automotive nervous system. Circulation 1966; 19:400–444.
63. Pendergast DR, Shindell D, Cerretelli P, Rennie DW. Role of central and peripheral adjustments in oxygen transport at the onset of exercise. Int J Sports Med 1980; 1:160–170.
64. Whipp BJ, Ward SA. Cardiopulmonary coupling during exercise. J Exp Biol 1982; 100:175–193.
65. Piiper J, Pendergast DR, Marconi C, Meyer M, Heisler N, Cerretelli P. Blood flow distribution in dog gastrocnemius muscle at rest and during stimulation. J Appl Physiol 1985; 58:2068–2074.
66. Sheriff DD, Rowell LB, Scher AM. Is rapid rise in vascular conductance at onset of dynamic exercise due to muscle pump? Am J Physiol 1993; 265:H1227–1234.
67. Berg BR, Cohen KD, Sarelius IH. Direct coupling between blood flow and metabolism at the capillary level in striated muscle. Am J Physiol 1997; 272:H2693–2700.
68. Welsh DG, Segal SS. Coactivation of resistance vessels and muscle fibers with acetylcholine release from motor nerves. Am J Physiol 1997; 273:H156–163.
69. Koller A, Sun D, Huang A, Kaley G. Corelease of nitric oxide and prostaglandins mediates flow-dependent dilation of rat gracilis muscle arterioles. Am J Physiol 1994; 267:H326–332.
70. Richardson RS, Poole DC, Knight DR, Kurdak SS, Hogan MC, Grassi B, Johnson EC, Kendrick K, Erickson BK, Wagner PD. High muscle blood flow in man: is maximal O_2 extraction compromised? J Appl Physiol 1993; 75:1911–1916.
71. Kurjiaka DT, Segal SS. Interaction between conducted vasodilation and sympathetic nerve activation in arterioles of hamster striated muscle. Circ Res 1995; 76:885–891.
72. Song H, Tyml K. Evidence for the sensing and integration of biological signals by the capillary network. Am J Physiol 1993; 265:H1235–1242.
73. Saito Y, Eraslan A, Hester RL. Importance of venular flow in the control of arteriolar diameter in the hamster cremaster muscle. Am J Physiol 1993; 265:H1294–1300.
74. Saito Y, Eraslan A, Hester RL. Role of EDRF in the control of arteriolar diameter during increased metabolism of striated muscle. Am J Physiol 1994; 267:H195–200.

75. Groebe K. Precapillary servo control of blood pressure and postcapillary adjustment of flow to tissue metabolic status. Circulation 1996; 94:1876–1885.
76. Knight DR, Schaffartzik W, Poole DC, Hogan MC, Wagner PD. Effect of hyperoxia on maximal leg O_2 supply and utilization in man. J Appl Physiol 1993; 75:2586–2594.
77. Wagner PD. Determinants of maximal oxygen transport and utilization. Ann Rev Physiol 1996; 58:21–50.
78. Richardson RS, Poole DC, Knight DR, Wagner PD. Red blood cell transit time in man: theoretical effect of capillary density. In: Hogan MC, Mathieu-Costello O, Poole DC, Wagner PD, eds. Oxygen Transport to Tissue XVI. New York: Plenum Press, 1993, pp 521–532.
79. Roca J, Agusti AG, Alonson A, Poole DC, Viegas C, Barbera JA, Rodriguez-Roisin R, Ferrer A, Wagner PD. Effects of training on muscle O_2 transport at $\dot{V}O_{2max}$. J Appl Physiol 1992; 73:1067–1076.
80. Clark A, Clark PAA. The end-points of the oxygen path: transport resistance in red cells and mitochondria. Adv Exp Med Biol 1986; 200:43–47.
81. Wittenburg BA, Wittenburg JB. Transport of oxygen in muscle. Ann Rev Physiol 1989; 51:857–878.
82. Groebe K, Thews G. Calculated intra- and extracellular gradients in heavily working red muscle. Am J Physiol 1990; 259:H84–92.
83. Richardson RS, Noyszewski EA, Kendrick KF, Leigh JS, Wagner PD. Myoglobin O_2 desaturation during exercise: evidence of limited O_2 transport. J Clin Invest 1995; 96:1916–1926.
84. Mathieu-Costello O. Capillary tortuosity and degree of contraction or extension of skeletal muscles. Microvasc Res 1987; 33:98–117.
85. Mathieu-Costello O, Ellis CG, Potter RF, Macdonald IC, Groom AC. Muscle capillary-to-fiber perimeter ratio: morphometry. Am J Physiol 1991; 261:H1617–1625.
86. Groom AC, Ellis CG, Potter RF. Microvascular architecture and red cell perfusion in skeletal muscle. Prog Appl Microcirc 1984; 5:64–83.
87. Poole DC, Mathieu-Costello O, West JB. Capillary tortuosity in rat soleus muscle is not affected by endurance training. Am J Physiol 1989; 256:H1110–1116.
88. Poole DC, Mathieu-Costello O. Capillary-fiber surface and mitochondrial volume relationship in soleus and plantaris muscles. Microcirculation 1996; 3:175–186.
89. Poole DC, Mathieu-Costello O. Effect of pulmonary emphysema on diaphragm capillary geometry. J Appl Physiol 1997; 82:599–606.
90. Poole DC, Musch TI, Kindig CA. In vivo microvascular structural and functional consequences of muscle length changes. Am J Physiol 1997; 272:H2107–2114.
91. Desjardins C, Duling BR. Heparinase treatment suggests a role for the endothelial cell glycocalyx in regulation of capillary hematocrit. Am J Physiol 1990; 258:H647–654.
92. Klitzman B, Duling BR. Microvascular hematocrit and red cell flow in resting and contracting striated muscle. Am J Physiol 1979; 237:H481–490.
93. Sarelius IH. Microcirculation in striated muscle after acute reduction in systemic hematocrit. Respir Physiol 1989; 78:7–17.
94. Federspiel WJ, Popel AS. A theoretical analysis of the effect of the particulate nature of blood on oxygen release in capillaries. Microvasc Res 1986; 32:164–189.

95. Federspiel WJ. Pulmonary diffusing capacity: implications of two-phase blood flow in capillaries. Respir Physiol 1978; 32:121–140.
96. Malvin GM, Wood SC. Effects of capillary red cell density on gas conductance of frog skin. J Appl Physiol 1992; 73:224–233.
97. Hogan MC, Willford DC, Keipert PE, Faithfull NS, Wagner PD. Increased plasma O_2 solubility improves O_2 uptake of in situ dog muscle working maximally. J Appl Physiol 1992; 73:2470–2475.
98. Sarelius IH. Cell flow path influences transit time through striated muscle capillaries. Am J Physiol 1986; 250:H899–907.
99. Wilson JR, Martin JL, Ferraro N, Weber KT. Effect of hydralazine on perfusion and metabolism in the leg during upright bicycle exercise in patients with heart failure. Circulation 1983; 68:425–432.
100. Ellis CG, Mathieu-Costello O, Potter RF, Macdonald IC, Groom AC. Effect of sarcomere length on total capillary length in skeletal muscle: in vivo evidence for longitudinal stretching of capillaries. Microvasc Res 1990; 40:63–72.
101. Welsh DG, Segal SS. Muscle length directs sympathetic nerve activity and vasomotor tone in resistance vessels of hamster retractor. Circ Res 1996; 79:551–559.
102. Wagner PD. The determinants of $\dot{V}_{O_2max}$. In: Appenzeller O, ed. Annals of Sports Medicine, Volume 4, part 4, New York: Oxford University Press, 1988, pp 196–212.
103. Gledhill N. Blood doping and related issues: a brief review. Med Sci Sports Exerc 1982; 14:183–189.
104. Stray-Gundersen J, Musch TI, Haidet GC, Swain DP, Ordway GA, Mitchell JH. The effect of pericardectomy on maximal oxygen consumption and maximal cardiac output in untrained dogs. Circ Res 1986; 58:523–530.
105. Gonzalez NC, Clancy RL, Wagner PD. Determinants of maximal oxygen uptake in rats acclimated to simulated altitude. J Appl Physiol 1993; 75:1608–1614.
106. Hogan MC, Roca J, Wagner PD, West JB. Limitation of maximal oxygen uptake and performance by acute hypoxia in dog muscle in situ. J Appl Physiol 1988; 65:815–821.
107. Wagner PD, Erickson BK, Kubo K, Hiraga A, Kai M, Yamaya Y, Richardson RS, Seaman J. Maximum O_2 transport and utilization before and after splenectomy. Equine Vet J 1995; 18:82–89.
108. Pugh LGCE. Cardiac output in muscular exercise at 5,800 m (19,000 ft). J Appl Physiol 1964; 19:441–447.
109. Wagner PD. Insensitivity of $\dot{V}_{O_2max}$ to hemoglobin-P_{50} at sea level and altitude. Resp Physiol 1997; 107:205–212.
110. Bebout DE, Story D, Roca J, Hogan MC, Poole DC, Gonzalez R, Ueno O, Haab P, Wagner PD. Effects of altitude acclimatization on pulmonary gas exchange during exercise. J Appl Physiol 1990; 67:2286–2295.
111. Drexler H, Faude F, Hoing S, Just H. Blood flow distribution within skeletal muscle during exercise in the presence of chronic heart failure: effect of milrinone. Circulation 1987; 76:1344–1352.
112. Kao AC, Van Trigt P, Shaeffer-McCall GS, Shaw JP, Kuzil BB, Page RD, Higginbotham MB. Central and peripheral limitations to upright exercise in untrained cardiac transplant recipients. Circulation 1994; 89:2605–2615.

113. Levy RD, Ernst P, Levine SM, Shennib H, Anzueto A, Bryan CL, Calhoon JH, Trinkle JK, Jenkinson SG, Gibbons WJ. Exercise performance after lung transplantation. J Heart Lung Transplant 1993; 12:27–33.
114. Marrades R, Roca J, Campistol JM, Diaz O, Barbera JA, Torregrosa JV, Masclans JR, Cobos A, Rodriguez-Roisin R, Wagner PD. Effects of erythropoietin on muscle O_2 transport during exercise in patients with chronic renal failure. J Clin Invest 1996; 97:2092–2100.
115. Scheiffer B, Wollert KC, Berchtold M, Saal K, Schieffer E, Hornig B, Riede UN, Drexler H. Development and prevention of skeletal muscle alterations after experimental myocardial infarction. Am J Physiol 1995; 269:H1507–1513.
116. Moore GE, Parsons B, Stray-Gundersen J, Painter PL, Brinker KR, Mitchell JH. Uremic myopathy limits aerobic capacity in hemodialysis patients. Am J Kidney Dis 1993; 22:277–287.
117. Sexton WL, Poole DC, Mathieu-Costello O. Microcirculatory structure-function relationships in skeletal muscle of diabetic rats. Am J Physiol 1994; 266:H1502–1511.
118. Kindig CA, Musch TI, Basaraba R, Poole DC. Imparied capillary hemodynamics in skeletal muscle of rats in chronic heart failure. J Appl Physiol 1999; 87:652–660.
119. Kindig CA, Sexton WL, Fedde MR, Poole DC. Skeletal muscle microcirculatory structure and function in diabetes. Respir Physiol 1998; 111:163–175.

19

Gas Exchange in Lung and Muscle at High Altitude

ROBERT B. SCHOENE

University of Washington
Seattle, Washington

I. Introduction

The transport of oxygen (O_2) from the air to the mitochondria is a complex, integrated process that is essential for the survival of organisms on this earth. In times of environmental and physiologic stress, redundancies and resilient adaptations in the system optimize the transport of this precious gas so that cellular respiration can proceed and the survival of the organism insured. Invoking these life-saving tactics may be immediate and short-lived or slow and ongoing responses. Nowhere in nature is there a more elegant example of these processes than at high altitude where the availability of O_2 is low and where humans sojourn for brief periods or for a lifetime.

This chapter will describe gas exchange of O_2 and carbon dioxide (CO_2) at the lung and the peripheral tissues in humans at high altitude and will refer briefly to the other aspects of integrated physiology, blood and circulation, that link these two ends of the gas exchange spectrum. Studies and observations of various species will be included to amplify understanding of humans.

II. The Problem

Successful O_2 delivery depends on both diffusion of the gas from the air to the blood in the lung and from the blood to the tissues in the periphery and transport of the gas by convection in the blood (Fig. 1). Diffusion requires: (1) permeability of the gas exchange interface which involves permissive solubility coefficients of the gases, (2) an adequate driving pressure for the gases from one media to another, (3) ample surface area for the gas exchange to take place, and (4) a diffusion distance for the gas that does not preclude equilibration of the gases from one phase to another. It is in number 2 that high altitude presents a formidable challenge both at the lung and the tissue. Additionally, the transport of O_2 from the lung to the tissues by convection is essential in the process and requires certain adaptations in the hypoxic environment to be successful. We will follow O_2's journey and begin with the air and lung.

III. The Lung

A. Overview

Transfer of oxygen from the alveolar air to the blood requires:

an adequate driving pressure for O_2 from the air to the blood,
sufficiently high surface area and low diffusion distance for gas exchange
an affinity of hemoglobin for O_2, and
an adequate time for equilibration of O_2 from air to blood as the red blood cells traverse the pulmonary capillary.

We will deal with each of these factors and the adaptations that occur at high altitude where the driving pressure for O_2 is less than it is at low altitude where there is a surfeit of O_2 available.

B. Alveolar Ventilation

The body's first defense against ambient hypoxia is an increase in alveolar ventilation. This response is mediated by a complex interaction of physiologic events initiated by stimulation of the carotid body by a low partial pressure of O_2 in the blood (1–3). This signal is transmitted to the brainstem from the carotid body, a highly metabolic organ exquisitely positioned and sensitized to sense the partial pressure of oxygen in the arterial blood (4–6). From the brainstem an efferent signal to the muscles of respiration which result in an increase in ventilation (Fig. 2). As one stays at high altitude, there is an ongoing adaptation that results in a decrease in alveolar PCO_2 and an increase in the alveolar PO_2 from a further increase in ventilation (7–11).

The higher P_{AO_2} results in a greater driving pressure for O_2 from the alveolus to the blood than would otherwise exist if there were not an increase in alveolar

Gas Exchange in Lung and Muscle at High Altitude 527

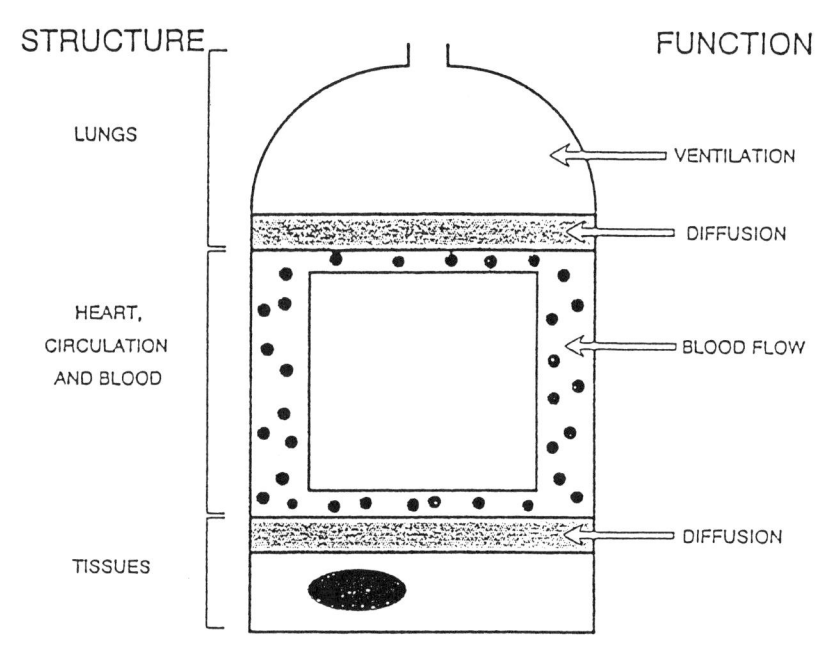

Figure 1 Schematic representation of oxygen transport pathway showing the integrated interaction of the four principal components of the convective and diffusive processes. (From Ref. 49.)

ventilation. As mentioned with continued stay at high altitude, there is further augmentation of ventilation and subsequently of alveolar P_{O_2}, thus further increasing the driving pressure at the air-blood interface. At moderate to extreme altitude, hyperventilation is essential to permit a viable level of O_2 to be transmitted to the blood (12). Without this response, life would not be possible. For instance, on the summit of Mt. Everest, the inspired partial pressure of O_2 is approximately 42 mm Hg. An extraordinary degree of hyperventilation is required to sustain life even on a transient basis (12,13). Actual measurements of alveolar gases on the summit in 1981 on the American Medical Research Expedition to Everest showed a P_{ACO_2} of 7.5–8.0 mm Hg and a P_{AO_2} of 32 mm Hg (12). This profound level of alveolar hypoxia makes the driving pressure for O_2 marginal for survival. Any impairment in gas exchange capabilities in the lung would make life tenuous. An intact and optimally brisk ventilatory response is, therefore, necessary in these environments. In fact, a number of studies in climbers who successfully have climbed to these altitudes have demonstrated that a greater than average hypoxic ventilatory response which is an inherent physiologic characteristic accentuated by the acclimatization process is an important trait in these individuals (14–17).

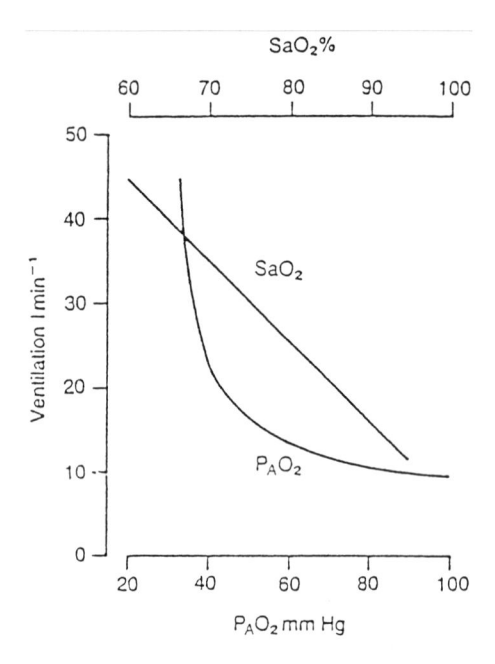

Figure 2 The hypoxic ventilatory response depicted schematically with ventilation plotted against P_{AO_2} and mm Hg Sa_{O_2} percent. (From Ref. 93.)

At even more modest altitudes, an increased ventilatory response and a more left-shifted oxygen-hemoglobin curve (OHC), which gives hemoglobin a greater affinity for oxygen, presumably conveys the improved oxygenation. The mechanism of a greater ventilatory response and higher arterial O_2 content may explain the better physical performance in humans at higher altitudes (13–17). Animals who live at high altitude or birds who migrate at extreme altitude have a left-shifted OHC that facilitates loading of O_2 from the air to hemoglobin, an elegant example of integrative physiology in which ventilation facilitates diffusion (18).

C. Pulmonary Diffusion and Gas Exchange

Alveolar ventilation results in an adequate alveolar partial pressure of O_2 for diffusion from the air to the blood, but the success of this transfer depends on a number of other factors. Because of the tremendous range of need for O_2 from rest to high levels of exercise, a large volume of gas must be exposed to a surface where diffusion of O_2 from the air to the blood can take place. The lung is well-designed for this purpose in that the alveolar-capillary interface provides a large surface area for gas exchange that is adaptable instantly to high levels of metabolic demand, such as in intense exercise.

O_2 flux depends on the demand for total body O_2 consumption which is proportional to the blood flow across the pulmonary capillary. The greater the ratio of diffusion capacity to perfusion, the more complete is the loading of O_2. Thus, with a decreased driving pressure for O_2 at high altitude, we encounter difficulties for gas exchange. Complete equilibration of O_2 from the air to the blood encounters several hurdles in that the driving pressure for O_2 from the air to the blood is less, transit time across the pulmonary capillary with exercise is shorter, and the loading of O_2 is impaired on the steep portion of the OHC (12,19).

The advantage conveyed to gas exchange at high altitude by an increase in alveolar partial pressure of O_2 from hyperventilation is in part offset by the inadequacy of the transit time of the red blood cell across the pulmonary capillary-alveolar interface. The degree to which oxygen is successful in getting from the alveolar air to the hemoglobin molecule is inversely related both to the altitude and the transit time in the pulmonary capillary, the latter of which is dependent on cardiac output (12,19) (Fig. 3a,b). On the other hand, the decrease in transit time from a higher cardiac output is, in part, offset by the limitation of maximum cardiac output during and after acclimatization to high altitude.

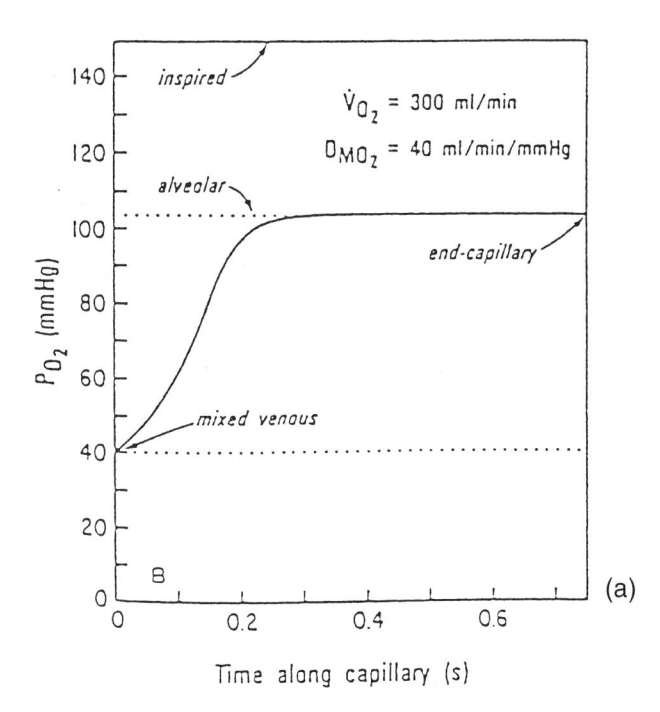

Figure 3 (a) Estimated time for transit of blood across the pulmonary capillary at sea level during rest demonstrating inadequate time for equilibration for oxygen from the air to the blood. (From Ref. 77.)

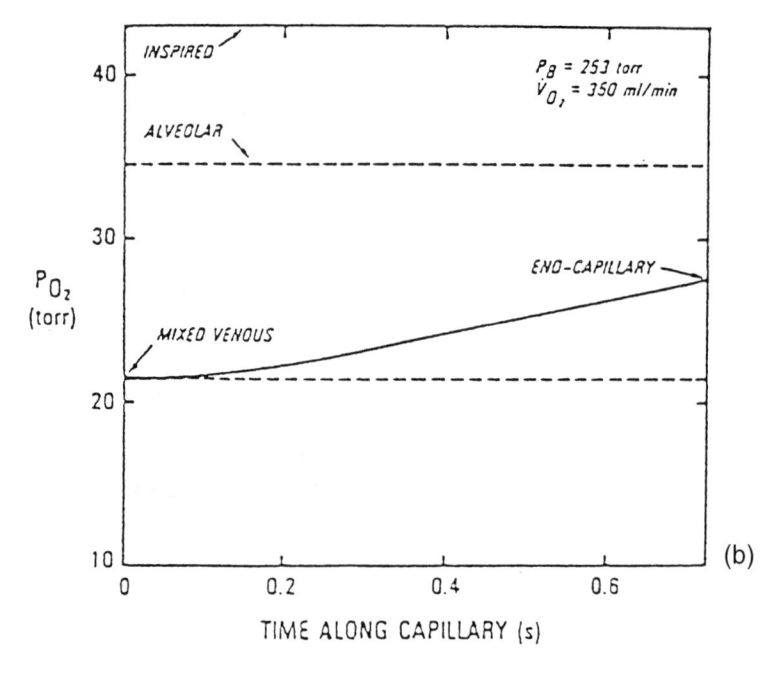

Figure 3 (b) Estimated time for transit of the red blood cell across the pulmonary capillary for an individual at rest on the summit of Mt. Everest. Because of the decreased driving pressure for oxygen from the air to the blood and inadequate time for equilibration, there is a diffusion limitation for oxygen. (From Ref. 77.)

Other factors play a role in the diffusion limitation for O_2 in the lung. The lower mixed venous partial pressure of O_2 during exercise at high altitude further slows the rate of equilibration which is further impaired by the fact that hemoglobin is also on the steep portion of the oxy-hemoglobin dissociation curve, making equilibration more difficult.

A number of studies in normal humans have both described and investigated the mechanism of impaired gas exchange at the lung especially during exercise. Arterial O_2 saturation decreases with exercise at high altitude, the greater degree of this drop the higher one goes (12,13,20–23) (Fig. 4).

Using the multiple inert gas elimination technique (MIGET), investigators have been able to quantitate this drop in arterial O_2 saturation by looking at the relationship of ventilation to perfusion as well as diffusion in the lung under hypoxic conditions. In acute hypobaric hypoxia to a simulated 15,000 feet altitude, Gale et al. (21), Torre-Bueno et al. (22), and Wagner et al. (23) used MIGET during high levels of exercise and documented both ventilation/perfusion (VA/Q) inequality and diffusion limitation in the lung which accounted for the worsening hypoxemia with increasing workloads. These studies were extended in Operation Everest II (OEII),

Gas Exchange in Lung and Muscle at High Altitude   531

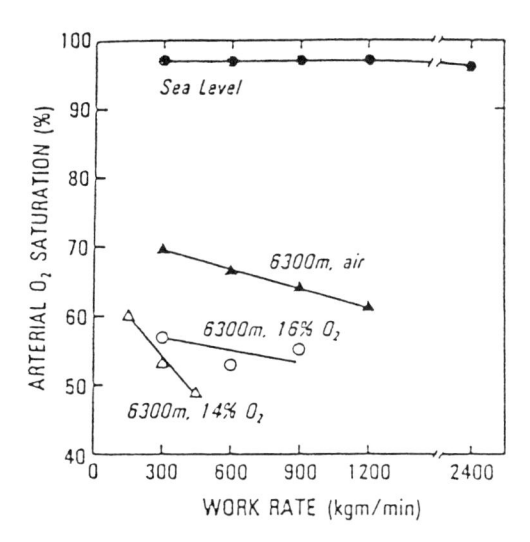

Figure 4 Decrease in arterial oxygen saturation with exercise as measured by ear oximetry with increasing work rates at sea level, 6300 meter altitude, and simulated 8800 meter altitude measured by breathing hypoxic gases at 6300 meters (16 and 14 percent oxygen respectively at a barometric pressure of 350 mm Hg.) (From Ref. 13.)

a project which over forty days simulated a climb of Mt. Everest in healthy male volunteers. Wagner et al. (19) again utilized MIGET to quantitate V_A/Q (Fig. 5) and diffusion (Fig. 6) up to a maximum exercise at a number of altitudes, including the summit (barometric pressure ~250 mm Hg). Diffusion limitation of oxygen became more pronounced the higher the subjects went while V_A/Q heterogeneity persisted. In addition, V_A/Q inequality contributed to hypoxemia and also correlated with the degree of pulmonary hypertension in these studies. The reasons for the improvement in V_A/Q heterogeneity at the highest altitudes is not clear, but may be secondary to transient interstitial lung edema at 6000 meters which clears upon further ascent. The increasing diffusion limitation was presumably secondary to the markedly decreased driving pressure for O_2 from the air to the blood.

Investigators speculated that these findings of V_A/Q mismatch at the intermediate altitudes were secondary to interstitial edema from high intravascular pressures (24–26). Not only were higher pulmonary artery pressures found in those with the most V_A/Q mismatch, but also an increase in pulmonary capillary wedge pressures evolved with higher levels of work and altitude (27). Some have attributed the increased wedge pressures not to left ventricular failure *per se* but to impaired left ventricular filling because of ventricular septal deviation from high right-sided pressures from the intense hypoxic pulmonary vasoconstriction.

Accentuated right-sided pressures are present in subjects with a previous history of high altitude pulmonary edema (HAPE) (28–30) (Fig. 7) and are thought

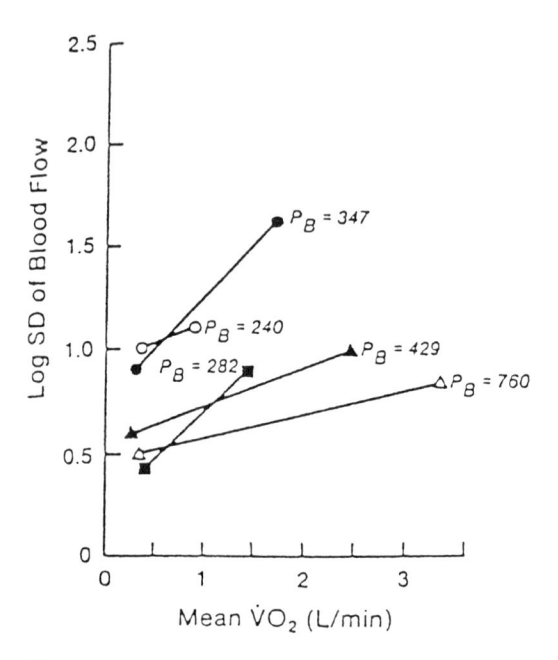

Figure 5 Data gathered during Operation Everest II investigating ventilation-perfusion inequality in the lung at different altitudes during the simulated ascent plotted against increasing oxygen uptake. V/Q inequality is expressed as the Log standard deviation of blood flow. V/Q inequality increased both with increasing altitude and increasing work rate. (From Ref. 19.)

to be responsible in part for the leak of fluid from the intra- to extra-vascular space in the lung (28–33). The increased pulmonary vascular response to hypoxia (HPVR) and exercise in these individuals is secondary to either an inherently greater HPVR and/or smaller lung volumes suggesting a limited pulmonary vascular bed to accommodate the high blood flow during exercise at high altitude. Whatever the mechanism interstitial edema must contribute to the impaired gas exchange found in these subjects.

A similar mechanism of high intravascular pressures leading to interstitial edema either from extravasation of fluid or hemorrhage from capillary rupture has been invoked in humans and other animals during high levels of exercise (31–40). This phenomenon occurs commonly in horses (32,33,35,36) and is secondary to overt bleeding in spite of the fact that they show little V_A/Q mismatch in the lung compared to other species including humans who show evidence of mild pulmonary hemorrhage after acute, intense exercise (37) and pigs who have perivascular edema after heavy exercise (39). Schaffartzik et al. (40) utilized intense exercise in humans and measured gas exchange with MIGET during recovery which was slower in the individuals with the higher aerobic capacity. They concluded that the impaired

Gas Exchange in Lung and Muscle at High Altitude

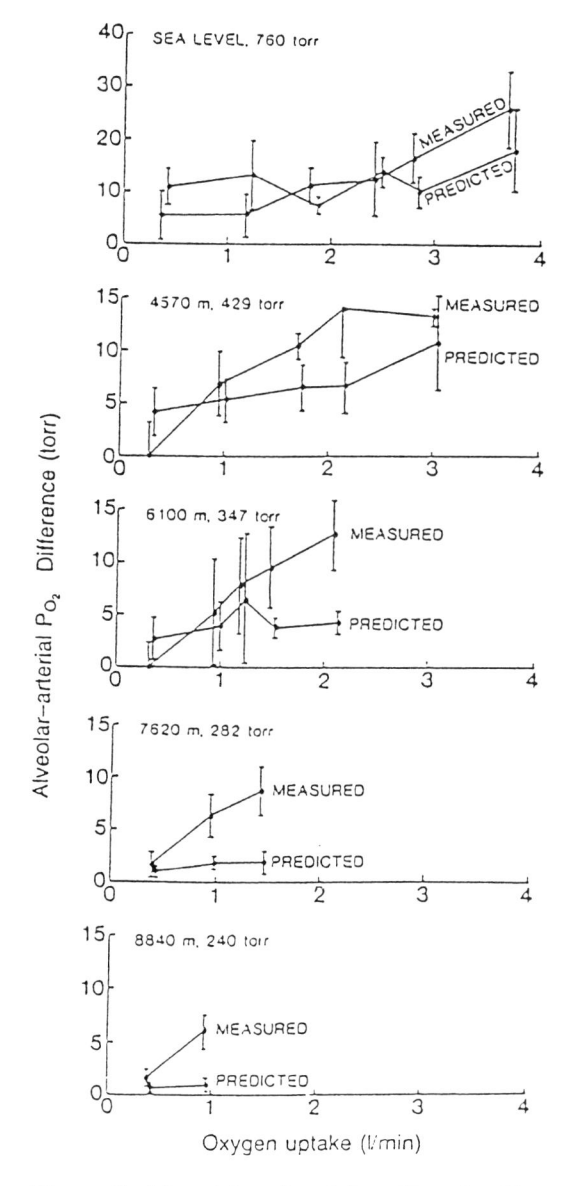

Figure 6 More data gathered from Operation Everest II, which demonstrate with each panel an increase in altitude from the top to the bottom panels from sea level to the simulated summit of Mt. Everest. Alveolar-arterial oxygen difference (mm Hg) with increasing work rates plotted against increasing work rates. The two lines in each graph demonstrate the measured (A-a) O_2 difference verses the predicted difference as measured with the multiple inert gas elimination technique which quantitates ventilation-perfusion inequality. The difference between the predicted and measured is therefore secondary to a diffusion limitation for oxygen from the air to the blood (From Ref. 19.)

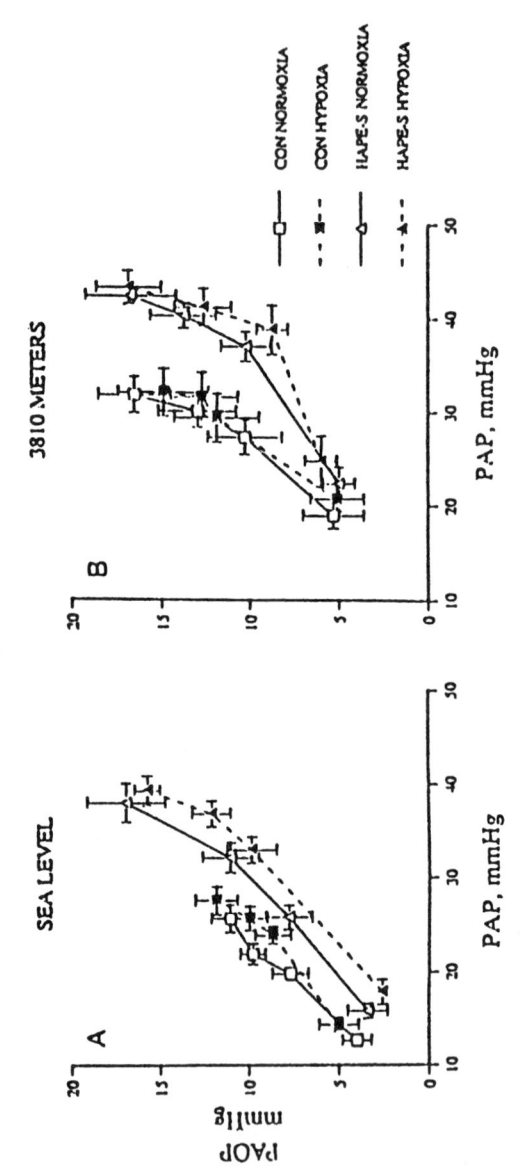

Figure 7 Pulmonary arterial occlusion pressure plotted against pulmonary artery pressure at sea level and 3810 meters altitude during exercise in control subjects and HAPE-susceptible subjects. The data support a greater propensity of the HAPE-susceptible subjects to have higher pulmonary intravascular pressures than control subjects. (From Ref. 30.)

gas exchange and slow recovery was most compatible with interstitial edema with slow clearing. Whatever the underlying dysfunction in the lung parenchyma in these observations, gas exchange is only worsened at high altitude where both exercise and a decreased driving pressure for oxygen play synergistic roles in impairing gas exchange in the lung.

IV. Gas Exchange in the Tissues

The transport of O_2 from the lung to the organs takes place by simple convection regulated by a complex mechanism of distribution of blood flow to the tissue beds finely-tuned for the demand for O_2 in a range of metabolic states from rest to exhaustive exercise. In health at sea level, this task is tricky enough, but in disease or at high altitude, it is virtually a matter of survival as the regulation of perfusion penuriously doles out just enough blood at just the right time to allow for adequate diffusion of O_2 from the blood to the tissues.

Although the process of O_2 transport in the tissues is often termed extraction, it is actually a more passive process of simple diffusion of gas from the blood to the mitochondria along a diffusion gradient from pre-capillary to post-capillary levels (Fig. 8). This process is not dissimilar from the lung, as described earlier. As in the lung, gas transfer is more successful the greater the driving pressure; thus, when the supply (i.e., blood flow) is not adequate, O_2 supply to the mitochondria is impaired. The process in the tissues is more complex than the lung (41,42,43,44) since there is greater heterogeneity in the manner in which different tissue beds receive perfusion and transport O_2 from the blood to the mitochondria. For instance, muscle cells have myoglobin which is thought to facilitate the journey of O_2 through the cytosol to the mitochondria. Physical function, therefore, depends on the adequacy of the O_2 supply and availability to the tissues, that is a function of, not one, but many links in the oxygen transport chain.

In healthy humans at low altitude, the convection of O_2 from the lung to the cells may be a major culprit in limiting exercise because of limitations of cardiac output as the demand for O_2 flux at high levels of work outstrips the supply (43,44). At low altitude where there is a surfeit of O_2 in the atmosphere and subsequently at the proximal end of the muscle capillary bed, there is a high driving pressure for O_2 diffusion; but as the demand for O_2 increases with exercise, there is a progressive decrease in O_2 content from the proximal to distal end of a muscle capillary and subsequent decrease in diffusion gradient. Furthermore, O_2 dissociation occurs on a steeper part of the oxygen-hemoglobin dissociation curve. Increased perfusion compensates in part and may paradoxically become an impairment as time available for gas exchange diminishes with greater blood flow (18,44). This impairment is offset only in part by a rightward shift of the oxygen-hemoglobin dissociation curve (Bohr effect) which results from acidosis and the efflux of CO_2 from the active muscle which facilitates unloading of oxygen from hemoglobin.

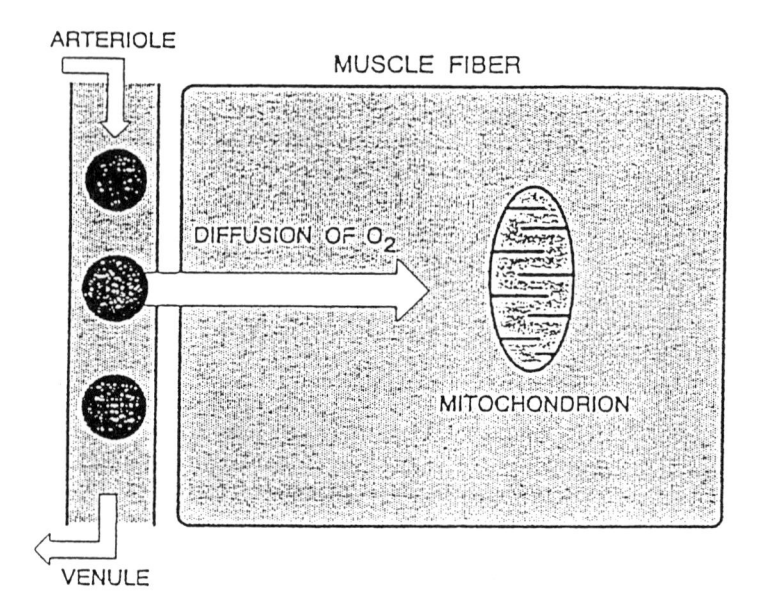

Figure 8 Schematic representation of oxygen transport in a skeletal muscle. Oxygen is supplied to the muscle by convection through the microcirculation from the arteriole to the venule across the muscle capillary bed. Oxygen diffuses from the red blood cell through the capillary, across the capillary wall to the muscle cell membrane which then diffuses in to the cytosol with facilitation by myoglobin to the mitochondrial membrane after which oxygen flux, depending on metabolic rate, occurs. (From Ref. 49.)

V. High Altitude

The process of gas exchange at high altitude is complicated by a number of factors, most of which were outlined earlier, but accentuated by the decreased O_2 content of the blood flowing to the tissues. In this section, factors affecting this process at high altitude will be discussed going from the flow of blood to the tissues to the unloading of and diffusion of O_2 to the mitochondria.

First, blood flow from the heart is necessary to carry O_2 to the tissues. The alterations of blood flow during exercise at high altitude compared to sea level and the potential heterogeneity of flow through the muscle beds will be discussed. Second, the surface area for gas exchange, including the quantity of red blood cells and capillary-muscle interface, is essential for O_2 availability to the tissues. Training and hypoxia may affect capillary and mitochondrial density and thus surface area for gas exchange and diffusion distance for O_2, respectively. Third, alterations in oxygen-hemoglobin dissociation may affect O_2 unloading to the tissues. Finally, O_2 must diffuse from blood to the cytosol to the mitochondria. It is this last crucial step that is affected most profoundly at high altitude.

VI. Blood Flow

At low and moderate altitude, cardiac output correlates with maximal O_2 consumption (45,46). It would thus seem logical that at very high altitudes an ability to maintain a high cardiac output would convey an advantage in work performance. Interestingly, with acclimatization, maximum heart rate and cardiac output drop at high altitude (12,20), and this phenomenon occurs especially at very high and extreme altitudes. Does this mean that cardiac performance limits exercise capacity or is the heart merely responding appropriately to the reduced demand for O_2 from peripheral sources? This question is one that is focus of ongoing debates.

The consensus is that at very high altitudes the healthy heart performs well (47) and by not reaching maximal sea level performance may in fact minimize deterioration of extraction of O_2 in the tissues and uptake by O_2 by the lungs as an increase in cardiac output would result in a briefer, inadequate time for O_2 extraction across the capillary-cell interface (51). This advantage of increased transit time is apparently balanced by the decrease in cardiac output and subsequent tissue blood flow (52).

In the working muscle bed, however, the effect of hypoxemia is to increase blood flow (53). Rowell et al. (54) made this observation in humans when they looked at blood flow in one and both quadriceps at maximal exercise during normoxia and hypoxia ($F_{IO_2} \sim 0.10$–0.11) (Fig. 9). They found both an increase in blood flow and an increase in arterial pressure. Rowell et al. (54) hypothesized that the baroreceptor response is invoked locally during hypoxic exercise and is mediated by the release of norepinephrine from the tissue beds. This response was necessary to maintain an adequate flow and pressure while increasing mean transit time of blood through the capillaries. They also found that one-legged exercise could utilize close to 75% of the blood flow that was measured in both legs suggesting that because of the limitation of the human heart, the capacitance for flow is underutilized in two-legged exercise.

However, the picture is far more complex. There must be an elegant regulation of blood flow in a heterogeneous pattern which increases blood flow to the tissues demanding an increase in O_2 flux while vasoconstricting other vascular beds to tissues that have a lower metabolic rate at the time. Further work is necessary to clarify the issue.

Looking further at gas exchange in exercising muscle, Richardson et al. (52) used a single-leg knee-extensor exercise protocol to rapid exhaustion to show that O_2 consumption increased in concert with blood flow and did not plateau even at maximal fatigue. With this technique, they achieved 80% more extraction than had been elicited with exercise protocols that were longer. These findings suggest that higher blood flow compensated for shorter transit times the tissue to extract oxygen and minimize the diffusion limitation of O_2. Of course, these experiments were done under normoxic conditions and did not test the limits of diffusion when hypoxemia was present such as at high altitude.

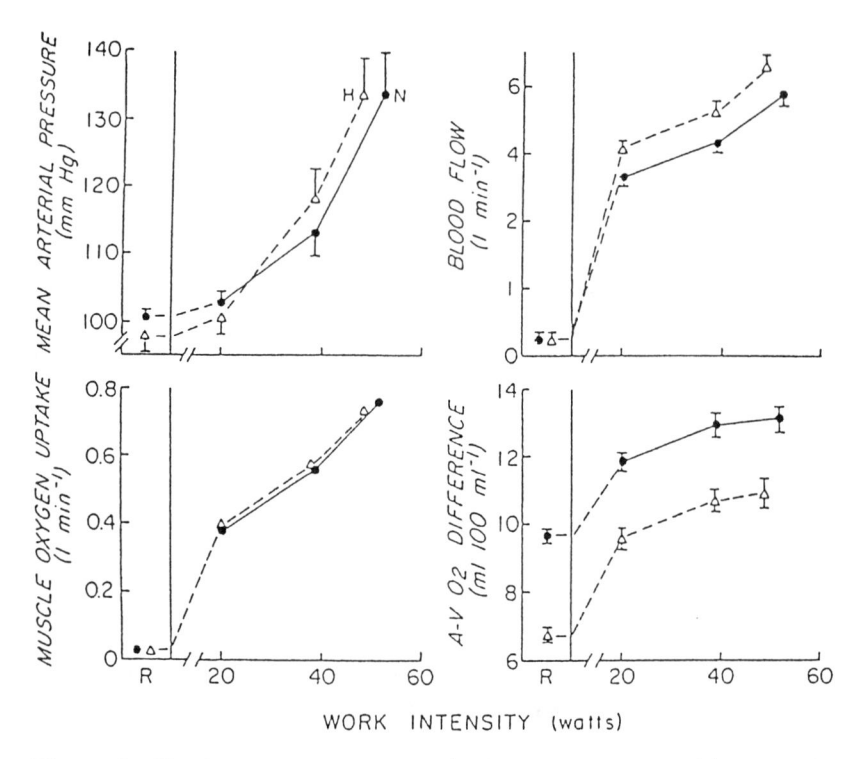

Figure 9 Circulatory responses to exercise by knee extensors with progressive work while breathing air (closed circles) and 10% oxygen (open triangles). Blood flow increases with hypoxemia at each workload. Oxygen uptake was similar at each workload in spite of a lower arterial oxygen content during hypoxemia which is secondary to increased blood flow. (From Ref. 51.)

In a later study, Richardson et al. (55) repeated the single-leg extensor exercise to maximum but used both normoxia and hypoxia ($F_{IO_2} = 0.12$). Unlike a previous study by Rowell et al. (54) who found that under hypoxia there was an increase in blood flow and a constant extraction of O_2, Richardson et al. (55) found that blood flow remained proportional to work rate while extraction maintained the work rate/oxygen consumption relationship. The explanation for these findings was not clear but suggested that difference in subjects' conditioning may have contributed to the invoking of different mechanisms to maintain O_2 flux. Adaptations to training include a proliferation of capillaries in the tissues as well as an increase of mitochondrial density, both of which result in an increased ability to extract and use O_2 in states of high metabolic demand.

In an earlier study by Hogan et al. (56), using an isolated canine gastocnemius muscle, maintained constant blood flow but altered the level of O_2 delivered to the muscle by changing the F_{IO_2} and found that the V_{O_2} max fell proportionally with muscle venous and calculated muscle capillary partial pressure of O_2 while the muscle diffusion capacity remained constant. These data suggest a fixed and thus limited diffusion capacity for O_2 of the muscle in the periphery under hypoxic conditions. Bender et al. (59) looked at the effect of 18 days of acclimatization at 4300 meters in seven male volunteers. O_2 delivery to the legs was measured during cycle ergometry under both normoxic and hypoxic conditions after return to sea level. They used indwelling arterial and venous catheters and found that maximum V_{O_2} was similar to pre-altitude exposure in spite of an increase in arterial oxygen content, arterial-venous extraction, and hemoglobin after acclimatization. There was, however, an increase in vascular resistance and decrease in blood flow and maintenance of comparable mixed venous P_{O_2} which suggested that acclimatization resulted in increased capability of the muscle bed to extract O_2 but a finely tuned integrative mechanism to match O_2 supply with demand. What is not clear is why, if the ability to extract is greater, the body does not permit a greater blood flow to increase performance.

What these experiments demonstrate is the body's resiliency to invoke different mechanisms to maintain O_2 flux when the energy requirement is increased. What is not known and what is an area of intense research in its embryonic phase is the regulation of blood flow at the microvascular level and tissue beds, its heterogeneity and the factors that regulate this flow and thus supply of O_2 with instantaneous adjustments depending on demand. The stress of hypoxia makes these questions even more fascinating, but perhaps the use of the hypoxic model may accentuate some of the adaptations and thus allow us to understand them more clearly.

Another important factor in the convective flow of O_2 to the tissues not only is distribution but the anatomy of microcirculation which supplies it. There has been intense interest in the effect of hypoxia and exercise on angiogenesis of the muscle capillaries. To ascertain whether vascular growth actually occurs or not is critical to the understanding of physical delivery of oxygen closer to the muscle membrane and subsequently to the mitochondria. The presumed effect of hypoxic exposure and exercise has been likened to the effect of endurance training on muscle capillaries and mitochondrial density.

There is abundant evidence that endurance training can alter capillary and mitochondrial distribution and proliferation (58–62). For instance, Crenshaw et al. (63) looked at the effect of extreme endurance training on capillary and mitochondrial distribution in human skeletal muscle. An increase in capillaries between muscle fibers as well as presence of subsarcolemmal mitochondria close to the capillaries which should facilitate diffusion of O_2 from the blood to the mitochondria was found. Intense exercise, however, is not necessary to induce these changes as was noted by Green et al. (64) who exercised subjects for only 10–12 days at a moderate level of exercise. They found an increase in capillary density around the type IIa, but not around the other fiber types. The study was more focused on the metabolic changes which showed suppression of glycolysis and glucose utilization as the muscle trained. In an elegant study looking at both the convective and diffusive characteristics of nine weeks of endurance training in humans, Roca et al. (65) found an increase in blood flow to the exercising leg after training both during normoxia and two levels of hypoxia ($F_{IO_2} = 0.15$ and 0.12). The techniques of the study did not permit differentiation between regulation of blood flow versus increase in capillary density. Whatever the mechanism, training induced improvement in O_2 flux by convection (as well as by diffusion) in both normoxic and hypoxic conditions.

In a prolonged progressive hypoxic experiment in a chamber simulating a climb to extreme altitude on Mt. Everest (OEII), Green et al. (66) documented an increase in capillary density in these subjects. A confounding variable in determination of the actual effect of the increase capillaries per fiber ratio in these prolonged hypoxic experiments is the fact that muscle fiber atrophy usually was found as well. From a diffusion standpoint, this makes for a shorter distance for diffusion of O_2 from the blood to the tissues, but whether this is a functionally beneficial adaptation is not known. As technology is now allowing, investigators can go from the descriptive phase to the mechanistic phase as the stimulus of exercise and hypoxia appear to increase messenger-RNA for vascular endothelial growth factor (VEGF) as recently reported by Hoppeler et al. (67). Investigators can now take advantage of the molecular adaptation to understand the mechanism by which these changes are made.

VII. The Role of Hemoglobin

Hemoglobin concentration in its O_2-carrying capacity plays a major role in convection of O_2 and the initial role of diffusion of O_2 to the working muscle. Except for a very small amount of O_2 that is dissolved in the plasma, hemoglobin far and away is the most important carrier of O_2 to the tissues. Alterations in hemoglobin concentration alter maximum O_2 consumption that emphasizes the important role of the carrier molecule for O_2 (68–70). To determine how much of a role hemoglobin concentration plays in convective versus diffusive roles of O_2 transport in maximum exercise in humans both normoxically and hypoxically, Schaffartzik et al. (42) took seven subjects from 3801 meters altitude for eight weeks to sea level and studied them both at their relative polycythemic level upon return from altitude as well as their previous sea level hemoglobin concentration. Reducing the hemoglobin concentration from 15.9 to 13.8 g/100ml decreased maximum workloads by approximately seven per cent both normoxically and hypoxically ($F_{IO_2} = 0.12$). Calculating the diffusion capacity of the muscle, the investigators found a predictable drop with the lower hemoglobin and found that O_2 delivery to the exercising leg was decreased by 154 and 83 cc's per minute in normoxia and hypoxia, respectively. They calculated that approximately "two-thirds of the fall in maximum O_2 consumption is attributable to the reduced convective transport of O_2 and of the muscle circulation and that the remaining one-third is accounted for by reduction of the overall muscle DO_2." Since O_2 must be offloaded from hemoglobin for diffusion into the muscle, clearly there's a quantitative relationship between the amount delivered to the tissues via convection and that which is subsequently delivered by diffusion.

In an attempt to look at the effect of more radical changes in hemoglobin or hematocrit, Gonzales et al. (71) studied acclimatized and unacclimatized rats varying their hematocrit from 60 to 45% and studied maximum exercise capacity. In all cases the increase in O_2 carrying capacity increased V_{O_2} max but less so in the acclimatized animals both during normoxia and hypoxia suggesting other compensatory mechanisms to optimize O_2 delivery. Of interest as well, was the increase in systemic vasoconstriction in the polycythemic animals which implies some effect eventually on tissue perfusion in the polycythemic state.

At some point an increase in hemoglobin in humans becomes a detriment to both exercise and mental performance. The profound polycythemia associated with chronic mountain sickness (72) and the substantial polycythemia of sojourners to extreme altitude actually results in a well-documented impairment of physical performance. In spite of an increase in O_2 carrying capacity, this impairment is thought to be secondary to an actual decrease in perfusion of the microcirculation secondary to the exponential increase in blood viscosity that occurs at hematocrits of approximately 60% and above.

In a remarkable study of high altitude natives living in the Peruvian Andes, by Winslow et al. (73) subjects with chronic mountain sickness whose hematocrits were greater than 65% prior to hemodilution to hematocrits of approximately 49%. Maximum O_2 consumption, heart rate, stroke volume, and a rightward shift of the ventilatory threshold was documented in the subjects' undergoing hemodilution. They studied a group of subjects and either by hemodilution or phlebotomy decreased their hematocrits from means of 67 to 49%. There was quite a bit of variability in the responses, some of which were not significant but suggestive. Work rate increased from 475 to 638 kpm/minute (N.S.), maximum heart rate from 138 to 162 bpm ($p < 0.05$) while maximum ventilation and VCO_2 did not change. Because of the potentially profound impairments that this population of patients has, it is difficult to ascertain the isolated role of hemoglobin in this study, but it raises some intriguing questions that deserve further investigation not only from a physiologic but also a clinical standpoint.

In a study in sojourners to extreme altitude, Sarnquist et al. (74) isovolemically hemodiluted mountaineers on Mt. Everest after their extreme altitude exposure. These investigators decreased the hematocrit level from close to 60% down to the low 50% level and did both maximum exercise and psychometric tests on these subjects. In spite of the decrease in hemoglobin concentration, V_{O_2} max did not decrease while psychometric function improved. This study suggests that the decrease in hemoglobin may have been compensated by increased cardiac output and tissue blood flow.

Of course, it is not clear where the impairment in O_2 transport is in these excessively polycythemic subjects. The impairment of perfusion to all of the microcirculation could impair gas exchange both at the lung and in the periphery, but these examples are in individuals who are either high altitude natives with maladaption to high altitude or sojourners at extreme altitude.

VIII. Oxygen-Hemoglobin Affinity

As we make the transition from convection to diffusion of O_2 from the blood to the tissues, we must consider the affinity of O_2 for hemoglobin and its affect on unloading and diffusion of O_2 to the tissues. Theoretically, the situation where there is a high affinity of hemoglobin for O_2, unloading of O_2 from the hemoglobin molecule to the tissues and subsequent O_2 flux in augmented metabolic states could be impaired. However, as has been well documented in animals who live at altitude and birds that migrate a phenomenal way at extreme altitude (75), markedly left-shifted OHCs have been documented. Of course, so far as gas exchange at the lung is concerned, at very high altitude where the driving pressure for O_2 from the air to the blood is much less, O_2 loading at the lung would be facilitated by a hemoglobin with a high affinity for O_2, i.e., a left-shifted oxy-hemoglobin disassociation curve. Severe degrees of respiratory alkalosis from hyperventilation in humans who climb to extreme altitude would also result in a left-shifted curve. Of course, the question arises as to the effect of this left-shifted curve on the unloading of O_2 to the tissues. An ideal system would bring blood to the exercising muscle where there's increased temperature and tissue acidosis such that the affinity for of hemoglobin for O_2 would decrease as the blood traverses the muscle capillary and thus facilitate unloading. In fact, in these extreme situations this is probably what happens.

In an attempt to look at this situation, Hogan et al. (76) maintained a constant blood flow and arterial O_2 content while perfusing an isolated canine gastrocnemius muscle which was isometrically, tetanically contracted with blood with both normal and increased oxygen-hemoglobin affinity. This experiment found that V_{O_2} max was impaired with a left-shifted curve suggesting that the avidity of hemoglobin for O_2 persisted during the perfusion of the muscle bed. In an attempt to find an optimal P50 partial pressure of oxygen where the arterial oxygen saturation is 50% (P50), Wagner (77) modeled OHCs at various altitudes including extreme altitudes of Mt. Everest. He found that with progressive increase in altitude the optimal P50 dropped but the overall V_{O_2} was relatively insensitive to such perturbations. This insensitivity stems from counter-balancing effects at the lung and tissues. Thus, a high affinity hemoglobin would favor O_2 uptake at the lung but impair unloading of O_2 at the tissues, and a low affinity hemoglobin would result in the opposite effects. Overall, these effects appear to balance over a wide range of P50. At least during hypoxia the theoretical model fits what is found in the field setting.

IX. Diffusion of Oxygen from Blood to the Tissue

From the earlier discussion one can see that acute and chronic adjustments are made in the O_2 transport system as the body becomes stressed with high altitude. Some of these adaptations are more successful than others, and there is no one single factor that limits O_2 delivery and physical performance at high altitude.

To understand O_2 delivery from the blood to the tissue and mitochondria has been problematic in that technology in the past has not allowed sophisticated investigations of this final step which actually is made up of a number of components in and of itself. In this regard, over the last decade, investigators have concentrated their effort on the peripheral diffusion of O_2 to the tissues to help understand overall limitations in exercise that occur at high altitude.

A proposed diffusion limitation for O_2 transport from the air to the blood on the summit of Mt. Everest was predicted by West and Wagner (11) and was further defined by the multiple inert gas elimination technique (see earlier discussion). A similar but more complicated process in reverse occurs in the muscle. Delivery of O_2 by convection to the tissues is followed by unloading of O_2 from the hemoglobin to the blood, diffusion of O_2 across the capillary membrane to the interstitium, then diffusion of O_2 from interstitial space across the cell membrane into the cytosol, a subsequent myoglobin-facilitated diffusion of O_2 through the cytosol to the mitochondrial membrane, and then utilization of O_2 in oxidative phosphorylation to produce energy in the form adenosine triphosphate (ATP). A curious quote by Wittenberg and Wittenberg (78) makes on wonder, therefore, why there is any limitation of energy production regardless of the supply of oxygen:

> There need be no unique rate-limiting step in normal working muscle. Oxygen delivery is not rate-limiting. The flows of oxygen, ATP, ADP, Pi, and substrate-donated electrons through the working muscle may better be regarded as a family of steady states, which when perturbed, will always return to their starting point by some kind of relaxation process, however complex. (79).

This may be true within the cell itself, but from a functional standpoint, it has long been observed that a decreased availability of O_2 in the air and within the blood delivering it to the cells, there is a decrease in energy output. The question arose: how much does a diffusion limitation in muscle contribute to this decrease energy output?

Intensification of the investigation of diffusion of O_2 in the peripheral tissues has occurred over the last ten years based on some observations of a rather fixed partial pressure of O_2 in the mixed venous blood of individuals exercising at moderate to extreme altitude. With increasing levels of exercise and thus O_2 demand, tissue extraction of O_2 increases according to the Fick principle, and with an estimation of O_2 diffusion capacity in the muscle membrane of approximately 100 cc/min/mm Hg, it was thought that the lowest partial pressure of O_2 in mixed venous blood that could be attained was approximately 15 mm Hg. Data obtained in OEII supported this prediction (22,23). A number of papers followed which discussed the theoretical reasons why extraction appeared to be limited (80–82). What must be noted, however, is that mixed venous blood is indeed just that, i.e., a summary of the mixing of effluent blood from many tissues, some of which have much higher extractions than others. For instance, the effluent blood coming directly from an intensely exercising muscle blood certainly can fall much lower than what is observed in mixed venous blood. But still, enough evidence supported the contention that for some reason even though there appears to be O_2 still available, i.e., in the mixed venous blood, there appears to be a limitation to its total extraction. The question then became where in the path from hemoglobin molecule to the mitochondria is the resistance to oxygen flux or is there merely homogeneous flow that is limited by the front-end convection process. Wagner (82) speculated that one of four possibilities for this limitation exists, the latter of two of which have negligible effect at Vo_2 max.

> A finite overall diffusion conductance for oxygen between hemoglobin and the mitochondria;
> Heterogeneity of perfusion with respect to local oxygen demand;
> Functional or structural shunts of arterial blood into the venous system;
> Direct diffusion of oxygen from pre-exchange arteries to post-exchange veins through muscle tissue.

Attention then focused on each of the steps of O_2's journey from hemoglobin to mitochondria.

The successful diffusion of O_2 from hemoglobin to the mitochondria depends both on "geography" and the laws of physics. Literally the distance for diffusion and the anatomic structures which support this and the driving pressures are critical elements. The wonderment about this phenomenon is not new. In 1919 Krogh (83) made the first important speculations about these structures and laws of diffusion. He considered both the distance for diffusion by looking at capillary-mitochondrial proximity and the diffusion coefficients for O_2. Although this concept has been rethought to a certain degree, his prescient speculations were brilliant and hold much value still today. In that light, once O_2 is dissociated from hemoglobin, the first barrier to O_2 transport is the capillary membrane. In that regard, O_2 flux across the capillary wall has been estimated and has been thought to be one of the least resistive barriers to O_2 diffusion in the overall spectrum of this last step (84–87). With such little resistance, it has been calculated that the pressure drop across the capillary wall necessary to provide O_2 under high metabolic demands would be 5–10 mm Hg or even less, 3–5 mm Hg (88). Thus, the total capillary surface area for gas exchange rather than the actual diffusion distance for O_2 is thought to be the critical element in successful O_2 availability to the mitochondria.

To elucidate the relationship of diffusion distance to O_2 flux, Bebout et al. (89) looked at trained versus untrained and immobilized muscle. Capillary proliferation is incurred by training and fiber atrophy by immobilization. They found that the increase of the capillary surface area augmented oxygen flux in a maximally exercised canine muscle, while decreased diffusion distance did not.

To investigate the effect of various degrees of arterial O_2, Hogan et al. (90) had done earlier work in which arterial and venous blood in a maximally exercised canine gastroctnemeous muscle was measured during electrical stimulation. The more hypoxic preparations fatigued earlier as venous partial pressure of O_2 decreased to approximately 11 mm Hg as maximum exercise was less compared to normoxia. Because there appeared to be differences in diffusion capacities during the various levels of hypoxemia in the previous study, Hogan et al. (56) repeated there studies only this time they maintained constant blood flow. In these studies the authors observed that as the arterial O_2 content and O_2 consumption dropped as did venous partial pressure of O_2 while extraction increased. Diffusion capacity for O_2 was calculated as being constant, but the authors felt that there was a limit to the extraction capabilities and thus a diffusion limitation.

Later studies turned to maximal leg exercise in humans. Richardson et al. (55) did maximal knee extensor exercises in humans both during normoxia and hypoxia. Arterial and venous oxygen partial pressures were measured as well as blood flow across this muscle bed. It was found that blood flow was similar in the two conditions but that work rate and oxygen consumption were lower in the hypoxic condition. They concluded with similar diffusion capacities and blood flows in the two preparations, yet with lower O_2 flux, the diffusibility of O_2 must play a critical role.

Two other factors come into play in the transport of O_2. They are the tissue cell membrane and the presence of myoglobin, which facilitates O_2 transport to the mitochondria. There is a fairly precipitous drop in O_2 gradient across the cell membrane with a rather constant, albeit lower, O_2 partial pressure across the cytoplasm to the mitochondria. This latter step is thought to be facilitated by the presence of myoglobin. Myoglobin enhances the flux of O_2 across the sarcoplasm in which there is both myoglobin-bound and free O_2. As O_2 demand increases, more O_2 is extracted from myoglobin as it flows into the mitochondria. There must be adequate levels of myoglobin present, and there must be the ability for myoglobin to bind and release O_2. It also must be able to diffuse within the sarcoplasm itself (78).

However, an intriguing article by Garry et al. (91) may revolutionize the thinking on the role of myoglobin in O_2 transport. They developed a gene-knockout mouse model without myoglobin. Mice were exercised and showed no impairment of performance compared to control animals. Both heart and striated (soleus) muscle were found to be depigmented but functionally normal. These findings raise new questions about the role of myoglobin and O_2 in metabolically active muscles.

In order to understand these steps more thoroughly, Richardson et al. (92) performed a study in humans who exercised maximally with leg extension ergometry during normoxia and hypoxia. Nuclear magnetic resonance spectroscopy was used to measure oxygen-myoglobin saturation, phosphoro-creatine, inorganic phosphate, and intracellular pH. Arterial and venous P_{O_2}'s as well as calculated mean capillary P_{O_2}'s were determined. At the highest of levels of work which were possible during hypoxia, the hypoxic exercise corresponded to 75% of the normoxic V_{O_2} max; whereas, under normoxia it reached approximately 95%. Arterial P_{O_2}'s and intracellular pH's were lower with hypoxia. Arterial P_{O_2}'s with normoxia were 115 and with hypoxia 46 mm Hg, while femoral venous P_{O_2}'s were 22 and 17, respectively. Large differences in P_{O_2} between blood and intracellular tissue with normoxia and hypoxia were found. Additionally, myoglobin desaturation occurred early on even at moderate work levels (20 s) were substantially lower during hypoxia than normoxia and did not decline much more up to maximum work. Where the myoglobin saturation was approximately 50%, the partial pressure of O_2 was about 3 mm Hg, being lower by approximately 1 mm Hg with hypoxia. Thus indicating that the greatest diffusion limitation was actually from the red blood cell to the sarcolemma, a distance of 1–5 μm, a barrier which therefore may play a great role in the resistive part of O_2 delivery to the mitochondria. Future innovations in technology will allow even greater resolution and thus understanding of this final critical step in O_2 transport.

X. Summary

This chapter has concentrated on both the "front end" and "back end" of O_2 delivery at high altitude. Both of these steps involve diffusion of O_2 from the air to the blood and subsequently from the blood to the mitochondria. The delivery of this blood by convection involves both macro and micro vasculature, the latter of which influences the availability and thus diffusion of O_2 on the periphery.

There is not just one step that appears to limit exercise performance at high altitude. What is impressive is not so much the limitation but the fact that the human body even functions at all. It is a tribute to the resiliency and resourcefulness of the physiological process that allows this to happen.

There is still much to be investigated. For with each answer comes further questions, and with technology comes the opportunity to answer these questions. In the future a better understanding of adaptation at the cellular and genetic level will be forthcoming, and an elucidation of heterogeneity of blood flow and tissue beds or lack thereof will become clear. What about the role of myoglobin? These are the primary areas of investigation, which are foreseen, in the next decade and beyond.

References

1. Boycott AE, Haldane JS. The effects of low atmospheric pressure on respiration. J Physiol (London) 1908; 37:355–377.
2. Rahn H, Otis AB. Man's respiratory response during and after aclimatization to high altitude. Am J Physiol 1946; 157:445–459.
3. Weil JV, Byrne-Quinn E, Sodal IE, et al. Hypoxic ventilatory response in normal man. J Clin Invest 1970; 49:1061–1072.
4. Lahiri S, Edelmann NH, Cherniak NS, Fishman AP. Roll of a carotid chemo reflex in respiratory aclimatization to hypoxia in goat and sheep. Respir Physiol 1981; 46:367–382.
5. McDonald DM. Peripheral chemoreceptors: structure-function relationships of the carotid body. In: Hornbein TF, ed. Regulation of Breathing. New York: Marcel Dekker, 1981: 105–319.
6. Vizek M, Pickett CK, Weil JV. Increased carotid body hypoxic sensitivity during aclimatization to hypobaric hypoxia. J Appl Physiol 1987; 63:2403–2410.
7. Lahiri S. Dynamic aspects of regulation of ventilation in man during aclimatization to high altitude. Respir Physiol 1972; 16:245–258.
8. Weil JV. Ventilatory control of high altitude. In: Fishman AP, Cherniak NS, Widdicome JG, eds. Handbook of Physiology: Section 3, The Respiratory System, Vol. 2, Control of Breathing, part 2. Bethesda, MD: American Physiologic Society, 1986, pp 703–708.
9. Schoene RB, Roach RC, Hackett PH, Sutton JR, Cymerman A, Houston CS. Operation Everest II: Ventilatory adaptation during gradual decompression to extreme altitude. Med Sci Sports Exerc 1990; 22:804–810.
10. Sato M, Severinghaus JW, Bickler P. Time course of augmentation and depression of hypoxic ventilatory response at altitude. J Appl Physiol 1994; 77:213–316.
11. Sato M, Serveringhaus JW, Powell FL, Xu FD, Spellman Jr. MJ. Augmented hypoxic ventilatory response in men at altitude. J Appl Physiol 1992; 73:101–107.
12. West JB, Hackett PH, Maret KH, Milledge JS, Peters Jr. RM, Pizzo CJ, Winslow RM. Pulmonary gas exchange on the summit of Mt. Everest. J Appl Physiol 1983; 55:678–687.
13. West JB, Boyer SJ, Graber DJ, Hackett PH, Maret KH, Milledge JS, Peters Jr. RM, Pizzo CJ, Samaja M, Sarnquist FH, Schoene RB, Winslow RM. Maximal exercise at extreme altitudes on Mt. Everest. J Appl Physiol 1983; 55:688–698.
14. Schoene RB. Control of ventilation in climbers to extreme altitude. J Appl Physiol 1982; 43:886–890.
15. Schoene RB, Lahiri S, Hackett PH, Peters Jr. RM, Milledge JS, Pizzo C, Boyers SJ, Graber DJ, Maret KH, West JB. Relationship of hypoxic ventilatory response to exercise performance on Mt. Everest. J Appl Physiol 1984; 46:1478–1483.
16. Matsuyama S, Kimura H, Sugita T, et al. Control of ventilation in extreme altitude climbers. J Appl Physiol 1986; 61:400–406.
17. Schoene RB. Hypoxic ventilatory response in exercise ventilation at sea level and high altitude. In: West JB, Lahiri S, eds. High Altitude and Man. Bethesda, MD: American Physiologic Society, 1984, pp. 19–30.

18. Piiper J, Sheid P. Model for capillary-alveolar equilibration with special reference to O2 uptake in hypoxia. Respir Physiol 1981; 46:193–208.
19. Wagner PD, Sutton JR, Reeves JT, Cymerman A, Groves DM, Malconian MK. Operation Everest II: pulmonary gas exchange during a simulated ascent of Mt. Everest. J Appl Physiol 1987; 63:2348–2359.
20. Sutton JR, Reeves JT, Wagner PD, Groves PM, Cymerman A, Malconian MK, Rock PD, Young PM, Walter SE, Hausten TS. Operation Everest II: Oxygen transport during exercise at extreme simulated altitude. J Appl Physiol 1988; 64:1309–1321.
21. Gale GE, Torre-Bueno J, Moon RE, Saltzman HA, Wagner PD. Ventilation-prefusion inequality in normal humans during exercise at sea level and simulated altitude. J Appl Physiol 1985; 58:978–988.
22. Torre-Bueno J, Wagner PD, Saltzman HA, Gale GE, Moon RE. Prefusion limitation in normal humans during exercise at sea level in simulated altitude. J Appl Physiol 1985; 58:989–995.
23. Wagner PD, Gale GE, Moon RE, Torre-Bueno J, Stolt BW, Saltzman HA. Pulmonary gas exchange in humans exercising at sea level in simulated high altitude. J Appl Physiol 1986; 61:260–273.
24. West JB, Tsukimoto K, Mathieu-Costello O, Prediletto R. Stress failure in pulmonary capillaries. J Appl Physiol 1991; 70:1731–1742.
25. West JB, Mathieu-Costello O. Structure, strength, failure, and remodeling of the pulmonary blood-gas barrier. Annu Rev Physiol 1999; 61:543–547.
26. West JB, Mathieu-Costello O. Strength of pulmonary blood-gas barrier. Respir Physiol 1992; 88:141–148.
27. Wagner PD. Elevated wedge pressure in HAPE-susceptible subjects during exercise. From proceedings of the Ninth International Hypoxia Symposium, Lake Louise, Canada, 1995. Queen City Printers Inc. Burlington Vermont.
28. Fred HL, Schmidt AM, Bates T, Hecht HH. Acute pulmonary edema of altitude clinical and physiologic observations. Circulation 1962; 25:929–937.
29. Hutgren H, Grover R, Hartley L. Abnormal circulatory responses to high altitude in subjects with a previous history of high altitude pulmonary edema. Circulation 1971; 44:759–770.
30. Eldridge MW, Podoloski A, Richardson RS, Johnson DH, Knight DR, Johnson AC, Hopkins SR, Michimata H, Grassi B, Finer J, Kurdak SS, Bickler PE, Wagner PD, Severinghaus JW. Pulmonary hemodynamic response to exercise in subjects with prior high altitude pulmonary edema. J Appl Physiol 1996; 81:911–921.
31. Mckechnie JK, Leary WP, Noakes TD, Kallmeyer JC, MacScarraigh ET, Olivier LR. Acute pulmonary edema in two athletes during a 90-km running race. S Af Med J 1979; 56:261–265.
32. Pascoe JR, Ferraro GL, Cannon JH, Arthur RM, Wheat JD. Exercise-induced pulmonary hemorrhage in racing horses: preliminary study. Am J Vet Res 1981; 42:703–707.
33. Whitwell KE, Greet TR. Collection and evaluation of tracheobronchial washes in the horse. Equin Vet J 1984; 16:499–508.
34. King RR, Raskin RE, Rosbolt JP. Exercise-induced pulmonary hemorrhage in the racing greyhound dog (abstract). J Vet Intern Med 1990; 4:130.

35. Erickson HH, Mcavoy JL, Westfall JA. Exercise-induced changes in the lung of shetland ponies: ultrastructure and morphomotry. J Submicrosc Cytol Pathol 1997; 29:65–72.
36. Seaman J, Erickson BK, Kubo K, Hiraja A, Kai M, Yamaya Y, Wagner PD. Exercise-induced ventilation/perfusion inequality in the horse. Equin Vet J 1995; 27:104–109.
37. Hopkins SR, Schoene RB, Henderson WR, Spragg RG, Martin TR, West JB. Intense exercise impairs the integrity of the pulmonary blood-gas in elite athletes. Am Rev Respir Crit Care Med 1997; 155:1090–1094.
38. Hopkins SR, Schoene RB, Henderson WR, Spragg RG, West JB. Sustained submaximal exercise does not alter the integrity of the lung blood-gas barrier in elite athletes. J Appl Physiol 1998; 84:1185–1189.
39. Schaffartzik W, Arcos JP, Tsukimoto K, Mathieu-Costello O, Wagner PD. Pulmonary interstitial edema in the pig after heavy exercise. J Appl Physiol 1993; 75:2535–2540.
40. Schaffartzik W, Poole DC, Derion T, Tsukimoto K, Hogan MC, Arcos JP, Bebout DE, Wagner PD. V sub A/Q distribution during heavy exercise and recovery in humans: implications for pulmonary edema. J Appl Physiol 1992; 72:1657–1667.
41. Roca J, Hogan MC, Story D, Bebout DE, Haab P, Gonzalez P, Ueno O, Wagner PD. Evidence for tissue diffusion limitation of VO2 max in normal man. J Appl Physiol 1989; 67:291–299.
42. di Prampero P, Ferretti G. Factors limiting maximal oxygen consumption in humans. Respir Physiol 1990; 80:113–128.
43. Saltin B, Gollnick PD. Skeletal muscle adaptability; significance for metabolism and performance. In: Peachey LD, Adrian RH, Geiger SR, eds. Handbook of Physiology. Skeletal Muscle. Bethesda, MD: American Physiologic Society, 1983: 561–631.
44. Wagner PD. Algebraic analysis of the determinants of VO2 max. Respir Physiol 1993; 93:221–237.
45. Astrand PO, Cuddy TE, Saltin B, Stenberg J. Cardiac output during sub maximal and maximal work. J Appl Physiol 1964; 19:268–273.
46. Blomqvist CG, Saltin B. Cardiovascular adaptations to physical training. An Rev Physiol 1983; 45:169–189.
47. Reeves JT, Groves BM, Sutton JR, Wagner PD, Cymerman A, Malconian MK, Rock PB, Young PM, Houston CS. Operation Everest II: preservation of cardiac function at extreme altitude. J Appl Physiol 1987; 63:531–539.
48. Richardson RS, Poole DC, Knight DR, Kurdak SS, Hogan MC, Grassi B, Johnson ES, Kendrick KF, Erickson BK, Wagner PD. High muscle blood flow in man: is maximal O2 extraction compromised? J Appl Physiol 1993; 74:1911–1916.
49. Wagner PD. Determinants of maximal oxygen transport and utilization. Ann Rev Physiol 1996; 58:21–50.
50. Rowell LB. Human Circulation: Regulation During Physical Stress. New York: Oxford University Press, 1986: 328–362.
51. Rowell LB, Saltin B, Kiens B, Christensen NJ. Is peak quadraceps blood flow in humans even higher during exercise with hypoxemia? Am J Physiol 1986; 251:H1038–H1044.
52. Richardson RS, Poole DC, Knight DR, Kurdak SS, Hogan MC, Grassi B, Johnson EC, Kendrick KF, Erickson BK, Wagner PD. High muscle blood flow in man: is maximal O2 extraction compromised? J Appl Physiol 1993; 75:1911–1916.

53. Richardson RS, Knight DR, Poole DC, Kurdak SS, Hogan MC, Grassi B, Wagner PD. Determinants of maximal exercise VO2 during single leg knee-extensor exercise in humans. J Appl Physiol 1995; 268:H1453–H1461.
54. Hogan MC, Bebout DE, Wagner PD, West JB. Maximal O2 uptake of *in situ* dog muscle during acute hypoxemia with constant perfusion. J Appl Physiol 1990; 69:570–576.
55. Bender PR, Groves BM, McCullough RE, McCullough RG, Wong SY, Hamilton AJ, Wagner PD, Cymerman A, Reeves JT. Oxygen transport to exercising leg and chronic hypoxia. J Appl Physiol 1988; 65:2592–2597.
56. Hermansen LE, Hultman E, Saltin B. Muscle glycogin during prolonged severe exercise. Acta Physiol Scand 1967; 71:129–139.
57. Hoppeler H, Luthi P, Claassen H, Weibel ER, Howald H. The ultra-structure of normal human skeletal muscle. Morphometric analysis on untrained men, women and well-trained orienteers. Pfluegers Arch 1973; 344:217–232.
58. Anderson P. Capillary density in skeletal muscle of man. Acta Physiol Scand 1975; 95:203–205.
59. Brodal P, Ingjer F, Hermansen L. Capillary supply of skeletal muscle fibers in untrained and endurance trained men. J Appl Physiol 1977; 232:H705–H712.
60. Schantz P, Hendrikssen J, Jansson E. Adaptation of human skeletal muscle to endurance training to long duration. Clin Physiol 1983; 3:141–151.
61. Crenshaw AG, Friden J, Thornell L, Hargens AR. Extreme endurance training; evidence of capillary and mitochondria compartmentalization in human skeletal muscle. Europ J Appl Physiol 1991; 63:173–178.
62. Green HJ, Jones S, Ball-Burnett ME, Smith D, Livesey J, Farrance BW. Early muscular and metabolic adaptations to prolonged exercise training in humans. J Appl Physiol 1991; 70:2032–2038.
63. Roca J, Agusti AGN, Alonso A, Poole DC, Viegas C, Barbera JA, Rodriguez-Roisin R, Ferrer A, Wagner PD. Effects of training of muscle O2 transport at VO2 max. J Appl Physiol 1992; 73:1067–1076.
64. Green HJ, Jones LL, Houston ME, Ball-Burnett ME, Farrance BW. Muscle energetics during prolonged cycling after exercise hypervolemia. J Appl Physiol 1989; 66:622–631.
65. Hoppeler H. In: Roach RC, Wagner PD, Huckett PH, eds. Hypoxia: Into the Next Millennium. New York: Kluwer Academic/Plenum Publishers, 1999, pp 277–286.
66. Woodson RD, Willis RE, Lenfant C. Effect of acute and established anemia on O2 transport at rest submaximal and maximal work. J Appl Physiol 1978; 44:36–43.
67. Stainsby WN, Schneider B, Welch HG. A pictographic essay on blood and tissue oxygen transport. Med Sci Sports Exer 1988; 20:213–221.
68. Horstman HD, Gleser M, Wolfe D, Tyron T, Delhunt J. Effects of hemoglobin reduction on VO2 max and related hemodynamics in exercising dogs. J Appl Physiol 1976; 37:97–102.
69. Gregg SG, Mazzeo RS, Budinger TF, Brookes GA. Acute anemia increases lactate production and decreases clearance during exercise. J Appl Physiol 1989; 67:756–764.
70. Gonzalez N, Erwig LP, Painter CF, Clancy RL, Wagner PD. Effect of hematocrit on systemic O2 transport and hypoxic and normoxic exercise in rats. J Appl Physiol 1984; 77:1341–1348.

71. Winslow RM, Monge CC. Hypoxia, polycythemia, in chronic mountain sickness. Baltimore, MD: Johns Hopkins University Press, 1987, pp 177–202.
72. Winslow RM, Monge CC, Brown EG, Klein HG, Sarnquist F, Winslow NJ, McKneally SS. Effects of hemodilution of O_2 transport in high-altitude polycythemia. J Appl Physiol 1985; 59:1495–1502.
73. Sarnquist FH, Schoene RB, Hackett PH, Townes BD. Hemodilution of polycythemic mountaineers: effects of exercise and mental function. Avit Environ Med 1986; 57:313–317.
74. Black CP, Tenney SM. Oxygen transport during progressive hypoxia in high-altitude and sea-level water foul. Respir Physiol 1980; 39:217–239.
75. Hogan MC, Bebout DE, Wagner PD. Effect of increased Hb-O2 infinity on VO2 max at constant O2 delivery in dog muscle *in situ*. J Appl Physiol 1991; 70:2656–2662.
76. Wagner PD. Insensitivity of Vo_2 max to hemoglobin-P50 at sea level an altitude. Respir Physiol 1997; 107:205–212.
77. West JB, Wagner PD. Predicted gas exchange on the summit of Mt. Everest. Respir Physiol 1980; 42:1–16.
78. Whittenberg BA, Whittenburg JB. Transport of oxygen in muscle. Ann Rev Physiol 1989; 51:857–878.
79. Fichera G, Sneider MA, Wyman J. On the existence of a steady state in a biological system. Proc Natl Acad Sci USA 1977; 74:4182–4814.
80. Wagner PD. Gas exchange in peripheral diffusion limitation. Med Sci Sports Exer 1992; 24:54–58.
81. Wagner PD. Limitations of oxygen transport to the cell. Intensive Care Med 1995; 21:391–398.
82. Wagner PD. Determinants of maximal oxygen transport in utilization. Ann Rev Physiol 1996; 58:21–50.
83. Krogh A. The number in distribution of capillaries in muscle with calculations of the pressure head necessary for supplying the tissue. J Physiol 1919; 52:409–415.
84. Kawashiro T, Nusse W, Shyde P. Determination of diffusivity of oxygen and carbon dioxide in respiring tissue. Results in rat skeletal muscle. Pflugers Arch 1975; 359:231–251.
85. Mahler M, Louy C, Homsher E, Peskoff A. Reappraisal of diffusion, solubility and consumption of oxygen in frog skeletal muscle, with applications to muscle energy balance. J Gen Physiol 1985; 86:105–134.
86. Hoppeler H, Linstedt SL. Malleability of skeletal muscle an overcoming limitations: Structural elements. J Exp Biol 1985; 115:355–364.
87. Coin DT, Olsen JS. The rate of oxygen uptake by human red blood cells. J Biol Chem 1979; 254:1178–1190.
88. Landis EM, Pappenheimer JR. Exchange of substances through the capillary walls. In: Hamilton WF, Dowe P, eds. Handbook of Physiology. Bethesda, MD: American Physiologic Society, 1963: 961–1034.
89. Bebout DE, Hogan MC, Hempleman SC, Wagner PD. Effects of training and immobilization on VO2 and DO2 in dog gastrocnemius muscle *in situ*. J Appl Physiol 1993; 74:1697–1703.
90. Hogan MC, Roca J, Wagner PD, West JB. Limitation of maximal O2 uptake and performance by acute hypoxia in dog muscle *in situ*. J Appl Physiol 1988; 65:815–821.

91. Richardson RS, Noyszewski EA, Kendrick KF, Leigh JS, Wagner PD. Myoglobin O_2 desaturation during exercise: Evidence of limited O_2 transport. J Clin Invest 1995; 96:1916–1926.
92. Garry DJ, Ordway GA, Lorenz JN, Radford NB, Chinn ER, Grange RW, Bassel-Duby R, Williams RS. Mice without myoglobin. Nature 1998; 395:905–908.
93. Ward MP, Milledge JS, West JB. High Altitude Medicine in Physiology. London: Chapman and Hall Medical, 1989: 73.

20

Systemic Gas Exchange and Exercise Performance in Chronic Pulmonary Disease

CHARLES G. GALLAGHER

St. Vincent's University Hospital
Dublin, Ireland

I. Introduction

Use of oxygen (O_2) and production of carbon dioxide (CO_2) by mitochondria are basic processes that enable life. These, in turn, require O_2 uptake from and CO_2 output to the external environment by the lungs and their transport between the lungs and the mitochondria. During steady-state conditions, O_2 use and CO_2 production are equal to O_2 uptake and CO_2 output, respectively. During non–steady-state conditions, they are different by amounts equal to the change in body (including lung) gas stores. Because exercise capacity is frequently measured during non–steady-state conditions, the terms O_2 uptake ($\dot{V}O_2$) and carbon dioxide output ($\dot{V}CO_2$) will be used for simplicity in this chapter.

When resting, normal humans use only a small fraction of the body's maximum potential for oxygen use and transport. While resting metabolic rate is frequently normal or slightly elevated in patients with chronic pulmonary disease, their maximal oxygen uptake ($\dot{V}O_{2max}$) is usually much lower than that in normal humans. This reduced $\dot{V}O_{2max}$ impairs exercise capacity and quality of life.

This chapter reviews respiratory, cardiovascular, and limb muscle function during exercise in patients with chronic pulmonary disease and discusses their possible role in the impaired $\dot{V}O_{2max}$ and exercise capacity. It focuses on patients with chronic obstructive pulmonary disease (COPD) and patients with interstitial lung disease (ILD). As reviewed elsewhere [1,2; Fig. 3], patients with COPD frequently have greater metabolic acidosis than normal subjects at the same $\dot{V}O_2$. This is probably a result of abnormal limb muscle and/or cardiovascular function, although hypoxia may have a role in some patients [2]. There are significant problems with current noninvasive methods of assessing metabolic acidosis during exercise in patients with chronic pulmonary disease [3–5]. This chapter does not review the important issue of metabolic acidosis during exercise in chronic pulmonary disease, and the interested reader is referred to recent reviews of that topic [1,2,6,7].

Understanding of the cardiorespiratory and metabolic responses to exercise is facilitated by examination of the determinants of $\dot{V}O_2$ and $\dot{V}CO_2$, as shown in the following equations. The cardiovascular responses are represented by Eq. (1) and (2):

$$\dot{V}O_2 = Q_T(CaO_2 - C\bar{v}O_2) \tag{1}$$

$$\dot{V}O_2 = (HR \cdot SV)(CaO_2 - CvO_2) \tag{2}$$

where Q_T is cardiac output, the product of stroke volume (SV) and heart rate (HR), and $CaO_2 - C\bar{v}O_2$ is the oxygen content difference between systemic arterial and mixed venous blood.

When inspired CO_2 concentration is zero or negligible, the respiratory response to exercise is best represented by:

$$\dot{V}A = 863\dot{V}CO_2/PaCO_2 \tag{3}$$

$$\dot{V}E = 863\dot{V}CO_2/PaCO_2(1 - V_{DS}/V_T) \tag{4}$$

Where $\dot{V}E$ is minute ventilation, the sum of alveolar ventilation ($\dot{V}A$) and dead space ventilation; $PaCO_2$ is arterial CO_2 partial pressure; and V_{DS}/V_T is the ratio of physiological dead space to tidal volume. Equations (3) and (4) are used because usually $\dot{V}E$ and $\dot{V}A$ are related more closely to $\dot{V}CO_2$ than to $\dot{V}O_2$. Increasing V_{DS}/V_T is a potent ventilatory stimulant; the possible mechanisms responsible for ventilatory stimulation with altered V_{DS}/V_T are discussed elsewhere [8,9].

The ratio of $\dot{V}CO_2$ to $\dot{V}O_2$ is defined as the respiratory exchange ratio (R):

$$R = \dot{V}CO_2/\dot{V}O_2 \tag{5}$$

Figure 1 shows the changes in respiratory and cardiovascular function from rest to maximal exercise in health, exemplified by the responses of five normal men [2]. Their average age was 40 years, and they took part in mild recreational exercise, but none was an athlete. There was a ninefold increase in $\dot{V}O_2$ from rest to maximum exercise. This was accommodated by increases in Q_T and $CaO_2 - C\bar{v}O_2$ of 2.7- and 1.8-fold, respectively. Because of the 35% increase in R, $\dot{V}CO_2$ increased 13-fold, which is greater than the increase in $\dot{V}O_2$. Because of the typical hyperventilation (caused by metabolic acidosis) at maximal exercise, the 16-fold increase in $\dot{V}A$ was even greater than the increase in $\dot{V}CO_2$. Because V_{DS}/V_T decreased by 47%, $\dot{V}E$ increased 12.5-fold (i.e., relatively less than the increase in $\dot{V}A$) from rest to maxi-

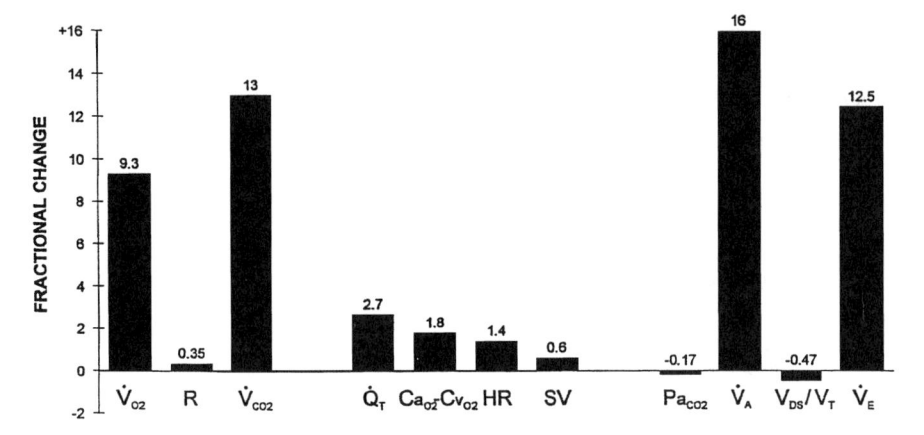

Gas Exchange and Exercise Performance in COPD 555

Figure 1 Fractional changes in cardiorespiratory function from rest to maximum exercise in five normal men aged 36–43 years. (From Ref. 4.)

mum exercise. These data are presented, not as predicted values, but to emphasize the major demands placed on cardiorespiratory function during exercise. The fractional increase in $\dot{V}_E$ was greater than that in $\dot{V}O_2$ because of the increase in R as well as the hyperventilation. In contrast, the increase in Q_T was much less than the increase in $\dot{V}O_2$. This is because essentially all of the increase in Q_T is directed to the working muscles, which increase their extraction of O_2 from arterial blood. The selective increase in blood flow to working muscles is caused by vasodilation in working muscles and vasoconstriction in ''nonexercising'' tissues. The net effect is that there is a much greater fractional increase in $\dot{V}_E$ than in Q_T from rest to maximal exercise (12.5- and 2.7-fold, respectively).

There is a small but significant increase in resting $\dot{V}O_2$ in COPD and ILD patients compared with normal subjects [4,10,11]. For this reason and because of the increased load on inspiratory muscles during exercise, one might therefore expect a higher $\dot{V}O_2$ for a given work rate during exercise. However, as reviewed elsewhere [4,12,13], this is not the case (Fig. 2). The reasons for this are unclear. Although it is possible that the delayed $\dot{V}O_2$ kinetics [13] compared with normal subjects might be responsible, this is not the only reason. $\dot{V}O_2$ during steady-state exercise was found to be normal in patients with chronic lung disease [4].

II. Respiratory Responses

Typical responses to exercise testing in patients with COPD are summarized in Table 1 and Figure 3 and are discussed in the following sections. Except for differing $PaCO_2$ responses, the responses of patients with ILD are fairly similar, but important differences are emphasized in the following sections.

OXYGEN UPTAKE ($\dot{V}O_2$) IN COPD

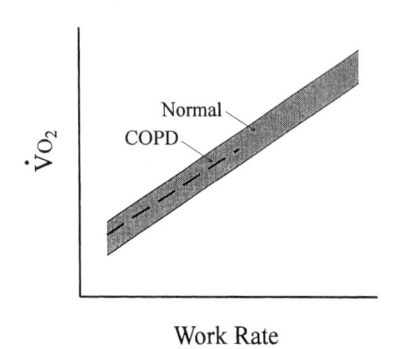

Figure 2 Comparison of oxygen uptake during progressive exercise in COPD patients and in normal humans. Peak oxygen uptake is reduced, but oxygen uptake at a given work rate is usually within normal limits in patients with COPD.

Table 1 Typical Responses to Exercise Testing in Patients with Chronic Obstructive Pulmonary Disease[a]

At maximal exercise:	At submaximal exercise:
Low peak $\dot{V}O_2$ and peak work rate	Normal or near normal $\dot{V}O_2$
Low $\dot{V}E$	High $\dot{V}E$
High $\dot{V}E$/MVV	High F, low V_T
Low V_T	High Pa_{CO_2}, low arterial Pa_{O_2}
Normal or slightly reduced V_T/VC ratio	Normal cardiac output (usually)
Low heart rate (usually)	High heart rate, low stroke volume
Low oxygen pulse	Increased metabolic acidosis
Reduced metabolic acidosis (usually)	

$\dot{V}O_2$, oxygen uptake; $\dot{V}E$, minute ventilation; MVV, maximum voluntary ventilation; V_T, tidal volume; VC, vital capacity; Pa_{CO_2}, arterial carbon dioxide partial pressure; Pa_{O_2}, arterial oxygen partial pressure.
[a]Data are shown in comparison to normal subjects of the same sex, age, and body size. See text for details.
Source: Ref. 4.

Figure 3

[Figure: six panels showing Ventilation, Arterial PO₂, Arterial PCO₂, Heart Rate, Lactic Acid, Dyspnea/Leg Discomfort plotted vs Oxygen Uptake, comparing COPD patients (shaded) with Normal (dashed). Ventilation panel marked FEV₁ × 35. PCO₂ panel labels COPD and Normal curves.]

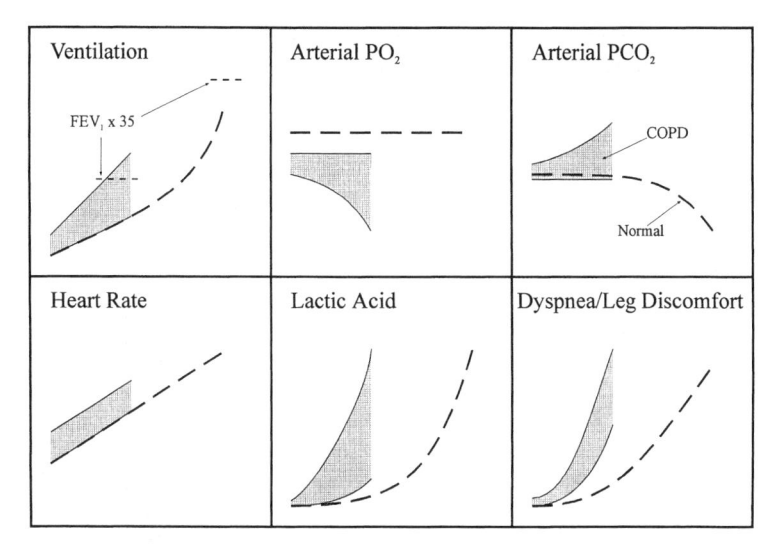

Oxygen Uptake

Figure 3 Schematic comparison of the range of responses of patients to progressive exercise compared with the average response in normal humans. See text for details.

A. Ventilation

Patients with chronic pulmonary disease have increased dead space ventilation at rest (Fig. 4). Furthermore, the normal decrease in relative dead space ventilation (VDS/VT) is attenuated or absent in chronic pulmonary disease [11,14–17]. The increased VDS/VT necessitates a greater total ventilation ($\dot{V}_E$) if $\dot{V}_A$ were to remain the same as in normal subjects [Eq. (4)]. The majority of patients with moderate or severe COPD and many with mild COPD have a lower $\dot{V}_A$ (and therefore a higher Pa_{CO_2}) than do normal humans at the same metabolic rate (Fig. 4). The decrease in $\dot{V}_A$ is usually significantly less than the increase in dead space ventilation. Therefore, patients with COPD usually have a higher $\dot{V}_E$ than normal humans at the same metabolic rate [18–20]. Patients with ILD also have higher $\dot{V}_E$ than do normal humans. Again, this is a result of elevated VDS/VT, although their $\dot{V}_A$ is frequently normal or near normal [11].

Even for patients with similar airway obstruction, there is frequently great variability in the increase in $\dot{V}_E$. This is caused by variability in both $\dot{V}_A$ and VDS/VT, but the relative importance of each of these is unclear. Variability in the ventilatory response to exercise is a significant contributor to variability in $\dot{V}_{O_2max}$ [18].

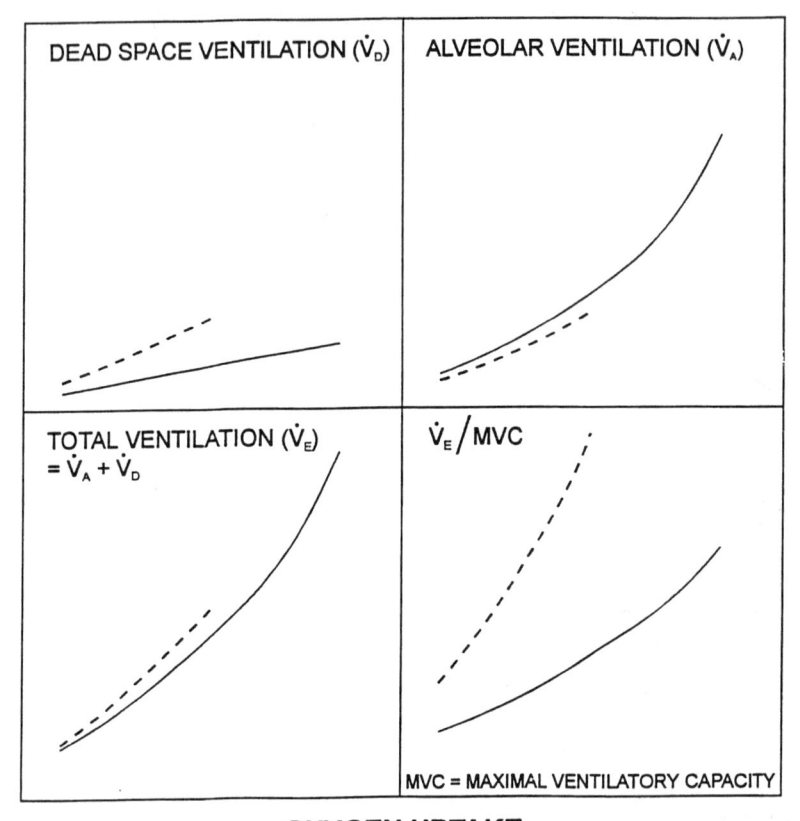

Figure 4 Schematic comparison of typical ventilatory changes during progressive exercise in patients with COPD and in normal humans. See text for details. (From Ref. 4.)

B. Breathing Pattern

Normal humans initially increase $\dot{V}_E$ during exercise by increasing both V_T and respiratory frequency (F). However, at high work rates, V_T usually remains constant at approximately 50–60% of vital capacity, and further increases in $\dot{V}_E$ are caused by increases in F alone [21–23]. The same general pattern usually occurs in patients with COPD and ILD [16,24,25]. However, V_T is less and F is greater than in normal humans at similar levels of $\dot{V}_E$, and peak V_T is also less. Such a low V_T–high F breathing pattern is not unique to COPD and ILD. Such a tachypneic breathing pattern is also observed in the vast majority of patients with different respiratory or cardiac conditions. A study [25] of patients with COPD, ILD, bronchial asthma, and heart disease found a strong linear correlation (R = 0.827; P < .0001) between peak exercise V_T and vital capacity when all patients were considered together (Fig. 5). There was no significant difference between the different groups. Therefore, differences in peak exercise V_T between different patients (whether with the same or different diseases) are largely caused by differences in severity of respiratory mechanical impairment, not differences in disease state. There is also a linear relation between peak exercise V_T and vital capacity in normal humans [21]. Therefore, the ratio of peak exercise V_T to vital capacity in COPD and ILD patients is usually similar to that of normal humans and patients with other cardiorespiratory diseases [17,25].

The increase in F during exercise in normal humans is a result of decreases in both inspiratory and expiratory durations. However, the fractional decrease in inspiratory duration is less than the fractional decrease in expiratory duration. Therefore, the ratio of inspiratory duration to total breath duration (inspiratory duty cycle) in normal humans increases from approximately 0.35 to 0.40 at rest to as high as 0.50 to 0.55 during heavy exercise [22,26,27]. However, patients with severe COPD often show little or no increase in the inspiratory duty cycle with exercise [28,29].

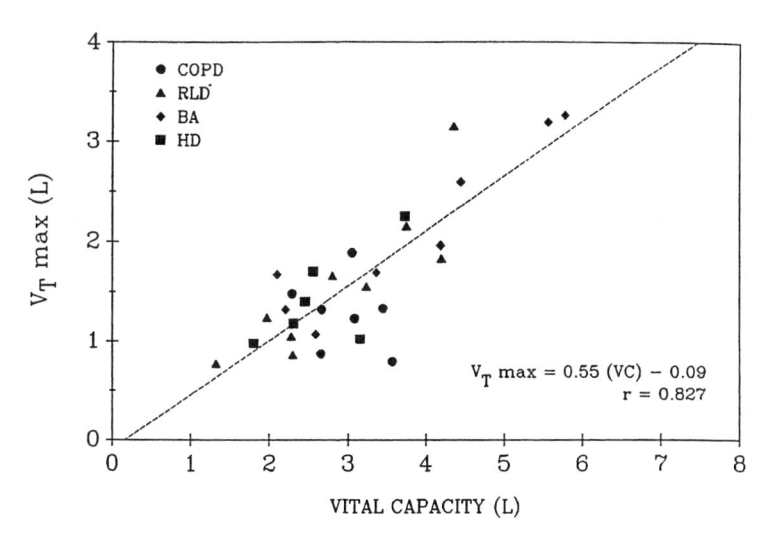

Figure 5 Relation between peak exercise tidal volume ($V_{T_{max}}$) and vital capacity (VC) for patients with chronic obstructive pulmonary disease, restrictive lung disease, heart disease, and bronchial asthma. Different symbols are used for the four patient groups. There was a significant linear relation between $V_{T_{max}}$ and VC (see regression line): $V_{T_{max}} = 0.55$ (VC) $- 0.09$ L (R = 0.827; P < .0001). (From Ref. 25.)

This is beneficial in allowing greater time for expiration, thus facilitating further increases in $\dot{V}_E$ [4]. Patients with less severe COPD and those with ILD often show some increase in the inspiratory duty cycle with exercise [4,11,30].

C. Lung Mechanics

The highest level of $\dot{V}_E$ (i.e., maximum ventilatory capacity [MVC]) that a subject can produce [8] is ultimately limited by the boundaries of the maximum inspiratory and expiratory flow volume curves, i.e., by the highest inspiratory and expiratory flow rates that can be generated. Therefore, examination of the maximum inspiratory and expiratory flow–volume curves is useful in assessing MVC and pulmonary mechanics during exercise. Patients with COPD have reduced maximum expiratory flow rates (MEF) at all lung volumes with lesser reductions in maximum inspiratory flow rates (MIF) [2]. The shape of the expiratory curve is distorted, but the shape of the inspiratory curve is essentially normal (Fig. 6). The reduction in MEF is caused by airway narrowing, which is caused partly by airway disease and partly by loss of lung recoil. In contrast, the reduction in MIF is caused by a combination of the increased inspiratory flow resistance and reduced inspiratory muscle strength. Because of the decrease in MIF and MEF, MVC in patients with COPD is reduced compared with that in normal humans. This, along with the elevated $\dot{V}_E$ response to exercise, means that the $\dot{V}_E$/MVC ratio is much higher during exercise in patients with COPD than in normal humans at the same work rate (Fig. 4).

Some, but not all, normal humans have expiratory flow limitation during exercise, but usually only at high work rates [31]. In contrast, patients with COPD usually demonstrate expiratory flow limitation at low work rates and frequently during most or all of expiration (Fig. 6) [32–35]. Some patients with severe COPD have expiratory flow limitation even at rest [2]. The development of expiratory flow limitation at low work rates constrains the ability of patients with COPD to further increase $\dot{V}_E$. Further increases in $\dot{V}_E$ can then be achieved by either: (1) increasing end-expiratory lung volume (EELV) so that MEF increases; or (2) further increasing inspiratory flow rate during exercise so that inspiratory time decreases and more time is available for expiration, i.e., the inspiratory duty cycle decreases or fails to increase.

Patients with COPD adopt both of these measures. EELV frequently increases above resting levels or stays the same in exercising COPD patients (Fig. 6). In contrast, EELV usually decreases significantly in normal humans [31,36], although it may increase in very fit subjects or the elderly when expiratory flow limitation develops during exercise. The increase in EELV seems to be a consequence of expiratory flow limitation. As previously discussed, patients with COPD usually have a lower inspiratory duty cycle than do normal humans during exercise. Adopting a short duty cycle is a useful strategy for increasing $\dot{V}_E$ when expiratory flow limitation occurs.

COPD PATIENT
FEV$_1$ = 1.91

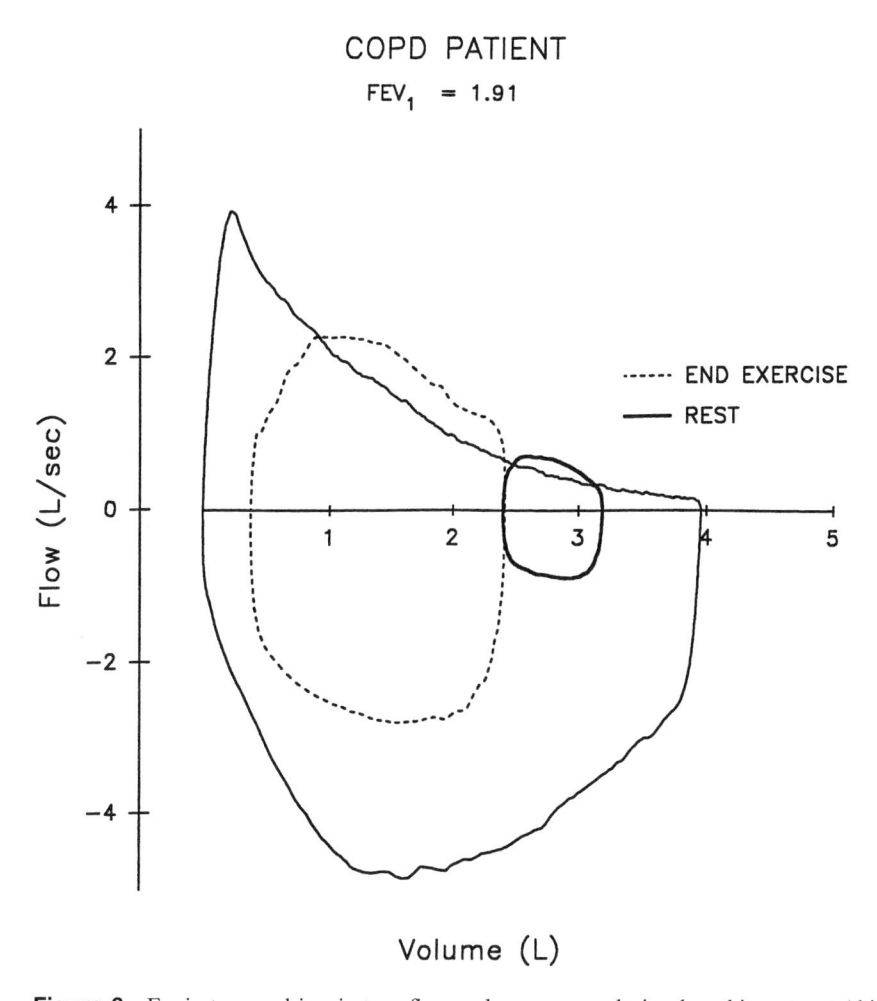

Figure 6 Expiratory and inspiratory flow–volume curves during breathing at rest (thick line) and maximum exercise (dashed line) as well as maximum flow–volume curves at rest (outer solid line) in a patient with moderate COPD. The patient exceeded his maximum expiratory flow volume curve at rest and during maximal exercise but did not reach his maximum inspiratory flow–volume curve. End-expiratory lung volume increased with exercise. (From Ref. 4.)

Some, but not all patients with ILD develop flow limitation during exercise (Fig. 7). In some cases, flow limitation develops even during submaximal exercise [37]. Not surprisingly, flow limitation most likely occurs in patients with a higher ventilatory response to exercise. Unlike normal subjects who usually decrease EELV and patients with COPD who increase EELV, patients with ILD typically have little

LUNG VOLUMES AND FLOW LIMITATION DURING EXERCISE IN ILD

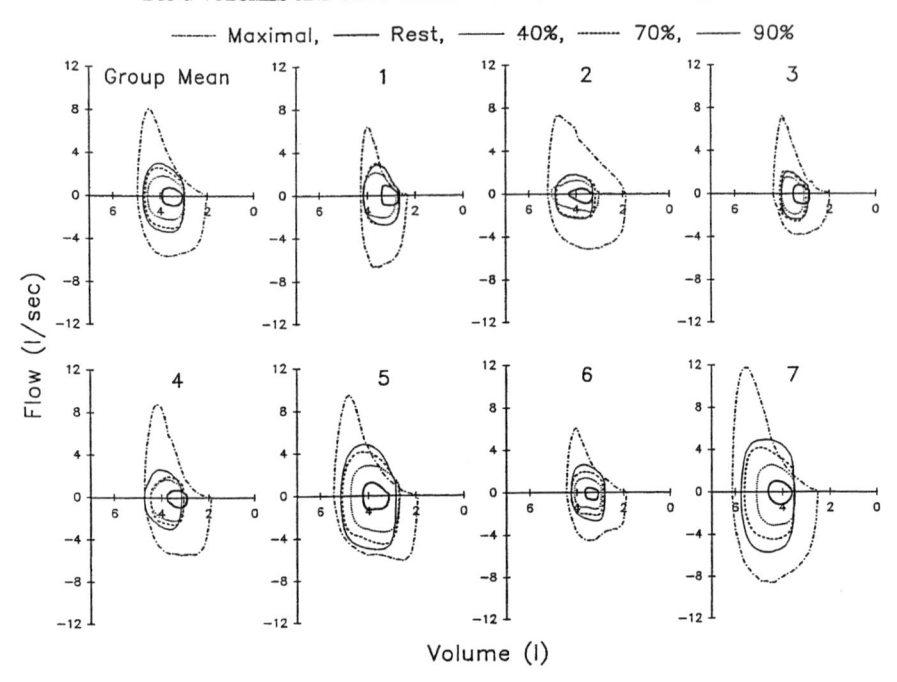

Figure 7 Flow volume curves at rest and at three work rates compared with maximum flow–volume curves for seven patients with interstitial lung disease. Group mean curves are also shown. Four patients reached or exceeded their expiratory flow volume curves during exercise. (From Ref. 37.)

or no change in EELV during exercise [37]. Clearly, expiratory flow limitation can account for the absence of the normal decrease in EELV in some patients. However, other patients with ILD without flow limitation who should be able to decrease EELV during exercise do not do so. It has been suggested that this lack of decrease in EELV in the absence of expiratory flow limitation may be a consequence of hypoxia [37].

Some patients with COPD or ILD have expiratory flow rates during exercise that exceed the maximum expiratory flow volume (MEFV) curve measured at rest [2,33,37]; some patients even exceed the MEFV curve during resting breathing. The possible reasons for this are listed in Table 2 and discussed below:

1. Thoracic gas compression: The development of positive intrathoracic pressure during expiration will compress alveolar gas; therefore, expired volume measured at the mouth will underestimate the reduction of lung gas volume [2]. Accordingly, flow volume curves with volume measured

Table 2 Reasons Why Expiratory Flow May Exceed Maximum Expiratory Flow Volume Curve

Thoracic gas compression
Errors in absolute lung volume
Airway narrowing after deep inspiration in maximum expiratory flow volume maneuvers
Nonuniform lung emptying
Bronchodilation during exercise

Source: Ref. 2.

at the mouth generally underestimate expiratory flow at a particular lung volume. This will be especially marked in patients with COPD because of their high volumes. Because of the greater intrathoracic pressure during MEFV maneuvers, this effect should be much greater with MEFV curves than during spontaneous breathing at rest or during exercise.

2. Errors in absolute lung volume during exercise so that the exercise flow–volume curve is placed incorrectly in relation to the MEFV curve.
3. Bronchoconstriction during the MEFV maneuvers caused by inspiring to total lung capacity; therefore, the MEFV would underestimate expiratory flow available for spontaneous breathing at rest or during exercise. This is the opposite of the airway hysteresis observed in normal humans.
4. Inhomogeneous lung emptying: In the presence of nonuniformity, maximal expiratory flow at a particular lung volume will vary with the time required to reach that volume. Thus, maximal flow should be less during MEFV maneuvers than during spontaneous expirations commencing below total lung capacity.
5. Bronchodilation during exercise: There is evidence that this may occur in patients with COPD [38]. This might be caused by altered airway mechanics or increase in respiratory recoil.

D. Respiratory Muscle Function

Patients with COPD have to generate much greater inspiratory muscle pressures than normal humans at similar work rates. Inspiratory muscle pressure is increased for five major reasons (Table 3). First, their EELV during exercise (and often also at rest) is significantly above the relaxation volume of the respiratory system. Because of this dynamic hyperinflation, they have to generate a certain inspiratory muscle pressure (equal to the combined recoil of the lungs and chest wall at that lung volume) before inspiratory flow can even begin. This threshold load persists throughout inspiratory flow. Therefore, because of dynamic hyperinflation, patients with COPD must generate inspiratory pressure during late expiration and for the

Table 3 Inspiratory Muscle Load During Exercise in Chronic Obstructive Pulmonary Disease

---
Inspiratory muscle pressure generated (P_{mus}) is elevated because of:
   Increased end expiratory lung volume (dynamic hyperinflation)
   Increased inspiratory resistance
   Increased minute ventilation
   Decreased lung compliance (frequency dependant)
   Chest wall distortion
Inspiratory pressure generating capacity (P_{max}) is decreased because of:
   Inspiratory muscle weakness
   Dynamic hyperinflation
   Therefore, the load (P_{mus}/P_{max}) on inspiratory muscles is much greater than in normal humans.

Source: Ref. 4.

duration of inspiratory flow that does not contribute directly to inspiration. It must be generated to overcome the threshold load before inspiration can even begin. If the increase in lung volume is large enough to decrease static lung compliance, dynamic hyperinflation will also increase the elastic load that the inspiratory muscles have to overcome [4]. Second, they have to generate greater inspiratory pressures for a given level of ventilation because of their increased inspiratory resistance. Third, patients with COPD have a greater $\dot{V}E$ at a given work rate than normal humans (Fig. 3), which further increases the demands on respiratory muscles during exercise. Fourth, the elastic load may be increased because of frequency dependence of compliance. Although static lung compliance is increased in COPD, dynamic compliance is significantly less than static compliance. The dynamic compliance of patients with COPD usually decreases even more as respiratory frequency increases with exercise [39]. Therefore, dynamic compliance during exercise can be significantly less in patients with COPD than in normal humans. Finally, the elastic load is also increased because of marked chest wall distortion during exercise.

Although the load on inspiratory muscles is markedly increased in patients with COPD, inspiratory muscle strength is decreased [40]. Their pressure-generating capacity is further reduced by the increase in EELV during exercise. Therefore, the stress on inspiratory muscles (i.e., the pressure generated as a fraction of pressure-generating capacity) is markedly increased in patients with COPD during exercise (Table 3). The decrease in Pa_{O_2} and increase in Pa_{CO_2}, which many patients develop during exercise, may further impair inspiratory muscle function.

Patients with ILD have to generate much greater inspiratory muscle pressures than normal humans during exercise because of their decreased lung compliance, increased $\dot{V}E$ [11] and the absence of the normal decrease in EELV [37]. In addition, their inspiratory muscle strength is sometimes reduced, especially in those with respiratory myopathy caused by high-dose corticosteroids [41]. Therefore, the stress on inspiratory muscles is much greater than normal in patients with ILD during exercise.

The lack of decrease in EELV in patients with ILD is not because of the absence of expiratory muscle recruitment. Marciniuk et al. [42] recently showed that patients with ILD progressively recruit expiratory muscles with increasing exercise intensity, but this is used to increase expiratory flow rates, not to decrease EELV.

E. Blood Gases

Pulmonary gas exchange in chronic pulmonary disease is reviewed in detail in Chapts. 8 and 9; therefore, only a very brief summary is given here.

At rest, patients with COPD usually have a lower Pao$_2$ and a similar or higher Paco$_2$ than do normal humans. As summarized in Figure 3, Pao$_2$ may decrease, remain the same, or even sometimes increase during exercise in patients with COPD. Oxygen desaturation during exercise is most prominent in patients with severe COPD [43,44]. The decrease in saturation is usually caused by both a widening of the alveolar–arterial Po$_2$ gradient and hypoventilation [45,46]. As previously discussed, the increase in total ventilation during exercise in COPD is usually less than the increase in dead space ventilation, resulting in alveolar hypoventilation. Even patients with mild COPD frequently have a higher Paco$_2$ than do normal humans, and when metabolic acidosis develops, the normal hyperventilation is attenuated or absent [6,15,30,47].

Patients with ILD typically experience a decrease in arterial Pao$_2$ during exercise that is often severe [11,48,49]. As reviewed elsewhere [11], Paco$_2$ typically remains relatively unchanged from rest to exercise in patients with ILD. The mechanisms of blood gas changes during exercise are reviewed in detail elsewhere [4].

III. Cardiovascular Responses

Normal humans have a linear increase in Q$_T$ in relation to $\dot{V}o_2$ as power output increases during incremental exercise. Such a linear increase in Q$_T$ is also observed in patients with COPD. Most published studies show that patients with COPD usually have a normal Q$_T$ at a given $\dot{V}o_2$ during exercise [17,20,50,51], but Q$_T$ at end exercise is reduced because of the low $\dot{V}o_{2max}$. This fact has often been used as evidence of normal cardiac function during exercise in COPD, but this is not valid because the $\dot{V}o_2$–Q$_T$ relation may be normal in the presence of cardiac dysfunction. Although the Q$_T$ response to exercise is usually normal, stroke volume is less, and heart rate is greater than in normal people at the same $\dot{V}o_2$ [16,20,50]. However, the slope of the heart rate–$\dot{V}o_2$ relation is usually normal in patients with COPD [16]. Heart rate at end exercise is usually less than normal, although it may be near normal or even normal in some patients with mild or moderate disease

[32,52]. Because the fractional reduction in maximal heart rate is less than that of peak $\dot{V}O_2$, oxygen pulse (i.e., $\dot{V}O_2$/heart rate) is low in patients with COPD at end exercise and at a given $\dot{V}O_2$ during exercise.

Because of their elevated pulmonary vascular resistance and normal Q_T response to exercise, patients with COPD have much higher pulmonary artery pressures during exercise than do normal humans [14,50,53]. This is the major reason for their right ventricular dysfunction, which occurs during exercise in most patients with moderate or severe COPD [53,54]. Right ventricular dysfunction also occurs frequently in patients with mild COPD [55]. Some COPD patients without evidence of primary cardiac disease develop left ventricular dysfunction during exercise [54–56].

The normal Q_T–$\dot{V}O_2$ relation during exercise implies that the O_2 content difference between arterial and mixed venous blood is normal or near normal. Several studies have shown that up to 70% of arterial oxygen content is extracted by the tissues at end exercise in patients with COPD [44,51,57], which is similar to that of normal untrained humans. However, there is also evidence that fractional oxygen extraction may be less than normal and mixed venous PO_2 may be greater than normal in some patients with COPD at end exercise [44,58]. This indicates either impaired oxygen uptake by working muscles and/or impairment of the normal redistribution of blood flow to working muscles during exercise.

As reviewed elsewhere [11], cardiovascular function is also abnormal in patients with ILD. They frequently have an elevated heart rate and reduced stroke volume, resulting in normal Q_T response to exercise. They lose the normal decrease in pulmonary vascular resistance with exercise and usually have elevated pulmonary artery pressures during exercise [11].

IV. Skeletal Muscle Responses

As previously discussed, there is good evidence of respiratory muscle dysfunction both at rest and during exercise in patients with chronic pulmonary disease. In contrast, little attention has traditionally been paid to the function of other skeletal muscles in these patients. However, in recent years, it has become clear that limb muscle function is frequently abnormal in patients with chronic pulmonary disease.

A number of studies have reported impaired limb muscle strength in COPD [59–62]. This involves both upper- and lower-limb muscle groups. In addition, significant correlations have been found between limb muscle strength and exercise performance in COPD [61]. Studies using magnetic resonance spectroscopy have documented abnormal limb muscle function, including premature intracellular acidosis, during exercise in patients with COPD, compared with normal subjects [62–65].

Studies of limb muscle biopsy samples have also shown abnormalities in COPD. Maltais et al. [7] found a significant reduction in oxidative enzyme activity.

They also found an inverse relation between oxidative enzyme activities and lactic acidosis in their patients. There was also evidence of muscle fiber type alterations in COPD with a decrease in the proportion of fatigue-resistant slow fibers [66].

As previously indicated, some patients with COPD have a higher than normal mixed venous P_{O_2} during exercise. Although this might be caused by defective uptake of O_2 by working muscles, it could also be caused by increased blood flow through nonexercising, less metabolically active tissues. The role of each of these remains to be clarified.

A. Mechanisms of Skeletal Muscle Dysfunction

The possible mechanisms underlying limb muscle dysfunction in chronic pulmonary disease include inactivity, hypoxia, impaired muscle perfusion, cytokine production, and medications, including corticosteroids [67]. Inactivity is frequent in chronic pulmonary disease and can definitely impair muscle function. Hypoxia may also directly impair muscle function. Although the available evidence suggests that limb muscle blood flow is normal or increased in COPD during exercise [57], it is still possible that abnormal distribution of blood flow within muscles could cause myopathy in some fibers. Malnutrition, especially protein malnutrition occurs in many patients with chronic lung disease and may impair muscle function [68]. Increased cytokine production may be myopathic and occurs in some patients with chronic pulmonary disease. High, and possibly low, doses of corticosteroids can cause profound myopathic changes, and inactivity may further predispose patients to steroid myopathy [41].

This discussion outlines mechanisms that may contribute to skeletal muscle dysfunction in chronic lung disease. It must be emphasized that, although there is considerable speculation, there are currently very little data on the respective importance of these potential mechanisms. There is a great need for research into the mechanisms of skeletal muscle dysfunction in chronic pulmonary disease and in chronic diseases in general.

V. Exercise Limitation

Until now, this chapter has discussed the major abnormalities in respiratory, cardiovascular, and skeletal muscle function during exercise. Many studies and review articles have posed the question, ''What limits exercise in chronic pulmonary disease?''. Before one can begin to address the issue of ''exercise limitation,'' one must clarify what is meant by that term.

In general terms, it is useful to consider exercise limitation in terms of the factors that cause a patient (or group of patients) to stop exercising. A number of points arise from that definition. First, such factors could be physiological, psychological (anxiety or poor motivation), or protocol/equipment-related (e.g., uncomfortable seat on a cycle ergometer), etc. For this discussion, we will assume that

Table 4 Potential Contributors[a] to Impaired Exercise Tolerance in Respiratory Disease

---
Ventilatory limitation
Hypoxia
Cardiovascular dysfunction
Limb muscle dysfunction

---
[a]Including symptoms related to these.

equipment factors are not important, although they sometimes are during clinical exercise testing. Second, the factors limiting exercise may vary considerably with the type of exercise. Although $\dot{V}O_{2max}$ in healthy humans is limited primarily by the ability to deliver oxygen to the working muscles [69], this is not the case during constant work rate (endurance) exercise. Even for the same type (e.g., maximum incremental) of exercise, significant differences occur depending on the muscles used (e.g., upper limb vs. lower limb, large muscle mass vs. small muscle mass). This issue is important because, although many studies have examined limitation of maximum incremental leg exercise, other forms of exercise, especially endurance exercise, are more important for patients. Third, the factors that limit exercise capacity may vary among patients, whether with the same or different underlying disease process. Although there are limited data regarding this issue, the factors limiting exercise probably vary markedly depending on the severity and duration of disease.

Finally, it should also be recognized that looking for the one cause of exercise limitation in a patient or group of patients is too simplistic. It is likely that a number of "defects" in the oxygen transport pathway, as well as symptoms related to these defects, may each contribute to the impaired exercise tolerance of patients. The issue is then to decide which "defects" contribute to exercise limitation and the quantitative importance of each. Correction of hypoxia improves $\dot{V}O_{2max}$ in patients with ILD, indicating that hypoxia contributes to their exercise limitation [70,71]. However, factors other than hypoxia also contribute to their limitation because $\dot{V}O_{2max}$ remains subnormal despite correction of hypoxia.

Most studies examining exercise limitation have used correlative, predictive, or interventional approaches. These approaches are briefly discussed in the following sections.

A. Correlative Approaches to Assessment

Many studies have used a correlative approach to examine exercise limitation. Although some such studies provide useful information, there are frequently major problems with this approach. Significant correlations do not prove causation, and the absence of correlation does not necessarily exclude it. The relatively weak correlation between forced expiratory volume in 1 second (FEV_1) and $\dot{V}O_{2max}$ in chronic pulmonary disease has frequently been cited as evidence against ventilatory limitation to maximal exercise performance. The maximum ventilation that can be achieved is dependent on inspiratory as well as expiratory mechanics, and the part of the expiratory flow volume loop represented by FEV_1 is different from that part used during exercise [8,37]. In addition, such analysis ignores the ventilatory response to exercise [18]. Therefore, even if respiratory mechanics were the sole cause of exercise limitation, one would not necessarily expect a strong correlation between FEV_1 and $\dot{V}O_{2max}$. Therefore, apart from the general point that correlations cannot prove causation, a plausible hypothesis must underly any correlation analysis. As discussed in Sec. D, ventilatory function is not the only important contributor to exercise limitation in chronic pulmonary disease, but that conclusion is not based on studies of the $\dot{V}O_{2max}$–FEV_1 correlation.

Great caution should also be used in interpreting correlations of linked variables. There is a strong linear relation between $\dot{V}O_2$ and Q_T during incremental exercise, and this correlation varies little between subjects. Therefore, there will be a significant correlation between $\dot{V}O_{2max}$ and maximum Q_T regardless of the cause or causes of reduced $\dot{V}O_{2max}$; if patients stop exercising because of ventilatory function or poor motivation, there will be a significant correlation between $\dot{V}O_{2max}$ and Q_T.

Care must also be taken regarding subjects included in a correlation analysis. If two groups of subjects (e.g., COPD and normals) differ from each other for two unrelated variables, there will usually be a significant correlation between those two variables if both patient groups are included together, even if there is no correlation for each group on its own.

B. Assessment by Markers

Using this approach, different investigators have looked for physiological changes that might cause or be a marker for a cause of exercise limitation. This approach can, of course, be applied to any physiological function. To assess whether ventilatory function limits exercise, many studies have compared $\dot{V}_E$ at end exercise ($\dot{V}_{Emax}$) to maximal voluntary ventilation (MVV) [72]; if V_{Emax} equaled or approached MVV, they reasoned that ventilatory function limited exercise. Other studies have looked for evidence of inspiratory muscle fatigue and/or expiratory flow limitation during exercise. If they were found, they concluded that they contributed to exercise limitation. Other studies have used an increase in Pa_{CO_2} during exercise as evidence that ventilatory function limited exercise. When hypoxia develops during exercise, it is assumed that this contributes to exercise limitation. If predicted maximum heart rate is not reached at end exercise, it has traditionally been assumed that there is significant cardiac reserve and that cardiac function does not limit exercise. With the recent interest in limb muscle function, this "marker" approach will be increasingly applied to limb muscle function.

This approach has significant advantages over the correlative approach. If one hypothesis is that inspiratory muscle fatigue limits exercise, it is important to know if it occurs. Whenever this approach is used, two general questions need to be addressed: (1) Is the "marker" a valid measure of the physiological change that we are interested in? and (2) does the presence of this physiological change mean that it contributes to exercise limitation?

With regard to the first question, many markers that have been examined in previous studies are not specific. Several studies of exercising patients with COPD found changes in the electromyographic frequency spectrum of the diaphragm or the development of abdominal paradox that were interpreted as evidence of inspiratory muscle fatigue [73–75]. However, neither of these changes is specific to fatigue [4,76]. As discussed elsewhere [2], many studies that assessed exercise limitation in COPD have expressed $\dot{V}_{Emax}$ as a fraction of measured or predicted MVV. Although such studies provide important information, they are of limited value in assessment of exercise limitation. This is because MVV varies significantly with V_T and EELV, and these can be different between the MVV maneuver and exercise. Second, the pattern of respiratory muscle activation during exercise is very different from (and more efficient than) that during MVV maneuvers in normal humans [77], and this is probably also the case for patients with COPD. Finally, resting MVV may underestimate MVV during exercise because of bronchodilatation during exercise. Studies that predict MVV from FEV_1 are less useful in this regard because such predictions are not precise. This is supported by the finding, as shown schematically in Figure 3, that $\dot{V}_{Emax}$ exceeds MVV predicted from FEV_1 in some patients; obviously, predicted MVV underestimates true MVV in them. Prediction of MVV may be improved by including inspiratory [78] as well as expiratory flow rates, but this does not solve the problem that MVV varies with V_T and EELV [8]. There is no one unique MVV for any patient. Studies that compare $\dot{V}_{Emax}$ to MVC for the same V_T and EELV or that compare exercise flow–volume loops to maximum flow–volume loops are likely to be more useful in assessment of ventilatory limitation to exercise [37].

With regard to the second question, it must be emphasized that finding an abnormal response to exercise does not imply that that abnormality contributes to exercise limitation. Finding an increase in Pa_{CO_2} during exercise usually implies abnormal control of breathing or respiratory mechanics during exercise, but it does not mean that exercise is limited by ventilatory function. Some patients with COPD show an increase in Pa_{CO_2} from rest to mild exercise when their ventilation is significantly less than that at maximal exercise. Clearly, their exercise was not limited (by ventilation or otherwise) at mild exercise when arterial Pa_{CO_2} first increased.

C. Interventional Assessment

This approach involves assessing the effect of a specific intervention on exercise performance. If correction of hypoxia improves exercise performance, this indicates that hypoxia contributes to exercise limitation. If inspiratory muscle function limits exercise tolerance, reduction of the load on inspiratory muscles should improve exercise performance [26,36,79,80]. To date, this approach has been applied largely to respiratory interventions, but it can (and should) be used in assessing cardiovascular and limb muscle limitation of exercise performance in patients with lung disease.

This approach has the major advantage that, unlike the other approaches previously discussed, it is a direct assessment of exercise limitation. The utility of this approach depends on how selective the intervention is. Correction of hypoxia by supplemental O_2 also depresses ventilation at a given work rate [9]. Therefore, when O_2 supplementation was shown to improve maximal exercise performance in patients with ILD, it was not clear whether this was caused by a correction of tissue hypoxia per se or by the decrease in ventilation [70]. It only became clear that the former was the case when the decrease in ventilation was prevented by the addition of external dead space [71].

D. Ventilatory Limitation of Exercise Performance

I define ventilatory function as limiting exercise performance when the patient is unable (including inability caused by symptoms) to provide the further increase in alveolar/total ventilation needed to exercise longer. Does ventilatory function limit exercise tolerance in patients with COPD? This issue has been reviewed elsewhere [2]. Most of the available evidence indicates that ventilatory function contributes to exercise limitation in patients with moderate or severe COPD. This conclusion is based on studies comparing flow volume curves during exercise to maximum flow volume curves and studies that altered ventilatory demand or respiratory mechanics during exercise. Although ventilatory function contributes to exercise limitation in COPD, it is not the only (and probably not the major) cause of exercise limitation. This is supported by, e.g., the observation that normalization or near normalization of lung mechanics by transplantation improves $\dot{V}O_{2max}$, but only to approximately 50% of predicted normal values [81–83].

Does ventilatory function contribute to exercise limitation in ILD? Based on examination of their exercise and maximum flow volume curves [37] and based on their ability to increase ventilation further with O_2 and dead space loading [71], patients with ILD usually have significant ventilatory reserve at end exercise. Therefore, ventilatory function does not normally limit their exercise tolerance [71].

E. Hypoxia

As previously discussed, most patients with ILD and many with COPD experience desaturation during exercise. Does hypoxia contribute to their exercise limitation? There is good evidence that hypoxia is a major contributor to exercise limitation in patients with ILD, and it probably also contributes to exercise limitation in patients with COPD who experience desaturation during exercise [71]. However, hypoxia is not the sole mechanism of exercise limitation, even in patients with ILD. Correction of hypoxia in ILD improves exercise performance but does not normalize it. Factors other than hypoxia clearly contribute to their impaired exercise performance.

F. Cardiovascular Function

As previously discussed, patients with COPD or ILD have abnormalities of right and left heart function during exercise. It has usually been assumed that cardiac function does not contribute to their exercise limitation, but this conclusion is based on fairly limited data at this time. This conclusion is usually based on studies that used a correlative or marker approach, and they are not definitive. In addition, although there are ample data on central cardiac function during exercise in lung disease, there are very few data on peripheral vascular function, including the distribution of blood flow during exercise. Further studies are needed to assess the role of cardiovascular function in exercise limitation in patients with chronic lung disease.

G. Skeletal Muscles

As previously discussed, recent studies have highlighted the high prevalence of limb muscle dysfunction in patients with COPD. At this time, there are insufficient data to indicate whether limb muscle dysfunction is an important contributor to exercise limitation, but it is likely to be. The persistent impairment in exercise capacity after normalization (or near normalization) of lung mechanics and gas exchange after transplantation [81–83] is probably related to limb muscle dysfunction; it is much less likely to be related to cardiovascular factors. Although myopathy that develops during or after transplantation (related to medications, etc.) may be important, it is probably not the sole cause for the myopathy and impaired exercise capacity in these patients. Studies to date suggest that exercise training after transplantation causes a relatively small improvement in exercise capacity, but further studies are needed.

Studies of exercise training have documented improved exercise capacity after training in patients with COPD [1,6], although this has not been found in all patients [84]. These studies are clearly of major clinical importance, and they also provide mechanistic insights. However, it should be emphasized that such training programs induce widespread physiological changes. Most studies of exercise training in COPD have used endurance training, usually of the lower limbs. Endurance exercise training is a complex process that induces alterations in cardiovascular, respiratory, hormonal, and neuromuscular function, as well as inducing muscle and metabolic changes. For example, ventilation, heart rate, and catecholamines decrease and stroke volume increases during heavy exercise after training. These widespread responses may be clinically beneficial, but these interactions must be borne in mind when using such studies to gain insight into the mechanisms of exercise limitation. If a specific ''limb-training'' protocol improves exercise performance, the role of physiological adaptations outside, as well as in, limb muscles in the improvement must be considered.

VI. Conclusion

Chronic obstructive pulmonary disease and ILD are systemic diseases with abnormal ventilatory, gas exchange, cardiovascular, skeletal muscle, and metabolic responses to exercise. There are considerable data concerning ventilatory, gas exchange, and central hemodynamic responses to exercise in chronic lung disease but, until now, few studies have examined the responses of skeletal muscles and the peripheral circulation to exercise in these patients. Recent studies provide strong evidence of skeletal muscle dysfunction in patients with chronic lung disease. Further research is needed to clarify the mechanisms underlying skeletal muscle dysfunction. Further work is also needed to dissect the respective roles of ventilatory, gas exchange, cardiovascular, and limb muscle function in exercise limitation in chronic lung disease.

Acknowledgment

The author thanks Ms. V. Hearn for preparing the manuscript.

References

1. Casaburi R. Exercise training in chronic obstructive lung disease. In: Principles and Practice of Pulmonary Rehabilitation, Philadelphia: WB Saunders, ed. 1993.
2. Gallagher CG. Exercise and chronic obstructive pulmonary disease. Med Clin N Am 1990; 74:619–641.
3. Belman MJ, Epstein LJ, Doornbos D, Elashoff JD, Koerner SK, Mohsenifar Z. Noninvasive determinations of the anaerobic threshold. Chest 1992; 102:1028–1034.
4. Gallagher CG. Exercise limitation and clinical exercise testing in chronic obstructive pulmonary disease. Clin Chest Med 1994; 15:305–326.
5. Sue DY, Wasserman K, Moricca RB, Casaburi R. Metabolic acidosis during exercise in patients with chronic obstructive pulmonary disease. Chest 1988; 94:931–938.
6. Casaburi R, Patessio A, Ioli F, Zanaboni S, Donner CF, Wasserman K. Reductions in exercise lactic acidosis and ventilation as a result of exercise training in patients with obstructive lung disease. Am Rev Respir Dis 1991; 143:9–18.
7. Maltais F, Simard A, Simard C, Jobin J, Desgagnes P, Leblanc P. Oxidative capacity of the skeletal muscle and lactic acid kinetics during exercise in normal subjects and in patients with COPD. Am J Respir Crit Care Med 1996; 153:288–293.
8. McParland C, Mink J, Gallagher CG. Respiratory adaptations to dead space loading during maximal incremental exercise. J Appl Physiol 1991; 70:55–62.

9. Syabbalo N, Zintel T, Watts R, Gallagher CG. Carotid chemoreceptors and respiratory adaptations to dead space loading during incremental exercise. J Appl Physiol 1993; 75:1378–1384.
10. Lanigan C, Moxham J, Ponte J. Effect of chronic airflow limitation on resting oxygen consumption. Thorax 1990; 45:388–390.
11. Marciniuk DD, Gallagher CG. Clinical exercise testing in interstitial lung disease. Clin Chest Med 1994; 15:287–303.
12. Levison H, Cherniack RM. Ventilatory cost of exercise in chronic obstructive pulmonary disease. J Appl Physiol 1968; 25:21–27.
13. Nery LE, Wasserman K, Andrews JD, Huntsman DJ, Hansen JE, Whipp BJ. Ventilatory and gas exchange kinetics during exercise in chronic airways obstruction. J Appl Physiol 1982; 53:1594–1602.
14. Agusti AGN, Barbera JA, Roca J, Wagner PD, Guitart R, Rodriguez-Roisin R. Hypoxic pulmonary vasoconstriction and gas exchange during exercise in chronic obstructive pulmonary disease. Chest 1990; 97:268–275.
15. Jones NL. Pulmonary gas exchange during exercise in patients with chronic airway obstruction. Clin Sci 1966; 31:39–50.
16. Nery LE, Wasserman K, French W, Oren A, Davis JA. Contrasting cardiovascular and respiratory responses to exercise in mitral valve and chronic obstructive pulmonary diseases. Chest 1983; 83:446–453.
17. Spiro SG, Hahn HL, Edwards RHT, Pride NB. An analysis of the physiological strain of submaximal exercise in patients with chronic obstructive bronchitis. Thorax 1975; 30:415–425.
18. Bauerle O, Younes M. Role of ventilatory response to exercise in determining exercise capacity in chronic obstructive pulmonary disease. J Appl Physiol 1995; 79:1870–1877.
19. Jones NL, Jones G, Edwards RHT. Exercise tolerance in chronic airway obstruction. Am Rev Respir Dis 1971; 103:477–491.
20. Marcus JH, McLean RL, Duffell GM, Ingram RH. Exercise performance in relation to the pathophysiologic type of chronic obstructive pulmonary disease. Am J Med 1970; 49:14–22.
21. Gallagher CG, Brown E, Younes MK. Breathing pattern during maximal exercise and during submaximal exercise with hypercapnia. J Appl Physiol 1987; 63:238–244.
22. McParland C, Krishnan B, Lobo J, Gallagher CG. Effect of physical training on breathing pattern during progressive exercise. Resp Physiol 1992; 90:311–323.
23. Syabbalo NC, Krishnan B, Zintel T, Gallagher CG. Differential ventilatory regulation during constant workrate exercise and maximal incremental exercise. Respir Physiol 1994; 97:175–187.
24. Gallagher CG, Younes M. Breathing pattern during and after maximal exercise in patients with chronic obstructive lung disease, interstitial lung disease, and cardiac disease, and in normal subjects. Am Rev Respir Dis 1986; 133:581–586.
25. Gowda K, Zintel T, McParland C, Orchard R, Gallagher CG. Diagnostic value of maximal exercise tidal volume. Chest 1990; 98:1351–1354.
26. Gallagher CG, Younes MK. Effect of pressure assist on ventilation and respiratory mechanics in heavy exercise. J Appl Physiol 1989; 66:1824–1837.

27. Younes M. Determinants of thoracic excursions during exercise. In: Exercise. Whipp BJ, Wasserman K (eds). New York: Marcel Dekker, 1991, pp 1–65.
28. Dodd DS, Brancatisano T, Engel LA. Chest wall mechanics during exercise in patients with severe chronic airflow obstruction. Am Rev Respir Dis 1984; 129:33–38.
29. Scano G, Gigliotti F, van Meerhaeghe A, De Coster A, Sergysels R. Influence of exercise and CO_2 on breathing pattern in patients with chronic obstructive lung disease (COLD). Eur Respir J 1988; 1:139–144.
30. Barbera JA, Roca J, Ramirez J, Wagner PD, Ussetti P, Rodriguez-Roisin R. Gas exchange during exercise in mild chronic obstructive pulmonary disease. Am Rev Respir Dis 1991; 144:520–525.
31. Johnson BD, Saupe KW, Dempsey JA. Mechanical constraints on exercise hyperpnea in endurance athletes. J Appl Physiol 1992; 73:874–886.
32. Babb TG, Viggiano R, Hurley B, Staats B, Rodarte JR. Effect of mild-to-moderate airflow limitation on exercise capacity. J Appl Physiol 1991; 70:223–230.
33. Grimby G, Stiksa J. Flow-volume curves and breathing patterns during exercise in patients with obstructive lung disease. Scand J Clin Lab Invest 1970; 25:303–313.
34. Leaver DG, Pride NB. Flow-volume curves and expiratory pressures during exercise in patients with chronic airways obstruction. Scand J Resp Dis 1971; 52:23–27.
35. Potter WA, Olafsson S, Hyatt RE. Ventilatory mechanics and expiratory flow limitation during exercise in patients with obstructive lung disease. J Clin Invest 1971; 50:910–919.
36. Krishnan B, Zintel T, McParland C, Gallagher CG. Lack of importance of respiratory muscle load in ventilatory regulation during heavy exercise. J Physiol (London) 1996; 490.2:537–550.
37. Marciniuk DD, Sridhar G, Clemens RE, Zintel TA, Gallagher CG. Lung volumes and expiratory flow limitation during exercise in interstitial lung disease. J Appl Physiol 1994; 77:963–973.
38. Dean NC, Stulbarg MS, Doherty JJ, Gold WM, Brown JK. Exercise-induced bronchodilatation in patients with severe COPD. Abstract. Am Rev Respir Dis 1989; 139:A85.
39. Suero JT, Woolf CR. Alterations in the mechanical properties of the lung during dyspnea in chronic obstructive pulmonary disease. J Clin Invest 1970; 49:747–751.
40. Rochester DF, Braun NMT. Determinants of maximal inspiratory pressure in chronic obstructive pulmonary disease. Am Rev Respir Dis 1985; 132:42–47.
41. Gallagher CG. Respiratory steroid myopathy. Am J Respir Crit Care Med 1994; 150:4–6.
42. Marciniuk DD, Harris-Eze AO, Clemens RE, Zintel TA, Gallagher CG. Respiratory muscles during exercise in interstitial lung disease (ILD). Abstract. Am J. Respir Crit Care Med 1996; 153:A653.
43. Owens GR, Rogers RM, Pennock BE, Levin D. The diffusing capacity as a predictor of arterial oxygen desaturation during exercise in patients with chronic obstructive pulmonary disease. N Engl J Med 1984; 310:1218–1221.
44. Raffestin B, Escourrou P, Legrand A, Duroux P, Lockhart A. Circulatory transport of oxygen in patients with chronic airflow obstruction exercising maximally. Am Rev Respir Dis 1982; 125:426–431.

45. Dantzker DR, D'Alonzo GE. The effect of exercise on pulmonary gas exchange in patients with severe chronic obstructive pulmonary disease. Am Rev Respir Dis 1986; 134:1135–1139.
46. Wagner PD, Dantzker DR, Dueck R, Clausen JL, West JB. Ventilation-perfusion inequality in chronic obstructive pulmonary disease. J Clin Invest 1977; 59:203–216.
47. Light RW, Mahutte CK, Brown SE. Etiology of carbon dioxide retention at rest and during exercise in chronic airflow obstruction. Chest 1988; 94:61–67.
48. Keogh BA, Lakatos E, Price D, Crystal RG. Importance of the lower respiratory tract in oxygen transfer. Am Rev Respir Dis 1984; 129:S76–S80.
49. Marciniuk D, Watts R, Gallagher CG. Dead space loading and exercise limitation in patients with interstitial lung disease. Chest 1994; 105:183–189.
50. Light RW, Mintz HM, Linden GS, Brown SE. Hemodynamics of patients with severe chronic obstructive pulmonary disease during progressive upright exercise. Am Rev Respir Dis 1984; 130:391–395.
51. Wehr KL, Johnson RL. Maximal oxygen consumption in patients with lung disease. J Clin Invest 1976; 58:880–890.
52. Matthews JI, Bush BA, Ewald FW. Exercise responses during incremental and high intensity and low intensity steady state exercise in patients with obstructive lung disease and normal control subjects. Chest 1989; 96:11–17.
53. Mahler DA, Brent BN, Loke J, Zaret BL, Matthay RA. Right ventricular performance and central circulatory hemodynamics during upright exercise in patients with chronic obstructive pulmonary disease. Am Rev Respir Dis 1984; 130:722–729.
54. Brown SE, Pakron FJ, Milne N, Linden GS, Stansbury DW, Fischer CE, Light RW. Effects of digoxin on exercise capacity and right ventricular function during exercise in chronic airflow obstruction. Chest 1984; 85:187–191.
55. Matthay RA, Berger HJ, Davies RA, Loke J, Mahler DA, Gottschalk A, Zaret BL. Right and left ventricular exercise performance in chronic obstructive pulmonary disease: radionuclide assessment. Ann Intern Med 1980; 93:234–239.
56. Butler J, Schrijen F, Henriquez A, Polu J-M, Albert RK. Cause of the raised wedge pressure on exercise in chronic obstructive pulmonary disease. Am Rev Respir Dis 1988; 138:350–354.
57. Roca J, Sala E, Marrades RM, Alonso J, Gonzalez de Suso JM, Moreno A, Barbera JA, Gomez FP, Iglesia R, Rodriguez-Roisin R, Wagner PD. Patients with chronic obstructive pulmonary disease show skeletal muscle disfunction during exercise. Abstract. Eur Res J 1997; 10:1695.
58. Oelberg D, Medoff B, Markowitz D, Ginns L, Systrom D. Impaired systemic oxygen extraction during incremental exercise in patients with chronic obstructive pulmonary disease. Abstract. Am J Respir Crit Care Med 1996; 153:A21.
59. Allard C, Jones NL, Killian KJ. Static peripheral skeletal muscle strength and exercise capacity in patients with chronic airflow limitation. Abstract. Am Rev Respir Dis 1989; 139:A90.
60. Bernard S, LeBlanc P, Whittom F, Carrier G, Jobin J, Belleau R, Maltais F. Peripheral muscle weakness in patients with chronic obstructive pulmonary disease. Am J Respir Crit Care Med 1998; 158:629–634.
61. Gosselink R, Troosters T, Decramer M. Peripheral muscle weakness contributes to exercise limitation in COPD. Am J Respir Crit Care Med 1996; 153:976–980.

62. Kutsuzawa T, Shioya S, Kurita D, Haida M, Ohta Y, Yamabayashi H. P-NMR study of skeletal muscle metabolism in patients with chronic respiratory impairment. Am Rev Respir Dis 1992; 146:1019–1024.
63. Mannix ET, Boska MD, Galassetti P, Burton G, Manfredi F, Farber MO. Modulation of ATP production by oxygen in obstructive lung disease as assessed by ^{31}P-MRS. J Appl Physiol 1995; 78:2218–2227.
64. Payen JF, Wuyam B, Levy P, Reutenauer H, Stieglitz P, Paramelle B, Le Bas JF. Muscular metabolism during oxygen supplementation in patients with chronic hypoxemia. Am Rev Respir Dis 1993; 147:592–598.
65. Wuyam B, Payen JF, Levy P, Bensaidane H, Reutenauer H, Le Bas JF, Benabid AL. Metabolism and aerobic capacity of skeletal muscle in chronic respiratory failure related to chronic obstructive pulmonary disease. Eur Respir J 1992; 5:157–162.
66. Satta A, Migliori G, Spanevello A, Neri M, Bottinelli R, Canepari M, Pellegrino M, Reggiani C. Fibre types in skeletal muscles of chronic obstructive pulmonary disease patients related to respiratory function and exercise tolerance. Eur Respir J. 1997; 10:2853–2860.
67. Marciniuk DD, Gallagher CG. Clinical exercise testing in chronic airflow limitation. Med Clin N Am 1996; 80:565–587.
68. Engelen MPKJ, Schols AMWJ, Baken WC, Wesseling GJ, Wouters EFM. Nutritional depletion in relation to respiratory and peripheral skeletal muscle function in outpatients with COPD. Eur Respir J 1994; 7:1793–1797.
69. Wagner PD. Determinants of maximal oxygen transport and utilization. Annu Rev Physiol 1996; 58:21–50.
70. Harris-Eze AO, Sridhar G, Clemens RE, Gallagher CG, Marciniuk, DD. Oxygen improves maximal exercise performance in interstitial lung disease. Am J Respir Crit Care Med 1994; 150:1616–1622.
71. Harris-Eze AO, Sridhar G, Clemens RE, Zintel TA, Gallagher CG, Marciniuk DD. Role of hypoxemia and pulmonary mechanics in exercise limitation in interstitial lung disease. Am J Resp Crit Care Med 1996; 154:994–1001.
72. Clark TJH, Freedman S, Campbell EJM, Winn RR. The ventilatory capacity of patients with chronic airways obstruction. Clin Sci 1969; 36:307–316.
73. Bye PTP, Esau SA, Levy RD, Shiner RJ, Macklem PT, Martin JG, Pardy RL. Ventilatory muscle function during exercise in air and oxygen in patients with chronic airflow limitation. Am Rev Respir Dis 1985; 132:236–240.
74. Grassino A, Gross D, Macklem PT, Roussos C, Zagelbaum G. Inspiratory muscle fatigue as a factor limiting exercise. Bull Europ Physiopath Resp 1979; 15:105–111.
75. Pardy RL, Rivington RN, Despas PJ, Macklem PT. The effects of inspiratory muscle training on exercise performance in chronic airflow limitation. Am Rev Respir Dis 1981; 123:426–433.
76. Tobin MJ, Perez W, Guenther SM, Lodato RF, Dantzker DR. Does rib cage-abdominal paradox signify respiratory muscle fatigue? J Appl Physiol 1987; 63:851–860.
77. Klas JV, Dempsey JA. voluntary versus reflex regulation of maximal exercise flow volume loops. Am Rev Respir Dis 1989; 139:150–156.
78. Dillard TA, Hnatiuk OW, McCumber TR. Spirometric determinants in chronic obstructive pulmonary disease patients and normal subjects. Am Rev Respir Dis 1993; 147:870–875.

79. Dolmage TE, Goldstein RS. Proportional assist ventilation and exercise tolerance in subjects with COPD. Chest 1997; 111:948–954.
80. O'Donnell DE, Sanii R, Younes M. Improvement in exercise endurance in patients with chronic airflow limitation using continuous positive airway pressure. Am Rev Respir Dis 1988; 138:1510–1514.
81. Evans A, Al-Himyary AJ, Hrovat MI, Pappagianopoulos P, Wain JC, Ginns LC, Systrom DM. Abnormal skeletal muscle oxidative capacity after lung transplantation by ^{31}P-MRS. Am J Respir Crit Care Med 1997; 155:615–621.
82. Hall M, Snell G, Side E, Esmore D, Walters E, Williams T. Exercise, potassium and muscle deconditioning post-thoracic organ transplantation. J Appl Physiol 1994; 77:2784–2790.
83. Williams T, Snell G. Early and long-term functional outcomes in unilateral, bilateral, and living-related transplant recipients. Clin Chest Med 1997; 18:245–257.
84. Babb TG, Long KA, Rodarte JR. The relationship between maximal expiratory flow and increases of maximal exercise capacity with exercise training. Am J Respir Crit Care Med 1997; 156:116–121.

Additional References

1. Borg GAV. Psychophysical bases of perceived exertion. Med Sci Sports Med 1982; 14:377–381.
2. Brown SE, Fischer CE, Stansbury DW, Light RW. Reproducibility of $V_{O_{2max}}$ in patients with chronic air-flow obstruction. Am Rev Respir Dis 1985; 131:435–438.
3. Brown SE, King RR, Temerlin SM, Stansbury DW, Mahutte CK, Light RW. Exercise performance with added dead space in chronic airflow obstruction. J Appl Physiol 1984; 56:1020–1026.
4. Carter R, Nicotra B, Blevins W, Holiday D. Altered exercise gas exchange and cardiac function in patients with mild chronic obstructive pulmonary disease. Chest 1993; 103:745–750.
5. Celli BR, Rassulo J, Make BJ. Dyssynchronous breathing during arm but not leg exercise in patients with chronic airflow obstruction. N Engl J Med 1986; 314:1485–1490.
6. Chen H-I, Dukes R, Martin BJ. Inspiratory muscle training in patients with chronic obstructive pulmonary disease. Am Rev Respir Dis 1985; 131:251–255.
7. Cheong TH, Magder S, Shapiro S, Martin JG, Levy RD. Cardiac arrhythmias during exercise in severe chronic obstructive pulmonary disease. Chest 1990; 97:793–797.
8. Cockcroft A, Beaumont A, Adams L, Guz A. Arterial oxygen desaturation during treadmill and bicycle exercise in patients with chronic obstructive airways disease. Clin Sci 1985; 68:327–332.
9. Dillard TA, Piantadosi S, Rajagopal KR. Prediction of ventilation at maximal exercise in chronic airflow obstruction. Am Rev Respir Dis 1985; 132:230–235.
10. Flynn MG, Barter CE, Nosworthy JC, Pretto JJ, Rochford PD, Pierce RJ. Threshold pressure training, breathing pattern, and exercise performance in chronic airflow obstruction. Chest 1989; 95:535–540.
11. Gimenez M, Servera E, Candina R, Mohan Kumar T, Bonnassis JB. Hypercapnia during maximal exercise in patients with chronic airflow obstruction. Bull Eur Physiopathol Respir 1984; 20:113–119.

12. Goldstein S, Askanazi J, Elwyn DH, Thomashow B, Milic-Emili J, Kvetan V, Weissman C, Kinney JM. Submaximal exercise in emphysema and malnutrition at two levels of carbohydrate and fat intake. J Appl Physiol 1989; 67:1048–1055.
13. Grimby G, Elgefors B, Oxhoj H. Ventilatory levels and chest wall mechanics during exercise in obstructive lung disease. Scand J Respir Dis 1973; 54:45–52.
14. Jones NL. Clinical Exercise Testing. 3rd ed. Philadelphia: WB Saunders, 1988.
15. Killian KJ, Leblanc P, Martin DH, Summers E, Jones NL, Campbell EJM. Exercise capacity and ventilatory, circulatory, and symptom limitation in patients with chronic airflow limitation. Am Rev Respir Dis 1992; 146:935–940.
16. Knox AJ, Morrison JFJ, Muers MF. Reproducibility of walking test results in chronic obstructive airways disease. Thorax 1988; 43:388–392.
17. Leblanc P, Bowie DM, Summers E, Jones NL, Killian KJ. Breathlessness and exercise in patients with cardiorespiratory disease. Am Rev Respir Dis 1986; 133:21–25.
18. Marrades RM, Roca J, Sala E, Moreno A, Alonso J, Gonzalez de Suso JM, Barbera JA, Iglesia R, Gomez F, Rodriguez-Roisin R, Wagner PD. Exercise training improves cellular bioenergetics in patients with chronic obstructive pulmonary disease (COPD). Eur Res J 1997; 10:1695.
19. McParland C, Resch EF, Krishnan B, Wang Y, Cujec B, Gallagher CG. Inspiratory muscle weakness in chronic heart failure: role of nutrition and electrolyte status and systemic myopathy. Am J Respir Crit Care Med 1995; 151:1101–1107.
20. Muza SR, Silverman MT, Gilmore GC, Hellerstein HK, Kelsen SG. Comparison of scales used to quantitate the sense of effort to breathe in patients with chronic obstructive pulmonary disease. Am Rev Respir Dis 1990; 141:909–913.
21. Owens MW, Kinasewitz GT and Strain DS. Evaluating the effects of chronic therapy in patients with irreversible air-flow obstruction. Am Rev Respir Dis 1986; 134:935–937.
22. Petrof BJ, Calderini E, Gottfried SB. Effect of CPAP on respiratory effort and dyspnea during exercise in severe COPD. J Appl Physiol 1990; 69:179–188.
23. Raimondi AC, Edwards RHT, Denison DM, Leaver DG, Spencer RG, Siddorn JA. Exercise tolerance breathing a low density gas mixture, 35% oxygen and air in patients with chronic obstructive bronchitis. Clin Sci 1970; 39:675–685.
24. Servera E, Gimenez M, Mohan-Kumar T, Candina R, Bonassis JB. Oxygen uptake at maximal exercises in chronic airflow obstruction. Bull Eur Physiopathol Resp 1983; 19:553–556.
25. Shuey CB, Pierce AK, Johnson RL. An evaluation of exercise tests in chronic obstructive lung disease. J Appl Physiol 1969; 27:256–261.
26. Sridhar G, Clemens R, Zintel T, Gallagher CG. Dead space loading and exercise limitation in moderate chronic obstructive pulmonary disease (COPD). Am Rev Resp Dis 1993; 147:A189.
27. Stubbing DG, Pengelly LD, Morse JLC, Jones NL. Pulmonary mechanics during exercise in subjects with chronic airflow obstruction. J Appl Physiol 1980; 49:511–515.
28. Swinburn CR, Wakefield JM, Jones PW. Performance, ventilation and oxygen consumption in three different types of exercise test in patients with chronic obstructive lung disease. Thorax 1985; 40:581–586.
29. Wasserman K, Hansen JE, Sue DY, Whipp BJ. Principles of Exercise Testing and Interpretation. 1st ed. Philadelphia: Lea & Febiger, 1987.

30. Weisman IM, Connery SM, Belbel RJ, Zeballos. The role of cardiopulmonary exercise testing in the selection of patients for cardiac transplantation. Chest 1992; 102:1871–1874.
31. Wijkstra P, van der Mark Th., Kraan J, van Altena R, Koeter G, Postma D. Effects of home rehabilitation on physical performance in patients with chronic obstructive pulmonary disease (COPD). Eur Respir J 1996; 9:104–110.
32. Wilson SH, Cooke NT, Moxham J, Spiro SG. Sternomastoid muscle function and fatigue in normal subjects and patients with chronic obstructive pulmonary disease. Am Rev Respir Dis 1984; 129:460–464.
33. Younes M. Interpretation of clinical exercise testing in respiratory disease. Clin Chest Med 1984; 5:189–206.

21

Cardiopulmonary and Peripheral Vascular Alterations in Chronic Congestive Heart Failure

DONNA M. MANCINI and AINAT BENIAMINOVITZ

New York Presbyterian Hospital, Columbia University
New York, New York

I. Introduction

Heart failure may be defined as the inability of the heart to adequately perfuse the metabolizing tissue. The clinical syndrome of congestive heart failure (CHF) involves a complex interplay of skeletal muscle and peripheral adaptations in conjunction with decreased myocardial performance. Evidence for a peripheral abnormality in CHF was first described 20 years ago by Zelis et al. [1]. In studies of peak reactive hyperemic blood flow response in volume-overloaded patients with rheumatic heart disease, marked reduction in peak forearm blood flow at rest, exercise, and in response to physiological maneuvers was observed in these patients compared with normal subjects. These findings suggested defects of the periphery rather than a simple central reduction in cardiac output response. Recent studies in cardiopulmonary exercise testing have also suggested a peripheral vasculature and skeletal muscle impairment in CHF. This review briefly outlines the cardiac adaptations and then focuses on the peripheral and pulmonary adaptations observed in patients with CHF. We also review potential benefits of exercise training in patients with this disease.

II. Pathophysiology of Heart Failure: Cardiac Adaptations

Cardiac failure is the final common pathway for a variety of diseases that results in myocyte loss or decreased function. In the presence of a reduced cardiac output, the heart is dependent on three principle compensatory mechanisms to maintain normal function [2]: (1) the Frank-Starling mechanism increases preload to sustain cardiac stroke volume; (2) myocardial hypertrophy occurs to increase the mass of contractile tissue; and (3) the sympathetic nervous system is activated to augment myocardial contractility. These compensatory mechanisms are limited and ultimately become detrimental, contributing to the progression of the disease process.

The development of myocardial hypertrophy is an adaptive mechanism that reduces the stress per unit area of muscle, which in turn permits the ventricle to sustain an excessive volume or pressure load. However, with prolonged loads and greater degrees of hypertrophy, this compensatory response becomes maladaptive, and the ventricular muscle fails. A model of right ventricular failure induced in mammalian species by pulmonary artery banding was one of the first models used to study ventricular hypertrophy [3,4]. In animals with both hypertrophy and failure, muscle function studies showed a reduction in the maximum velocity of shortening below values obtained in muscles from normal animals. Smaller mechanical changes were observed in animals with hypertrophy alone. The contractile performance of the intact right ventricle of these same animals also showed depressed function that paralleled the muscle studies. At equivalent end-diastolic fiber lengths, the wall force developed by the right ventricle was significantly lower than normal in animals with heart failure. When end-diastolic volume was increased or reduced in the animals with heart failure, the relationship between end-diastolic volume and stroke volume was shifted downward and to the right of the normal curve. Ventricular performance is thus preserved in the face of reduced contractility by increasing end-diastolic pressure, volume, and fiber length. Interestingly, muscle studies from animals with chronic volume overload [5] showed that no change in contractility or changes in the pressure–volume relationship occurred. Thus, the nature of the stress underlying the hypertrophic response seems to determine whether contractility is affected.

From several animal models of heart failure, it becomes evident that the time between the creation of the hemodynamic load and the appearance of myocardial failure depends on the type of overload created (pressure or volume), the abruptness with which it is applied, and the severity of the imposed overload [2]. Hypertrophy initially serves to normalize performance, whereas ventricular failure ensues in most, but not all, instances.

A. Myocardial Cell Abnormalities

In conjunction with the morphological changes that occur in CHF, changes occur on a cellular level as well. Adenosine triphosphate (ATP) is the high-energy phosphate-containing compound directly used for excitation and contraction in muscle cells. The myocardial cell must continually resynthesize ATP to maintain normal pump function and cellular viability. There are conflicting results as to whether ATP concentrations are reduced in the failing heart. In a rat model of moderate heart failure, the ATP concentration is identical to that in normal rat hearts [6], but in the severely failing hamster heart, the ATP concentration was 28% lower than age-matched controls [7].

Myocardial biopsy specimens from patients with cardiomyopathy provides evidence that the capacity for ATP resynthesis via the creatine kinase system is compromised in heart failure. These samples show decreases of 30–50% in the tissue activity of creatine kinase and in tissue content of the guanidino substrate for the reaction [8,9]. Similar observations of decreased activity of creatine kinase and the decreased guanidino pool have been found in animal models [10].

^{31}Phosphorus (^{31}P) magnetic resonance spectroscopy (MRS) spectra studies of the failing myocardium in humans have shown that phosphocreatine (PCr) is decreased in failing myocardium [11,12]. These studies report lower PCr/ATP resonance area ratios in the ^{31}P MRS spectra. Ingwall [13] has been instrumental in linking myocardial contractile dysfunction to these cellular biochemical abnormalities. Her group observed decreased contractile function in several animal models of heart failure, such as the hypertensive rat heart, the cardiomyopathic Syrian hamster heart, the infarcted rat heart, and the chemically mediated turkey model of cardiomyopathy. In these hearts, the isovolumic contractile performance was impaired compared with age-matched hearts of normal animals. In concert with the impaired contractility, the tissue content of PCr, the short-term energy supply of the cell, was lower in the severely failing mammalian myocardium regardless of the cause of the failure.

B. Neurohormonal Receptors in the Failing Heart

Adrenergic activation in CHF is well documented by the numerous studies that have shown elevated serum levels of norepinephrine in heart failure patients as well as a significant positive correlation between severity of heart failure and norepinephrine concentrations [14,15]. The SOLVD (studies of left ventricular dysfunction) registry substudy showed a 35% increase in plasma norepinephrine even in patients with asymptomatic left ventricular dysfunction [16], arguing for early activation of the adrenergic axis. Activation of the renin–angiotensin system also occurs in heart failure. Assessment of plasma renin and aldosterone levels similarly indicates that the activation occurs early in the course of CHF [15].

Most of the studies of receptor abnormalities in CHF have focused on the β-adrenergic receptors. The normal human heart expresses a mixed population of β-adrenergic receptor subtypes, with 70–80% being β_1 and the remainder β_2. In CHF, the degree of downregulation of the β_1 subunit [17] correlates with the severity of the heart failure [18]. In conjunction with downregulation, several alterations in the β-adrenergic/G protein signal transduction pathways occur in the chronically failing human heart. In ischemic cardiomyopathy, there is uncoupling of the β_1 receptor from its signal transduction pathway, whereas β_2 uncoupling occurs with all forms of cardiomyopathy [18]. Uncoupling is achieved by phosphorylation of the β-receptor. In heart failure, the kinases responsible for phosphorylating the β-receptors are unregulated [19], the activity of the inhibitory G protein is increased [20], and adenylyl cyclase activity is decreased in heart failure [18]. Other counterregulatory hormones also limit the β-receptor/G protein signal transduction pathway during heart failure. A decrease in β-adrenergic responsiveness by nitric oxide [21] or a decrease in neuronal norepinephrine release by natriuretic peptides [22] are two such examples.

C. Exercise and Congestive Heart Failure: Decreased Cardiac Output Response

Physical exercise involves the interaction of the respiratory, cardiac, and vascular systems to meet the increased metabolic demands of the skeletal muscles. Although each system can theoretically be the limiting step to maximal physical performance, exercise capacity is primarily limited by the cardiac output response in normal humans [1,2].

Decreased exercise capacity in patients with heart failure has been traditionally attributed to a decreased cardiac output response to exercise that leads to skeletal muscle underperfusion and intramuscular lactic acidosis [23,24]. This is based on observations that patients with heart failure show reduced cardiac output responses to exercise. In 1981, Weber et al. [25] performed exercise hemodynamic measurements and ventilatory gas measurements during progressive treadmill exercise in 40 patients with heart failure. This represented the first large application of the measurement of peak oxygen consumption in patients with heart failure as a noninvasive method for characterizing cardiac reserve and functional status in these patients. They found that with worsening heart failure, the cardiac output response is markedly diminished, and they were able to group patients into four classes (groups A to D) on their cardiac output response to exercise. A patient with severe heart failure may only increase his cardiac output twofold versus the normal individual, who can increase his cardiac output response by approximately fivefold.

Recently, we performed a similar analysis in a larger series of 65 patients using bicycle exercise [26]. Twenty-nine percent of patients had New York Heart Association class II, 65% had class III, and 6% had class IV heart failure symptomatology. Our results are concordant with the initial observations of Weber et al. [25]. A series of lines are generated with a progressively lower cardiac index as a function of percent maximum oxygen consumption ($\dot{V}O_{2max}$) as the peak $\dot{V}O_2$ declines. We also observed a highly significant correlation between peak cardiac output and peak $\dot{V}O_2$ similar to prior reports. Thus, in this and other studies, there is a significant correlation between the peak $\dot{V}O_2$ and cardiac output.

Recently, Wilson et al. [27,28] reported that 56% of patients with heart failure had a normal cardiac output response to exercise using the following formula:

cardiac output = 0.5 $\dot{V}_{O_{2max}}$ + 3. Wilson et al. hypothesized that in these patients, peripheral factors rather than central hemodynamic response seemed to constitute the major limitation to exercise performance. Although Wilson et al. concluded that more than half of their population had a normal cardiac output response to exercise, the peak cardiac output of this patient cohort was only 8.5 L/min. In normal subjects from which Wilson et al. primarily derived their formula, more than 95% achieved a peak cardiac output substantially above this value. Thus, in terms of absolute cardiac output, the exercise response in patients with heart failure is markedly abnormal, although like the normal subjects, it can be described by a similar linear equation. Because $\dot{V}_{O_2}$ is the product of the cardiac output and the arteriovenous oxygen difference, the relationship between $\dot{V}_{O_2}$ and cardiac output should be linear with the arteriovenous difference describing the slope. Higginbotham et al. [29] described this relationship during bicycle exercise in 102 normal subjects. A similar relation was observed in patients with heart failure in our recent study [26]. Indeed, the slopes of the two equations were the same, with the normal and heart failure groups described by different segments of the same line. Deviations from this line are likely a result of differences on the arteriovenous oxygen difference, which depends primarily on muscle metabolic function.

III. Peripheral Vascular and Skeletal Muscle Adaptations in Congestive Heart Failure

Although peak $\dot{V}_{O_2}$ is clearly dependent on the cardiac output response to exercise, patients with similarly reduced left ventricular ejection fractions have a wide range of exercise capacity. Moreover, several investigators have demonstrated that therapeutic interventions that acutely enhance exercise hemodynamic measurements do not increase exercise capacity [30,31]. For example, dobutamine is a potent positive inotropic agent with combined β_1 and β_2 agonist activity. Administered at rest and during exercise, it results in significant hemodynamic benefits. With dobutamine therapy, pulmonary capillary wedge pressure is decreased and cardiac index increased at rest and throughout exercise. However, despite a substantial hemodynamic improvement, peak $\dot{V}_{O_2}$ is minimally increased in these patients. The augmented cardiac output is presumably directed by peripheral vasodilation to the metabolically nonactive vascular beds. This results in an increased cardiac output during exercise with a narrowing of the arterial-venous oxygen difference (A-$\dot{V}_{O_2}$). Blood flow to the exercising muscles is not increased; therefore, maximal oxygen uptake remains essentially unchanged. Alternatively, an increase in skeletal muscle perfusion may occur with dobutamine and may not be used because of regional vascular abnormalities.

Although a decreased cardiac output is paramount to skeletal muscle fatigue observed in CHF, there is experimental evidence that primary skeletal muscle and vascular abnormalities exist. Indeed, the peripheral circulation undergoes substantial transformations during the progression of CHF with an alteration of regional vascular control. Abnormalities of forearm and calf circulation to a variety of vasodilator stimuli, including vasodilating drugs, reactive hyperemia, and exercise, have been well documented and are reviewed in Sections III.A and III.B. The resulting changes in the peripheral circulation play an integral role in the development of symptoms in patients with left ventricular dysfunction. In the following section, we describe the vascular and skeletal muscle changes observed in human CHF.

A. Vascular Endothelial Abnormalities

The endothelium is an important modulator of vascular tone. It releases relaxing and constricting factors both at rest and during exercise in response to neurotransmitters, hormones, or physical stimuli such as shear stress. In both animal and human models of CHF, the responses to endothelium-mediated vasodilation are blunted. In a canine pacing model of heart failure [32], local administration of acetylcholine, an endothelium-dependent vasodilator, resulted in blunted vasodilatory responses compared with normal dogs. Reduced endothelial-dependent dilation in the aorta of rats with an ischemic cardiomyopathy has also been shown [33]. Kubo et al. [34] demonstrated that endothelium-dependent vasodilation is attenuated in patients with heart failure. Forearm blood flow assessed by plethysmography was measured at rest and during intra-arterial infusions of methacholine and nitroprusside. Metacholine releases endothelium-derived relaxing factor through stimulation of muscarinic receptors. Nitroprusside results in relaxation of vascular smooth muscle. Forearm blood flow responses to two doses of metacholine was attenuated in subjects with heart failure when compared with normal age-matched subjects. Forearm blood flow responses to intra-arterial nitroprusside administration tended to be lower in patients with heart failure than in normal subjects, but the reduction was less marked than that observed with methacholine. Thus, endothelial-derived vasodilation seemed more abnormal than vascular smooth muscle vasodilation in patients with heart failure. In contrast, Katz et al. [35] showed that the impairment of the peripheral circulation was not limited to the vascular endothelium [35]. The vasodilatory responses in the lower limb circulation was reduced to both acetylcholine and nitroglycerin in patients with CHF compared with normal subjects. Both of these studies did suggest a reduced stimulated release of nitric oxide in response to acetylcholine. Basal release of nitric oxide from peripheral vessels in patients with heart failure may also be altered. Some studies suggest an increased basal release, whereas others demonstrate no change or a reduction.

Change in sheer stress is an important determinate of endothelial function. In normal vasculature, changes in sheer stress on the endothelial cell that accompany alterations in blood flow serve to enhance vasodilation via release of nitric oxide and prostaglandins [35,36]. As is discussed in Section V, aerobic training normalizes endothelial function in patients with CHF, probably via a mechanism of increased shear stress. In canine models of heart failure, the vascular responses to low-dose acetylcholine are amplified by pretreatment with indomethacin [32]. These alterations in vascular reactivity in CHF have been postulated to be adaptive in that they function to maintain shear stress close to control levels [37].

Endothelial dysfunction seems to be a time-dependent alteration. With increasing severity of CHF, there is a deterioration of endothelial vascular function. In rats with early stages of heart failure, vascular endothelial function was preserved, whereas in more severe stages, an impairment was noted [38]. Concentrations of circulating cytokines such as tumor necrosis factor alpha (TNF-α) are elevated in severe heart failure. TNF-α impairs stimulated release of endothelium-derived relaxing factor (EDRF). Plasma levels of TNF in patients with heart failure are correlated with the degree of endothelial dysfunction assessed by infusion of acetylcholine [39]. Chronically decreased skeletal muscle perfusion, increased tissue angiotensin-converting enzyme activity, increased oxygen free-radical formation, and increased endothelial vasoconstriction agents are other potential mechanisms that are involved in the development of endothelial dysfunction in these patients.

B. Vascular Smooth Muscle

In a series of elegant studies, Teerlink et al. [40] and Zelis et al. [41,42] demonstrated that fluid and sodium retention can impair arteriolar vasodilatation in humans. Rhythmic grip exercise of three different intensities was performed in seven patients with right heart failure caused by rheumatic heart disease and 22 control subjects with forearm blood flow measured using venous plethysmography [40]. Forearm blood flow was reduced at rest and each level of exercise in patients with heart failure. Forearm oxygen extraction calculated from brachial venous and systemic arterial blood was also found to be consistently increased. This type of small muscle mass exercise does not require any significant increase in cardiac output, thus the difference in forearm perfusion is not related to central hemodynamic factors and implied peripheral changes.

Using a canine model of heart failure produced by rapid ventricular pacing, Zelis et al. [41] measured the arterial sodium content in the aorta and femoral artery in control animals and those with heart failure. A significant increase in the arterial sodium content in the animals with heart failure was demonstrated. Zelis et al. postulated that arteriolar stiffness from increased salt and water content resulted in an abnormal vasodilatory response in heart failure. Longhurst et al. [43] showed a similar deficiency in the forearm vasculature responses to static exercise.

The fixed vasodilatory capacity of the skeletal bed in CHF during exercise was demonstrated in a study comparing one-versus two-leg bicycle exercise. In contrast to normal controls, patients with severe CHF were unable to augment maximal limb blood flow during one-leg bicycle exercise over that reached during two-leg bicycle exercise [44].

Regional specificity of the peripheral circulation abnormality has been demonstrated in patients with CHF. A comparison of peak reactive hyperemia between the forearms and calves of these patients demonstrated abnormal calf flow only [45].

Furthermore, only calf peak reactive hyperemia correlated to peak $\dot{V}O_2$. Selective deconditioning may be responsible for these regional differences. As CHF worsens, there is decreased use of lower extremities, but upper-extremity use remains relatively preserved.

During exercise, peripheral vasoconstriction is increased to prevent systemic hypotension in patients given the decreased increase in cardiac output [46]. Tissue hypoxia and enhanced sympathetic and angiotensin activation in CHF are two proposed mechanisms mediating abnormal peripheral vasoconstriction in CHF (47). Institution of sympathetic and renin–angiotensin blockade do not completely reverse the peripheral derangements observed in CHF, although they modify it.

C. Abnormalities in Skeletal Muscle Composition and Function in CHF

Metabolic abnormalities during exercise have been described using ^{31}P MRS, a technology that permits noninvasive monitoring of PCr, inorganic phosphate, ATP, and pH in working muscle. During exercise, adenosine diphosphate (ADP) is a key stimulant to mitochrondrial oxidative phosphorylation. The inorganic phosphorous to PCr (Pi/PCr) ratio correlates closely with ADP concentration. By monitoring changes in the Pi/Pcr ratio at different work levels, alterations in the control of oxidative phosphorylation can be detected. Exercise also activates glycolysis, producing an increase in intracellular lactate concentration and a decrease in intracellular pH. By monitoring changes in muscle pH during exercise, changes in glycolytic activity can be detected. The metabolic behavior of both the forearm and calf muscle during exercise in patients with heart failure has been examined. Abnormal skeletal muscle metabolism, i.e., reduced oxidative metabolism with earlier shift to glycolytic metabolism, has been demonstrated in patients with heart failure using ^{31}P MRS [48–54]. Specifically, patients with heart failure have a more pronounced increase in the Pi/Pcr ratio and a more rapid decrease in local pH than do normal subjects performing comparable workloads. As is discussed in the following paragraphs of this section, these abnormalities seem to be independent of total limb perfusion [49,53,54], histochemical changes [51], muscle mass [52], or severe tissue hypoxia [55].

Using plethysmography to measure forearm blood flow, no significant difference between forearm blood flows was observed during forearm exercise in patients and control subjects, despite the presence of significant metabolic abnormalities. This suggested that these metabolic abnormalities were not flow-mediated [56]. Massie et al. [57] performed similar studies with identical results. They demonstrated persistent metabolic abnormalities in patients with CHF compared with normal subjects during ischemic exercise, i.e., exercise performed during arterial occlusion. Moreover, acutely increasing cardiac output with therapeutic agents such as dobutamine did not improve the metabolic abnormalities observed in these patients [57].

To provide simultaneous monitoring of cellular metabolism and oxygenation, we have coupled ^{31}P MRS to near-infrared spectroscopy. Near-infrared absorption enables the assessment of changes in tissue oxygenation at the level of small blood vessels, capillaries, and intracellular sites of oxygen uptake by monitoring the difference in absorption of oxygenated and deoxygenated hemoglobin at 760 and 850 nm of light [53,56]. Calf exercise was performed in normal subjects and patients with heart failure [55] using this combined approach of ^{31}P MRS and near-infrared spectroscopy. We were able to demonstrate that during exercise with minimal cardiovascular stress, the metabolic abnormalities observed in patients with heart failure occur despite what seems to be adequate muscle oxygenation.

In this study, we also measure ^{1}Hydrogen (^{1}H) proton spectroscopy to assess the development of deoxymyoglobin during exercise. ^{1}H MRS allows in vivo detection of deoxygenated myoglobin. Myoglobin, an oxygen-binding protein located exclusively in the skeletal muscle, functions as an additional intracellular source of oxygen and facilitates the transfer of oxygen to mitochondria. Similar to hemoglobin, the oxymyoglobin dissociation curve follows a hyperbolic function of oxygen pressure. However, myoglobin binds oxygen at low pressures much more readily than hemoglobin. The 50% desaturation of myoglobin does not occur until approximately 2.5 mm Hg at 37°C [58–62]. Therefore, significant deoxygenation of myoglobin does not occur until the partial pressure of tissue oxygen decreases to below 2.5 mm Hg [58,59]. In rapidly metabolizing muscle, such as occurs during exercise, a steep oxygen gradient develops between myoglobin deoxygenation and cytochrome AA3, the rate-limiting step of mitochondrial respiration. A coherent relationship occurs between deoxygenated myoglobin and AA3 during high metabolic activity, enabling myoglobin to serve as a noninvasive indicator of tissue hypoxia [60].

Proton resonances from oxygenated myoglobin are usually concealed under the water peak. However, with deoxygenation, the electron spin of the ferrous ion changes from a low to a high spin state. A paramagnetic shift occurs, making protons from deoxygenated myoglobin visible at approximately 70 ppm from the water peak . Thus, in vivo monitoring of deoxymyoglobin provides a noninvasive probe by which to assess severe tissue hypoxia. In this study, 16 patients with heart failure and seven normal subjects performed supine calf plantarflexion. At maximal exercise, only three patients and four of the normal subjects showed deoxymyoglobin signal during low-level exercise. The absence of deoxymyoglobin signal during the small muscle mass exercise in patients with CHF and the normal muscle oxygenation throughout exercise indicates that the ^{31}P metabolic abnormalities in these patients do not result from inadequate oxygen availability. As previously discussed, prior studies demonstrated similar tissue perfusion via venous plethysmography between normal subjects and those with heart failure. However, whether maldistribution of blood flow occurred, resulting in ischemia to exercising muscle, remained unclear. This study [55] excludes this hypothesis and demonstrates that the metabolic changes are not from severe tissue hypoxia during small muscle mass exercise. In numerous prior observations, as in this study, intracellular pH was significantly decreased during exercise in patients with heart failure. Therefore, a reduction in pH occurred in the presence of significant oxygen cellular reserve. Reduction in intracellular pH with lactate formation is often viewed as an indicator of tissue hypoxia. The absence of significant deoxymyoglobin signal in the majority of subjects suggests that muscles produce and release lactate under aerobic conditions. This phenomenon would occur if mitochondrial flavin adenine dinucleotide failed to reoxidize the proton shuttle of the mitochondrial membrane at a rate sufficient to keep cytosolic nicotinamide adenine dinulceotide/reduced nicotinamide adenine dinucleotide [NADH+H^{+}]/[NAD] normal. The redox state of the cytosol would become reduced. NADH accumulation in the cytosol would result in pyruvate oxidation of NADH to NAD, with the subsequent accumulation of lactate acid [61]. These results are consistent with those of Connett et al. [62], who demonstrated formation of lactate without myoglobin desaturation in a canine gracilis muscle preparation. These metbolic changes occur despite adequate oxygen stores during exercise.

Muscle biopsy studies have also demonstrated histochemical abnormalities. A variety of histochemical changes were initially described by Lipkin et al. [63] and included fiber atrophy and decrease in oxidative enzymes. In percutaneous calf muscle biopsy specimens obtained from 22 patients with heart failure, a significant increase in percentage type IIb fibers (i.e., glycolytic, fast twitch, easily fatiguable fibers), type II fiber atrophy, and a reduction in a lipolytic enzyme based in the mitochondria (i.e., β-hydroxyl coenzyme A dehydrogenase) was described [64]. Sullivan et al. [65] further expanded these findings and described a reduction in oxidative and glycolytic enzymes. Mitochrondrial changes, including decrease in the volume and surface density of cristae, were described by Drexler et al. [66]. The vascularity of skeletal muscles has been assessed using capillary-to-fiber ratios. The results of these studies have been conflicting. Some investigators have reported a decrease in all measures of capillary density [65,66]. In our study, we found a normal capillary-to-fiber ratio [67].

In addition to fiber atrophy noted on muscle biopsy, patients also show generalized muscle atrophy, again consistent with inactivity and deconditioning. Anthropomorphic measurements performed using Lange (Cambridge Science Instruments, Cambridge, MA) calipers to measure skinfold fat thickness, arm circumference, and 24-hour urine collections for creatinine to estimate total muscle mass were performed in 62 patients with heart failure. Patients with heart failure had adequate fat stores, but 60% had evidence of significant muscle loss. Calf muscle volume was also assessed with magnetic resonance imaging (MRI) in 15 patients with heart failure and 10 control subjects. MRI studies showed a reduced muscle volume in patients with heart failure. Significant water and/or fat infiltration was also noted in the muscle sections of these patients [68]. In this study, we were able only to demonstrate a modest correlation between the calf muscle mass measurements and the MRS metabolic changes. Moreover, measurement of the time constant of recovery of Pcr, another index of oxidative metabolism that is independent of work intensity and muscle mass, was significantly reduced in patients with heart failure compared with normal subjects, further supporting that the metabolic changes are not the result of muscle atrophy. Other investigators using MRI and dual-energy x-ray absorptiometry have confirmed our findings of reduced leg mass in these patients [69].

Abnormalities of skeletal muscle strength and performance would be anticipated in light of the significant skeletal muscle atrophy observed in these patients. However, the results of assessment of muscle strength by several groups of investigators is conflicting. Quadricep muscle strength has been most widely assessed. Early studies in small numbers of patients using the twitch interpolation technique to circumvent subjective differences and insure maximal effort demonstrated a reduction in maximal isometric strength [70]. Moreover, these studies suggested that maximal strength was correlated with peak $\dot{V}O_2$. However, other studies have failed to demonstrate a decrease in maximal isometric or isokinetic quadricep strength [70]. A correlation between quadricep muscle size and maximal strength has been demonstrated in normal subjects and in patients with CHF [70]. This suggests that weaker subjects have less muscle mass, although strength/ unit area of muscle may be normal.

The impact of muscle mass on peak $\dot{V}O_2$ has been investigated. We demonstrated a weak but significant correlation with total skeletal muscle mass derived from equations using 24-hour urinary protein measurements [67]. Jondeau et al. [71] contrasted peak $\dot{V}O_2$ consumption during combined upper-arm and maximal leg exercise. In normal subjects, the addition of more muscle mass via arm exercise did not increase peak exercise performance, and $\dot{V}O_2$ remained unchanged. Thus, cardiac output response to exercise rather than amount of exercising muscle seems to determine peak $\dot{V}O_2$. However, in patients with severe CHF, the addition of upper-arm exercise significantly increased peak $\dot{V}O_2$. The importance of skeletal muscle mass in limiting peak $\dot{V}O_2$ is suggested by this study. An alternative hypothesis is that the peripheral vasodilatory abnormalities in these patients resulted in a physiological shunt to the upper-arm musculature, resulting in higher peak $\dot{V}O_2$ with combined arm and leg exercise.

What elicits the intrinsic skeletal muscle changes in patients with heart failure is unkown, but the leading speculation is that these changes are most likely caused by deconditioning. Several recent studies demonstrate that aerobic training can improve maximal exercise capacity in patients with heart failure by 15–30% [72,73]. These studies are discussed in Section V. Other factors in addition to deconditioning may contribute to the intrinsic skeletal muscle changes. Caloric protein malnutrition may occur; increased tissue necrosis factor, elevated serum cortisol, and chronic skeletal muscle underperfusion may also contribute to skeletal muscle changes.

In many patients with heart failure, intrinsic skeletal muscle changes may represent the primary determinate of exercise performance. Wilson et al. [74] studied 34 patients with heart failure and six normal subjects with determinations of exercise hemodynamic measurements and leg blood flow. All patients showed a reduced exercise capacity with peak $\dot{V}O_2$ less than 18 mL/kg/min; however, approximately 25% had normal leg blood flow. Although all of these patients showed normal leg blood flow, lactate release was abnormal [74]. This implies that their exercise limitation is most probably caused by intrinsic skeletal muscle changes rather than limited cardiac output response.

The limb skeletal muscles in patients with heart failure have been the most intensely investigated. Whether a generalized skeletal muscle defect occurs or regional changes occur was not clear. In some patients with cardiomyopathies, it has been suggested that a generalized myopathic process occurs. However, a recent study would not support a generalized myopathic process. We examined the histochemical changes of the diaphragm in heart failure. Unlike the limb musculature, the histochemical changes elicited in the diaphragm of patients with heart failure included an increase in the activity of citrate synthase, a decrease in the activity of lactate dehydrogenase, an increase in myosin heavy chain type I isomer, and a significant decrease in myosin heavy chain type II B isomer. These changes were consistent with a shift from glycolytic to oxidative metabolism and mimicked those observed with endurance exercise. Presumably, these changes reflected the adapatation of the diaphragm to a chronically increased work of breathing observed in patients with heart failure. These findings imply that skeletal muscle changes are not generalized, but are organ-specific [75].

D. Alterations of the Skeletal Muscle and Peripheral Vasculature in Peripheral Vascular Disease

Similar derangements in skeletal muscle and the peripheral vasculature are observed in chronic arterial occlusive disease [76–78]. Percutaneous needle biopsies of the quadriceps femoris or the gastrocnemius muscles were performed in 31 patients with chronic arterial occlusive disease immediately before and 1 week to 3 months after revascularization [76]. Seven patients undergoing elective hip surgery were chosen as controls. Significantly decreased levels of ATP and total adenine nucleotides were observed in the muscle biopsy specimens of patients with peripheral vascular disease compared with controls. Energy charge potential, which reflects the relative concentration of ATP, ADP, and AMP, as well as the ATP-to-ADP ratio, and both PCr and creatine were significantly decreased in muscle samples from the patients with peripheral vascular disease. Furthermore, the degree of ischemia inversely correlated with levels of ATP, energy charge potential, and the ATP/ADP ratios. Neither consistent nor significant normalization of muscle high-energy phosphates was demonstrated after arterial reconstruction in this sudy. The authors postulated that this was probably caused by concomitant injury during surgery. However, it is more intriguing to postulate that similar to CHF, the alterations that occur in the skeletal muscle caused by the "arterioscelortic syndrome" are not solely a result of reduced skeletal muscle perfusion.

Histochemical studies investigating the calf muscle of patients with peripheral vascular disease have shown conflicting results. Early reports described an increase in oxidative and glycolytic enzyme activity in the calf muscle of patients with peripheral vascular disease versus control subjects [79]. An increase in type 1 fibers and in the number and size of mitochondria was also observed, although electron microscopy of mitochondria showed structural abnormalities [80]. More recent studies suggest that with increased severity of the disease the oxidative potential of the muscle is reduced. Gastrocnemius biopsy specimens from 82 patients with peripheral vascular disease and 19 normal subjects were examined. The cross-sectional area of type 1 and 2 muscle fibers was reduced compared with normal subjects. A decrease in absolute capillary numbers/muscle fiber was also reported. Aerobic enzymes were significantly reduced, and anaerobic enzyme levels seemed to be increased [81]. The muscle atrophy and enzymatic changes were consistent with deconditioning and very similar to what has been described in patients with heart failure. Henriksson et al. [80] also reported muscle atrophy and a reduction in oxidative enzymes in patients with peripheral vascular disease. They also concluded that the low oxidative potential of the gastrocnemuis muscle was probably a consequence of a low level of physical activity [80].

Metabolic studies have demonstrated that the muscle of patients with severe peripheral vascular disease during low-level exercise has a significantly greater depletion of Pcr and a greater decrease in intracellular pH [82]. Recovery of PCr after exercise is also prolonged in these patients, similar to patients with CHF. Interestingly, no significant correlations could be made between claudication pain and intracellular pH and/or the concentration of inorganic phosphorus. Thus, a shift from oxidative to glycolytic metabolism in the calf muscle of patients with peripheral vascular disease was observed, similar to that observed in patients with heart failure.

Ample evidence for endothelial dysfunction in peripheral vascular disease is present as well. The effects of atherosclerosis on the vasoconstrictor responses in the hindlimb resistance vessels of monkeys is one such example. Vasoconstrictor responses to serotonin were increased in the atherosclerotic monkeys compared with the decreased response observed in controls. Also with atherosclerosis, the vasoconstrictor effects of the large-limb arteries to serotonin were markedly enhanced [83]. Studies of normal and arteriosclerotic rabbits have shown that there is an attenuation of endothelium-dependent relaxation of the smooth muscle to EDRF [84]. In these studies, the level of nitric oxide recovered was increased in the athersclerotic rabbits even though the vasorelaxant effect of EDRF was reduced. Furthermore, acetylcholine stimulated an additional release of EDRF, but the biological activity was minimal. This suggested that the formation of nitric oxide was normal in the endothelium of athersclerotic vessels, but the EDRF generated from nitric oxide was impaired.

The technique of transcutaneous oxygen partial pressure (PO_2) measurements enables the evaluation of the microcirculation of the skin. Using this technique, Matsen et al. [85] showed that the transcutaneous PO_2 level was lower in the foot of patients with peripheral arterial disease and that the reduction was correlated to the severity of disease. However, Bongard and Krahenbuhl [86] could not find any realtionship between skin blood flow as evaluated by the xenon-133 clearance method.

Morphological changes of the vasculature are also observed in peripheral vascular disease. As the arterial circulation worsens, the number and definition of capillaries observed microscopically declines [87]. Total skin microcirculation was evaulated by laser Doppler fluxmetry, and the blood flow in the "nutritional" skin capillaries by dynamic capillaroscopy [88] was simulatenously used to study the nailfold microcirculation in the big toe of 12 legs with various degrees of peripheral vascular disease and of 10 healthy subjects. The resting blood flow to the nutritional capillaries was similar in patients and controls, whereas the total skin blood flow was significantly increased in the patients with peripheral vascular disease than the normal subjects. However, post–occlusive reactive hyperemic response was impaired for both nutritional capillary and total skin blood flow in the group with peripheral vascular disease. The ratio between nutritional capillary and total blood flow was also examined in these patients to evaluate how much of the skin blood flow reached the nutritional capillaries in the ischemic area. A marked decrease of this ratio was found in patients with peripheral vascular disease, indicating a maldistribution of blood between non-nutritional and nutritional skin vessels of the ischemic area. This maldistribution of blood flow has also been demonstrated by other groups using strain gauge plethysmography [89,90]. In these studies, a significantly higher resting skin blood flow was present in clinically ischemic feet compared with normal subjects.

The technique of near-infrared spectroscopy has also been applied to the study of skeletal muscle oxygenation in patients with peripheral vascular disease [82]. Patients with intermittent claudication demonstrate an earlier decrease in calf muscle oxygenation compared with normal subjects during treadmill exercise [91]. In patients with chronic subclavian artery occlusion, delayed oxygenation recovery time after forearm occlusion is observed [92].

IV. Pulmonary Adaptation in Congestive Heart Failure

Congestive heart failure affects lung function through several mechanisms, including a chronic increase in pulmonary venous pressure, decrease in cardiac output, and pulmonary parenchyma compression and/or displacement.

Chronic pulmonary venous hypertension develops in patients with heart failure. Engorgement of the entire pulmonary circulation occurs with histological changes observed in the arteries, veins, and capillaries. In the pulmonary arterial circulation, both the media and intima of the vessels are affected. Media changes include hypertrophy from chronic vasoconstriction and peripheral extension of smooth muscle into intra-acinar arterioles, causing the "muscularization" of arterioles. Intimal fibroproliferative changes occur from growth of the smooth muscle cell and myofibroblasts derived from the media. Release of platelet-derived smooth muscle growth factors may stimulate these changes, which may be cellular or fibrotic, eccentric or concentric, laminar or nonlaminar. Microcirculatory histopathological changes also occur and include engorged, distended alveolar capillaries, hemorrhagic alveolar edema, and focal clusters of alveolar hemosiderin-laden macrophages. Accumulation of edema in the pleura and interstitial space leads to lymphatic dilatation. Pulmonary veins also become dilated and develop medial hypertrophy. As medial hypertrophy becomes prominent, a distinct external membrane forms, resulting in "arterialization of veins." Dilatation of interstitial and pleural lymphatics is also observed with focal alveolar hemosiderosis. Bronchial veins also become congested and dilated because of increased flow through bronchopulmonary anastomoses.

Increased capillary pressure results in increased transudation of fluid through the capillary wall to the extravascular space. There is little interstitial space in the alveolus, where fluid can accumulate. Because the pressure in the adjacent tissue surrounding bronchi and vessels is lower than in the alveolar interstitium, flow of fluid is promoted away from the alveolar wall to the peribronchial interstitium. Lung lymphatic vessels are located in this extra-alveolar interstitial space and thereby provide a mechanism for the removal of fluid. As a consequence of this increased peribronchial interstitial pressure from fluid accumulation, the diameter of the small bronchioles are decreased, resulting in increased airflow resistance. Furthermore, reflex bronchoconstriction also occurs from activation of J fibers, small nonmyelinated nerve fibers located in the alveolar interstitium, which are stimulated by the interstitial edema. Pulmonary arteriolar constriction also results from J-fiber activation [93–96].

The histopathological changes that result from pulmonary venous hypertension depend on both the severity and chronicity of the hypertension. Many of the changes are reversible over months to years after the stimulus for the chronic pulmonary venous hypertension is removed. The reversal of these changes has been studied in patients with mitral stenosis who undergo valvuloplasty and/or mitral valve replacement as well as in patients who undergo cardiac transplantation. Levine et al. [97] described progressive improvement in pulmonary vascular resistance after percutaneous mitral valvuloplasty. In these 14 patients with critical mitral stenosis, an immediate decrease in pulmonary vascular resistance was observed, with further improvement in most patients. Similarly, Camara et al. [98] described the long-term results of mitral valve surgery in 88 patients with severe pulmonary hypertension. In 14 patients, right heart catherization was performed a mean of 24 months after surgery. Systolic pulmonary pressure decreased from a preoperative mean of 101 to 41 mm Hg. Thus, although pulmonary hypertension was significantly relieved by surgery, the patients remained with moderate pulmonary hypertension. Persistent pulmonary function abnormalities have been reported in patients after mitral valvotomy despite successfully lowered pulmonary pressures and may, in part, be caused by irreversible histopathological changes. In lung biopsy specimens obtained from 15 adolescents at the time of mitral valvotomy, excessive deposition of connective tissue was observed in alveolar walls [99]. Excessive deposition of connective tissue resulted in compression of adjacent peripheral airways. Intra-acinar vessels also showed severe intimal fibrosis with dense adventitial connective tissue. Thus, although it is presumed that the increase in airways resistance in patients with mitral stenosis is caused by mucosal swelling from bronchial edema, persistent abnormalities may result from the marked increase in connective tissue. The time course for the resolution of pulmonary hypertension in patients with heart failure was assessed in heart transplant recipients. In 24 transplant recipients, mean pulmonary arterial pressure decreased from 38 mm Hg preoperatively to 22 mm Hg at 2 weeks postoperatively. It remained unchanged at 1-year follow-up evaluation. Thus, there is a rapid resolution of moderately elevated pulmonary arterial pressures after cardiac transplantation [100].

A. Pulmonary Function Test Abnormalities in Congestive Heart Failure

A variety of pulmonary function test abnormalities have been described in patients with heart failure, including decreased lung volume, increased resistance in peripheral airways, decreased respiratory muscle strength, and decreased lung compliance. Several investigators have recently reported on pulmonary function test abnormalities in patients with heart failure and have described restrictive abnormalities with or without diffusion defects. They have emphasized that these abnormalities are more marked in patients with a history of smoking [101–106]. The ultimate effect of these pulmonary alterations, i.e., loss of volume, decreased lung compliance, and increased airway resistance, results in an increased work of breathing.

B. Dyspnea

Dyspnea is a frequent symptom in patients with heart failure. During exercise, patients clearly experience a greater sense of dyspnea than do normal subjects at any given workload. In patients with acute heart failure, a rapid increase in pulmonary capillary wedge pressure results in interstitial fluid edema, decreased lung compliance, and activation of juxtapulmonary capillary receptors, leading to tachypnea and breathlessness. In patients with chronic heart failure, the role of increased intrapulmonary vascular pressure is not as clear. Several studies of stable ambulatory patients with heart failure have been unable to demonstrate a correlation between exertional dyspnea and pulmonary capillary wedge pressure at rest and with exercise [107–110]. Moreover, acute therapeutic interventions that suppress the increase in pulmonary pressures during exercise do not acutely alter the ventilatory response [109].

An excessive ventilatory response to exercise is a consistent finding in patients with heart failure. With increasing severity of CHF, the ventilatory response is increased. The increase in ventilation during exercise does not seem to be related to acute increases in intrapulmonary pressure [110]. Moreover, acute therapeutic interventions such as prazosin and dobutamine, which acutely lower resting and exercise pulmonary capillary wedge pressures, do not affect the ventilatory response to exercise. Early lactic acidosis is one proposed mechanism for this, although the immediate onset of the excessive ventilatory response and failure to alter this response with dichloroacetate makes this unlikely [111]. However, the two therapeutic interventions that have been shown to attenuate this excessive ventilatory response, i.e., aerobic training [112–115] and cardiac transplantation [116], both affect either intrinsic skeletal muscle enzymatic activity or oxygen delivery. Thus, in part, the excessive ventilatory response is derived from changes that occur in the skeletal muscles.

Attenuated pulmonary perfusion leading to ventilation–perfusion ($\dot{V}/\dot{Q}$) mismatching is another possible mechanism for the increased ventilatory response [112,117]. Rubin and Brown [117] were the first to suggest that an increased minute ventilation during exercise was closely related to an increase in physiological dead space. More recently, Sullivan et al. [113] measured the hemodynamic, ventilatory, and metabolic responses to maximal upright bicycle exercise in patients with heart failure and in control subjects. Measurement of arterial blood gases and expired gas analysis made possible the examination of the individual components of the modified alveolar gas (Bohr) equation and, therefore, derivation of physiological dead space. These investigators demonstrated that the excess ventilation was almost entirely derived by an increase in dead space ventilation. The ratio of dead space ventilation to tidal volume ($\dot{V}_D/\dot{V}_T$) normally decreases hyperbolically during progressive incremental exercise. Although $\dot{V}_D/\dot{V}_T$ decreased with exercise in patients with heart failure, the $\dot{V}_D/\dot{V}_T$ ratio was increased in patients at rest and during exercise compared with normal subjects. Dead space per breath almost doubled in patients with exercise. Carbon dioxide production, tidal volume, and alveolar ventilation were comparable. The ventilatory equivalent for carbon dioxide consumption ($\dot{V}_E/\dot{V}_{CO_2}$) was increased at rest and throughout exercise in patients with heart failure and was not related to peak pulmonary capillary wedge pressure, pulmonary artery pressure, arterial lactate, or tidal volume. However, $\dot{V}_E/\dot{V}_{CO_2}$ was correlated with the maximal increase in dead space. Arterial carbon dioxide partial pressure (P_{CO_2}) was not different in cardiac or control subjects at any level of exercise, indicating that there was no alteration in the arterial P_{CO_2} set point.

A potential mechanism for the increase in physiological dead space ventilation in these patients is pulmonary hypoperfusion with resultant $\dot{V}/\dot{Q}$ mismatching. Thus, regional ventilation and perfusion may occur in the lower lungs and result in excess physiological dead space ventilation in patients with severe heart failure [118]. However, recent investigators have demonstrated both an improved and worsened $\dot{V}/\dot{Q}$ mismatch during exercise in patients with heart failure [119].

Although ventilation during exercise is primarily driven by carbon dioxide production, at end exercise a steeper increase in $\dot{V}_E/\dot{V}_{CO_2}$ relation is observed. This abrupt change in slope presumably develops as a response to the development of lactic acidosis. However, other non–carbon dioxide stimuli such as muscle ergoreflexes, potassium, or central command may also be contributing to the uncoupling of $\dot{V}_E$ and $\dot{V}_{CO_2}$ [120]. Both animal and human studies suggest that exercise hyperkalemia may contribute to the control of breathing during exercise [120]. However, a recent study that investigated the effect of aerobic training on exercise induced hyperkalemia in patients with chronic heart failure failed to demonstrate a significant improvement in ventilation during submaximal exercise despite improved potassium homeostasis [121].

Ergoreceptors are unmyelinated and small myelinated afferents in muscle sensitive to metabolic changes related to skeletal muscle work. They have been shown to be responsible for the early circulatory response to exercise, including activation of the sympathetic vasoconstrictor drive. Sterns et al. [122] have demonstrated that the sympathetic responses to exercise generated by muscle metaboreceptors are impaired in CHF. Muscle sympathetic nerve activity of the peroneal nerve was measured in nine subjects with heart failure and eight age-matched control subjects during static exercise for 2 minutes and during a period of post–hand-grip regional circulatory arrest. Circulatory occlusion isolates the metaboreceptor contribution to sympathetic nervous system responses. Muscle sympathetic nerve activity was similar during static exercise for the two groups, whereas there was a marked attenuation in muscle sympathetic activity in the CHF group during post–hand-grip circulatory arrest (15% increase in the heart failure group vs. 57% increase in the control subjects). Recently, the ventilatory and hemodynamic response to dynamic hand grip during a 3-minute period of circulatory occlusion was compared in heart failure and normal subjects before and after a training regimen [123]. Patients showed an overactivation compared with normal subjects, i.e., a 87% versus 55% increase in minute ventilation, 100% versus 54% increase in diastolic pressure, and an 108% versus 49% increase in leg vascular resistance. Aerobic training reduced the ergoreflex contribution in the CHF subjects. This attenuation may be caused by a lessening of intramuscular pH with training.

C. Respiratory Muscle Perfusion

The effect of heart failure on respiratory muscle perfusion has not been well studied. The diaphragm, the major respiratory muscle, has a complex and generous blood supply provided by the internal mammary, intercostal, and phrenic arteries and the costophrenic arcades. Because of its rich vascularization, the diaphragm is thought to never become ischemic. Most animal studies of CHF that look specifically at diaphragmatic perfusion support this premise [124–126]. However, the accessory muscles of respiration are not endowed with such a generous blood supply. Serratus anterior muscle oxygenation during maximal bicycle exercise was compared by near-infrared spectroscopy in 10 patients with heart failure and in seven age-matched normal subjects [127]. Minimal change in absorption at 760 to 800 nm absorption occurred in normal subjects during exercise, whereas patients with heart failure showed progressive respiratory muscle deoxygenation throughout exercise. This demonstrated that accessory respiratory muscle deoxygenation occurs during exercise in patients with heart failure and suggests that respiratory muscle ischemia may be occurring.

Subjects with mitral stenosis also have an increased work of breathing and limited capacity to increase perfusion to the respiratory muscles. Similar to patients with heart failure, patients with mitral stenosis demonstrated accessory respiratory muscle deoxygenation during bicycle exercise [128]. Monitoring of both accessory respiratory and leg muscle oxygenation with near-infrared spectroscopy during bicycle exercise before, 48 hours, and 3 months after valvuloplasty in 11 patients with mitral stenosis showed a decrease in accessory respiratory muscle deoxygenation 48 hours after valvuloplasty, whereas leg muscle oxygenation and maximal exercise performance remained unaltered. Thus, the acute symptomatic improvement experienced by these patients seemed to be a result of better pulmonary perfusion via an improved cardiac output response to exercise.

Changes in respiratory muscle deoxygenation has been shown to correlate with ratings of perceived dyspnea in patients with heart failure [129]. After cardiac transplantation, the sensation of dyspnea is greatly ameliorated. However, measurement of the tension index remains markedly abnormal after heart transplantation both at rest and during exercise. Thus, the sensation of dyspnea does not seem to be determined by the actual work performed. In posttransplant patients, accessory respiration muscle deoxygenation using near-infrared spectroscopy during exercise was no longer detected. This suggests that the relief of exertional dyspnea is achieved by other mechanisms, such as improved respiratory muscle perfusion. Work of breathing probably remains elevated because of chronic fibrotic changes in the lung that do not resolve after transplant.

D. Airflow Obstruction

Pulmonary function test abnormalities in patients with decompensated heart failure suggest the presence of airflow obstruction. Cabanes et al. [130] described bronchial hyperresponsiveness in patients with severely impaired left ventricular function after inhalation of the cholinergic agonist methacholine. Inhalation of the vasoconstrictive α-adrenergic agonist methoxamine prevented the methacholine-induced bronchial obstruction, suggesting that bronchial edema was partially causative for the bronchial hyperreactivity. In a subsequent study, Cabanes et al. [131] went on to demonstrate significant improvement in submaximal and maximal exercise performance after inhalation of methoxamine in patients with heart failure limited by dyspnea. In this study, Cabanes et al. performed two exercise protocols with and without pretreatment with methoxamime. In both the submaximal and maximal exercise protocols, they were able to demonstrate a significant improvement in exercise duration with methoxamine. These findings suggest a limitation to airflow during exercise in patients with heart failure limited by dyspnea.

Other investigators have examined agents such as ipratropium bromide and salbutamol on pulmonary pressures and pulmonary function tests in patients with heart failure. Ipratropium is an inhaled anticholingeric bronchodilator. Kindman et al. [132] studied the acute effects of this agent in 29 patients awaiting cardiac transplantation. Significant increases in forced expiratory volume in 1 second, forced expiratory flow (midexpiratory phase), and maximum voluntary ventilation were demonstrated. Uren et al. [133] reported significant improvement in bronchodilation at rest after inhalation of both the β-2 agonist salbutamol and ipratropium. Small but significant increases in $\dot{V}O_{2max}$ after inhalation of both ipratropium and salbutamol versus placebo were also described [133]. These findings suggest that bronchoconstriction contributes to exercise limitation in patients with heart failure.

E. Respiratory Muscle Function

Recent studies have described an increase in diaphragmatic work in patients with heart failure. The tension time index is the product of the force of contraction and duration of contraction per breath. This value gives the work or $\dot{V}O_2$ of the diaphragm/breath. In patients with heart failure, this is significantly elevated at rest and throughout exercise, with levels at peak exercise approaching the fatigue threshold [129]. However, measurement of maximal transdiaphragmatic pressure before and after exercise using supramaximal bilateral transcutaneous phrenic nerve stimulation in normal subjects and in those with heart failure did not demonstrate any evidence of low-frequency respiratory muscle fatigue. Maximal transdiaphragmatic pressure was derived before and after exercise from analysis of 6 to 12 twitches obtained at functional residual capacity using the twitch interpolation technique of Bigland-Ritchie.

Some investigators have demonstrated reduced resting maximal inspiratory and expiratory mouth pressures consistent with respiratory muscle weakness. Hammond et al. [134] measured maximal inspiratory and expiratory mouth pressure and maximal hand-grip force in 16 patients with CHF and in 18 normal subjects. Maximal respiratory pressures were significantly reduced. Hand-grip force was less dramatically reduced, suggesting greater respiratory muscle weakness [134].

Further evidence that respiratory muscle weakness and airflow obstruction may limit the maximal exercise capacity of patients with heart failure is derived from an exercise study whereby the work of breathing was acutely reduced in patients with CHF by inhalation of a gas mixture lighter than air and with greater laminar flow, i.e., helium–oxygen mixture [135]. Fifteen patients with CHF and nine age-matched normal subjects in a single, blind, randomized manner underwent two maximal cardiopulmonary exercise tests, inhaling room air and/or a 79% helium/21% oxygen mixture. In normal subjects, there was no significant difference in peak oxygen uptake, exercise duration, or peak minute. In contrast, the patients with CHF exercised an average of 146 seconds longer with the helium mixture.

Similar to normal subjects, their peak $\dot{V}O_2$ and peak minute ventilation were unchanged. This study demonstrated that in patients with CHF, respiratory muscle work and/or airflow obstruction contributes to limiting exercise performance.

F. Respiratory Muscle Endurance

As respiratory muscle strength tends to be reduced, the work of breathing increased, and respiratory muscle perfusion inadequate, it is not surprising that the endurance of these muscles would be compromised. Respiratory muscle endurance can be assessed by measuring maximal sustainable ventilatory capacity using progressive isocapnic hyperpnea [136]. Maximal sustainable ventilatory capacity is determined using a rebreathing circuit. Airflow through the circuit is adjusted using a graduated flowmeter. Airflow enters a 5-L anesthesia bag, which is then passed into a 6-L mixing chamber and then to the patient via a two-way nonrebreathing Hans Rudolph valve. The subject is instructed to adjust his or her breathing so that the 5-L bag remains collapsed. Exhaled air is then recirculated via a variable flow carbon dioxide scrubber circuit. Inspiratory and expiratory flow rates are monitored with pneumotachographs interfaced in the airflow circuit. Isocapnia and normoxia were maintained throughout the test by the addition of carbon dioxide or oxygen as needed. Both maximal voluntary ventilation and maximal sustainable ventilatory capacity were significantly reduced in patients with heart failure compared with normal subjects, suggesting that respiratory muscle endurance is reduced in these patients. Maximal sustainable ventilatory capacity averaged only 50 L/min versus 90 L/min in normal subjects. Interestingly, the maximal sustainable ventilatory capacity in both the normal subjects and those with heart failure paralleled peak ventilation achieved during maximal exercise testing.

Selective respiratory muscle training [137] in patients with heart failure improved respiratory muscle endurance and strength. More importantly, it enhanced both submaximal and maximal exercise capacity in these patients, again suggesting a pulmonary limitation to maximal exercise performance. This study is discussed in greater detail in Section V.

G. Summary

In final analysis, what is the limiting factor for maximal exercise capacity in patients with heart failure? There is no simple answer. Rather than grouping patients into one pattern, there are probably subgroups that may be primarily limited by one factor more than another. Some patients may primarily be limited by a reduced cardiac output response, and in other subgroups, pulmonary factors or muscle deconditioning may be predominant. It is important to emphasize that the exercise response of a patient with heart failure needs careful analysis to determine which factor may constitute the major limitation. Then, appropriate therapeutic interventions can be tailored to the patient to enhance their exercise performance. For example, patients who seemed limited by intrinsic skeletal muscle changes will benefit more from aerobic training than from drugs that increase blood flow. Another element that impacts on the exercise response of these patients is the chronicity of their disease. For example, in an individual with severe heart failure from a recent extensive myocardial infarction, it is unlikely that exercise will be limited by vascular or skeletal muscle changes that occur only after a period of significant disability.

In summary, exercise capacity in patients with heart failure is limited not only by changes that affect the ability to increase cardiac output, but also by changes that occur in the blood vessels, the muscles, and the lungs as a consequence of their disease.

V. Exercise Training in Congestive Heart Failure

Exercise training has long been advocated as a means to delay aging and decrease cardiovascular mortality in normal subjects. The evidence to support either one of these outcomes in normal or disease states is lacking. However, aerobic training can confer a multitude of significant hemodynamic, morphological, and metabolic changes in humans.

Many of the central and peripheral changes induced by aerobic training may have a marked therapeutic effect in patients with heart failure. Potential advantages of training in heart failure include central hemodynamic changes such as an increase in stroke volume, a potential increase in contractility, alteration of autonomic tone with a decrease in sympathetic stimulation, an improvement in endothelial and vascular function with a decrease in peripheral vascular resistance, muscle enzymatic changes with an increased oxidative capacity, and decrease in lactate production.

There is a growing literature on the benefits of aerobic training in these patients. However, many questions remain, such as which mode of training is optional for these patients and the effect of training on long-term morbidity and mortality.

Initial studies by Letac et al. [138], Lee et al. [139], Williams et al. [140], and Cohn et al. [141] established the safety of training in this population. They also demonstrated that patients with reduced left ventricular function can demonstrate the hallmarks of training, i.e., improvement in work capacity with a concomitant decrease in heart rate. These studies did not investigate the physiological mechanisms underlying the improved work state.

Using an ischemic rat model of heart failure, Musch et al. [142] studied the effects of endurance training. Fifty rats underwent thoracotomy. A sham procedure was performed in 25 animals. In the remaining 25 rats, the left anterior descending artery was ligated. These groups were then randomized to sedentary versus trained protocol. The training protocol consisted of 60-minute sessions of treadmill exercise 5 days a week for 10–12 weeks. Parameters studied included infarct size, $\dot{V}O_2$, heart rate and blood pressure response, rest and exercise hemodynamic measurements, succinate dehydrogenase activity in the soleus and plantaris muscle, lactate levels, and regional perfusion of the skeletal muscle, renal and splanchnic beds. After the training program in the rats with heart failure, $\dot{V}O_2$ was higher, succinate dehydrogenase activity increased, and lactate levels decreased during submaximal exercise. No differences were observed in regional perfusion or in hemodynamic measurements. In this rat model of heart failure, all derived benefits were from peripheral mechanisms.

Recent studies by Sullivan et al. [143], Coats et al. [144], Hambrecht et al. [145] and Hornig et al. [146] have attempted to characterize the physiological mechanisms for the clinical improvement in patients with heart failure. Sullivan et al. studied 12 patients with heart failure with a mean $\dot{V}O_2$ of 16.3 mL/kg/min and an ejection fraction 21% [143]. Aerobic training was performed 3–5 hours a week for 6 months. Hemodynamic measurements, skeletal muscle perfusion, $\dot{V}O_2$, and left ventricular ejection fraction were measured before and after training. With training, peak $\dot{V}O_2$ increased 23% from 16.8 to 20.6 mL/kg/min. Peak cardiac output, peak arterial-venous oxygen difference (A-$\dot{V}O_2$), and peak leg blood flow also significantly increased. Ejection fraction was unchanged. Training decreased leg lactate production. Leg blood flow during submaximal exercise did not increase, suggesting that the major benefit derived from training was via increased oxygen extraction by the skeletal muscles. The largest proportion of the increase in $\dot{V}O_2$ was derived from peripheral adaptation with a possible small central contribution.

Coats et al. [144] performed a controlled crossover home-based trial of 8 weeks of exercise training in 17 patients with stable, moderate to severe CHF. Peak $\dot{V}O_2$ increased from 13.2 to 15.6 mL/kg/min. He also studied the effect of training on autonomic tone by measuring heart rate variability and radiolabeled norepinephrine spillover. After training, these measurements demonstrated a shift from sympathetic to enhanced vagal activity. Other investigators have demonstrated a decrease in serum catecholamine levels both at rest and during submaximal exercise in these patients after aerobic training [145,147].

Two recent studies using selective arm training [148,149] and another study [150] using aerobic exercise have demonstrated an improvement but not normalization in the metabolic abnormalities observed with exercise in patients with heart failure. Percutaneous muscle biopsy specimens of the vastus lateralis were obtained before and after 6 months of aerobic training in 22 patients. Aerobic training increased the volume density of mitochondria. Staining for cytochrome c oxidase–positive mitochondria was used as a qualitative index of oxidative enzyme activity in skeletal muscle. This measurement was also significantly increased with training. Thus, aerobic training in patients with heart failure results in improved skeletal muscle oxidative function [145].

The effect of aerobic training on endothelial function has also recently been studied in this patient population [146]. Isolated forearm training using hand-grip exercise was performed for 4 weeks in 12 patients with chronic heart failure. Flow-dependent dilatation of the radial artery was assessed using a high-resolution ultrasound system. Measurements were performed at rest, during reactive hyperemia, during an intra-arterial infusion of sodium nitroprusside, an endothelial independent vasodilator, and after an intra-arterial infusion of N-monomethyl-L-arginine, an inhibitor of endothelial synthesis and release of nitric oxide. The impaired flow-dependent dilatation observed in the patients with heart failure was improved by training. N-monomethyl-L-arginine attenuated this improvement implying that the normalization of flow-dependent dilatation with training resulted from enhanced endothelial release of nitric oxide. This is an important finding in that it may indicate that, with training, there is an improvement in skeletal muscle perfusion. In addition, improvement in the endothelial function of large conduit vessels may decrease impedance to the failing left ventricle and thus improve left ventricular ejection fraction. At this point, other investigators have demonstrated increases in skeletal muscle leg perfusion and cardiac output at maximal but not during submaximal activity.

Many questions remain regarding the value of exercise training in these patients. Indeed, it is not clear even what mode of training would be most advantageous. A study by Jugdutt et al. [147] suggested that a 12-week exercise training program in patients after extensive anterior infarctions can further distort left ventricular shape, increase infarct expansion, reduce scar thickness, and reduce ejection fraction. Endurance training in rats after large myocardial infarctions resulted in reduced survival and left ventricular dilatation [148]. The recent "exercise in anterior myocardial infarction" trial by Italian investigators randomized 93 patients within 2 months of their anterior wall myocardial infarction to a 6-month exercise training versus sedentary protocol [149]. Echocardiographic indices of ventricular size and function were obtained before and at the completion of the study. In this study, where the majority of the patients had ejection fractions greater than 40%, exercise training did not produce greater ventricular dilatation or reduction in ejection fraction compared with the control group. In a subgroup analysis including 30 patients with ejection fractions less than 40%, no echocardiographic evidence of deterioration of left ventricular function was observed. However, in this group, mean left ventricular ejection fraction was still high, averaging 35%, and only a small percent of patients were maintained on angiotensin-converting enzyme inhibitors. The question as to the effect of prolonged exercise training on cardiac remodeling in this subcategory deserves further investigation.

The response to aerobic training is variable. Compliance with the training regimen is the most frequently sited marker to predict success. However, recent studies suggest that the initial cardiac output response to maximal exercise may determine the response to exercise training. Wilson et al. [150] studied 32 patients with heart failure with hemodynamic measurements during treadmill exercise before enrollment in a rehabilitation program. Using the formula $Co = 0.5 \dot{V}O_2 + 3$, he divided the patients into two groups: normal and reduced cardiac output response to exercise [150]. Twenty-one of the 32 patients had a "normal" cardiac output response to exercise. All of these patients tolerated training, and nine patients achieved therapeutic benefit with training defined as a more than 10% increase in both peak $\dot{V}O_2$ and anaerobic threshold. In contrast, the patients with a reduced cardiac output response had a high drop out rate during training because of exhaustion, and only one patient benefited from training. Although interesting, this conclusion is based on a derived formula that is flawed, as previously discussed. Moreover, the findings of this study are not consistent with the findings of most clinicians and/or prior referenced studies.

To circumvent the potential deleterious effect on high-intensity aerobic training, a few studies have focused on either low-intensity or specific muscle training. Studies that focus on small muscle mass training, which does not stress the cardiovascular system, may have the added advantage of inducing peripheral skeletal muscle changes without adverse cardiac effects.

Belardinelli et al. [151] investigated the value of low-intensity exercise training in 27 patients with chronic heart failure randomized to training versus control groups. The exercise prescription in this study called for 3 weekly training sessions of bicycle exercise at 40% of peak $\dot{V}O_2$ for 8 weeks. Peak $\dot{V}O_2$, serum catecholamines, lactate, and vastus lateralis skeletal muscle biopsies were performed before and after training. Peak $\dot{V}O_2$ increased and serum lactate and catecholamine levels decreased during submaximal exercise, and the volume density of mitochondria were enhanced at the conclusion of the study only in the trained group. Similarly, Demopoulos et al. [152] demonstrated the value of low-intensity training in patients with severe CHF. Using a semirecumbent stationary bicycle, patients trained below 50% of peak $\dot{V}O_2$ 1 hour per day, four times per week for 3 months. Peak $\dot{V}O_2$ increased from 11.5 to 15 mL/kg/min. Peak reactive hyperemia of the calf, but not the forearm muscle increased with training. In this study, left ventricular diastolic wall stress was measured during bicycle exercise at low ($< 50\%$) and more conventional training workloads (70–80% peak $\dot{V}O_2$). Diastolic wall stress was significantly reduced at the lower than at the conventional training rates in these patients.

We performed selective respiratory muscle training in 14 patients with class II–IV congestive heart failure [153]. Six patients dropped out early in the training period and formed a comparison group. Respiratory muscle strength, respiratory muscle endurance, and submaximal and maximal exercise capacity were measured before and after 3 months of training. The training protocol combined both endurance and strength training. Submaximal and maximal exercise performance was increased in the trained group but not in the comparison group. Perceived dyspnea during submaximal exercise was also significantly reduced with selective respiratory muscle training.

In summary, exercise training seems to have benefits for individuals with CHF, but the optimal regimen and the long-term effects of such programs remain to be resolved. Future studies investigating the clinical benefit of low-intensity exercise training and/or regional muscle group training in patients with heart failure seem warranted.

References

1. Zelis R, Mason DT, Braunwald E. A comparison of peripheral resistance vessels in normal subjects and in patients with congestive heart failure. J Clin Invest 1968; 47:960–961.
2. Strobeck JE, Sonnenblick EH. Pathophysiology of heart failure: deficiency in cardiac contraction. In: Cohn JN, ed. Drug Treatment of Heart Failure. Seacaucus: Advanced Therapeutics Communications International, 1988, pp 13–48.
3. Spann JF Jr., Bucino RA, Sonnenblick EH, Braunwald E. Contractile state of cardiac muscle obtained from cats with experimentally produced ventricular hypertrophy and heart failure. Circ Res 1967; 21:341–354.
4. Span JF Jr., Covell JW, Eckberg DL, Ross J Jr., Braunwald E. Contractile performance of the hypertrophied and chronically failing cat ventricle. Am J Physiol 1972; 223:1150–1155
5. Cooper G IV, Puga F, Zujko KJ, Harrison CE, Coleman HN 3d. Normal myocardial function and energetics in volume-overload hypertrophy in the cat. Circ Res 1973; 32:140–148.
6. Neubauer S, Horn M, Naumann A, Tian R, Hu K, Laser M, Friedrich J, Gaudron P, Schnackerz K, Ingwall JS. Impairment of energy metabolism in intact myocardium of rat hearts with chronic myocardila infarction. J Clin Invest 1995; 95:1092–1100.
7. Nascimben L, Friedrich J, Liao R, Pauletto P, Pessina AC, Ingwall JS. Enalapril treatment increases cardiac performance and energy reserve via the creatine kinase reaction in myocardium of Syrian myopathic hamsters with advanced heart failure. Circulation 1995; 91:1824–1833.
8. Nascimben L, Pauletto P, Pessina AC, Reis I, Ingwall JS. Decreased energy reserve may cause pump failure in human dilated cardiomyopathy. Circulation 1991; 84:II–563.
9. Van der Laarse A, Hollaar L, Kor SW, Van den Eijnde S, Souverijn JH, Hedenmaeker PJ, Bruschke AV. Myocardial creatine kinase-MB concentration in normal and explanted human hearts with acute myocardial infarction. Clin Physiol Biochem 1992; 9:11–17.
10. Ingwall JS. Is the failing myocardium energy starved? Heart Failure 1994; 3:128–136.
11. Conway MA, Allis J, Ouwerkerk R, Niioka T, Rajagopauen B, Radda GK. Detection of low phosphocreatine to ATP ratio in failing hypertrophied human myocardium by ^{31}P magnetic resonance spectroscopy. Lancet 1991; 338:973–976.
12. Hardy CJ, Weiss RG, Bottomley PA, Gertenblith G. Altered myocardial high-energy phosphate metabolites in patients with dilated cardiomyopathy. Am Heart J 1991; 122:795–801.
13. Ingwall JS. ATP synthesis in the normal and failing heart. In: Poole-Wilson PA, Colucci WS, Massie BM, Chatterjee K, Coats AJS, eds. Heart Failure. New York: Churchill Livingstone, 1997, pp 75–85.
14. Thomas JA, Marks BH. Plasma norepinephrine in congestive heart failure. Am J Cardiol 1978; 41:233–243.
15. Levine TB, Francis GS, Goldsmith SR, Simon AB, Cohn JN. Activity of the sympathetic nervous system and renin-angiotensin system assessed by plasma hormone

levels and their relation to hemodynamic abnormalities in congestive heart failure. Am J Cardiol 1982; 49:1659–1666.
16. Francis GS, Benedict C, Johnstone EE, Kirlin PC, Nicklas J, Liang CS, Kubo SH, Rudin-Toretsky E, Yusef S. Comparison of neuroendocrine activation in patients in patients with left ventricular dysfunction with and without congestive heart failure: a substudy of the studies of left ventricular dysfunction (SOLVD). Circulation 1990; 82:1724–1729.
17. Bristow MR, Ginsberg R, Fowler M, Minobe W, Rasmussen R, Zera P, Menlove R, Shah P, Jamieson S, Stinson EB. Beta$_1$ and beta$_2$ adrenergic receptor subtype populations in normal and failing human ventricular myocardium. Circ Res 1986; 59:297–309.
18. Bristow MR, Anderson FL, Port JD, Skerl L, Hershberger RE, Larrabee P, O'Connell JB, Renlund DG, Volkman K, Murray J, Feldman AM. Differences in beta-adrenergic neuroeffector mechanisms in ischemic versus idiopathic dilated cardiomyopathy. Circulation 1991; 84:1024–1039.
19. Ungerer M, Bohm M, Elce S, Erdmann E, Lohse MJ. Altered expression of beta-adrenergic receptor kinase and beta$_1$ adrenergic recptors in the failing human heart. Circulation 1993; 87:454–463.
20. Feldman AM, Gates AE, Veazey WB, Hershberger RE, Bristow MR, Baughman KL, Baumgartner WA, Van Dop C. Increase of the M_r 40,000 pertussis toxin substrate (G protein) in the failing human heart. J Clin Invest 1988; 82:189–197.
21. Hare JM, Loh E, Creager MA, Colucci WS. Nitric oxide inhibits the positive iontropic response to beta-adrenergic stimulation in humans with left ventricular dysfunction. Circulation 1995; 92:2198–2203.
22. Munzel T, Kurz S, Holtz J, Busse R, Steinhaur H, Just H, Drexler H. Neurohormonal inhibition and hemodynamic unloading during prolonged inhibition of ANF degradation in patients with severe chronic heart failure. Circulation 1992; 86:1089–1098.
23. Wasserman K, Hansen J, Sue D, Whipp B. Principles of Exercise Testing and Interpretation. Philadelphia: Lea and Febiger, 1987, pp 1–45.
24. Weber K, Janicki J. Cardiopulmonary Exercise Testing: Physiologic Principles and Clinical Applications. Philadelphia: WB Saunders, 1986.
25. Weber K, Kinasewitz G, Janicki J, Fishman A. Oxygen utilization and ventilation during exercise in patients with chronic cardiac failure. Circulation 1982; 65:1213–1223.
26. Mancini D, Katz S, Donchez L, Aaronson K. Coupling of hemodynamic measurements with oxygen consumption during exercise does not improve risk stratification in patients with heart failure. Circulation 1996; 94:2492–2496.
27. Wilson J, Rayos G, Yeoh TK, Gothard P. Dissociation between peak exercise oxygen consumption and hemodynamic dysfunction in potential heart transplant candidates. J Am Coll Cardiol 1995; 26:429–435.
28. Wilson J, Rayos G, Yeoh TK, Gothard P, Bak K. Dissociation between exertional symptoms and circulatory function in patients with heart failure. Circulation 1995; 92:47–53.
29. Higginbotham M, Morris K, Williams R, McHale P, Coleman R, Cobb F. Regulation of stroke volume during submaximal and maximal upright exercise in normal man. Circ Res 1986; 58(2):281–291.

30. Maskin C, Forman R, Sonnenblick E, LeJemtel T: Failure of dobutamine to increase exercise capacity despite hemodynamic improvement in severe chronic heart failure. Am J Cardiol 1983; 51:177–182.
31. Wilson J, Martin J, Schwartz D, Ferraro N: Exercise tolerance in patients with heart failure: role of impaired nutritive flow to skeletal muscle. Circulation 1984; 69:1079–1087.
32. Kaiser L, Spickard RC, Olivier NB. Heart failure depresses endothelium-dependent responses in canine femoral artery. Am J Physiol 1989; 256:H962–H967.
33. Yang BC, Khan S, Mehta JL. Blockade of platlet-mediated relaxation in rat aortic rings exposed to xanthine-xanthine oxidase. Am J Physiol 1994; 266:H2212–H2219.
34. Kubo SH, Rector TS, Bank AJ, Williams RE, Heifetz SM. Endothelium-dependent vasodilation is attenuated in patients with heart failure. Circulation 1991; 84:1589–1596.
35. Katz SD, Biasucci L, Sabba C, Strom JA, Jondeau G, Galavo M, Solomon S, Nikolic SD, Forman R, LeJemtel TH. Impaired endothelium-mediated vasodilation in the peripheral vasculature of patients with congestive heart failure. J Am Coll Cardiol 1992; 19:918–925.
36. Moncada S, Radomski MW, Palmer RMJ. Endotthelium-derived relaxing factor: identification as nitric oxide and role in the control of vascular tone and platelet function. Biochem Pharmacol 1988; 37:2495–2501.
37. Koller A, Sun D, Huang A, Kaley G. Corelease of nitric oxide and prostaglandins mediates flow-dependent dilation of rat gracilis muscle arterioles. Am J Physiol 1994; 267:H326–H332.
38. Koller A, Kaley G. Endothelial regulation of wall shear stress and blood flow in skeletal muscle microcirculation. Am J Physiol 1991; 260:H862–H868.
39. Katz SD, Rao R, Berman JW, Schwarz M, Demopoulos L, Bijou R, LeJemtel TH. Pathophysiological correlates of increased serum tumor necrosis factor in patients with congestive heart failure: relation to nitric oxide-dependent vasodilation in the forearm circulation. Circulation 1994; 90:12–16
40. Teerlink JR, Clozel M, Fischli W, Clozel J-P. Temporal evolution of endothelial dysfunction in a rat model of chronic heart failure. J Am Coll Cardiol 1993; 22:615–620.
41. Zelis R, Mason D, Braunwald E, Winterhalter M, King C. A comparison of the effects of vasodilator stimuli on peripheral resistance vessels in normal subjects and in patients with congestive heart failure. J Clin Invest 1968; 47:960–970.
42. Zelis R, Delea C, Coleman H, Mason D. Arterial sodium content in experimental congestive heart failure. Circulation 1970; 61:213–216.
43. Longhurst J, Gifford W, Zelis R. Impaired forearm oxygen consumption during static exercise in patients with congestive heart failure. Circulation 1976; 54:477–480.
44. LeJemtel TH, Maskin CS, Lucido D, Chadwick BJ. Failure to augment maximal limb blood flow in response to one-leg versus two-leg exercise in patients with severe heart failure. Circulation 1986; 74:245–251.
45. Marshall JM. Skeletal muscle vasculature and systemic hypoxia. News in Physiological Sciences 1995; 10:274–280.
46. Jondeau G, Katz SD, Toussaint J-F, Dobourg O, Monrad ES, Bourdarias JP, LeJemtel TH. Regional specificity of peak hyperemic responses in patients with conges-

tive heart failure: correlation with peak aerobic capacity. J Am Coll Cardiol 1993; 22:1399–1402.
47. Drexler H, Hayoz D, Munzel T, Hornig B, Just H, Brunner HR, Zelis R. Endothelial function in chronic heart failure. Am J Cardiol 1991; 69:1596–1601.
48. Wilson JR, Fink L, Maris J, Ferraro N, Power-Vanwart J, Eleff S, Chance B: Evaluation of energy metabolism in skeletal muscle of patients with heart failure with gated phosphorus-31 nuclear magnetic resonance. Circulation 1985; 71:57–62.
49. Weiner DH, Fink LI, Maris J, Jones RA, Chance B, Wilson JR. Abnormal skeletal muscle bioenergetics during exercise in patients with heart failure: role of reduced muscle blood flow. Circulation 1986; 73:1127–1136.
50. Mancini DM, Ferraro N, Tuchler M, Chance B, Wilson JR. Calf muscle metabolism during leg exercise in patients with heart failure: A ^{31}P NMR study. Am J Cardiol 1988; 62:1234–1240.
51. Mancini DM, Coyle E, Coggan A, Beltz J, Ferraro N, Montain S, Wilson JR. Contribution of intrinsic skeletal muscle changes to ^{31}P NMR skeletal muscle metabolic abnormalities in patients with heart failure. Circulation 1989; 80:1338–1346.
52. Mancini DM, Reichek N, Chance B, Lenkinski R, Mullen J, Wilson JR. Contribution of skeletal muscle atrophy to exercise intolerance and altered muscle metabolism in heart failure. Circulation 1992; 85:1364–1373.
53. Massie B, Conway M, Yonge R, Frostick S, Ledingham J, Sleight P, Radda G, Rajagopalan B. Skeletal muscle metabolism in patients with congestive heart failure: relation to clinical severity and blood flow. Circulation 1987; 76:1009–1019.
54. Massie B, Conway M, Rajagopalan B, Yonge R, Frostick S, Ledingham J, Sleight P, Radda G. Skeletal muscle metabolism during exercise under ischemic conditions in congestive heart failure: evidence for abnormalities unrelated to blood flow. Circulation 1989; 78:320–326.
55. Mancini D, Wilson JR, Bolinger L, Li H, Kendrick K, Chance B, Leigh JS. In vivo magnetic resonance spectroscopy measurement of deoxymyoglobin during exercise in patients with heart failure: demonstration of abnormal muscle metabolism despite adequate oxygenation. Circulation 1994; 90:500–508.
56. Weiner D, Fink L, Maris J, Jones R, Chance B, Wilson JR. Abnormal skeletal muscle bioenergetics during exercise in patients with heart failure: role of reduced muscle blood flow. Circulation 1986; 73:1127–1136.
57. Massie B, Conway M, Rajagopalan B, Yonge R, Frostick S, Ledingham J, Sleight P, Radda G. Skeletal muscle metabolism during exercise under ischemic conditions in congestive heart failure: evidence for abnormalities unrelated to blood flow. Circulation 1988; 78:320–326.
58. Wittenberg B, Wittenberg J. Role of myoglobin in the oxygen supply to red skeletal muscle. J Biol Chem 1975; 250:9038-9043.
59. Cole R. Myoglobin function in exercising skeletal muscle. Science 1982; 216:523–525.
60. Chance B. Metabolic heterogeneities in rapidly metabolizing tissues. J Appl Cardioil 1989; 4:207–221.
61. Wasserman K, Hansen J, Sue D, Whipp B. Principles of exercise testing and interpretation. Philadelphia: Lea & Febiger, 1987, pp 3–22.
62. Connett R, Gayeski T, Honig C. Lactate accumulation in fully aerobic working dog gracilis muscle. Am J Physiol 1984; 246:H120–H128.

63. Lipkin D, Jones D, Round J, Poole-Wilson P. Abnormalities of skeletal muscle in patients with chronic heart failure. Int J Cardiol 1988; 18:187–195.
64. Mancini DM, Coyle E, Coggan A, Beltz J, Ferraro N, Montain S, Wilson JR. Contribution of intrinsic skeletal muscle changes to ^{31}P NMR skeletal muscle metabolic abnormalities in patients with heart failure. Circulation 1989; 80:1338–1346.
65. Sullivan M, Green H, Cobb F. Skeletal muscle biochemistry and histology in ambulatory patients with long-term heart failure. Circulation 1990; 81:518–527.
66. Drexler H, Riede U, Munzel T, Konig H, Funke E, Just H. Alterations of skeletal muscle in chronic heart failure. Circulation 1992; 85:1751–1759.
67. Mancini DM, Walter G, Reichek N, Lenkinski R, McCully KK, Mullen JL, Wilson JR. Contribution of skeletal muscle atrophy to exercise intolerance and altered muscle metabolism in heart failure. Circulation 1992; 85:1364–1373.
68. Miyagi K, Asanol H, Ishizak S, Kameyama T, Sassayama S. Loss of skeletal muscle mass is a major determinant of exercise tolerance in chronic heart failure. Abstract. Circulation 1991; 84(Suppl II):74.
69. Buller N, Jones D, Poole-Wilson P. Direct measurement of skeletal muscle fatigue in patients with chronic heart failure. Br Heart J 1991; 65:20–24.
70. Minotti J, Pillay P, Oka R, Wells L, Christoph I, Massie BM. Skeletal muscle size: relationship to muscle function in heart failure. J Appl Physiol 1993; 75:373–381.
71. Jondeau G, Katz S, Zohman L, Goldberger M, McCarthy M, Bourdarias JP, LeJemtel TH. Active skeletal muscle mass and cardiopulmonary reserve: failure to attain peak aerobic capacity during maximal bicycle exercise in patients with severe congestive heart failure. Circulation 1992; 86:1351–1356.
72. Sullivan M, Higginbotham M, Cobb F. Exercise training in patients with severe left ventricular dysfunction: hemodynamic and metabolic effects. Circulation 1988; 78:506–515.
73. Coats A, Adamopoulos S, Radaelli A, McCance A, Meyer T, Bernardi L, Solda P, Davey P, Ormerod O, Forfar C, Conway J, Sleight P. Controlled trial of physical training in chronic heart failure. Circulation 1992; 85:2119–2131.
74. Wilson J, Mancini D, Dunkman W. Exertional fatigue due to skeletal muscle dysfunction in patients with heart failure. Circulation 1993; 87:470–475.
75. Mancini DM, Coyle E, Cogga A, Beltz J, Ferrano N, Montain S, Wilson JR. Contribution of intrinsic skeltal muscle changes to ^{31}P NMR skeletal muscle metabolic abnormalities in patients with heart failure. Circulation 1989; 80:1338–1346.
76. Todd GJ, Van De Wiele B, Askanzi J, Yoshikawa K, Elwyn DH, Kinney JM, Reemtsma K. Muscle high energy phosphated in chronic peripheral vascular disease. J Surg Res 1988; 44:277–283.
77. Pernow B, Saltin B, Wahren J, Cronestrand R. Muscle metabolism during exercise n patients with occlusive arterial disease: effect of reconstructive surgery. Scand J Clin Lab Invest 1973; 128:21–25.
78. Shepard JT, Cohen RA, Katusic ZS. Endothelium dysfunction in vascular disease. In: Clement DL, Shepard JT, eds. Vascular Diseases in the Limbs. St. Louis: Mosby-Year Book, 1993, pp 23–29.
79. McCully K, Halber C, Posner J. Exercise induced changes in oxygen saturation in the calf muscles of elderly subjects with peripheral vascular disease. J Gerontol Biol Sci 1994; 49:B128–B134.

80. Henriksson J, Nygaard E, Anderson J, Eklof B. Enzyme activities, fiber types, and capillarization in calf muscles of patients with intermittent claudication. Scand J Clin Lab Invest 1980; 40:361–369.
81. Kurosawa Y, Iwane H, Hamaoka T, Murase N, Sako T, Higuchi H. The effects of peripheral vascular disease on muscle oxygenation and energy metabolism. Abstract. Med Sci Sport Exerc 1996; 28:562.
82. Hands LJ, Bore PJ, Galloway G, Morris PJ, Radda GK. Muscle metabolism in patients with peripheral vascular disease investigated by ^{31}P nuclear magnetic resonance spectroscopy. Clin Sci 1986; 71:283–290.
83. Heistad DD, Armstrong ML, Piegors DJ, Mark AL. Augmented responses to vasoconstrictor stimuli in hypercholesterolemic and atherosclerotic monkeys. Circ Res 1984; 54:711–718.
84. Harrison DG, Minor RL, Guerra R, Quillen JE, Sellke FW. Endothelial dysfunction in arteriosclerosis. In: Rubanyi GM, ed. Cardiovascular significance of endothelium-derived vasoactive factors. New York: Futura Publishing Company, 1991, pp 263–280.
85. Matsen FA, Wyss CR, Pedegana LR, Krugmire RB Jr., Simmons CW, King RV, Burgess EM. Transcutaneous oxygen tension measurement in peripheral vascular disease. Surg Gynecol Obstet 1980; 150:525–528.
86. Bongard O, Krahenbuhl B. Pedal blood flow and transcutaneous Po_2 in normal subjects and in patients suffering from severe arterial occlusive disease. Clin Physiol 1984; 4:393–401.
87. Fagrell B, Lundberg G. A simplified evaluation of of vital capillary microscopy for predicting skin viability in patients with severe arterial insufficiency. Clin Physiol 1984; 4:403–411.
88. Bongard O, Fagrell B. Discrepancies between total and nutritional skin microcirculation in patients with peripheral arterial occlusive disease (PAOD). Vasa 1990; 19:105–111.
89. McEvan A, Ledingham I. Blood flow characteristics and tissue nutrition in apparently ischaemic feet. Br Med J 1971; 3:220–224.
90. Morris-Jones W, Preston E, Greaney M, Duleep K. Gangrene of the toes with palpable peripheral pulses. Ann Surg 1981; 193:462–466.
91. Clyne C, Mears H, Weller R, O'Donnel T. Calf muscle adaptation to peripheral vascular disease. Circ Res 1985; 19:507–512.
92. Holm J, Jorntorp B, Scherston T. Metabolic activity in human skeletal muscle: effect of peripheral arterial insufficiency. Eur J Clin Invest 1972; 2:321–325.
93. Edward W. Pathology of pulmonary hypertension. In: Kapoor A, Laks H, Schroeder J, Yacoub M, eds. Cardiomyopathies and Heart-Lung Transplantation. New York: McGraw Hill, 1991, pp 377–402.
94. Edwards W. Pathology of pulmonary hypertension. Cardiovasc Clin 1988; 18:321–359.
95. Waagenwoort C, Waagenwoort N. Pathology of Pulmonary Hypertension, New York: Wiley, 1977, pp 1–290.
96. Fuster V, Dines D, Rodarte J, McGoon D. The Heart and the Lungs: Relationships Between Disease of the Heart and Disease of the Lungs in Cardiology: Fundamental and Practice. St. Louis: Mosby Year Book, 1991, pp 2037–2049.

97. Levine M, Weinstein J, Diver D, Berman A, Wyman R, Cunningham M, Safian R, Grossman W, McKay R. Progressive improvement in pulmonary vascular resistance after percutaneous mitral valvuloplasty. Circulation 1989; 79:1061–1067.
98. Camara M, Aris A, Padro J, Caralps JM. Long term results of mitral valve surgery in patients with severe pulmonary hypertension. Ann Thorac Surg 1988; 45:133–136.
99. Haworth S, Hall S, Patel M. Peripheral pulmonary vascular and airway abnormalities in adolescents with rheumatic mitral stenosis. Int J Cardiol 1988; 18:405–416.
100. Bhatia S, Kirshenbaum J, Shemin R, Cohn L, Collins J, DiSesa V, Young P, Mudge G, St John-Sutton M. Time course of resolution of pulmonary hypertension and right ventricular remodeling after orthotopic cardiac transplantation. Circulation 1987; 76:819–826.
101. Kindman LA, Vagelos R, Willson K, Prikazky L, Fowler M. Abnormalities of pulmonary function in patients with congestive heart failure, and reversal with ipratropium bromide. Am J Cardiol 1994; 73:258–262.
102. Collins J, Clark T, Brown D. Airway function in healthy subjects and patients with left heart disease. Clin Sci Mol Med 1975; 49:217–228.
103. Kindman A. Pulmonary abnormalities in congestive heart failure: a therapeutic opportunity? In: Kennedy GT, Crawford MH, eds. Congestive Heart Failure: Current Clinical Issues. Futura: Armonk, 1994, pp 39–50.
104. Wright R, Levine M, Bellamy P, Simmons M, Batra P, Stevenson L, Walden J, Laks H, Tashkin D. Ventilatory and diffusion abnormalities in potential heart transplant recipients. Chest 1990; 98:816–820.
105. Kraemer M, Kubo S, Rector T, Brunsvold N, Bank A. Pulmonary and peripheral vascular factors are important determinants of peak exercise oxygen uptake in patients with heart failure. J Am Coll Cardiol 1993; 21:641–648.
106. Hosenpud J, Stibolt T, Atwal K, Shelley D. Abnormal pulmonary function specifically related to congestive heart failure: comparison of patients before and after transplantation. Am J Med 1990; 88:493–496.
107. Fink L, Wilson JR, Ferraro N. Exercise ventilation and pulmonary artery wedge pressure in chronic stable congestive heart failure. Am J Cardiol 1986; 57:249–253.
108. Weber K, Kinasewitz G, Janicki J, Fishman A. Oxygen utilization and ventilation during exercise in patients with chronic cardiac failure. Circulation 1982; 65:1213–1223.
109. Franciosa J, Leddy C, Wilen M, Schwartz D. Relation between hemodynamic and ventilatory responses in determining exercise capacity in severe congestive heart failure. Am J Cardiol 1984; 53:127–134.
110. Hughes J, Glazier J, Rosenzweig D, West J. Factors determining the distribution of pulmonary blood flow in patients with raised pulmonary venous pressure. Clin Sci 1969; 37:847–858.
111. Sullivan M, Higginbotham M, Cobb F. Increased exercise ventilation in patients with chronic heart failure: intact ventilatory control despite hemodynamic and pulmonary abnormalities. Circulation 1988; 77:552–559.
112. Wilson JR, Mancini DM, Ferraro N, Egler J. Effect of dichloroacetate on the exercise performance of patients with heart failure. J Am Coll Cardiol 1988; 12:1464–1469.

113. Sullivan M, Higginbotham M, Cobb F: Exercise training in patients with severe left ventricular dysfunction: hemodynamic and metabolic effects. Circulation 1988; 78:506–515.
114. Sullivan M, Higginbotham M, Cobb F. Exercise training in patients with chronic heart failure delays ventilatory anaerobic threshold and improves submaximal exercise performance. Circulation 1989; 79:324–329.
115. Coats A, Adamopoulos S, Radaelli A, McCance A, Meyer T, Bernardi L, Solda P, Davey P, Ormerod O, Forfar C, Conway J, Sleight P. Controlled trial of physical training in chronic heart failure. Circulation 1992; 85:2119–2131.
116. Marzo KP, Wilson JR, Mancini DM. Effects of cardiac transplantation on ventilatory response to exercise. Am J Cardiol 1992; 69:547–553.
117. Rubin S, Brown H. Ventilation and gas exchange during exercise in severe chronic heart failure. Am Rev Respir Dis 1984; 129(Suppl):S63–S64.
118. Wada O, Asanoi H, Miyagi K, Ishizaka S, Kameyama T, Seto H, Sasayama S. Importance of abnormal lung perfusion in excessive exercise ventilation in chronic heart failure. Am Heart J 1993; 125:790–798.
119. Uren NG, Simon W, Davies AG, Irwin SL, Jordan L, Hilson AJW, Agnew JE, Lipkin DP. Regional ventilation-perfusion mismatch and exercise capacity in chronic heart failure (abstract). Circulation 1991; 84(Suppl II):II-7.
120. Mancini D, LaManca J, Donchez L, Henson D, Levine S. The sensation of dyspnea during exercise is not determined by the work of breathing in patients with heart failure. J Am Coll Cardiol 1996; 28:391–395.
121. Barlow C, Qayyum M, Davey P, Conway J, Paterson D, Robbins P. Effect of physical training on exercise-induced hyperkalemia in chronic heart failure. Circulation 1994; 89:1144–1152.
122. Sterns DA, Ettinger SM, Gray KS, Whisler SK, Mosher TJ, Smith MB, Sinoway LI. Skeletal muscle meta-baroreceptors exercise responses are attenuated in heart failure. Circulation 1991; 84:2034–2039.
123. Clark AL, Poole-Wilson PA, Coats AJS. Exercise limitation in chronic heart failure: central role of the periphery. J Am Coll Cardiol 1996; 28:1092–1102.
124. Fixler D, Atkins J, Mitchell J, Horwitz L. Blood flow to respiratory, cardiac, and limb muscles in dogs during graded exercise. Am J Physiol 1976; 231:1515–1519.
125. Reid M, Johnson R. Efficiency, maximal blood flow and aerobic work capacity of the canine diaphragm. J Appl Physiol 1983; 54:763–772.
126. Musch T. Elevated diaphragmatic blood flow during submaximal exercise in rats with CHF. Am J Physiol 1993; 265:H1721–1726.
127. Mancini D, Nazzaro D, Ferraro N, Chance B, Wilson JR. Demonstration of respiratory muscle deoxygenation during exercise in patients with heart failure. J Am Coll Cardiol 1991; 18:492–498.
128. Marzo K, Herrmann H, Mancini DM. Effect of balloon mitral valvuloplasty on exercise capacity, ventilation, and skeletal muscle oxygenation. J Am Coll Cardiol 1993; 21:856–865.
129. Mancini DM, Henson D, LaManca J, Levine S. Respiratory muscle function and dyspnea in patients with chronic congestive heart failure. Circulation 1992; 86:909–918.

130. Cabanes L, Weber S, Matran R, Regnard J, Richard M, Degeorges M, Lockhart A. Bronchial hyperresponsiveness to methacholine in patients with impaired left ventricular function. N Engl J Med 1989; 320:1317–1322.
131. Cabanes L, Costes F, Weber S, Regnard J, Benvenuti C, Castaigne A, Guerin F, Lockhart A. Improvement in exercise performance by inhalation of methoxamine in patients with impaired left ventricular function. N Engl J Med 1992; 326:1661–1665.
132. Kindman A, Vagelos R, Willson K, Prikazky L, Fowler. Abnormalities of pulmonary function in patients with congestive heart failure, and reversal with ipratropium bromide. Am J Cardiol 1994; 73:258–262.
133. Uren N, Davies S, Jordan S, Lipkin D. Inhaled bronchodilators increase maximum oxygen consumption in chronic left ventricular failure. Eur Heart J 1993; 14:744–750.
134. Hammond M, Bauer K, Sharp J, Rocha R. Respiratory muscle strength in congestive heart failure. Chest 1990; 98:1091–1094.
135. Mancini D, Donchez, Levine S. Acute unloading of the work of breathing extends exercise duration in patients with heart failure. J Am Coll Cardiol 1997; 29:590–596.
136. Mancini DM, LaManca J, Levine S, Henson D. Respiratory muscle endurance is decreased in patients with heart failure. Circulation 1992; 86(Suppl):I-515A.
137. Mancini DM, Henson D, LaManca J, Donchez L, Levine S. Benefit of selective respiratory muscle training on exercise capacity in patients with congestive heart failure. Circulation 1995; 91:320–329.
138. Letac B, Cribier A, Desplances JF: A study of LV function in coronary patients before and after physical training. Circulation 1977; 56:375–378.
139. Lee AP, Ice R, Blessey R, Sanmarco ME. Long-term effects of physical training on coronary patients with impaired ventricular function. Circulation 1979; 60:1519–1526.
140. Williams RS, McKinnis R, Cobb F, Higginbothham MB, Wallace AG, Coleman RE, Califf RM. Effects of physical conditioning on left ventricular ejection fraction in patients with coronary artery disease. Circulation 1984; 70:69–75.
141. Cohn E, Williams R, Wallace A. Exercise responses before and after physical conditioning in patients with severely depressed left ventricular ejection fraction. Am J Cardiol 1982; 49:296–300.
142. Musch T, Moore R, Leathers D, Bruno A, Zelis R. Endurance training in rats with chronic heart failure induced by myocardial infarction. Circulation 1986; 74:431–441.
143. Sullivan M, Higginbotham M, Cobb F. Exercise training in patients with severe left ventricular dysfunction: hemodynamic and metabolic effects. Circulation 1988; 78:506–515.
144. Coats A, Adamopoulos S, Radaelli A, McCance A, Meyer T, Bernardi L, Solda P, Davey P, Ormerod O, Forfar C, Conway J, Sleight P. Controlled trial of physical training in chronic heart failure. Circulation 1992; 85:2119–2131.
145. Hambrecht R, Niebauer J, Fiehn E, Kalberer B, Offner B, Hauer K, Riede U, Schlierf G, Kubler W, Schuler G. Physical training in patients with stable chronic heart failure: effects on cardiorespiratory fitness and ultrastructural abnormalities of leg muscles. J Am Coll Cardiol 1995; 25:1239–1249.

146. Hornig B, Maier V, Drexler H. Physcial training improves endothelial function in patients with heart failure. Circulation 93:210–214, 1996.
147. Jugdutt B, Michorowski B, Kappagoda C: Exercise training after anterior Q wave myocardial infarction: importance of regional left ventricular function and topography. J Am Coll Cardiol 1988; 12:362–372.
148. Gaudron P, Hu K, Schamberger R, Budin M, Walter B, Ertl G. Effect of endurance training early or late after coronary artery occlusion on left ventricular remodeling, hemodynamics, and survival in rats with chronic transmural myocardial infarction. Circulation 1994; 89:402–412.
149. Giannuzzi P, Tavazzi L, Temporelli PL, Corra U, Imparato A, Gattone M, Giordano A, Sala L, Schweiger C, Malinverni C. Long-term physical training and left ventriuclar remodeling after anterior myocardial infarction: results of the exercise in anterior myocardial infarction (EAMI) trial. J Am Coll Cardiol 1993; 22:1821–1829.
150. Wilson J, Groves J, Rayos G. Circulatory status and response to cardiac rehabilitation in patients with heart failure. Circ 1996; 94:1567–1572.
151. Belardinelli R, Georgiou D, Scocco V, Barstow TJ, Purcaro A. Low intensity exercise training in patients with chronic heart failure. J Am Coll Cardiol 1995; 26:975–982.
152. Demopoulos L, Bijou R, Fergus A, Jones N, Strom J, LeJemtel T. Exercise training in patients with severe congestive heart failure: enhancing peak aerobic capacity while minimizing the increase in ventricular wall stress. J Am Coll Cardiol 1997; 29:597–603.
153. Mancini DM, Henson D, La Manca J, Donchez L, Levine S: Benefit of selective respiratory muscle training on exercise capacity in patients with chronic congestive heart failure. Circulation 1995; 91:320–329.

22

Role of Hemoglobin in the Delivery of Oxygen to Tissues

ROBERT M. WINSLOW

Sangart, Inc.
San Diego, California

I. Introduction

The principal molecular mechanisms underlying the blood oxygen (O_2) equilibrium curve (OEC; Fig. 1) have been described in detail [1]. Traditional discussions of the importance of this curve have focused on its cooperative nature, the fact that it steepens in its midportion such that small changes in O_2 partial pressure P_{O_2} effect large changes in total blood oxygen content. Such shifts are mediated by "allosteric effectors," e.g., hydrogen ion (H^+), carbon dioxide (CO_2), 2,3-diphosphoglycerate (2,3-DPG) and Cl^-. Nitric oxide (NO) has been proposed recently as a physiologically important allosteric effector [2]. Less well described than the structural basis of this cooperative curve are the physiological implications of its regulation.

The relationship between blood O_2 content and P_{O_2} has been recognized for more than a century. In 1932, Hurtado [3] argued that the small right shift in the hemoglobin OEC, which he believed occurred in high-altitude natives, increased O_2 extraction from the blood and was therefore an adaptive advantage. Using arterial and mixed venous P_{O_2} values (Pa_{O_2} and $P\bar{v}_{O_2}$, respectively) measured in such natives, Hurtado asserted that the right-shifted curve (higher P50* lower O_2

---

*P50 = O_2 partial pressure at half hemoglobin saturation

Human Blood Oxygen Equilibrium Curve

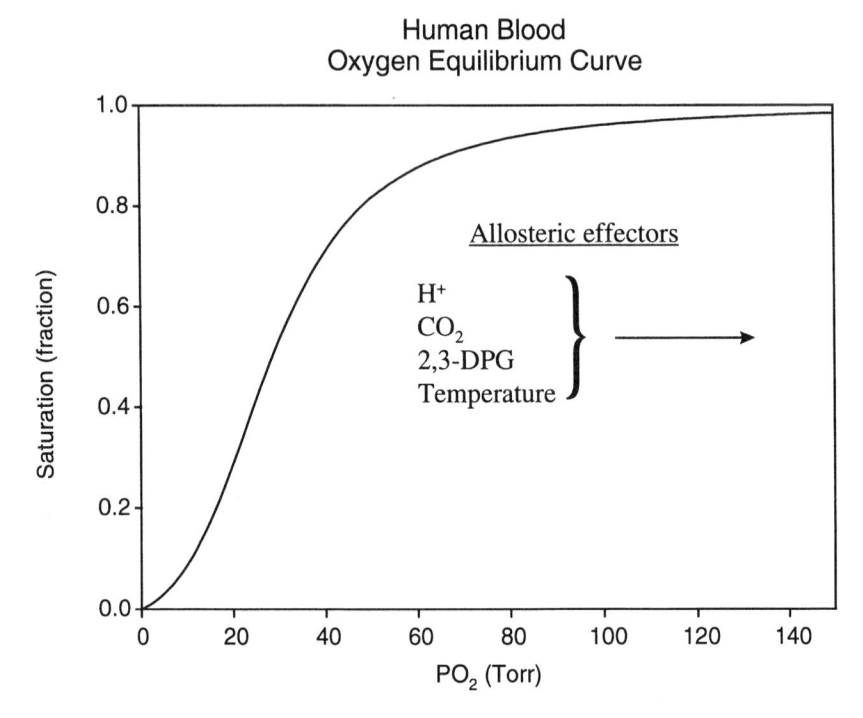

Figure 1 The human blood oxygen equilibrium curve. The unique feature of this curve is its steepness ("cooperativity") in its midportion, at oxygen partial pressure (P_{O_2}) values encountered in the tissues. This means that small changes in oxygen concentration (P_{O_2}) are translated into large changes in hemoglobin saturation. Some of the effectors that can alter the position of the curve are shown.

affinity) resulted in greater unloading of O_2 in tissues. This concept has persisted in the standard physiology textbooks to the present time, even though more modern measurements have shown that even in high-altitude natives, the shape and position of the blood OEC are remarkably constant [4]. Only when humans are exposed to extreme altitude (>5,400 m above sea level) does the in vivo OEC shift, but toward higher, not lower, affinity [5]. This increase in affinity at extreme altitude is the result of alkalosis and is critical to maintenance of arterial O_2 saturation at such altitudes.

Many advances in the understanding of the delivery of O_2 to tissues have been made in the intervening years since Hurtado's chapter was published in the *Handbook of Physiology* [6]. Recently, direct measurements of local P_{O_2} in individual vessels and adjacent tissue has permitted the "mapping" of O_2 transfer at different levels of the circulation [7,8]. In addition, new roles for hemoglobin, such as its possible role in NO metabolism [2,9], have suggested a tighter link between O_2 transport by hemoglobin and control of microvascular blood flow.

Cell-free hemoglobin has been proposed as a substitute for transfusions [10]. Many of these solutions are highly vasoactive, and their development has focused attention again on the mechanisms of control of vascular tone. Central in this development is the role of NO, the putative endothelium-derived relaxing factor (EDRF), because NO binds to hemoglobin with very high affinity. In addition, the presence of cell-free hemoglobin in the plasma space has important consequences for O_2 transport because of "facilitated" diffusion. Thus, the physiological importance of the OEC is again a subject of intense interest. The availability of these new solutions provides an exciting opportunity to study the effects of O_2 affinity, viscosity, oncotic pressure, and diffusion in addition to NO scavenging. Furthermore, many of these properties can be altered in systematic ways to test specific hypotheses.

The hypothesis explored in this chapter is that the main importance of the shape and position of the hemoglobin OEC is to maintain tissue perfusion at optimal levels. This is distinct from the conventional view, in which convective O_2 delivery to tissues is simply viewed as the product of cardiac output and the arterial–mixed venous O_2 content difference.

A. Traditional Views of Oxygen Affinity

The traditional view is that shifting the OEC to the right facilitates O_2 unloading in tissue sites. However, in certain situations, the opposite could be true. For example, Barcroft [11] believed that increased O_2 affinity was important in the adaptation to high altitude. His reasoning was based on analogy with the placental circulation, where fetal blood has a higher affinity than that of the mother to facilitate transfer of O_2 from the maternal to fetal circulation. Chemical modification of hemoglobin to increase its affinity conveys superior survival on hypoxic rats [12], and mutant hemoglobins with increased affinity may precondition subjects to hypoxia [13]. On the summit of Mt. Everest, the P50 of whole blood was found to be approximately 19 mm Hg, protecting arterial saturation [5].

A more rational view of the role of O_2 affinity in altitude acclimatization was proposed some time ago by Kleeberg et al. [14], who observed an immediate alkalosis in acute hypoxia, increasing affinity via the Bohr effect, followed by an increase in 2,3-DPG, which gradually shifts the OEC back to its "normal" position. The previously cited studies in both high-altitude natives and mountain climbers at extreme altitude seem to confirm this general picture.

There are two sides to the traditional O_2 affinity problem: increased affinity will promote O_2 uptake in the lung, but decreased affinity could promote O_2 unloading in the tissues. The key is the balance between the ability of the lung to oxygenate the blood and the demand for O_2 in the tissue. In other words, if ambient O_2 supply and lung function are normal, the O_2-unloading advantage of a high P50 can be beneficial to the tissues. When O_2 is limited, an increased P50 can inhibit uptake of O_2 in the lung, decreasing convective O_2 delivery. In the tissues, when O_2 consumption ($\dot{V}_{O_2}$) is low, a right shift of the OEC should result in an increased $P\bar{v}_{O_2}$. But when $\dot{V}_{O_2}$ is high and tissue P_{O_2} is low, then the P50 will be less relevant because all OECs converge at low P_{O_2}.

Under extremely hypoxic conditions, where the gradient for diffusion of O_2 between the alveolus and blood is reduced, a decreased P50 is beneficial, as observed in climbers on the summit of Mt. Everest [5] and in animals [15]. The situation in tissues may be different. There, the gradient for O_2 diffusion widens under stress, for example, in extreme exercise where tissue P_{O_2} decreases. Examination of the OEC would suggest that when the curve is right-shifted (low affinity), O_2 should be delivered at higher P_{O_2}.

The limits of P50 in normoxia can be set by observation of subjects with mutant hemoglobins. Carriers of hemoglobins whose P50 is approximately 20 mm Hg develop mild polycythemia [16], as do those with P50s of approximately 70 mm Hg [17], indicating insufficient delivery of O_2 to the renal erythropoietin (EPO) sensor in both cases.

Experimental confirmation of these limits has been difficult, and the results have been controversial. Martin et al. [18] showed that O_2 could be delivered satisfactorily to a working heart by blood with a P50 of 13 mm Hg, but Hogan et al. [19] found that maximal $\dot{V}_{O_2}$ of dog gastrocnemius muscle was 17% decreased when perfused with low-P50 blood, and Woodson et al. [20] observed a 24% decreased in dog brain $\dot{V}_{O_2}$ when perfused with carbamylated blood (P50 = 18 mm Hg).

Studies in dogs with induced myocardial infarction have shown that even small increases in P50 can result in diminution of the necrotic tissue [21,22]. Exchange transfusion in piglets [23] with cells whose P50 was almost 50 mm Hg showed that cardiac output decreased linearly with the P50 increase, whereas $\dot{V}_{O_2}$ and $P\bar{v}_{O_2}$ remained unchanged. Studies of increased P50 with perhaps the least confounding factors have been conducted with the strong allosteric effector RSR-13 [24]. This drug increased the P50 of dog red blood cells by 12.3 ± 0.9 mm Hg, decreasing arterial O_2 saturation to 90–92% and increasing tissue P_{O_2} from 35.5 ± 11.6 to 44.1 ± 15.2 mm Hg. Although the O_2 extraction at critical O_2 delivery ($\dot{Q}_{O_2}$) was not significantly increased, tissue P_{O_2}, measured with muscle surface electrodes, was 30–40% higher. However, below critical $\dot{Q}_{O_2}$, the tissue P_{O_2} did not differ from controls, suggesting that the increase in P50 did not increase diffusive O_2 transport to tissues. The qualitative explanation for these results is that when O_2 demand is high relative to the supply and O_2 extraction is maximal, the position of the OEC has minimal effect on overall tissue oxygenation because all OECs, regardless of P50, converge at low P_{O_2}. An additional explanation for the effect of increased P50 to increase O_2 extraction is that flow heterogeneity (the shunting of arteriolar blood to venules) could limit extraction [24,25]. Thus, the most logical conclusion from this very large body of work conducted over several decades is that autoregulatory mechanisms that control microperfusion of capillary beds apparently maintain a relationship between O_2 supply and demand that is held very constant.

Kohzuki et al. [26] perfused dog gastrocnemius muscle with red blood cells of varying P50 and found that the high affinity cells led to a faster increase in developed tension in the muscle, a lower peak tension, and faster rate of decline during the early fatigue period. They also found a flow-rate dependence of these parameters with both high- and low-affinity red blood cells. They concluded that both red blood cells at both flow rates delivered sufficient O_2 to the exercising muscle; therefore, the limitation to maximal O_2 delivery in exercising muscle is likely limited by both red blood cell transit times and O_2-releasing mechanisms. In a similar study, Liard and Kunert [27] performed exchange transfusion in dogs with red blood cells loaded with inositol hexaphosphate (IHP) to increase their P50. They found that animals responded with reduced cardiac output and increased peripheral resistance, suggesting vasoconstriction as a result of the increased O_2 availability. These studies show how remarkably well the O_2 transport system regulates itself to ensure that adequate O_2 delivery is maintained. They also show that because of this highly efficient regulation, alteration of any single component of the system, such as P50, is met with multiple physiological responses, clouding simple interpretations of the results.

To summarize this brief review, it seems that simple statements about the relative benefits of shifts of the OEC are naive. More properly, it should be appreciated that a large number of interacting variables act in concert to assure that tissue O_2 delivery is optimal under a wide variety of conditions. How this optimum is achieved in a specific vascular bed, and the role of hemoglobin in the process, is of interest in view of the remarkable intricacy of hemoglobin function and the fact that this essential protein is conserved in some form throughout the animal kingdom. The mechanisms that come into play to assure tissue oxygenation are highly redundant, as is expected for any process that is essential to life. If blood flow regulation is an important factor, then physiological experiments with altered P50 red blood cells are likely to be difficult to interpret because compensation in numerous components of the O_2 transport system will occur.

B. Structural and Functional Basis of the Oxygen Equilibrium Curve

Human hemoglobin is a tetrameric protein of molecular mass 64,000 D. It is composed of 2 α chains and 2 β chains, each of which bears an iron-containing heme group. These subunits interact in such a way that O_2 binding is "cooperative." Several small molecules bind to hemoglobin at nonheme sites, producing structural changes in the molecule that alter O_2 binding. These effects are called "allosteric." The principal allosteric effectors within the red blood cell are H^+, 2,3-DPG, and CO_2. Other effectors, Cl^- and adenosine triphosphate (ATP), also decrease O_2 affinity, but their physiological roles are minor. The recently reported [2] allosteric effects of NO are of potential importance because this molecule is also a potent vasorelaxant (EDRF). The OEC is very sensitive to temperature.

The OEC was described mathematically in the pioneering work of Adair [28], who recognized that hemoglobin was made up of four subunits, each of which could bind a single O_2 molecule. He described an equation based on the stepwise equilibrium binding of four O_2 molecules:

$$Y = \frac{a_1 p + 2a_2 p^2 + 3a_3 p^3 + 4a_4 p^4}{4(1 + a_1 p + a_2 p^2 + a_3 p^3 + a_4 p^4)} \tag{1}$$

where Y is the fractional saturation of hemoglobin with O_2, p is the partial pressure of O_2, and the a's are related to the four O_2 equilibrium constants such that $K_1 = a_1$, and for the remaining a's, $K_i = a_i/a_{i-1}$. The new parameters (a's) are called Adair parameters. This equation is very useful in making physiological calculations, and values for whole blood have been determined with a high degree of precision [29] (Table 1). The detailed effects of the principal allosteric effectors on the Adair constants have also been determined [30].

Since the elucidation of the exact structure of hemoglobin, several mechanistic theories for the influence of the allosteric effectors have been proposed [31]. Monod et al. [32] proposed the most successful of these, based on the structural work of Bolton and Perutz [33], who described two conformations for hemoglobin, corresponding to deoxyhemoglobin and oxyhemoglobin. According to the two-state model, hemoglobin can exist in either R (oxy, relaxed) or T (deoxy, tense) conformation, each with its unique O_2 affinity. The ratio of these constants is approximately 0.01 for human hemoglobin A, i.e., the O_2 affinity of molecules in the R conformation is 100 times greater than the affinity of those in the T conformation. The essence of the allosteric theory is that the equilibrium between the two conformations in the deoxy state,

$$Hb^R \longleftrightarrow Hb^T \tag{2}$$

given by the allosteric constant,

$$L = \frac{[Hb^T]}{[Hb^R]} \tag{3}$$

Table 1 Oxygenation Parameters for Normal Human Blood

a_1 ($\times 10^{-1}$)	0.151 ± .015
a_2 ($\times 10^{-3}$)	0.972 ± .078
a_3 ($\times 10^{-5}$)	0.170 ± .085
a_4 ($\times 10^{-5}$)	0.167 ± 0.0003
n_{max} (Hill's parameter)	2.6
P50 (mm Hg), male	28.8

Conditions: pH, 7.4; P_{CO_2}, 40; 2,3-DPG/Hb, 0.88.
Source: Ref. 29.

is influenced by a number of allosteric effectors. These small molecules react with hemoglobin at nonheme sites in such a way as to stabilize the T conformation. Thus, the overall reactivity of a mixture of R and T hemoglobin molecules toward O_2 will depend on the position of the R–T equilibrium. Monod et al. [32] related the allosteric constant L to P_{O_2} (p) and to the fractional saturation of hemoglobin with O_2 (Y):

$$Y = \frac{LK_T p(1 + K_T p)^3 + K_R p(1 + K_R p)^3}{L(1 + K_T p)^4 + (1 + K_R p)^4} \tag{4}$$

Of fundamental importance in this model is that the T state is physically constrained by salt and hydrogen bonds to a much greater degree than is the R state. With successive oxygenation of the heme groups, some of these bonds break, and the stability of the T structure decreases; as a result, the molecules undergo a transition to the R state, accompanied by the release of the constraints and an increase in O_2 affinity. For deoxyhemoglobin, the equilibrium is almost entirely on the T side. It is the shift from T to R during oxygenation that accounts for cooperativity. For normal hemoglobin, most of the molecules probably shift from T to R between binding of the second and third O_2 molecules; hence, the OEC is steepest in its middle portion.

Bohr et al. [34] observed that the position of the blood OEC along the abscissa was affected by changes in CO_2 partial pressure (P_{CO_2}), i.e., when pH was lowered (or P_{CO_2} increased), the O_2 affinity of the blood decreased (increased P50). The separate effects of H^+ and CO_2 have been elucidated [35]. They are qualitatively similar, but the effect of H^+ (now properly called the ''pH Bohr effect'') is much stronger than the CO_2 effect in lowering O_2 affinity.

According to the two-state model of hemoglobin function, H^+ shifts the R–T equilibrium toward T, stabilizing that structure. The stereochemical interpretation of this phenomenon is that H^+ participates in opening and closing salt bridges involving the carboxy-terminal residues. The pK values of the imidazoles of histidine HC3(146)β and of valine NA1(1)α are lowered in oxyhemoglobin as a result of the rupture of the salt bridges in which they participate. This change in pK leads to a release of protons during the transition from T to R. Experiments with mutant and chemically modified hemoglobins suggest that these groups account for approximately two thirds of the Bohr effect [36].

The normal intracellular constituent 2,3-DPG (and, to a lesser extent, ATP) is very important in the regulation of the blood OEC [37]. 2,3-DPG is present in normal human red blood cells and is a metabolic intermediate in the glycolytic pathway. Under conditions of diminished O_2 availability (such as anemia or hypoxia), its concentration increases and the blood OEC moves to the right. This is usually considered to facilitate transfer of O_2 to the tissues. The regulatory mechanisms that govern the concentration of 2,3-DPG in the red blood cells are not completely understood, but alkalosis in response to hyperventilation is probably an important factor [38].

The effect of 2,3-DPG can be explained in terms of two-state theory of hemoglobin function. 2,3-DPG can bind to deoxyhemoglobin in a molar ratio of 1:1; by doing this, it further constrains the T conformation, leading to a further shift of the R–T equilibrium toward T and a lowering of O_2 affinity. Salt bridges involving the free amino groups of valine NAl(1)β and the imidazoles of histidine H21(143)β are probably the most important binding sites [39]. In deoxyhemoglobin, 2,3-DPG lies in the central cavity of the molecule and is coordinated to the aforementioned groups, as well as to the α-amino groups of lysine EF6(82)β. On transition to the R structure, the valines move apart, the H helices move together, and 2,3-DPG drops out. Like the effects of the other salt bridges in the deoxy structure, 2,3-DPG increases the Bohr effect.

Carbon dioxide can bind to the α-amino groups of the amino-terminal amino acids with a resultant decrease of O_2 affinity [40]. This binding is diminished in the presence of 2,3-DPG because both 2,3-DPG and CO_2 can bind to the β-chain amino-terminal amino group. Such competition does not occur for the α-chain amino-terminus because 2,3-DPG does not bind there.

The rates of O_2 uptake and release by red blood cells and hemoglobin solutions have been studied in vitro in rapid mixing experiments [41] and in an artificial capillary system [42,43]. These studies suggest that the position of the OEC will have little influence on the rate of O_2 uptake where alveolar P_{O_2} is normal but may affect the rate of O_2 release where tissue O_2 consumption is high. Diffusion of O_2 through a layer of unstirred plasma surrounding the red blood cell membrane is critical to the rates of exchange, but the significance of this effect in vivo (or the loss of this effect in the case of cell-free O_2 carriers) is still not fully appreciated. However, it seems that the reaction of O_2 with hemoglobin itself is not rate-limiting [41].

Nitric oxide can bind to the heme groups of hemoglobin with very high affinity. Recently, binding of NO to the sulfhydryl group of β93Cys (to form SNO-Hb) was also described [2]. These investigators found an increase of SNO-Hb in the lung as hemoglobin is oxygenated, and a decrease of SNO-Hb in tissues as O_2 is given up (Table 2). They proposed that NO might in this way also be a potent

Table 2 Endogenous Levels of SNO-Hb and Fe_{II}-Hb in the Rat

Blood	SNO-Hb (mmol/L)	Hb(Fe_{II})NO (mmol/L)
Arterial	311 ± 55[a]	536 ± 99[b]
Venous	32 ± 14	894 ± 126

[a] $P < .05$ vs. venous.
[b] $P < .05$ for paired samples vs. venous.
Source: Ref. 2.

facilitator of O_2 delivery to tissues, effecting vasodilation at the points where O_2 demand is high. Thus, the allosteric effects of NO binding to β93Cys could be an allosteric mechanism linking O_2 demand and blood flow.

The reactivity of β93Cys with various alkylating agents is increased when hemoglobin is oxygenated, and Jia et al. [2] showed that S-nitrosylation at this highly conserved site is also O_2-dependent (Fig. 2). These investigators found that the rates of S-nitrosylation are markedly greater when hemoglobin is in the oxy (R) conformational state and that the rates were still greater when pH was greater than 7.4. They suggested that at the high pH, β93Cys is more exposed, making it more reactive. The structural hypothesis is that β93Cys is normally partially screened by the C-terminal residue, β146His, but at high pH, the salt bridge that constrains the residue (β94Asp–β146His) is loosened. As Fig. 2 shows, the rate of release of NO from SNO-Hb is slow when a receptor molecule is not present. In red blood cells, this role could be filled by glutathione, which is present in high concentration. It remains to be seen whether the transport of NO as SNO-Hb is of physiological importance. Figure 3 shows the interactions of the various forms of NO–hemoglobin proposed by Gow and Stamler [44].

C. Regulatory Implications of Low Oxygen Solubility

Critical to an understanding of the role of the OEC in regulating O_2 transport to tissues is the extremely low solubility of O_2 in aqueous solution. The solubility coefficient (α) for O_2 in plasma is 1.2074 μmol/L/mm Hg [29]. To put this figure in perspective, consider a sample of blood that contains 15 g of hemoglobin per 100 mL (i.e., 15 g/dL). The molecular weight of each hemoglobin subunit is 16,100 g/mol, so the hemoglobin concentration in this sample of blood is 9.32 mmol/L (heme basis). At 100 mm Hg P_{O_2}, when this hemoglobin is completely saturated (see Fig. 1), the plasma O_2 concentration is 0.12074 mmol/L, or only 1.3% of the total O_2 carried in the blood.

The implications of this remarkable feature of blood come into clearer focus when the actual P_{O_2} values at various levels of the circulation are considered. Direct measurements of P_{O_2} in vessels of different size in experimental animals are now available [8,45]. Studies in the awake hamster skinfold model show that significant decreases in P_{O_2} occur in arterioles, even before blood reaches capillaries (Fig. 4). The movement of O_2 from vessels of any size to tissue is a function of the O_2 concentration gradient between the vessel and tissue. Figure 2 shows that even when the tissue P_{O_2} is zero, this gradient will not be more than 0.064 mmol/L, whereas the gradient between red blood cells and plasma would be 8.68 mmol/L, 135 times greater. Oxygen does not diffuse from red blood cells to plasma along this steep gradient because it is bound to hemoglobin inside the red blood cell according to the OEC. Oxyhemoglobin cannot diffuse in the plasma space because it is contained within the red blood cell membrane.

Thus, although the red blood cell acts as a reservoir of O_2, the actual movement of O_2 from vessels to tissue is driven by small gradients. The importance of

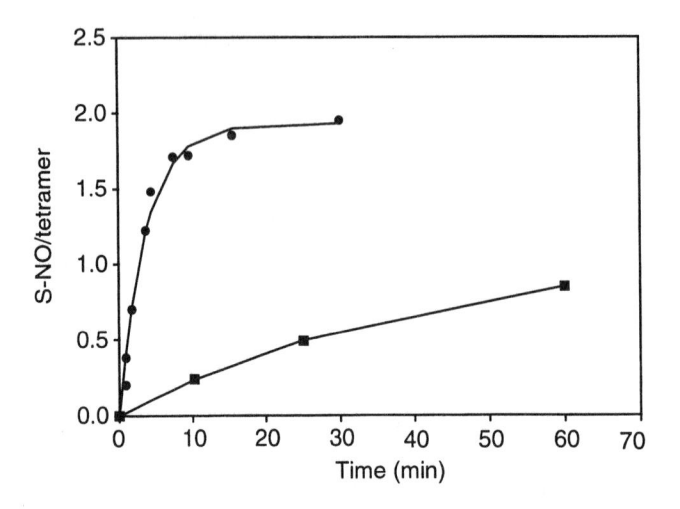

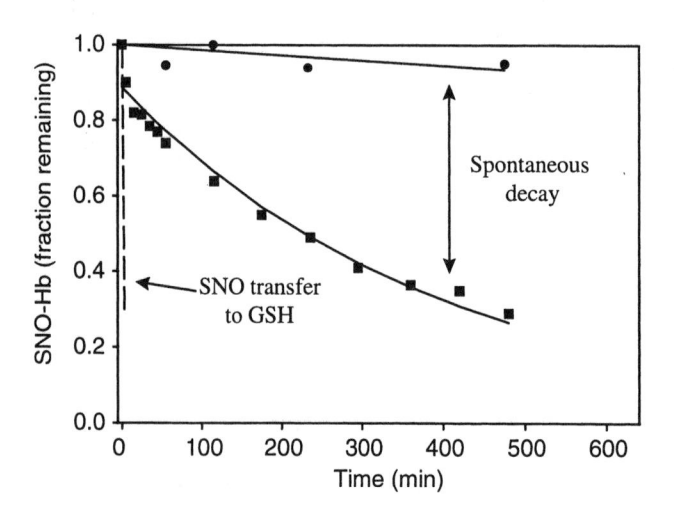

Figure 2 Time courses of on (top) and off (bottom) reactions of nitric oxide (NO) with β93Cys of human hemoglobin. Oxygenation accelerates the rat of the on reaction, and deoxygenation accelerates the off reaction. The spontaneous dissociation is very slow to the rate in the presence of a carrier molecule such as glutathione. (Modified from Ref. 2.)

this fact is that even very small shifts of the OEC within a vessel will have profound effects on the vessel/tissue O_2 diffusion gradient. For example, consider the case in which the vessel P_{O_2} is 28.5 mm Hg (arterioles; Fig. 4). The hemoglobin saturation is 0.5, the oxyhemoglobin concentration is 4.55 mmol/L, and the plasma O_2 concentration is 0.034 mmol/L. Using values for normal blood [46], we can

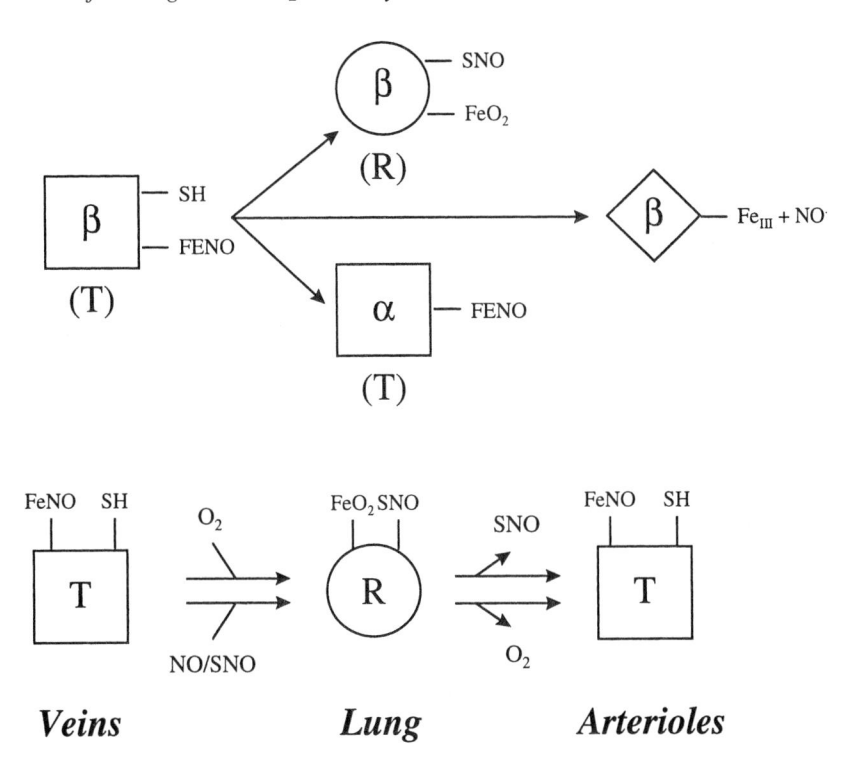

Figure 3 Proposed allosteric mechanisms by which nitric oxide (NO) and oxygen can interact to produce local vasorelaxation and increased blood flow in areas of tissue in which oxygen demand is high. NO, scavenged in tissue and bound to heme, migrates to the β93Cys sulfhydryl group in the lung in response to the T → R switch. This NO would then become available in tissue and relax arterioles when oxygen is reduced and the R → T transition occurs. (From Ref. 44.)

calculate that the P_{CO_2} increases from 40 to 51.8 mm Hg in the tissues, which causes a shift in pH from 7.40 to 7.34. This results in an increase of P50 from 28.8 to 30.8 mm Hg, but the fractional saturation would decrease from 0.49 to 0.45. This 4% decrease in the hemoglobin saturation would decrease red blood cell O_2 concentration to 4.19 mmol/L but increase plasma O_2 concentration from 0.034 to 0.38 mmol/L. This would have the effect of increasing the O_2 diffusion gradient 63-fold from 0.006 mmol/L to 0.37 mmol/L. Thus, the combination of the very low solubility of O_2 and the unique shape and position of the blood OEC and its sensitivity to H^+ (the Bohr effect) provide the basis for a powerful mechanism for the regulation and maintenance of tissue O_2 levels. A further aspect of this example is the fact that the solubility coefficient for CO_2 is 20 times higher than it is for O_2, and the reaction with carbonic anhydrase is essentially instan-

O₂ Distribution

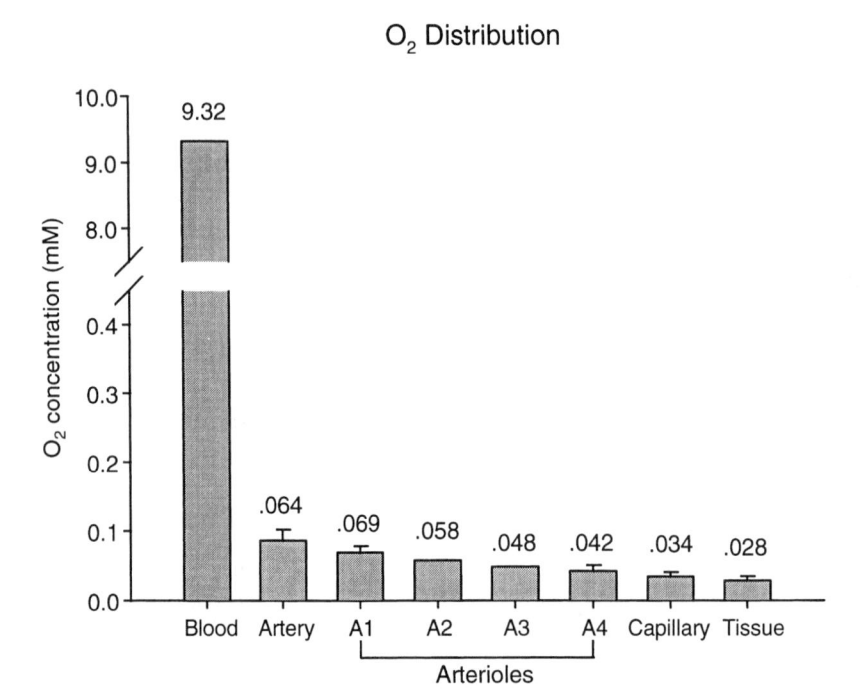

Figure 4 Concentrations of oxygen in the various levels of the circulation. At an oxygen partial pressure of 100 mm Hg, only 1.3% of the total oxygen is carried dissolved in the plasma. Yet the diffusion of oxygen from plasma to the tissues is proportional to the difference in oxygen concentration between those two spaces. The data in this figure (8) suggest that this gradient is very small. In contrast, if even a very small fraction of the red blood cell oxygen dissociates, the gradient can become many times greater.

taneous. Therefore, when CO_2 enters blood in the tissues, its value will increase rather quickly.

However, complicating these considerations is the fact that the systemic and microvascular hematocrits are not equal. For eample, Lindbom et al. [47] observed that when rabbits were hemodiluted with dextran to reduce the systemic hematocrit from a mean of 36 ± 4% to 17 ± 2%, capillary hematocrit decreased by only 14.1 ± 2.5% to 11.4 ± 5.1%. Thus, at the capillary level, the difference between the red blood cell reserve and plasma O_2 concentration is much less than shown in Fig. 4 and apparently is maintained rather constant over a range of systemic hematocrit values. The mechanism of the discrepancy between microvascular and systemic hematocrits is still not completely explained, but at least part of the difference seems to be caused by the Fåhraeus effect, whereby red blood cells traverse capillary beds faster than the corresponding volume of plasma.

II. Autoregulation of Tissue Oyxgen Delivery

Recruitment of perfused capillaries in response to increased O_2 demand was proposed almost 80 years ago by Krogh [48]. Underlying this proposed mechanism is the fact that at rest, only a fraction of capillaries are perfused, and when O_2 demand increases, more capillaries are open to flow, increasing the total perfusion of the tissue and the surface area available for O_2 diffusion. Many studies in the years since Krogh's article have been aimed at understanding the mechanisms for this control, but only recently have the precise experimental techniques been available for microscopic P_{O_2} measurements.

In the context of the present discussion, autoregulation maintains tissue P_{O_2} by regulation of blood flow. It is known that local blood flow is regulated in very complex ways and by different mechanisms in different tissues. Here we are concerned with the linkage between tissue O_2 demand and the delivery of O_2 by hemoglobin and the integration of this mechanism with the regulation of blood flow. Neurogenic and myogenic vasoactivity known to occur in larger vessels may be regulated by different, central mechanisms [49]. Furthermore, autoregulation is important in maintaining capillary hydrostatic pressure, which is important for fluid balance, and in protecting capillary integrity, which is important in all tissues, especially the brain and lung.

Experimental observation of capillary density or red blood cell flow velocity in response to P_{O_2} is limited because accurate control of Pa_{O_2} in small animals is technically difficult. However, Lindbom et al. [50] approached this problem by adjusting the P_{O_2} of the superfusate in a microscopic field of rabbit tenuissimus muscle and found a remarkable dependence of capillary density on P_{O_2} (Fig. 5). Their data show an almost linear decrease in capillary density as P_{O_2} increased from 0 to 150 mm Hg, with essentially no capillaries flowing at the highest P_{O_2}. As capillary density decreases, there is a small decrease in mean red blood cell flow velocity that partially offsets the reduced perfusion. These investigators emphasized that the sensitivity of the microvasculature to alterations in O_2 availability seems to be greatest within the normal tissue P_{O_2} range. From the total capillary density in the fields of view in their experiments, they were able to estimate that an increase in P_{O_2} from 22 to 35 mm Hg resulted in a reduction of total blood flow from 7.5 to 5.6 mL/min/100 g. In studies of the mechanism of capillary reduction in response to lowered P_{O_2}, Lindbom and Arfors [51] subsequently observed that, rather than control by precapillary "sphincters," a graded increase in resistance in all terminal arterioles leads to reduced flow in downstream capillaries.

In a completely separate model, Mouren et al. [52] showed that the coronary circulation constricts in response to high Pa_{O_2} in a manner that is independent of cyclooxygenase or lipoxygenase products, NO, or free radicals, and that in this model, vasoconstriction is mediated by closure of ATP-sensitive K^+ channels.

Clearly, control of vascular tone is a complex phenomenon and likely to be different in different vascular beds. Figure 6 shows a schematic representation of the

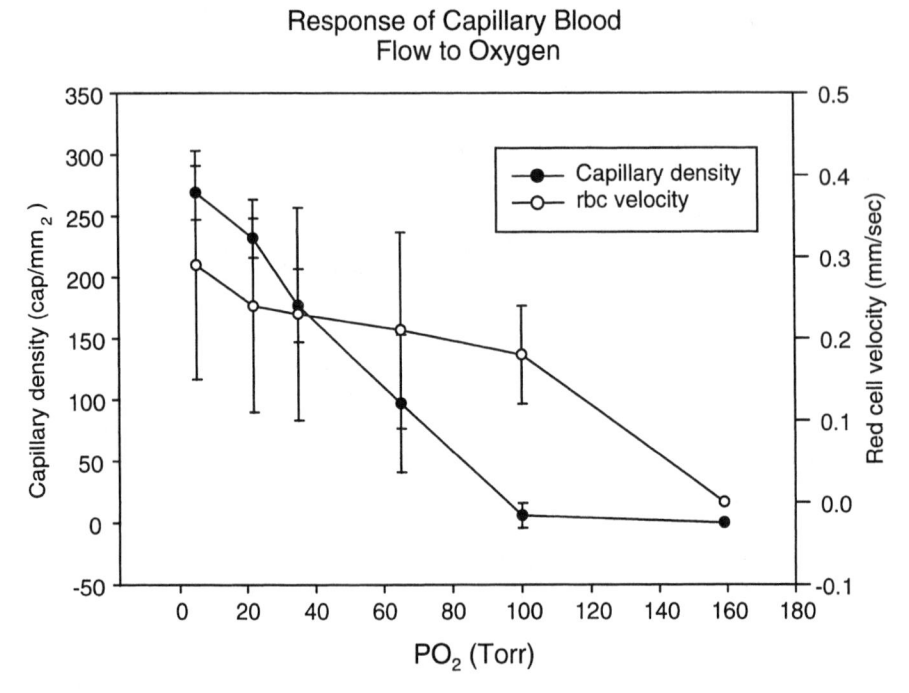

Figure 5 Response of rabbit skeletal muscle capillary blood flow to oxygen levels. The oxygen in the fluid superfusing a skin window preparation was controlled at various levels, and the number of flowing capillaries and red blood cell velocity in the open capillaries were counted. Capillary density shows a striking dependence on oxygen partial pressure, whereas red blood cell velocity shows somewhat in the open vessels. (Data from Ref. 50.)

arterial blood supply in the rat skeletal muscle. Although vascular tone is nonuniform along the various levels of the arterial circulation, systematic measurements have shown that the highest tone in the arterioles occurs at the transition from the arcade arterioles to the transverse arterioles [53]. These vessels have significantly greater nerve density, and their diameters range from 10 to 35 μm (Table 3). Saltzman et al. [54] have shown that major reduction of pressure occurs along these vessels, which are encased in a single continuous smooth muscle layer and are capable of closing their lumen, thus exerting total control over capillary blood flow. It seems, then, that in the rat spinotrapezius muscle, the overall flow of blood to the muscle is controlled by a central neural mechanism in the proximal supply arteries (200–300 μm), but that the transverse arterioles (5–35 μm) control blood flow to individual capillary beds. Ping and Johnson [55] found that without sympathetic nerve stimulation, all orders of arterioles, except first-order, dilated in reaction to pressure reduction. With sympathetic nerve stimulation, dilation was enhanced in

Role of Hemoglobin in O_2 Delivery

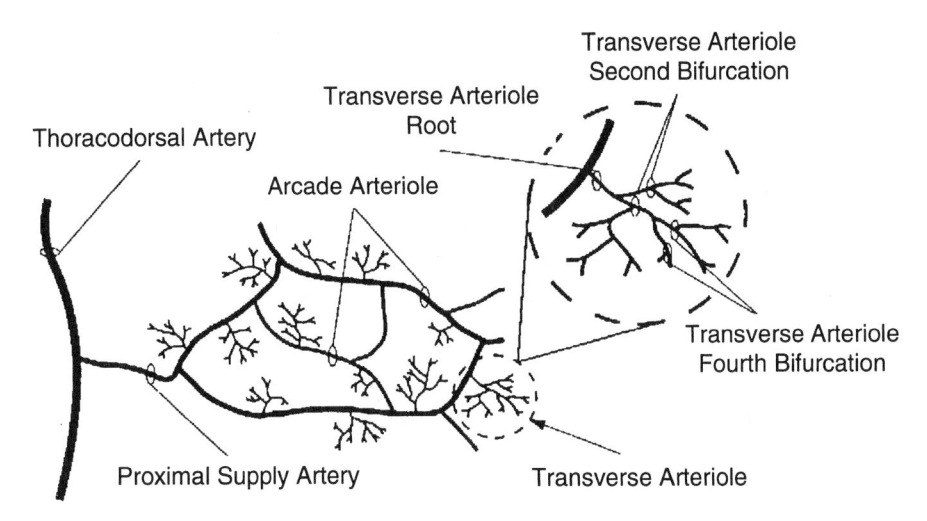

Figure 6 Tracing of the branched vessels in rat skeletal muscle. The diameters of the vessels at the various levels and their degree of adrenergic innervation are given in Table 1. (From Ref. 53.)

all six orders of arterioles, and flow increased significantly. Calculated wall shear stress for first-, second-, and third-order arterioles decreased significantly during pressure reduction.

These studies seem to argue in favor of two complementary but balancing components in autoregulation: one mediated by the sympathetic nervous system with 200–300-μm vessels and the other by a local endothelium-mediated mech-

Table 3 Diameter and Relative Innervation of Arterioles in Skeletal Muscle of Wistar-Kyoto Rats

Vessel	Diameter (μm)	Mean plexus length per surface area ± SD (μm/μm^2)
Artery	400–500	0.083 ± .019
Proximal supply artery	200–300	0.063 ± .014
Arcade arteriole	20–60	0.063 ± .023
Transverse arteriole root	10–35	[a]0.095 ± .043
Transverse arteriole, 2nd bifurcation	5–10	0.044 ± .041
Transverse arteriole, 4th bifurcation	5–10	0.019 ± .025
Capillary	5	0

[a] $P < .001$ compared with Arcade arterioles.
Source: Ref. 53.

anism in the 30–50-μm vessels. It is the latter point of regulation at which the hemoglobin OEC is likely to directly offset local tissue perfusion.

Another indication of the importance of the OEC in the local regulation of vascular tone is the observation by Smiesko et al. [56] that dilation of arcading arterioles in rat mesentery followed local vasooclusion. These investigators found that vasodilation closely correlated ($r = 0.96$) with a delay of 7.7 seconds. Increased red blood cell flow velocity decreases O_2 release in a flowing vessel [57], indicating a potent flow-dependent mechanism for regulating O_2 delivery to tissue.

Our main concern is with the nature of the control of the small (30–50 μm) vessels, which seem to control capillary blood flow. The transverse arterioles (10–35 μm) are known to be sensitive to myogenic mechanisms as well as P_{O_2} [50], but the larger arcade (20–60 μm) vessels may be more sensitive to myogenic and flow-dependent mechanisms, such as EDRF [56,58].

III. Nitric Oxide as the Endothelium-Derived Relaxing Factor

If the OEC plays an important role in regulation of local blood flow in 30–50-μm vessels, the next question concerns the mechanism of this interaction, i.e., does the mechanism involve O_2 signaling directly or is some other molecule, such as EDRF, the primary mediator? It is known that endothelium is capable of producing a factor(s) with vasorelaxant properties (EDRF) [59]. Pharmacological studies have tentatively identified EDRF as NO [60], although other nitrosylated compounds, primarily nitrosothiols, have also been proposed for this role. For example, Feelisch et al. [61] compared a number of compounds in their half-life and reactivity with hemoglobin to add circumstantial evidence to the argument that NO is, in fact, EDRF (Table 4).

The identity of NO as EDRF was based, in large part, on experiments in which aortic strips were superfused with hemoglobin solutions, showing that in this case, vasorelaxation was inhibited, presumably because of the scavenging of NO by hemoglobin. The NO–HbFe$_{II}$ reaction is well studied, and it is known that NO binds at the heme iron of hemoglobin with very high affinity [62].

If NO is EDRF, there are many aspects of its effects that remain to be explained. NO exists in solutions as NO$^{\cdot}$, and it is a highly reactive species, capable of reacting with HbFe$_{II}$ (at heme sites), with β93Cys (a nitrosyl reaction), and with molecular O_2. Because the half-life of NO$^{\cdot}$ is only a few seconds, it has been extremely difficult to show in a definitive way all of its physiological functions. The thiols listed in Table 1 can inactivate NO at low concentrations, but at high concentrations can act as NO donors. The latter possibility was suggested by Jia et al. [2], who proposed that NO, generated in the lung, could be transported to tissue sites as S-nitrosohemoglobin, where it then would be available to donate NO. Key to this proposed mechanism is the concept of O_2 as an allosteric effector

Table 4 EDRF Candidates

Compound	Half-life in bioassay (seconds)	Oxyhemoglobin *IC50[a] (nmol/L)
EDRF	3–5	25
NO	3–5	25
S-nitrosocysteine	4–6	40
S-nitrosystamine	4–6	40
Dinitrosyl-iron-cysteine complex	Not measurable	> 100
Hydroxylamine	Not measurable	> 300
Sodium nitroxyl	Not measurable	> 300

[a]Concentration of oxyhemoglobin at which the compound is 50% inhibited.
EDRF, endothelin-derived relaxing factor; NO, nitric oxide.
Source: Ref. 61.

of NO binding, i.e., in the deoxy (T) state, NO is more likely to dissociate from S-nitrosohemoglobin than in the oxy (R) state (Fig. 2). Jia et al. [2] showed that the S-nitrosohemoglobin concentration is significantly different in the arterial and mixed venous circulation of the rat (Table 2).

Nitric oxide is produced in endothelial cells and diffuses outward to react with the heme group of guanylate cyclase in myocytes of vascular smooth muscle and in platelets in the vessels [63]. NO can stimulate the activity of guanylate cyclase in smooth muscle up to 200-fold [64]. This reaction results in a shift in the equilibrium between bound and free calcium such that vasorelaxation occurs. The diffusion of NO through aqueous solution is limited by its redox reaction with free O_2, which occurs rapidly and results in the production of nitrite:

$$4NO + O_2 + H_2O \rightarrow 4H^+ + 4NO_2^- \tag{5}$$

The equilibrium equation for this reaction is:

$$\frac{d[NO]}{dt} = k[NO]^2[O_2] \tag{6}$$

Kharitonov et al. [65] studied this reaction in the stopped-flow apparatus and reported a value of k of 6.3 ($\pm$0.4) $\times$ 10^6 (mol/L^{-1})2 s^{-2}. Using this value of k, Eq. (3), and concentrations of NO and O_2 of 100 nm and 230 μmol/L, respectively, these investigators calculated the simple half-life (i.e., the time for halving the concentration of NO concentration) to be approximately 2 hours. They went on to speculate that even if the concentration reached the level of 4 μmol/L, the half-life of NO would be approximately 3 minutes for the autoxidation [Eq. (2)] reaction. Therefore, the oxidation reaction is probably so slow that it will not impede the diffusion of NO from its site of synthesis in the endothelium to either its target, guanylate cyclase, or to red blood cells in the vessels.

The novel mechanism proposed by Stamler et al. to explain this observation of increased SNO-Hb in the arterial blood compared with venous blood proposes that when O_2 demand is high, NO promotes the local release of O_2. One difficulty with this proposal was that it seemed to require the generation of NO in the lung, which could then bind to β93Cys. However, the mechanism was attractive because it linked the allosteric transition of hemoglobin to the regulation of blood flow. The same investigators subsequently proposed that the source of NO in the lung was, in fact, hemoglobin itself: that when deoxy hemoglobin combines with O_2, the allosteric T–R transition favors a migration of heme-bound NO to the sulfhydryl-bound NO. Thus, hemoglobin can scavenge NO in tissue sites with very high affinity, carrying to it the lung, where some of it redistributes to SNO and is now available to be released in tissues, where it can act as a vasodilator [44].

There are two unresolved issues in regard to this mechanism that will require additional experimentation. First, NO is bound to heme as NO˙ but to β93Cys at NO^-, which has to be converted to NO˙ in the transition to heme-binding. One candidate for the electron acceptor in this conversion is O_2 itself. The second problem is that the NO released from SNO may require a carrier molecule that is itself diffusible and that can reach vascular smooth muscle in a manner to act as a vasorelaxant. There are a number of thiol-containing proteins in plasma that could fill this role. In the red blood cell, glutathione could serve this purpose (Fig. 2). In the case of cell-free hemoglobin, hemoglobin itself could act as such a transporter (see Section IV.D).

IV. Cell-Free Hemoglobin: New Tools to Study Oxygen Transport

Cell-free hemoglobin, modified to reduce its rate of clearance, is an attractive candidate for a "blood substitute" [10]. Developing these solutions has been costly, and many problems in their clinical implementation remain to be solved. But the fact that so many of their physical properties (e.g., viscosity, O_2 affinity, and other solution properties) make them interesting probes of the microvascular O_2 transport mechanisms.

The loose interface between $\alpha\beta$ dimers is of critical importance for hemoglobin-based blood substitutes. The equilibrium constant for this dissociation reaction is 10^{-6} mol/L for oxyhemoglobin, which means that as hemoglobin concentration decreases, the relative proportion of dimeric molecules increases. These dimers are very quickly and efficiently filtered in the glomerulus of the kidney. Mechanisms to remove dimers that are present when mild hemolysis occurs include haptoglobin binding, which can remove free hemoglobin in concentrations up to 200 mg/dL. When this threshold is exceeded, renal clearance of hemoglobin is very high, and renal toxicity may result.

A. Brief Description of Available Solutions

Many chemical modifications of hemoglobin have been devised (Table 5). The purposes of these modifications are to prevent tetramar–dimer dissociation, modulate O_2 affinity, and prolong vascular retention. They take advantage of several reactive sites on the surface of hemoglobin, in its internal cavity, and at the amino terminus.

Internally Cross-Linked Hemoglobins

One of the most useful model hemoglobins for experimentation ($\alpha\alpha$-hemoglobin) incorporates a single covalent cross-link between α-deoxyhemoglobin lysine α99 residues with the reagent 3,5-bis(dibromosalicyl)fumarate [66]. This single modification at once binds $\alpha\beta$ dimers together and reduces the O_2 affinity of cell-free molecules to approximately that of intact human red blood cells. When cross-linking is conducted with oxygenated hemoglobin, the dimensions of the internal cavity change enough so that the reaction occurs between β82 lysines. In this case, the final cross-linked product has a much higher O_2 affinity than that of the deoxy cross-linked product. This material can also be produced easily but has been less well studied because its O_2 affinity has been traditionally thought to be too high to be physiologically or clinically useful.

A unique class of cross-linkers, trimesic acid derivatives, result in three-point reactions [67]. In early reports, the resulting modified hemoglobins that result seem to be stable, and the reaction seems to have a high degree of specificity.

A variation on this 64,000-kd-molecular-weight hemoglobin is the genetically produced "rHb1.1" [68], in which cross-linking is performed genetically. In this case, two α chain genes are introduced into the *Escherichia coli* genome such that when they are transcribed, a single gene product results in which one α chain

Table 5 Classes of Hemoglobin-Based Products

Class	Examples	Intravascular persistence (hours)	Oncotic pressure	Viscosity	Vasoactivity
Cross-linked tetramers	HemeAssist[a] Optro[a]	~12	Low	Low	Marked
Polymerized tetramers	HemoPure[b] HemoLink[c] PolyHeme[d]	~12–24	Low	Low	Moderate
Surface-modified tetramers	PHP[e] PEG–hemoglobin[f]	~24–48	Moderate to high	Moderate to high	Mild

[a]Baxter, Round Lake, IL. [b]BioPure, Cambridge, MA. [c]Hemosol, Toronto, Canada. [d]Northfield, Chicago, IL. [e]Apex Bioscience, Research Triangle Park, NC. [f]Enzon, Piscataway, NJ.
PHP, pyridoxal hemoglobin polyoxyethylene; PEG, polyethylene glycol.

is contiguous with the other (dialpha peptide). A second mutation (Presbyterian, β108 Asn → Lys) is also engineered into rHb1.1. The purpose of this mutation is to lower the O_2 affinity such that the P50 of the final product is 33 mm Hg (control, 28 mm Hg). Thus, the product has a molecular weight of 64,000 kd and does not dissociate in to dimers. Its physiological properties are similar to $\alpha\alpha$-hemoglobin.

Other cross-linking agents are analogs of 2,3-DPG. Nor-formyl pyridoxal phosphate (NFPLP), a prototype of such a cross-linker, binds in the 2,3-DPG "pocket" between β chains and has the dual effects of preventing dimerization and reducing O_2 affinity. This product has been extensively studied [69], but, unfortunately, the cross-linker itself is difficult to synthesize, and scale-up has not been achieved practically.

All of the internally cross-linked hemoglobins share certain properties in common. Their molecular weight is close to that of native hemoglobin (64,000 d), they have very low viscosity, close to that of plasma, and short vascular retention times (approximately 12 hours). The colloid osmotic (oncotic) pressure of these hemoglobins is somewhat higher than human blood at an equivalent hemoglobin concentration; therefore, most have been formulated at lower concentration so that they will be isooncotic. All of the products seem to show some degree of vasoactivity when injected into animals.

Polymerized Hemoglobins

Perhaps the greatest experience is with polymerized hemoglobin. Sehgal et al. [70] reported polymerization of pyridoxalated human hemoglobin with the bifunctional reagent glutaraldehyde. Subsequently, these products have been extensively developed and are currently being studied in advanced clinical trials. The product has a molecular weight distribution between 120,000 and 600,000 d, a P50 of 16 mm Hg, a Bohr effect reduced by half, reduced cooperativity, and viscosity approximately half that of whole blood. In addition, many variations on the polymerization reaction have been developed with different cross-linking agents and different source hemoglobins, such as bovine. Although direct comparisons have not been reported, polymerized hemoglobins seem to be somewhat less vasoactive than intramolecular cross-linked hemoglobins.

Conjugated Hemoglobins

Conjugated hemoglobins are those to which some modifying molecule has been attached to the surface. Modifying groups include polyethylene glycol [71], polyoxyethylene [72], or dextran [73]. These products have increased molecular weights, depending on the number and size of the modifying groups, but are relatively easy to produce. Increasing the molecular size may also increase the hydration shell around the protein molecule in the case of polyoxyethylene and polyethylene glycol, and may thereby restrict the reaction of hemoglobin with other molecules in the cell-free environment. The products may show high viscosity and oncotic pressure out of proportion to their molecular mass [74].

Finally, nonspecific reagents can react with any of the 44 ϵ-amino lysine groups on the surface of hemoglobin or the four amino-terminal groups. Such bifunctional reactants include glutaraldehyde and ring-opened sugars (e.g., raffinose) and have been used in at least two of the products presently in clinical trials. Although the modification reactions are clearly understood, chemically, the extent of reaction can sometimes be difficult to control, and a range of product molecular weights may result [75].

Surface-modified hemoglobins, especially those modified with polyethylene glycol, seem to be the least vasoactive of the hemoglobin derivatives [76]. However, they tend to have high viscosity and oncotic pressure compared with the other types of modified hemoglobins. They also have the largest intravascular retention, with half-times of disappearance up to 2 days.

B. Vasoactivity

Vasoconstriction is one of the most perplexing problems in the development of a safe and efficacious red blood cell substitute. When infused into animals and humans, many hemoglobin-based solutions produce significant hypertension, increased vascular resistance, and decreased O_2 transport. This phenomenon has been observed in both the systemic and pulmonary circulations in models of clinical use [77,78] and in humans [79].

A common explanation for the vasoactivity is the avidity with which hemoglobin combines with NO, the EDRF. However, the NO affinity of model hemoglobins does not correlate with the effect on mean arterial blood pressure in rats [80], and it is possible that oversupply of O_2 due to diffusion of oxyhemoglobin or removal of NO due to diffusion of HbNO also plays an additional, if not exclusive, role.

C. Viscosity

Traditional thought concerning blood viscosity predicts that reduced viscosity should reduce vascular resistance to flow and increase cardiac output. The exponential dependence of viscosity on hematocrit is well known, and in pathological conditions, such as ischemia, better oxygenation of tissues by blood with lower hematocrit can be demonstrated [81], establishing that in the case of red blood cell O_2 transport, flow can be more important than O_2 content.

Early studies with cell-free hemoglobin [82,83] were aimed at developing solutions with low viscosity at low shear rates. Experiments do couple hemoglobin with hydroxyethylstarch showed that such conjugates had increased viscosity relative to hemoglobin alone and therefore were predicted to be unfavorable as plasma expanders. Recent work by Intaglietta et al. [84] has suggested that perhaps this is, in fact, incorrect. Instead, they have proposed that microvascular viscosity is related to maintenance of a certain level of wall shear stress [58] on the endothelium, and, when this is altered (e.g., in hemodilution or hemorrhage), control of vasoactive substances such as endothelin and prostaglandins might be potent regulators of capillary perfusion [85]. Viscosity of cell-free hemoglobin also directly affects the diffusion of oxyhemoglobin in solution.

D. Facilitated Diffusion

As predicted [86–88], O_2 transport by cell-free hemoglobin is clearly different from O_2 transport by red blood cells. Rosen et al. [89] found that when animals were exchange-transfused with hemoglobin solutions, cardiac output did not change as predicted on the basis of blood viscosity, even when total hemoglobin content was accounted for. Gould et al. [90] could not distinguish between the possibility that O_2 transport was so efficient that increased cardiac output was not necessary, and the possibility that cardiac output was limited by increased peripheral resistance. The work of the United States Army group [77] with hemoglobin solutions and that of Liard et al. [27] with inositol hexaphosphate (IHP)-loaded red blood cells supports the latter interpretation.

Attempts to demonstrate augmented transport by O_2 diffusion in vivo by cell-free hemoglobin have been unsuccessful [91–93]. In normal blood, O_2 moves from the red blood cell to the vessel wall by simple diffusion. When hemoglobin is present in the plasma space, O_2 can also move bound to hemoglobin as oxyhemoglobin (Fig. 7). This second process is called "facilitated diffusion" [94].

Arterioles, particularly at the A2/A3 level, have been shown, unexpectedly, to consume large amounts of O_2 by a novel technique to measure O_2 concentration in localized areas of the microcirculation [45], indicating that they are capable of prodigious metabolic activity. Innervation of these arterioles is particularly dense [53], which suggests that they regulate downstream capillary blood flow. Increasing the O_2 available to these arterioles would be expected to be a potent stimulus to engage mechanisms that regulate the delivery of O_2 to capillary beds (autoregulation). The exact biochemical mechanism(s) that underlie these events could be mediated by O_2- or NO-sensitive pathways. The presence of hemoglobin, free in the plasma space, as in a blood substitute, will predictably engage these mechanisms because of its capacity for facilitated diffusion.

The transport of O_2 in the blood by two pathways (O_2 and oxyhemoglobin diffusion) can be expressed mathematically as the transport (flux, $-J$) of O_2 to the vessel wall, which is the sum of the diffusion of free (O_2) and chemically bound oxygen (oxyhemoglobin):

$$-J = \frac{D_{O_2}\alpha \Delta P_{O_2}}{\Delta X} + \frac{D_{HbO_2}[Hb]_T \Delta Y}{\Delta X} \tag{7}$$

where D_{O_2} and D_{HbO_2} are the diffusion constants for O_2 and cell-free oxyhemoglobin, respectively, α is the solubility of O_2 in plasma, ΔP_{O_2} is the difference in P_{O_2} inside and outside the vessel, ΔY is the gradient of hemoglobin saturation from the center of the vessel to its wall, and $[Hb]_T$ is the total cell-free hemoglobin concentration. D_{O_2} and D_{HbO_2} have been measured experimentally in static solution (Table 6). The distance for diffusion, ΔX, is considered to be the same for the two molecules, O_2 and oxyhemoglobin.

Role of Hemoglobin in O_2 Delivery

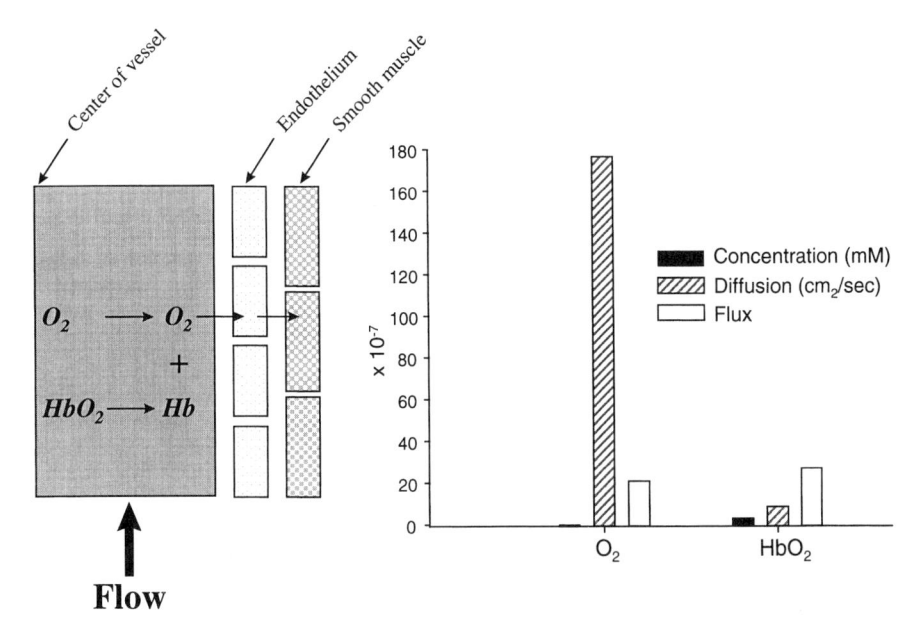

Figure 7 Facilitated diffusion. The figure shows the movement of free, dissolved oxygen and oxyhemoglobin. The right panel shows graphically the relationships in Table 6. When hemoglobin is present in the plasma space, the contribution to the total oxygen flux to tissues at oxygen partial pressure of 100 mm Hg is doubled compared with the normal situation in which oxygen is transported dissolved in plasma. This remarkable fact is caused by the very low solubility of oxygen in plasma.

Table 6 shows that D_{HbO_2} is approximately 1/20 of D_{O_2}. However, because the solubility of O_2 in plasma is low ($\alpha = 1.2074$ μmol/L/mm Hg), and D_{O_2} is relatively high, when plasma hemoglobin concentration is only 3 mmol/L (4.83 g/dL) at P_{O_2} of 100 mm Hg, the product of diffusion and concentration [the numerators in Eq. (1)] for free O_2 and oxyhemoglobin are nearly equal. Thus, plasma hemoglobin contributes as much O_2 as dissolved O_2, effectively doubling the amount of O_2

Table 6 Oxygen Flux, the Product of Oxygen and Oxyhemoglobin Diffusion

	Concentration at 100 mm Hg (mmol/L)	Diffusion constant[a] (cm^2/sec)	Flux (concentration × diffusion)
Oxygen	0.1207	177 × 10^{-7}	2.48 × 10^{-6}
Oxyhemoglobin	3	9.15 × 10^{-7}	2.74 × 10^{-6}

[a]Mean values from Wittenberg (94) and Bouwer et al. (95).

available from red blood cells. These relationships are shown quantitatively in Fig. 7.

Further analysis of Eq. (7) provides a conceptual framework on which to consider strategies to defeat this mechanism. The gradient along which oxyhemoglobin diffuses is $[Hb]_T \Delta Y$ and the distance through which oxyhemoglobin must diffuse (ΔX_{HbO_2}). The quantity ΔY at a given P_{O_2} is the slope of the OEC at that P_{O_2} and is dependent on the shape of the curve (a property of the hemoglobin molecule) and its position (i.e., P50).

V. Summary and Hypothesis: The OEC Is a Critical Link in Oxygen Signal Transduction

The control of O_2 delivery to tissues is complex and highly redundant. It seems that the vasculature of tissues is excessive in regard to O_2 demand. Thus, Skinner [96] estimated that if the vascular beds of all tissues were maximally dilated, the amount of blood flow required to sustain a blood pressure of 100 mm Hg would be in the range of 40–50 L/min, whereas the maximal human cardiac output is only approximately about 25 L/min. Thus, the distribution of blood flow must be peripherally regulated, and shunting or heterogeneity of flow must be essential to any comprehensive description of O_2 delivery to tissue.

It is likely that blood flow is controlled by a balance of central and local regulatory mechanisms. We hypothesize that the central mechanism, mediated by chemoreceptor activity, probably acts through myogenic mechanisms at the arterial/arteriolar level, whereas local mechanisms are mediated by the ability of hemoglobin to regulate the vessel/tissue O_2 gradient. These latter mechanisms may also include hemoglobin–NO interactions and, in the case of cell-free hemoglobin, facilitated diffusion as well.

The hypothesis has been suggested that blood flow is regulated to maintain tissue P_{O_2} in myocardium [49]. Thus, when O_2 demand increases, extraction also increases because of perfusion of capillary beds previously without flow. Granger et al. [97] suggested that the terminal arterioles are more sensitive to tissue P_{O_2} than are the larger vessels; hence, relatively small changes in their diameter could have large effects on capillary perfusion.

The role of O_2 as a vasoconstrictor is a critical concept. Vasoconstriction at the arteriolar level will have two distinct effects: the number of functional capillaries will be reduced, and the flow velocity through the patent vessels will be increased. Both will reduce tissue P_{O_2}. Johnson and colleagues cited earlier literature to support the idea that dilation of the pial vessels after pressure reduction is abolished when O_2-rich solutions are superfused over the tissue [49,55], and similar findings were reported by Sullivan and Johnson [98,99]. More recent studies by Lindom et al. [47,50,51] add further evidence that O_2 is a vasoconstrictor.

Thus, a very attractive hypothesis is that when O_2 demand is high, the OEC shifts to the right, releasing O_2 and steepening the vessel/tissue diffusion gradient.

The role, if any, of NO in the link between O_2 demand and local blood flow is not yet clearly defined. The postulated allosteric mechanisms [2,9,44] are persuasive but not yet compelling. Much work needs to be performed to fully understand the physiological importance of these mechanisms.

These discussions of the effect of O_2 on local regulation of blood flow do not shed light on possible mechanisms of control. In other words, how is a signal (increased tissue O_2 demand) transduced into a response (increased capillary blood flow)? Attempts to show that O_2 directly affects arteriolar diameter (100) were only partially successful, in that such constriction could be seen only at relatively high PaO_2. Possible metabolites that could be formed or released in response to O_2 demands include prostaglandins [101] with vasodilator properties that tend to reduce basal vascular tension. It is difficult to design experiments that can be unambiguously interpreted because perturbation of O_2 delivery (e.g., hematocrit hemoglobin changes) also affect viscosity. In turn, local shear forces are now known to be transduced into local metabolic changes in endothelial cells.

Understanding how the local supply of O_2 to tissues is modulated by its interaction with hemoglobin is critical to the understanding of a wide variety of processes of biological and clinical importance. For example, vascular endothelial growth factor is a strong determinant of the rate of tumor growth, and its expression is mediated, at least in part, by a hypoxia inducible factor (HIF-1) [102]. The regulation of cerebral blood flow by O_2 and CO_2 may also be linked to NO metabolism by the effects of hypoxia on NO synthase [103]. Finally, the expression of erythropoietin is linked to O_2 supply through HIF-1–mediated mechanisms that are being studied intensively [104,105].

Thus, although the blood OEC has been studied for more than a century, its intricacies and implications for understanding basic physiological and biochemical processes are still yielding exciting new insights. It is even possible that if the role of the OEC is better understood, new useful transfusion products might be designed to benefit patients.

Acknowledgment

The author acknowledges with gratitude the many helpful discussions with Drs. Marcos Intaglietta, Paul Johnson, Kim Vandegriff, and Ron Rohlfs, and the expert assistance of Renee Schad in preparation of the manuscript. This work was supported in part by grant no. 5 P01 HL48018 from the National Institutes of Health, National Heart, Lung and Blood Institute, Bethesda, MD.

References

1. Winslow RM, Vandergriff KD. Oxygen-hemoglobin dissociation curve. In: Crystal RG, West JB, Barnes PJ, Weibel ER, eds. The Lung: Scientific Foundation. 2nd ed. Philadelphia: Raven, 1997, pp 1625–1632.

2. Jia L, Bonaventura J, Stamler JS. S-nitrosohaemoglobin: a dynamic activity of blood involved in vascular control. Nature 1996; 380:221–226.
3. Hurtado A. Studies at high altitude: blood observations in the Indian natives of the Peruvian Andes. Am J Physiol 1932; 100:487–505.
4. Winslow RM, Monge CC, Statham NJ, Gibson CG, Charache S, Whittembury J, Moran O, Berger RL. Variability of oxygen affinity of blood: human subjects native to high altitude. J Appl Physiol 1981; 51:1411–1416.
5. Winslow RM, Samaja M, West JB. Red cell function at extreme altitude on Mount Everest. J Appl Physiol 1984; 56:109–116.
6. Hurtado A. Animals in high altitudes: resident man. In: Handbook of Physiology. Adaptation to the Environment. Washington, DC: American Physiological Society, 1964.
7. Kerger H, Torres Filho IP, Rivas M, Intaglietta M. Systemic and subcutaneous microvascular oxygen tension in conscious Syrian golden hamsters. Am J Physiol 1995; 268:H802–H810.
8. Torres Filho IP, Kerger H, Intaglietta M. Po_2 measurements in arteriolar networks. Microvasc Res 1996; 51:202–212.
9. Stamler J, Jia L, Eu JP, McMahon TJ, Demchenko IT, Bonaventura J, Gernert K, Piantadosi CA. Blood flow regulation by S-nitrosohemoglobin in the physiological oxygen gradient. Science 1997; 276:2034–2037.
10. Winslow RM. Hemoglobin-Based Red Cell Substitutes. Baltimore: Johns Hopkins University Press, 1992.
11. Barcroft J. Features in the Architecture of Physiological Function. London: Cambridge University Press, 1934.
12. Eaton JW, Skelton TD, Berger E. Survival at extreme altitude: protective effect of increased hemoglobin-oxygen affinity. Science 1974; 185:743–744.
13. Hebbel RP, Eaton JW, Kronenberg RS, Zanjani ED, Moore LG, Berger E. Human llamas: adaptation to altitude in subjects with high hemoglobin oxygen affinity. J Clin Invest 1978; 62:593–600.
14. Kleeberg UR, Ruhle KH, Schilling M, Freitag M, Schlehe H, Konietzko N, Matthys H. Adaptation of the oxygen affinity of haemoglobin in acute hypoxia. Eur J Clin Invest 1974; 4:45–51.
15. Stein JC, Ellsworth ML. Capillary oxygen transport during severe hypoxia: role of hemoglobin oxygen affinity. J Appl Physiol 1993; 75:1601–1607.
16. Charache S, Weatherall DJ, Clegg JB. Polycythemia associated with a hemoglobinopathy. J Clin Invest 1966; 45:813–822.
17. Reissmann KR, Ruth WE, Nomura T. A human hemoglobin with lowered oxygen affinity and impaired heme-heme interactions. J Clin Invest 1961; 40:1826–1833.
18. Martin JL, Duvelleroy M, Teisseire B, Duruble M. Effect of an increase in HbO_2 affinity on the calculated capillary recruitment of an isolated rat heart. Pflugers Arch 1979; 382:57–61.
19. Hogan MD, Bebout DE, Wagner PD. Effect of increased O_2 affinity on $\dot{V}o_2$max at constant O_2 delivery in dog muscle in situ. J Appl Physiol 1991; 70:2656–2662.
20. Woodson RD, Fitzpatrick JH, Costello DJ, Gilboe DD. Increased blood oxygen affinity decreases canine brain oxygen consumption. J Lab Clin Med 1982; 100:411–424.

21. Pantely GA, Oyama AA, Metcalfe J, Lawson MS, Welch JE. Improvement in the relationship between flow to ischemic myocardium and the extent of necrosis with glycolytic intermediates that decrease blood oxygen affinity in dogs. Circ Res 1981; 49:395–404.
22. Rude RE, Tumas J, Gunst M, Kloner RA, DeBoer LW, Maroko PR. Effects of ortho-iodo sodium benzoate on acute myocardial ischemia, hemodynamic function, and infarct size after coronary artery occlusion in dogs. Am J Cardiol 1983; 51:1422–1427.
23. Teisseire BP, Ropars C, Vallez MO, Herigault RA, Nicolau C. Physiological effects of high-P50 erythrocyte transfusion on piglets. Am Physiol Soc 1985; 58:1810–1817.
24. Curtis SE, Walker TA, Bradley WE, Cain WM. Raising P50 increases tissue Po_2 in canine skeletal muscle but does not affect critical O_2 extraction ratio. J Appl Physiol 1997; 83:1681–1689.
25. Walley KR. Heterogeneity of oxygen delivery impairs oxygen extraction by peripheral tissues: theory. J Appl Physiol 1996; 81:885–894.
26. Kohzuki H, Enoki Y, Matsumura K, Sakata S, Shimizu S. Flow-dependent influence of high-O_2-affinity erythrocytes on peak $\dot{V}o_2$ in exercising muscle in situ. J Appl Physiol 1996; 80:832–838.
27. Liard JF, Kunert MP. Hemodynamic changes induced by low blood oxygen affinity in dogs. Am J Physiol 1993; 264:R396–R401.
28. Adair GS. The hemoglobin system VI: the oxygen dissociation curve of hemoglobin. J Biol Chem. 1925; 63:529–545.
29. Winslow RM, Swenberg ML, Berger RL, Shrager RI, Luzzana M, Samaja M, Rossi-Bernardi L. Oxygen equilibrium curve of normal human blood and its evaluation by Adair's equation. J Biol Chem 1977; 252:2331–2337.
30. Winslow RM, Samaja M, Winslow NJ, Rossi-Bernardi L, Shrager RI. Simulation of the continuous O_2 equilibrium curve over the physiologic range of pH, 2,3-diphosphoglycerate, and pCO_2. J Appl Physiol 1983; 54:524–529.
31. Antonini E, Brunori M. Hemoglobin and Myoglobin in Their Reactions with Ligands. New York: Elsevier Science, 1971.
32. Monod J, Wyman J, Changeaux J. On the nature of allosteric transitions: a plausible model. J Mol Biol 1965; 12:88–118.
33. Bolton W, Perutz MF. Three dimensional fourier synthesis of horse deoxyhemoglobin at 2 Angstrom units resolution. Nature (London) 1970; 228:551–552.
34. Bohr C, Hasselbalch KA, Krogh A. Uber einen in biologischer Bezeihung wichtigen Einfluss, den die Kohlensaurespannung des Blutes auf dessen Saurstoffbindung. Scand Arch Physiol 1904; 16:402–412.
35. Kilmartin JV, Rossi-Bernardi L. Interaction of hemoglobin with hydrogen ions, Carbon dioxide, and organic phosphates. Physiol Rev 1973; 53:836–890.
36. Kilmartin JV, Fogg J, Rossi-Bernardi L. Identification of the high and low affinity CO_2-binding sites of human haemoglobin. Nature (London) 1975; 256:759–761.
37. Benesch R, Benesch RE. The effect of organic phosphates from the human erythrocyte on the allosteric properties of hemoglobin. Biochem Biophys Res Comm 1967; 26:162–167.
38. Lenfant C, Sullivan K. Adaptation to high altitude. N Engl J Med 1971; 284:1298–1309.

39. Arnone A. X-ray diffraction study of binding of 2,3-diphosphoglycerate to human deoxyhemoglobin. Nature (London) 1972; 237:146–149.
40. Kilmartin JV, Fogg J, Luzzana M, Rossi-Bernardi L. Role of the α-amino groups of the α and β chains of human hemoglobin on oxygen-linked binding of carbon dioxide. J Biol Chem 1973; 248:7039–7043.
41. Vandegriff KD, Olson JS. Morphological and physiological factors affecting oxygen uptake and release by red blood cells. J Biol Chem 1984; 259:12619–12627.
42. Boland EJ, Nair PK, Lemon DD, Olson JS, Hellums JD. An in vitro capillary system for studies on microcirculatory O_2 transport. J Appl Physiol 1987; 62:791–797.
43. Lemon DJ, Nair PK, Boland EF, Olson JS, Hellums JD. Physiological factors affecting O_2 transport by hemoglobin in an in vitro capillary system. J Appl Physiol 1987; 62:798–806.
44. Gow AJ, Stamler JS. Reactions between nitric oxide and haemoglobin under physiological conditions. Nature 1998; 391:169–173.
45. Torres Filho IP, Intaglietta M. Microvessel Po_2 measurement of phosphorescence decay method. Am J Physiol 1993; 265:H1434–H1438.
46. Winslow RM. A model for red cell O_2 uptake. Int J Clin Monit Comput 1985; 2:81–93.
47. Lindbom L, Mirhashemi S, Intaglietta M, Arfors K-E. Increase in capillary blood flow and relative haematocrit in rabbit skeletal muscle following acute normovolaemic anaemia. Acta Physiol Scand 1988; 134:503–512.
48. Krogh A. The supply of oxygen to the tissues and the regulation of the capillary circulation. J Physiol (London) 1919; 52:457–474.
49. Johnson PC. Brief review: autoregulation of blood flow. Circ Res 1986; 59:483–495.
50. Lindbom L, Tuma RF, Arfors KE. Influence of oxygen on perfusion capillary density and capillary red cell velocity in rabbit skeletal muscle. Microvasc Res 1980; 19:197–208.
51. Lindbom L, Arfors K-E. Mechanism and site of control for variation in the number of perfused capillaries in skeletal muscle. Int J Microcirc Clin Exp 1985; 4:121–127.
52. Mouren S, Souktani R, Beaussier M, Abdenour L, Arthaud M, Duvelleroy M, Vicaut E. Mechanisms of coronary vasoconstriction induced by high arterial oxygen tension. Am J Physiol 1997; 41:H67–H75.
53. Schmid-Schonbein GW, Zweifach BW, DeLano FA, Chen PCY. Microvascular tone in a skeletal muscle of spontaneously hypertensive rats. Hypertension 1987; 9:164–171.
54. Saltzman D, DeLano FA, Schmid-Schonbein GW. The microvasculature in skeletal muscle. VI. Adrenergic innervation of arterioles in normotensive and spontaneously hypertensive rats. Microvasc Res 1992; 44:263–273.
55. Ping P, Johnson PC. Arteriolar network response to pressure reduction during sympathetic nerve stimulation in cat skeletal muscle. Am J Physiol 1994; 266:H1251–H1259.
56. Smiesko V, Lang DJ, Johnson PC. Dilator response of rat mesenteric arcading arterioles to increased blood flow velocity. Am J Physiol 1989; 257:H1958–H1965.
57. Tsai AG, Intaglietta M. Local tissue oxygenation during constant red blood cell flux: a discrete source analysis of velocity and hematocrit changes. Microvasc Res 1989; 37:308–322.

Role of Hemoglobin in O_2 Delivery 645

58. Koller A, Kaley G. Endothelial regulation of wall shear stress and blood flow in skeletal muscle microcirculation. Am J Physiol 1991; 260:H862–H868.
59. Furchgott RF, Zawadzki JV. The obligatory role of endothelial cells in the relaxation of arterial smooth muscle by acetylcholine. Nature 1980; 288:373–376.
60. Palmer RMJ, Ferrige A, Moncada S. Nitric oxide release accounts for the biological activity of endothelium-derived relaxing factor. Nature 1987; 327:524–526.
61. Feelisch M, tePoel M, Zamora R, Deussen A, Moncada S. Understanding the controversy over the identity of EDRF. Nature 1994; 368:62–65.
62. Gibson QH. The kinetics of reactions between haemoglobin and gases. In: Butler JAV, Katz B, eds. Progress in Biophysics and Biophysical Chemistry. New York: Pergamon Press, 1959, pp 1–54.
63. Lancaster JR. Simulation of the diffusion and reaction of endogenously produced nitric oxide. Proceedings of the National Academy of Science (PNAS) 1994; 91:8137–8141.
64. Moncada S, Palmer RMJ, Higgs EA. Nitric oxide: physiology, pathophysiology, and pharmacology. Pharmacol Rev 1991; 43:109–142.
65. Kharitonov VG, Sundquist AR, Sharma VS. Kinetics of nitric oxide autoxidation in aqueous solution. J Biol Chem 1994; 269:5881–5883.
66. Walder JA, Zaugg RH, Walder RY, Steele JM, Klotz IM. Diaspirins that cross-link β chains of hemoglobin: bis(3,5-dibromosalicyl) succinate and bis(3,5-dibromosalicyl) fumarate. Biochemistry 1979; 18:4265–4270.
67. Kluger R, Wodzinska J, Jones RT, Head C, Fujita TS, Shih DT. Three-point crosslinking: potential red cell substitutes from the reaction of trimesoyl tris(methyl phosphate) with hemoglobin. Biochemistry 1992; 31:7551–7559.
68. Gerber MJ, Stetler GI, Templeton D. Recombinant human hemoglobin designed for use as an oxygen delivering therapeutic. In: Tsuchida E, ed. Artificial Red Cells. New York: Wiley, 1995, pp 187–197.
69. Bakker JC, Berbers GA, Bleeker WK, den Boer PJ, Biessels PT. Preparation and characterization of crosslinked and polymerized hemoglobin solutions. Biomater Artif Cells Immobil Biotechnol 1992; 20:233–241.
70. Sehgal LR, Rosen AL, Gould S, Sehgal H, Dalton L, Mayoral J, Moss G. In vitro and in vivo characteristics of polymerized pyridoxylated hemoglobin solution. Fed Proc 1979; 39:718.
71. Nho K, Glower D, Bredehoeft S, Shankar H, Shorr R, Abuchowski A. PEG-bovine hemoglobin: safety in a canine dehydrated hypovolemic-hemorrhagic shock model. Biomater Artif Cells Immobil Biotechnol 1992; 20:511–524.
72. Iwasaki K, Ajisaka K, Iwashita Y. Modification of human hemoglobin with polyethylene glycol: a new candidate for blood substitute. Biochem Biophys Res Comm 1983; 113:513–518.
73. Chang JE, Wong JTF. Synthesis of soluble dextran-hemoglobin complexes of different molecular sizes. Can J Biochem 1977; 55:398–403.
74. Vandegriff KD, McCarthy M, Rohlfs RJ, Winslow RM. Colloid osmotic properties of modified hemoglobins: chemically cross-linked versus polyethylene glycol surface-conjugated. Biophys Chem 1997; 69:23–30.
75. Marini MA, Moore GL, Fishman RM, Jesse R, Medina F, Snell SM, Zegna AI. Reexamination of the polymerization of pyridoxylated hemoglobin with glutaraldehyde. Biopolymers 1990; 29:871–882.

76. Winslow RM, Gonzales A, Gonzales M. Physiologic effects of hemoglobin-based oxygen carriers compared to red blood cells in acute hemorrhage. Blood 1996; 88:626a.
77. Hess JR, MacDonald VW, Brinkley WW. Systemic and pulmonary hypertension after resuscitation with cell-free hemoglobin. J Appl Physiol 1993; 74:1769–1778.
78. Keipert PE, Gonzales A, Gomez CL, MacDonald VW, Hess JR, Winslow RM. Acute changes in systemic blood pressure and urine output of conscious rats following exchange transfusion with diaspirin-crosslinked hemoglobin solution. Transfusion 1993; 33:701–708.
79. Kasper S-M, Walter M, Grune F, Bischoff A, Erasmi H, Buzello W. Effects of a hemoglobin-based oxygen carrier (HBOC-201) on hemodynamics and oxygen transport in patients undergoing preoperative hemodilution for elective abdominal aortic surgery. Cardiovasc Anesth 1996; 83:921–927.
80. Rohlfs RJ, Vandegriff KD, Winslow RM. The reaction of nitric oxide with cell-free hemoglobin based oxygen carriers: physiological implications. In: Winslow RM, Vandegriff KD, Intaglietta M, eds. Advances in Blood Substitutes: Industrial Opportunities and Medical Challenges. Boston: Birkhäuser, 1997, pp 298–327.
81. Stucker O, Trouve R, Vicaut E, Charansonney O, Teisseire B, Durele M, Duvelleroy M. Effects of different hematocrits on the isolated working rabbit heart reperfused after ischemia. Clin Exp 1985; 2:325–335.
82. Usami S, Chien S, Gregersen MI. Hemoglobin solution as a plasma expander: effects on blood viscosity. Proc Soc Exp Biol Med 1971; 136:1232–1235.
83. Cerny LC, Stasiw DM, Cerny EL. Biophysical properties of resuscitation fluids. Crit Care Med 1982; 10:254–260.
84. Intaglietta M, Johnson PC, Winslow RM. Microvascular and tissue oxygen distribution. Cardiovasc Res 1996; 32:632–643.
85. Kuchan MJ, Frangos JA. Shear stress regulates endothelin-1 release via protein kinase C and cGMP in cultured endothelial cells. Am J Physiol 1993; 264:H150–H156.
86. Homer LD, Weathersby PK, Kiesow LA. Oxygen gradients between red blood cells in the microcirculation. Microvasc Res 1981; 22:308–323.
87. Federspiel WJ, Popel AS. A theoretical analysis of the effect of the particulate nature of blood on oxygen release in capillaries. Microvasc Res 1986; 32:164–189.
88. Page TC, McKay CB, Light WR, Hellums JD. Experimental simulation of oxygen transport. In: Winslow RM, Vandegriff KD, Intaglietta M, eds. Blood Substitutes: New Challenges. Boston: Birkhäuser, 1996, pp 132–145.
89. Rosen AL, Gould S, Sehgal LR, Noud G, Sehgal HL, Rice DL, Moss GS. Cardiac output response to extreme hemodilution with hemoglobin solutions of various P50 values. Crit Care Med 1979; 7:380–384.
90. Gould SA, Rosen AL, Sehgal L, Noud G, Sehgal H, DeWoskin R, Levine H, Kerstein M, Rice C, Moss GS. The effect of altered haemoglobin-oxygen affinity on oxygen transport by haemoglobin solution. J Surg Res 1980; 28:246–251.
91. Biro GP, Anderson PJ, Curtis SE, Cain SM. Stroma-free hemoglobin: its presence in plasma does not improve oxygen supply to the resting hindlimb vascular bed of hemodiluted dogs. Can J Physiol Pharmacol 1991; 69:1656–1662.

92. Hogan MC, Wilford DC, Keipert PE, Faithfull NS, Wagner PD. Increased plasma O_2 solubility improves O_2 uptake of in situ dog muscle working maximally. J Appl Physiol 1992; 361:2460–2475.
93. Hogan MC, Kurdak SS, Richardson RS, Wagner PS. Partial substitution of red blood cells with free hemoglobin does not improve maximal O_2 uptake of working in situ dog muscle. Adv Exp Med Biol 1994; 361:375–378.
94. Wittenberg JB. Myoglobin-facilitated oxygen diffusion: role of myoglobin in oxygen entry into muscle. Physiol Rev 1970; 50:559–636.
95. Bouwer STH, Hoofd L, Kreuzer F. Diffusion coefficients of oxygen and hemoglobin measured by facilitated oxygen diffusion through hemoglobin solutions. Biochim Biophys Acta 1997; 1338:127–136.
96. Skinner NS. Blood flow regulation as a factor in regulation of tissue O_2 delivery. Chest 1972; 61:13S–14S.
97. Granger HL, Goodman AH, Granger DN. Role of resistance and exchange vessels in local microvascular control of skeletal muscle oxygenation in the dog. Circ Res 1976; 38:379–385.
98. Sullivan SM, Johnson PC. Effects of oxygen on blood flow autoregulation in cat sartorius muscle. Am J Physiol 1981; 241:H804–H815.
99. Sullivan SM, Johnson PC. Effects of oxygen on arteriolar dimensions and blood flow in car sartorius muscle. Am J Physiol 1981; 241:H547–H556.
100. Jackson WF, Duling BR. The oxygen sensitivity of hamster cheekpouch arterioles: in vitro and in situ studies. Circ Res 1983; 53:515–525.
101. Busse R, Forstermann U, Matsuda H, Pohl U. The role of prostaglandins in endothelium-mediated vasodilatory response to hypoxia. Pflugers Arch 1984; 401:77–83.
102. Mazure NM, Chen EY, Laderoute KR, Giaccia AJ. Induction of vascular endothelial growth factor by hypoxia is modulated by a phosphatidylinositol 3-kinase/Akt signaling pathway in Ha-ras-transformed cells through a hypoxia inducible factor-1 transcriptional element. Blood 1997; 90:3322–3331.
103. Schmetterer L, Findl O, Strenn K, Graselli U, Eichler HG, Wolzt M. Role of NO in the O_2 and CO_2 responsiveness of cerebral and ocular circulation in humans. Am J Physiol 1997; 273:R2005–R2012.
104. Goldberg MA, Schneider TJ. Similarities between the oxygen-sensing mechanisms regulating the expression of vascular endothelial growth factor and erythropoietin. J Biol Chem 1994; 269:4355–4359.
105. Huang LE, Bunn HF. Regulation of erythropoietin gene expression. Curr Opin Hematol 1995; 2:125–131.

23

Integrated Gas Exchange Response: Chronic Renal Failure

GEOFFREY E. MOORE

University of Pittsburgh
Pittsburgh, Pennsylvania

I. Introduction

This chapter addresses oxygen (O_2) transport in end-stage renal disease (ESRD) with an emphasis on physical activity (i.e., exercise). Integrated O_2 transport is complex enough, even without the superimposition of an end-stage metabolic disease. The combination of the two is remarkably difficult to comprehend as a whole. Unfortunately, this review may seem superficial in some parts, but in many areas there is not much known about the physiology. The reader must bear these caveats in mind.

End stage renal disease pathophysiology of O_2 transport in the resting state sets the stage for O_2 transport during exercise. From the level of the molecule up to subcellular, organ, and whole-organism levels, O_2 supply/use matching is a finely regulated system that maintains near homeostasis during widely varying external conditions, even in ESRD. This system tightly links blood oxygenation and O_2 delivery to the metabolic requirements of tissues, and the relatively minor metabolic demand during rest requires but a fraction of total capacity for O_2 delivery. In medically stable patients with ESRD, it is self-evident that O_2 supply is adequate to meet use while at rest: (1) central venous oxygen partial pressure (P_{O_2}) $\gg$ Km of mitochondrial cytochromes for O_2; (2) brain oxygenation is adequate to sustain life; (3) central venous lactate is not elevated; and (4) there is no evidence of peripheral O_2 insufficiency (e.g., gangrene). It then follows that, in the context of O_2 supply/use sufficiency, exercise is the condition of more interest for freely roaming, medically stable people. Because functional capacity and quality of life are, however, markedly diminished by ESRD, the following discussion of integrated O_2 transports is mostly about limitations of exercise tolerance, although there are some sections that discuss resting physiology [1].

We consider the effects of uremia on the O_2 transport pathway and the effects of dialysis on O_2 transport. This review emphasizes pathophysiology in hemodialysis patients because more is known about them, and more patients are treated with hemodialysis than with other forms of renal replacement therapy. There is very little literature on exercise in persons on peritoneal dialysis, some of which is reviewed in this chapter. Readers interested in renal transplantation must look for information elsewhere, as this material is beyond the scope of this chapter. Unfortunately, the author is not aware of a comprehensive discussion of O_2 transport after renal transplantation.

A. Renal Disease Conditions

Briefly, consider the range of renal disease from insufficiency to failure. Patients whose creatinine clearance is progressively deteriorating have a condition called chronic renal insufficiency (CRI). In general, a person must lose more than 95% of the normal creatinine clearance capacity before some form of renal replacement therapy is needed. In the United States, approximately one third of dialysis patients developed ESRD because of diabetes, and another one fourth of dialysis patients developed ESRD because of hypertension. These causes of ESRD are worth mentioning, because they mean that most ESRD patients have serious and severe cardiovascular comorbidities. Some O_2 transport studies have specifically studied patients with CRI, but most such research has involved patients with ESRD. As might be expected, exercise research findings in CRI typically parallel ESRD but are less severe. For a discussion on general pathophysiology of exercise in ESRD, the reader is referred to the original review by Painter [2].

For individuals who develop ESRD, there are now three methods of renal replacement: hemodialysis, peritoneal dialysis, and renal transplantation. In the absence of one of these treatments, a person with ESRD would die in a few days. Hemodialysis and peritoneal dialysis are used to remove solutes and water that are normally excreted by the kidneys. These two treatments are commonly referred to as dialysis, although technically they consist of both dialysis (i.e., solute passing down a concentration gradient across a semipermeable membrane) and ultrafiltration (i.e., water filtering down a pressure gradient across this membrane). The dialysis component is used to control osmotic content of blood, mostly waste nitrogen (urea) and other small molecules; the filtration component is used to control water balance. In hemodialysis, a semipermeable membrane divides blood from dialysate, which flow in countercurrent paths. In peritoneal dialysis, the dialysate is instilled into the abdominal cavity through a surgically implanted tube, wherein the peritoneal surface serves as the semipermeable membrane; the dialysate is allowed to dwell in the abdominal cavity for a time and is then drained. By manipulating the parameters of a dialysis treatment, a nephrologist independently controls dialysis and filtration. Except where stated, in this chapter, the term *dialysis* is used to mean the combination of dialysis and filtration, either through hemodialysis or peritoneal dialysis.

B. Painter/Hanson Paradigm

It has been thought that most of the O_2 transport system, including cardiac, vascular, and muscular aspects of O_2 transport, are adversely affected by ESRD, as illustrated in the model by Painter and Hanson [3] (Fig. 1). This chapter builds on the Painter/Hanson paradigm; therefore, it is useful to discuss this model. The organization of this model is conceptually a sequential system that has been exceptionally useful, because it simplifies an extremely complex problem into more solvable components. On the foundations of the Painter/Hanson paradigm, research has improved our understanding of physiological dysfunctions in ESRD. We now know the whole O_2 transport pathway is affected, and we further understand some interactions between physiological systems and effects of therapy on pathophysiology.

Consider, for a moment, the physiological essentials of activities of daily living. People readily perform activities easily supported by aerobic metabolism, but usually shy away from intense activities that require a large anaerobic component. Strength is another important aspect of daily living, particularly so for persons who are weakened by chronic diseases. Weak, unsupple muscles cannot do much work, whether aerobic or anaerobic, and thus weakness limits ability to perform activities of daily living. Finally, activities of daily living require endurance so that exertion can be maintained to completion of a task. Many patients with chronic disease also have become deconditioned to a point where they have little endurance. Thus, rehabilitation of persons with ESRD is largely a problem of low aerobic capacity, weakness, and limited endurance.

Although this three-part problem may sound simple, exercise intolerance of renal failure is, in fact, an extremely complex problem because of metabolic disturbances of uremia, abnormalities in O_2 transport, muscle contractility problems, and increased fatigue. Together, these disturbances markedly diminish functional capacity in patients with renal failure. Furthermore, at least in dialysis patients, the interindividual variability is large. Reasons for this are unclear; perhaps it is a result of multiple underlying pathophysiologies leading to ESRD, variability in secondary complications of ESRD, or combinations thereof. This complex situation highlights some shortcomings of the Painter/Hanson paradigm, which focuses exclusively on

Normal   **Renal Failure**

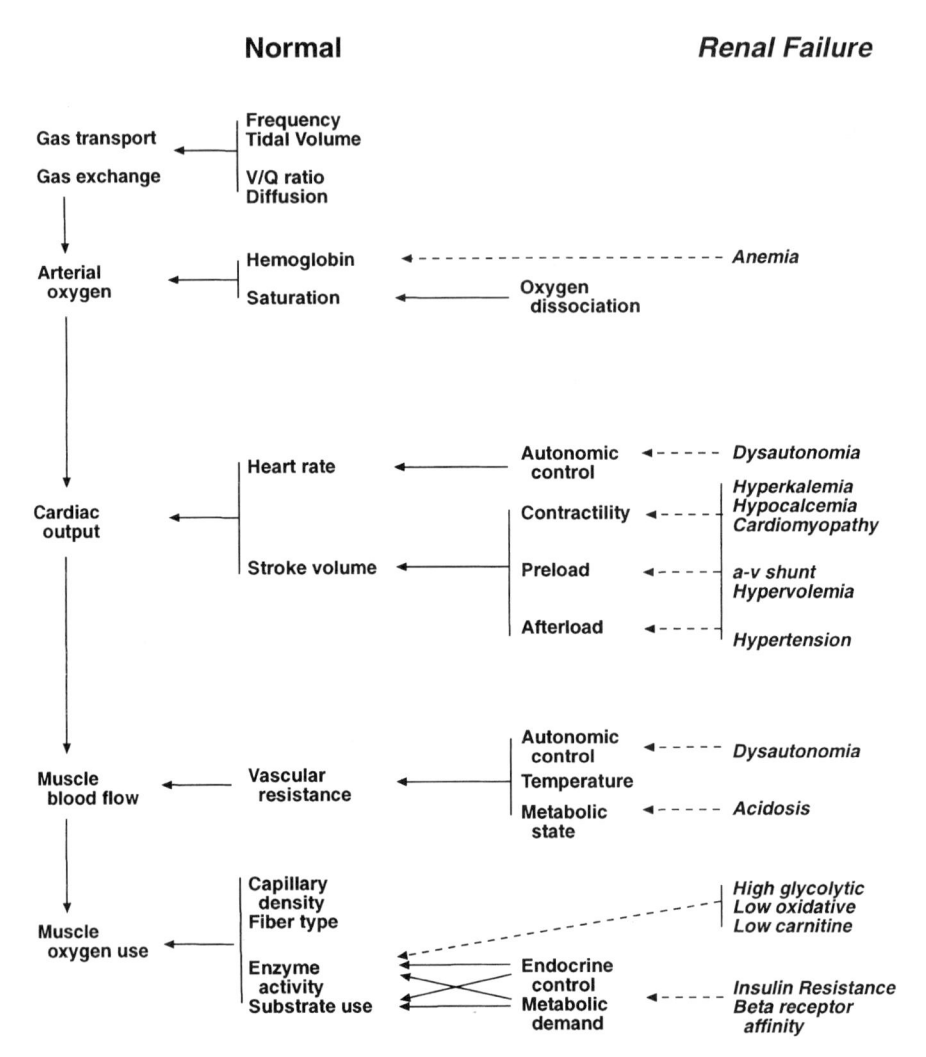

```
Gas transport ←── | Frequency
                  | Tidal Volume
Gas exchange      | V/Q ratio
     │            | Diffusion
     ▼
Arterial      ←── | Hemoglobin   ←-------------------- Anemia
oxygen            |                    Oxygen
                  | Saturation    ←──  dissociation
     │
     ▼
                  | Heart rate    ←──  Autonomic     ←----- Dysautonomia
                  |                    control
                  |                                         Hyperkalemia
Cardiac       ←── |                    Contractility ←----- Hypocalcemia
output            |                                         Cardiomyopathy
                  |
                  | Stroke volume ←──  Preload       ←----- a-v shunt
                  |                                         Hypervolemia
                  |
                  |                    Afterload     ←----- Hypertension
     │
     ▼
                                       Autonomic     ←----- Dysautonomia
                                       control
Muscle        ←── | Vascular      ←──  Temperature
blood flow        | resistance
                                       Metabolic     ←----- Acidosis
                                       state
     │
     ▼
                  | Capillary
                  | density                                 High glycolytic
                  | Fiber type    ←-------------------      Low oxidative
Muscle        ←── |                                         Low carnitine
oxygen use        | Enzyme             Endocrine
                  | activity           control
                  | Substrate use ←──  Metabolic     ←----- Insulin Resistance
                                       demand               Beta receptor
                                                            affinity
```

Figure 1 The Painter/Hanson model for effects of renal failure on oxygen transport physiology. Headings indicate the nature of the underlying columns. Note the lack of depicted interactions between systems.

mechanisms of O_2 transport. In the model, O_2 pathways are independent from each other, and there is little that reflects weakness, lack of endurance, altered control mechanisms, or how therapy for ESRD affects O_2 transport. This chapter discusses research findings on these issues, concluding with an updated model and a summary of our understanding of exercise intolerance in ESRD.

II. Oxygen Transport Factors Affecting Aerobic Capacity

Section II discusses the path of O_2 transport from lung to muscle mitochondrion in persons with ESRD.

A. Pulmonary

Renal failure adversely affects lung function, and there are a few mechanisms by which gas exchange could be affected in a severely afflicted patient: phrenic neuropathy/alveolar hypoventilation, reduced diffusional capacity, and ventilation–perfusion ($\dot{V}/\dot{Q}$) inequalities. For the most part, these problems have been studied only during rest, but these abnormalities also might limit aerobic capacity, particularly in patients with a long history of smoking. Most of the pulmonary literature on ESRD patients deals with interactions of pulmonary function with hemodialysis treatments. This became an issue because it was widely observed that dialysis patients often become hypoxemic during and/or after hemodialysis. The data suggest this is probably a self-limited phenomenon that has clinical concern only for persons with severe lung disease. It remains speculative whether these abnormalities are relevant during free-roaming physical activity performed between the dialysis treatments.

Phrenic Neuropathy

Phrenic neuropathy could, in theory, cause a pulmonary limitation to O_2 transport through perceived dyspnea or respiratory fatigue. Phrenic nerve latency is prolonged in hemodialysis patients (i.e., there is a delay in appearance of the reflection wave through the reflex arc after an electrical stimulation of the nerve) [4]. This suggests that phrenic nerve conduction is impaired, a possibility supported by good correlation with abnormally slow peroneal nerve conduction velocity [4]. Whether phrenic neuropathy causes respiratory fatigue or a respiratory limitation to exercise is not known, although it might be in a patient with diabetes and/or who's been on dialysis for many years. There is evidence that hemodialysis acutely decreases minute ventilation while increasing inspiratory occlusion pressure and causing an upward shift in the expired volume ($\dot{V}_E$)/carbon dioxide partial pressure (P_{CO_2}) curve; this suggests that dialysis patients have some neuromuscular hypoexcitability that requires increased central command for any given $\dot{V}_E$ [5]. Nonetheless, this problem is probably not clinically meaningful (nerve latency studies did not include measurement of P_{CO_2} to confirm this point) [4].

Low Diffusional Conductance

Dialysis patients with no known lung problems have measurably reduced diffusing capacity, or carbon monoxide (CO) transfer function (D_{LCO}) [6]. D_{LCO} is reduced in hemodialysis patients (group average of 30.4 mL CO/min/mm Hg vs. a laboratory standard of 40.1 mL CO/min/mm Hg), probably because of a cumulative effect of bioincompatibly with the cuprophan membranes in some dialyzers [7]. Bioincompatibility causes granulocytes to adhere to pulmonary endothelium [7]. It has been suggested that chronic exposure to pulmonary granulocyte sequestration causes pulmonary fibrosis, with subsequent reduction in DLCO and restrictive lung disease [8]. Polysulfone dialysis membranes are less immunostimulatory than cuprophan membranes; therefore, use of dialyzers made from polysulfone might stop or at least retard this progressive process [7,9]. The inflammatory process also affects children; children on hemodialysis have forced expiratory volume in 1 second (FEV_1) and vital capacity that are approximately 80% of age-predicted values [10]. DLCO is reduced by approximately 5% of normal for each year of dialysis with a cuprophan dialyzer [7].

Interstitial fluid in the lungs (from fluid retention) might also decrease DLCO and vital capacity, in proportion to the amount of excess fluid in the lungs. But because reduction in DLCO is proportional to the number of years on dialysis, whereas interstitial fluid is unrelated to years on dialysis, it is not thought that fluid retention routinely reduces DLCO, although it may do so in dialysis patients who present with acute congestive heart failure.

Peritoneal dialysis may also adversely affect pulmonary function, although not by the most obvious possible mechanism: mechanical pressure on the diaphragm and reduced lung volumes. Two liters of intraperitoneal dialysate volume (a typical burden) has no clinical effect on spirometry [11]. Rather, DLCO is diminished in peritoneal dialysis patients, despite the absence of any immunological stimulation by dialysis membranes [6]. Anemia of renal failure contributes to the diminished diffusional conductance (see Section II.B), but anemia is probably not a complete explanation [6,12]. There is more to learn about pulmonary diffusional abnormalities in dialysis patients.

Dead Space

Despite the effects of dialysis on lung function, dialysis patients apparently have normal dead space, because the ratio of the cost of ventilation to carbon dioxide elimination [$\dot{V}_{CO_2}$], i.e. ($\dot{V}_E/\dot{V}_{CO_2}$), is identical to that of normal controls [13]. Other investigators have used the multiple inert gas technique to study lung function during dialysis and also found no change in dead space [14]. In comparison, patients with congestive heart failure have an increased ratio of the cost of ventilation to oxygen uptake, i.e. ($\dot{V}_E/\dot{V}_{O_2}$), which is caused by a larger-than-normal dead space [13].

Ventilation/Perfusion

There is no evidence of chronic $\dot{V}/\dot{Q}$ abnormalities in dialysis patients [14,15]. Indeed, during dialysis, $\dot{V}/\dot{Q}$ matching improves and the alveolar–arterial (A–a) O_2

gradient narrows, if anything, and only after dialysis does the A–a gradient widen [15]. Hemodialysis is actually associated with an improvement in $\dot{V}/\dot{Q}$ matching, although dialysis causes a decrease in both alveolar ventilation and cardiac output [14,16].

In summary, one cannot firmly conclude that pulmonary pathophysiology does not limit aerobic capacity in dialysis patients, because no study has looked at exercise while controlling for the cumulative effects of the multiple potential pulmonary limitations to exercise. Studies with data collected at rest all suggest that lung function is only slightly subnormal, despite a gradual long-term reduction in D$_{LCO}$. If the A–a O_2 gradient does not widen and there is no arterial desaturation during exercise (anecdotally true for most dialysis patients), then it is unlikely that pulmonary gas exchange limits O_2 transport in dialysis patients. Patients on dialysis who also have severe chronic obstructive pulmonary disease, however, may not fare as well and may show a pulmonary limitation to exercise (personal observation).

B. Blood: Oxygen Carrying Capacity

The lung transfers O_2 to red blood cells, which is the next part of the O_2 pathway that will be considered here. Almost all dialysis patients become very anemic (excluding those with polycystic kidneys), because they lose the main source of the hormone, erythropoietin (Epo), that stimulates production of red blood cells. Normally, approximately 85% of endogenous Epo is created by the juxtaglomerular apparatus; therefore, this source of Epo is lost in ESRD [17]. It is largely for this reason that dialysis patients are anemic, although reduced red blood cell longevity also contributes. Recombinant human Epo is very effective at increasing hematocrit, and there was great hope that administration of Epo to dialysis patients would relieve morbidity associated with ESRD. Epo does improve quality of life in dialysis patients and reduces the severity of left ventricular hypertrophy [18–22]. In the last decade, however, most Epo research in dialysis patients has been on the use of Epo to increase hematocrit, red blood cell mass, and exercise intolerance.

Initial data suggested that Epo works wonderfully well to improve exercise intolerance in dialysis patients. Some patients on Epo can increase peak $\dot{V}O_2$ ($\dot{V}O_{2peak}$) by up to 40% [23]. However, most patients fail to obtain such a large increase and have an "on-Epo" $\dot{V}O_{2peak}$ of $\leq$ 24 mL/kg/min [18,24–27]. The ventilatory threshold undergoes similar benefit but remains around 16 mL O_2/kg/min [23,24,26]. Researchers and clinicians have been slow to recognize that Epo therapy does not follow our common-sense notions about aerobic capacity and that exercise intolerance must be more complex than simply a matter of O_2-carrying capacity.

The problem is that the on-Epo ranges are similar to $\dot{V}O_2$ values reported before Epo was in use [28–34]. One striking finding is that the increase in $\dot{V}O_{2peak}$ after Epo therapy does not correlate with the increase in hemoglobin [18,24,25].

This contrasts with the strong correlation between hemoglobin and maximum $\dot{V}O_2$ ($\dot{V}O_{2max}$) in normal persons who undergo blood doping [35]. Moreover, the increase in $\dot{V}O_{2peak}$ is inversely proportional to $\dot{V}O_{2peak}$ before the start of Epo therapy (Fig. 2) [25]. This very robust inverse correlation is in stark contrast to the lack of correlation with change in hemoglobin. There have even been some patients treated with Epo whose $\dot{V}O_{2peak}$ did not increase at all, despite substantial increases in hematocrit [24,36,37]. One is forced to conclude that the usefulness of Epo is determined more by the integrated response to exercise than by the anemia.

The lack of correlation between changes in $\dot{V}O_{2peak}$ and in hemoglobin cannot be overstated. The increase in $\dot{V}O_{2peak}$ after Epo is not simply a consequence of increased O_2-carrying capacity, which may only be important in patients who are extremely anemic (hemoglobin level < 8 g/dL) [38]. There are two implications: (1) hemoglobin is not a good measure of the effectiveness of Epo in dialysis patients; and (2) O_2-carrying capacity (arterial O_2 content) is not a strong determinant of $\dot{V}O_{2peak}$ in dialysis patients—at least not once hemoglobin level is greater than 8–10 g/dL. The complexity of this issue is discussed in greater detail in Section III on integrated physiology.

C. Cardiac Abnormalities

There are four common cardiac abnormalities in ESRD: left ventricular hypertrophy (LVH), coronary artery disease (CAD), incompetent chronotropic response to exercise, and congestive heart failure. There are many other abnormalities, of course, but these four are prevalent. Here each is considered briefly.

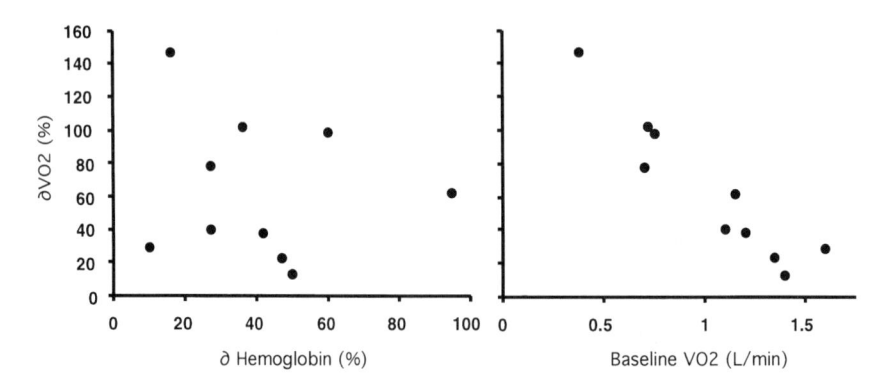

Figure 2 Correlates of percent increase in peak oxygen consumption ($\dot{V}O_{2peak}$) in dialysis patients after erythropoietin therapy. Data show the change in hemoglobin (i.e., the primary effect of erythropoietin) has no relationship to the increase in $\dot{V}O_{2peak}$. Rather, the increase in $\dot{V}O_{2peak}$ is inversely related to the baseline $\dot{V}O_{2peak}$. These data suggest that patients with a $\dot{V}O_{2peak}$ greater than 1.7 L/min may not increase $\dot{V}O_{2peak}$ from erythropoietin therapy. (From Ref. 25. Reproduced with permission of S. Karger AG, Basel.)

Left Ventricular Hypertrophy

Patients with ESRD commonly have LVH as a compensatory change caused by an increased pumping load on the heart. Preload, the volume of venous blood returning to the heart, is increased because of fluid retention between dialysis treatments. This causes increased cardiac filling pressures, stroke volumes, and blood pressure. In addition, many patients with ESRD have hypertension as their main underlying cause of renal failure. In such patients, the resistance to cardiac output, or afterload, is also increased. The long-term compensatory response for these loads is LVH and a thickening of the cardiac walls. Although LVH does not directly diminish O_2 transport, it does make such persons more vulnerable to myocardial ischemia during exercise and can cause impaired ventricular filling (i.e., diastolic dysfunction). Epo therapy reduces the severity of LVH, but preliminary data unfortunately suggest that Epo does not increase peak cardiac output [25,39].

Coronary Artery Disease

Coronary artery disease is very common in ESRD, and cardiovascular disease is the most common cause of death for dialysis patients [40]. Nonetheless, exercise-induced electrocardiogram abnormalities and angina are not that common in dialysis patients (personal observation). The main reason why exercise electrocardiograms have a low predictive value in dialysis patients is that most patients have extremely limited functional capacity, do not surpass their ischemic threshold, and so do not achieve a high enough heart rate to show ischemia. Furthermore, there is reasonable concern that negative test results are false negatives because few patients exceed 85% of age-predicted heart rate, which is one criteria for exercise tests to be valid. It is not clear whether the low functional capacity limits the heart rate response or whether the abnormal heart rate response limits functional capacity [41,42]. Either way, CAD is probably not a factor limiting O_2 transport in most dialysis patients, despite its high prevalence.

Subnormal Peak Chronotropic Response

As a whole, dialysis patients have a peak heart rate that is approximately 75–80% of their age-predicted maximum [2,43,44]. The mechanism(s) behind this abnormality is (are) not fully understood, although data from transplant recipients show that peak heart rate is normalized almost immediately after transplantation [28]. This suggests some circulating factor(s) is (are) responsible. Such factors could affect the chronotropic response by inhibiting volitional effort, blocking response to sympathetic drive, or blocking release of parasympathetic (vagal) tone. As previously noted, some authorities suspect that the chronotropic response is low because the patients cannot create enough skeletal muscle demand for blood flow [41]. This is certainly plausible, although it downplays the high resting sympathetic drive and any subsequent downregulation of cardiac responsiveness to catecholamine stimulation [45]. In addition, it does not explain a lot of ESRD patients who obviously try hard during exercise tests, but who fail to achieve an age-predicted heart rate (personal observation). Whatever the mechanism(s) behind chronotropic limitation, the net effect is an abnormally low peak heart rate and low peak cardiac output [29].

Congestive Heart Failure

Our last cardiac consideration is heart failure. Until recently, most clinicians would ascribe this to the fluid overload (i.e., under filtration), but it is now known that heart failure can be partially caused by underdialysis. Patients who are underdialyzed can present with frank congestive heart failure, even without excess fluid weight [46]. It is thought this is caused by abnormalities in calcium, because myocardial contractility increases during hemodialysis due to an increase in ionized serum calcium [47,48]. Alternatively, this phenomenon of "underdialysis heart failure" may lend support to the idea of a circulating cardiac inhibitor. Irrespective of the mechanism(s) involved, heart failure superimposed on renal failure can severely limit functional capacity.

D. Vasculature Conductance and Resistance Vessels

The determinants of $\dot{V}_{O_2}$ in the Fick equation (heart rate, stroke volume, arterial O_2 content, and venous O_2 content) do not include a parameter for how the O_2 gets to tissues, which is a role of the vasculature. The vasculature does play a role in $\dot{V}_{O_2}$, in part through the effects of afterload on cardiac output, and in part through diffusion effects that are ultimately reflected in venous O_2 content. Thus, conductance and resistance vessels are intimately involved in determining afterload and blood flow through tissues. Epo studies have shown that generating $\dot{V}_{O_2}$ is not as simple as merely increasing arterial O_2 content. One must also consider the effects of the circulation, and in dialysis patients, that also means considering the effects of vascular pathophysiology.

Peripheral Vascular Disease

The vascular tree of patients with ESRD has not been as well studied as the heart or blood, but vascular abnormalities considerably diminish O_2 transport in many dialysis patients. Peripheral arterial atherosclerosis is very common in ESRD, partly because of hypercholesterolemia commonly associated with renal failure and partly because of underlying diabetes and hypertension. In addition to atherosclerotic obstruction of conductance vessels, data from Epo studies suggest that resistance vessels are also involved. The interactions of resistance-vessel abnormalities with target organ damage (secondary to longstanding hypertension and/or diabetes) remain obscure. Hypercholesterolemia reduces the acetylcholine-mediated production of nitric oxide in resistance vessels [49,50]. Little work has been conducted in this area with ESRD patients; therefore, one can only presume that such pathological structure or function would add to O_2 transport problems.

E. Tissue

Having considered convective O_2 supply abnormalities, the capillary bed where diffusion of O_2 to tissues occurs will now be examined. For the sake of interest in exercise, and perhaps in part because of the nature of biopsies of skeletal muscle compared with vital organs, skeletal muscle serves as a paradigm tissue in studying the microvasculature.

Capillary/Myofiber Dissociation

One important sequelae of ESRD is loss of capillaries and, even worse, dissociation of capillaries and myofibers (i.e., loss of homogeneity in the capillary/myofiber distribution). Dialysis patients lose capillaries in gastrocnemius, vastus lateralis, rectus femoris, biceps, deltoid, and triceps; therefore, capillaries are probably diminished in all skeletal muscles [51–55]. Moreover, capillaries and myofibers seem to lose their stoichiometric association, creating heterogeneity of capillary/fiber distributions within the muscle (Figure 3 photomicrograph) [56]. This must be particularly detrimental to diffusion of O_2 across the capillary/muscle interface [56,57]. Dialysis patients do have lower diffusional O_2 conductance (Dm_{O2}) than similarly sedentary controls, due, only in part, to the lower hemoglobin in dialysis patients [76]. Abnormal capillarity could help explain a low Dm_{O2}, because some myofibers have no blood supply and suffer from a perfusion/use inequality [59].

Uremic Myopathy

The dysfunctional regulation of capillary to myofibers (by whatever process governs the number of capillaries for each myofiber) yields an abnormal capillary/myofiber interface, but this is not the complete extent of muscle tissue abnormalities. Myocytes also become markedly abnormal in ESRD, characterized by changes collectively called "uremic myopathy" [54,60]. In many ways, these changes are nonspecific and difficult to distinguish from myopathies found in other chronic diseases (e.g., congestive heart failure). Uremic myopathy characteristics include generalized fiber atrophy (and especially type II fibers), moth-eaten fibers, mitochondrial myopathy (i.e., mitochondrial swelling and ragged red fibers), fiber rarefaction and distortion, Z band degeneration, lipid inclusions, and numerous other pathological changes [55,60]. In many biopsy specimens, the fibers show wide variability in size and shape, suggesting heterogeneity in structure and perhaps function [51,53,55,56]. It is thought that these degenerative changes contribute to muscle weakness; therefore, exercise intolerance is probably not simple deconditioning.

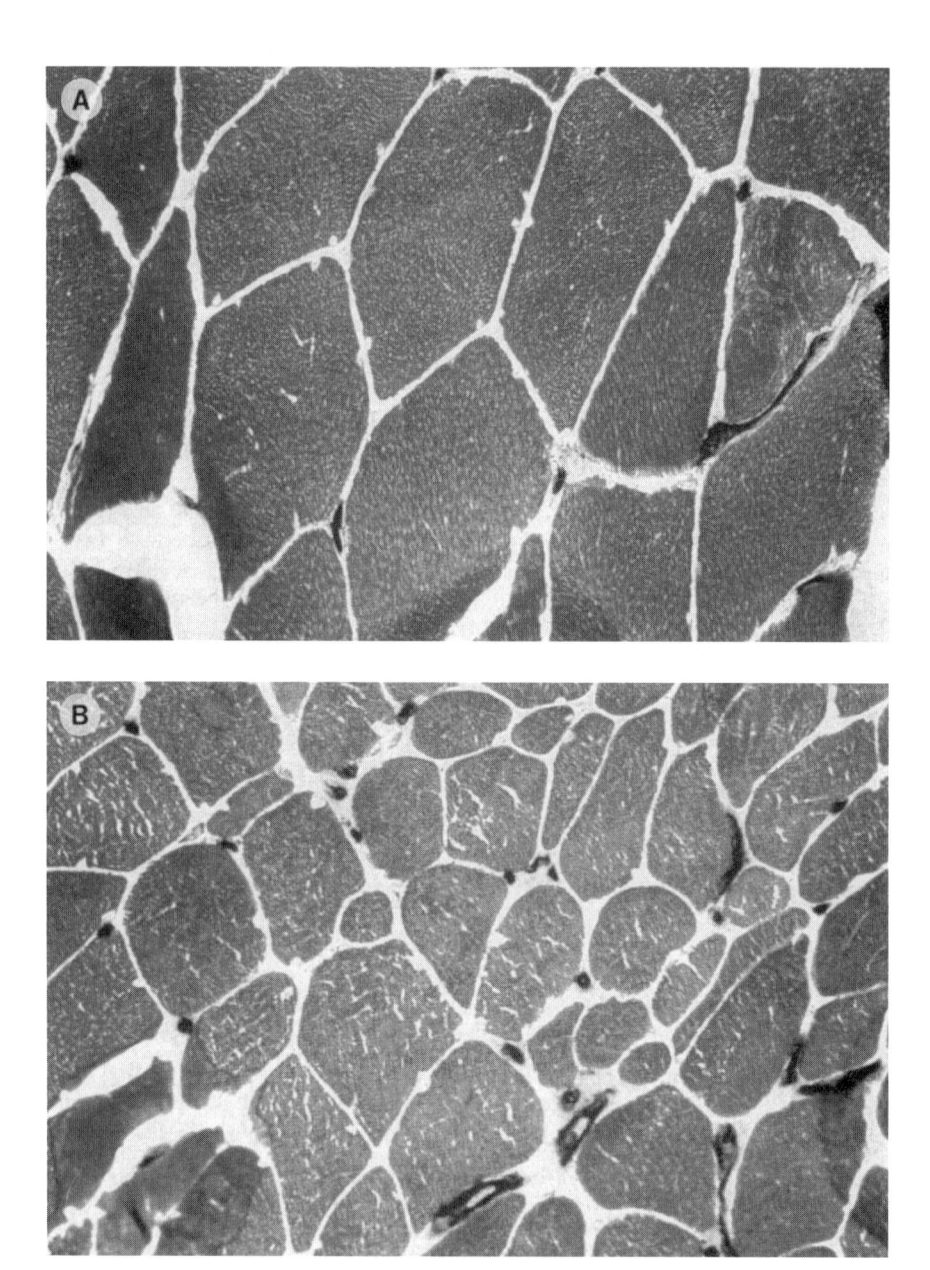

Figure 3 Biopsy specimens of rectus femoris from dialysis patients; capillary endothelium is darkened with Ulex B stain. Note variability in fiber size and angular shapes, heterogeneity of capillary/fiber relationships, and absence of capillaries for some fibers.

Muscle Weakness

Strength is an important determinant of aerobic power; without strong muscle contractions, there can be little demand for O_2. Therefore, it is perhaps not surprising that skeletal muscle weakness in dialysis patients is closely linked to $\dot{V}O_{2peak}$, more so than O_2-carrying capacity. $\dot{V}O_{2peak}$ correlates closely with isokinetic cycling power ($r = 0.84$) and isokinetic knee extension ($r = 0.68$), but not with hematocrit or hemoglobin concentration ($r = 0.35$ and 0.33, respectively) [61]. Thus, factors leading to weakness (hyperparathyroidism, deconditioning, loss of membrane potential, sarcopenia, uremic myopathy) probably reduce aerobic capacity in dialysis patients.

Muscle Adenosine Triphosphate Metabolism

The effects of uremic myopathy on skeletal muscle energy metabolism are not clear. Most studies suggest abnormal activity in glycolytic (e.g., phosphorylase, phosphofructokinase) and oxidative enzymes (e.g., citrate synthase), but the changes are not uniformly up or down. This may be a consequence of fairly small numbers of subjects or of the muscles selected for biopsy. Vastus lateralis glycolytic enzymes are sometimes two or three times normal: in one study, phosphorylase was found to be 8.4 ± 0.6 versus 4.1 ± 0.7 nmol/mg/min, and protein kinase was 147 ± 21 versus 52 ± 5 nmol/mg/min [62]. Other studies have claimed depressed glycolytic enzymes, although some of this may be species differences (some of these data were from rats) [62,63]. Insulin resistance may be a part of this phenomenon (see Section V.D) [64]. In oxidative enzymes, vastus lateralis oxidative capacity seems to be near normal in comparison to trained endurance athletes (19.5 ± 5.7 vs. 28.3 ± 7.1 $\mu L\ O_2$/g/hr) [60]. Our studies found rectus femoris succinate dehydrogenase was approximately half that of normal subjects, but these were not controlled comparisons (personal observation). The variability in enzyme activities are confusing, but seem to diminish the likelihood of clinical significance.

Muscle Lipid Metabolism

Carnitine is a critically important compound involved in fat metabolism and as a scavenger for acyl moieties. Abnormal carnitine levels play a role in the low exercise tolerance of dialysis patients. The mechanisms of these carnitine effects are not fully clear, but very long-term dialysis is associated with a reduction in muscle carnitine, as well as a change in the composition of muscle acylcarnitines (i.e., acyl groups bound to carnitine) [65–68]. Muscle carnitine correlates with the time to exhaustion in dialysis patients but does not correlate with aerobic capacity [65]. Therefore, it seems logical that carnitine supplementation increases exercise tolerance in dialysis patients, although the associated increase in $\dot{V}O_{2peak}$ is only 10% [65,69,70]. Because abnormal muscle carnitine can limit aerobic capacity in some dialysis patients, there is probably a small but highly variable benefit of carnitine supplementation to dialysis patients as a group: some individuals may particularly benefit, but others may not benefit at all.

III. Integrated Oxygen Transport

In dialysis patients, the interconnectedness of O_2 transport physiology is most thoroughly understood in relation to hemoglobin, because recombinant Epo has provided a tool to modulate hemoglobin as a control variable. In addition, exercise training and manipulations of the environmental conditions have been studied. Before reviewing these subjects, the physiological interface between the circulation and tissue demand for O_2, as modeled by circulation/contraction coupling, is considered.

A. Circulation/Contraction Coupling

Some investigators now believe that O_2 transport in dialysis patients is heavily determined by abnormalities in the capillary/myofiber interface, which consists of the capillary cells, interstitial space, and sarcolemma. At maximal exercise in normal muscle, this region creates the single largest Po_2 gradient in the pathway (75–90 mm Hg, arterial; approximately 40 mm Hg, mean capillary), and thus represents the highest impedance to O_2 transfer in the O_2 transport pathway [71]. The myocyte's oxidative machinery generates an O_2 gradient across this interface by lowering the intracellular Po_2, which makes O_2 diffuse down the gradient from red blood cell to mitochondrion; the circulatory supply of O_2 increases in an amount needed to maintain the Po_2 gradient. When the circulation cannot meet the demand, either $\dot{V}o_{2max}$ is reached or circulatory decompensation occurs.

In contrast to the high O_2 impedance (or low O_2 transfer function), there is very little impedance to O_2 transfer inside a normal myocyte [71]. This is thought to be because myoglobin has a high O_2 transfer function from mitochondria out to the sarcolemma [72]. Many investigators have partially blamed the low aerobic capacity of dialysis patients on low mitochondrial oxidative enzyme activities [63]. However, this model diminishes the importance of: (1) myoglobin's high O_2 transfer function; and (2) the substantial impedance to O_2 transfer at the capillary/myofiber interface. Normal skeletal muscle has several-fold excess oxidative potential (relative to total cardiac oxygen output) [73]. A 50% reduction in O_2-consuming enzyme activity should still leave myocytes enough capacity to generate a Po_2 gradient, even if the capillary/myofiber interface is normal. It must be relatively easy to create a gradient when there is subnormal diffusing capacity because of capillary rarefaction.

The author's view is that the real myocyte issue is probably not enzyme activity, but whether there is enough aerobic demand to generate a complete Po_2 gradient, i.e., a mitochondrial Po_2 at some near-zero value that is effectively transmitted by myoglobin to the sarcolemma. If so, then there is "enough" oxidative capacity to exceed O_2 supply. The leg blood flow/nuclear magnetic resonance spectroscopy findings support this view with convincing data that O_2-carrying capacity is not related to the $\dot{V}O_{2peak}$ limit in dialysis patients. Myocytes in ESRD patients have more than enough capacity to create a PO_2 gradient, or they would not become so acidotic and adenosine triphosphate (ATP)-depleted. The findings from Marrades et al. [76] show that dialysis patients are, in fact, O_2 supply-dependent after Epo therapy (Fig. 2). Following this line of reasoning, intramyocyte abnormalities must not be a limiting factor.

There are also some conflicting views with regard to oxidative metabolism in skeletal muscle of dialysis patients, mostly centering around the postexercise rate of phosphocreatine (PCr) regeneration during recovery. Some data show that PCr regeneration is normal (i.e., despite any abnormalities in oxidative enzyme activities, the ability to make ATP is unaffected), and some data suggest that PCr regeneration is subnormal (i.e., oxidative ability to make ATP is depressed) [57,74–78]. There are conflicting data on the effect of Epo therapy on PCr regeneration, with some evidence showing that Epo has no effect, and other data showing that Epo improves the oxidative ability to generate ATP [76,77]. However, the differences in these studies may not be that meaningful because: (1) these differences resolve when pH is taken into account; and (2) there is sufficient oxidative reserve to satisfy nicotinamide adenine dinucleotide (NAD)-linked ATP generation [76,79].

Several lines of evidence supporting the existence of O_2 supply limitation have been discussed, including regulation of blood flow. Post-Epo data show that leg blood flow decreases and vascular resistance increases with increasing hematocrit. Abnormal regulation of blood flow in resistance vessels is likely, because it has been shown that dialysis patients have markedly abnormal endothelial function [80–83]. Therefore, although capillary/myofiber dissociation creates an anatomic perfusion/use inequality, there is also potential for function perfusion/use inequality [59,84,85]. In summary, it seems likely that O_2 supply limitation in dialysis patients is partly a product of the structural and functional abnormalities in the capillary/myofiber interface.

B. Erythropoietin

The factors that increase $\dot{V}O_{2peak}$ after Epo are complex, but are probably not changes in central circulation. Preliminary data indicate that peak cardiac output does not increase after Epo therapy [37,39]. Nonetheless, Epo profoundly improves hemodynamic function by several mechanisms. Epo decreases resting cardiac index, LVH (including diameter, wall thickness, and mass), and reduces ischemic ST segment changes during exercise testing [24,26,86–88].

However, Epo increases systemic vascular resistance and is associated with exacerbation of hypertension in approximately 20% of patients [89]. It was thought that severe anemia caused tissue to be relatively ''hypoxic,'' which then stimulated vasodilation, all of which was improved by Epo [89]. But recent data show that in vitro artery segments, taken from surgical specimens and then incubated with Epo, decrease their release of prostacyclin (a vasorelaxing compound) and increase release of prostaglandin F_2, thromboxane B_2, and endothelin (vasoconstricting compounds) [80,90]. Thee is also suggestion that Epo improves responsiveness to sympathetic stimulation [91]. Furthermore, rat data suggest that the increase in systemic vascular resistance has nothing to do with so-called hypoxic stimulation, nor a change in vasoconstrictor balance, but rather is a consequence of an acquired resistance to nitric oxide–mediated vasodilation [92]. Together, these findings suggest that Epo directly affects vascular regulation of blood flow.

The alteration of blood flow by Epo provides a reason for the disappointing increase in $\dot{V}o_{2peak}$ after Epo therapy: O_2 delivery to muscle increases by only a small fraction of the increase in O_2-carrying capacity. In one study, leg O_2 delivery increased approximately 37% after a 69% increase in hemoglobin, suggesting that only half of the increase in O_2-carrying capacity is delivered to exercising muscle [58]. Indeed, the change in O_2 delivery explained almost all of the whole-body increase in $\dot{V}o_{2peak}$ after Epo (which increased 33%) [58].

Epo also increases Dm_{O2} in skeletal muscle, although sedentary hemodialysis patients on Epo still have a lower Dm_{O2} than sedentary controls (Fig. 3) [58]. The increase in O_2 extraction means that there has to be an increase in O_2 diffusion for any given O_2 supply, which can be expressed as the ratio: $Dm_{O2}/(\beta \times \dot{Q}o_2)$. The reader should refer to Chapter 1 for a general discussion of O_2 extraction, but, briefly, β is the slope of the oxyhemoglobin dissociation curve, when $\beta = (Cao_2 - Cfvo_2)/(Pao_2 - Pfvo_2)$. Thus, β is the change in blood oxygen content per change in driving pressure. In the group of dialysis patients that were studied before and after Epo, a 31% increase in Dm_{O2} and a 65% increase in β (caused by the increase in hemoglobin concentration) were offset by a 13% decrease in blood flow. This comparison of sedentary controls versus dialysis patients shows that, even after adjustment for anemia, dialysis patients have reduced muscle O_2 conductance [58].

In a separate Epo study by the same investigators, nuclear magnetic resonance spectroscopy was used to compare myocyte ATP metabolism with convective and diffusive O_2 transport. In this latter study, however, a decrease in leg blood flow offset the increase in O_2 content, so leg O_2 delivery and $\dot{V}o_{2peak}$ remained constant. Moreover, a 50% increase in hemoglobin (after Epo) had no effect on intracellular ATP metabolism [76]. Several studies show that intracellular pH and ATP/adenosine diphosphate ratios decrease more rapidly in ESRD patients than in normal persons [57,75,76]. All of these findings support the existence of O_2 supply limitation in dialysis patients.

In the subset of patients who increase muscle O_2 supply after Epo, anaerobic contribution to energy metabolism decreases, but not as much as one might expect. Lactate production decreases with an increase in hemoglobin from approximately

8 to 10 g/dL, but there is no further change in lactate metabolism when hemoglobin increases to greater than 10 g/dL [38]. It is worth noting that peak exercise lactate is not highly elevated in most dialysis patients, even in the most anemic conditions (hemoglobin levels ≤ 8 g/dL). The average peak lactate of 4.6 mmol/L is comparable to steady-state exercise for trained athletes [38]. However, peak exercise lactate can be very high (> 10 mmol/L) in some dialysis patients; therefore, there is great interindividual variability (personal observation). The reason for this is not clear, but there may be volitional factors because some patients are unable to push themselves to very intense exercise and a "true" $\dot{V}O_{2max}$. It may also be related to insulin resistance effects on glycolytic metabolism (see Section V.D).

For completeness, the effect of Epo on oxyhemoglobin dissociation curves should be mentioned. Epo causes a statistically significant decrease in hemoglobin binding affinity for O_2, mediated through 2,3-diphosphoglycerate, but there is no evidence that this has a functionally meaningful clinical effect [93]. It is likely that the relative contribution of this change is miniscule in comparison to other pathophysiological phenomena (such as decreased blood flow).

In aggregate, Epo studies suggest there are two main factors limiting $\dot{V}O_{2peak}$ in dialysis patients: (1) low O_2 delivery because of low blood flow; and (2) skeletal muscle O_2 transport limitation. This explains the lack of correlation with hemoglobin in patients on Epo (for hemoglobin levels > 8 g/dL), because Epo not only increases hemoglobin, it also reduces the vasodilatory response to exercise. This counteracts the increase in O_2-carrying capacity and blunts the increase in O_2 delivery, and it is changes in O_2 delivery, not arterial O_2 content, that have close association with changes in $\dot{V}O_{2peak}$.

C. Exercise Training

There are relatively few exercise training studies in ESRD patients because such studies are difficult to perform. Early studies showed that whole-body $\dot{V}O_{2peak}$ increases 20–40% after training [30,32–34]. More recent studies in dialysis patients have been less impressive than the earlier studies, showing that $\dot{V}O_{2peak}$ usually increases less than 20%, and there are even patients whose $\dot{V}O_{2peak}$ does not improve at all [56,94]. Exercise training in transplant recipients show that improvements in $\dot{V}O_{2max}$ are related to increases in skeletal muscle strength [95]. Perhaps this is also true for dialysis patients. It is unclear why it seems more difficult for today's dialysis patients to achieve big increases in $\dot{V}O_{2peak}$ than it was 10 or 15 years ago. One possibility is that experience with this population has grown and investigators are more comfortable with these patients; therefore, inclusion/exclusion criteria are more relaxed, and "sicker" subjects are being enrolled. It is possible that routine use of Epo has increased the average $\dot{V}O_{2peak}$ of the dialysis population, with hemoglobin levels now in the 10–12-g/dL range (rather than 8–10 g/dL), and that this makes it harder to show improvement in $\dot{V}O_{2peak}$. The latter idea seems unlikely, because pretraining $\dot{V}O_{2peak}$ does not seem to be meaningfully higher now than it was 15 years ago. One thing is clear: some patients can train very hard and not increase $\dot{V}O_{2peak}$.

The only published study to investigate the determinants of $\dot{V}O_{2peak}$ failed to show a mean increase after training [56]. In this study, in which average training heart rates were greater than 80% of peak heart rate, $\dot{V}O_{2peak}$ went from 14.8 ± 0.9 to 16.8 ± 1.3 mL/kg/min ($P < .1$); 6 of 11 subjects improved, but 5 of 11 had no real change in $\dot{V}O_{2peak}$. Peak power output increased, nonetheless, from 60 ± 4 W to 70 ± 6 W ($P < .05$), and heart rates were lower for any given submaximal workload. Of those who increased $\dot{V}O_{2peak}$, the mechanism of improvement was always a widening of the arteriovenous O_2 difference. There were no changes in peak heart rate, stroke volume, or arterial O_2 content; therefore, all of the improvement came about through adaptations in the peripheral circulation. Any subject who could not improve the peripheral O_2 extraction did not improve $\dot{V}O_{2peak}$, although everyone experienced increases in endurance and submaximal measures of performance [56].

One important point from exercise training studies is that $\dot{V}O_{2peak}$ is not the only important outcome parameter. Exercise training almost always improves endurance and work efficiency, even when there is no change in $\dot{V}O_{2peak}$. The mechanisms for these other improvements remain obscure.

D. Altitude Exposure

One interesting study looked at the effects of altitude exposure on dialysis patients [96]. With prolonged exposure to altitude, dialysis patients showed seemingly paradoxical findings when contrasted to studies with normal persons. The dialysis patient's peak exercise blood lactate increased, along with aerobic capacity, during a 2-week stay at 2000 m [96]. This phenomenon may be explained by the study design. If, like most dialysis patients, the subjects showed no plateau in O_2 uptake, the tests were really measuring $\dot{V}O_{2peak}$ (this was not clearly described). In addition, the study was conducted on a group of dialysis patients vacationing in the Alps. This was very likely a coordinated social effort through a dialysis center, so that patients who otherwise were not inclined to travel could go on vacation (making arrangements for dialysis treatments can be intimidating). Given the tendency of dialysis patients toward a sedentary lifestyle, it seems likely they were more physically active on vacation than at home. Therefore, the higher lactate level may have been a result of the dialysis patients increasing their activity and vitality, were more motivated, or had a small training effect, and thus were able to go further during the exercise tests. These altitude findings should be confirmed by more well-controlled studies before their paradoxical data are accepted.

IV. Interactions Between Systems

Having looked at recent developments in our understanding of O_2 transport in ESRD, the recent advances in our understanding of the interactions between dysfunctional O_2 transport and the effects treatments of ESRD have on O_2 transport will now be considered.

A. Effects of ESRD Therapy on Oxygen Transport

Fluid Overload

Fluid overload is ubiquitous in dialysis patients because they produce little or no urine. Hemodialysis patients are more affected by intermittent fluid overload than are peritoneal dialysis patients, because hemodialysis patients have 2 days between treatments, and peritoneal dialysis patients have very frequent (or even continuous) treatment. Fluid overload may reduce diffusional conductance of O_2 in all tissues because of increased interstitial water (in which O_2 is poorly soluble). This potential problem has not been routinely studied, because study eligibility criteria almost always include being in a well-managed clinical condition. For this reason, research findings may not always mimic real-world situations.

The other aspect of fluid overload affecting O_2 transport is that cardiac preload is increased, sometimes to the point of frank congestive heart failure (right-sided, or left- and right-sided). This is usually mild heart failure, but can be more severe after major holidays, missed dialysis sessions, or other situations where dietary intake of salt is high for the amount of time between treatments.

Calcium

Dialysis patients commonly have abnormal calcium metabolism because of secondary hyperparathyroidism. Increases in serum calcium during dialysis cause an increase in myocardial contractility [48]. Decreases in intravascular fluid volume during dialysis leads to reduction in cardiac preload and a reduced Frank-Starling effect [47,97]. The decreased Frank-Starling effect is counteracted by the calcium-mediated increase in contractility, which maintains hemodynamic stability. Dialysis has prolonged beneficial effects on cardiac function in persons with heart failure; therefore, dialysis may have other positive effects in addition to fluid and electrolyte balance [98,99]. Dialysis of uremic patients also improves contractility of skeletal muscle [100]. Dialysis thus stabilizes cardiac output and improves contractile function of skeletal muscle.

Nitric Oxide

Exercise researchers have been clarifying the role of nitric oxide on vascular function, but research on nitric oxide as a mediator of O_2 transport in dialysis patients is lacking. Nitric oxide metabolism is markedly affected by the dialysis procedure, which causes an abrupt and several-fold increase in circulating nitric oxide [101]. The magnitude of this increase is partly dependent on the type of dialysis membrane used (with cuprophane causing more nitric oxide release than polysulfone or polyacrylonitrile membranes) [101]. Whether chronic exposure to high nitric oxide levels alters vascular smooth muscle biology over the long term or whether there is a differential effect from the type of membrane is not known. A great deal remains to be learned about the role of nitric oxide in regulating blood flow in dialysis patients. Epo therapy causes an acquired resistance to nitric oxide–mediated vasodilation in a rat model (see Section III.A) [92].

Bicarbonate

Bicarbonate dialysate is superior to acetate dialysate solutions because it causes fewer autonomic side effects [102]. In part, this may be a result of the treatment of metabolic acidosis of uremia. Metabolic acidosis is a pivotal factor in lean body mass wasting and the sacropenia commonly observed in dialysis patients [103]. Low-protein diets prescribed to dialysis patients ameliorate the side effects of nitrogen load, but low-protein intake contributes to sarcopenia. Bicarbonate therapy to reduce the magnitude of acidosis can reduce muscle wasting [103]. Maintenance of muscle mass is critically important in the patient's ability to generate force and a high O_2 uptake; therefore, use of bicarbonate might be important in retaining normal O_2 transport. As in many of the other domains mentioned herein, this issue has not yet been studied.

V. Systemic Factors

After looking at O_2 transport from a reductionist perspective, it is prudent to regain a more comprehensive or "holistic" perspective because the exercise response in ESRD does not fully follow traditional dogmas. Some dialysis patients fare well with exercise training, but some can exercise train very hard, or use Epo to achieve a big increase in hematocrit, and yet not improve their aerobic capacity. Systemic sequelae of ESRD may be one reason for this physiological heterogeneity between dialysis patients. This final section considers the interactions of regulatory processes on O_2 transport systems.

A. Emotive Factors

When thinking about exercise intolerance and integrated O_2 transport, it is easy to overlook the fact that many patients with renal failure just do not feel very good [1]. It is not easy to do vigorous exercise testing when one does not feel well. Most patients can give maximal efforts anyway, but some cannot muster the motivation to perform hard physical work. Furthermore, many renal failure patients suffer from depression [1,104,105]. Although psychological problems might not have a direct effect on O_2 transport, it is likely that they contribute to a lower peak work rate and a more sedentary lifestyle. The effects of psychological problems on O_2 transport are not really known, but should be considered when interpreting exercise data from some patients. In addition, it is not known how much this problem influences the exercise research data, but it probably has some confounding effects.

B. Central Command

Sympathetic Overstimulation

Dialysis patients often have central command abnormalities involving neuroendocrine and autonomic regulation. Dialysis patients who still have their failed kidneys have much higher resting mean sympathetic nerve activity than do normal persons (58 ± 3 vs. 23 ± 3 efferent bursts/min); however, nephrectomized dialysis patients have normal mean sympathetic nerve activity [45]. It is therefore believed that nonfunctioning kidneys are a cause of excess sympathetic stimulation. Because only a small minority of dialysis patients have undergone nephrectomy, the majority of patients have sympathetic hyperactivity. Among exercise researchers, debate exists about whether exercise involves a phenomenon of "functional sympatholysis," which occurs when skeletal muscle metabolically overrides sympathetic drive that would otherwise cause vasoconstriction [106–108]. Until this debate is resolved in normal subjects, the effects in dialysis patients will remain unclear. Nonetheless, sympathetic hyperactivity in ESRD surely presents an obstacle to increasing muscle blood flow during exercise.

Neuropathy

Patients who have been on dialysis for a long time are at increased risk for developing symptomatic neuropathy. In dialysis patients who are not diabetic, the large myelinated fibers are more profoundly affected by uremic neuropathy than the small unmyelinated fibers [109]. In contrast, diabetic dialysis patients have neuropathy that affects all fibers, large and small. Furthermore, there are both sympathetic and parasympathetic abnormalities in the majority of diabetic dialysis patients [110]. In addition, neuropathy is generally worse in patients who have been on dialysis for longer than 10 years [111]. As a consequence, dialysis patients, whether diabetic or not, frequently suffer from orthostatic intolerance, volatile changes in blood pressure, and subnormal cardiac chronotropic response to exercise. Simultaneous kidney/pancreas transplantation is thought to stabilize and perhaps improve this neuropathy, but transplantation of kidney or pancreas alone does not stabilize polyneuropathy [112].

A small percentage (approximately 10%) of dialysis patients have autonomic dysfunction severe enough to cause hemodynamic instability (such as dialysis-induced hypotension). This group can be further subdivided into those who regain blood pressure after an intravenous saline infusion and those who remain hypotensive despite a saline infusion. The mechanism causing responsiveness to saline is not clear but seems to be related to autonomic dysfunction. In particular, electrocardiogram R-to-R intervals during Valsalva maneuver show lower variability in volume-nonresponsive dialysis patients in comparison to volume-responsive patients and normal controls [113]. Unfortunately, this group difference is not a helpful distinction, because a substantial number of dialysis patients have responses comparable to normals. Indeed, dialysis-induced hypotension is thought to be similar to vasodepressor syncope in normal subjects [114]. The balance of vasoconstrictors and vasodilators in dialysis patients is not fully understood.

Baroreflex

Arterial baroreceptor function in ESRD is markedly abnormal in almost all dialysis patients. This has been attributed to autonomic neuropathy in the afferent baroreflex arc, as well as to elevated serum norepinephrine [110,115,116]. Furthermore, dialysis patients who still have their dysfunctional kidneys (the vast majority of patients) have a several-fold elevation of sympathetic nervous activity [45]. Thus, it is generally believed that neurohumoral control of vasoreactivity is impaired in the majority of patients. Such an abnormality may partly explain an inability of dialysis patients to achieve more complete O_2 extraction after Epo therapy, as many patients have whole-body O_2 extraction ratios that decrease to less than 0.5 [39]. What needs to be developed is an integrated understanding of baroreflex and vasoconstrictor/vasodilator control in the context of O_2 delivery.

C. Hyperparathyroidism

Hyperparathyroidism is a well-known secondary problem of uremia, classically associated with muscle and bone weakness. The final activation step in vitamin D metabolism occurs in the kidneys; therefore, persons with ESRD lack sufficient 1,25-hydroxy-vitamin-D_3 and become hypocalcemic. The resulting muscle weakness reduces the ability of skeletal muscle to create metabolic demand for O_2 uptake. Hypocalcemia also reduces contractility in the heart and can result in heart failure [46]. Thus, uncontrolled secondary hyperparathyroidism seems likely to contribute to low aerobic capacity in some patients. Because there are now good pharmacological options for managing secondary hyperparathyroidism, this problem should be less frequently encountered than in the past.

D. Insulin Resistance

Uremia causes a form of insulin resistance, and some dialysis patients also have β cell resistance to glucose, as well as an abnormal response to growth hormone [117]. These defects in glucose metabolism reduce pyruvate dehydrogenase flux

[64,118]. Because uremia does not alter insulin receptor binding or tyrosine kinase activity, there seems to be an insulin-specific, postreceptor defect in the activation of pyruvate dehydrogenase [64]. Thus, insulin resistance may play a limiting role in energy metabolism of dialysis patients, involving the metabolic link between glycolytic (i.e., O_2-independent) and Krebs cycle (i.e., O_2-dependent) pathways. This may explain the paradox of higher-than-normal blood lactate during submaximal exercise, but lower-than-normal blood lactate at peak exercise [38]. Because exercise activates pyruvate dehydrogenase in uremia, exercise training might counteract these abnormalities [64]. Insulin resistance is associated with hypertension and may play a role in linking glucose metabolism to vasodilation [119–121]. How this fact adds to the complexity of glycogen metabolism in ESRD is not clear.

E. Endothelins

Endothelins (ETs) are a small family of polypeptide isoforms with extremely potent vasoconstrictor properties. ETs are produced by vascular endothelial cells and are named ET-1, ET-2, and ET-3 [80]. ETs play a critical role in the control of systemic vascular resistance, and thus in regulation of blood flow to tissues. Dialysis patients have remarkably high ET-1 levels, on the order of three to six times higher than normal controls; ET-2 and ET-3 levels are less elevated, typically twice that of normal controls [81,122–124].

Endothelin 1 is correlated with systolic and diastolic blood pressure and, more importantly, may participate in regulation of blood flow during exercise. In normal subjects performing high-intensity submaximal one-legged exercise, ET-1 was extremely elevated in the nonexercised leg, suggesting that ET-1 participates in shunting blood flow away from less active muscle during exercise [125]. This author could find no studies assessing the role of ETs in limiting O_2 transport in dialysis patients, but the integral role of ET-1 in regulating blood flow makes it a likely candidate as a factor contributing to the low $\dot{V}O_{2peak}$ in dialysis patients.

F. Uremic Toxins

Patients with ESRD have circulating compounds known collectively as "uremic toxins" [126]. Very little is known about uremic toxins, in part because there are dozens (if not hundreds) of these so-called "middle molecules." They are called middle molecules because they are too large to be efficiently cleared by dialysis, and it is for this reason that they remain in the blood.

Uremic toxins retain biologic activity that can be ergolytic. Undialyzed uremic patients have a low electrochemical potential across the resting sarcolemma, such that the resting potential is lower than activation threshold [100]. The cause of this problem is not well understood, although it involves calcium; the normal action potential is restored by appropriate dialysis [100]. Therefore, one reason

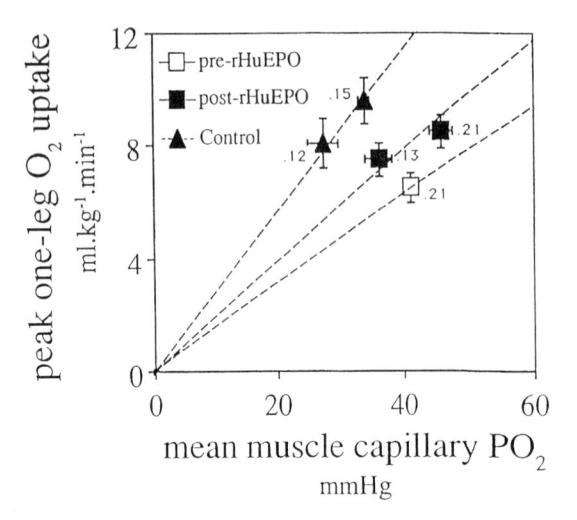

Figure 4 Relationships of one-legged oxygen uptake to mean muscle capillary oxygen partial pressure in dialysis patients versus sedentary controls; dialysis patients were studied before and after treatment with recombinant human erythropoietin (rHuEPO). The inspired oxygen fraction (F$_{IO_2}$) of each measurement is indicated adjacent to each plotted point; dashed lines indicate muscle oxygen conductance of each study group. Data show that before erythropoietin therapy, dialysis patients had lower muscle oxygen conductance than normal subjects, and that increasing hematocrit with erythropoietin increased but did not normalize muscle oxygen conductance.

undialyzed uremic patients are weak may be that muscle is decoupled from neural excitation. If one were to try to measure $\dot{V}O_{2max}$ in an undialyzed uremic person, it would surely be very low, and it is even doubtful such a person could perform an exercise test.

It is not known whether the molecules responsible for loss of electrochemical membrane potential are circulating in underdialyzed uremic persons. One probable uremic toxin is endogenous ouabain, which is a digoxin-like (or ouabain-like) compound detectable in up to two thirds of dialysis patients [127,128]. Endogenous ouabain has been anecdotally associated with bradycardic episodes and thus may have some cardiovascular role mediated through alteration of sodium-potassium ATPase (Na-K-ATPase) function and membrane potential.

G. Bone and Connective Tissue

Few people think of connective tissues as limiting O$_2$ transport, but, in fact, there are some limitations related to bone disease. Muscle acts through tendons, ligaments, and joints by pulling on bone. Therefore, diseases of tendons, bones, cartilage, and ligaments can reduce aerobic capacity if they prevent the muscle from pulling with great force. In renal failure, there are some bone and connective tissue sequelae that can be devastating and thereby severely limit $\dot{V}O_{2peak}$. The main conditions worth mentioning are renal osteomalacia/secondary hyperparathyroidism, stress fractures, destructive arthritis (gout in particular), aluminum bone disease, and tendon avulsions [129]. Renal osteodystrophy from hyperparathyroidism has been included by some authorities as a main contributor to weakness of uremic myopathy [63]. Even if bone involvement is not directly involved in uremic myopathy (hyperparathyroidism seems a sufficient cause), bone does play a role as a reservoir of calcium. Unfortunately, these connective-tissue problems are common, and there often is no satisfactory solution; many patients become more inactive and deconditioned as a result of their bone and joint problems (personal observation).

VI. Conclusions

Having considered a bewildering number of factors contributing to the low $\dot{V}O_{2peak}$ in dialysis patients, we still cannot say what limits whole-body O_2 transport in any given patient. Looking at the original Painter/Hanson model, we can now see some interactions across physiological systems due to the effects of ESRD therapies and to cell–cell signaling/cytokines/hormones (Fig. 5). In addition, we see that low $\dot{V}O_{2peak}$ is largely a problem of: (1) weak patients who cannot generate a high mitochondrial demand for O_2; (2) low peak-exercise muscle blood flow, related to a low peak cardiac output/heart rate and an inability to redistribute blood flow to exercising muscle; and (3) low diffusional O_2 conductance in muscle (DmO_2). However, these three factors cannot be blindly applied to all dialysis patients because heterogeneity in this population means that a single paradigm cannot account for all patients. Some patients may have O_2 transport limited by being too weak and frail to perform much physical activity and thus be ''demand limited,'' but some patients may have O_2 transport limited by poor blood flow regulation or O_2 diffusion and thus be ''supply limited.'' In conclusion, we can make some reasonably conservative speculations:

1. Oxygen transport to and from air to tissues is remarkably complicated in renal failure patients. There is virtually no organ system left unaffected by renal failure, and many of them directly and/or indirectly affect O_2 transport. Even organs not traditionally thought to limit O_2 transport, such as the lungs, are affected by ESRD and thus may be important in some patients.
2. Oxygen transport is altered in ESRD, but the effects are generally not clinically meaningful at rest. At peak exercise, O_2 delivery to skeletal muscle is decidedly subnormal because of low peak heart rate, low O_2-carrying capacity of blood, and perhaps because of subnormal redistribution of blood flow.

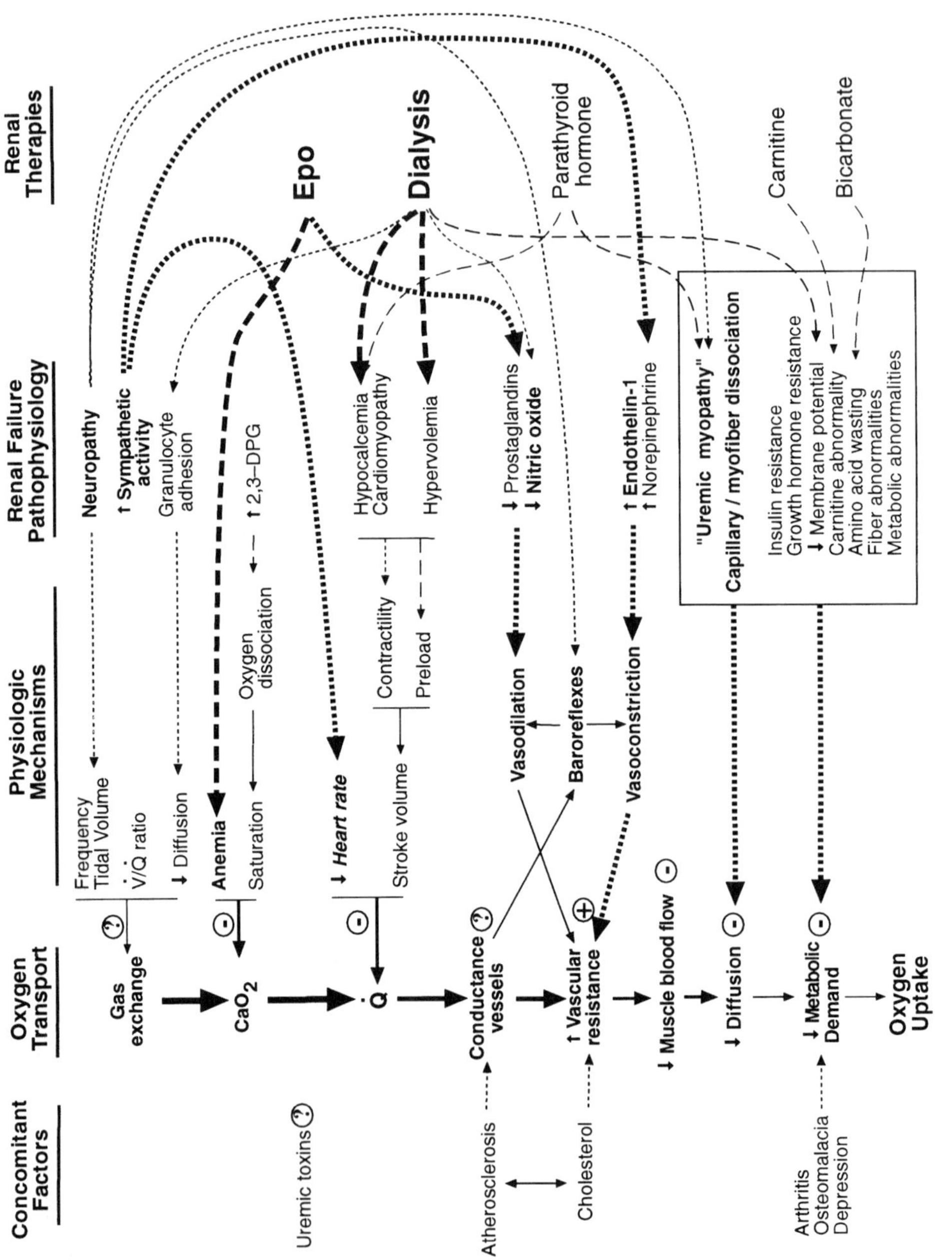

Concomitant Factors
Oxygen Transport
Physiologic Mechanisms
Renal Failure Pathophysiology
Renal Therapies
Uremic toxins
Atherosclerosis
Cholesterol
Arthritis
Osteomalacia
Depression
Gas exchange
CaO2
Q
Conductance vessels
↑ Vascular resistance
↓ Muscle blood flow
↓ Diffusion
↓ Metabolic Demand
Oxygen Uptake
Frequency
Tidal Volume
V/Q ratio
↓ Diffusion
Anemia
Saturation
↓ Heart rate
Stroke volume
Oxygen dissociation
Contractility
Preload
Vasodilation
Baroreflexes
Vasoconstriction
Neuropathy
↑ Sympathetic activity
Granulocyte adhesion
↑ 2,3–DPG
Hypocalcemia
Cardiomyopathy
Hypervolemia
↓ Prostaglandins
↓ Nitric oxide
↑ Endothelin-1
↑ Norepinephrine
"Uremic myopathy"
Capillary / myofiber dissociation
Insulin resistance
Growth hormone resistance
↓ Membrane potential
Carnitine abnormality
Amino acid wasting
Fiber abnormalities
Metabolic abnormalities
Epo
Dialysis
Parathyroid hormone
Carnitine
Bicarbonate

Figure 5 Modified Painter/Hanson model for effects of renal failure on oxygen transport physiology; underlying structure of the columns and rows remain from the original model (see Fig. 1). Factors of major importance now appear in boldface type; dashed arrows show mechanisms that substantially alter oxygen transport in end-stage renal disease; arrows with a "+" indicate mechanisms that improve oxygen transport; arrows with a "−" show mechanisms that reduce oxygen transport; arrows with a "?" show mechanisms where the affect on oxygen transport is not clear. Erythropoietin (Epo) has a trophic effect on erythrogenesis, improving anemia and increasing arterial oxygen content; Epo adversely effects prostaglandin/nitric oxide–mediated vasodilation, reducing peripheral-blood flow; Epo reduces left ventricular hypertrophy (LVH), mechanism unknown. Dialysis has multiple effects, only some are shown: it transiently alters pulmonary function (see text); improves hypocalcemia and myocardial contractility; improves hypovolemia and cardiac congestion; releases vasodilatory substances (acutely); and reduces uremic toxins and effects thereof. Exercise training improves peripheral metabolism/oxygen use, affective disorders, and perhaps vasomotor regulation. Parathyroid hormone has normalizing effects on hypocalcemia and musculoskeletal function. Atherosclerosis and hypercholesterolemia decrease convective blood flow to tissues. Sympathetic hyperactivity increases vasoconstriction and heart rate and resolves after nephrectomy. Bicarbonate and carnitine improve peripheral tissue metabolism. Skeletal and affective disorders decrease tolerance of physically stressful activities. Interactions between systems seems to occur mostly in the periphery via vasomotor control of vascular resistance and through therapies affecting metabolic control.

3. Whether before or after the introduction of Epo, $\dot{V}O_{2peak}$ is low in ESRD when compared with age- and gender-matched normal subjects. Even after treatment with Epo, $\dot{V}O_{2peak}$ is generally less than 24 mL/kg/min and more than 2 standard deviations below normal. If Epo is to achieve its maximal theoretical benefit, we must know how to improve O_2 delivery to muscle (both convectively to the vascular bed and across the capillary/myofiber interface).
4. Circulation/contraction coupling seems to be an important contributor to the low $\dot{V}O_{2peak}$ based on studies of exercise training, muscle strength, whole-body and leg O_2 transport, and skeletal muscle energy metabolism. Despite evidence for abnormalities in some metabolites (e.g., carnitine), the probable main culprits are anatomic and functional abnormalities in the capillary/myofiber interface, as well as overall muscle weakness.
5. Given the anatomic and functional abnormalities highlighted in the microcirculation and resistance vessels, it seems probable that neurohumoral and cell-signaling mechanisms are involved in the dysfunctional circulation/contraction interaction (e.g., ET-1, nitric oxide).
6. Exercise training and Epo usually, but not always, increase $\dot{V}O_{2peak}$. Why some patients do not respond to exercise and Epo is unknown.
7. The complexity and number of problems makes it improbable that solving any one problem will make a very big difference (e.g., the experience with exercise and Epo); therefore, any truly beneficial solution must take an integrated approach. Nonetheless, exercise training and Epo help patients maintain independence, improve quality of life, and lower risk of comorbidity. These latter findings are not directly related to O_2 transport and therefore were not discussed herein, but they highlight the continued importance of research on the mechanisms of exercise intolerance in ESRD.

Acknowledgment

The author thanks Drs. Patricia Painter, Loren Bertocci, and William Haskell for their support and reviews of this chapter.

References

1. Evans RW, Manninen DL, Garrison LP, Hart LG, Blagg CR, Gutman RA, Hull AR, Lowrie EG. The quality of life of patients with end-stage renal failure. N Engl J Med 1985; 312:553–559.
2. Painter PL. Exercise in end-stage renal disease. Exerc Sports Sci Rev 1988; 16:305–339.

3. Painter P, Hanson P. A model for clinical exercise prescription: application to hemodialysis patients. J Cardiopulmonary Rehabil 1987; 7:177–189.
4. Zifko U, Auinger M, Albrecht G, Kastenbauer T, Lahrmann H, Grisold W, Wanke T. Phrenic neuropathy in chronic renal failure. Thorax 1995; 50:793–794.
5. Sebert P, Bellet M, Girin E, Cledes J, Barthelemy L. Ventilatory and occlusion pressure responses to hypercapnia in patients with chronic renal failure. Respiration 1984; 45:191–196.
6. Bush A, Gabriel R. Pulmonary function in chronic renal failure: effects of dialysis and transplantation. Thorax 1991; 46:424–428.
7. Moinard J, Guenard H. Membrane diffusion of the lungs in patients with chronic renal failure. Eur Resp J 1993; 6:225–230.
8. Kolb G, Hoffken H, Muller T, Havemann K, Joseph K, Lange H. Kinetics of pulmonary leukocyte sequestration in man during hemodialysis with different membrane-types. Int J Artif Organs 1990; 13:729–736.
9. Kolb G, Fischer W, Muller T, Hoffken H, Joseph K, Lange H, Havemann K. Granulocyte-related bioincompatibility of hemodialysis: inhibition of oxidative metabolism, degranulation reaction, enzyme release and leukocyte sequestration in the lung. Int J Artif Organs 1989; 12:294–298.
10. Paul K, Mavridis G, Bonzel KE, Scharer K. Pulmonary function in children with chronic renal failure. Eur J Pediatr 150; 1991; 11:808–812.
11. Beasley CR, Ripley JM, Smith DA, Neale TJ. Pulmonary function in chronic renal failure patients managed by continuous ambulatory peritoneal dialysis. N Z Med J 1986; 99:313–315.
12. Dujic Z, Eterovic D, Tocilj J. Pulmonary function in chronic renal failure: effects of dialysis and transplantation. Thorax 1992; 47:763.
13. Lewis NP, Macdougall IC, Willis N, Henderson AH. The ventilatory cost of exercise compared in chronic heart failure and chronic renal anaemia. Q J Med 1992; 83:523–531.
14. Romaldini H, Rodriguez Roisin R, Lopez FA, Ziegler TW, Bencowitz HZ, Wagner PD. The mechanisms of arterial hypoxemia during hemodialysis. Am Rev Respir Dis 1984; 129:780–784.
15. Pitcher WD, Diamond SM, Henrich WL. Pulmonary gas exchange during dialysis in patients with obstructive lung disease. Chest 1989; 96:1136–1141.
16. Blanchet F, Kanfer A, Cramer E, Benyahia A, Georges R, Mery JP, Amiel C. Relative contribution of intrinsic lung dysfunction and hypoventilation to hypoxemia during hemodialysis. Kidney Int 1984; 26:430–435.
17. Erslev AJ, Wilson J, Caro J. Erythropoietin titers in anemic, nonuremic patients. J Lab Clin Med 1987; 109:429–433.
18. CESG. Association between recombinant human erythropoietin and quality of life and exercise capacity in patients receiving haemodialysis. Br Med J 1990; 300:573–578.
19. Radermacher J, Koch KM. Treatment of renal anemia by erythropoietin substitution: the effects on the cardiovascular system. Clin Nephrol 1995; 44(Suppl 1):S56–S60.
20. Juric M, Rupcic V, Topuzovic N, Jakic M, Brlosic R, Rusic A, Karner I, Stipanic S, Kes P. Haemodynamic changes and exercise tolerance in dialysis patients treated with erythropoietin. Nephrol Dial Transplant 1995; 10:1398–1404.

21. Morris KP, Skinner JR, Hunter S, Coulthard MG. Cardiovascular abnormalities in end stage renal failure: the effect of anaemia or uraemia? Arch Dis Childhood 1994; 71:119–122.
22. Wizemann V, Schafer R, WK. Follow-up of cardiac changes induced by anemia compensation in normotensive hemodialysis patients with left-ventricular hypertrophy. Nephron 1993; 64:202–206.
23. Mayer G, Thum J, Cada EM, Stummvoll HK, Graf H. Working capacity is increased following recombinant human erythropoietin treatment. Kidney Int 1988; 34:525–528.
24. Metra M, Cannella G, La Canna G, Guaini T, Sandrini M, Gaggiotti M, Movilli E, Dei Cas L. Improvement in exercise capacity after correction of anemia in patients with end-stage renal failure. Am J Cardiol 1991; 68:1060–1066.
25. Lundin AP, Akerman MJ, Chesler RM, Delano BG, Goldberg N, Stein RA, Friedman EA. Exercise in hemodialysis patients after treatment with recombinant human erythropoietin. Nephron 1991; 58:315–319.
26. MacDougall IC, Lewis NP, Saunders MJ, Cochlin DL, Davies ME, Hutton RD, Fox KA, Coles GA, Williams JD. Long-term cardiorespiratory effects of amelioration of renal anemia by erythropoietin. Lancet 1990; 335:489–493.
27. Robertson HT, Haley NR, Guthrie M, Cardenas D, Eschbach JW, Adamson JW. Recombinant erythropoietin improves exercise capacity in anemic hemodialysis patients. Am J Kidney Dis 1990; 15:325–332.
28. Painter PL, Messer-Rehak D, Hanson P, Zimmerman SW, Glass NR. Exercise capacity in hemodialysis, CAPD, and renal transplant patients. Nephron 1986; 42:47–51.
29. Moore GE, Brinker KR, Stray-Gundersen J, Mitchell JH. Determinants of $\dot{V}O_{2peak}$ in patients with end-stage renal disease: on and off dialysis. Med Sci Sports Exerc 1993; 25:18–23.
30. Lundin AP, Stein RA, Frank F, La Belle P, Berlyne GM, Krasnow N, Friedman EA. Cardiovascular status in long-term hemodialysis patients: an exercise and echocardiographic study. Nephron 1981; 28:234–238.
31. Lundin AP, Stein RA, Brown CD, La Belle P, Kalman FS, Delano BG, Heneghan WF, Lazarus NA, Krasnow N, Friedmen EA. Fatigue, acid-base and electrolyte changes with exhaustive treadmill exercise in hemodialysis patients. Nephron 1987; 46:57–62.
32. Zabetakis PM, Gleim GW, Pasternak FL, Saraniti A, Nicholas JA, Michelis MF. Long-duration submaximal exercise conditioning in hemodialysis patients. Clin Nephrol 1982; 18:17–22.
33. Shalom R, Blumenthal JA, Williams RS, McMurray RG, Dennis VW. Feasibility and benefits of exercise training in patients on maintenance dialysis. Kidney Int 1984; 25:958–963.
34. Goldberg AP, Geltman EM, Hagberg JM, Gavin JR III, Delmez JA, Carney RM, Naumowicz A, Oldfield MH, Harter HR. Therapeutic benefits of exercise training for hemodialysis patients. Kidney Int 1983; 24(Suppl 16):S303–309.
35. Robertson RJ, Gilcher R, Metz KF, Skrinar GS, Allison TG, Bahnson HT, Abbott RA, Becker R, Falkel FE. Effect of induced erythrocythemia on hypoxia tolerance during physical exercise. J Appl Physiol Respir Environ Exercise Physiol 1982; 53:490–495.

36. Ross DL, Grabeau GM, Smith S, Seymour M, Knierim N, Pitetti KH. Efficacy of exercise for end-stage renal disease patients immediately following high-efficiency hemodialysis: a pilot study. Am J Nephrol 1989; 9:376–383.
37. Thompson JR, Stray-Gundersen J. Cardiovascular adaptations in maximal exercise among patients with end-stage renal disease after graded increases in hemoglobin (abstract). J Am Soc Nephrol 1991; 2:389.
38. Meierhenrich R, Jedicke H, Voigt A, Lange H. The effect of erythropoietin on lactate, pyruvate and excess lactate under physical exercise in dialysis patients. Clin Nephrol 1996; 45:90–97.
39. Painter P, Moore GE. The impact of recombinant erythropoietin therapy on exercise capacity in hemodialysis patients. Adv Renal Replacement Ther 1994; 1:55–65.
40. System USRD. USRDS 1993 Annual Data Report. Bethesda, MD: National Institutes of Health, NIDDK, March 1993.
41. Noakes TD, Diesel W. $\dot{V}O_{2peak}$ and end-stage renal disease (letter). Med Sci Sports Exerc 1993; 25:1429–1430.
42. Moore GE, Mitchell JH. $\dot{V}O_{2peak}$ and end-stage renal disease (response to letter). Med Sci Sports Exerc 1993; 25:1430–1431.
43. Barnea N, Drory Y, Iaina A, Lapidot C, Reisin E, Eliahou H, Kellerman JJ. Exercise tolerance in patients on chronic hemodialysis. Israel J Med Sci 1980; 16:17–21.
44. Ulmer HE, Greimer H, Schuler HW, Scharer K. Cardiovascular impairment and physical working capacity in children with chronic renal failure. Acta Paediatr Scand 1978; 67:43–48.
45. Converse RLJ, Jacobsen TN, Toto RD, Jost CM, Cosentino F, Fouad-Tarazi F, Victor RG. Sympathetic overactivity in patients with chronic renal failure. N Engl J Med 1992; 327:1912–1918.
46. Wong CK, Pun KK, Cheng CH, Lau CP, Leung WH, Chan WK, Yeung DW. Hypocalcemic heart failure in end-stage renal disease. Am J Nephrol 1990; 10:167–170.
47. Nixon JV, Mitchell JH, McPhaul JJ, Henrich WL. Effect of hemodialysis on left ventricular function. J Clin Invest 1983; 71:377–384.
48. Henrich WL, Hunt JM, Nixon JV. Increased ionized calcium and left ventricular contractility during hemodialysis. N Engl J Med 1984; 310:19–23.
49. Gilligan DM, Guetta V, Panza JA, Garcia CE, Quyyumi AA, Cannon RO. Selective loss of microvascular endothelial function in human hypercholesterolemia. Circulation 1994; 90:35–41.
50. Casino PR, Kilcoyne CM, Quyyumi AA, Hoeg JM, Panza JA. The role of nitric oxide in endothelium-dependent vasodilation of hypercholesterolemic patients. Circulation 1993; 88:2541–2547.
51. Ahonen R. Light microscopic study of striated muscle in uremia. Acta Neuropathol (Berl) 1980; 49:51–55.
52. Ahonen R. Striated muscle ultrastructure in uremic patients and in renal transplant recipients. Acta Neuropathol (Berl) 1980; 50:163–166.
53. Floyd M, Ayyar DR, Barwick DD, Hudgson P, Weightman D. Myopathy in chronic renal failure. Q J Med 1974; 43:509–524.
54. Lazaro RP, Kirshner HS. Proximal muscle weakness in uremia: case reports and review of the literature. Arch Neurol 1980; 37:555–558.

55. Bautista J, Gil-Necija E, Castilla J, Chinchon I, Rafel E. Dialysis myopathy: report of 13 cases. Acta Neuropathol (Berl) 1983; 61:71–75.
56. Moore GE, Parsons DB, Painter PL, Brinker KR, Stray-Gundersen J, Mitchell JH. Uremic myopathy limits aerobic capacity of hemodialysis patients. Am J Kidney Dis 1993; 22:277–287.
57. Moore GE, Bertocci LA, Painter PL. ^{31}P-Magnetic resonance spectroscopy assessment of subnormal oxidative metabolism of skeletal muscle in renal failure patients. J Clin Invest 1993; 91:420–424.
58. Marrades RM, Roca J, Campistol JM, Diaz O, Barbera JA, Torregrosa JV, Masclans JR, Cobos A, Rodriguez-Roisin R, Wagner PD. Effects of erythropoietin on muscle O_2 transport during exercise in patients with chronic renal failure. J Clin Invest 1996; 97:2092–2100.
59. Piiper J. Modelling of oxygen transport skeletal muscle: blood flow distribution, shunt, and diffusion. In: Goldstick TK, ed. Oxygen Transport to Tissue. New York: Plenum Press, 1992, pp 3–10.
60. Diesel W, Emms M, Knight BK, Noakes TD, Zyl Smit RV, Kaschula ROC, Sinclair-Smith CC. Morphologic features of the myopathy associated with chronic renal failure. Am J Kidney Dis 1993; 22:677–684.
61. Diesel W, Noakes TD, Swanepoel C, Lambert M. Isokinetic muscle strength predicts maximum exercise tolerance in renal patients on chronic hemodialysis. Am J Kidney Dis 1990; 16:109–114.
62. Hörl WH, Sperling J, Heidland A. Enhanced glycogen turnover in skeletal muscle of uremic rats: cause of uncontrolled actomyosin ATPase? Am J Clin Nutr 1978; 31:1861–1864.
63. Brautbar N. Skeletal myopathy in uremia: abnormal energy metabolism. Kidney Int 1983; 24(Suppl 16):S81–83.
64. Contreras I, Caro JF, Aveledo L, Diaz K, Durrego P, Weisinger JR. In chronic uremia, insulin activates receptor kinase but not pyruvate dehydrogenase. Nephron 1992; 61:77–81.
65. Hiatt WR, Koziol BJ, Shapiro JI, Brass EP. Carnitine metabolism during exercise in patients on chronic hemodialysis. Kidney Int 1992; 41:1613–1619.
66. Golper TA, Wolfson M, Ahmad S, Hirschberg R, P K, Katz LA, Nicora R, Ashbrook D, Kopple JD. Multicenter trial of L-carnitine in maintenance hemodialysis patients. I. Carnitine concentrations and lipid effects. Kidney Int 1990; 38:904–911.
67. Bartel LL, Hussey JL, Shrago E. Effect of dialysis on serum carnitine, free fatty acids, and triglyceride levels in man and the rat. Metabolism 1982; 31:944–947.
68. Savica V, Bellinghieri G, DiStefano C, Corvaja E, Consolo F, Corsi M, Maccari F, Spagnoli LG, Villaschi S, Palmieri G. Plasma and muscle carnitine levels in hemodialysis patients with morphological-ultrastructural examination of muscle samples. Nephron 1983; 35:232–236.
69. Siami G, Clinton ME, Mrak R, Griffis J, Stone W. Evaluation of the effect of intravenous L-carnitine therapy on function, structure and fatty acid metabolism of skeletal muscle in patients receiving chronic hemodialysis. Nephron 1991; 57:306–313.
70. Ahmad S, Robertson HT, Golper TA, Wolfson M, Kurtin P, Katz LA, Hirschberg R, Nicora R, Ashbrook DW, Kopple JD. Multicenter trial of L-carnitine in maintenance

hemodialysis patients. II. Clinical and biochemical effects. Kidney Int 1990; 38:912–918.
71. Gayeski TEJ, Honig CR. O_2 gradients from sarcolemma to cell interior in a red muscle of maximal $\dot{V}O_2$. Am J Physiol 1986; 251:789–799.
72. Wittenberg BA, Wittenberg JB. Effects of carbon monoxide on isolated heart muscle cells. Res Rep Health Eff Inst 1993; 62:1–21.
73. Saltin B, Strange S. Maximal oxygen uptake: old and new arguments for a cardiovascular limitation. Med Sci Sports Exerc 1992; 24:30–37.
74. Thompson CH, Kemp GJ, Taylor DJ, Ledingham JG, Radda GK, Rajagopalan B. Effect of chronic uraemia on skeletal muscle metabolism in man. Nephrol Dial Transplant 1993; 8:218–222.
75. Thompson CH, Kempm GJ, Green YS, Rix LK, Radda GK, Ledingham JG, Skeletal muscle metabolism in uremic rats: a ^{31}P-magnetic resonance study. Nephron 1993; 63:330–334.
76. Marrades RM, Alonso J, Roca J, Gonzalez de Suso JM, Campistol JM, Barberal JA, Diaz O, Torregrosa JV, Masclans JR, Rodriguez-Roisin R, Wagner PD. Cellular bioenergetics after erythropoietin therapy in chronic renal failure. J Clin Invest 1996; 97:2101–2110.
77. Park JS, Kim SB, Park SK, Lim TH, Lee DK, Hong CD. Effect of recombinant human erythropoietin on muscle energy metabolism in patients with end-stage renal disease: a ^{31}P-nuclear magnetic resonance spectroscopic study. Am J Kidney Dis 1993; 21:612–618.
78. Durozard D, Pimmel P, Baretto S, Caillette A, Labeeuw M, Baverel G, Zech P. ^{31}P-NMR spectroscopy investigation of muscle metabolism in hemodialysis patients. Kidney Int 1993; 43:885–892.
79. Cooper JM, Petty RKH, Hayes DJ, Challiss RAJ, Brosnan MJ, Shoubridge EA, Radda GK, Morgan-Hughes JA, Clark JB. An animal model of mitochondrial myopathy: a biochemical and physiological investigation of rats treated in vivo with the NADH CoQ reductase inhibitor, diphenyleneiodonium. J Neurol Sci 1988; 83:335–347.
80. Takahashi K, Totsune K, Mouri T. Endothelin in chronic renal failure. Nephron 1994; 66:373–379.
81. Deray G, Carayon A, Maistre G, Benhmida M, Masson F, Barthelemy C, Petitclerc T, Jacobs C. Endothelin in chronic renal failure. Nephrol Dial Transplant 1992; 7:300–305.
82. Haaber AB, Eidemak I, Jensen T, Feldt-Rasmussen B, Strandgaard S. Vascular endothelial cell function and cardiovascular risk factors in patients with chronic renal failure. J Am Soc Nephrol 1995; 5:1581–1584.
83. Nakayama M, Yamada K, Yamamoto Y, Yokoyama K, Nakano H, Kubo H, Shigematsu T, Kawaguchi Y, Sakai O. Vascular endothelial dysfunction in patients on regular dialysis treatment. Clin Nephrol 1994; 42:117–120.
84. Piiper H. Diffusion limitation of oxygen in heterogeneous lung and tissue models. In: Erdmann W, Bruley DF, eds. Oxygen Transport to Tissue. New York: Plenum Press, 1992, pp 623–627.
85. Piiper H. Oxygen supply by perfusion and diffusion in heterogeneous tissue models. In: Erdmann W, Bruley DF, eds. Oxygen Transport to Tissue. New York: Plenum Press, 1992, pp 319–323.

86. Morris KP, Skinner JR, Hunter S, Coulthard MG. Short term correction of anaemia with recombinant human erythropoietin and reduction of cardiac output in end stage renal failure. Arch Dis Child 1993; 68:644–648.
87. Wizemann B, Kaufmann J, Kramer W. Effect of erythropoietin on ischemia tolerance in anemic hemodialysis patients with confirmed coronary artery disease. Nephron 1992; 62:161–165.
88. Nonnast-Daniel B, Schaffer J, Frei U. Hemodynamics in hemodialysis patients treated with recombinant human erythropoietin. Contrib Nephrol 1989; 76:283–289.
89. Dunn CJ, Markham A. Epoetin beta: a review of its pharmacological properties and clinical use in the management of anaemia associated with chronic renal failure [review]. Drugs 1996; 51:299–318.
90. Bode Böger SM, Böger RH, Kuhn M, Radermacher J, Frolich JC. Endothelin release and shift in prostaglandin balance are involved in the modulation of vascular tone by recombinant erythropoietin. J Cardiovasc Pharmacol 1992; 20(Suppl 12):S25–28.
91. Hand LJ, Bore PJ, Galloway G, Morris PJ, Radda GK. Muscle metabolism in patients with peripheral vascular disease investigated by ^{31}P nuclear magnetic resonance spectroscopy. Clin Sci 1986; 71:283–290.
92. Vaziri ND, Zhou XJ, Naqvi F, Smith J, Oveisi F, Wang ZQ, Purdy RE. Role of nitric oxide resistance in erythropoietin-induced hypertension in rats with chronic renal failure. Am J Physiol 1996; 271(1 Pt 1):E113–122.
93. Monti JP, Brunet P, Baz M, Klinkmann H, Berland Y, Merzouk T, Elsen R, Crevat A. 2,3 diphosphoglycerate haemoglobin binding in uraemic patients treated with erythropoietin: a ^{31}P nuclear magnetic resonance study. Nephrol Dial Transplant 1993; 8:223–226.
94. Painter PL. Personal communication, May 1997.
95. Kempeneers G, Noakes TD, van Zyl-Smydt R, Myburgh KH, Lambert M, Adams B, Wiggins T. Skeletal muscle limits the exercise tolerance of renal transplant recipients: effects of a graded exercise training program. Am J Kidney Dis 1990; 16:57–65.
96. Mairbäurl H, Schobersberger W, Hasibeder W, Knapp E, Hopferwieser T, Humpeler E, Loeffler HD, Wetzels E, Wybitul K, Baumgartl P, Dittrich P. Exercise performance of hemodialysis patients during short-term and prolonged exposure to altitude. Clin Nephrol 1989; 32:31–39.
97. Martin Malo A, Aljama P, Pasalodos J, Sancho M, Valles E, Moreno E, Gomez J, Perez R, Burdiel L, Andres E. Effects of haemodialysis and haemofiltration on myocardial function. Contrib Nephrol 1984; 41:403–408.
98. Forslund T, Riddervold F, Fauchald P, Torvik D, Fyhrquist F, Simonsen S. Hormonal changes in patients with severe congestive heart failure treated by ultrafiltration. Nephrol Dial Transplant 1992; 7:306–310.
99. Blake P, Paganini EP. Refractory congestive heart failure: overview and application of extracorporeal ultrafiltration. Adv Renal Replacement Ther 1996; 3:166–173.
100. Cotton JR, Woodard T, Carter NW, Knochel JP. Resting skeletal muscle membrane potential as an index of uremic toxicity. J Clin Invest 1979; 63:501–506.
101. Rysz J, Luciak M, Kedziora J, Blaszczyk J, Sibinska E. Nitric oxide release in the peripheral blood during hemodialysis. Kidney Int 1997; 51:294–300.

102. Velez RL, Woodard TD, Henrich WL. Acetate and bicarbonate hemodialysis in patients with and without autonomic dysfunction. Kidney Int 1984; 26:59–65.
103. Price SR, Mitch WE. Metabolic acidosis and uremic toxicity: protein and amino acid metabolism. Semin Nephrol 1994; 14:232–237.
104. Hart LG, Evans RW. The functional status of ESRD patients as measured by the sickness impact profile. J Chron Dis 1987; 40(Suppl 1):117S–130S.
105. Evans RW. Recombinant human erythropoietin and the quality of life of end-stage renal disease patients: a comparative analysis. Am J Kidney Dis 1991; 18:62–70.
106. Shoemaker JK, Pandey P, Herr MD, Silber DH, Yang QX, Smith MB, Gray K, Sinoway LI. Augmented sympathetic tone alters muscle metabolism with exercise: lack of evidence for functional sympatholysis. J Appl Physiol 1997; 82:1932–1938.
107. Hansen J, Thomas GD, Harris SA, Parsons WJ, Victor RG. Differential sympathetic neural control of oxygenation in resting and exercising human skeletal muscle. J Clin Invest 1996; 98:584–596.
108. Thomas GD, Hansen J, Victor RG. ATP-sensitive potassium channels mediate contraction-induced attenuation of sympathetic vasoconstriction in rat skeletal muscle. J Clin Invest 1997; 99:2603–2609.
109. Angus-Leppan H, Burke D. The function of large and small nerve fibers in renal failure. Muscle Nerve 1992; 15:288–294.
110. Trojaborg W, Smith T, Jakobsen J, Rasmussen K. Cardiorespiratory reflexes, vibratory and thermal thresholds, sensory and motor conduction in diabetic patients with end-stage nephropathy. Acta Neurol Scand 1994; 90:1–4.
111. Bazzi C, Pagani C, Sorgato G, Albonico G, Fellin G, D'Amico G. Uremic polynephropathy: a clinical and electrophysiological study in 135 short- and long-term hemodialyzed patients. Clin Nephrol 1991; 35:176–181.
112. Trojaborg W, Smith T, Jakobsen J, Rasmussen K. Effect of pancreas and kidney transplantation on the neuropathic profile in insulin-dependent diabetics with end-stage nephropathy. Acta Neurol Scand 1994; 90:5–9.
113. Stojceva Taneva O, Masin G, Polenakovic M, Stojcev S, Stojkovski L. Autonomic nervous system dysfunction and volume nonresponsive hypotension in hemodialysis patients. Am J Nephrol 1991; 11:123–126.
114. Converse RLJ, Jacobsen TN, Jost CM, Toto RD, Grayburn PA, Obregon TM, Fouad-Tarazi F, Victor RG. Paradoxical withdrawal of reflex vasoconstriction as a cause of hemodialysis-induced hypotension. J Clin Invest 1992; 90:1657–1665.
115. Baldamus CA, Mantz P, Kachel HG, Koch KM, Schoeppe W. Baroreflex in patients undergoing hemodialysis and hemofiltration. Contrib Nephrol 1984; 41:409–414.
116. Ewing DJ. Cardiovascular reflexes and autonomic neuropathy. Clin Sci Mol Med 1978; 55:321–327.
117. Defronzo RA. Pathogenesis of glucose intolerance in uremia. Metabolism 1978; 27:1866–1880.
118. Cecchin F, Ittoop O, Sinha MK, Caro JF. Insulin resistance in uremia: insulin receptor kinase activity in liver and muscle from chronic uremic rats. Am J Physiol 1988; 254(4 Pt 1):E394–401.
119. Baron AD. The coupling of glucose metabolism and perfusion in human skeletal muscle: the potential role of endothelium-derived nitric oxide. Diabetes 1996; 45(Suppl 1):S105–S109.

120. Baron AD. Hemodynamic actions of insulin. Am J Physiol 1994; 267(2 Pt 1): E187–E202.
121. Baron AD, Brechtel G. Insulin differentially regulates systemic and skeletal muscle vascular resistance. Am J Physiol 1993; 265(1 Pt 1):E61–E67.
122. Miyauchi T, Sugishita Y, Yamaguchi I, Ajisaka R, Tomizawa T, Onizuka M, Matsuda M, Kono I, Yanagisawa M, Goto K, Suzuki N, Matsumoto H, Masaki T. Plasma concentrations of endothelin-1 and endothelin-3 are altered differently in various pathophysiological conditions in humans. J Cardiovasc Pharmacol 1991; 17(Suppl 7):S394–397.
123. Predel HG, Meyer-Lehnert H, Backer A, Stelkens H, Kramer HJ. Plasma concentrations of endothelin in patients with abnormal vascular reactivity: effects of ergometric exercise and acute saline loading. Life Sci 1990; 47:1837–1843.
124. Saito Y, Kazuwa N, Shirakami G, Mukoyama M, Arai H, Hosoda K, Suga S, Ogawa Y, Imura H. Endothelin in patients with chronic renal failure. J Cardiovasc Pharmacol 1991; 17(Suppl 7):S437–439.
125. Maeda S, Miyauchi T, Sakane M, Saito M, Maki S, Goto K, Matsuda M. Does endothelin-1 participate in the exercise-induced changes of blood flow distribution of muscles in humans? J Appl Physiol 1997; 82:1107–1111.
126. Daugirdas JT, Ing TS. Physiologic principles. In: Handbook of Dialysis. Boston: Little, Brown, 1994, pp 13–29.
127. Valdes RJ, Graves SW, Becker SL. Protein binding of endogenous digoxin-immunoreactive factors in human serum and its variation with clinical condition. J Clin Endocrinol Metab 1985; 60:1135–1143.
128. Hamlyn JM, Blaustein MP, Bova S, DuCharme DW, Harris DW, Mandel F, Mathews WR, Ludens JH. Identification and characterization of a ouabain-like compound from human plasma. Proc Natl Acad Sci USA 1991; 88:6259–6263.
129. Murphey MD, Sartoris DJ, Quale JL, Pathria MN, Martin NL. Musculoskeletal manifestations of chronic renal insufficiency [review]. Radiographics 1993; 13:357–379.

24

Multiple Organ Failure

ARI UUSARO

Kuopio University Hospital
Kuopio, Finland

JAMES A. RUSSELL

St. Paul's Hospital
Vancouver, British Columbia, Canada

I. Introduction

Critically ill patients usually do not die as a result of the disease that led to admission to the intensive care unit (ICU). Furthermore, the mortality of single-organ failure, such as acute respiratory distress syndrome (ARDS), decreased over the last decade (1). Improved technology and pharmacology of critical care may prolong survival of patients. However, despite these advances, progressive or sequential organ dysfunction has become a major cause of morbidity and mortality in modern critical care. Multiple system organ failure (MSOF) has emerged as the most common pattern of deterioration leading to death of critically ill patients.

II. Definitions and Epidemiology of Multiple Organ Dysfunction/Failure

Tilney et al. (2) first introduced the term "sequential system failure" in 1973 to describe progressive MSOF after abdominal aortic aneurysmectomies. Shock caused by massive acute blood loss led to the postoperative failure of multiple initially uninvolved organs. Later, the terms "multiple organ failure" and "multiple system organ failure" were introduced (3).

The terms "organ failure" versus "organ dysfunction" require definition. Organ failure describes the presence of severe organ dysfunction that requires significant life support and is associated with significant morbidity and mortality. There is a lack of consensus to precisely define organ failure, and different criteria have been used. Organ dysfunction and multiple organ dysfunction syndrome (MODS) define the dynamic process of organ dysfunction and a range of severity from mild to extreme (4). Severe organ dysfunction defines profound failure of an organ (e.g., oliguric renal failure) that requires full active support. Mild to moderate organ dysfunction may not result in clinical findings (e.g., mildly to moderately elevated serum creatinine level). Several scoring systems have been described that quantify the severity of MODS (Table 1). An example of dichotomous (organ failure present/absent) classification of organ failures is shown in Table 2. An example of a dynamic and more recent classification of the severity of organ failures is shown in Table 3.

One key element of MODS is development of progressive physiological dysfunction in two or more organ systems after an acute threat to systemic homeostasis (4). There are numerous initiating events of MSOF/MODS, such as shock, sepsis, trauma, aspiration, and pancreatitis. Sepsis is the most frequent initiator of multiple organ failure (11). Regardless of the initiating event, the syndrome of MSOF/MODS generally follows a common course: cardiovascular and lung function usually deteriorates early, whereas hepatic, intestinal, neurological, coagulation, and renal dysfunction usually occurs later (12).

Table 1 Commonly Used Multiple System Organ Failure or Organ Dysfunction Scoring Systems

Organ system[a]	Fry et al. (5)	Knaus et al. (6)	Marshall et al. (7)	Hebert et al. (8)	Le Gall et al. (9)	Vincent et al. (10)
Respiratory	x	x	x	x	x	x
Cardiovascular		x	x	x	x	x
Renal	x	x	x	x	x	x
Hepatic	x		x	x	x	x
Neurologic		x	x	x	x	x
Coagulation		x	x	x	x	x
Gastrointestinal	x					

[a]Organ systems that are evaluated in various organ dysfunction scoring systems. Most organ system dysfunction scoring systems use similar variables to assess respiratory (arterial oxygen partial pressure/fraction of inspired oxygen), renal (creatinine), hepatic (bilirubin), coagulation (platelets), and neurological (Glasgow Coma score) dysfunction. Cardiovascular dysfunction is assessed by different methods in different scoring systems. Gastrointestinal dysfunction is not assessed in recently described scoring systems.

Table 2 Example of a Dichotomous Classification of Organ System Failures

Respiratory failure (presence of one or more of the following):
  Respiratory rate $\leq$ 5/min or $\geq$ 49/min
  $P_{aCO_2} \geq$ 50 mm Hg
  $A_aD_{O_2} \geq$ 350 mm Hg ($A_aD_{O_2} = 713 \times F_{IO_2} - P_{aCO_2} - P_{aO_2}$)
  Dependent on ventilator on the fourth day of OSF, not applicable for the initial 72 hours of OSF.
Cardiovascular failure (presence of one or more of the following):
  Heart rate $\leq$ 54/min
  Mean arterial blood pressure $\leq$ 49 mm Hg
  Ventricular tachycardia and/or ventricular fibrillation
  Serum pH $\leq$ 7.24 with $P_{aCO_2} \leq$ 49 mm Hg
Renal failure (presence of one or more of the following)[a]:
  Urine output $\leq$ 479 mL/24 hr or $\leq$ 159 mL/8 hr
  Serum BUN $\geq$ 100 mg/100 mL
  Serum creatinine $\geq$ 3.5 mg/100 mL
Neurological failure:
  Glasgow Coma Score $\leq$ 6 (in the absence of sedation at any point in day)
Hematologic failure (presence of one or more of the following):
  WBC count $\leq$ 1000/μL
  Platelet count $\leq$ 20,000/μL
  Hematocrit $\leq$ 20%

OSF, organ system failure; P_{aCO_2}, arterial carbon dioxide partial pressure; $A_aD_{O_2}$, alveolar–arterial oxygen difference, F_{IO_2}, fraction of inspired oxygen; P_{aO_2}, arterial oxygen partial pressure; BUN, blood urea nitrogen; WBC, white blood cell.
Excluding patients on chronic dialysis before hospital admission.
Source: Data from Ref. 6.

Multiple system organ failure is important because of its high mortality, high costs, and large resource consumption. The mortality of MSOF ranges from 20% to 100% depending on the number of organ failures. In general, there is a direct association between the number of organ failures and increasing mortality (Fig. 1) (6,8,13–16). MSOF develops in 10–15% of ICU admissions and is responsible for most of the ICU deaths (up to 80%), and it is estimated that up to half of ICU costs are attributed to caring for patients who have MSOF (12,13,17–20).

III. Hypothesis

The pathogenesis and pathophysiology of multiple organ dysfunction in critically ill patients is not fully understood and is probably multifactorial. However, because cells need oxygen for maintenance of function and because prolonged cell hypoxia leads to cell death, it has been hypothesized that tissue hypoxia causes MSOF in critical illness. The purpose of this chapter is to review critically the evidence for and against this hypothesis.

Table 3 Example of a Dynamic Classification of the Severity of Organ Dysfunction

Organ system	Score 1	Score 2	Score 3	Score 4
Respiratory: Pao_2/Fio_2 (mm Hg)	< 400	< 300	< 200 (respiratory support)	< 100 (respiratory support)
Cardiovascular: hypotension	MAP < 70 mm Hg	Dopamine < 5 or dobutamine (any dose)	Dopamine > 5, epinephrine ≤ 0.1 or norepinephrine ≤ 0.1	Dopamine > 15, epinephrine > 0.1, or norepinephrine > 0.1
Renal: creatinine, mg/dL (μmol/L) or urine output	1.2–1.9 (110–170)	2.0–3.4 (171–299)	3.5–4.9 (300–440) or < 500 mL/d	> 5.9 (> 440) or < 200 mL/d
Neurologic	13–14	10–12	6–9	< 6
Hepatic: bilirubin, mg/dL (μmol/L)	1.2–1.9 (20–32)	2.0–5.9 (33–101)	6.0–11.9 (102–204)	> 12.0 (> 204)
Coagulation: platelets ($\times 10^3/\mu$L)	< 150	< 100	< 50	< 20

Adrenergic drugs infused for at least 1 hour (doses are in μg/kg/min). Score of 1 indicates mild organ dysfunction and score of 4 indicates the most severe organ failure. A score of 0 indicates normal organ function. The worst value for each organ system is recorded on each day. Pao_2, arterial oxygen partial pressure; Fio_2, fraction of inspired oxygen; MAP, mean arterial pressure.
Source: Data from Ref. 10.

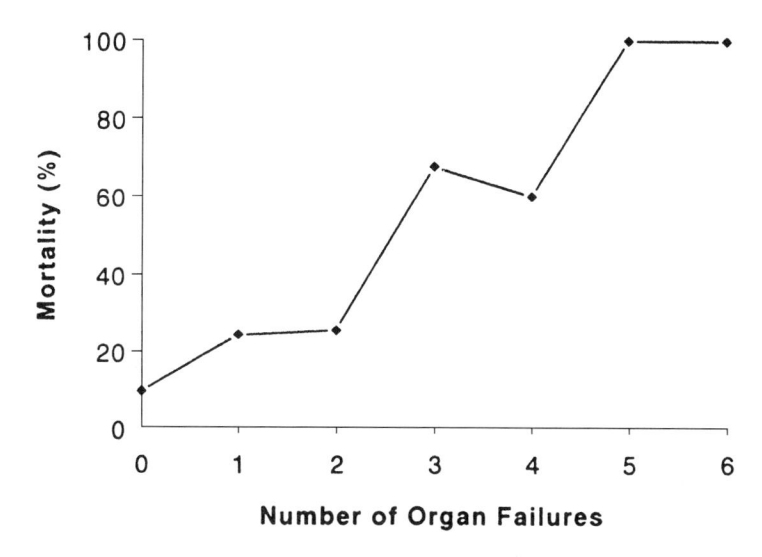

Figure 1 Mortality per number of organ system failures of patients who had sepsis syndrome. There was a significant linear increase in mortality with each additional organ system failure. Mortality rate ranged from 10% for zero organ system failures to 100% for five or six organ system failures. (From Ref. 8.)

IV. Mechanisms of Imbalance Between Oxygen Delivery and Consumption that Could Cause Multiple System Organ Failure

Cells depend on a continuous supply of oxygen to mitochondria for the generation of adenosine triphosphate (ATP). If cellular oxygen tension and supply is limited, oxidative ATP synthesis decreases, and ATP must be produced by anaerobic glycolysis (21). The ATP yield of anaerobic glycolysis (2 mol ATP/mole glucose) is small in comparison to oxidative phosphorylation (36 mol ATP/mole glucose) (21). There are several mechanisms of cellular damage secondary to hypoxia, including cellular acidosis, formation of oxygen-free radicals, increase in intracellular calcium concentration, and degradation of membrane phospholipids (22). The mechanisms of impaired oxygen delivery (D_{O_2}) that could cause MSOF are reviewed in this section.

A. Global Oxygen Delivery Could Be Impaired: Anemic, Hypoxemic, and Stagnant Hypoxia

Global D_{O_2} is defined as the product of cardiac output (CO) and arterial oxygen content (Ca_{O_2}) according to the following formula:

$$D_{O_2} = CO \times Ca_{O_2} \times 10$$

where CO is expressed as liters per minute, and CaO_2 is expressed as milliliters per 100 ml).

CaO_2 is calculated as:

$$CaO_2 = (Hb \times 1.34 \times SaO_2) + (PaO_2 \times 0.0031)$$

where Hb is hemoglobin concentration, SaO_2 is arterial oxygen saturation, and PaO_2 is arterial partial pressure of oxygen. Dissolved oxygen ($PaO_2 \times 0.0031$) is approximately 1% of total of oxygen content and can usually be ignored in the clinical setting.

According to these formulas, global DO_2 could be impaired because of anemia, hypoxemia, or reduced CO.

Anemia

Anemia lowers oxygen-carrying capacity of the blood. In chronic anemia, a compensatory increase in CO and low blood viscosity usually prevent tissue hypoxia (23). In critically ill patients, the optimum hemoglobin or hematocrit is not known (24). If tissue perfusion is adequate, experimental studies indicate that very low hematocrit levels are well tolerated (25). However, the effects of anemia on tissue oxygenation in critically ill patients are not straightforward because several factors can alter affinity of hemoglobin for oxygen and consequently alter unloading capacity of oxygen from hemoglobin at the tissue level. For example, hydrogen ion, carbon dioxide, temperature, and increased 2,3-diphosphoglycerate (2,3-DPG) decrease affinity of hemoglobin for oxygen and shift the oxyhemoglobin dissociation curve to the right (26). A shift to the right increases oxygen availability to tissues at a given oxygen tension. Although there is some evidence that critically ill patients tolerate moderate anemia without increased mortality or morbidity, outcome may be worse for anemic critically ill patients with impaired cardiovascular reserve (27).

Hypoxemia

Hypoxemia, defined as decreased PaO_2, is a common finding in critically ill patients. Hypoxemia may be caused by low partial pressure of oxygen (PO_2) in the inspired air (e.g., high altitude), diffusion impairment, ventilation–perfusion ($\dot{V}/\dot{Q}$) mismatch, and intrapulmonary right to left shunt of blood. Increased intrapulmonary shunt and increased $\dot{V}/\dot{Q}$ mismatch are the most important mechanisms for hypoxemia in the critically ill patient (28). In most critically ill patients, hypoxemia can be improved by aggressive cardiopulmonary support, and even in severe ARDS, patients rarely die of refractory hypoxemia (29).

Stagnant Hypoxia

Stagnant hypoxia is caused by decreased blood flow. Tissue hypoxia may develop despite adequate hemoglobin concentration and arterial blood oxygenation if blood flow is inadequate to meet oxygen demand. Hypovolemic, cardiogenic, and obstructive shock are characterized by low CO syndrome: there is peripheral vasoconstriction, oliguria, tachycardia and widened arteriovenous oxygen difference caused by increased oxygen extraction. Septic shock is an example of distributive shock, which is characterized by increased CO, low systemic vascular resistance, hypotension and usually narrowed arteriovenous oxygen difference caused by maldistribution of blood flow. The potential role of vascular obstruction in septic shock is controversial and is discussed in Sections B and C.

B. Impaired Blood Flow Distribution Between Organs

Critical illness and therapy such as mechanical ventilation alter blood flow distribution between organs. Impaired blood flow distribution between organs may induce tissue hypoxia in critically ill patients. In shock, blood flow to vital organs, such as heart and brain, is preserved, whereas blood flow to the gastrointestinal tract, skin, and muscle is decreased.

The splanchnic circulation is important in the regulation of circulating blood volume and systemic blood pressure (30). In acute hypovolemia, splanchnic blood volume and blood flow are markedly reduced to maintain perfusion of heart and brain (31–33).

The effects of sepsis on splanchnic blood flow are controversial because of limited clinical studies and differences between studies of models of sepsis. In general, hypovolemic models of endotoxic shock show decreased splanchnic blood flow, whereas hyperdynamic models of endotoxic shock find increased splanchnic blood flow (34,35). In healthy humans, a bolus of endotoxin roughly doubles splanchnic blood flow without any change in heart rate and systemic blood pressure (36). Septic patients have nearly double the splanchnic blood flow of normal subjects (37,38).

Respiratory failure, mechanical ventilation, and associated therapy such as sedation and paralysis change respiratory muscle blood flow, Do_2, and oxygen consumption ($\dot{V}o_2$). Increased respiratory muscle work increases respiratory muscle oxygen demand and $\dot{V}o_2$, and this increased oxygen demand must be met by increased respiratory muscle blood flow to avoid anaerobic metabolism (39,40). For example, cardiogenic shock induced by cardiac tamponade in spontaneously breathing dogs increases respiratory muscle oxygen demand such that the respiratory muscles receive approximately 21% of CO during spontaneous breathing (41). After institution of paralysis and mechanical ventilation, respiratory muscle blood flow decreases to 3% of CO (41). There is indirect evidence from human studies that this redistribution of blood flow to respiratory muscles is at least, in part, from splanchnic circulation. More specifically, Mohsenifar et al. (42) have shown that gastric mucosal perfusion as measured by gastric mucosal pH (pH_i) could be used to predict success of weaning from mechanical ventilation. They found that patients in whom gastric mucosal pH_i decreased during weaning had increased risk of failure to wean from mechanical ventilation. This suggests that blood flow was redistributed away from the gut to the respiratory muscles, causing gastric mucosal acidosis in patients who subsequently failed to wean.

Respiratory support of critically ill patients may alter both global blood flow and blood flow distribution between organs. Although positive end-expiratory pressure (PEEP) increases PaO_2, PEEP may decrease global DO_2 because of decreased CO (43). PEEP also changes distribution of blood flow between organs in animal models of critical illness (44–48). Positive pressure ventilation reduces gut and hepatic blood flow (45,47). High levels of PEEP (> 20 cm H_2O) decrease hepatic, renal, pancreatic, and colonic blood flow, whereas brain and cardiac perfusion are maintained (46). Sepsis modifies the PEEP-induced changes in organ perfusion such that PEEP only decreases hepatic, pancreatic, and splenic blood flow in septic sheep. Volume resuscitation does not restore normal blood flow distribution (46). Hypocapnia decreases hepatic arterial blood flow without affecting hepatic function, and mild hypercapnia increases hepatic blood supply (49).

C. Impaired Blood Flow Distribution Within Organs

The distribution of blood flow within organs is under precise control to maintain the balance of DO_2 to oxygen demand. Hemorrhagic shock changes the distribution of blood flow within organs such as the heart, kidneys, and gut. Sepsis impairs the normal distribution of blood flow within organs such as the heart, kidneys, and gut, and also alters the normal redistribution of blood flow that occurs in shock. The abnormal distribution of blood flow during sepsis, as indicated by abnormal distribution of blood transit times, could explain the oxygen extraction defect of sepsis. The abnormal distribution of blood flow within organs during sepsis could be explained by endothelial injury, decreased erythrocyte and leukocyte deformability, microvascular obstruction, and changes in concentration of local and systemic vasoactive substances.

Impaired blood flow distribution within organs may cause local imbalance of DO_2 and oxygen demand, leading to tissue hypoxia. During hemorrhagic shock, blood flow redistributes within organs. For example, in the heart, there is redistribution of blood flow from the endocardium to the epicardium during hemorrhagic shock, which causes subendocardial patchy necrosis (50,51). In the kidney, during hypovolemic shock there is redistribution of renal blood flow from outer to inner cortex and medulla, which, if severe, causes ischemic damage (52). In experimental hemorrhagic shock, cerebral perfusion was unchanged, supporting the concept of maintaining perfusion of brain in hemorrhagic shock (53–55). Gut blood flow decreases dramatically in hemorrhage or cardiogenic shock, and the decrease is out of proportion to the decrease in total CO (56–58). Inferior mesenteric artery resistance increases up to four times more than total vascular resistance in hemorrhagic shock (56,59).

Sepsis impairs the normal redistribution of blood flow within organs during shock. The impaired redistribution of blood flow during septic shock could contribute to local tissue hypoxia and organ dysfunction. In a canine septic model, myocardial blood flow redistributed so that in some regions blood flow increased, and in other regions blood flow decreased (60). Sepsis also impairs renal blood flow redistribution. In sepsis, the normal distribution of blood flow from cortex to medulla is impaired such that the cortical/juxtamedullar blood flow ratio declines, and there is underperfusion of the renal cortex (61,62).

Divergent results have been obtained in numerous studies on the effect of sepsis on mesenteric blood flow. Divergent findings may be a result of differences in species, adequacy of resuscitation and the magnitude of the insult (63). In general, splanchnic blood flow is decreased in hypodynamic models of sepsis but preserved or increased in hyperdynamic models (64,65). Although splanchnic blood flow is similarly increased in several different animal models of hyperdynamic sepsis, marked decreases in gut blood flow have also been observed despite hyperdynamic circulation (63). Clinical studies of gut blood flow in septic patients also suggest impaired gut blood flow distribution (38,66). Endotoxemia changes the distribution of gut red blood cell transit times: there is greater dispersion of distribution of transit times, suggesting that sepsis induces regions of slow flow (which could cause local tissue hypoxia) and very rapid flow (which could cause shunting of blood and increases venous oxygen tension). The changes in transit times induced by endotoxin could account for the impaired oxygen extraction in the gut (67,68).

There is an oxygen extraction defect in animal models of sepsis. Acute bacteremia and acute endotoxemia increase the critical Do_2 and decrease the critical oxygen extraction ratio (69–72).

There are several possible mechanisms for oxygen extraction defects. Abnormal redistribution of blood flow within organs could be a mechanism of impaired oxygen extraction in sepsis. Maintenance of high perfused capillary density is important in regulating oxygen extraction by keeping oxygen diffusion distances small (73). Recently, perfused capillary density was demonstrated to be decreased in sepsis (74). As the density of perfused capillaries decreases, the average distance for oxygen diffusion increases, which impairs oxygen extraction. Increased heterogeneity of blood flow distribution and capillary transit times within an organ is one possible mechanism for an oxygen extraction defect (67,68,75). Poorly perfused capillaries have high capillary oxygen extraction ratios. On the other hand, well-perfused capillaries have decreased capillary oxygen extraction ratios because capillary Do_2 exceeds local tissue oxygen demand. Endothelial injury, microvascular obstruction, decreased blood cell deformability, and release of vasoactive mediators are all potential causes of increased dispersion of capillary transit times during sepsis. Endothelial injury in sepsis impairs precapillary arteriolar regulation, which could increase dispersion of capillary transit times (76–78). Rheological alterations such as decreased erythrocyte and leukocyte deformability during sepsis may also alter microvascular hemodynamics and distribution of blood flow within organs (79). Capillaries may be obstructed by surrounding edema, platelet and thrombin plugs, and leukocytes (80). Microembolization causes mechanical obstruction of capillary beds and activates synthesis of mediators such as arachidonic acid metabolites. Synthesis and release of vasoactive mediators may aggravate the effects of pure mechanical obstruction by inducing inappropriate vasodilation and vasoconstriction (81,82).

Vascular reactivity to metabolic feedback could be disturbed in sepsis, and this could lead to uncoupling of local Do_2 and demand and, thus, impaired blood flow distribution. The normal distribution of blood flow within organs is normally controlled by inputs from the sympathetic nervous system and by systemic and local vasoactive mediators (83,84). α-Receptor blockade impairs the normal oxygen extraction capability of tissues, indicating that adrenergic α tone is important in the normal blood flow distribution during hemorrhagic shock.

D. Increased Oxygen Demand

Tissue hypoxia may also develop because of increased tissue oxygen demand if this is not met by increased Do_2. Examples of increased oxygen damand in the critically ill patient include increased body temperature in febrile patients, the effects of inadequate sedation, and the effects of increased respiratory muscle work in patients who have acute respiratory failure (40,41,85,86). Fever increases $\dot{V}o_2$ by approximately 5% for each degree celsius increase of temperature.

Increased respiratory muscle work during acute respiratory failure increases the proportion of blood flow to respiratory muscles from 3% to 25% (41). Mechanical ventilation of dogs in acute respiratory failure and shock decreased the proportion of blood flow to respiratory muscles from 25% to 2–3% (41). Sedation and paralysis of critically ill, mechanically ventilated patients significantly decrease global $\dot{V}o_2$, presumably because of decreased respiratory muscle and possibly skeletal muscle $\dot{V}o_2$ (87). Common therapeutic interventions in the critically ill, such as sedation and physiotherapy, may change oxygen uptake and increase the risk of imbalance between Do_2 and demand (86–89). Finally, adrenergic agents can increase oxygen demand and $\dot{V}o_2$ because of a thermogenic effect. Dobutamine may increase oxygen consumption in healthy volunteers up to 20%; however, the increase in oxygen demand caused by dobutamine may be less in critically ill patients (90–92). If local blood flow does not increase enough to match increased oxygen demand induced by the drug, tissue hypoxia can develop. This is one possible mechanism to explain the development of gastric mucosal hypoxia in response to vasoactive drugs despite increased gut blood flow (93,94).

During human sepsis and septic shock, splanchnic oxygen demand is increased and may jeopardize splanchnic oxygenation (37,38,95,96). Administration of endotoxin increases splanchnic $\dot{V}o_2$ and splanchnic tumor necrosis factor release in healthy volunteers (36). Although splanchnic blood flow distribution is similar in patients with trauma and those who have sepsis, $\dot{V}o_2$ of the splanchnic region of septic patients is significantly greater than splanchnic $\dot{V}O_2$ in patients with trauma (95).

V. The Oxygen Delivery/Consumption Relationship: Physiology

Regardless of the underlying cause, irreversible shock causes acute respiratory, renal, hepatic, and cardiovascular failure. However, the focus of this section is not to review severe shock. Instead, the focus is on tissue hypoxia and especially occult tissue hypoxia as a mechanism of MSOF. Literature for and against occult tissue hypoxia as a cause of MOSF is reviewed. However, before that, we briefly review basic physiology and pathophysiology of the relationship between DO_2 and $\dot{V}O_2$. It is important to understand this background to understand the rationale of clinical trials of increased DO_2 in critically ill patients and to understand studies of the role of tissue hypoxia as a cause of MSOF.

The whole-body DO_2/oxygen consumption relationship is biphasic. Global DO_2 is the product of CO and CaO_2. As DO_2 decreases, $\dot{V}O_2$ is maintained relatively constant (plateau phase) until the so-called critical DO_2 is reached. Below the critical DO_2, $\dot{V}O_2$ decreases as DO_2 decreases. This is called physiological dependence of $\dot{V}O_2$ on DO_2 (Fig. 2). Arterial lactate levels begin to increase as DO_2 decreases below the critical DO_2 because of the onset of anaerobic metabolism.

Oxygen consumption is maintained constant as DO_2 decreases because of a progressive increase in the extraction of oxygen by tissues. The extraction of oxygen may be expressed as the oxygen extraction ratio (O_2ER). The O_2ER is calculated as the arterial–mixed venous oxygen content difference divided by the CaO_2. The critical O_2ER is the O_2ER at the critical DO_2 point. Below the critical O_2ER, the O_2ER continues to increase but not enough to maintain a constant $\dot{V}O_2$ (Fig. 2).

Normal animals have critical DO_2 of 5–10 mL/kg/min and the normal critical O_2ER in approximately 0.5–0.8 (69–71,97,98). Until recently, the normal critical DO_2 and O_2ER had not been determined in individual humans. Instead, the critical points were calculated from pooled data from studies of cardiac surgical patients (99,100). The pooled normal critical DO_2 was approximately 8 mL/kg/min. However, we have previously discussed in detail the potential errors that can occur when using pooled data (101). Therefore, recently Ronco et al. (102) conducted a study designed to determine the critical DO_2 and O_2ER in individual humans. In this study, critically ill patients were studied when their attending physicians and families had agreed to stop life support. After informed consent was obtained from the families, life support was gradually withdrawn in a standardized protocol in each patient. Arterial lactate, DO_2 and $\dot{V}O_2$ were determined throughout the period of withdrawal of life support at 5- to 20-minute intervals. Vasopressors were withdrawn first, followed by decrease in fraction of inspired oxygen (FIO_2),

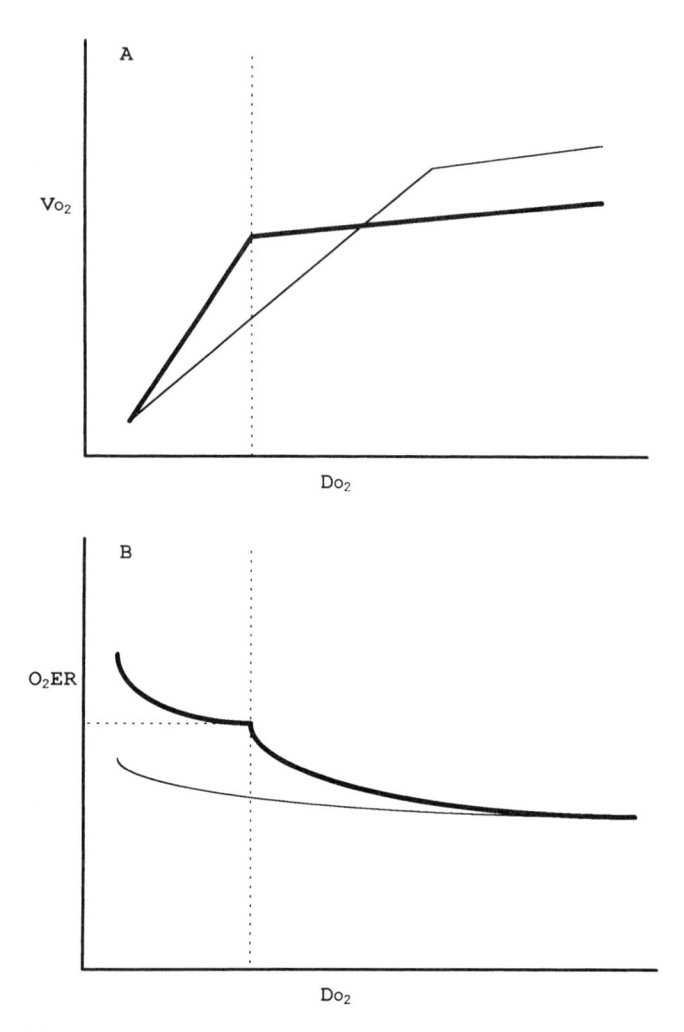

Figure 2 (A) Relationship of oxygen delivery (Do_2) and oxygen consumption ($\dot{V}o_2$) in normal (heavy line) and pathological (narrow line) conditions. Normally, as Do_2 decreases, $\dot{V}o_2$ is maintained at a relatively constant level. Below the critical Do_2 (dashed line for normal condition), $\dot{V}o_2$ decreases as Do_2 decreases, because $\dot{V}o_2$ is physiologically dependent on Do_2. Compared with the physiological relationship of Do_2 and $\dot{V}o_2$, pathological dependence of $\dot{V}o_2$ on Do_2 is characterized by a much wider range of dependence and by a higher critical Do_2. (B) Relationship of Do_2 and the oxygen extraction ratio (O_2ER). Normally, as Do_2 decreases, the O_2ER increases to maintain $\dot{V}o_2$ at a relatively constant level. The critical O_2ER is the O_2ER at the critical Do_2. Below the critical Do_2, O_2ER continues to increase but not enough to maintain $\dot{V}o_2$. Pathological dependence of $\dot{V}o_2$ on Do_2, is characterized by a failure of the O_2ER to increase adequately (as Do_2 decreases) to maintain $\dot{V}o_2$. In pathological conditions, there is often a small but inadequate increase of O_2ER as Do_2 decreases.

Multiple Organ Failure 697

and then mechanical ventilation was discontinued. $\dot{V}O_2$ was determined by indirect calorimetry. In this study, the critical DO_2 was 4.5 mL/kg/min, much lower than expected in the critically ill, and the critical O_2ER was 0.6, higher than expected. There were also no differences between septic and nonseptic patients in the critical DO_2 or critical O_2ER (Fig. 3). In addition, there were no differences in critical DO_2 and O_2ER between patients who had normal arterial lactate and those who had increased arterial lactate at the beginning of the protocol. This study suggested that the normal critical DO_2 and O_2ER of humans are approximately 5 mL/kg/min and 0.6, respectively (102).

Pathological dependence of $\dot{V}O_2$ on DO_2 is characterized by three differences from the physiological relationship. First, $\dot{V}O_2$ is dependent on DO_2 over a much wider range of DO_2 and at much higher values of DO_2. Thus, the critical DO_2 is higher in pathological dependence of $\dot{V}O_2$ on DO_2. Second, the critical O_2ER is lower in pathological dependence of $\dot{V}O_2$ on DO_2. This suggests that there is decreased ability of the tissues to increase the extraction of oxygen as DO_2 is decreased. The third difference between these relationships is that the plateau phase of $\dot{V}O_2$ is higher in the pathological relationship than in the physiological relationship, which is consistent with a state of increased oxygen demand (Fig. 2). Animal models of critical illness have shown pathological dependence of $\dot{V}O_2$ on DO_2, and in these studies, the critical DO_2 is increased to approximately 12 mL/kg/min (from approximately 7 mL/kg/min in control), and critical O_2ER is decreased to approximately 0.5 (from approximately 0.75 in control) (69,71). The possible mechanisms responsible for the impaired extraction ability were discussed previously in Section IV.

VI. Evidence for Occult Tissue Hypoxia as a Cause of Multiple System Organ Failure

This section reviews literature examining the relationship between tissue hypoxia and MSOF. More specifically, we review pathological dependence of $\dot{V}O_2$ on DO_2, hyperlactatemia, and gastric mucosal acidosis (as assessed by gastric tonometry) as potential indicators of tissue hypoxia in relation to MSOF. We then review the evidence in randomized control trials that supranormal DO_2 decreases MSOF. Finally, we review animal models for evidence of occult tissue hypoxia as a cause of MOSF.

Comparison between survivors and nonsurvivors of critical illness could potentially provide information of the impact of tissue hypoxia as a cause of MSOF. Several studies have shown that survivors have higher DO_2 and $\dot{V}O_2$ compared with nonsurvivors (103–105). In addition, Russell et al. (105) found that MSOF developed in 63% of the nonsurvivors and in none of the survivors with ARDS. This raises the question, did nonsurvivors have occult tissue hypoxia (because they had lower DO_2 and $\dot{V}O_2$), that led to MSOF? However, these studies do not indicate that

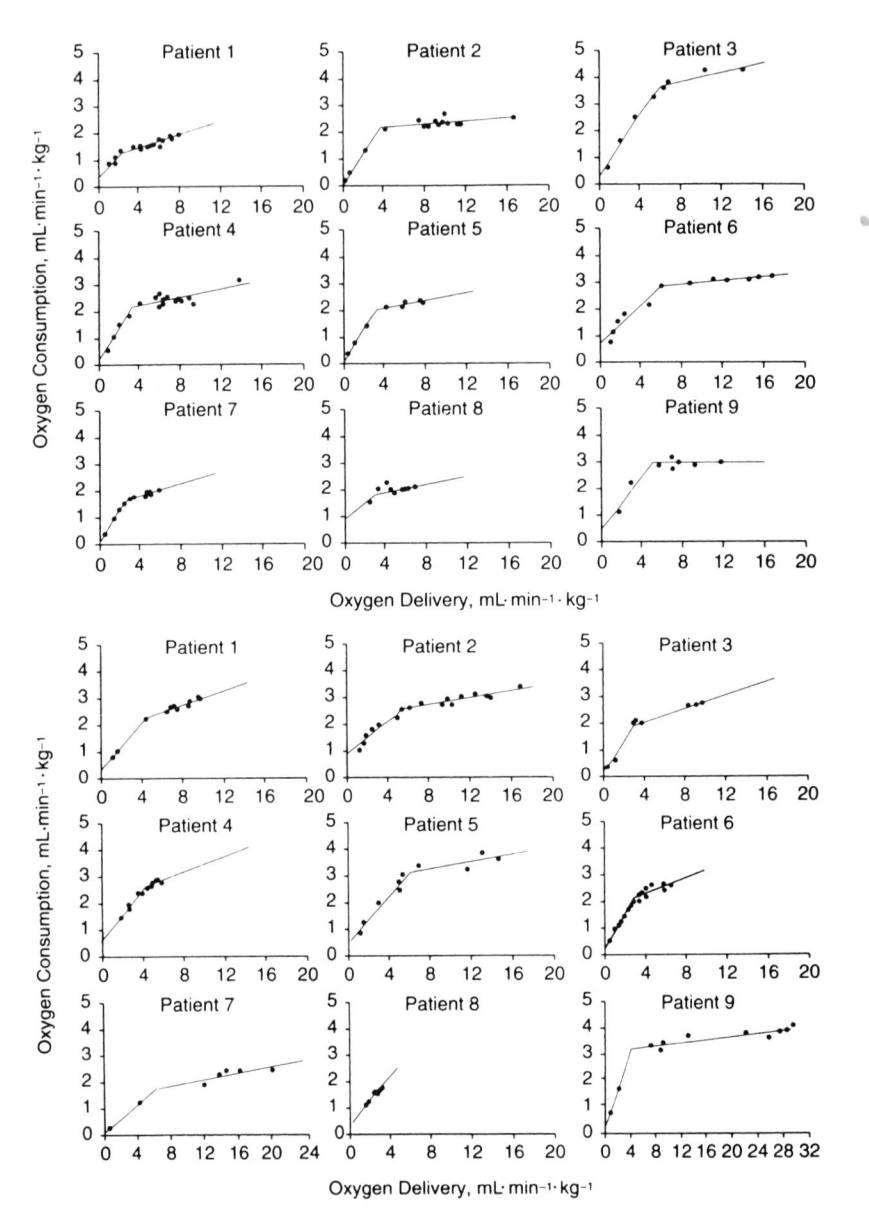

Figure 3 The relationship between oxygen delivery (Do$_2$) and oxygen consumption (V̇o$_2$) for septic (top) and nonseptic (bottom) critically ill patients. Points represent discrete measurements of Do$_2$ and V̇o$_2$, whereas the two lines superimposed in each patient represent the two best-fit linear regression lines. In all patients but one (patient no. 8, nonseptic), a biphasic relationship between Do$_2$ and V̇o$_2$ was found. There were no differences in critical Do$_2$ threshold, critical oxygen extraction ratio, and maximal oxygen extraction ratio between septic and nonseptic patients. (From Ref. 102.)

the nonsurvivors were hypoxic, because lower D_{O_2} and $\dot{V}_{O_2}$ alone do not indicate tissue hypoxia. We cannot conclude a causal relationship between tissue hypoxia and MSOF from these studies.

A. Pathologic Dependence of Oxygen Consumption on Oxygen Delivery

An artificial dependence of $\dot{V}_{O_2}$ on D_{O_2} due to methodological problems, such as mathematical coupling of shared measurement error, counfounds interpretation of clinical studies in which calculated $\dot{V}_{O_2}$ was used. In addition, it is not clear whether there is pathological dependence of measured $\dot{V}_{O_2}$ on D_{O_2} and, thus, whether there is occult tissue hypoxia. In our review, none of the studies of pathological dependence of $\dot{V}_{O_2}$ on D_{O_2} that used measured $\dot{V}_{O_2}$ examined relationship to MSOF. Even in studies of $D_{O_2}/\dot{V}_{O_2}$ that used calculated $\dot{V}_{O_2}$, few studied the relationship to MSOF (105). We conclude that there is little to no evidence in the literature of D_{O_2}–$\dot{V}_{O_2}$ dependence of an association between tissue hypoxia and MSOF.

Pathological dependence of $\dot{V}_{O_2}$ on D_{O_2} despite normal biochemical markers of tissue oxygenation, such as arterial lactate, could indicate occult tissue hypoxia, which may contribute to the development of organ failure. Pathological dependence of $\dot{V}_{O_2}$ on D_{O_2} may be shown by altering D_{O_2} and measuring the corresponding changes in $\dot{V}_{O_2}$.

The clinical studies that show pathological dependence of $\dot{V}_{O_2}$ on D_{O_2} were led by the pivotal study of Danek et al. (106). They showed that $\dot{V}_{O_2}$ was dependent on D_{O_2} in patients who had ARDS but not in a control group of critically ill, mechanically ventilated patients who did not have ARDS. Subsequently, there was a flourish of very similar clinical studies that asked the question, "Is $\dot{V}_{O_2}$ pathologically dependent on D_{O_2} in critical illness?" (107–112). In these studies, D_{O_2} was altered by PEEP (to decrease CO and D_{O_2}), infusion of volume (to increase CO and D_{O_2}), prostacyclin (a vasodilator), blood transfusion (to increase hemoglobin concentration and thus D_{O_2}), and dobutamine (an inotrope that increases CO and D_{O_2}). In these studies using widely varied techniques to change D_{O_2}, the results and conclusions of the investigators were remarkably similar: $\dot{V}_{O_2}$ was pathologically dependent on D_{O_2}, suggesting covert oxygen debt (Table 4). However, the number of patients in these studies varied between 10 and 73, and some of the studies did not include a control group. In addition, the development of multiple organ failure was not addressed in these studies. There are also methodological problems, such as use of calculated $\dot{V}_{O_2}$ and mathematical coupling of shared measurement error.

B. Lactate

Here we review briefly the biochemistry and physiology of lactate production and clearance and studies of the association between hyperlactatemia and MSOF, and we conclude that lactate is moderately accurate predictor of MSOF, especially after trauma and hemorrhage.

Table 4 Representative Studies that Used Calculated Oxygen Consumption Showing Pathological Dependence of Oxygen Consumption on Oxygen Delivery

Reference	Year	No. of patients	D_{O_2} manipulation	Controls
Danek et al. (106)	1980	29	PEEP	Non-ARDS
Mohsenifar et al. (107)	1983	12	Random	None
Kaufman et al. (108)	1984	21	Random	CHF
Astiz et al. (109)	1987	10	Fluid	Septic shock
Bihari et al. (110)	1987	27	Prostacyclin	Survivors vs. nonsurvivors
Fenwick et al. (111)	1990	32	Transfusion	Normal vs. high lactate
Vincent et al. (112)	1990	73	Dobutamine	Normal vs. high lactate

D_{O_2}, oxygen delivery; PEEP, positive end-expiratory pressure; ARDs, acute respiratory distress syndrome; CHF, congestive heart failure.

Although lactate is a normal by-product of metabolism, elevated lactate levels may indicate anaerobic metabolism and tissue hypoxia and may thus be associated with hypoxic organ failure. The anaerobic metabolic pathway known as glycolysis is the first step of glucose metabolism and occurs in the cytoplasm of virtually all cells. The end product of glycolysis is pyruvate. Pyruvate diffuses into the mitochondria and is metabolized to carbon dioxide by the more energy-efficient metabolic pathway, the Krebs cycle. The metabolism of glucose to pyruvate results in chemical reduction of the enzyme cofactor nicotinamide adenine dinucleotide (NAD^+, oxidized form) to its reduced form (NADH). The intramitochondrial process known as the electron transport chain then oxidizes NADH to NAD^+ using molecular oxygen. Tightly coupled to this reaction is a process termed oxidative phosphorylation, which produces ATP, the major source of energy to drive intracellular chemical reactions (113). Under steady-state conditions, pyruvate is in equilibrium with lactate and with NAD^+ and NADH, facilitated by the enzyme lactate dehydrogenase (LDH). During cellular anoxia, the mitochondrial arm of the pathway ceases to function, and pyruvate formed in the glycolysis is instead metabolized by LDH to lactate. Lactate leaves the cell and accumulates in the extracellular fluid. Some tissues such as myocardium can take up and use lactate as a substrate for oxidative metabolism. The liver and kidney take up and convert lactate to glucose. However, when tissue hypoxia is sufficiently severe, lactate production exceeds lactate use, and the result is hyperlactatemia (113).

The specific sources of excess lactate production in severe perfusion failure are not known, but lactic acidosis usually indicates generalized tissue hypoxia (114,115). The potential organ sources of excess lactate production during tissue hypoxia include the lung, gut, muscle, and other organs. Normally, lungs do not produce lactate, but in disease, lungs are a source of lactate production (116–119). In patients with acute lung injury and ARDS, lungs produced excess lactate compared with patients without lung injury (120–122). In patients with multiple organ failure and hepatic involvement, the hepatosplanchnic bed was the main source of lactate, whereas lungs were the main source of lactate in patients with multiple organ failure and ARDS (122).

Several studies show a relationship between elevated lactate concentration and mortality (123). In patients with shock, survival decreased from 90% to 10% as lactate concentration increased from 2.0 to 8.0 mmol/L (115). Increased mortality of patients with hyperlactatemia has been widely reported. Furthermore, patients with chronic liver disease who have decreased lactate clearance also have a relationship between increased lactate and increased mortality (124–126). In addition, the persistence of hyperlactatemia is associated with increased mortality (127–129).

There are studies, mainly in surgical and trauma patients, that investigated the association of hyperlactatemia and the development of multiple organ failure (130–135). In general, these studies show an association between increased lactate and development of MSOF. In 92 surgical patients who had polytrauma or major hemorrhage, changes in lactate levels predicted the development of multiple organ failure (132). In 39 severely injured patients, elevated lactate levels at 12 and 24 hours after injury were associated with the development of MSOF (131). Elevated lactate levels at days 2, 3, and 4 identified patients who ultimately developed MSOF after multiple trauma (133). Sauaia et al. (130) observed that lactate level greater than 2.5 mmol/L at the day of admission was independently associated with MSOF after severe trauma. Initial and highest lactate levels and the duration of hyperlactatemia were significantly higher in trauma patients who developed organ failures (MSOF not addressed) compared with trauma patients who did not (134). Lactate levels, and especially the duration of hyperlactatemia, were good predictors of the development of MSOF in patients who had septic shock (Fig. 4) (135). Cairns et al. (136) found that lactate levels were significantly higher 12 hours after injury in patients who developed MSOF as compared with those who did not, despite no differences between groups in global $\dot{D}o_2$ or $\dot{V}o_2$ and supranormal levels of $\dot{D}o_2$ in both groups. They used near-infrared spectroscopy to study local oxygen supply (tissue oxyhemoglobin [Hbo_2]) and mitochondrial $\dot{V}o_2$ (cytochrome a,a$_3$) of the upper arm. They found decoupled Hbo_2 and a,a$_3$, a sign of mitochondrial oxidative dysfunction, in 89% of patients who ultimately developed MSOF, compared with 13% in patients who did not develop MSOF (136). Hence, there may be flow-independent impairment in mitochondrial oxygen use after trauma, and this may lead to elevated lactate levels and MSOF.

It is important to emphasize that most of the patients in the aforementioned studies had major trauma, hemorrhage, and/or hypovolemia; in these patients, hyperlactatemia was associated with the development of MSOF. It is likely that hyperlactatemia is an indicator of anaerobic metabolism in this patient population. Thus, because hyperlactatemia likely indicates anaerobic metabolism and tissue hypoxia in patients who have trauma and major hemorrhage, the association of hyperlactatemia and MSOF suggests an association between tissue hypoxia and

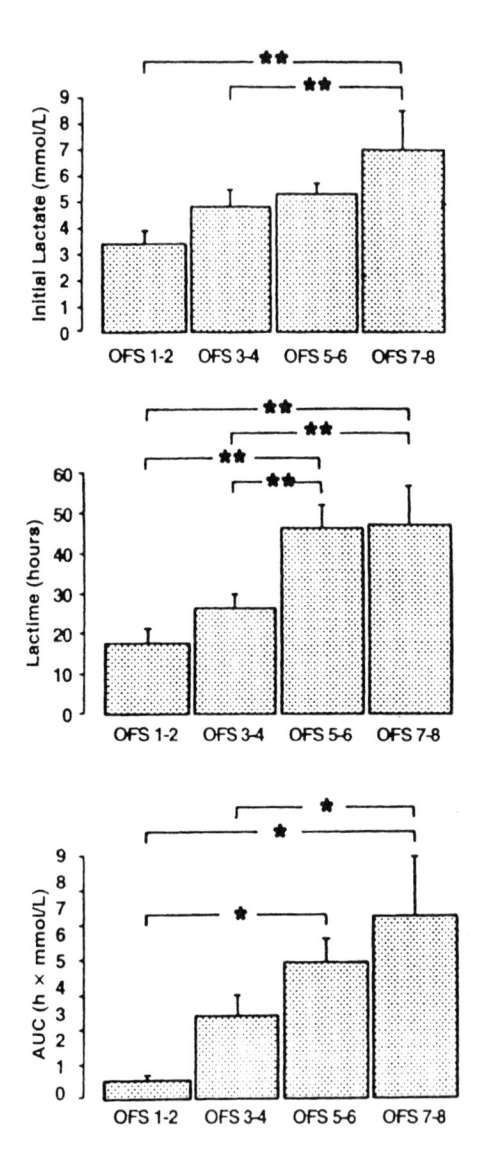

Figure 4 Initial blood lactate level, time during which blood lactate exceeded 2.0 mmol/L (lactime), and area under the curve (AUC) according to the organ failure score (OSF) (mean ± SE of the mean). *$P < .01$. The AUC for abnormal (> 2.0 mmol/L) lactate levels was calculated using initial and final lactate levels and assuming a linear regression, according to the equation: AUC = 0.5 × lactime × (initial lactate + final lactate) − 2 × lactime. (From Ref. 135.)

MSOF in these patients. However, there are several nonhypoxic causes of elevated lactate levels that may be important in other conditions such as sepsis, which makes hyperlactatemia more difficult to interpret in sepsis.

C. Gastric Tonometry

Gastric tonometry is a relatively new method to assess gastric mucosal and splanchnic perfusion. Monitoring splanchnic perfusion may be of specific value in critically ill patients because the gut participates in the regulation of blood volume and systemic blood pressure; in shock, perfusion of vital organs such as the brain and heart is maintained at the expense of gut; and splanchnic hypoxia may be associated with the development of multiple organ failure (30–32, 137–139).

Gut mucosal blood flow and the different metabolic requirements of the different layers of the gut wall make the surface of the mucosa especially vulnerable to hypoperfusion and ischemia. The artery and vein of the intestinal villus run in parallel, but their blood flows run in opposite directions. The artery forms a dense capillary network close to the top of the villus. This anatomic arrangement allows countercurrent exchange of oxygen from the artery to the vein along their course within the villus (140). This results in a descending gradient of tissue P_{O_2} from the base of the villus to its tip that is inversely related to the blood flow. In addition, the lower P_{O_2} at the tip makes the villus susceptible to tissue hypoxia if vasoconstriction occurs. Furthermore, the high metabolic demand of the mucosa, up to 80% of the total gut $\dot{V}_{O_2}$ increases the risk of mucosal hypoxia (141).

Gastric tonometry has been extensively reviewed elsewhere (142,143). Briefly, gastric tonometry uses a nasogastric tube that has a silicone balloon at the tip. The silicone balloon is freely permeable to CO_2, whereas a sampling tube is impermeable to CO_2. After tonometer insertion into the stomach, the tonometer balloon is filled with saline. It is assumed that as CO_2 of the gastric mucosa diffuses into the saline, equilibrium will be achieved between tissue CO_2 and saline CO_2. In addition, it is assumed that the bicarbonate concentration in the mucosa is the same as in the arterial blood. The carbon dioxide partial pressure (P_{CO_2}) of the saline is determined, and a simultaneous arterial blood sample is obtained to measure the systemic arterial bicarbonate concentration. pH_i can be calculated by applying a modified Henderson-Hasselbalch equation:

$$pH_i = 6.1 + \log(\text{arterial } HCO_3^- / \text{tonometer } CO_2 \times 0.03 \times k)$$

where k is a time-dependent equilibrium constant that corrects for the time the saline has been in the balloon in equilibrium with gastric lumen and gastric mucosal CO_2.

Under normal conditions, tissue C_{O_2} is generated as an end product of aerobic metabolism. CO_2 production increases during hypoxia as anaerobically generated ATP undergoes hydrolysis, resulting in the cellular accumulation of hydrogen ions. Excess tissue C_{O_2} is produced by the buffering action of bicarbonate on hydrogen ions: $H^+ + HCO_3^- \leftrightarrow H_2O + CO_2$. Thus, it is assumed that excess mucosal C_{O_2} is an indicator of local acidosis caused by tissue hypoxia. Gastrointestinal tonometry has been validated by comparing tonometer pH$_i$ with direct gastric intramucosal pH measured by microelectrodes (144,145). Antonsson et al. (145) demonstrated a correlation between the two methods in pigs after administration of endotoxin, partial vascular occlusion, and total vascular occlusion. However, the gastric tonometry pH$_i$ underestimated the decrease in pH$_i$ during total and partial vascular occlusion (145).

We believe systemic arterial-mucosal Co_2 gap best reflects mucosal oxygenation because: (1) HCO_3^- of the gastric mucosa is not always in equilibrium with the systemic arterial CO_3^-; (2) remote systemic changes in acid-base status influence and confound the interpretation of pH$_i$; and (3) gastric mucosal Co_2 can increase because of decreased mucosal blood flow and not because of mucosal hypoxia (146). The potential pitfalls of gastric tonometry are discussed in Section VII.

Several clinical studies show that gut is sensitive to hypovolemia. In human volunteers, for example, a 15% reduction in circulating blood volume resulted in a 40% reduction in splanchnic blood volume, whereas heart rate, blood pressure, and CO remained unchanged (31). Hypovolemia, simulated by using lower-body negative pressure application, decreased CO and gastric mucosal blood flow, as measured by laser Doppler flowmetry, despite unchanged arterial pressure in human volunteers (33). After multiple injuries, hepatic blood flow is depressed after 12 hours and increases progressively thereafter during the first week; delayed liver dysfunction correlates with the degree of hepatic hypoperfusion (147).

Several reports show an association between gastric mucosal acidosis, mortality, and MSOF. At least four recent studies have found an association between gastric mucosal acidosis and MSOF in critically ill adults. Two studies were specifically designed to investigate prediction of MODS by gastric tonometry (148,149). In a study of 30 critically ill patients with sepsis, pH$_i$, measured within 24 hours after the onset of sepsis, was a better predictor of MODS than oxygen-derived variables or lactate levels (148). In a series of 79 patients who underwent trauma, patients who had pH$_i$ less than 7.25 at 24 hours after trauma were 4.5 times more likely to develop multiple organ failure compared with patients who had pH$_i$ greater than 7.25 (149). It is interesting to note that in the latter study, mucosal-arterial Co_2 gap was not predictive of death or development of multiple organ failure. In 51 patients undergoing elective major surgery (mainly cardiovascular), gastric mucosal acidosis developed by the end of surgery in 32 patients, and 7 of these patients developed postoperative multiple organ failure (150). In 19 patients with pH$_i$ greater than 7.32, there were no patients with multiple organ failure. Doglio et al. (151) observed that patients who had abnormal pH$_i$ at the time of ICU admission had higher number of organ failures compared with those with normal pH$_i$ (> 7.35) (151). Thus, these four studies suggest an association between gastric mucosal acidosis and MSOF. However, none of these studies addresses the question, Does gastric mucosal acidosis (and tissue hypoxia) cause MSOF?

In a small randomized study of DO_2 in 27 patients, 6 of the 8 patients who developed MODS had pH_i less than 7.3 at 24 hours after admission (152). Gutierrez et al. conducted a randomized clinical trial of gastric tonometry in 260 critically ill ICU patients (153). Patients admitted to the ICU had a gastric tonometer inserted and then were divided into two strata: normal pH_i (> 7.35) and low pH_i (< 7.35). Then, within each stratum, patients were randomized to ongoing management using normalization of gastric pH_i or conventional clinical management. In patients who had a low pH_i on admission, there was no difference in mortality between treatment groups. In patients who had a normal pH_i on admission, those randomized to gastric tonometer management had a significantly lower mortality than did those who received conventional clinical treatment (153). Unfortunately, this report provided no data of the incidence of MSOF in these patients.

Based on these few studies available, there seems to be an association between gastric mucosal acidosis and MOSF. However, to our knowledge there are no studies that prove that gastric mucosal acidosis causes MSOF.

D. Randomized Control Trials of Supranormal Oxygen Delivery: Effects on Multiple Organ Failure

Several observations led to the hypothesis that increasing DO_2 to high levels (supranormal DO_2) decreases the incidence of MSOF. First, survivors of critical illness have higher cardiac index, DO_2, and $\dot{V}O_2$ than do nonsurvivors of critical illness (103,105). Second, survivors of critical illness who have higher levels of DO_2 and $\dot{V}O_2$ also have significantly less MSOF (105). Third, clinical studies suggest that the critical DO_2 of critically ill patients is higher than that of normal subjects. Finally, animal models of critical illness such as bacteremia and endotoxemia also suggest that the critical DO_2 is increased in sepsis, a common admission diagnosis and common complication of critical illness.

Rigorous randomized, controlled, clinical trials of supranormal DO_2 are the best way to evaluate the possible causal relationship between tissue hypoxia and MSOF. If supranormal DO_2 decreases the incidence of MSOF compared with normal DO_2, it is possible that tissue hypoxia contributes to the development of MSOF. There are at least nine randomized, controlled, clinical trials of supranormal DO_2 compared with normal DO_2 (Table 5). However, in all of these studies, survival was the major endpoint (153–161). None of the randomized, controlled, clinical trials rigorously evaluated the incidence of MSOF. There are five randomized, controlled, clinical trials of supranormal DO_2 in which the development of single-organ failure or MSOF was reported (154–156,160,161). In three of these studies, there is at least some evidence that tissue hypoxia might be related to organ failure (154–156). The first randomized, controlled, clinical trial of Shoemaker et al. (154) randomized 88 high-risk surgical patients to supranormal DO_2 end points of cardiac index greater than 4.5 L/min/m², DO_2 greater than 600 mL/min/m², and $\dot{V}O_2$ greater than 170 mL/min/m² versus normal clinical end points (154). They observed that the

Table 5 Randomized Controlled Trials of Supranormal Versus Normal Oxygen Delivery

Reference	Year	Patients	No. of patients	Mortality (%) Controls	Mortality (%) Interventions	P value
Shoemaker et al. (154)	1988	Surgical	88	28	4	<.05
Bone et al. (158)	1989	ARDS	100	48	60	NS
Fleming et al. (155)	1992	Trauma	67	44	24	NS
Tuchschmidt et al. (157)	1992	Septic shock	51	72	50	NS
Boyd et al. (156)	1993	Surgical	107	22	6	<.05
Gutierrez et al. (153)	1992	Critical, pH$_i$ normal	141	53	28	<.05
	1992	Critical, pH$_i$ low	119	37	36	NS
Yu et al. (159)	1993	Critical	67	34	34	NS
Hayes et al. (160)	1994	Critical	109	34	54	<.05
Gattinoni et al. (161)	1995	Critical	503	48	49	NS

ARDS, acute respiratory distress syndrome; NS, not significant.

average number of complications, including poorly defined single-organ failures, was lower in patients who received supranormal Do_2 compared with controls. In another study of 67 patients after severe trauma, Fleming et al. (155) observed that the number of poorly defined single-organ failures per patient was less in protocol patients (0.79 ± 0.68 vs. 1.74 ± 0.64 in controls) who received supranormal Do_2 than in controls. However, this study was not truly randomized because treatment was allocated by day of admission. In a third randomized, controlled, clinical trial of high-risk surgical patients (n = 107), there was no overall difference in the number of postoperative single-organ failures between the supranormal Do_2 group and control group (156). Nine of the 12 patients in the control group who died had MODS, compared with two of three patients in the protocol group.

According to studies reviewed here, supranormal Do_2 may be associated with reduced incidence of multiple organ failure, suggestive of the hypothesis of tissue hypoxia causing organ failures. However, not all studies of supranormal Do_2 confirm this. Furthermore, there is an alternative hypothesis to explain how catecholamines have beneficial effects not related to Do_2. These issues are discussed in Section VII.

E. Animal Models

Although tissue hypoxia has been suspected to cause multiple organ failure, it is interesting to note that experimental models of multiple organ failure are not based on tissue hypoxia. In addition, animal studies of oxygen transport are usually of short duration; therefore, the impact of tissue hypoxia on the development of multiple organ failure is impossible to evaluate. The most frequently used models of multiple organ failure use endotoxin, proinflammatory cytokines, and intravenous or intraperitoneal administration of bacteria or chemicals such as zymosan to induce MSOF (162,163). We are not aware of experimental studies that have linked occult tissue hypoxia and the development of multiple organ failure. In contrast, one elegant experimental study suggests that occult tissue hypoxia may not be responsible for the development of organ failure in a canine model of sepsis and septic shock (164). In this 3-week study, the investigators compared septic and control animals and repeatedly measured and calculated $\dot{V}o_2$ after Do_2 was increased by volume loading. They also measured lactate levels and assessed organ failures. Ten of the 16 septic animals and none of the six controls died (Fig. 5). Interestingly, at all time points studied, both before and after volume infusion, levels of Do_2 or $\dot{V}o_2$ did not differ between septic and control animals, nor did they differ between septic survivors and nonsurvivors (Fig. 6). In addition, despite significant mortality, reduction in cardiovascular function, and metabolic acidosis, septic animals in this study had lactate levels similar to those of nonseptic controls. However, septic animals had more organ failures compared with nonseptic animals. The investigators of the study questioned that $\dot{V}o_2$ reflects pathogenetic mechanism in sepsis and septic shock, and they also questioned the use of $\dot{V}o_2$ as a target of therapeutic

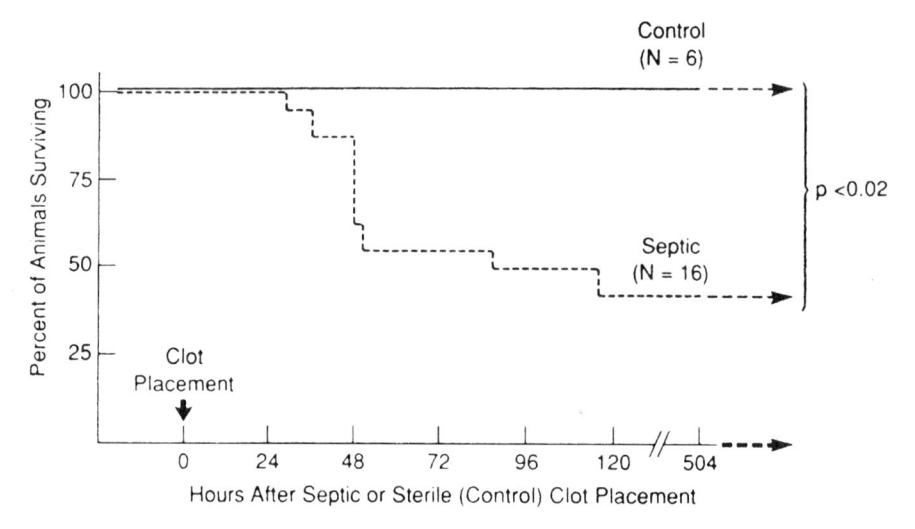

Figure 5 Percentage of control (n = 6) and septic (n = 16) animals surviving over time (hours) after surgery. At the surgical procedure, either a clot infected with *Escherichia coli* (septic animals) or a sterile clot (controls) was implanted intraperitoneally. By day 21, 100% of control animals and 37.5% of the septic animals survived. (From Ref. 164.)

interventions (164). The study also failed to confirm that inadequate Do_2 in sepsis causes MSOF. Using the same experimental procedure (intraperitoneal *Escherichia coli*–infected clot), the same investigators improved survival and prevented multiple organ dysfunction in their 28-day experiment by infusing a tyrosine kinase inhibitor, tyrphostin, which has no effect on oxygen transport (163). The latter study supports the hypothesis that occult tissue hypoxia is of limited importance in the pathophysiology of multiple organ failure.

VII. Evidence Against Occult Tissue Hypoxia as a Cause of Multiple System Organ Failure

This section reviews evidence that occult tissue hypoxia may not be the cause of multiple organ failure in critically ill patients. Although pathological dependence of $\dot{V}o_2$ on Do_2 has been suggested to indicate occult tissue hypoxia, we review the methodological problems of studies showing pathological dependence of $\dot{V}o_2$ on Do_2. We review studies in which no dependence was found. We then address lactic acidosis, because high circulating lactate levels are often considered indicative of tissue hypoxia. There are several nonhypoxic mechanisms for hyperlactatemia, especially in patients with sepsis. We then review gastric tonometry and some important methodological problems with the technique. Although gastric mucosal acidosis is associated with increased mortality and the development of multiple

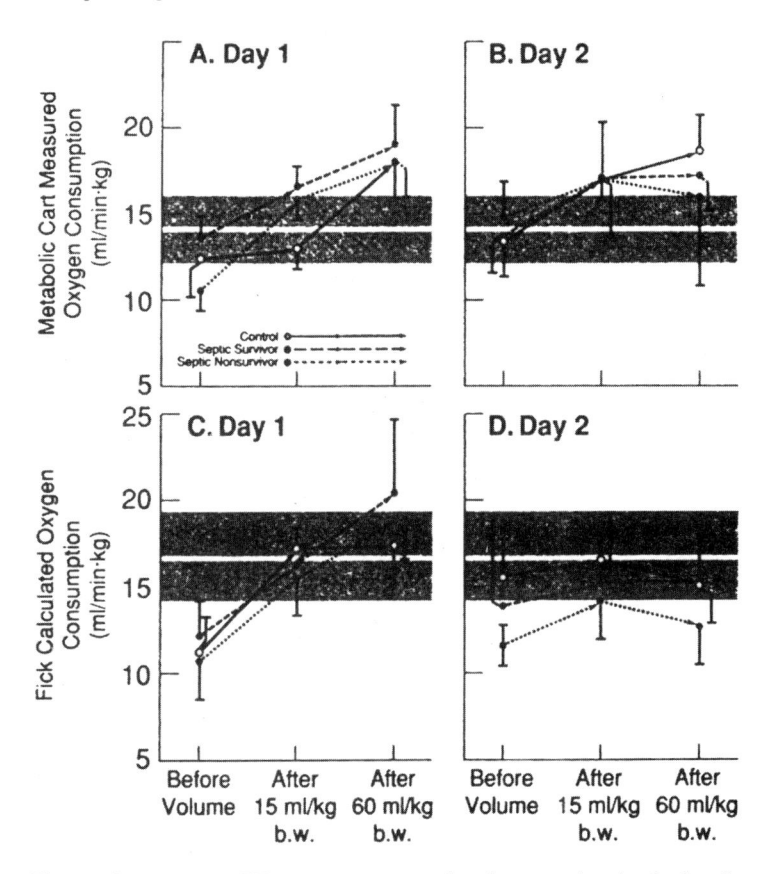

Figure 6 Mean (± SE) oxygen consumption (measured and calculated) on day 1 (A and C) and day 2 (B and D) in control animals, septic survivors, and septic nonsurvivors. The origin of the arrow represents the mean of each measure before volume infusion, and the tip represents the mean after volume infusion. The left-hand arrow for each point demonstrates the change with the initial 15-mL/kg body weight infusion, and the right hand arrow represents the final change after both 15-mL/kg body weight and 45-mL/kg body weight infusions (total, 60 mL/kg body weight). Oxygen consumption (either measured or calculated) did not differ between septic and control animals, nor did it differ between septic survivors or nonsurvivors. Volume infusion increased oxygen delivery similarly in each group (data not shown). The gray bars are "normal" ranges for each measure. (From Ref. 164.)

organ failure (148–151), these methodological problems influence interpretation of these studies. Finally, we review evidence that there may be methodological problems with the randomized studies that have shown beneficial effects of supranormal Do_2 on MSOF in critically ill patients. We also review studies that have not been able to confirm these beneficial effects of supranormal Do_2 on MSOF.

A. Methodological Problems in Studies of Global Oxygen Delivery and Consumption

Methodological problems in studies of global D_{O_2} and $\dot{V}_{O_2}$ may explain many of the findings of pathological dependence of $\dot{V}_{O_2}$ on D_{O_2}. Thus, abnormal dependence of $\dot{V}_{O_2}$ on D_{O_2} may represent merely methodological problems and not covert oxygen debt. The first potential methodological problem is that oxygen demand of critically ill patients can vary considerably. As a result, increased oxygen demand can cause a secondary increase in D_{O_2}, e.g., during exercise (85–88,165). Several studies have clearly shown that oxygen demand of critically ill patients varies with changes during routine ICU interventions (88,165), with sedation (86), with changes in mechanical ventilation (87), and by cooling of febrile patients (85). During exercise, oxygen demand increases, leading to increased $\dot{V}_{O_2}$ and D_{O_2}.

Some studies of $\dot{V}_{O_2}$ and D_{O_2} that showed pathological dependence of $\dot{V}_{O_2}$ on D_{O_2} collected data over extended periods or were not careful to control oxygen demand. Thus, the positive slope of $\dot{V}_{O_2}$ and D_{O_2} may indicate increases of D_{O_2} in response to increased oxygen demand rather than pathological dependence of $\dot{V}_{O_2}$ on D_{O_2}.

Primary changes in oxygen demand also influence the $D_{O_2}/\dot{V}_{O_2}$ relationship of individual organs. For example, increased renal blood flow increases glomerular filtration, which, in turn, increases metabolic work of reabsorption and thus $\dot{V}_{O_2}$ without any defect of tissue oxygenation (166). In other words, there is a positive slope of the renal $D_{O_2}/\dot{V}_{O_2}$ relationship without renal hypoxia. Similarly, increased hepatic blood flow augments the delivery of metabolic substrates to the liver, and $\dot{V}_{O_2}$ increases (167). When the $D_{O_2}/\dot{V}_{O_2}$ relationship is examined, there is a linear relationship of hepatic D_{O_2} and $\dot{V}_{O_2}$ that can be misinterpreted as pathological dependence of $\dot{V}_{O_2}$ on D_{O_2} but, in fact, does not represent tissue hypoxia.

Metabolic activity may also be downregulated in tissues if oxygen availability is reduced, a phenomenon called *oxygen conforming*. Cultured hepatocytes and cardiac myocytes reduce their metabolic activity and oxygen demand without cellular injury during reductions of oxygen availability (168,169). This seems to be a normal adaptive response to states of decreased oxygen availability, which protects cells from hypoxic injury. Patients with stable aortic stenosis who do not seem to have tissue hypoxia increase both D_{O_2} and $\dot{V}_{O_2}$ after aortic valvuloplasty (170). Reversal of oxygen conforming behavior has been proposed as the mechanism. Furthermore, stable patients with chronic obstructive pulmonary disease and obstructive sleep apnea increase their $\dot{V}_{O_2}$ when D_{O_2} is increased by passive leg elevation (171,172). These patients do not have tissue hypoxia but, rather, could have reversal of oxygen-conforming behavior.

The second problem in many of the studies of $\dot{V}_{O_2}$ and D_{O_2} that potentially counfounds the interpretation of the results is the problem of mathematical coupling of shared measurement error (101,173). In many clinical studies of $\dot{V}_{O_2}$ and D_{O_2}, $\dot{V}_{O_2}$ and D_{O_2} were calculated from a common set of variables:

$$D_{O_2} = (Q \times Hb \times 1.34 \times Sa_{O_2}) + (Q \times Pa_{O_2})$$
$$\dot{V}_{O_2} = (Q \times Hb \times 1.34 \times (Sa_{O_2} - S\bar{v}_{O_2})) + (Q \times (Pa_{O_2} - P\bar{v}_{O_2}))$$

where Q is cardiac output, Sa_{O_2} and $S\bar{v}_{O_2}$ are the arterial and mixed venous oxygen saturations, respectively, Hb is hemoglobin concentration, 1.34 is the binding constant of oxygen to hemoglobin, and Pa_{O_2} and $P\bar{v}_{O_2}$ are the arterial and mixed venous oxygen tensions, respectively. Cardiac output is most commonly measured by the thermodilution method, and hemoglobin, Sa_{O_2}, $S\bar{v}_{O_2}$, Pa_{O_2}, and $P\bar{v}_{O_2}$ are measured using commonly available blood gas analyzers and oximeters. It is evident that the two equations share these variables: Q, Hb, Sa_{O_2} and Pa_{O_2}. Therefore, errors in the measurement of any one of these variables will show in the D_{O_2} and in the $\dot{V}_{O_2}$ calculations and would cause errors in their respective calculations. As a result, there is an artifactual relationship of D_{O_2} and $\dot{V}_{O_2}$ that is explained by the coupling of shared measurement error rather than by the presence of pathological dependence of $\dot{V}_{O_2}$ and D_{O_2}, and covert oxygen debt.

There have been attempts to evaluate and solve the problem of mathematical coupling of shared measurement error, but the proposed solution may not exclude mathematical coupling of shared measurement error as a cause of pathological dependence of $\dot{V}_{O_2}$ on D_{O_2} (174). Because the methodological problems of studies of D_{O_2} and $\dot{V}_{O_2}$ have been recently reviewed elsewhere, these problems are not reviewed here in detail (175).

Mathematical coupling of shared measurement error can be avoided in studies of the relationship of $\dot{V}_{O_2}$ and D_{O_2} by determining $\dot{V}_{O_2}$ and D_{O_2} with mathematically independent techniques. Over the past years, an increasing number of investigators have designed and successfully completed elegant studies of $\dot{V}_{O_2}$ and D_{O_2} in which $\dot{V}_{O_2}$ and D_{O_2} were determined independently (102,173,176–184). More specifically, $\dot{V}_{O_2}$ has been measured by analysis of respiratory gases, and D_{O_2} has been calculated using thermodilution CO and Ca_{O_2} as previously described. The results of these studies are strikingly similar: if $\dot{V}_{O_2}$ and D_{O_2} are determined independently, $\dot{V}_{O_2}$ is not pathologically dependent on D_{O_2} (Table 6). Furthermore, in studies in which $\dot{V}_{O_2}$ was determined both by Fick and respiratory gas analysis techniques, pathological dependence of $\dot{V}_{O_2}$ on D_{O_2} was associated with Fick but not with respiratory gas–determined $\dot{V}_{O_2}$. Recently, a consensus conference on tissue hypoxia concluded that finding an increase in $\dot{V}_{O_2}$ subsequent to an increase in D_{O_2} in and of itself is insufficient to indicate tissue hypoxia (185). Thus, the use of changes in $\dot{V}_{O_2}$ in response to changes in D_{O_2} is not particularly useful in the care of critically ill patients to detect occult tissue hypoxia. In summary, based on studies of global D_{O_2} and $\dot{V}_{O_2}$, covert oxygen debt has not been convincingly demonstrated.

B. Hyperlactatemia May Not be Caused by Tissue Hypoxia

Although hyperlactatemia has been used as a global marker of inadequate D_{O_2} to tissues and evidence of anaerobic metabolism secondary to tissue hypoxia, there are

Table 6 Representative Studies that Used Measured Oxygen Consumption and Do Not Show Pathological Dependence of Oxygen Consumption on Oxygen Delivery

Reference	Year	No. of patients	DO_2 manipulation	Controls
Lutch and Murray (176)	1972	19	PEEP	Normal, COPD, ALI
Annat et al. (177)	1986	8	PEEP + fluid	ARDS
Carlile and Gray (178)	1989	9	PEEP	ALI
Vermeij et al. (179)	1990	20	—	Abdominal surgery/sepsis
Ronco et al. (180)	1991	14	Transfusion	ARDS: normal vs. high lactate
Ronco et al. (181)	1993	14	Dobutamine	Sepsis: normal vs. high lactate
Ronco et al. (102)	1993	19	Life support discontinued	Dying patients: septic and nonseptic
Manthous et al. (182)	1993	10	Dobutamine	Septic shock
Marik and Sibbald (183)	1993	23	Transfusion	Sepsis
Phang et al. (173)	1994	17	Dobutamine	ARDS
Mira et al. (184)	1994	17	MAST + dobutamine	Sepsis: normal vs. high lactate

DO_2, oxygen delivery; PEEP, positive end-expiratory pressure; MAST, military antishock trousers; COPD, chronic obstructive pulmonary disease; ALI, acute lung injury; ARDS, acute respiratory distress syndrome.

also several nonhypoxic mechanisms of hyperlactatemia. Because high circulating lactate levels are associated with increased morbidity and mortality, lactate may be merely an indicator of poor prognosis, not tissue hypoxia, especially in patients with sepsis. Some studies found a poor relationship between lactate levels and MSOF (148).

Briefly, the nonhypoxic mechanisms of hyperlactatemia are as follows. Delayed clearance of lactate can cause hyperlactatemia without cellular hypoxia. Because the liver and kidney are the major organs of lactate clearance and because dysfunction of these organs is so prevalent in the critically ill patient, delayed clearance of lactate may be a frequent contributor to the hyperlactatemia of critical illness (186,187). We are unaware of studies using infusion of radiolabelled lactate in the critically ill to define the prevalence and severity of impaired lactate clearance during critical illness.

Although true anatomic shunts in peripheral tissues have not been demonstrated in sepsis, physiological shunts could develop because of pathological vasodilation. Furthermore, other capillaries could have decreased perfusion and conductive flow of oxygen such that adjacent tissue is hypoxic and is generating lactate. However, the low-flow state, especially during the early phase of sepsis, may cause sequestration of lactate in tissues, and systemic arterial plasma lactate could remain normal. During volume resuscitation, increased flow could "flush" lactate from the periphery to the central circulation, and increased conductive flow of oxygen could reverse tissue hypoxia. Thus, a "lactate hangover" could occur during reversal of tissue hypoxia.

Dysfunction of pyruvate dehydrogenase (PDH) can be induced in models of sepsis. PDH converts pyruvate to oxaloacetate, permitting pyruvate to enter the Kreb's cycle. Dysfunction of PDH causes accumulation of pyruvate and lactate and the lactate/pyruvate (L/P) ratio remains normal, indicating aerobic metabolism. PDH activity is decreased in muscle of septic rats and can be partially reversed by dichloracetate (188,189). Curtis and Cain (190) have shown that endotoxemic dogs develop lactic acidosis that is not secondary to tissue hypoxia but, rather, is caused by inactivation of PDH because dichloracetate, a PDH activator, reverses the lactic acidosis without changing Do_2 or $\dot{V}o_2$ globally or regionally (gut and hindlimb). Another nonhypoxic mechanism of hyperlactatemia is caused by increased protein breakdown (catabolism) in critical illness. Catabolism causes release of amino acids that are converted to increased pyruvate and lactate levels with normal L/P ratio indicating aerobic metabolism (191).

Stress increases aerobic glycolysis because of a primary abnormality of glycolysis (rather than accelerated anaerobic glycolysis). Accelerated aerobic glycolysis in excess of oxidative metabolism needs causes pyruvate to accumulate and convert to lactate and alanine (i.e., normal L/P ratio). Endotoxin increases mRNA synthesis and synthesis of a glucose transporter protein. This glucose transporter protein moves from its intracellular site to the plasma membrane and increases cellular glucose uptake and release of lactate and pyruvate (192,193). Increased glucose transporter protein and increased release of pyruvate and lactate has been described in muscle and liver of septic rats (194).

Changes in acid-base homeostasis are common in critically ill patients and may have a major impact on blood lactate levels. Respiratory alkalosis increases lactate levels (187,195). The mechanism seems to be increased peripheral lactate production, because hepatic lactate use increases. The acute effects of metabolic alkalosis, induced by an infusion of buffer base, are less consistent, although an increase in blood lactate is usually observed (187).

Vasoactive drugs infused to critically ill patients may also increase lactate levels by nonhypoxic mechanisms. Adrenaline infusion in healthy volunteers has major effects on carbohydrate metabolism and causes a small increase in plasma lactate that is probably mediated by β_2-adrenoreceptors (196–198). Increased skeletal muscle glycogenolysis increases peripheral lactate production. Splanchnic glucose production and lactate extraction are also increased, probably secondary to increases in hepatic glycogenolysis and gluconeogenesis (199). However, worsening tissue perfusion and deleterious effects on tissue oxygenation in response to adrenaline infusion cannot be excluded in critically ill patients. Adrenaline infusion decreased portal venous and total hepatic blood flow and increased mesenteric vascular resistance and lactate levels in experimental models and caused lactic acidosis in critically ill patients with severe sepsis (200,201).

Recent evidence suggests that sepsis causes lactic acidosis without high-energy phosphate depletion, indicating absence of tissue hypoxia. Several investigators have used phosphorus-31 nuclear magnetic resonance spectroscopy to measure intracellular levels of phosphate (P_i), ATP, and phosphocreatine. Cellular hypoxia rapidly decreases phosphocreatine and ATP and increases P_i (194). Animal models of sepsis, including endotoxemia and cecal ligation and perforation, produced lactic acidosis without decreasing phosphocreatine or ATP in skeletal muscle (202,203).

C. Lactate and the Oxygen Delivery/Consumption Relationship

As previously discussed, dependence of global $\dot{V}O_2$ on DO_2 has been used in clinical studies to identify occult tissue hypoxia. In studies in which $\dot{V}O_2$ and DO_2 are both calculated using common variables (CO and CaO_2), patients who have increased lactate levels have pathological dependence of $\dot{V}O_2$ on DO_2, whereas patients who have normal lactate levels do not (111,112). In contrast, in several studies in which $\dot{V}O_2$ and DO_2 were determined independently, increased lactate level did not predict pathological dependence of $\dot{V}O_2$ on DO_2 (102,173,180,181). Increased lactate level did not predict pathological dependence of $\dot{V}O_2$ on DO_2 in patients who had sepsis, in whom DO_2 was increased using dobutamine, and in patients who had ARDS, in whom DO_2 was increased using blood transfusion and dobutamine.

We determined the critical DO_2 in humans by measuring DO_2 and $\dot{V}O_2$ during withdrawal of inotropes and mechanical ventilation in patients for whom ICU care was discontinued. The critical DO_2 was 4.5 mL/kg/min and was not different between patients who had increased baseline plasma lactate levels and those who did not. Furthermore, many patients had increased lactate levels at the onset of study, and although DO_2 decreased, lactate remained elevated but unchanged until the critical DO_2 was reached when lactate increased dramatically. This later increase of lactate could be a result of lactate release from hypoxic tissues and/or decreased lactate clearance. The last result reinforces that critically ill patients can have hyperlactatemia without dependence of $\dot{V}O_2$ on DO_2 (102). Thus, lactate could have been increased because of nonhypoxic causes of hyperlactatemia.

To summarize, hyperlactatemia is a nonspecific finding in critically ill patients. Hyperlactatemia could indicate hypoxic mechanisms, nonhypoxic mechanisms, or both. Unfortunately, hyperlactatemia is neither specific nor sensitive for tissue hypoxia. Although hyperlactatemia, especially of long duration, is associated with increased mortality in many studies and also with increased incidence of organ failures in some studies, this by itself does not prove that death or organ failure are caused by tissue hypoxia.

D. Methodological Problems with the Use of Gastric Tonometry

Gastric tonometry is used to calculate pH_i, and low pH_i is traditionally considered to indicate gastric mucosal hypoxia. There are a number of studies showing that the risk of death is increased in patients with low pH_i. In addition, there are some studies that show that low pH_i is associated with the development of multiple organ failure in critically ill patients (148–151). However, because of methodological problems of the gastric tonometry technique, it may be difficult to conclude that low pH_i is caused by gastric mucosal hypoxia. Patients may have gastric mucosal acidosis and they may develop organ failures, but this may be unrelated to tissue hypoxia. The methodological problems of the tonometry technique are reviewed next.

Gastric mucosal CO_2 and arterial bicarbonate HCO_3^- (representing gastric mucosal HCO_3^-) are needed for the calculation of pH_i. The technique relies heavily on the correct calibration and maintenance of the blood gas analyzer used. Analysis of gastric PCO_2 with various blood gas analyzers contributes to errors in the calculated pH_i (204–206). In addition, sampling technique and delay in the analysis of PCO_2 affect calculated pH_i (207).

Back-diffusion of CO_2, generated by the reaction between secreted H^+ and HCO_3^-, can cause erroneously low values of pH_i. Histamine receptor blockers (H_2-blockers) have been recommended to reduce generation of intraluminal CO_2 and to improve the reproducibility of measurements of pH_i (208,209). The recommendation is based on studies performed in healthy volunteers, but recent studies in critically ill patients contradict those in healthy volunteers (210,211). In critically ill patients, the use of H_2-blockers may have no effect on calculated gastric pH_i.

The function of gastric mucosa may be disturbed, and the acid secretion defect may explain the lack of need of H_2-blockers in the critically ill (212). However, it is possible that the use of H_2-blockers modifies normal values for pH_i, although this has not been confirmed in critically ill patients (213).

Enteral feeding decreases gastric pH_i by stimulating secretion of hydrogen ions, which are then buffered by bicarbonate secreted by the nonparietal gastric cells generating CO_2 (214). Therefore, discontinuation of enteral feeding for at least 1 hour before measurements are taken has been recommended when measuring gastric pH_i.

Another potential source of error when assuming low pH_i represents mucosal hypoxia arises from the fact that not all excess CO_2 in tissues during low flow is generated because of anaerobic metabolism. During tissue hypoxia, production of CO_2 increases as anaerobically generated ATP undergoes hydrolysis and fixed acids such as lactic acid are produced, resulting in the cellular accumulation of hydrogen ions. In hypoxic tissues, CO_2 is produced by the buffering action of bicarbonate on hydrogen ions: $H^+ + HCO_3^- \leftrightarrow H_2O + CO_2$.

Normally, CO_2 is produced in cells by aerobic metabolism, and it diffuses freely down its concentration gradient into the interstitium. Dissolved CO_2 in interstitial fluid can diffuse freely across the vascular endothelium into the vascular space. CO_2 is transported in erythrocytes and plasma to the lungs, where it is eliminated by ventilation. Normally, the body is an open system for CO_2, and CO_2 in blood and tissues is tightly regulated by ventilation. Decreased ventilation increases venous and arterial P_{CO_2}, which alters the diffusion rate of CO_2 from the interstitium to plasma and therefore rapidly increases interstitial P_{CO_2}.

During metabolic steady-state, gastric mucosal P_{CO_2} reflects the balance between CO_2 production by tissue and CO_2 removal by gastric blood flow. Therefore, gastric P_{CO_2} can increase because of decreased gastric blood flow (stagnant flow) without implying anaerobic production of CO_2. To reemphasize, even if CO_2 is being produced by normal aerobic metabolism without anaerobic generation of CO_2, the gastric P_{CO_2} increases to abnormal levels if gastric blood flow decreases. If gastric blood flow decreases further, such that gastric D_{O_2} decreases below the critical D_{O_2}, CO_2 can then be liberated from HCO_3^- by anaerobic synthesis of fixed acids such as lactic acid (215). In addition, tissue CO_2 is also influenced by decreasing CO_2 production. As D_{O_2} decreases below the critical D_{O_2}, $\dot{V}_{O_2}$ decreases progressively (physiological dependence of $\dot{V}_{O_2}$ on D_{O_2}). Therefore, CO_2 production also decreases below the critical D_{O_2}. Decreased CO_2 production will tend to decrease the gastric P_{CO_2}.

In addition to problems in evaluating tissue CO_2, there may also be problems with the assumption that HCO_3^- of the gastric mucosa is in equilibrium with the systemic arterial HCO_3^- when gastric mucosal pH_i is calculated. This assumption may not always be true. For example, when gastric mucosal blood flow decreases in shock, the gastric tissue HCO_3^- may be significantly lower than the systemic arterial HCO_3^-. Use of systemic HCO_3^- to calculate gastric pH_i would therefore overestimate the gastric pH_i. In rats with induced peritonitis, intramural HCO_3^- exceeded arterial HCO_3^- before and during the first 120 minutes that followed onset of peritonitis (216). Administration of bicarbonate increases arterial bicarbonate and may correct calculated gastric pH_i despite the presence of mucosal acidosis (217).

Recent studies suggest that gastric mucosal acidosis may not indicate mucosal hypoperfusion and hypoxia. Endotoxin administration with fluid resuscitation decreased pH_i, but at the same time there was a redistribution of blood flow from the muscularis to the gut mucosa, and blood flow to the mucosa actually increased (218). In another study in pigs, infusion of endotoxin increased ileal mucosal hydrogen ion concentration and induced mucosal acidosis (219). However, at the same time, mucosal Po_2 increased significantly, suggesting that hypoxia was not responsible for the mucosal acidosis. These results suggest that gastric mucosal acidosis during endotoxemia is not caused by gastric mucosal hypoperfusion. Increased nitric oxide synthesis induced by endotoxin was suggested as a mechanism of mucosal acidosis. Because nitric oxide alters the ATP content of intestinal epithelial cells, the generation of protons derived from ATP degradation could cause tissue acidosis (218). Thus, nitric oxide overproduction could cause both tissue acidosis by a direct cellular mechanism and the vasodilation during septic shock.

As derangements in cellular energy metabolism have been demonstrated in models of sepsis, uncoupling of oxidative phosphorylation, inhibition of mitochondrial respiration, and reduced availability of substrates for oxidative metabolism were postulated as mechanisms to explain mucosal acidosis in the absence of hypoxia (219).

The interpretation of clinical studies of gastric tonometry is also difficult because normal values for gastric pH_i have not been established. In patients with cardiac disease, mean pH_i was 7.52, with an SD of 0.10. A pH_i less than 7.32, two SDs below the group mean, was considered evidence of intramucosal acidosis (220). In addition, higher normal limits for pH_i, such as 7.35, have been used in clinical studies (153). In healthy volunteers, mean pH_i was 7.30 without H_2-blockers and 7.39 with H_2-blockers (208). In a recent study in healthy volunteers, the mean pH_i was 7.23 and increased to 7.31 after administration of ranitidine (213).

Gastric mucosal pH is also complicated by remote systemic acidosis and alkalosis, extremely common disorders in the critically ill. Indeed, Boyd et al. (221) presented data suggesting that systemic acid base deficit/excess was as predictive of outcome of the critically ill as was gastric tonometry pH_i. The use of pH gap (gastric mucosal–arterial pH) has been recommended to solve this problem (222). However, gastric mucosal–arterial Pco_2 difference was found to be a more reliable index of gastric oxygenation than pH_i alone or pH gap (223). Therefore, gastric mucosal–arterial Pco_2 difference was recommended for use in future studies of gastric tonometry (146). It has been suggested that the gastric arterial CO_2 difference increases to approximately 25–35 mm Hg during stagnant gastric blood flow and that levels greater than 25–35 mm Hg indicate anaerobic generation of CO_2 (215).

If pH$_i$ is so complex physiologically, how do we interpret studies showing that abnormally low gastric pH$_i$ is associated with increased mortality and morbidity in critically ill patients? One interpretation is that decreased pH$_i$ can be caused by systemic respiratory and/or metabolic acidosis, both of which are associated with increased mortality. Another interpretation is that decreased gastric blood flow, even without tissue hypoxia and anaerobic metabolism, increases gut permeability and endotoxin translocation and amplifies the systemic inflammatory response syndrome, all of which increase mortality and morbidity. The observation that increased gut permeability and systemic endotoxemia preceed the development of gastric mucosal acidosis in patients undergoing cardiopulmonary bypass supports this view (224). Finally, another interpretation is that many of the patients in these studies who had very abnormal gastric pH$_i$ also had tissue hypoxia, and therefore had higher mortality and morbidity.

E. Methodological Problems with Randomized Control Trials of Supranormal Oxygen Delivery

Although there is some evidence that increasing Do_2 may improve outcome of critically ill patients, this has not been confirmed in studies of supranormal Do_2, and there is also evidence that increasing Do_2 may be detrimental. Methodological problems in some of the studies of supranormal Do_2 may also limit interpretation of the results.

In the first randomized, controlled, clinical trial of supranormal Do_2, Shoemaker et al. (154) showed that the number of single-organ failures was lower in patients who received supranormal Do_2 compared with controls. In a study of high-risk surgical patients, mortality was lower in those who were randomized to supranormal Do_2, and the leading cause of death was multiple organ failure (156). Hayes et al. (160) studied a heterogeneous group of 100 critically ill patients who were randomized either to supranormal Do_2 or control group because they did not achieve supraphysiological treatment goals (cardiac index $>$ 4.5 L/min/m^2, Do_2 $>$ 600 mL/min/m^2, and V̇o_2 $>$ 170 mL/min/m^2) after fluid resuscitation alone. In the treatment group, dobutamine was administered (5 to 200 μg/kg/min) to increase the cardiac index and Do_2 until all three goals had been achieved simultaneously, unless side effects of the drug appeared. The aim was to achieve target values as soon as possible after enrollment and to continue until death or apparent resolution of the acute illness. Although it was estimated that 260 patients would be needed for the study to demonstrate a 15% reduction in mortality rate, the study was discontinued after enrollment of 109 patients because of excess mortality in the protocol arm. The in-unit mortality rate was 30% in the control group, compared with 50% in the protocol group. The in-hospital mortality rate was 34% (the same as the predicted risk of death) in the control group, compared with 54% (predicted risk of death, 34%) in the treatment group. Interestingly, although high doses of dobutamine were used, the excess deaths in the treatment group were not caused by cardiac events, but were attributed to development of multiple organ failure (160).

The largest study thus far of supranormal D_{O_2} was reported by Gattinoni et al. (161). They conducted a multicenter study of 762 heterogeneous critically ill patients randomly allocated to one of the three groups designed to achieve different hemodynamic goals: (1) normal cardiac index (2.5 to 3.5 L/min/m^2; control group); (2) supranormal cardiac index (> 4.5 L/min/m^2; cardiac index group); and (3) a normal mixed venous oxygen saturation (> 70%; the oxygen saturation group). In addition, predefined standard intensive care (e.g., urine output > 0.5 mL/kg/hr) was maintained for all patients. Therapy consisted of volume expansion, transfusion, inotropes, vasodilators, and vasopressors. Hemodynamic treatment aimed at achieving the study target was mandatory for 5 days. The primary end points of the study were mortality up to discharge from the ICU, mortality 6 months after randomization, and morbidity among survivors as estimated by the number of dysfunctional organ systems. There were no differences in ICU mortality (48%, 49%, and 52%, respectively) or 6-month mortality (62%, 62%, and 64%, respectively) among the three groups. Importantly, there were also no differences in the number of organ failures between the groups. Because all patients did not achieve the intended goals of the treatment, subgroup analysis was performed to include only patients who had reached the end points of resuscitation. There was no difference in outcome among groups of patients who had reached the end points of therapy. There were also no diagnostic subgroups of patients who did benefit from supranormal D_{O_2} (161). Thus, the large multicenter trial of supranormal D_{O_2} found no effect on multiple organ failure, suggesting that MSOF is not caused by tissue hypoxia or that supranormal D_{O_2} does not reverse or prevent tissue hypoxia.

Timing of intervention may be important in explaining why some studies of supranormal D_{O_2} have shown benefit, whereas others have not. One interpretation of the results of these studies is that supranormal D_{O_2} may be effective in randomized controlled trials if therapy is delivered early to prevent tissue hypoxia in patients at risk. In contrast, trials in critically ill patients who have ARDS, septic shock, or signs of tissue hypoxia present already at the time of the intervention show no effect or even adverse effects of the intervention. This is supported by a recent meta-analysis of studies of the effects of supranormal D_{O_2} on mortality in critically ill patients (225). The relative risk of death was 0.20 (95% confidence interval, 0.07 to 0.55) if therapy was initiated preoperatively compared with a relative risk of 0.98 (95% confidence interval, 0.79 to 1.22) if therapy was initiated after ICU admission.

We and other investigators have reviewed some of the methodological problems with randomized trials (225,226). For example, there have been deficiencies in the blinding of randomization, in patient selection, in assuring that the patients are comparable at baseline, and in describing cointerventions. In addition, some of the trials did not have a clear definition of the clinical protocols and algorithms used to increase D_{O_2} and in some of the studies, statistical analysis was not performed on an intent-to-treat basis. There is also a problem of crossovers in some of the studies and an absence of prestudy sample size estimates in several studies. In general, the quality of randomized controlled trials of Do_2 is variable, which is why drawing reliable inferences from them may be difficult (225).

F. Potential Effects of Catecholamines on Inflammation

The beneficial or detrimental effects of catecholamines in clinical trials are usually attributed to effects on tissue oxygenation. However, there are other potential mechanisms of action that could be important in critically ill patients. Recent evidence suggests that catecholamines have effects on inflammation because they modify the levels of pro-inflammatory and anti-inflammatory cytokines. In studies that found benefit of supranormal Do_2 on organ failures, the group that received supranormal Do_2 received higher doses and more catecholamines. It is possible that the mechanism of benefit in the supranormal Do_2 group may not be reversal of hypoxia, but could be anti-inflammatory actions of catecholamines.

There are pro-inflammatory cytokines such as tumor necrosis factor (TNF) and interleukin (IL)-6, and anti-inflammatory cytokines such as IL-10 (227). MODS or failure could be caused by uncontrolled systemic inflammatory response and excessive cytokine action (228). It has been suggested that if the balance between pro-inflammatory and anti-inflammatory cytokines is disturbed, these mediators may be harmful (229).

In patients with sepsis, persistently high levels of cytokines, especially TNF and IL-6, are associated with the development of multiple organ failure and death (Fig. 7) (230). Multiple organ failure is also the most important cause of death in high-risk surgical patients (156). Interestingly, both elective and emergency surgery are associated with release of TNF and IL-6, and the greater the surgical trauma is, the greater the release (231–233).

Boyd et al. (156) randomized high-risk surgical patients to a supranormal Do_2 group (using dopexamine) or a normal Do_2 group (156). Dopexamine increased Do_2 significantly compared with baseline in the supranormal group and compared with the control group. However, there was no increase in global $\dot{V}o_2$, nor was there a difference in $\dot{V}o_2$ between the supranormal Do_2 and control groups. However, the mortality rate was lower in the supranormal group by 75%, and the deaths in the control group were a result of development of multiple organ failure (156). If occult tissue hypoxia was reversed by the increased Do_2 caused by dopexamine, then one would have expected increased $\dot{V}o_2$. Could dopexamine have exerted its benefit through an entirely different mechanism—an anti-inflammatory mechanism—rather than a hypoxia prevention mechanism?

Vasoactive drugs modulate cytokine production in vitro and in vivo. Norepinephrine inhibits lipopolysaccharide-induced TNF-α production (234–236). This inhibitory effect is likely β-receptor–mediated. In a recent human study, adrenaline started 3 hours before lipopolysaccharide challenge inhibited in vivo TNF appearance and increased IL-10 release (Fig. 8) (237). Because IL-10 is a cytokine with

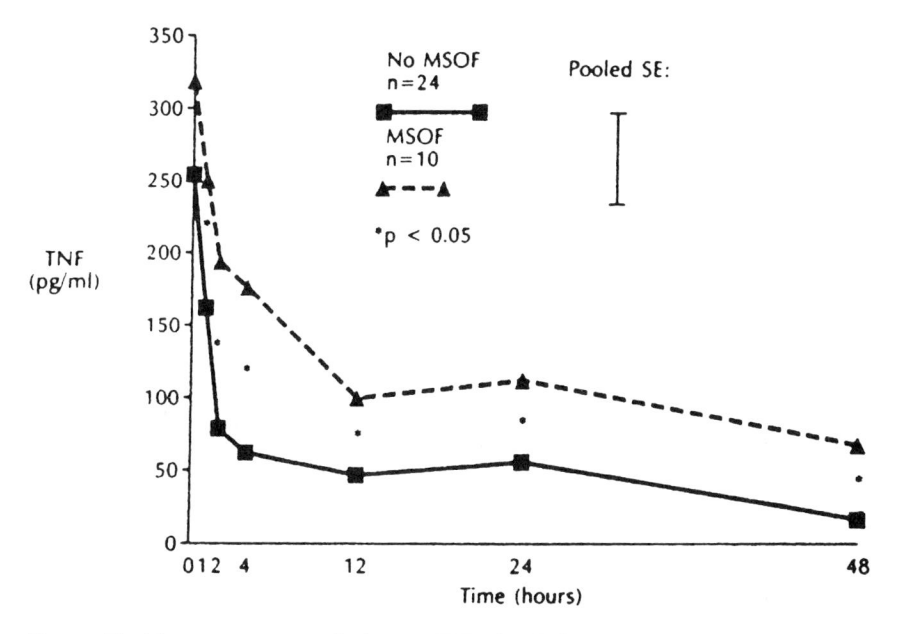

Figure 7 Mean tumor necrosis factor (TNF) levels in septic shock patients who subsequently developed or did not develop multiple system organ failure (MSOF). Note the persistent elevation in TNF levels in septic patients with MSOF. (From Ref. 230.)

anti-inflammatory properties and because low levels of IL-10 are associated with more severe organ injury, the investigators concluded that adrenaline may have a net anti-inflammatory effect on the cytokine network early in the course of systemic inflammation (237,238). Although dobutamine is probably the most widely used catecholamine in critical care, we are not aware of studies that have examined the effects of dobutamine on cytokine production.

Phosphodiesterase inhibitors also modify cytokine production in vitro and in vivo. Pentoxifylline inhibited TNF and IL-6 activity in a dose-related fashion in whole blood incubated with endotoxin (239). In endotoxemic mice, both pentoxifylline and amrinone increased survival and decreased TNF production (240,241). Human studies confirm the anti-inflammatory effects of phosphodiesterase inhibitors. In healthy volunteers challanged with endotoxin, a 4-hour infusion of pentoxifylline, started 30 minutes before endotoxin injection, totally blocked endotoxin-induced TNF but had no effect on IL-6 synthesis (242).

Vasoactive drugs may also modify inflammation by other mechanisms than simply inhibition of cytokine production. Leukocyte–endothelial interactions play a critical role in the development of organ failure (243). Leukocyte adherence to activated endothelium is a critical early step for initiation of release of neutrophil products. Cytokines stimulate endothelial cells to increase expression of

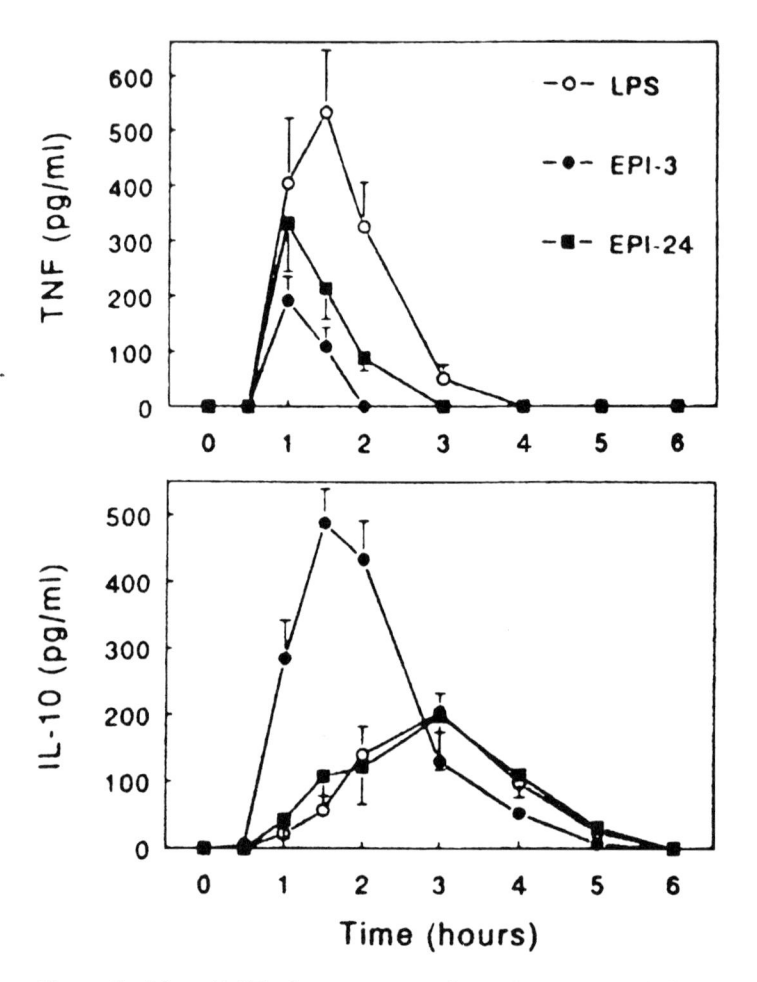

Figure 8 Mean (± SE) plasma concentrations of tumor necrosis factor (TNF; top) and interleukin (IL)-10 (bottom) after intravenous injection of lipopolysaccharide (LPS) at t = 0. LPS, subjects injected with LPS only (n = 6); EPI-3, subjects infused with epinephrine (30 ng/kg/min) from t = −3 to 6 hours (n = 5); EPI-24, subjects infused with epinephrine (30 ng/kg/min) from −24 to 6 hours (n = 6). EPI-3 attenuated the LPS-induced increase in TNF levels and potentiated the increase in IL-10 levels (both $P < .0005$ vs. LPS only). EPI-24 only reduced TNF levels ($P = .05$ vs. LPS only), without any effect on IL-10 release. (From Ref. 237.)

surface adhesion molecules, such as E-selectin, intercellular adhesion molecule-1, and vascular cell adhesion molecule-1. Amrinone pretreatment significantly decreases cytokine-induced upregulation of these adhesion molecules (244). Pretreatment with dopexamine attenuates leukocyte adherence to postcapillary venules in rats during endotoxemia (245). Therefore, it is possible that inotropes have beneficial effects on organ function and survival through some other effects than their effects on oxygen transport.

VIII. Alternative Mechanisms of Multiple Organ Failure

There are several nonhypoxic mechanisms of multiple organ failure. For example, Tighe et al. (246) measured systemic and hepatic blood flow and Do_2 in pigs with peritonitis (246). CO was increased by more than 25% by administrating either dobutamine, dopexamine, or colloid before the induction of fecal peritonitis. Before infection, CO, $\dot{V}o_2$, and hepatic blood flow was increased by dopexamine, dobutamine, and volume infusion, and Do_2 was increased in the dobutamine and dopexamine groups. There were no significant differences between hepatic hemodynamic or oxygen transport variables in any of the groups during the infection period. Hepatic ultrastructure was well maintained in the dopexamine group, whereas considerable deterioration was observed in the volume, dobutamine, and control groups (246). There was no relationship between changes in Do_2 or $\dot{V}o_2$ and the degree of protection of the hepatic ultrastructure. Because increasing CO and $\dot{V}o_2$ before and during infection was protective only when dopexamine was administered, the investigators speculated that dopexamine may have an unexpected anti-inflammatory effect (246).

Because there is a lot of controversy regarding the impact of occult tissue hypoxia in the development of multiple organ failure, a number of alternative mechanisms have been proposed. These other mechanisms that could cause multiple organ failure, such as ischemia–reperfusion injury, leukocyte activation, leukocyte–endothelial interactions, and cytokine actions, are reviewed next.

Reperfusion after ischemia causes tissue injury. Although ischemia-induced tissue hypoxia can lead to irreversible tissue injury if the period of ischemia is sufficiently prolonged, much of the tissue damage frequently occurs after oxygenation is restored rather than during the period of ischemia. More specifically, ischemic tissues in a variety of organs are vulnerable to xanthine oxidase-mediated reperfusion injury (247–249). Xanthine oxidase has been found in vascular endothelium as well as the gut epithelium. Under normal conditions, it exists predominantly as xantine dehydrogenase; however, with ischemia, xanthine dehydrogenase is converted to xanthine oxidase. At the same time, breakdown of ATP increases the level of purine metabolites, hypoxanthine and xanthine. With reperfusion, oxygen becomes available, and the xanthine oxidase-dependent oxidation of hypoxanthine and xanthine generates a burst of reactive oxygen metabolites such as hydroxyl radical (·OH), that cause tissue injury (247). Reperfusion injures cells directly. After reoxygenation, reactive oxygen metabolites within cells may damage cell and organelle membranes, denature proteins, and disrupt the chromosomes. In addition, oxidants may escape from cells and injure adjacent cells as well as enter the circulation. Although this cellular damage may occur in all cells, endothelial cells in the microvasculature seem to be especially affected; hence, microcirculatory disruption is a prominent feature of severe reperfusion injury (250). It is interesting to note that the crucial step, the conversion of xanthine dehydrogenase to xanthine oxidase, takes only 10 seconds in intestinal tissue, 8 minutes in cardiac muscle, and approximately 30 minutes in the liver, spleen, kidney, and lung (251). This may explain the different relative susceptibility of these organs to ischemia–reperfusion-mediated tissue injury.

Reperfusion injury also stimulates inflammation. Polymorphonuclear leukocytes are required for the full expression of ischemia–reperfusion injury; oxidant injury seems to rapidly activate polymorphonuclear leukocytes (252,253). Macrophages are also stimulated by reperfusion. Reactive oxygen metabolites enhance proinflammatory cytokine production, i.e., TNF, IL-1, and IL-6. It is likely that these and other cytokines play an important role in amplifying the inflammatory response to ischemia and reperfusion. Among the many actions of the proinflammatory cytokines are direct cytotoxicity, polymorphonuclear leukocyte activation, and the stimulation of additional production of reactive oxygen metabolites (250).

A number of stimuli after shock and trauma may prime and activate leukocytes, including ischemia, reactive oxygen metabolites, and cytokines (254). Activated leukocytes can produce cellular injury by release of lysosomal enzymes and cytokines. Normally, circulating neutrophils do not adhere to vascular endothelium, and neutrophil adhesion to vascular endothelium is a key element in injury and inflammatory response (255,256). When the endothelium is activated, e.g., by cytokines, neutrophils adhere to the endothelial surface (255). Neutrophil adherence is facilitated by adhesion molecules expressed on neutrophils and endothelial cells (255). The adherence of neutrophils to vascular endothelial surfaces creates a microenvironment into which activated neutrophils release products that cause endothelial damage, leading to increase in microvascular permeability and widespread edema. Excessive aggregation of neutrophils within the microvasculature can also lead to focal ischemia and organ dysfunction. It has been proposed that gut ischemia/reperfusion, secondary to splanchnic hypoperfusion, is responsible for creating the local inflammatory environment that primes circulating neutrophils to adhere to endothelial cell surfaces (257).

Cytokines are another potential cause of MSOF, and an anticytokine hypothesis has dominated clinical trials in sepsis for several years. The hypothesis is that overproduction and persistently high levels of proinflammatory cytokines, such as IL-1, TNF, IL-6, and IL-8, cause multiple organ failure (230,258). Cytokines increase the production of secondary mediators such as nitric oxide, arachidonic acid metabolites, bradykinin, and histamine. These secondary mediators activate neutrophils and endothelial cells to perpetuate tissue injury. However, cytokines are necessary for the immune response, and there are anti-inflammatory as well as pro-inflammatory cytokines. In addition, none of the attempts to modulate the biological activity of cytokines with antibodies has been successful in improving outcome in several clinical trials.

In summary, there are many other potential causes for the development of multiple organ failure than occult tissue hypoxia, and only some of them have been discussed here. One event may activate several other pathways, which in turn may reactivate the release of mediators that cause MSOF.

IX. Facilitative Role for Tissue Hypoxia in MSOF

The role of occult tissue hypoxia as a cause of multiple organ failure is not clear, and it is unlikely that occult tissue hypoxia alone is responsible for the development of organ failure. However, we suggest that tissue hypoxia may play a role in the development of organ failure because tissue hypoxia could be an important component of a "two-hit" model of multiple organ failure. According to this two-hit model, tissue hypoxia alone is not sufficient to cause organ failure, but instead may have a facilitative role.

The two-hit phenomenon in MSOF describes the biological phenomenon in which an initial insult, the first hit, primes the host such that a second insult (the second hit) amplifies the host's response greatly (12). Because several clinical conditions may precede multiple organ failure, the first hit could be infection, inflammation, dead/injured tissue, or inadequate tissue perfusion. The second hit could be another insult, such as infection, anesthesia, and hypotension (259).

The gut is particularly vulnerable to hypoxia because of redistribution of blood flow to vital organs such as the heart and brain. Gut is also particularly sensitive to ischemia–reperfusion injury (251). Furthermore, postischemic gut also serves as a priming bed for circulating neutrophils (257). In animal model studies, gut ischemia–reperfusion or intraperitoneal endotoxin alone did not induce organ failure. However, the sequential insults of gut ischemia–reperfusion and endotoxin caused organ damage and increased mortality (Fig. 9) (257). Neutrophil priming occurred in the gut at 90 minutes of reperfusion. Further studies are required to confirm the two-hit model hypothesis.

X. Summary

We have reviewed the evidence for and against the hypothesis that occult tissue hypoxia causes multiple organ failure. We have reviewed several lines of evidence in attempting to link tissue hypoxia and multiple organ failure, including the dependence of $\dot{V}O_2$ on DO_2, the value of hyperlactatemia and gastric tonometry in assessing tissue oxygenation, and the randomized controlled trials of supranormal

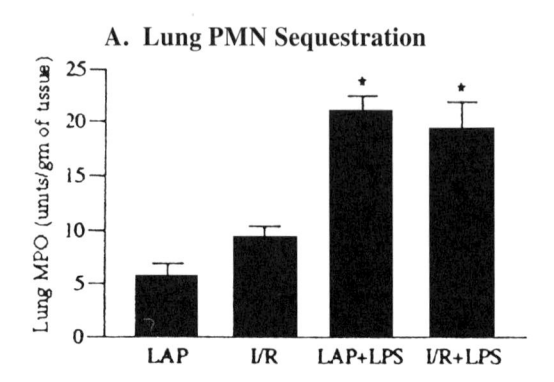

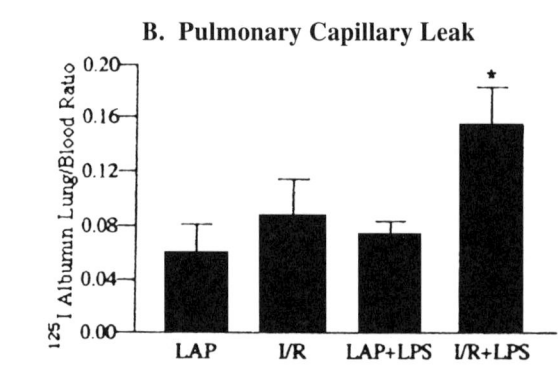

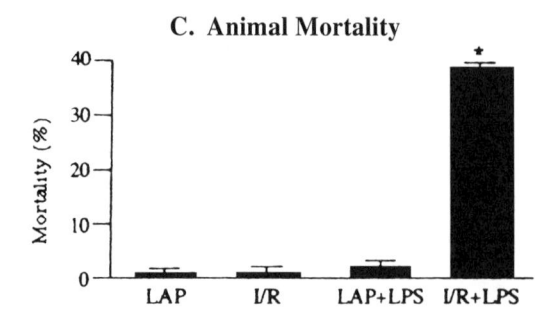

Figure 9 (A) Lung myeloperoxidase (MPO), (B) ^{125}I albumin lung/blood ratio, and (C) animal mortality at 18 hours of reperfusion. LAP, sham laparotomy; I/R (ischemia–reperfusion), 45 minutes of intestinal ischemia; LAP + LPS, laparatomy plus endotoxin (lipopolysaccharide [LPS]) 6 hours later; I/R + LPS, I/R plus LPS 6 hours later. $^*P < .05$ compared with LAP, I/R, and LAP + LPS. (From Ref. 257.)

DO_2 and the effects on the incidence of multiple organ failure. Despite our efforts, we were unable to definitively show that occult tissue hypoxia causes multiple organ failure. There are few animal models of multiple organ failure, and virtually all have a nonshock mechanism.

The association between high lactate or gastric mucosal acidosis and development of multiple organ failure suggests, but does not prove occult tissue hypoxia. It is most likely that the pathophysiology of multiple organ failure is multifactorial. The two-hit model of multiple organ failure is a relatively new approach to explain the pathophysiology of organ failure. We suggest that occult tissue hypoxia may cause multiple organ failure by the two-hit hypothesis, although each of the two hits may be nonhypoxic.

We recommend potentially fertile areas for future investigation to test the hypothesis that occult tissue hypoxia causes multiple organ failure. It would be useful to re-evaluate the timing of intervention and also the target patient population in randomized controlled trials of supranormal DO_2. We believe that a preoperative strategy to optimize DO_2 in a homogeneous group of high-risk elective surgical patients requires further studies. Second, we suggest that the potential effect of splanchnic tissue hypoperfusion on outcome should be tested. If gastric tonometry is to be used, gastric-arterial CO_2 gradient, instead of pH_i, should be used as the variable to trigger additional treatment. The additional treatment should also be directed by clear, reproducible algorithms. Finally, the two-hit model of multiple organ failure and the role of different hits, such as tissue hypoxia, require futher evaluation. Finally, we propose that the anti-inflammatory and pro-inflammatory effects of catecholamines require further studies as an influence on MSOF.

References

1. Milberg JA, Davis DR, Steinberg KP, Hudson LD. Improved survival of patients with acute respiratory distress syndrome (ARDS): 1983-1993. JAMA 1995; 273: 306–309.
2. Tilney NL, Bailey GL, Morgan AP. Sequential system failure after rupture of AAA: an unsolved problem in postoperative care. Ann Surg 1973; 178:117–122.
3. Eiseman B, Beart R, Norton L. Multiple organ failure. Surg Gynecol Obstet 1977; 144:323–326.
4. Bone RC, Balk RA, Cerra FB, Dellinger RP, Fein AM, Knaus WA, Schein RM, Sibbald WJ. Definitions for sepsis and organ failure and quidelines for the use of innovative therapies in sepsis. Chest 1992; 101:1644–1655.
5. Fry DE, Pearlstein L, Fulton RL, Polk HC Jr. Multiple system organ failure: the role of uncontrolled infection. Arch Surg 1980; 115:136–140.
6. Knaus WA, Draper EA, Wagner DP, Zimmerman JE. Prognosis in acute organ-system failure. Ann Surg 1985; 202:685–693.
7. Marshall JC, Cook DJ, Christon NV, Bernard GR, Sprung CL, Sibbald WJ. Multiple organ dysfunction score: a reliable descriptor of a complex clinical outcome. Crit Care Med 1995; 23:1638–1652.

8. Hebert PC, Drummond AJ, Singer J, Bernard GR, Russell JA. A simple multiple system organ failure scoring system predicts mortality of patients who have sepsis syndrome. Chest 1993; 104:230–235.
9. Le Gall J-R, Klar J, Lemeshow S, Saulnier F, Alberti C, Artigas A, Teres D. The logistic organ dysfunction system: a new way to assess organ dysfunction in the intensive care unit. JAMA 1996; 276:802–810.
10. Vincent J-L, Moreno R, Takala J, Willatts S, De Mendonca A, Bruining H, Reinhart CK, Suter PM, Thijs LG. The SOFA (Sepsis-related Organ Failure Assessment) score to describe organ dysfunction/failure. Intensive Care Med 1996; 22:707–710.
11. Marshall JC, Sweeney D. Microbial infection and the septic response in critical surgical illness: sepsis, not infection, determines outcome. Arch Surg 1990; 125: 17–23.
12. Deitch EA. Multiple organ failure: pathophysiology and potential future therapy. Ann Surg 1992; 216:117–134.
13. Tran DD, Groeneveld ABJ, van der Meulen J, Nauta JJP, van Schijndel RS, Thijs LG. Age, chronic disease, sepsis, organ system failure, and mortality in a medical intensive care unit. Crit Care Med 1990; 18:474–479.
14. DeCamp MM, Demling RH. Post-traumatic multisystem organ failure. JAMA 1988; 260:530–534.
15. Faist E, Baue AE, Dittmer H, Heberer G. Multiple organ failure in polytrauma patients. J Trauma 1983; 23:775–787.
16. Pine RW, Wertz MJ, Lennard ES, Dellinger EP, Carrico CJ, Minshew BH. Determinants of organ malfunction or death in patients with intra-abdominal sepsis. Arch Surg 1983; 118:242–249.
17. Baue AE. Multiple, progressive, or sequential systems failure: a syndrome of the 1970's. Arch Surg 1975; 110:779–781.
18. Madoff RD, Sharpe SM, Fath JJ, Simmons RL, Cerra FB. Prolonged surgical intensive care. Arch Surg 1985; 120:698–702.
19. Rapoport J, Teres D, Lemeshow S, Avrunin JS, Haber R. Explaining variability of cost using a severity-of-illness measure for ICU patients. Med Care 1990; 28:338–348.
20. Oye RK, Bellamy PE. Patterns of resource consumption in medical intensive care. Chest 1991; 99:685–689.
21. Gutierrez G, Lund N, Bryan-Brown CW. Cellular oxygen utilization during multiple organ failure. Crit Care Clin 1989; 5:271–287.
22. Gutierrez G. Cellular energy metabolism during hypoxia. Crit Care Med 1991; 19:619–626.
23. Finch CA, Lenfant C. Oxygen transport in man. N Engl J Med 1972; 286:407–415.
24. Hebert PC, Wells G, Marshall J, Martin C, Tweeddale M, Pagliarello G, Blajchman M. Transfusion requirements in critical care: a pilot study. JAMA 1995; 273:1439–1444.
25. Levine E, Rosen A, Sehgal L, Gould S, Sehgal H, Moss G. Physiologic effects of acute anemia: implication for a reduced transfusion trigger. Transfusion 1992; 30:11–16.
26. Tremper KK, Barker SJ. Blood-gas analysis. In: Hall JB, Schmidt GA, Wood LDH, eds. Principles of Critical Care. New York: McGraw-Hill, 1992, pp 181–196.

27. Hebert PC, Wells G, Tweeddale M, Martin C, Marshall J, Pham BA, Blajchman M, Schweitzer I, Pagliarello G. Does transfusion practice affect mortality in critically ill patients? Am J Respir Crit Care Med 1997; 155:1618–1623.
28. Nunn JF. Applied Respiratory Physiology. London: Butterworths, 1987.
29. Montgomery AB, Stager MA, Carrico CJ, Hudson LD. Causes of mortality in patients with the adult respiratory distress syndrome. Am Rev Respir Dis 1985; 132:485–489.
30. Rowell LB, Brengelman GL, Blackmon JR, Twiss RD, Kusumi F. Splanchnic blood flow and metabolism in heat-stressed man. Appl Physiol 1968; 24:475–484.
31. Price HL, Deutsch S, Marshall BE, Stephen GW, Behar MG, Neufeld GR. Hemodynamic and metabolic effects of hemorrhage in man with particular reference to the splanchnic circulation. Circ Res 1966; 18:469–474.
32. Edouard AR, Degremont A-C, Duranteau J, Pussard E, Berdeaux A, Samii K. Heterogeneous regional vascular responses to simulated transient hypovolemia in man. Intensive Care Med 1994; 20:414–420.
33. Duranteau J, Sitbon P, Vicaut E, Descorps-Declere A, Vugue B, Samii K. Assessment of gastric mucosal perfusion during simulated hypovolemia in healthy volunteers. Am J Respir Crit Care Med 1996; 154:1653–1657.
34. Lang CH, Bagby GJ, Ferguson JL, Spitzer JJ. Cardiac output and redistribution of organ blood flow in hypermetabolic sepsis. Am J Physiol 1984; 246:R331–337.
35. Xu D, Qi L, Guillory D, Cruz N, Berg R, Deitch EA. Mechanisms of endotoxin-induced intestinal injury in a hyperdynamic model of sepsis. J Trauma 1993; 34:676–683.
36. Fong Y, Marano MA, Moldaver LL, Wei H, Calvano SE, Kenney JS, Allison AC, Cerami A, Shires GT, Lowry SF. The acute splanchnic and peripheral tissue metabolic response to endotoxin in humans. J Clin Invest 1990; 85:1896–1904.
37. Dahn MS, Lange P, Wilson RF, Jacobs LA, Mitchell RA. Hepatic blood flow and splanchnic oxygen consumption measurements in clinical sepsis. Surgery 1990; 107:295–301.
38. Ruokonen E, Takala J, Kari A, Saxen H, Mertsola J, Hansen EJ. Regional blood flow and oxygen transport in septic shock. Crit Care Med 1993; 21:1296–1303.
39. Cherniac RM. The oxygen consumption and efficiency of the respiratory muscles in health and emphysema. J Clin Invest 1959; 38:494–499.
40. Field S, Kelly SM, Macklem PT. The oxygen cost of breathing in patients with cardiorespiratory disease. Am Rev Resp Dis 1982; 126:9–13.
41. Viires N, Sillye G, Aubier M, Rassidakis A, Roussos C. Regional blood flow distribution in dog during induced hypotension and low cardiac output: spontaneous breathing versus artificial ventilation. J Clin Invest 1982; 72:935–947.
42. Mohsenifar Z, Hay A, Hay J, Lewis MI, Koerner SK. Gastric intramucosal pH as a predictor of success or failure in weaning patients from mechanical ventilation. Ann Intern Med 1993; 119:794–798.
43. Suter PM, Fairley HB, Isenberg MD. Optimum end-expiratory airway pressure in patients with acute pulmonary failure. N Engl J Med 1975; 292:284–288.
44. Manny J, Justice R, Hetchman HB. Abnormalities in organ blood flow and its distribution during positive end-expiratory pressure. Surgery 1979; 85:425–432.
45. Matuschak GM, Pinsky MR, Rogers RM. Effects of positive end-expiratory pressure on hepatic blood flow and performance. J Appl Physiol 1987; 62:1377–1383.

46. Berstein AD, Gnidec AA, Rutledge FS, Sibbald NJ. Hyperdynamic sepsis modifies a PEEP-mediated redistribution in organ blood flows. Am Rev Respir Dis 1990; 141:1198–1208.
47. Geiger K, Georgieff M, Lutz H. Side effects of positive pressure ventilation on hepatic function and splanchnic circulation. Int J Clin Monit Comput 1986; 69: 103–106.
48. Arvidsson D, Almquist P, Haglund U. Effects of positive end-expiratory pressure on splanchnic circulation and function in experimental peritonitis. Arch Surg 1991; 126:631–636.
49. Fujita Y, Sakai T, Ohsumi A, Takaori M. Effects of hypocapnia and hypercapnia on splanchnic circulation and hepatic function in the beagle. Anesth Analg 1989; 69:152-157.
50. Carlton EL, Selinger SL, Utley J, Hoffman JIE. Intramyocardial distribution of blood flow in hemorrhagic shock in anesthetized dogs. Am J Physiol 1976; 230:41–49.
51. Archie JP, Mertz WR. Myocardial oxygen delivery after experimental shock. Ann Surg 1978; 187:205–210.
52. Ratcliffe PJ, Moonen CTW, Holloway PA, Ledingham JG, Radda GK. Acute renal failure in hemorrhagic hypotension: cellular energetics and renal function. Kidney Int 1986; 30:355–360.
53. Wyler F, Neutze JM, Rudolp Am. Effects of endotoxin on distribution of cardiac output in unanesthetized rabbits. Am J Physiol 1970; 219:246–251.
54. Kreimeier U, Brückner WB, Niemczyk S, Messmer K. Hyperosmotic saline dextran for resuscitation from traumatic-hemorrhagic hypotension: effect on regional blood flow. Circ Shock 1990; 32:83–99.
55. Miller CF, Breslow MJ, Shapiro RM, Traystman RF. Role of hypotension in decreasing cerebral blood flow in porcine endotoxemia. Am J Physiol 1987; 253:H956–H964.
56. Bailey RW, Morris JB, Hamilton SR, Bulkley GB. The pathogenesis of non-occlusive ischaemic colitis. Ann Surg 1986; 203:590–599.
57. McNeill JR, Stark RD, Greenway CV. Intestinal vasoconstriction after hemorrhage: roles of vasopressin and angiotensin. Am J Physiol 1970; 219:1342–1347.
58. Carter EA, Tompkins RG, Yarmush ML, Walker WA, Burke JF. Redistribution of blood flow after thermal injury and hemorrhagic shock. J Appl Physiol 1988; 65:1782–1788.
59. Schlictig R, Kramer DJ, Pinsky MR. Flow redistribution during progressive hemorrhage is a determinant of critical O_2 delivery. J Appl Physiol 1991; 70:169–178.
60. Groeneveld ABJ, van Lambalgen AA, van den Bos GC, Bronsveld W, Thijs LG. Maldistribution of heterogeneous coronary blood flow during canine endotoxin shock. Cardiovasc Res 1991; 25:80–88.
61. van Lambalgen AA, van Kraats AA, van den Bos GC, Stel HV, Straub J, Donker AJ, Thijs JG. Renal function and metabolism during endotoxemia in rats: role of hypoperfusion. Circ Shock 1991; 35:164–173.
62. Ravikant T, Lucas CE. Renal blood flow distribution in septic hyperdynamic pigs. J Surg Res 1977; 22:294–298.
63. Fink MP. Gastrointestinal mucosal injury in experimental models of shock, trauma, and sepsis. Crit Care Med 1991; 19:627–641.

64. Brondveld W, Lambalgen AA, van der Bos GC, Thijs LG, Koopman PAR. Regional blood flow and metabolism in canine endotoxin shock before, during, and after infusion of glucose-insulin-potassium (GIK). Circ Shock 1986; 18:31–42.
65. Bressack MA, Morton NS, Hortop J. Group B streptococcal sepsis in the piglet: effect of fluid therapy on venous return, organ edema and organ blood flow. Circ Res 1987; 61:659–669.
66. Marik PE, Mohedin M. The contrasting effects of dopamine and norepinephrine on systemic and splanchnic oxygen utilization in hyperdynamic sepsis. JAMA 1994; 274:1354–1357.
67. Humer MF, Phang PT, Friesen BP, Allard MF, Goddard CM, Walley KR. Heterogeneity of gut capillary transit times and impaired gut oxygen extraction in endotoxemic pigs. J Appl Physiol 1996; 81:895–904.
68. Walley KR. Heterogeneity of oxygen delivery impairs oxygen extraction by peripheral tissues: theory. J Appl Physiol 1996; 81:885–894.
69. Nelson DPG, Beyer C, Samsel RW, Wood LDH, Schumacker PT. Pathologic supply dependence of O_2 uptake during bacteremia in dogs. J Appl Physiol 1987; 63:1487–1492.
70. Nelson DPC, King CE, Dodd SL, Schumacker PT, Cain SM. Systemic and intestinal limits of O_2 extraction in the dog. J Appl Physiol 1987; 63:387–394.
71. Nelson DPG, Samsel RW, Wood LDH, Schumacker PT. Pathologic supply dependence of systemic and intestinal O_2 uptake during endotoxemia. J Appl Physiol 1988; 64:2410–2419.
72. Samsel RW, Nelson DPG, Sanders WM, Wood LDH, Schumacker PT. Effect of endotoxin on systemic and skeletal muscle O_2 extraction. J Appl Physiol 1988; 65:1377–1382.
73. Tenney SM. A theoretical analysis of the relationship between venous blood and mean tissue oxygen pressures. Respir Physiol 1974; 20:283–296.
74. Lam C, Tyml K, Martin C, Sibbald W. Microvascular perfusion is impaired in a rat model of normotensive sepsis. J Clin Invest 1994; 94:2077–2083.
75. Honig CR, Odoroff CL. Calculated dispersion of capillary transit times: significance for oxygen exchange. Am J Physiol 1981; 240:H199–H208.
76. Altura BM, Gebrewold A, Burton RW. Reactive hyperemic responses of single arterioles are attenuated markedly after intestinal ischemia, endotoxemia and traumatic shock: possible role of endothelial cells. Microcirc Endothelium Lymphatics 1985; 2:3–14.
77. Song H, Tyml K. Evidence for sensing and integration of biological signals by the capillary network. Am J Physiol 1993; 265:H1235–H1242.
78. Tyml K, Budreau CH. Heterogeneity of microvascular response to ischemia in skeletal muscle. Int J Microcirc Clin Exp 1988; 7:205–221.
79. Puranapanda V, Hinshaw LB, O'Rear EA, Chang AC, Whitsett TL. Erythrocyte deformability in canine septic shock and the efficacy of pentoxifylline and leukotriene antagonist. Proc Soc Exp Biol Med 1987; 185:206–210.
80. Goddard CM, Allard MF, Hogg JC, Herbertson MJ, Walley KR. Prolonged leukocyte transit time in coronary microcirculation of endotoxemic pigs. Am J Physiol 1995; 269:H1389–1397.
81. Cain SM, King CE, Chapler CK. Effects of time and microembolization on O_2 extraction by dog hindlimb in hypoxia. J Crit Care 1988; 3:89–95.

82. Ellsworth ML, Goldfarb RD, Alexander RS. Microembolization induced oxygen utilization impairment in the canine gracilis muscle. Adv Shock Res 1981; 5:89–94.
83. Moncada S, Palmer RM, Higgs EA. Nitric oxide: physiology, pathophysiology, and pharmacology. Pharmacol Rev 1991; 43:109–142.
84. Cohen RA, Shepherd JT, Vanhoutte PM. Inhibitory role of the endothelium in the response of isolated coronary arteries to platelets. Science 1983; 221:273–274.
85. Manthous CA, Hall JB, Olson D, Singh M, Chatila W, Pohlman A, Kushner R, Schmidt GA, Wood LDG. Effect of cooling on oxygen consumption in febrile critically ill patients. Am J Respir Crit Care Med 1995; 151:10–14.
86. Boyd O, Grounds M, Bennett D. The dependency of oxygen consumption on oxygen delivery in critically ill postoperative patients is mimicked by variations in sedation. Chest 1992; 101:1619–1624.
87. Manthous CA, Hall JB, Kushner R, Schmidt GA, Russo G, Wood LDG. The effect of mechanical ventilation on oxygen consumption in critically ill patients. Am J Respir Crit Care Med 1995; 151:210–214.
88. Weissman C, Kemper M. The oxygen uptake-oxygen delivery relationship during ICU interventions. Chest 1991; 99:430–435.
89. Weissman C, Kemper M, Damask MC, Askanazi J, Hyman AI, Kinney JM. Effect of routine intensive care interactions on metabolic rate. Chest 1984; 86:815–818.
90. Bhatt S, Hutchinson R, Tomlinson B, Oh T, Mak M. Effects of dobutamine on oxygen supply and uptake in healthy volunteers. Br J Anaesth 1992; 69:298–303.
91. Green C, Frazer R, Underhill S, Maycock P, Fairhurst J, Campbell I. Metabolic effects of dobutamine in normal man. Clin Sci 1992; 82:77–83.
92. Uusaro A, Hartikainen J, Parviainen M, Takala J. Metabolic stress modifies the thermogenic effect of dobutamine in man. Crit Care Med 1995; 23:674–680.
93. Uusaro A, Ruokonen E, Takala J. Gastric mucosal pH does not reflect changes in splanchnic blood flow after cardiac surgery. Br J Anaesth 1995; 74:149–154.
94. Parviainen I, Ruokonen E, Takala J. Dobutamine-induced dissociation between changes in splanchnic blood flow and gastric intramucosal pH after cardiac surgery. Br J Anaesth 1995; 74:277–282.
95. Dahn MS, Lange P, Lobdell K, Hans B, Jacobs LA, Mitchell RA. Splanchnic and total body oxygen consumption differences in septic and injured patients. Surgery 1987; 101:69–80.
96. Wilmore DW, Goodwin CW, Aulick LH, Powanda MC, Mason AD, Pruitt BA Jr. Effect of injury and infection on visceral metabolism and circulation. Ann Surg 1980; 192:491–500.
97. Cain SM. Oxygen delivery and uptake in dogs during anemic and hypoxic hypoxia. J Appl Physiol 1977; 42:228–234.
98. Gutierrez G, Warley AR, Dantzker DR. Oxygen delivery and utilization in hypothermic dogs. J Appl Physiol 1986; 63:1487–1492.
99. Komatsu T, Shibutani K, Okamoto K, Kumar V, Kubal K, Sanchala V, Lees DE. Critical level of oxygen delivery after cardiopulmonary bypass. Crit Care Med 1987; 15:194–197.
100. Shibutani K, Komatsu T, Kubal K, Sanchala V, Kumar V, Bizarri DV. Critical level of oxygen delivery in anesthetized man. Crit Care Med 1983; 11:640–643.

101. Russell JA, Phang PT. The oxygen delivery consumption controversy: approaches to management of the critically ill. Am J Respir Crit Care Med 1994; 149:533–537.
102. Ronco JJ, Fenwick JC, Tweeddale MG, Wiggs BR, Phang PT, Cooper DJ, Cunningham KF, Russell JA, Walley KR. Identification of the critical oxygen delivery for anaerobic metabolism in critically ill septic and nonseptic humans. JAMA 1993; 270:1724–1730.
103. Shoemaker WC, Appel PL, Kram HB. Tissue oxygen debt as a determinant of lethal and nonlethal postoperative organ failure. Crit Care Med 1988; 16:1117–1120.
104. Shoemaker WC, Appel PL, Kram HB. Role of oxygen debt in the development of organ failure, sepsis, and death in high-risk surgical patients. Chest 1992; 102:208–215.
105. Russell JA, Ronco JJ, Lockhat D, Belzberg A, Kiess M, Dodek PM. Oxygen delivery and consumption and ventricular preload are greater in survivors than in nonsurvivors of the adult respiratory distress syndrome. Am Rev Respir Dis 1990; 141:659–665.
106. Danek SJ, Lynch JP, Weg JG, Dantzker DR. The dependence of oxygen uptake on oxygen delivery in the adult respiratory distress syndrome. Am Rev Respir Dis 1980; 122:387–395.
107. Mohsenifar Z, Goldbach P, Tashkin DP, Campisi DJ. Relationship between oxygen consumption and oxygen delivery in adult respiratory distress syndrome. Chest 1983; 84:267–271.
108. Kaufman BS, Rackow EC, Galk JL. The relationship between oxygen delivery and consumption during fluid resuscitation of hypovolemic and septic shock. Chest 1984; 85:336–340.
109. Astiz ME, Rackow EC, Falk JL, Kaufman BS, Weil MH. Oxygen delivery and consumption in patients with hyperdynamic septic shock. Crit Care Med 1987; 15:26–28.
110. Bihari D, Smithies M, Gimson A, Tinker J. The effects of vasodilation with prostacyclin on oxygen delivery and uptake in critically ill patients. N Engl J Med 1987; 317:397–403.
111. Fenwick JC, Dodek PM, Ronco JJ, Phang PT, Wiggs BR, Russell JA. Increased concentrations of plasma lactate predict pathologic dependence of oxygen consumption on oxygen delivery in patients with adult respiratory distress syndrome. J Crit Care 1990; 5:81–86.
112. Vincent JL, Roman A, DeBacker D, Kahn RJ. Oxygen uptake/supply dependence: effects of short-term dobutamine infusion. Am Rev Respir Dis 1990; 142:2–7.
113. Kruse JA, Carlson RW. Lactate metabolism. Crit Care Clin 1987; 5:725–746.
114. Arieff AI, Graf L. Pathophysiology of type A hypoxic lastic acidosis in dogs. Am J Physiol 1987; 253:271–276.
115. Weil MH, Afifi AA. Experimental and clinical studies on lactate and pyruvate as indicators of the severity of acute circulatory failure. Circulation 1970; 41:989–994.
116. Strauss B, Caldwell PRB, Fritss HW Jr. Observations on a model of proliferative lung disease: I. Transpulmonary arteriovenous differences in lactate, pyruvate and glucose. J Clin Invest 1970; 49:1305–1310.
117. Sayeed MM. Pulmonary cellular dysfunction in endotoxin shock: metabolic and transport derangements. Circ Shock 1982; 9:335–355.

118. Mitchel AM, Cournaud A. The fate of circulating lactic acid in the human lung. J Clin Invest 1955; 34:471–476.
119. Harris P, Bailey T, Bateman M. Lactate, pyruvate, glucose and free fatty acid in mixed venous and arterial blood. J Appl Physiol 1963; 18:933–936.
120. Brown SD, Clark C, Gutierrez G. Pulmonary lactate release in patients with sepsis and the adult respiratory distress syndrome. J Crit Care 1996; 11:2–8.
121. Kellum JA, Kramer DJ, Lee K, Mankad S, Bellomo R, Pinsky MR. Release of lactate by the lung in acute lung injury. Chest 1997; 111:1301–1305.
122. Douzinas EE, Tsidemiadou PD, Pitaridis MT, Andrianakis I, Bobota-Chloraki A, Katsouyanni K, Sfyras D, Malagari K, Roussos C. The regional production of cytokines and lactate in sepsis-related multiple organ failure. Am J Respir Crit Care Med 1997; 155:53–59.
123. Broder G, Weil MH. Excess lactate: an index of reversibility of shock in human patients. Science 1964; 143:1457–1459.
124. Vitek V, Cowley RA. Blood lactate in the prognosis of various forms of shock. Ann Surg 1971; 173:308–313.
125. Bakker J, Coffernils M, Leon M, Gris P, Vincent JL. Blood lactate levels are superior to oxygen-derived variables in predicting outcome in human septic shock. Chest 1991; 99:956–962.
126. Kruse JA, Zaidi SAJ, Carlson R. Significance of blood lactate levels in critically ill patients with liver disease. Am J Med 1987; 83:77–82.
127. Vincent JL, Dufaye P, Berre J, Leeman M, Degante SP, Kahn RJ. Serial lactate determinations during circulatory shock. Crit Care Med 1983; 11:449–451.
128. Falk JL, Rackow EC, Laevy J, Astiz ME, Weil MH. Delayed lactate clearance in patients surviving circulatory shock. Acute Care 1985; 11:212–215.
129. Parker MM, Shelhamer JH, Natanson C, Alling DW, Parillo JE. Serial cardiovascular variables in survivors and nonsurvivors of human septic shock: heart rate as an early predictor of prognosis. Crit Care Med 1987; 15:923–929.
130. Sauaia A, Moore EA, Moore EE, Haenel JB, Read RA, Lezotte DC. Early predictors of postinjury multiple organ failure. Arch Surg 1994; 129:39–45.
131. Moore FA, Haenel JB, Moore EE, Whitehill TA. Incommensurate oxygen consumption in response to maximal oxygen availability predicts postinjury multiple organ failure. J Trauma 1992; 33:58–65.
132. Cerra FB, Negro F, Abrams J. APACHE II score does not predict multiple organ failure or mortality in postoperative surgical patients. Arch Surg 1990; 125:519–522.
133. Roumen RMH, Redl H, Schlag G, Sandtner W, Koller W, Goris RJA. Scoring systems and blood lactate concentrations in relation to the development of adult respiratory distress syndrome and multiple organ failure in severely traumatized patients. J Trauma 1993; 35:349–355.
134. Manikis P, Jankowski S, Zhang H, Kahn RJ, Vincent JL. Correlation of serial blood lactate levels to organ failure and mortality after trauma. Am J Emerg Med 1995; 13:619–622.
135. Bakker J, Gris P, Coffernils M, Kahn RJ, Vincent JL. Serial blood lactate levels can predict the development of multiple organ failure following septic shock. Am J Surg 1996; 171:221–226.

136. Cairns CB, Moore FA, Haenel JB, Gallea BL, Ortner JP, Rose SJ, Moore EE. Evidence for early supply independent mitochondrial dysfunction in patients developing multiple organ failure after trauma. J Trauma 1997; 42:532–536.
137. Bulkley GB, Oshima A, Bailey RW. Pathophysiology of hepatic ischemia in cardiogenic shock. Am J Surg 1986; 151:87–97.
138. Arvidsson D, Rasmunssen I, Almquist P, Niklansson F, Haglund U. Splanchnic oxygen consumption in septic and hemorrhagic shock. Surgery 1991; 109:190–197.
139. Meakins JL, Marshall W. The gastrointestinal tract: the "motor" of MOF. Arch Surg 1986; 121:197–201.
140. Lundgren O, Haglund U. The pathophysiology of the countercurrent exchanger. Life Sciences 1978; 23:1411–1422.
141. Bohlen HG. Intestinal tissue Po_2 and microvascular responses during glucose exposure. Am J Physiol 1980; 238:H164–H171.
142. Arnold J, Hendriks J, Bruining H. Tonometry to assess the adequacy of splanchnic oxygenation in the critically ill patient. Intensive Care Med 1994; 20:452–456.
143. Groeneveld ABJ, Kolkman JJ. Splanchnic tonometry: a review of physiology, methodology, and clinical applications. J Crit Care 1994; 9:198–210.
144. Fiddian-Green RG, Pittenger G, Whitehouse WM. Back diffusion of CO_2 and its influence on the intramural pH in gastric mucosa. J Surg Res 1982; 33:39–48.
145. Antonsson JB, Boyle CC, Kruithoff KL, Wang H, Sacristan E, Rothschild HR, Fink MP. Validation of tonometric measurement of gut intramural pH during endotoxemia and mesenteric occlusion in pigs. Am J Physiol 1990; 259:G519–523.
146. Russell JA. Gastric tonometry: does it work? Intensive Care Med 1997; 23:3–6.
147. Gottlieb ME, Sarfeh IJ, Stratton H, Goldman ML, Newell JC, Shah DM. Hepatic perfusion and splanchnic oxygen consumption in patients postinjury. J Trauma 1983; 23:836–843.
148. Marik PE. Gastric intramucosal pH: a better predictor of multiorgan dysfunction and death than oxygen derived variables in patients with sepsis. Chest 1993; 104:225–229.
149. Miller PR, Chang MC, Meredith JW. Comparison of pH_i and mucosal-arterial CO_2 gap as predictors of outcome in trauma patients. Chest 1996; 110:138S.
150. Mythen MG, Webb AR. Intra-operative gut mucosal hypoperfusion is associated with increased post-operative complications and cost. Intensive Care Med 1994; 20:99–104.
151. Doglio GR, Pusajo JF, Egurrola MA, Bonfigli GC, Parra C, Vetere L, Hernandez MS, Fernandez S, Palizas F, Gutierrez G. Gastric mucosal pH as a prognostic index of mortality in critically ill patients. Crit Care Med 1991; 19:1037–1040.
152. Ivature RR, Simon RJ, Havriliak D, Garcia C, Greenbarg J, Stahl WM. Gastric mucosal pH and oxygen consumption indices in the assessment of adequacy of resuscitation after trauma: a prospective, randomized study. J Trauma 1995; 39:128–136.
153. Gutierrez G, Palizas F, Doglio G, Wainsztein N, Gallesio A, Pacin J, Dubin A, Schiavi E, Jorge M, Pusajo J, Klein F, San Roman E, Dorfman B, Shottlender J, Giniger R. Gastric intramucosal pH as a therapeutic index of tissue oxygenation in critically ill patients. Lancet 1992; 339:195–199.

154. Shoemaker WC, Appel PL, Kram HB, Waxman K, Lee TS. Prospective trial of supranormal values of survivors as therapeutic goals in high-risk surgical patients. Chest 1988; 94:1176–1186.
155. Fleming A, Bishop M, Shoemaker W, Appel P, Sufficool W, Kuvhenguwha A, Kennedy F. Prospective trial of supranormal values as goals of resuscitation in severe trauma. Arch Surg 1992; 127:1175–1181.
156. Boyd O, Grounds RM, Bennett ED. A randomized clinical trial of the effect deliberate perioperative increase of oxygen delivery on mortality in high-risk surgical patients. JAMA 1993; 270:2699–2707.
157. Tuchschmidt J, Fried J, Astiz M, Rackow E. Elevation of cardiac output and oxygen delivery improves outcome in septic shock. Chest 1992; 102:216–220.
158. Bone RC, Slotman G, LISAA nimet. Randomized double-blind, multicenter study of prostaglandin E_1 in patients with the adult respiratory distress syndrome. Chest 1989; 96:114–119.
159. Yu M, Levy MM, Smith P, Takiguchi SA, Miyasaki A, Myers SA. Effect of maximizing oxygen delivery on morbidity and mortality rates in critically ill patients: a prospective, radomized, controlled study. Crit Care Med 1993; 21:830–838.
160. Hayes MA, Timmins AC, Yau EHS, Palazzo M, Hinds CJ, Watson D. Elevation of systemic oxygen delivery in the treatment of critically ill patients. N Engl J Med 1994; 330:1717–1722.
161. Gattinoni L, Brazzi L, Pelosi P, Latini R, Tognoni G, Pesenti A, Fumagalli R. A trial of goal-oriented hemodynamic therapy in critically ill patients. N Engl J Med 1995; 333:1025–1032.
162. Steinberg S, Flynn W, Kelley K, Bitzer L, Sharma P, Gutierrez C, Baxter J, Lalka D, Sands A, van Liew J, Hasset J, Beam T, Flint L. Development of a bacteria-independent model of the multiple organ failure syndrome. Arch Surg 1989; 124:1390–1395.
163. Sevransky JE, Shaked G, Novogrodsky A, Levitzki A, Gazit A, Hoffman A, Elin RJ, Quezado ZMN, Freeman BD, Eichacker PQ, Danner RL, Banks SM, Bacher J, Thomas III ML, Natanson C. Tyrphostin AG 556 improves survival and reduces multiorgan failure in canine *Escherichia coli* peritonitis. J Clin Invest 1997; 99:1966–1973.
164. Eichacker PQ, Hoffman WD, Danner RL, Banks SM, Richmond S, Fitz Y, Natanson C. Serial measurements of total body oxygen consumption in an awake canine model of septic shock. Am J Respir Crit Care Med 1996; 154:68–75.
165. Weissman C, Kemper BA, Elwyn DH, Askanazi J, Hyman AI, Kinney JM. The energy expenditure of the mechanically ventilated critically ill patients. Chest 1986; 89:254–259.
166. Schlichtig R, Kramer DJ, Boston R, Pinsky MR. Renal O_2 consumption during progressive hemorrhage. J Appl Physiol 1991; 70:1957–1962.
167. Samsel RW, Cherqui D, Pietrabissa A, Sanders WM, Roncella M, Edmond JC, Schumacker PT. Hepatic oxygen and lactate extraction during stagnant hypoxia. J Appl Physiol 1991; 17:186–193.
168. Arai AE, Pantely GA, Anselone CG, Bristow J, Bristow JD. Active downregulation of myocardial energy requirements during prolonged moderate ischemia in swine. Circ Res 1991; 69:1458–1469.

169. Schumacker PT, Chandel N, Agusti AGN. Oxygen conformance of cellular respiration in hepatocytes. Am J Physiol 1993; 265:L395–L402.
170. Schumacker PT, Soble JS, Feldman T. Oxygen delivery and uptake relationships in patients with aortic stenosis. Am J Respir Crit Care Med 1994; 149:1123–1131.
171. Albert RK, Schrijen F, Poincelot F. Oxygen consumption and transport in stable patients with chronic obstructive pulmonary disease. Am Rev Respir Dis 1986; 134:678–682.
172. Williams AJ, Mohsenifar Z. Oxygen supply dependence in patients with obstructive sleep apnea and its reversal after therapy with nasal continuous positive airway pressure. Am Rev Respir Dis 1989; 140:1308–1311.
173. Phang PT, Cunningham KF, Ronco JJ, Wiggs BR, Russell JA. Mathematical coupling explains dependence of oxygen consumption on oxygen delivery in ARDS. Am J Respir Crit Care Med 1994; 150:318–323.
174. Stratton HH, Feustel PJ, Newell JC. Regression of calculated variables in the presence of shared measurement error. J Appl Physiol 1987; 62:2083–2093.
175. Baigorri F, Russell JA. Oxygen delivery in critical illness. Crit Care Clin 1996; 12:971–994.
176. Lutch JS, Murray JF. Continuous positive-pressure ventilation: effects on systemic oxygen transport and tissue oxygenation. Ann Intern Med 1972; 76:193–202.
177. Annat G, Viale JP, Percival C, Froment M, Motin J. Oxygen delivery and uptake in the adult respiratory distress syndrome. Am Rev Respir Dis 1986; 133:999–1001.
178. Carlile PV, Gray BA. Effect of opposite changes in cardiac output and arterial P_{O_2} on the relationship between mixed venous P_{O_2} and oxygen transport. Am Rev Respir Dis 1989; 140:891–898.
179. Vermeij CG, Feenstra BWA, Bruining HA. Oxygen delivery and uptake in postoperative and septic patients. Chest 1990; 98:415–420.
180. Ronco JJ, Phang PT, Walley KR, Wiggs B, Fenwick JC, Russell JA. Oxygen consumption is independent of changes in oxygen delivery in severe adult respiratory distress syndrome. Am Rev Respir Dis 1991; 143:1267–1273.
181. Ronco JJ, Fenwick JC, Wiggs BR, Phang PT, Russell JA, Tweeddale MG. Oxygen consumption is independent of increases in oxygen delivery by dobutamine in septic patients who have normal or increased plasma lactate. Am Rev Respir Dis 1993; 147:25–31.
182. Manthous CA, Schumacker PT, Pohlman A, Schmidt GA, Hall JB, Samsel RW, Wood LDH. Absence of supply dependence of oxygen consumption in patients with septic shock. J Crit Care 1993; 8:203–211.
183. Marik PE, Sibbald WJ. Effect of stored-blood transfusion on oxygen delivery in patients with sepsis. JAMA 1993; 269:3024–3029.
184. Mira JP, Fabre JE, Baigorri F, Coste J, Annat G, Artigas A, Nitemberg G, Dhainaut JF. Lack of oxygen supply dependence in patients with severe sepsis: a study of oxygen delivery increased by military antishock trouser and dobutamine. Chest 1994; 106:1524–1531.
185. Consensus Conference. Tissue hypoxia: how to detect, how to correct, how to prevent. Am J Respir Crit Care Med 1996; 154:1573–1578.
186. Rowell LB, Kraning KK, Evans TO. Splanchnic removal of lactate and pyruvate during prolonged exercise in man. J Appl Physiol 1966; 21:1773–1783.

187. Goldstein PJ, Simmons DH, Tashkin DP. Effect of acid-base alterations on hepatic lactate utilization. J Physiol (Lond) 1972; 223:261–278.
188. Vary TC, Siegel JH, Nakatami T, Sato T, Aoyama H. Effect of sepsis on activity of pyruvate dehydrogenase complex in skeletal muscle and liver. Am J Physiol 1986; 250:E634–640.
189. Vary TC, Siegel JH, Tall BD, Morris JG. Metabolic effects of partial reversal of pyruvate dihydrogenase activity in sepsis. Circ Shock 1988; 24:3–18.
190. Curtis SE, Cain SM. Regional and systemic oxygen delivery uptake relations and lactate flux in hyperdynamic endotoxin-treated dogs. Am Rev Respir Dis 1992; 145:348–354.
191. Garber AJ, Karl IE, Kipnis DM. Alanine and glutamine synthesis and release from skeletal muscle. J Biol Chem 1976; 251:836–843.
192. Zeller WP, The SM, Sweet M. Altered glucose transporter in RNA abundance in a rat model of endotoxic shock. Biochem Biophys Res Comm 1991; 176:535–540.
193. Widnell CC, Baldwin SA, Danies A, Martin S, Pasternak CA. Cellular stress induces a redistribution of the glucose transporter. FASEB J 1990; 4:1634–1637.
194. Hotchkiss RS, Karl IE. Reevaluation of the role of cellular hypoxia and bioenergetic failure in sepsis. JAMA 1992; 267:1503–1510.
195. Huckabee WE. Relationships of pyruvate and lactate during anaerobic metabolism: I. Effects of infusion of pyruvate or glucose and of hyperventilation. J Clin Invest 1958; 37:244–254.
196. Clutter W, Bier D, Shah S, Cryer P. Epinephrine plasma metabolic clearance rates and physiologic threshold for metabolic and hemodynamic actions in man. J Clin Invest 1980; 66:94–101.
197. Lundholm G, Svendmyr N. Influence of adrenaline on blood flow and metabolism in the human forearm. Acta Physiol Scand 1965; 65:344–351.
198. Ensinger H, Lindner K, Dirks B, Kilian J, Grunert A, Ahnefeld F. Adrenaline: relationship between infusion rate, plasma concentration, metabolic and haemodynamic effects in volunteers. Eur J Anaesthesiol 1992; 9:435–446.
199. Bearn A, Billing B, Sherlock S. The effect of adrenaline and noradrenaline on hepatic blood flow and splanchnic carbohydrate metabolism in man. J Physiol 1951; 115:430–441.
200. Cheung P-Y, Barrington KL, Pearson RJ, Bigam DL, Finer NN, van Aerde JE. Systemic, pulmonary and mesenteric perfusion and oxygenation effects of dopamine and epinephrine. Am J Respir Crit Care Med 1997; 155:32–37.
201. Day NPJ, Phu NH, Bethell DP, Mai NTH, Chau TTH, Hien TT, White NJ. The effects of dopamine and adrenaline infusions on acid-base balance and systemic haemodynamics in severe infection. Lancet 1996; 348:219–223.
202. Jepson MM, Cox M, Bates PC, Rothwell NJ, Stock MJ, Cady EB, Millward DJ. Regional blood flow and skeletal muscle energy status in endotoxemic rats. Am J Physiol 1987; 252:E581–E587.
203. Jacobs DO, Maris J, Fried R, Settle RG, Rolandelli RR, Korunda MJ, Chance B, Rombeau JL. In vivo phosphorus 31 magnetic spectroscopy of rat hind limb, skeletal muscle during sepsis. Arch Surg 1988; 123:1425–1428.
204. Riddington DW, Venkatesh KB, Clutton-Brock T, Bion J. Measuring carbon dioxide tension in saline and alternative solutions: quantification of bias and precision in two blood gas analyzers. Crit Care Med 1994; 22:96–100.

205. Knichtwitz G, Mertes N, Kuhlmann M. Improved P_{CO_2} measurement in six standard blood gas analyzers using a phosphate-buffered solution for gastric tonometry. Anaesthesia 1995; 50:532–534.
206. Takala J, Parviainen I, Siloaho M, Ruokonen E, Hämäläinen E. Saline P_{CO_2} is an important source of error in the assessment of gastric intramural pH. Crit Care Med 1994; 22:1877–1879.
207. Wood PR, Lawler PGP. Measurement technique and variation in intramucosal pH. Br J Anaesth 1996; 76:563–564.
208. Heard SO, Helsmoortel CM, Kent JC, Shahnarian A, Fink PM. Gastric tonometry in healthy volunteers: effects of ranitidine on calculated intramural pH. Crit Care Med 1991; 19:271–274.
209. Kolkman JJ, Groeneveld AB, Meuwissen SG. Effect of ranitidine on basal and bicarbonate enhanced intragastric P_{CO_2}: a tonometric study. Gut 1994; 35:737–741.
210. Maynard N, Atkinson S, Mason R, Smithies M, Bihari D. Influence of intravenous ranitidine on gastric intramucosal pH in critically ill patients. Crit Care Med 1994; 22:A79.
211. Baigorri F, Calvet X, Duarte M, Saura P, Jubert P, Royo C, Joseph D, Artigas A. Effect of ranitidine treatment in gastric intramucosal pH determinations in critical patients. Intensive Care Med 1994; 20(Suppl 2):S2.
212. Higgins D, Mythen MG, Webb AR. Low intramucosal pH is associated with failure to acidify the gastric lumen in response to pentagastrin. Intensive Care Med 1994; 20:105–108.
213. Parviainen I, Väisänen O, Ruokonen E, Takala J. Effect of nasogastric suction and ranitidine on the calculated gastric intramucosal pH. Intensive Care Med 1996; 22:319–323.
214. Marik PE, Lorenzana A. Effect of tube feeding on the measurement of gastric intramucosal pH. Crit Care Med 1996; 24:1498–1500.
215. Schlictig R, Bowles SA. Distinguishing between aerobic and anaerobic appearance of dissolved CO_2 in intestine during low flow. J Appl Physiol 1994; 76:2443–2451.
216. Desai VS, Weil MH, Tang W, Yang G, Bisera J. Gastric intramural P_{CO_2} during peritonitis and shock. Chest 1993; 104:1254–1258.
217. Benjamin E, Polokoff E, Oropello JM, Leibowitz AB, Iberti TJ. Sodium bicarbonate administration affects the diagnostic accuracy of gastrointestinal tonometry in acute mesenteric ischemia. Crit Care Med 1992; 20:1181–1183.
218. Revelly J-P, Ayuse T, Brienza N, Fessler HE, Robotham JL. Endotoxic shock alters distribution of blood flow within the intestinal wall. Crit Care Med 1996; 24:1345–1351.
219. VanderMeer TJ, Wang H, Fink MP. Endotoxemia causes ileal mucosal acidosis in the absence of mucosal hypoxia in a normodynamic porcine model of septic shock. Crit Care Med 1995; 23:1217–1226.
220. Fiddian-Green RG, Baker S. Predictive value of the stomach wall pH for complications after cardiac surgery: comparison with other monitoring. Crit Care Med 1987; 15:153–156.
221. Boyd O, Mackay CJ, Lamb G, Bland JM, Grounds RM, Bennett ED. Comparison of clinical information gained from routine blood-gas analysis and from gastric tonometry for intramural pH. Lancet 1993; 341:142–145.

222. Fiddian-Green RG. Gastric intramucosal pH, tissue oxygenation and acid-base balance. Br J Anaesth 1995; 74:591–606.
223. Schlichtig R, Mehta N, Gayowski TJP. Tissue-arterial P_{CO_2} difference is a better marker of ischemia than intramural pH (pH_i) or arterial pH–pH_i difference. J Crit Care 1996; 11:51–56.
224. Riddington DW, Venkatesh B, Boivin CM, Bonser RS, Elliott TSJ, Marshall T, Mountford PJ, Bion JF. Intestinal permeability, gastric intramucosal pH, and systemic endotoxemia in patients undergoing cardiopulmonary bypass. JAMA 1996; 275:1007–1012.
225. Heyland DK, Cook DJ, King D, Kernerman P, Brun-Buisson C. Maximizing oxygen delivery in critically ill patients: a methodologic appraisal of the evidence. Crit Care Med 1996; 24:517–524.
226. Russell JA. Quantitative assessment of randomized controlled trials of increased oxygen delivery in critically ill adults. Am Rev Respir Dis 1993; 147:A616.
227. Bone RC. Toward a theory regarding the pathogenesis of the systemic inflammatory response syndrome: what we do and do not know about cytokine regulation. Crit Care Med 1996; 24:163–172.
228. Beal AL, Cerra FB. Multiple organ failure syndrome in the 1990s: systemic inflammatory response and organ dysfunction. JAMA 1994; 271:226–233.
229. Bone RC. Immunologic dissonance: a continuing evolution in our understanding of the systemic inflammatory response syndrome (SIRS) and the multiple organ dysfunction syndrome (MODS). Ann Intern Med 1996; 125:680–687.
230. Pinsky MR, Vincent J-L, Deviere J, Alegre M, Kahn RJ, Dupont E. Serum cytokine levels in human septic shock: relation to multiple-system organ failure and mortality. Chest 1993; 103:565–575.
231. Cruickshank AM, Fraser WD, Burns HJG, van Damme J, Shenkin A. Response of serum interleukin-6 in patients undergoing elective surgery of varying severity. Clin Sci 1990; 79:161–165.
232. Tang GJ, Kuo CD, Yen TC, Kuo HS, Yien HW, Lee TY. Perioperative plasma concentrations of tumor necrosis factor-alpha and interleukin-6 in infected patients. Crit Care Med 1996; 24:423–428.
233. Kragsbjerg P, Holmberg H, Vikerfors T. Serum concentrations of interleukin-6, tumour necrosis factor-alpha, and C-reactive protein in patients undergoing major operations. Eur J Surg 1995; 161:17–22.
234. van der Poll T, Jansen J, Endert E, Sauerwein HP, van Deventer SJH. Noradrenaline inhibits lipopolysaccharide-induced tumor necrosis factor and interleukin-6 production in human whole blood. Infect Immun 1994; 62:2046–2050.
235. Hu X, Goldmuntz EA, Brosnan CF. The effect of norepinephrine on endotoxin-mediated macrophage activation. J Neuroimmunol 1991; 31:35–42.
236. Severn A, Rapson NT, Hunter CA. Regulation of tumor necrosis factor production by adrenaline and β-adrenergic agonists. J Immunol 1992; 148:3441–3445.
237. van der Poll T, Coyle SM, Barbosa K, Braxton CC, Lowry SF. Epinephrine inhibits tumor necrosis factor-α and potentiates interleukin 10 production during human endotoxemia. J Clin Invest 1996; 97:713–719.
238. Donnelly SC, Strieter RM, Reid P, Kunkel SL, Burdick MD, Armstrong I, Mackenzie A, Haslett C. The association between mortality rates and decreased concen-

trations of interleukin-10 and interleukin-1 receptor antagonist in the lung fluid of patients with the adult respiratory distress syndrome. Ann Intern Med 1996; 125:191–196.
239. Barton MH, Moore JN. Pentoxifylline inhibits mediator synthesis in an equine in vitro whole blood model of endotoxemia. Circ Shock 1994; 44:216–220.
240. Schade UF. Pentoxifylline increases survival in murine endotoxin shock and decreases formation of tumor necrosis factor. Circ Shock 1990; 31:171–181.
241. Giroir BP, Beutler B. Effect of amrinone on tumor necrosis factor production in endotoxic shock. Circ Shock 1992; 36:200–207.
242. Zabel P, Wolter DT, Schonharting MM, Schade UF. Oxpentifylline in endotoxemia. Lancet 1989; ii:1474–1478.
243. Adams DH, Nash GB. Disturbance of leucocyte circulation and adhesion to the endothelium as factors in circulatory pathology. Br J Anaesth 1996; 77:17–31.
244. Fortenberry JD, Huber AR, Owens ML. Inotropes inhibit endothelial cell surface adhesion molecules induced by interleukin-1β. Crit Care Med 1997; 25:303–308.
245. Schmidt W, Schmidt H, Hacker A, Gebhard M-M, Martin E. Influence of dopexamine on leukocyte adherence and vascular permeability in postcapillary venules during endotoxemia. Crit Care Med 1997; 25(Suppl 1):A42.
246. Tighe D, Moss R, Heywood G, Al-Saady N, Webb A, Bennett D. Goal-directed therapy with dopexamine, dobutamine and volume expansion: effects of systemic oxygen transport on hepatic ultrastructure in porcine sepsis. Crit Care Med 1995; 23:1997–2007.
247. Moore FA, Moore EE. Evolving concepts in the pathogenesis of postinjury multiple organ failure. Surg Clin North Am 1995; 75:257–277.
248. Nielsen VG, Tan S, Weinbroum A, McCammon AT, Samuelson PN, Gelman S, Parks DA. Lung injury after hepatoenteric ischemia-reperfusion: role of xanthine oxidase. Am J Respir Crit Care Med 1996; 154:1364–1369.
249. Nielsen VG, Tan S, Baird MS, McCammon AT, Parks DA. Gastric intramucosal pH and multiple organ injury: impact of ischemia-reperfusion and xanthine oxidase. Crit Care Med 1996; 24:1339–1344.
250. Waxman K. Shock: ischemia, reperfusion, and inflammation. New Horiz 1996; 4:153–160.
251. McCord JM. Oxygen-derived free radicals in post-ischemic tissue injury. N Engl J Med 1985; 312:159–163.
252. Goldman G, Welbourn R, Klausner JM, Kobzik L, Valeri CR, Shepro D, Hechtman HB. Mast cells and leukotrienes mediate neutrophil sequestration and lung edema after remote ischemia in rodents. Surgery 1992; 112:578–586.
253. Punch J, Rees R, Cashmer B, Oldham K, Wilkins E, Smith Jr DJ. Acute lung injury following reperfusion after ischemia in the hind limb of rats. J Trauma 1991; 31:760–765.
254. Partnick DA, Moore FA, Moore EE, Barnett CC Jr, Silliman CC. Neutrophil priming and activation in the pathogenesis of postinjury multiple organ failure. New Horiz 1996; 4:194–210.
255. Pastores S, Katz DP, Kvetan V. Splanchnic ischemia and gut mucosal injury in sepsis and the multiple organ dysfunction syndrome. Am J Gastroent 1996; 91:1697–1710.

256. Cipolle MD, Pasquale MD, Cerra FB. Secondary organ dysfunction: from clinical perspectives to molecular mediators. Crit Care Clin 1993; 9:261–298.
257. Moore EE, Moore FA, Franciose RJ, Kim FJ, Biffl WL, Banerjee A. The postischemic gut serves as a priming bed for circulating neutrophils that provoke multiple organ failure. J Trauma 1994; 37:881–887.
258. Livingston DH, Mosenthal AC, Deitch EA. Sepsis and multiple organ dysfunction syndrome: a clinical-mechanistic overview. New Horiz 1995; 3:257–266.
259. Biffl WL, Moore EE. Splanchnic ischemia/reperfusion and multiple organ failure. Br J Anaesth 1996; 77:59–70.

Author Index

Italic numbers give the page on which the complete reference is listed.

A

Aaronson K, 583, 585, *607*
Abassi Z, 455, *465*
Abbott RA, 655, *678*
Abboud FM, 370, *379*
Abdel-Latif M, 360, *377*
Abdenour L, 629, *644*
Abrams J, 701, *734*
Abramson MJ, 200, *224*
Abrouk F, 251, *260*
Abuchowski A, 636, *645*
Acero AL, 394, *406*
Achten E, 98, *116*
Ackerson L, 263, 265, 269, 276, *281*
Adachi H, 341, *354*
Adair GS, 621, *643*
Adamopoulos S, 591, 597, 603, *610*, *613*, *614*
Adams B, 665, *682*
Adams DH, 721, *741*
Adams JM, 92, *115*
Adamson JW, 655, *678*
Adelstein AM, 200, *224*
Adnot S, 231, 254, *258*, *261*, 314, *327*
Adrian ED, 397, *407*
Affi AA, 699, 700, *733*

Agmon Y, 455, 456, 458, 460, 461, 463, *466*, *467*
Agnew JE, 597, *613*
Agusti AG, 312, *327*, 496, 508, 511, 514, *521*
Agusti AGN, 136, *146*, 216, *227*, 231, 232, 234, 235, 238, 246, *257*, *258*, 263, 264, 265, 266, 267, 268, 269, 271, 272, 273, 274, 275, 277, 278, 279, 280, *281*, *282*, *283*, 539, *550*, 557, 566, *574*, 710, *737*
Agusti C, 264, 265, 268, 280, *282*
Agusti-Vidal A, 242, *259*, 263, 268, 269, 279, 280, *281*
Ahmad S, 660, *680*
Ahnefeld F, 714, *738*
Ahonen R, 659, *679*
Aigner F, 192, *197*
Ajisaka R, 670, *683*
Akamine S, 254, *261*
Akerman MJ, 655, 656, 657, *677*
Aksnes G, 170, *175*
Alazraki NP, 291, *300*
Albert RK, 57, 73, *110*, *112*, 122, *143*, 317, *328*, 566, *576*, 710, *737*
Alberti C, 686, *728*
Albonico G, 669, *683*

743

Albrecht G, 653, *676*
Alegre M, 720, 721, 724, *740*
Alejandro A, 595, *612*
Alexander JI, 192, *197*
Alexander JK, 160, *173*
Alexander RS, 694, *732*
Alexander SC, 436, *445*
Alfrey CP, 166, *174*
Al-Himyary AJ, 271, *283*
Al-Himyary AJ, 571, 572, *578*
Alijama P, 667, *682*
Allan PL, 183, *195*
Allard C, 566, *576*
Allard MF, 360, 373, 375, *377*, *380*, 414, 423, 425, *431*, 693, 694, *731*
Allen GM, 202, *224*
Allen PS, 30, 31, *42*, *43*
Allis J, 583, *606*
Allison AC, 691, *729*
Allison TG, 655, *678*
Almquist P, 692, 703, *730*, *735*
Alonso A, 539, *550*
Alonso J, 662, 664, *680*
Alonson A, 496, 508, 511, 514, *521*
Alonzo J, 566, *576*
Al-Saady N, 722, *741*
Altemeier WA, 125, 126, 133, *144*, *145*
Altura BM, 693, *731*
Amato MB, 305, 313, 321, *324*, *329*
Ambrosino N, 271, *283*
Amery A, 481, 482, *519*
Amiel C, 655, *677*
Amis TC, 74, *112*, 125, *144*
Andersen JB, 231, 236, 237, *257*
Andersen P, 31, *43*, 383, 385, 386, 390, 392, 398, 400, *401*
Anderson FL, 583, *607*
Anderson J, 593, *611*
Anderson P, 539, *550*
Anderson PJ, 638, *646*
Anderson SD, 206, *225*
Andersson T, 188, *196*
Andres E, 667, *682*
Andrews JD, 555, *574*
Andrianakis I, 701, *734*
Andrivet P, 231, 254, *258*, *261*
Andronikou S, 152, *172*

Angell JJE, 341, *354*
Angus GE, 238, *259*
Angus-Leppan H, 669, *682*
Anjou-Lihnkskog E, 190, *197*
Annat G, 711, 712, *737*
Anrep GV, 387, *403*
Anselone CG, 710, *736*
Anthonisen NR, 67, 74, *111*, *112*, 136, *147*, 207, *226*
Antonini E, 622, *643*
Antonsson JB, 101, *117*, 704, *735*
Anzuetto A, 319, *329*, 515, *523*
Aoyama H, 713, 714, *738*
Appel P, 705, 706, 707, *736*
Appel PL, 697, 705, 706, 718, *733*, *736*
Arai H, 670, *683*
Archer BT, 106, *118*
Archer SL, 310, *326*
Archie JP, 101, *115*, 692, *730*
Arcos J, 480, 485, *519*
Arcos JP, 532, *549*
Ardell JL, 122, 125, 133, *143*, *144*
Arfors KE, 373, *380*, 421, *432*, 628, 629, 630, 640, *644*
Argov Z, 31, *42*
Aria AE, 710, *736*
Arieff AI, 104, *118*, 699, 700, *733*
Armando MC, 93, *115*
Armstrong A, 397, *407*
Armstrong I, 721, *740*
Armstrong JB, 396, *406*
Armstrong ML, 593, *611*
Armstrong RB, 46, 91, *108*, *115*, 385, 400, *401*
Arnold J, 703, *735*
Arnone A, 624, *644*
Arthaud M, 629, *644*
Arthur PG, 31, 39, *42*, *43*
Arthur RM, 532, *548*
Artigas A, 304, 305, *323*, 686, 711, 712, 715, 717, *728*, *737*, *739*
Arvidsson D, 692, 703, *730*, *735*
Asanoi H, 597, *613*
Asanol H, 590, *610*
Ashbaugh DG, 304, 305, *323*
Ashbrook D, 660, *680*
Ashbrook DW, 660, *680*

Author Index

Asitz M, 705, 707, 720, *736*
Askanazi J, 591, *610*, 694, 710, *732*, *736*
Asmussen E, 158, *173*
Astin TW, 220, *228*
Astiz ME, 699, 700, 701, *733*, *734*
Astrand PO, 470, 474, 476, 488, *517*, 537, *549*
Astrup J, 436, *445*
Atkins J, 598, *613*
Atkins JL, 452, 458, 463, *465*
Atkins N, 85, *114*
Atkinson DE, 30, 37, *42*
Atkinson S, 715, 717, *739*
Atwal K, 596, *612*
Aubier M, 691, 694, *729*
Auger WR, 296, *302*
Auinger M, 653, *676*
Aukburg SJ, 57, 66, 67, *110*, *111*
Aukland K, 451, *465*
Aulick LH, 694, *732*
Aulie A, 122, *143*
Austrian R, 269, *282*
Avalli L, 305, *324*
Aveledo L, 660, 670, *680*
Avrunin JS, 687, *728*
Ayres SM, 297, *302*
Ayus J, 463, *467*
Ayuse T, 716, 717, *739*
Ayyar DR, 659, *679*

B

Babb TG, 560, 566, 572, *575*, *578*
Babcock MA, 480, *519*
Bacchus AN, 360, 370, *377*, *379*
Bache RJ, 337, 344, *353*, *355*, 376, *381*, 470, 488, 491, 492, 493, 494, 495, *517*
Bacher J, 707, 708, *736*
Bacic B, 101, 103, *117*
Backer A, 670, *683*
Baehr PH, 458, *466*
Baer RW, 368, 369, *378*, *379*
Bagby GH, 691, *729*
Baglioni S, 304, 305, *323*, *324*
Bahnson HT, 655, *678*
Bai TR, 245, *260*

Baier H, 222, *228*
Baigorri F, 711, 712, 715, 717, *737*, *739*
Bailey GL, 685, *727*
Bailey RW, 692, 703, *730*, *735*
Bailey T, 700, *734*
Bainton CR, 152, *172*
Baiocchi S, 271, *283*
Baird MS, 722, *741*
Bak K, 583, *607*
Baken WC, 567, *577*
Baker S, 716, *739*
Bakker GJ, 396, *406*
Bakker J, 701, 703, *734*
Bakker JC, 636, *645*
Balaban RS, 30, 36, *42*, 452, *465*
Baldamus CA, 669, *683*
Baldwin SA, 713, *738*
Balice-Gordon RJ, 396, *406*
Balk RA, 686, *727*
Ball SCJ, 67, *111*
Ball WC, 121, *143*
Ballard RD, 205, *225*
Ball-Burnett ME, 539, *550*
Ballester E, 211, 213, 214, 218, 220, *226*, *227*, *228*, 235, 243, 245, 253, *258*, *260*, *261*
Ballett B, 352, *357*
Banerjee A, 724, 725, 726, *742*
Bank A, 596, *612*
Bank AJ, 586, 587, *608*
Bankir L, 448, 450, *465*
Banks SM, 707, 708, 709, *736*
Barbas CS, 305, 313, 321, *324*, *329*
Barbee RW, 337, *353*
Barbera J, 320, *329*
Barbera JA, 4, 20, *26*, *27*, 139, *147*, 217, 221, 222, *227*, *228*, 231, 232, 234, 235, 236, 238, 241, 243, 246, 250, 254, *258*, *259*, *260*, *261*, 263, 264, 268, 272, 273, 277, *281*, 307, *325*, 496, 508, 511, 514, 515, *521*, *523*, 539, *550*, 557, 560, 565, 566, *574*, *575*, *576*, 659, 662, 663, 664, *679*, *680*
Barbosa K, 720, 721, 722, *740*
Barcroft J, 8, *26*, 156, *172*, 619, *642*
Baretto S, 662, *681*
Barker BR, 106, *118*

Barker SJ, 100, 101, *117*, 690, *728*
Barlow C, 125, *144*, 598, *613*
Barman SA, 122, 125, 133, *143*
Barnard P, 152, 161, *172*, *173*
Barnea N, 657, *679*
Barnes PJ, 199, 217, 222, *223*, *227*, *228*
Barnes SD, 311, *326*
Barnett CC, 724, *741*
Baron AD, 670, *683*
Barrington KL, 714, *738*
Barstow TJ, 470, 476, *517*, 605, *615*
Bartel LL, 660, *680*
Barthelemy C, 662, 663, 670, *681*
Barthelemy L, 653, *676*
Bartkett D, 156, *173*
Bartkowski R, 57, 66, *110*
Bartlett RH, 317, 318, *328*, 341, *354*
Barton ED, 107, *118*, 388, 392, 397, *404*, 487, 503, *520*
Barton MH, 721, *741*
Barwick DD, 659, *679*
Basaraba R, 515, *523*
Basaraba RJ, 73, *112*
Bass H, 207, *226*
Bassel-Duby R, 388, *404*, 546, *552*
Bassingthwaighte JB, 122, 125, *144*, 363, 370, *377*, *379*, 421, *431*
Bateman M, 700, *734*
Bates DV, 67, 74, 82, *111*, *112*, *113*, 121, *143*, 207, *226*
Bates ER, 292, *301*
Bates JH, 125, *144*
Bates PC, 714, *738*
Bates T, 531, 532, *548*
Batra P, 596, *612*
Batra S, 363, *378*
Baudinette RV, 55, *109*
Baue AE, 687, *728*
Bauer C, 464, *467*
Bauer K, 599, 600, *614*
Bauer M, 441, *445*
Bauerffeind P, 94, *115*
Baugham RP, 319, *329*
Baughman KL, 583, *607*
Baum M, 305, 306, 313, 314, *324*, *327*
Bauman A, 200, *224*
Baumgardner JE, 57, 66, 67, *110*, *111*

Baumgartl H, 451, 452, 462, *465*
Baumgartl P, 665, 666, *682*
Baumgartner WA, 583, *607*
Bautista J, 659, *679*
Baverel G, 662, *681*
Baxter J, 707, *736*
Baylis C, 456, *466*
Baz M, 663, 664, *682*
Bazzi C, 669, *683*
Beal AL, 720, *740*
Beall GN, 207, 209, *226*
Beam T, 707, *736*
Bearn A, 714, *738*
Beart R, 685, *727*
Beasley CR, 654, *677*
Beaussier M, 629, *644*
Beaver WL, 46, *108*, 484, *519*
Bebout DE, 15, 20, *27*, 107, *118*, 388, 389, 390, 392, 397, *403*, *404*, *405*, 487, 497, 503, 515, *519*, *520*, 522, 532, 535, 537, 538, 542, 545, *549*, 550, *551*, 620, *642*
Bebout E, 480, 485, *519*
Bebrewold A, 693, *731*
Beck IT, 417, *431*
Beck KC, 126, *145*, 166, *174*, 183, *195*
Becker CJ, 359, 361, 371, *376*, 414, *431*
Becker H, 310, 312, 320, *325*
Becker LB, 376, *381*
Becker R, 655, *678*
Becker SL, 671, *684*
Beer G, 398, *407*
Beeri R, 458, 463, *466*, *467*
Beglioomini E, 286, 290, 291, 292, *300*
Begofsky EH, 98, *116*
Behar MG, 691, 703, 704, *729*
Behn M, 142, *147*
Beiser GD, 488, *520*
Belardinelli R, 605, *615*
Bellamy P, 596, *612*
Bellamy PE, 687, *728*
Bellamy RF, 368, 369, *378*
Belleau R, 566, *576*
Bellemare F, 202, *224*
Bellet M, 653, *676*
Bellinghieri G, 660, *680*
Bellomo R, 701, *734*

Author Index

Belman MJ, 554, *573*
Beltz J, 588, 590, 591, *609, 610*
Belzberg A, 697, 699, 705, *733*
Benabid AL, 271, *282*, 566, *577*
Benard SL, 73, *112*
Bencowitz HZ, 318, *328*, 654, 655, *677*
Bender PR, 538, 545, *550*
Bendixen HH, 184, *195*
Benedict C, 583, *607*
Benesch R, 623, *643*
Benesch RE, 623, *643*
Bengali ZK, 238, *259*
Benhmida M, 662, 663, 670, *681*
Beninati W, 318, *328*
Benito S, 252, *261*
Benjamin E, 716, 717, *739*
Bennett D, 694, 710, 722, *732, 741*
Bennett ED, 351, *357*, 705, 707, 716, 720, *736, 739*
Bennett LR, 207, 209, *226*
Bensaidane H, 271, *282*, 566, *577*
BenSasson SA, 458, *466*
Benumof J, 191, *197*
Benvenuti C, 599, *614*
Benyahia A, 655, *677*
Benzer H, 192, *197*, 314, *327*
Benzi RH, 376, *381*
Beoucif S, 320, *329*
Berbers GA, 636, *645*
Berchtold M, 515, *523*
Berdeaux A, 691, 703, *729*
Berg B, 185, 190, *196, 197*
Berg BR, 397, *407*, 492, 494, *520*
Berg H, 177, 178, *193*
Berg R, 691, *729*
Berger E, 152, *172*, 619, *642*
Berger EM, 152, *172*
Berger HJ, 566, *576*
Berger RL, 618, 622, 625, *642, 643*
Berggren SM, 178, *193*
Bergman NA, 184, *195*
Bergofsky EH, 297, *302*
Bergstrom M, 184, *195*
Berk JL, 345, *355*
Berland Y, 663, 664, *682*
Berlyne GM, 655, 665, *678*
Berman A, 595, *612*

Berman JW, 587, *608*
Bern RM, 98, *116*
Bernard GR, 304, 305, *323*, 686, 687, 689, *727, 728*
Bernard S, 125, *144*, 566, *576*
Bernard SL, 73, *112*, 122, 125, *143, 144*
Bernardi L, 591, 597, 603, *610, 613, 614*
Berne RM, 340, *354*, 360, 370, *377, 379*, 390, 394, 395, *404*
Berrayah L, 142, *148*
Berre J, 351, *356*, 701, *734*
Berstein AD, 692, *730*
Bert P, 149, *171*
Bertocci LA, 659, 664, *679*
Bertram H, 451, 462, *465*
Bessman SP, 39, 40, *44*, 387, *403*
Bethell DP, 714, *738*
Better O, 455, *465*
Betts DF, 36, *43*
Beutler B, 721, *741*
Beyer C, 349, *356*, 425, *432*, 693, 695, 697, *731*
Beyers N, 375, *380*
Bhatia S, 596, *612*
Bhatt S, 694, *732*
Bhatt SB, 351, *356*
Bianconcini M, 36, *43*
Biasucci L, 586, 587, *608*
Bickler PE, 531, 532, 534, *548*
Bier D, 714, *738*
Biessels PT, 636, *645*
Biffl WL, 724, 725, 726, *742*
Bigam DL, 714, *738*
Bigaud M, 424, *432*
Bigelow DB, 304, 305, *323*
Bihari D, 348, 351, *356*, 699, 700, 715, 717, *733, 739*
Bihari DJ, 334, 347, *353*
Bijou R, 587, 605, *608, 615*
Billing B, 714, *738*
Bindslev L, 181, 182, 192, *194, 197*
Binger CA, 156, *172*
Bion J, 715, *738*
Bion JF, 718, *740*
Birder LA, 375, *381*
Birnbaum ML, 152, 156, *172*
Biro GP, 638, *646*

Bischoff A, 637, *646*
Bisera J, 716, 717, *739*
Bishop JM, 82, 84, *113*, 142, *147*, 229, 257, 353, *357*
Bishop M, 705, 706, 707, *736*
Bismar H, 428, *434*
Bitterman PB, 263, 269, 278, *281*
Bitzer L, 707, *736*
Bizarri DV, 695, *732*
Bjertnaes LJ, 189, *196*
Black CP, 541, *551*
Blackmon JR, 691, 703, *729*
Blagg CR, 650, 668, *676*
Blais L, 200, *224*
Blajchman M, 690, *729*
Blake P, 667, *682*
Blakemore WS, 83, *113*
Blanchet F, 655, *677*
Bland JM, 716, *739*
Blaszczyk J, 667, *682*
Blaustein MP, 671, *684*
Bleeker WK, 636, *645*
Blessey R, 602, *614*
Block EH, 394, 396, *405*
Blomqvist CG, 85, *114*, 537, *549*
Blomqvist H, 255, *261*
Blum AL, 94, *115*
Blum H, 36, *43*
Blume FD, 152, *172*
Blumenthal JA, 655, 665, *678*
Bobota-Chloraki A, 701, *734*
Bock AV, 156, *172*
Bockman EL, 383, *401*
Bode Boger SM, 663, *681*
Bodine SC, 396, *406*
Boerboom LE, 369, *379*
Boger RH, 663, *681*
Bohlen HG, 411, *430*, 703, *735*
Bohm M, 583, *607*
Bohr C, 79, *112*, 623, *643*
Boivin CM, 718, *740*
Boivin JF, 200, *224*
Boland EF, 624, *644*
Boland EJ, 624, *644*
Bolas NM, 36, *43*
Bolinger L, 588, 589, *609*
Bolton DPG, 478, 480, 481, 482, *519*

Bolton W, 622, *643*
Bombino M, 304, 305, *324*
Bonaventura J, 617, 618, 621, 624, 626, 632, 633, 641, *642*
Bone RC, 303, 311, 312, 313, *323*, 686, 705, 720, *727*, *736*, *740*
Bonfigli GC, 704, 709, 715, *735*
Bongard O, 594, *611*
Bongiorno PF, 341, *354*
Bonser RS, 718, *740*
Bonzel KE, 654, *677*
Boon P, 98, *116*
Bore P, 593, 594, *611*
Bore PJ, 663, *681*
Bosch J, 264, *281*
Boska MD, 566, *577*
Bosken C, 246, *260*
Bosken CH, 238, 245, *259*, *260*
Boston R, 710, *736*
Bottinelli R, 567, *577*
Bottomley PA, 583, *606*
Bouby N, 448, 450, *465*
Boucot NG, 82, *113*
Bouman LN, 488, *520*
Bourdarias JP, 588, 591, *608*, *610*
Bouwer STH, 639, *647*
Bova S, 671, *684*
Bower JS, 286, 290, 291, 292, 297, 298, 298, *300*, *301*, *302*
Bowles SA, 104, *117*, 716, *739*
Boycott AE, 526, *547*
Boyd O, 351, *357*, 694, 705, 707, 710, 716, 720, *732*, *736*, *739*
Boyer SJ, 152, *172*
Boyers SJ, 527, *547*
Boyle CC, 704, *735*
Boylew JB, 101, *117*
Bracamonte M, 207, 209, *226*
Bradley WE, 620, *643*
Brancatisano T, 560, *575*
Branwald E, 295, *302*
Brasch F, 130, *145*
Brass EP, 660, 670, *680*
Bratel T, 254, *261*
Braun NMT, 564, *575*
Braunwald E, 285, *300*, 364, *378*, 488, *520*, 581, 582, 584, 587, *606*, *608*

Author Index

Brautbar N, 660, 661, *680*
Braverman LE, 152, *172*
Braxton CC, 720, 721, 722, *740*
Brazzi L, 313, *327*, 705, 718, 719, *736*
Brdiczka D, 39, 40, *44*
Brebos J, 207, 209, *226*
Brechtel G, 670, *683*
Bredehoeft S, 636, *645*
Bredle DL, 345, *355*, 426, *433*
Brengleman GL, 691, 703, *729*
Brenner BM, 448, 454, *465*
Brenner M, 424, *432*
Brent BN, 566, *576*
Breslow MJ, 692, *730*
Bressack MA, 693, *731*
Brezis M, 447, 448, 451, 454, 455, 456, 457, 458, 460, 461, 462, 463, 464, *465, 466, 467*
Brezus N, 451, 452, 456, *465, 466*
Brian JE, 437, *445*, 449
Brienza A, 251, *261*, 313, *327*
Brienza N, 251, *261*, 716, 717, *739*
Brigham KL, 304, 305, *323*, 426, *433*
Brinker KR, 515, *523*, 655, 658, 659, 665, *678, 679*
Brinkley WW, 637, 638, *646*
Briscoe WA, 67, *111*, 229, *257*
Brismar B, 178, 180, 181, 182, 183, 184, 185, 186, 190, *193, 194, 195, 196, 197*
Bristol DG, 93, *115*
Bristow JD, 710, *736*
Bristow MR, 583, 584, *607*
Britton J, 200, *224*
Brlosic R, 655, *677*
Brochard L, 252, *261*, 305, 314, 320, 322, *324, 327, 329*
Brodal P, 539, *550*
Broder G, 701, *734*
Brody MJ, 93, *115*
Broman H, 264, 267, 271, 272, 274, 275, 278, *282*
Broman L, 190, *197*, 264, 267, 271, 272, 274, 275, 278, *282*
Broman M, 190, *197*
Brondveld W, 693, *731*
Bronikowski TA, 57, *110*
Bronsveld W, 693, *730*

Brook CJ, 303, 305, 307, 311, 312, *323*
Brooke MH, 483, *519*
Brookes GA, 540, *550*
Brooks GA, 39, 40, *44*, 472, 483, *518, 519*
Brosnan CF, 720, *740*
Brosnan MJ, 662, *681*
Brown AC, 209, *226*
Brown CD, 655, *678*
Brown D, 596, *612*
Brown DW, 142, *147*
Brown E, 558, 559, *574*
Brown EG, 541, *551*
Brown GS, 29, *42*
Brown H, 597, *613*
Brown JH, 132, *145*
Brown JK, 563, *575*
Brown MD, 389, *404*
Brown R, 209, *226*
Brown SD, 701, *734*
Brown SE, 565, 566, *576*
Brown TR, 30, 31, *42*
Bruckner WB, 692, *730*
Bruining H, 686, 688, 703, *728, 735*
Bruining HA, 105, *118*, 711, 712, *737*
Brun BC, 307, 312, 313, *324*
Brun-Buisson C, 231, *258*, 286, 290, 291, 292, *300*, 719, 720, *740*
Brundage BH, 297, *302*
Brunet F, 359, 361, 373, 374, *377*
Brunet P, 663, 664, *682*
Brunner HR, 588, *609*
Bruno A, 602, *614*
Bruno F, 313, *327*
Brunsvold N, 596, *612*
Brunton J, 209, *226*
Bruroni M, 622, *643*
Bruschi C, 271, *283*
Bruschke AV, 583, *606*
Brussel T, 192, *198*
Bryan AC, 204, *225*, 307, 314, *324*
Bryan C, 183, *195*
Bryan CL, 515, *523*
Buchanan JW, 70, *111*
Buchbinder M, 296, *302*
Bucino RA, 582, 584, *606*
Buckberg GD, 101, *115*

Buckey JC, 165, *174*
Budin M, 603, 605, *615*
Budinger TF, 540, *550*
Buell MG, 417, *431*
Buerk D, 394, *406*
Buffington CW, 370, *379*
Buist AS, 67, *111*, 136, *147*, 200, 209, 224, 226
Bulkley GB, 692, 703, 730, *735*
Buller N, 591, *610*
Bunn HF, 641, *647*
Buono MJ, 487, *520*
Burdeau CH, 693, *731*
Burdick MD, 721, *740*
Burdiel L, 667, *682*
Burger EJ, 67, *111*
Burgess EM, 593, *611*
Burgos F, 4, *26*, 139, *147*, 231, 236, 243, *258*
Burke D, 669, *682*
Burke JF, 692, *730*
Burke R, 396, 397, 398, 400, *406*
Burke RE, 397, *407*
Burke TV, 206, *225*
Burki NK, 206, *225*
Burnham M, 184, *195*
Burns HJG, 720, 721, 724, *740*
Burpo RP, 85, *114*
Burri PH, 156, *172*
Burrows B, 229, *257*
Bursztein S, 46, *108*
Burton G, 566, *577*
Burton RW, 693, *731*
Bush A, 653, *676*
Bush BA, 566, *576*
Busse R, 583, *607*, 641, *647*
Butland B, 200, *224*
Butler GC, 472, *518*
Butler J, 566, *576*
Butler JE, 202, *224*
Butler N, 200, *224*
Butt AY, 241, *259*
Buzello W, 637, *646*
Bye PTP, 206, *225*, 570, *577*
Bylin G, 137, *147*, 210, 211, 218, *226*, 242, *260*

Bynner J, 200, *224*
Byrne-Quinn E, 526, *547*

C

Cabanes L, 599, *614*
Cabral A, 352, *357*
Cada EM, 655, *677*
Cade JF, 203, *224*
Cady EB, 714, *738*
Caeser J, 95, *115*
Cahoon RL, 160, *173*
Cai GZ, 319, *329*
Caillette A, 662, *681*
Cain SM, 93, 104, 105, *115*, *118*, 334, 339, 340, 341, 343, 344, 345, 346, 347, 348, 349, 350, 351, 352, *353*, *354*, *355*, *356*, *357*, 360, 361, 371, 377, *380*, 414, 425, 426, 427, *431*, *432*, *433*, 638, *646*, 693, 694, 695, 713, 714, *731*, *732*, *738*
Cain WM, 620, *643*
Cairns CB, 701, *735*
Caldini P, 286, 290, *301*
Caldwell JH, 370, *379*
Caldwell PRB, 699, 700, *733*
Calhoon JH, 515, *523*
Califf RM, 602, *614*
Callegari G, 271, *283*
Calvano SE, 691, *729*
Calvet X, 715, 717, *739*
Calvin JE, 294, *301*
Camara M, 595, *612*
Cameron PD, 183, *195*
Campagne P, 152, *172*
Campbell EJM, 202, *224*, 569, *577*
Campbell I, 694, *732*
Campbell JA, 98, *116*
Campbell JC, 85, *114*
Campbell JE, 202, *224*
Campisi DJ, 427, *433*, 699, 700, *733*
Campistol JM, 515, *523*, 659, 662, 663, 664, *679*, *680*
Cander L, 85, *114*
Canepari M, 567, *577*
Cannella G, 655, 662, *677*

Cannon JH, 532, *548*
Cannon RO, 659, *679*
Capen RL, 57, 60, 66, *110*
Cappelletti G, 304, 305, *323*
Carayon A, 662, 663, 670, *681*
Carcelen A, 152, *172*
Cardenas D, 655, *678*
Cardus J, 4, 20, *26*, *27*, 139, *147*, 231, 236, 243, 250, *258*, *260*, 307, *325*
Carlet J, 304, 305, *323*
Carli A, 359, 361, 373, 374, *377*
Carlile PV, 711, 712, *737*
Carlin J, 200, *223*
Carlsen E, 87, *114*
Carlson R, 701, *734*
Carlson RW, 428, *433*, 699, 700, *733*
Carlton EL, 692, *730*
Carney RM, 655, 665, *678*
Carny CK, 90, *115*
Caro J, 655, *677*
Caro JF, 660, 670, *680*, *683*
Carpenter DO, 400, *407*
Carrasco DI, 475, *518*
Carrico CJ, 307, 311, 312, *324*, 687, *728*
Carrier G, 566, *576*
Carrington CB, 263, 278, *280*
Carroll JE, 483, *519*
Carter EA, 692, *730*
Carter NW, 667, 671, *682*
Caruthers SD, 122, 125, 133, *143*
Carvalho CR, 321, *329*
Casaburi R, 271, 272, *283*, 470, 474, 476, 481, 482, 483, 484, 487, 507, *517*, *518*, *520*, 554, 572, *573*
Cashmer B, 724, *741*
Caspari W, 150, *171*
Cassino PP, 659, *679*
Castagna J, 470, 481, *518*
Castaing Y, 231, 235, 236, 243, 251, 253, 256, *257*, *258*, *260*, *261*, 285, 286, 290, 291, 292, *300*
Castiagne A, 599, *614*
Castilla J, 659, *679*
Castle BL, 166, *175*
Catena R, 375, *380*
Cattaert A, 481, 482, *519*

Caulfield JB, 346, *355*, 370, *379*
Cave CB, 125, *144*
Cecchin F, 670, *683*
Cederlund T, 180, *194*
Celli BR, 177, *193*
Cera FB, 428, 429, *434*
Cerami A, 691, *729*
Ceretelli P, 397, *407*
Cerny LC, 637, *646*
Cerra FB, 686, 687, 701, 720, 724, *727*, *728*, *734*, *740*, *742*
Cerretelli P, 14, *26*, 159, *173*, 470, 472, 478, 484, 485, 486, 487, 489, 491, *517*, *520*
Cerveri I, 142, *148*
Chabrier PE, 231, *258*
Chadwick BJ, 587, *608*
Chakrabarti NK, 189, *196*
Challiss RAJ, 662, *681*
Chan L, 463, *467*
Chanaud CM, 397, *407*
Chance B, 30, *42*, 105, *118*, 588, 589, 598, *609*, *613*, 714, *738*
Chandel N, 710, *737*
Chang AC, 694, *731*
Chang JE, 636, *645*
Chang MC, 704, 709, 715, *735*
Chang WK, 658, 670, *679*
Changeaux J, 622, 623, *643*
Chaniotakis M, 125, *144*
Chapler CK, 339, 340, 341, 343, 344, 345, 346, 352, *354*, *355*, *357*, 694, *731*
Chapman JB, 364, 365, *378*
Charache S, 618, 620, *642*
Charansonney O, 637, *646*
Chatila W, 694, 710, *732*
Chau TTH, 714, *738*
Chen CL, 191, *197*
Chen DG, 344, *355*
Chen EY, 641, *647*
Chen L, 189, *197*
Chen PCY, 630, 631, 638, *644*
Chen RYZ, 342, 343, *355*
Chen TL, 191, *197*
Chen W, 437, *445*
Cheney FW, 309, *325*

Cheng CH, 658, 670, *679*
Cherniack RM, 263, 265, 269, 276, *281*, 555, *574*, 691, *729*
Cherniak NS, 526, *547*
Chernick V, 287, *301*
Cherqui D, 414, *431*, 710, *736*
Chesler RM, 655, 656, 657, *677*
Cheung PY, 714, *738*
Chevalier PA, 125, *144*
Chi MM, 387, 389, *403*
Chien S, 101, *115*, 342, 343, *355*, 637, *646*
Chilian WM, 370, *379*
Chin ER, 388, *404*
Chinchon I, 659, *679*
Chinn ER, 546, *552*
Chirtel SJ, 337, *353*
Chiu LK, 342, *355*
Choen G, 191, *197*
Chopin C, 105, *118*, 351, *356*
Christensen E, 396, 397, *406*
Christensen NJ, 386, 391, *402*, 537, 538, *549*
Christon NV, 686, 687, *727*
Christoph I, 591, *610*
Chung KF, 217, 222, *227*
Chung Y, 106, *118*
Chuong CJ, 56, *110*
Chuong CJC, 56, *109*, *110*
Cilley RE, 341, *354*
Cinnella G, 251, *261*
Cinotti L, 251, *260*
Cipolle MD, 724, *742*
Claassen H, 91, *115*, 152, *172*, 387, 389, *403*, 539, *550*
Clancy RL, 511, *522*, 540, *550*
Clark A, 15, 23, *26*, 27, 30, *42*, 496, *521*
Clark AL, 598, *613*
Clark BJ, 105, *118*
Clark C, 701, *734*
Clark CH, 428, *434*
Clark CM, 36, *43*
Clark DF, 136, *147*
Clark JB, 662, *681*
Clark P, 15, *26*, 388, 392, *403*
Clark PAA, 23, *27*, 496, *521*
Clark RA, 254, *261*

Clark T, 596, *612*
Clark TJH, 569, *577*
Clarke RO, 166, *175*
Clausen J, 181, *194*
Clausen JL, 8, *26*, 230, 231, 235, *257*, 565, *576*
Clausen JP, 386, *402*
Cledes J, 653, *676*
Clegg JB, 620, *642*
Clelland CA, 241, *259*
Clemens RE, 272, 273, 276, *283*, 561, 562, 564, 565, 568, 569, 570, 571, *575*, *577*
Clerbaux T, 309, *325*
Cline F, 73, *112*
Clinton ME, 660, *680*
Closset J, 293, 294, *301*
Clozel JP, 370, *379*
Clozel M, 587, *608*
Clutter W, 714, *738*
Clutton-Brock T, 715, *738*
Clyne C, 594, *611*
Coats A, 591, 597, 603, *610*, *613*, *614*
Coats AJS, 598, *613*
Cobb F, 585, 590, 591, 597, 602, 603, *607*, *610*, *612*, *613*, *614*
Cobos A, 217, 222, *227*, 515, *523*, 659, 662, 663, 664, *679*
Cochrane JE, 472, *518*
Cockroft D, 200, *224*
Coffernils M, 701, 703, *734*
Coggan A, 588, 590, 591, *609*, *610*
Cohen A, 152, *172*
Cohen KD, 492, 494, *520*
Cohen P, 105, *118*
Cohen PJ, 436, *445*
Cohen RA, 591, *610*, 694, *732*
Cohn E, 602, *614*
Cohn JN, 583, *606*
Cohn L, 596, *612*
Coin DT, 544, *551*
Coker PJ, 122, 125, 133, *143*
Colbebatch HJH, 136, *147*
Colby TV, 263, 265, 269, 276, *281*
Cole R, 589, *609*
Cole RP, 388, 392, 397, *404*
Coleman H, 587, *608*

Author Index

Coleman HN, 582, 584, *606*
Coleman R, 585, *607*
Coleman RE, 602, *614*
Coleridge HCG, 370, *379*
Coleridge HM, 370, *379*
Collard P, 204, *225*
Colley PS, 309, *325*
Collins J, 596, *612*
Collins RM, 371, *380*
Colucci WS, 583, *607*
Comino EJ, 200, *224*
Comroe JH, 87, 88, *114*, 342, 344, *354*
Conley KE, 387, 389, *403*
Connett R, 589, 590, *609*
Connett RJ, 30, 39, 40, *42*, *44*, 101, *117*, 483, *519*
Connolly H, 342, 344, *354*
Connolly HV, 411, 422, 425, *430*, *432*
Consolazio FC, 158, *173*
Consolo F, 660, *680*
Constantine HP, 87, *114*
Conteras I, 660, 670, *680*
Conti G, 252, *261*
Converse RL, 669, *683*
Converse RLJ, 658, 668, 669, *679*
Conway J, 591, 597, 598, 603, *610*, *613*, *614*
Conway JH, 142, *147*
Conway M, 588, 589, *609*
Conway MA, 583, *606*
Cook DJ, 686, 687, 719, 720, 727, *740*
Cook DL, 321, *329*
Cook W, 237, *259*
Cooke A, 8, *26*
Cooper DJ, 360, 371, *377*, *380*, 428, *434*, 695, *733*
Cooper G, 364, 366, *378*, 582, 584, *606*
Cooper JM, 662, *681*
Cora U, 603, 605, *615*
Coremans JMCC, 105, *118*
Cornil A, 256, *261*
Cornish ER, 67, *111*
Corsi M, 660, *680*
Corte P, 217, 222, *227*
Corvaja E, 660, *680*
Cosentino F, 658, 668, 669, *679*
Cosio MG, 238, *259*

Coste J, 711, 712, *737*
Costello DJ, 620, *642*
Costes F, 599, *614*
Costin JC, 338, *353*
Cotes J, 136, *146*
Cotton DJ, 84, 85, *113*
Cotton JR, 667, 671, *682*
Coulson RL, 359, *376*
Coulthard MG, 655, 662, *677*, *681*
Cournand A, 63, 67, *111*, 229, *257*, 269, *282*, 700, *734*
Coutu RE, 263, 278, *280*
Covert D, 125, *144*
Cowley RA, 701, *734*
Cox M, 714, *738*
Coxson HO, 375, *380*
Coyle E, 588, 590, 591, *609*, *610*
Coyle EM, 483, *519*
Coyle SM, 720, 721, 722, *740*
Craig DB, 184, *195*
Cramer E, 655, *677*
Crank J, 57, 66, *110*
Crapo JD, 52, *109*
Crapo RO, 142, *148*
Craw MR, 87, *114*
Crawford AB, 163, *174*
Crawford ABH, 208, *226*
Cre ME, 229, *257*
Creager MA, 583, *607*
Crecelius CA, 460, *467*
Cremona G, 241, 254, *259*, *261*
Crenshaw AG, 539, *550*
Crevat A, 663, 664, *682*
Crevey BJ, 292, 297, 298, *301*, *302*
Cribier A, 602, *614*
Crim C, 319, *329*
Crine GJ, 321, *329*
Crog J, 451, *465*
Cronestrand R, 591, *610*
Cross KW, 229, *257*
Crotti S, 304, *324*
Crouser ED, 426, *433*
Cruickshank AM, 720, 721, 724, *740*
Cruz JC, 159, *173*
Cruz N, 691, *729*
Cruz OL, 55, 91, *109*, *115*
Cryer P, 714, *738*

Crystal GJ, 360, *377*
Crystal RG, 263, 265, 269, 273, 276, 278, *280*, *281*, 565, *576*
Cuddy TE, 537, *549*
Cumming G, 51, 54, 57, 66, *109*, *110*
Cumming K, 51, *109*
Cunningham DJC, 478, 480, 481, 482, *519*
Cunningham KF, 360, *377*, 428, *434*, 695, 697, 698, 711, 712, 715, *733*
Cunningham M, 595, *612*
Cunnion RE, 360, 373, 374, *377*
Cureton KA, 475, *518*
Curtis SE, 93, 104, 105, *115*, *118*, 346, 350, 351, 352, *355*, *356*, *357*, 425, 426, *432*, 620, 638, *643*, *646*, 713, 714, *738*
Curzen NP, 350, *356*
Custead W, 347, *355*, 427, *433*
Cvinsky AS, 90, *115*
Cymerman A, 23, *27*, 136, *146*, 156, 158, 159, 160, 170, *173*, *175*, 526, 529, 530, 531, 532, 533, 537, 538, 545, *547*, *548*, *549*, *550*

D

DaCosta J, 205, *225*
DaCosta LR, 417, *431*
Dahl R, 222, *228*
Dahlback M, 212, *227*
Dahn MS, 691, 694, 695, *729*, *732*
Dai X, 344, *355*
Dai XZ, 376, *381*
Dall'Ava-Santucci J, 359, 361, 373, 374, *377*
D'Alonzo GE, 231, 236, 248, *257*, 286, 287, 288, 290, 291, 292, 297, *300*, *302*, 565, *576*
Dalton L, 636, *645*
Daly MDeB, 341, 342, *354*, *355*
Damask MC, 694, *732*
Dambrosio M, 305, *324*
Damgaard-Pedersen K, 184, *195*
D'Amico G, 669, *683*
Damon DN, 390, 392, 393, 394, 398, 399, *404*, *405*
D'Andrea L, 304, 315, 317, *324*, *328*
Danek SJ, 347, *356*, 427, *433*, 699, 700, *733*
Danforth JM, 375, *381*
Danies A, 713, *738*
Danner RL, 707, 708, 709, *736*
Danson J, 67, *111*
Dantzker DR, 8, *26*, 134, *146*, 179, 190, *194*, 210, *226*, 230, 231, 235, 236, 248, 250, *257*, *260*, 285, 286, 287, 288, 290, 291, 292, 297, 298, 298, *300*, *301*, *302*, 303, 305, 307, 309, 310, 311, 312, 313, *323*, *324*, 325, *326*, 347, 349, *356*, 427, 428, *433*, *434*, 565, 570, *576*, *577*, 695, 699, 700, *732*, *733*
Darmon PL, 305, *324*
D'Assler YM, 98, *116*
Daugherty MO, 192, *197*
Daugirdas JT, 671, *683*
Daut J, 340, *354*
Davey P, 591, 597, 598, 603, *610*, *613*, *614*
Davidson JW, 375, *380*
Davies AG, 597, *613*
Davies NJH, 181, 184, *194*, *195*, 318, *328*
Davies RA, 566, *576*
Davies S, 599, 600, *614*
Davis DM, 370, *379*
Davis DR, 685, *727*
Davis JA, 557, 558, 565, *574*
Davis JW, 366, *378*
Davis K, 321, *329*
Davis MJ, 370, *379*
Daviskas E, 206, *225*
Dawson A, 158, *173*
Dawson CA, 57, *110*
Day NPJ, 714, *738*
De Backer D, 351, *356*
De Coster A, 560, *575*
De Deyn PP, 98, *116*
De Mendonca A, 686, 688, *728*
De Prampero P, 535, 540, *549*

De RM, 130, *145*
Dean GW, 70, *111*, 166, *174*
Dean NC, 563, *575*
DeBacker D, 425, *432*, 699, 700, 714, *733*
DeBoer LW, 620, *643*
DeCamp MM, 687, *728*
Dechamps P, 311, *326*
Dechert R, 318, *328*
Decramer M, 229, *256*, 566, *576*
Decroly P, 311, *326*
Defouilloy C, 231, 254, *258*, *261*
Defronzo RA, 670, *683*
Defrozo RA, 46, *108*
Degante SP, 701, *734*
Degeorges M, 599, *614*
DeGraff AC, 152, 156, *172*
Degremont AC, 691, 703, *729*
DeGroot WF, 203, *225*
Dehart P, 286, 290, 291, *300*, 303, 305, 307, 311, 312, *323*
Deheinzellin D, 305, 313, 321, *324*, *329*
Dei Cas L, 655, 662, *677*
Deitch EA, 687, 691, 724, 725, *728*, *729*, *742*
Delaney JP, 417, *431*
Delano BG, 655, 656, 657, *677*, *678*
DeLano FA, 630, 631, 638, *644*
Delashaw JB, 393, 394, 398, 399, *405*
Delclaux C, 314, 320, 322, *327*, *329*
Delcroix M, 286, 287, 288, 289, 290, 291, 292, 293, 294, 295, *300*, *301*
Delea C, 587, *608*
Delehunt J, 383, 391, *401*
Delhunt J, 540, *550*
D'Elia J, 464, *467*
Delille F, 309, 313, *325*
Dellinger RP, 321, *329*, 686, 687, *727*, *728*
Dellsperger KC, 370, *379*
Delmez JA, 655, 665, *678*
Delp MD, 385, 400, *401*, 470, 488, 491, 492, 493, 494, 495, *517*
Demaison L, 360, *377*
Demchenko IT, 618, 641, *642*
Demling RH, 687, *728*

Demopoulos L, 587, 605, *608*, *615*
Dempsey JA, 136, *146*, 152, 156, *172*, 386, *401*, 480, 484, 485, *519*, 560, 570, *575*, *577*
den Boer PJ, 636, *645*
Dennis VW, 655, 665, *678*
Denny E, 52, *109*
Denolin H, 298, 299, *302*
Denton RM, 36, *43*
Deray G, 662, 663, 670, *681*
Derdak S, 318, *328*
Derion T, 139, *147*, 480, 485, *519*, 532, *549*
Dervin G, 294, *301*
Desai VS, 716, 717, *739*
Descorps-Declere A, 691, *729*
Desgagnes P, 271, *283*, 554, 566, *573*
Desjardin JA, 205, *225*
Desjardins C, 390, 391, 392, *404*, *405*, 503, *521*
Despas PJ, 570, *577*
Desplances JF, 602, *614*
Detre KM, 297, *302*
Detusch S, 691, 703, 704, *729*
Deusch E, 427, *433*
Deussen A, 632, 633, *645*
Deutschman RA, 162, 164, 166, *173*, *174*
Deviere J, 720, 721, 724, *740*
DeWoskin R, 638, *646*
Dhainaut JF, 359, 361, 373, 374, *377*, 711, 712, *737*
Dhillon DP, 254, *261*
Di Stefano A, 200, *224*
Diament ML, 205, *225*
Diamond SM, 654, *677*
Diaz de Atauri MJ, 254, *261*
Diaz K, 660, 670, *680*
Diaz O, 4, 20, *26*, *27*, 139, *147*, 217, 222, 227, 231, 236, 243, *258*, 264, *281*, 515, *523*, 659, 662, 663, 664, *679*, *680*
Didier EP, 181, 183, *194*, *195*
Die TG, 142, *147*
Dierckx RA, 98, *116*
Diesel W, 20, *27*, 657, 660, 662, 669, *678*, *679*, *680*

Dietrich HH, 370, *379*, 391, *405*
Dillard TA, 570, *577*
Dinda PK, 417, *431*
Dines D, 595, *611*
Dinh-Xuan AT, 241, 254, *259*, *261*
Dinour D, 456, *466*
Dinur D, 451, 452, 456, *465*
DiPrampero PE, 152, *172*, 470, 472, 478, 484, 485, 486, 487, 489, *517*
Dirks B, 714, *738*
DiSesa V, 596, *612*
DiStefano C, 660, *680*
Dittmer H, 687, *728*
Dittrich P, 665, 666, *682*
Diver D, 595, *612*
Diza O, 243, *260*
Dlay J, 470, *518*
Dling BR, 90, *115*
Dnour D, 455, *466*
Dobourg O, 588, *608*
Dobson GP, 31, 36, *42*, *43*
Dodd DS, 560, *575*
Dodd LR, 392, *405*
Dodd S, 480, 484, 485, *519*
Dodd SL, 360, 361, 371, *377*, *380*, 414, 426, *431*, 693, 695, *731*
Dodek PM, 697, 699, 700, 705, 714, *733*
Doerschuk CM, 375, *380*, 425, *432*
Doggart JH, 156, *172*
Doglio G, 428, *434*, 705, 706, *735*
Doglio GR, 704, 709, 715, *735*
Doherty JJ, 563, *575*
Dolan S, 318, *328*
Dole WP, 370, *379*
Dollery CT, 71, 73, *112*, 121, 132, *143*, *145*, 188, *196*
Dolmage TE, 571, *578*
Dolovich MB, 74, *112*, 164, *174*, 183, *195*
Domino KB, 310, 312, 317, *325*, *327*
Donald AW, 269, *282*
Donchez L, 583, 585, 598, 601, 605, *607*, *613*, *614*, *615*
Donker AJ, 693, *730*
Donnell D, 222, *228*
Donnelly SC, 721, *740*

Donner CF, 554, 572, *573*
Doornbos D, 554, *573*
Dora K, 470, 493, 494, *518*
Dorfman B, 428, *434*, 705, 706, *735*
Dorinsky PM, 426, *433*
Dormer AE, 82, *113*
Dornhorst AC, 229, *256*
Douglas AR, 49, *108*
Douglas NJ, 206, *226*
Douzinas EE, 701, *734*
Downs JB, 312, 313, 314, 315, 320, 321, *327*, *329*
Draper EA, 686, 687, *727*
Drazenovic R, 425, *432*
Drexler H, 375, *381*, 515, *522*, *523*, 583, 588, 590, 603, *607*, *609*, *610*, *614*
Driscoll TB, 166, *174*
Drory Y, 657, *679*
Drown C, 483, *519*
Drummond AJ, 686, 687, 689, *728*
Drummond GB, 183, *195*
Duarte M, 715, 717, *739*
Dubin A, 428, *434*, 705, 706, *735*
DuCharme DW, 671, *684*
Dudley GA, 399, *407*
Dueck R, 8, *26*, 181, 184, *194*, *195*, 230, 231, 235, *257*, 311, *326*, 565, *576*
Dufaye P, 701, *734*
Duffell GM, 557, 565, *574*
Dujic Z, 654, *677*
Duleep K, 594, *611*
Dulfano MJ, 205, *225*
Duling BR, 98, 101, *116*, *117*, 340, *354*, 370, *379*, 386, 390, 391, 392, 393, 394, 395, 397, 398, 399, 400, *402*, *404*, *405*, *406*, *407*, 470, 493, 494, 503, *518*, *521*, 641, *647*
Duncker DJ, 337, *353*, 470, 488, 491, 492, 493, 494, 495, *517*
Dunkman W, 591, *610*
Dunlop RS, 30, *42*
Dunn CJ, 662, *681*
Dupont E, 720, 721, 724, *740*
Dupuis BA, 105, *118*, 351, *356*
Dupuy PM, 222, *228*
Duranteau J, 691, 703, *729*
Durele M, 637, *646*

Author Index

Duroux P, 237, *259*, 286, 289, *301*, 566, 575
Durozard D, 662, *681*
Durrego P, 660, 670, *680*
Duruble M, 620, *642*
Dutton R, 347, *355*, 427, *433*
Dutton RE, 427, *433*
Duvelleroy M, 620, 629, 637, *642*, *644*, *646*
Duxson MJ, 397, *407*
Dwarkin LD, 448, 454, *465*

E

Early PJ, 96, 97, *116*
Eastham CL, 370, *379*
Eaton JW, 152, *172*, 619, *642*
Eberl S, 207, 209, *226*
Eckberg DL, 582, 584, *606*
Edelmann NH, 526, *547*
Edgerton VR, 396, *406*
Edmond JC, 710, *736*
Edouard R, 691, 703, *729*
Edwards AD, 105, *118*
Edwards J, 424, *432*
Edwards RHT, 557, 559, 565, *574*
Edwards W, 595, *611*
Edyvean J, 162, *174*
Effros RM, 470, *518*
Egashira K, 375, *381*
Egginton S, 389, *404*
Egler J, 597, *612*
Egurrola MA, 704, 709, 715, *735*
Ehrlich W, 368, 369, *378*
Eichacker PQ, 708, 709, *736*
Eichler HG, 641, *647*
Eidemak I, 662, *681*
Einstein R, 386, *401*
Eiseman B, 685, *727*
Eisenstein BL, 310, 312, 317, *325*, *327*
Eklof B, 593, *611*
Eklund A, 264, 267, 271, 272, 274, 275, 278, *282*
Eknoyan G, 463, *467*
Elashoff JD, 554, *573*
Elazarian L, 463, *467*

Elbeery JR, 366, *378*
Elce S, 583, *607*
Eldred E, 397, *407*
Eldridge MW, 531, 532, 534, *548*
Eleff S, 588, *609*
Eliahou H, 657, *679*
Eliasen K, 231, 236, 237, *257*
Elin RJ, 707, *736*
Ellerin L, 437, 440, *445*
Ellinger DC, 31, *43*
Elliott AR, 122, 123, *144*, 149, 162, 163, 164, 166, 168, 169, 170, *171*, *173*, *174*, *175*
Elliott TSJ, 718, *740*
Ellis CG, 390, 391, 392, 393, 394, *404*, *405*, 425, *432*, 500, 509, 513, *521*, *522*
Ellsworth ML, 101, *115*, 390, 391, 393, 394, 395, *404*, *405*, 620, *642*, 694, *732*
Elsen R, 663, 664, *682*
Elwyn DH, 591, *610*, 710, *736*
Ely SW, 370, *379*
Elzinga G, 359, *376*
Emerson CG, 394, 395, 399, *406*
Emery NJ, 73, *112*, 122, *143*
Emmett B, 39, *43*
Emms M, 20, *27*, 657, *679*
Emond JC, 414, *431*
Endert E, 720, *740*
Engberg G, 184, 185, 188, 189, *195*, *196*
Engel LA, 67, *111*, 162, 163, 169, *174*, 208, *226*, 560, *575*
Engelen MPKJ, 567, *577*
Engelman E, 345, *355*
English AW, 396, *406*
English DR, 373, *380*
English M, 347, *355*, 427, *433*
Enoka RM, 394, 396, 397, 400, *406*
Enoki Y, 620, *643*
Enquist BJ, 132, *145*
Ensinger H, 714, *738*
Entman ML, 375, *381*
Eovell JW, 582, 584, *606*
Eppenberger HM, 39, 40, *44*
Epstein F, 454, 455, 458, *465*
Epstein FH, 447, 448, 451, 452, 456, 457, 458, 460, 462, 463, *465*, *466*, *467*
Epstein LJ, 554, *573*

Epstein RM, 191, *197*
Epstein S, 85, *114*
Epstein SE, 488, *520*
Eraslan A, 494, *520*
Erasmi H, 637, *646*
Erdmann E, 583, *607*
Erecinska M, 414, *431*, 483, *519*
Erhardt JC, 370, *379*
Erickson BK, 46, 72, *108*, 494, 495, 507, 511, 514, *520*, *522*, 532, 537, *549*
Erickson HH, 73, *112*, 122, *143*, 471, 472, 474, 492, *518*, 532, *548*
Eriksen EF, 456, *466*
Eriksson E, 90, *114*, 394, 396, *405*, *406*
Ernst P, 200, *224*, 515, *523*
Erslev AJ, 655, *677*
Ertl G, 603, 605, *615*
Erwig LP, 540, *550*
Esau SA, 570, *577*
Eschbach JW, 655, *678*
Escourrou P, 237, *259*, 566, *575*
Esmore D, 571, 572, *578*
Espersen K, 177, 178, *193*
Estenne M, 162, *174*
Eterovic D, 654, *677*
Etherington PJ, 350, *356*
Ettiner SM, 598, *613*
Eu JP, 618, 641, *642*
Euler US, 318, *328*
Evans A, 571, 572, *578*
Evans AB, 271, *283*
Evans JW, 22, *27*, 135, 139, *146*, 166, *175*, 230, *257*
Evans RW, 650, 668, *676*, *682*
Evans TO, 713, *737*
Evans TW, 350, *356*
Evelieght MC, 309, 313, *325*
Ewald FW, 566, *576*
Ewing DJ, 669, *683*

F

Fabbri LM, 200, *224*
Faber JE, 386, *402*
Fabre JE, 711, 712, *737*
Fagard R, 481, 482, *519*

Fahey JT, 341, *354*
Fahir LE, 76, *112*
Fairhurst J, 694, *732*
Fairley HB, 692, *729*
Faist E, 687, *728*
Faithfull NS, 503, 504, *522*, 638, *647*
Falconer T, 30, *42*
Falk JL, 699, 700, 701, *733*, *734*
Falke K, 304, 305, *323*
Falke KJ, 130, *145*, 254, *261*, 310, 312, 313, 315, 317, 319, 320, *325*, *326*, *327*, *328*, *329*
Falkel FE, 655, *678*
Falsetti HL, 370, *379*
Fan FC, 342, 343, *355*
Fanfulla F, 142, *148*
Fang HK, 360, *377*
Faraci FM, 437, *445*, 449
Farber MO, 566, *577*
Fargrell B, 594, *611*
Farhi LE, 126, *145*
Farmer C, 318, *328*
Farquhar I, 425, *432*
Farrance BW, 539, *550*
Fastenow C, 93, *115*
Fath JJ, 687, *728*
Fauchald P, 667, *682*
Faucher PE, 487, *520*
Faude F, 515, *522*
Faulkner JA, 383, 387, 389, 396, *401*, *403*, *406*
Fawcett WJ, 348, *356*
Fedde MR, 73, *112*, 122, *143*, 471, 474, 515, *518*, *523*
Federspiel W, 388, 392, *403*
Federspiel WJ, 15, *26*, 56, 92, *109*, *110*, 391, *405*, 503, 504, *521*, *522*, 638, *646*
Fedullo FF, 296, *302*
Feelisch M, 632, 633, *645*
Feenstra BWA, 711, 712, *737*
Fein A, 286, *300*
Fein AM, 686, *727*
Feinberrg H, 360, *377*
Feldman AM, 583, *607*
Feldman T, 710, *737*
Feldt-Rasmussen B, 662, *681*

Author Index

Felez MA, 217, 222, *227*, 243, *260*, 264, *281*
Felicetti G, 271, *283*
Fellin G, 669, *683*
Feneley MP, 366, *378*
Fenn WO, 150, *171*
Fenwick JC, 360, *377*, 427, 428, *433*, *434*, 695, 699, 700, 711, 712, 714, *733*, *737*
Fergus A, 605, *615*
Ferguson JL, 691, *729*
Fernandes EDO, 305, 313, *324*
Fernandez S, 704, 709, 715, *735*
Ferrandis J, 204, *225*
Ferrano N, 591, *610*
Ferrans VJ, 263, 269, 278, *281*
Ferraro GL, 532, *548*
Ferraro N, 508, *522*, 585, 588, 590, 596, 597, 598, *608*, *609*, *610*, *612*, *613*
Ferrer A, 216, *227*, 231, 234, 235, *258*, 264, *281*, 496, 508, 511, 514, *521*, 539, *550*
Ferrer M, 243, *260*
Ferretti G, 535, 540, *549*
Ferrige A, 632, *645*
Fessler HE, 716, 717, *739*
Feustel PJ, 427, *433*, 711, *737*
Fichera G, 543, *551*
Fiddian-Green RG, 98, 101, *116*, *117*, 704, 716, 717, *735*, *739*, *740*
Fiehn E, 603, *614*
Field S, 691, 694, *729*
Figl EO, 370, *379*
Filler J, 229, *257*
Filley GF, 82, *113*
Fimmel CJ, 94, *115*
Finch CA, 690, *728*
Findl O, 641, *647*
Finer J, 531, 532, 534, *548*
Finer NN, 714, *738*
Fink GD, 93, *115*
Fink L, 588, 589, 596, *609*, *612*
Fink LI, 588, *609*
Fink MP, 428, 429, *434*, 693, 704, 716, *730*, *735*, *739*
Fink PM, 715, 717, *739*
Finkel MS, 375, *381*

Finley TN, 131, *145*, 287, *301*
Fiore T, 251, *261*, 313, *327*
Firedrick J, 583, *606*
Firesen BP, 373, *380*
Fischer CE, 566, *576*
Fischer W, 654, *677*
Fischli W, 587, *608*
Fishman A, 583, 596, *607*, *612*
Fishman AP, 297, *302*, 310, *325*, 526, *547*
Fishman RM, 637, *645*
Fitz Y, 708, 709, *736*
FitzGerald MP, 150, *171*
FitzGerald MX, 263, 278, *280*
Fitzgerald RD, 304, *323*
Fitzgerald-Finch A, 375, *380*
Fitzpatrick JH, 620, *642*
Fixler D, 598, *613*
Fixler DE, 101, *115*
Flannery EM, 200, *224*
Flatebo T, 122, 125, *143*, *144*
Fleckenstein JL, 106, *118*
Fleming A, 705, 706, 707, *736*
Flenley DC, 206, *226*
Fletcher CM, 229, *257*
Flick MR, 426, *433*
Flint A, 263, 265, 269, 276, *281*
Flint L, 707, *736*
Floyd M, 659, *679*
Flynn W, 707, *736*
Fogg J, 623, *643*
Folkow B, 386, 387, *402*, *403*, 411, 412, *430*
Fong Y, 691, *729*
Forbes HS, 156, *172*
Foresman B, 349, *356*, 427, *433*
Forfar C, 591, 597, 603, *610*, *613*, *614*
Forman R, 585, 586, *608*
Formichi B, 286, 290, 291, 292, *300*
Fornai E, 286, 290, 291, 292, *300*
Forrester T, 391, *405*
Forster HV, 152, 156, *172*
Forster RE, 8, *26*, 31, *42*, 55, 82, 83, 84, 85, *109*, *113*, *114*
Forstermann U, 641, *647*
Forsulund T, 667, *682*
Fort P, 318, *328*

Fortenberry JD, 722, *741*
Fortune JB, 209, 222, *226*
Fouad-Tarazi F, 658, 668, 669, *679, 683*
Fournier M, 396, *406*
Fourrier F, 351, *356*
Fowler M, 583, *607*
Fowler WS, 66, 67, *111*, 180, *194*
Fox E, 105, *118*
Fox PT, 440, *445*
Fracchia C, 271, *283*
Frackowiak RS, 98, *116*
Franciosa J, 596, *612*
Franciose RJ, 724, 725, 726, *742*
Francis GS, 583, *606, 607*
Frangos JA, 638, *646*
Frank F, 655, 665, *678*
Franke RE, 82, *113*
Frans A, 204, *225*, 309, *325*
Fraser S, 392, 393, *405*
Fraser WD, 720, 721, 724, *740*
Fratacci MD, 254, *261*
Frazer R, 694, *732*
Fred HL, 531, 532, *548*
Freedman S, 569, *577*
Freeman BD, 707, 708, *736*
Frei U, 662, *681*
Freitag M, 619, *642*
French W, 487, 507, *520*, 557, 558, 565, *574*
Freyschuss U, 218, *227*
Friberg L, 96, *116*
Friden J, 539, *550*
Fridrich P, 304, *323*
Fried J, 705, 707, 720, *736*
Fried JC, 350, 352, *356*
Fried R, 714, *738*
Friedman EA, 655, 656, 657, 665, *677, 678*
Friedman M, 222, *228*
Friedrich J, 583, *606*
Frierson JL, 386, 390, 392, 394, 398, *401, 405*
Friesen BP, 360, *377*, 414, 423, 425, *431*, 693, *731*
Friesenecker B, 427, *433*
Fritss HW, 699, 700, *733*

Froese AB, 183, *195*, 307, 314, *324*
Frolich JC, 663, *681*
Frolicher DA, 314, *327*
From AHL, 30, *42*
Froment M, 711, 712, *737*
Fromm RE, 424, *432*
Frostell C, 184, 192, *195*, *197*, 255, *261*
Frostell CG, 222, *228*, 320, *329*
Frostick S, 588, 589, *609*
Frumin MJ, 191, *197*
Fuchs S, 451, 455, 458, 460, 462, 463, *465, 466, 467*
Fuglevand AJ, 396, 397, 398, 399, 400, *405*
Fuhrman FA, 413, *430*
Fujita TS, 635, *645*
Fujita Y, 692, *730*
Fukuchi Y, 208, *226*
Fulmer JD, 263, 265, 269, 273, 276, 278, *280, 281*
Fumagalli R, 304, 305, 313, *324, 327*, 705, 718, 719, *736*
Fung YC, 52, *109*
Fung YCB, 53, *109*
Funk CI, 30, *42*
Funke E, 590, *610*
Funkquist B, 184, *195*
Furchgott RF, 241, *259*, 346, *355*, 632, *645*
Fuster V, 595, *611*
Futaki S, 376, *381*
Fyhrquist F, 667, *682*

G

Gabriel R, 653, *676*
Gadek JE, 263, 269, 278, *281*, 319, *329*
Gaensler EA, 263, 278, *280*
Gaesser GA, 95, *116*, 470, 472, 474, 475, 476, 478, 482, 483, 494, 509, *517, 518, 519*
Gaffney A, 165, *174*
Gaggiotti M, 655, 662, *677*
Galassetti P, 566, *577*
Galavo M, 586, *608*

Gale GE, 8, 26, 82, *113*, 136, *146*, 248, *260*, 267, 272, 274, 275, 277, 279, *283*, 530, 537, 544, *548*
Gall SA, 366, *378*
Gallagher CG, 265, 271, 272, 273, 276, 282, *283*, 554, 555, 556, 557, 558, 559, 560, 561, 562, 563, 564, 565, 567, 568, 569, 570, 571, *573*, *574*, *575*, *576*, *577*
Gallea BL, 701, *735*
Gallesio A, 428, *434*, 705, 706, *735*
Galloway G, 593, 594, *611*, 663, *681*
Galvas PE, 396, *406*
Gandevia SC, 202, *224*
Gans C, 396, *406*
Garber AJ, 713, 714, *738*
Garcia C, 705, *735*
Garcia CE, 659, *679*
Garcia-Palmer FJ, 271, *283*
Garfinkel A, 397, *407*
Garrison LP, 650, 668, *676*
Garver KA, 317, 318, *328*
Gary DJ, 388, *404*, 546, *552*
Gaskell WH, 387, *402*
Gasparetto A, 252, *261*
Gass CL, 29, *42*
Gatecel C, 320, *329*
Gates AE, 583, *607*
Gattinoni L, 304, 305, 313, 315, 317, *323*, *324*, *327*, *328*, 705, 718, 719, *736*
Gattone M, 603, 605, *615*
Gaudron P, 583, 603, 605, *606*, *615*
Gauger P, 318, *328*
Gauger PC, 318, *328*
Gaughan EM, 73, *112*, 122, *143*
Gavin JR, 655, 665, *678*
Gayeski T, 589, 590, *609*
Gayeski TE, 30, *42*, 372, 373, *380*
Gayeski TEJ, 15, 23, *26*, *27*, 39, 40, *44*, 101, *117*, 388, 392, *403*, 470, 483, 496, 497, 498, 499, 500, 503, 504, 506, *518*, *519*, 661, *680*
Gayowski TJP, 717, *740*
Gazit A, 707, *736*
Gea J, 264, 265, 266, 267, 268, 269, 272, 273, 274, 275, 278, 279, *281*, 312, *327*

Gebhard MM, 722, *741*
Gehr P, 55, *109*
Geiger K, 692, *730*
Geiger PJ, 39, 40, *44*, 387, *403*
Geltman EM, 655, 665, *678*
Georges R, 655, *677*
Gerber MJ, 635, *645*
Germann R, 427, *433*
Gernert K, 618, 641, *642*
Gerogiou D, 605, *615*
Gerola A, 360, *377*
Gertenblith G, 583, *606*
Gesser BP, 456, *466*
Gheorghiu D, 30, 31, *42*, *43*
Ghesquire J, 481, 482, *519*
Ghezzo H, 136, *147*, 238, *259*
Ghofrani HA, 319, *329*
Giaccia AJ, 641, *647*
Gianello-Netto A, 286, 290, 291, 292, *300*
Giannuzzi P, 603, 605, *615*
Gibboe DD, 620, *642*
Gibbons WJ, 515, *523*
Gibbs CL, 364, 365, *378*
Gibson CG, 618, *642*
Gibson J, 229, *256*
Gibson QH, 632, *645*
Gifford W, 587, *608*
Gigliotti F, 560, *575*
Gilbert E, 310, 311, 321, *326*, 345, *355*
Gilcher R, 655, *678*
Giles G, 200, *223*
Gillam PMS, 121, *143*
Gilligan DM, 659, *679*
Gilmour I, 184, *195*
Gil-Necija E, 659, *679*
Gimferrer JM, 241, *259*
Gimson A, 348, 351, *356*, 699, 700, *733*
Ginger R, 428, *434*, 705, 706, *735*
Ginns L, 566, *576*
Ginns LC, 271, *283*, 571, 572, *578*
Ginsberg R, 583, *607*
Giordano A, 603, 605, *615*
Giotto G, 251, *260*
Girin E, 653, *676*

Giroir BP, 721, *741*
Givertz MM, 583, *607*
Gladden LB, 474, *518*
Glaister DH, 165, *174*
Glass NR, 655, 657, *678*
Glaubermann B, 462, *467*
Glazier J, 597, *612*
Gledhill N, 511, *522*
Gleim GW, 655, 665, *678*
Glenny RW, 73, 101, *112*, *115*, 122, 125, 126, 131, 133, *143*, *144*, *145*, *146*, 166, *175*
Gleser M, 383, 391, *401*, 540, *550*
Glower D, 636, *645*
Gnidec AA, 692, *730*
Gobel FL, 364, *378*
Gobran S, 57, 66, 67, *110*, *111*
Gockel B, 192, *198*
Goda F, 101, 103, *117*
Godbey PS, 57, 66, *110*
Goddard CM, 360, 373, 375, *377*, *380*, 414, 423, 425, *431*, 693, 694, *731*
Goerg R, 142, *147*
Goergieff M, 692, *730*
Goetz AE, 133, *145*
Gold AJ, 319, *329*
Gold WM, 563, *575*
Goldbach P, 427, *433*, 699, 700, *733*
Goldberg AP, 655, 665, *678*
Goldberg MA, 641, *647*
Goldberg N, 655, 656, 657, *677*
Goldberger M, 591, *610*
Goldfarb RD, 694, *732*
Goldhaber SZ, 295, *302*
Goldman G, 724, *741*
Goldman ML, 704, *735*
Goldmuntz EA, 720, *740*
Goldring RM, 297, *302*
Goldsmith SR, 583, *606*
Goldstein PJ, 713, 714, *738*
Goldstein RS, 571, *578*
Goljan EF, 385, 400, *401*
Gollnick PD, 387, 389, 392, 400, *402*, 470, 471, 504, 513, *517*, 535, *549*
Golper TA, 660, *680*
Gomez C, 271, *283*
Gomez CL, 637, *646*

Gomez FP, 222, *228*, 231, 234, 241, 246, *258*, *259*, 566, *576*
Gomez J, 667, *682*
Gonyea WJ, 396, *406*
Gonzales A, 637, *646*
Gonzales M, 637, *646*
Gonzalez de Suso JM, 566, *576*, 662, 664, *680*
Gonzalez N, 540, *550*
Gonzalez NC, 511, *522*
Gonzalez P, 535, *549*
Gonzalez R, 107, *118*, 388, 389, 390, 392, *403*, 515, *522*
Goodman AH, 339, *354*, 386, *401*, 414, *431*, 640, *647*
Goodwin CW, 694, *732*
Gopda F, 101, *117*
Gorczynski RJ, 390, 392, 394, 397, *404*, *407*
Gore RW, 411, *430*
Goresky CA, 371, 373, *380*
Gorewit RC, 93, *115*
Gosselink R, 566, *576*
Gothard P, 583, *607*
Goto K, 670, *683*
Goto Y, 364, 365, 375, 376, *378*, *380*, *381*
Gottfried SB, 251, *261*
Gottlieb I, 186, *194*
Gottlieb ME, 704, *735*
Gottschalk A, 566, *576*
Goudot B, 309, 313, *325*
Gould S, 636, 638, *645*, *646*, 690, *728*
Gow AJ, 625, 627, 634, 641, *644*
Gowda K, 558, 559, *574*
Grabeau GM, 656, *678*
Graber DJ, 527, *547*
Graf H, 655, *677*
Graf L, 699, 700, *733*
Graham BL, 84, *113*
Graham JA, 57, *110*
Graham SA, 412, *430*
Grange RW, 388, *404*, 546, *552*
Granger DN, 93, 94, *115*, 339, *354*, 386, *401*, 413, 414, *431*, 640, *647*
Granger HJ, 339, *354*, 386, *401*, 410, 413, 414, 415, *430*, *431*

Author Index

Granger HL, 640, *647*
Grant BJ, 209, 222, *226*
Grant BJB, 203, *224*
Granton JT, 321, *329*, 375, *380*
Graselli U, 641, *647*
Grasi M, 142, *148*
Grasi V, 136, *147*
Grassi B, 389, 392, 393, *404*, 471, 472, 474, 488, 492, 494, 495, 507, 511, *518*, *520*, 531, 532, 534, 537, *548*, *549*
Grassino A, 67, *111*, 570, *577*
Graves SW, 671, *684*
Gray AT, 79, *112*
Gray BA, 711, 712, *737*
Gray K, 668, *682*
Gray KS, 598, *613*
Gray SD, 387, 389, 392, *403*, *404*, *405*
Grayburn PA, 669, *683*
Grayson J, 375, *380*
Greaney M, 594, *611*
Greaves IA, 136, *147*
Green C, 694, *732*
Green H, 590, *610*
Green HJ, 539, *550*
Green YS, 662, 664, *680*
Greenbarg J, 705, *735*
Greenfeld Z, 460, 461, 463, *467*
Greenfield LJ, 287, *301*
Greenleaf JF, 122, *143*
Greenletch D, 85, *114*
Greenway CV, 94, *115*, 412, *430*, 692, *730*
Greet TR, 532, *548*
Gregersen MI, 637, *646*
Gregg DE, 360, 371, *377*
Gregg SG, 540, *550*
Gregory AH, 106, 107, *118*
Gregory TJ, 319, *329*
Greimer H, 657, *679*
Grene R, 179, 190, *194*
Griberg O, 101, 103, *117*
Griffis J, 660, *680*
Grimby G, 560, 562, *575*
Grimminger F, 310, 312, 319, 321, *326*, *327*, *328*, *329*

Grinberg OY, 101, *117*
Gris P, 701, 703, *734*
Grissom RT, 463, *467*
Griswold W, 653, *676*
Groebe K, 90, 98, *114*, *116*, 470, 494, 496, 497, 498, 499, 500, 503, 504, 506, *518*, *521*
Groeneveld AB, 715, 717, *739*
Groeneveld ABJ, 687, 693, 703, *728*, *730*, *735*
Grois RJA, 701, *734*
Grone HJ, 456, *466*
Groom AC, 363, *378*, 392, 393, *405*, 500, 509, 513, *521*, *522*
Gross D, 570, *577*
Gross GJ, 376, *381*
Grossman W, 285, *300*, 595, *612*
Grounds M, 694, 710, *732*
Grounds RM, 351, *357*, 705, 707, 716, 720, *736*, *739*
Grover R, 531, 532, *548*
Grover RF, 142, *147*, 152, 156, *172*
Groves BM, 23, *27*, 136, *146*, 156, 158, 159, 160, 170, *173*, *175*, 297, *302*, 529, 531, 532, 533, 537, 538, 545, *548*, *549*, *550*
Groves J, 603, 605, *615*
Groves PM, 530, 537, *548*
Grune F, 637, *646*
Grunert A, 714, *738*
Gruning T, 317, *328*
Grynberg A, 360, *377*
Guaini T, 655, 662, *677*
Guenard H, 231, 235, 236, 243, 251, 253, 256, *257*, *258*, *260*, *261*, 286, 290, 291, 292, *300*
Guenther SM, 570, *577*
Guerin F, 599, *614*
Guerra R, 593, *611*
Guery B, 105, *118*
Guetta V, 659, *679*
Guevera L, 95, *115*
Guiliani R, 251, *261*, 313, *327*
Guillory D, 691, *729*
Guinard N, 320, *329*
Guintini C, 286, 290, 291, 292, *300*
Guire KE, 341, *354*

Guitart R, 220, *228*, 231, 232, 234, 235, 238, 246, 253, *257*, *258*, *261*, 264, *281*, 557, 566, *574*
Guiterrez G, 106, *118*, 349, *356*, 427, 428, *433*, *434*, 701, *734*
Gumina RJ, 376, *381*
Gunnarsson L, 178, 179, 181, 184, 185, 190, *193*, *196*, *197*
Gunst M, 620, *643*
Gunther A, 319, *328*, *329*
Gunther K, 340, *354*
Guntupalli KK, 319, *329*
Guppy M, 29, *42*
Gupta RG, 263, 278, *280*
Gurbanov K, 455, *465*
Gurdjian F, 309, 313, *325*
Gustavsson H, 178, 179, 181, 184, *193*
Guthrie M, 655, *678*
Gutierrez C, 707, *736*
Gutierrez G, 394, *406*, 690, 695, 704, 705, 706, 709, 715, *728*, *732*, *735*
Gutman RA, 650, 668, *676*
Guy HJ, 139, *147*, 149, 162, 163, 164, 166, 169, *171*, *173*, *174*, *175*, 478, 492, 494, 505, 511, *519*
Guy HJB, 122, *144*
Guyton GP, 39, *44*
Guzman SV, 287, *301*
Gys T, 98, *116*

H

Haab P, 107, *118*, 388, 389, 390, 392, *403*, 515, *522*, 535, *549*
Haaber AB, 662, *681*
Habbick B, 200, *224*
Haber R, 687, *728*
Hachenberg T, 192, *198*
Hacker A, 722, *741*
Hackett P, 161, *173*
Hackett PH, 152, *172*, 526, 527, 529, 530, 537, 541, *547*, *551*
Haenel JB, 701, *734*, *735*
Hagberg J, 483, *519*
Hagberg JM, 655, 665, *678*

Hagemann LP, 440, *445*
Haglund U, 692, 703, *730*, *735*
Hahn HL, 557, 559, 565, *574*
Hahn SM, 310, *325*
Haida M, 271, *282*, 566, *577*
Haidet GC, 511, *522*
Haisjackl M, 427, *433*
Haj Yehia A, 456, *466*
Hakim TS, 70, *111*, 166, *174*
Halasz NA, 192, 193, *197*
Halber C, 593, *610*
Haldane J, 79, *113*
Haldane JS, 526, *547*
Haley NR, 655, *678*
Halicka HD, 387, *403*
Hall JB, 428, *434*, 694, 710, 711, 712, *732*, *737*
Hall M, 571, 572, *578*
Hall S, 596, *612*
Hallemans R, 231, 236, 256, *257*, *261*, 292, *301*, 310, 311, 312, *326*
Haller RG, 106, *118*
Halliday FC, 348, *356*
Hamalainen E, 715, *739*
Hamaoka T, 593, *611*
Hambraeus-Jonzon K, 192, *197*
Hambrecht R, 603, *614*
Hamilton AJ, 538, 545, *550*
Hamilton SR, 692, *730*
Hamilton WD, 205, *225*
Hamlyn JM, 671, *684*
Hamm CR, 122, 125, 133, *143*, *144*
Hammerle AF, 304, *323*
Hammersen F, 90, *114*
Hammond JW, 152, 156, *172*
Hammond M, 599, 600, *614*
Hammond MD, 79, *112*, 136, *146*, 315, *327*
Hance AJ, 263, 269, 278, *281*
Hand LJ, 663, *681*
Handon P, 386, *401*
Hands L, 593, 594, *611*
Hanger CC, 57, *110*
Hanley FL, 368, *379*
Hans B, 694, 695, *732*
Hansen J, 583, 589, *607*, *609*, 668, *682*

Author Index

Hansen JE, 268, 272, *282*, *283*, 457, *466*, 470, 474, 476, 481, 482, *518*, 555, *574*, 691, 693, 694, *729*
Hanson CW, 130, *145*
Hanson J, 130, *145*
Hanson P, 650, 651, 655, 657, *676*, *678*
Hanson PG, 136, *146*
Hanson WL, 57, *110*
Hanstock CC, 31, *43*
Hardy CJ, 583, *606*
Hare JM, 583, *607*
Harf A, 252, *261*, 307, 309, 312, 313, *324*, *325*
Hargens AR, 539, *550*
Harman J, 36, *43*
Harms CA, 386, *401*, 480, *519*
Harris CW, 158, *173*
Harris DC, 463, *467*
Harris DW, 671, *684*
Harris P, 700, *734*
Harris SA, 668, *682*
Harris-Eze AO, 272, 273, 276, *283*, 565, 568, 571, *575*, *577*
Harrison CE, 582, 584, *606*
Harrison DG, 370, *379*, 593, *611*
Harrop G, 156, *172*
Harsi TR, 122, 125, 133, *143*
Hart LG, 650, 668, *676*, *682*
Harter HR, 655, 665, *678*
Hartikainen J, 694, *732*
Harting I, 271, *283*
Hartley L, 531, 532, *548*
Hartley LH, 159, *173*
Hartridge H, 8, *26*
Harvey RB, 363, *377*
Hasibeder W, 427, *433*, 665, *682*
Haslett C, 721, *740*
Hasselbalch KA, 623, *643*
Hasselbalch SG, 440, *445*
Hasset J, 707, *736*
Hata K, 366, 375, *378*, *380*
Hatch DJ, 180, *194*
Hatcher JD, 342, *355*
Hatt RE, 186, *194*
Hattler BC, 375, *381*
Hattner RS, 122, *143*
Hauer K, 603, *614*

Haupt MT, 428, *433*
Hauser DL, 321, *329*
Haussener V, 55, *109*
Hausten TS, 530, 537, *548*
Havermann K, 654, *676*, *677*
Havriliak D, 705, *735*
Haworth S, 596, *612*
Hay A, 691, 694, *729*
Hay J, 691, 694, *729*
Hayashi T, 364, *378*
Hayes DJ, 662, *681*
Hayes MA, 705, 718, 719, *736*
Hayford-Welsing EJ, 85, *114*
Hayoz D, 588, *609*
Haywood JR, 93, *115*
Head C, 635, *645*
Heard SO, 715, 717, *739*
Hebbel RP, 152, *172*, 619, *642*
Heberer G, 687, *728*
Hebert PC, 686, 687, 689, 690, *728*, *729*
Hecht HH, 531, 532, *548*
Hechtman HB, 294, *301*, 724, *741*
Heckmann U, 451, 462, *465*
Heckscher T, 207, *226*
Hedenmaeker PJ, 583, *606*
Hedenstierna G, 137, *147*, 178, 179, 180, 181, 182, 183, 184, 185, 186, 188, 189, 190, 192, *193*, *194*, *195*, *196*, *197*, 210, 211, 212, 213, 215, 218, 222, *226*, 227, 242, 254, 255, *259*, *260*, *261*, 264, 265, 267, 269, 272, 274, 275, 278, *281*, *282*, 311, 313, *326*
Hedley-Whyte J, 184, *195*
Hedlin G, 218, *227*
Hedstrand U, 205, *225*
Hegewald DP, 142, *148*
Heidelmeyer CF, 130, *145*, 319, 320, *329*
Heidland A, 660, *680*
Heifetz SM, 586, 587, *608*
Heigenhauser GF, 383, *401*
Heigenhauser GJF, 61, 85, *111*, 484, 485, 486, 487, *519*
Heiman M, 85, *114*
Heisler N, 14, *26*, 397, *407*, 491, *520*
Heistad DD, 437, *445*, 449, 593, 594, *611*

Heldin G, 218, 227
Hellums JD, 624, 644
Helms NJ, 85, 114
Helsmoortel CM, 715, 717, 739
Helums JD, 638, 646
Hempel FG, 105, 118
Hempleman SC, 15, 27, 79, 112, 545, 551
Hendenstrom H, 213, 227
Henderson AH, 654, 677
Henderson AM, 164, 174
Henderson JAM, 122, 143, 183, 195
Henderson KS, 136, 146
Henderson WR, 532, 549
Hendriks J, 703, 735
Hendrikssen J, 539, 550
Heneghan WF, 655, 678
Henneman E, 400, 407
Henning SL, 373, 380
Henrich WL, 654, 657, 667, 677, 679, 682
Henrikesson J, 271, 282, 593, 611
Henriksson-Larsen K, 400, 407
Henriquez A, 566, 576
Henry JW, 297, 302
Henry RL, 200, 224
Henson D, 598, 599, 600, 601, 605, 613, 614, 615
Her B, 351, 356
Herazo LF, 79, 85, 112, 114
Herbecq P, 351, 356
Herbertson MJ, 360, 373, 374, 375, 377, 380, 694, 731
Herbison GP, 200, 224
Herigault R, 254, 261, 310, 312, 314, 326, 327
Herigault RA, 620, 643
Herman B, 320, 322, 329
Hermansen L, 539, 550
Hermansen LE, 538, 550
Hernandez MS, 704, 709, 715, 735
Heron MI, 397, 407
Herpai Z, 417, 431
Herpin D, 204, 225
Herr MD, 668, 682
Herrmann H, 599, 613
Hershberger RE, 583, 607

Hertle FH, 142, 147
Herve P, 286, 289, 301
Heslet L, 231, 236, 237, 257
Hess JR, 637, 638, 646
Hester RL, 494, 520
Hetchman HB, 692, 729
Hewlett AM, 186, 196
Hey EN, 478, 480, 481, 482, 519
Heyland DK, 719, 720, 740
Heyman SN, 451, 452, 454, 455, 456, 458, 460, 462, 463, 464, 465, 466, 467
Heymann MA, 101, 115
Heywood G, 722, 741
Hiatt WR, 660, 670, 680
Hickey MS, 366, 378
Hida W, 220, 228
Hien TT, 714, 738
Higenbottam TW, 231, 234, 235, 241, 254, 258, 259, 261, 320, 329
Higgenbottam T, 229, 256
Higginbotham M, 585, 591, 597, 603, 607, 610, 612, 613, 614
Higginbotham MB, 515, 522, 602, 614
Higgins D, 716, 739
Higgs EA, 633, 645, 694, 732
Higuchi H, 593, 611
Hildebrandt J, 317, 318, 328
Hill AV, 470, 518
Hillman J, 345, 355
Hilsenbeck S, 192, 193, 198
Hilson AJW, 597, 613
Hinder RA, 94, 115
Hinds CJ, 705, 718, 719, 736
Hinshaw LB, 694, 731
Hintz CS, 387, 389, 403
Hiraga A, 46, 72, 108, 511, 514, 522, 532, 549
Hirata S, 364, 378
Hirooka Y, 375, 381
Hirschberg R, 660, 680
Hirschl RB, 317, 318, 328
Hisano R, 364, 365, 366, 378
Hite RD, 319, 329
Hlastala MP, 4, 26, 73, 79, 112, 122, 125, 143, 144, 290, 301, 307, 310, 311, 312, 317, 324, 325, 327, 328
Hnatiuk OW, 570, 577

Hochachka PW, 29, 30, 31, 36, 37, 39, *41*, *42*, *43*, *44*
Hock C, 440, *445*
Hodges MR, 310, *326*
Hodson WA, 79, *112*
Hodson WH, 287, *301*
Hoeg JM, 659, *679*
Hoeppeler H, 387, 389, *403*
Hoffken H, 654, *676*, *677*
Hoffman A, 455, *465*, 707, *736*
Hoffman EA, 54, *109*, 183, *195*
Hoffman JIE, 101, *115*, 368, 369, 370, *378*, *379*, 692, *730*
Hoffman WD, 708, 709, *736*
Hoford JD, 54, *109*
Hogan MC, 15, 20, *27*, 31, 39, *42*, *43*, 95, 107, *116*, *118*, 388, 389, 390, 392, 393, 397, *403*, *404*, *405*, 472, 474, 476, 478, 480, 485, 487, 488, 492, 494, 495, 497, 503, 504, 505, 507, 509, 511, 514, 515, *518*, *519*, *520*, *522*, 532, 535, 537, 538, 542, 545, *549*, *550*, *551*, 638, *647*
Hogan MD, 620, *642*
Hogan RA, 359, 361, 371, *376*, 414, *431*
Hogg JC, 200, *224*, 238, 242, 245, 246, *259*, *260*, 375, *380*, 694, *731*
Hogg W, 209, *226*
Hoing S, 515, *522*
Holden JE, 36, *43*
Hollaar L, 583, *606*
Holland RAB, 87, *114*
Hollander AP, 488, *520*
Holloway PA, 692, *730*
Holm J, 594, *611*
Holm L, 410, 413, *430*
Holmberg H, 720, *740*
Holmgren A, 190, *197*, 264, 267, 271, 272, 274, 275, 278, *282*
Holtz J, 583, *607*
Homans DS, 376, *381*
Homer LD, 390, 391, 395, *404*, 638, *646*
Homsher E, 544, *551*
Hong CD, 662, *681*
Honig C, 589, 590, *609*
Honig CR, 15, 23, *26*, *27*, 30, 39, 40, *42*, *44*, 101, *117*, 372, 373, *380*, 386, 388,

[Honig CR]
390, 392, 394, 398, *401*, *403*, *405*, 470, 483, 496, 497, 498, 499, 500, 503, 504, 506, *518*, *519*, 661, *680*, 693, *731*
Hooder RV, 321, *329*
Hoofd L, 470, *518*, 639, *647*
Hoopes PJ, 101, 103, *117*
Hopferwieser T, 665, *682*
Hopkins SR, 130, *145*, 531, 532, 534, *548*, *549*
Hoppeler H, 55, 91, *109*, *115*, 152, *172*, 387, 389, 394, *402*, *403*, 470, 480, 495, 496, 497, 511, 514, *517*, 539, 540, 544, *550*, *551*
Hopper J, 200, *223*
Horl WH, 660, *680*
Hormann C, 305, 306, 313, *324*
Horn M, 583, *606*
Hornblad Y, 264, 265, 267, 269, 272, 274, 275, 278, *282*
Hornig B, 515, *523*, 588, 603, *609*, *614*
Horsfield K, 51, 53, 54, 57, 66, *109*, *110*
Horstman DH, 383, 391, *401*
Horstman HD, 540, *550*
Hortop J, 693, *731*
Horwitz L, 598, *613*
Horwitz RI, 200, *224*
Hosenpud J, 596, *612*
Hosoda K, 670, *683*
Hotchkiss RS, 428, *434*, 714, *738*
Housely F, 203, 208, *224*
Houssay HEJ, 229, *257*
Houston CS, 23, *27*, 150, 160, 161, *171*, *173*, 526, 537, *547*, *549*
Houston ME, 539, *550*
Howald H, 152, *172*, 539, *550*
Howard P, 229, *256*
Hrager RI, 622, *643*
Hrovat MI, 271, *283*, 571, 572, *578*
Hrycko JN, 318, *328*
Hsia CCW, 56, 61, 79, 85, *109*, *110*, *111*, *112*, *114*, 484, 485, 486, 487, *519*, *520*
Hu K, 583, 603, 605, *606*, *615*
Hu X, 720, *740*
Huang A, 493, *520*, 587, *608*
Huang AH, 370, *379*

Huang CH, 191, *197*
Huang FY, 191, *197*
Huang L, 101, *117*
Huang LE, 641, *647*
Huang YT, 85, *114*
Hubens A, 98, *116*
Huber AR, 722, *741*
Hubmayr RD, 125, *144*
Huckabee WE, 714, *738*
Hudgel DW, 203, *224*
Hudgson P, 659, *679*
Hudlicka O, 389, *404*
Hudson L, 304, 305, *323*
Hudson LD, 307, 311, 312, 319, *324*, *329*, 685, *727*
Huet Y, 286, 290, 291, 292, *300*, 310, 312, *326*
Hughes J, 597, *612*
Hughes JMB, 74, *112*, 271, *282*
Hughson RL, 472, *518*
Hulands GH, 179, 186, 190, *194*, *196*
Hull AR, 650, 668, *676*
Hultman E, 538, *550*
Hultsch E, 191, *197*
Hulund H, 451, 452, *465*
Humer MF, 360, 373, *377*, *380*, 414, 423, 425, *431*, 693, *731*
Humpeler E, 665, *682*
Hunninghake GW, 263, 269, 278, *281*
Hunstman DJ, 555, *574*
Hunt JM, 657, 667, *679*
Hunter CA, 720, *740*
Hunter S, 655, 662, *677*, *681*
Hurford WE, 39, *44*
Hurley B, 560, 566, *575*
Hurtado A, 617, 618, *642*
Hus R, 390, 395, *404*
Hussey JL, 660, *680*
Hutchinson R, 694, *732*
Hutchinson RC, 351, *356*
Hutgren H, 531, 532, *548*
Huyghebaert MF, 359, 361, 373, 374, *377*
Hyatt J, 100, 101, *117*
Hyatt RE, 560, *575*
Hyers TM, 319, 321, *329*
Hyland RH, 204, *225*
Hyman AI, 694, 710, *732*, *736*

I

Iacovoni VE, 210, *226*
Iadecola C, 444, *445*
Iaina A, 657, *679*
Ibels LS, 460, *467*
Iberall AS, 394, 396, *405*
Iberti TJ, 716, 717, *739*
Ice R, 602, *614*
Igarashi Y, 364, 365, *378*
Iglesia R, 222, *228*, 243, *260*, 566, *576*
Ihre E, 215, *227*
Iliff LD, 179, 190, *194*
Imparato A, 603, 605, *615*
Ince C, 105, *118*
Ing TS, 671, *683*
Ingjer F, 539, *550*
Ingram RH, 131, *145*, 557, 565, *574*
Ingwall JS, 583, *606*
Inman WHW, 200, *224*
Inou T, 375, *381*
Inoue C, 220, *228*
Inoue H, 220, *228*
Intaglietta M, 101, *117*, 618, 625, 628, 632, 637, 638, 640, *642*, *644*, *646*
Ioli F, 554, 572, *573*
Ippolito EL, 251, *261*
Irwin SL, 597, *613*
Isabey D, 252, *261*
Isenberg MD, 692, *729*
Ishizak S, 590, *610*
Ishizaka S, 597, *613*
Ito BR, 370, *379*
Ittoop O, 670, *683*
Ivature RR, 705, *735*
Iversen K, 360, 373, 374, *377*
Iversen PO, 122, 132, *143*, *145*
Iwane H, 593, *611*
Iwasaki K, 636, *645*
Iwashita Y, 636, *645*

J

Jackson D, 160, *173*
Jackson JC, 317, 318, *328*
Jackson WF, 400, *407*, 641, *647*

Author Index

Jacob TD, 375, *381*
Jacobs C, 662, 663, 670, *681*
Jacobs DO, 714, *738*
Jacobs LA, 691, 694, 695, *729, 732*
Jacobsen NO, 456, *466*
Jacobsen TN, 658, 668, 669, *679, 683*
Jakic M, 655, *677*
Jakobsen J, 669, *683*
Jakobsson P, 271, *282*
James A, 246, *260*
James PE, 101, *117*
Jamieson JD, 142, *147*
Jamieson S, 583, *607*
Jamieson SW, 296, *302*
Jamison RL, 450, *465*
Janicki J, 583, 596, *607, 612*
Janicki JS, 364, *378*
Jankowski S, 701, *734*
Jansen J, 720, *740*
Jansson E, 539, *550*
Janvier R, 271, *283*
Jardin F, 309, 313, *325*
Jarhult J, 345, *355*
Jarnberg PO, 186, *194*
Jaspar N, 310, 312, *326*
Jedicke H, 656, 664, 670, *678*
Jelicks LA, 39, 40, *43*
Jeneson JAL, 36, *43*
Jenkins M, 200, *223*
Jenkinson SG, 515, *523*
Jenni R, 152, *172*
Jennings DB, 342, *355*
Jensen RL, 142, *148*
Jensen T, 662, *681*
Jepson MM, 714, *738*
Jernudd-Wilhelmsson Y, 264, 265, 267, 269, 272, 274, 275, 278, *282*
Jesse R, 637, *645*
Jia L, 617, 618, 621, 624, 626, 632, 633, 641, *642*
Jiang J, 101, 103, *117*
Jiang ZL, 53, *109*
Jianhua L, 106, 107, *118*
Jobin J, 271, *283*, 554, 566, *573, 576*
Jobsis F, 105, *118*
Jobsis-Vandervliert FF, 105, *118*
Jodal M, 427, *433*
Johannessen NW, 177, 178, *193*

Johannigman J, 318, *328*
Johansson H, 190, *197*
Johns RA, 192, *197*
Johnson PC, 101, *117*
Johnson A, 289, *301*
Johnson AC, 531, 532, 534, *548*
Johnson BD, 480, *519*, 560, *575*
Johnson DH, 531, 532, 534, *548*
Johnson EC, 130, *145*, 494, 495, 507, 511, *520*, 537, *549*
Johnson ES, 537, *549*
Johnson FL, 85, *114*
Johnson K, 317, 318, *328*
Johnson PC, 411, *430*, 629, 630, 632, 637, 640, *644, 646, 647*
Johnson R, 598, *613*
Johnson RG, 36, *43*
Johnson RL, 56, 61, 74, 79, 83, 84, 85, *109, 110, 111, 112, 113, 114*, 152, 156, *172*, 209, *226*, 484, 485, 486, 487, *519*, 565, 566, *576*
Johnstone EE, 583, *607*
Jondeau G, 586, 588, 591, *608, 610*
Jones AM, 470, 476, *517*
Jones D, 590, 591, *610*
Jones DP, 388, 392, *403*, 414, *431*
Jones HA, 74, *112*
Jones LL, 539, *550*
Jones N, 605, *615*
Jones NL, 49, 61, 85, *108, 111*, 229, *257*, 484, 485, 486, 487, *519*, 557, 565, 566, *574, 576*
Jones PW, 229, *257*
Jones R, 588, 589, *609*
Jones RA, 588, *609*
Jones RT, 635, *645*
Jones S, 539, *550*
Jones T, 98, *116*
Jordan L, 597, *613*
Jordan S, 599, 600, *614*
Jorfeldt L, 271, *282*, 394, *406*
Jorge M, 428, *434*, 705, 706, *735*
Jorgensen CR, 364, *378*
Jorntorp B, 594, *611*
Joseph D, 715, 717, *739*
Joseph K, 654, *676, 677*
Jost CM, 658, 668, 669, *679, 683*
Jost U, 451, 462, *465*

Jover L, 241, *259*
Jubert P, 715, 717, *739*
Jue T, 39, 40, *44*, 106, *118*
Jugdutt B, 603, 605, *615*
Jukes MGM, 478, 480, 481, 482, *519*
Julian MW, 426, *433*
Julou-Schaeffer G, 424, *432*
Juno P, 184, *195*
Juric M, 655, *677*
Just H, 375, *381*, 515, *522*, 583, 588, 590, *607*, *609*, *610*
Justice R, 692, *729*

K

Kachel HG, 669, *683*
Kafer ER, 189, *196*
Kahn RJ, 351, *356*, 699, 700, 701, 703, 714, 720, 721, 724, *733*, *734*, *740*
Kai H, 375, *381*
Kai M, 46, 72, *108*, 511, 514, *522*, 532, *549*
Kairalla RA, 305, 313, 321, *324*, *329*
Kaiser KG, 318, *328*
Kaiser L, 586, 587, *608*
Kal JE, 360, *377*
Kalberer B, 603, *614*
Kaley G, 493, *520*, 587, *608*, 632, 637, *645*
Kallmeyer JC, 532, *548*
Kalman FS, 655, *678*
Kameyama T, 590, 597, *610*, *613*
Kamimura CT, 373, *380*
Kaminski N, 456, *466*
Kampe M, 213, *227*
Kampp M, 418, *431*
Kanai AJ, 375, *381*
Kanber GJ, 142, *147*
Kaneko K, 164, *174*
Kanenko K, 122, *143*
Kanfer A, 655, *677*
Kao AC, 515, *522*
Kapitan K, 212, *227*
Kapitan KS, 136, 139, *146*, *147*, 296, *302*
Kappagoda C, 603, 605, *615*

Kari S, 691, 693, 694, *729*
Karl IE, 428, *434*, 713, 714, *738*
Karmeli F, 456, *466*
Karner I, 655, *677*
Kaschula ROC, 20, *27*, 657, *679*
Kasper SM, 637, *646*
Kassab GS, 53, *109*
Kastenbauer T, 653, *676*
Katayama Y, 254, *261*
Katsouyanni K, 701, *734*
Katusic ZS, 591, *610*
Katz DP, 724, *741*
Katz LA, 660, *680*
Katz LN, 360, *377*
Katz S, 583, 585, 591, *607*, *610*
Katz SD, 587, 588, *608*
Kaufman BS, 699, 700, *733*
Kaufmann J, 662, *681*
Kawaguchi O, 375, 376, *380*, *381*
Kawaguchi Y, 662, *681*
Kawashiro T, 544, *551*
Kayar SR, 387, 389, 394, *402*, *403*
Kazaglis J, 425, *432*
Kazerooni EA, 317, 318, *328*
Kazuwa N, 670, *683*
Kedziora J, 667, *682*
Keens TG, 204, *225*
Keipert PE, 503, 504, *522*, 637, 638, *646*, *647*
Kellerman JJ, 657, *679*
Kelley K, 707, *736*
Kelley VE, 456, *466*
Kellogg DL, 336, *353*
Kellum JA, 701, *734*
Kelly D, 93, *115*, 350, *356*
Kelly GE, 49, *108*
Kelly J, 125, *144*
Kelly SM, 691, 694, *729*
Kelman GR, 61, *111*, 203, *224*
Kely D, 425, *432*
Kemp GJ, 662, *680*
Kempeneers G, 665, *682*
Kemper BA, 710, *736*
Kemper M, 694, 710, *732*
Kempm GJ, 662, 664, *680*
Kendrick K, 494, 495, 507, 511, *520*, 588, 589, *609*

Kendrick KF, 15, *26*, 39, 40, *44*, 497, *521*, 537, 545, *549*, *552*
Kennedy F, 705, 706, 707, *736*
Kennedy FG, 388, 392, *403*, 414, *431*
Kennedy TC, 136, *147*
Kenney JS, 691, *729*
Kenny D, 376, *381*
Kent J, 30, *42*
Kent JC, 715, 717, *739*
Keogh BA, 263, 269, 278, *281*, 565, *576*
Kerb W, 20, *27*
Kerber RE, 370, *379*
Kerger H, 618, 625, 628, *642*
Kernerman P, 719, 720, *740*
Kerstein M, 638, *646*
Kes P, 655, *677*
Kety SS, 67, 96, 97, *111*, *116*, 435, 436, *444*
Keyeux A, 204, *225*
Khalabeigui F, 364, *378*
Khan S, 586, 587, *608*
Kharitonov VG, 633, *645*
Khouri EM, 360, 371, *377*
Kiel JW, 411, *430*
Kiens B, 386, 391, *402*, 537, 538, *549*
Kiesow LA, 390, 391, 395, *404*, 638, *646*
Kiess M, 697, 699, 705, *733*
Kilbourn RG, 352, *357*
Kilcoyne CM, 659, *679*
Kilian J, 714, *738*
Killer A, 493, *520*, 632, 637, *645*
Killian KJ, 566, *576*
Kilmartin JV, 623, 624, *643*, *644*
Kim FJ, 724, 725, 726, *742*
Kim SB, 662, *681*
Kim SJ, 360, *377*
Kim WD, 238, *259*
Kimmich HP, 49, *108*
Kimura H, 152, *172*, 527, *547*
Kinasewitz G, 583, 596, *607*, *612*
Kindig CA, 502, 504, 509, 510, 515, *521*, *523*
Kindman A, 596, 599, 600, *612*, *614*
King C, 587, *608*
King CE, 346, *355*, 360, 361, 371, *377*, *380*, 414, 426, *431*, 693, 694, 695, *731*
King D, 719, 720, *740*

King FW, 142, *147*
King GG, 207, 209, *226*
King M, 238, *259*
King RB, 370, *379*, 421, *431*
King RR, 532, *548*
King RV, 593, *611*
King TE, 263, 265, 269, 276, *281*
King TKC, 229, *257*
Kingaby GP, 166, *175*
King-Van Vlack CE, 352, *357*
Kinney JM, 591, *610*, 694, 710, *732*, *736*
Kipnis DM, 713, 714, *738*
Kirk KR, 57, *110*
Kirklin JK, 370, *379*
Kirlin PC, 583, *607*
Kirshenbaum J, 596, *612*
Kirshner HS, 659, *679*
Kirtz W, 450, *465*
Kiser R, 203, *225*
Kjellmer I, 386, *402*
Klar J, 686, *728*
Klas JV, 570, *577*
Klausner JM, 724, *741*
Kleeberg UR, 619, *642*
Klein F, 428, *434*, 705, 706, *735*
Klein HG, 541, *551*
Klein T, 456, *466*
Kleinerman J, 238, *259*
Kleinsasser A, 310, 321, *326*
Klinkmann H, 663, 664, *682*
Klitzman B, 390, 391, 392, 394, 397, *404*, 407
Kloner RA, 620, *643*
Klotz IM, 635, *645*
Kluger R, 635, *645*
Knabb RM, 360, 370, *377*, *379*
Knapp E, 665, *682*
Knaus W, 286, 290, 291, 292, *300*
Knaus WA, 686, 687, *727*
Knichtwitz G, 715, *739*
Knierim N, 656, *678*
Knight BK, 20, *27*, 657, *679*
Knight DR, 20, *27*, 95, *116*, 310, *325*, 471, 472, 476, 478, 488, 492, 494, 495, 505, 507, 509, 511, *518*, *519*, *520*, *521*, 531, 532, 534, 537, *548*, *549*
Knochel JP, 667, 671, *682*

Knopp TJ, 181, 184, *194*, *195*
Knudson DE, 136, *147*
Knudson RJ, 136, *147*
Kobzik L, 724, *741*
Koc D, 304, *323*
Koch KM, 655, 669, *677*, *683*
Koeppe RA, 318, *328*
Koerner SK, 297, *302*, 554, *573*, 691, 694, *729*
Kohzuki H, 620, *643*
Kolb G, 654, *676*, *677*
Kole YMM, 98, *116*
Kolkman JJ, 703, 715, 717, *735*, *739*
Koller A, 587, *608*
Koller W, 314, *327*, 701, *734*
Komaru T, 370, *379*
Komatsu T, 695, *732*
Komhoff M, 456, *466*
Kone BC, 456, *466*
Konertz W, 192, *198*
Konietzko N, 619, *642*
Konig H, 590, *610*
Kono I, 670, *683*
Kontos HA, 158, *173*
Koopman PAR, 693, *731*
Kopple JD, 660, *680*
Kor SW, 583, *606*
Korgh A, 544, *551*
Korthuis RJ, 337, *353*, 470, 488, 491, 492, 493, 494, 495, *517*
Korunda MJ, 714, *738*
Kosonen J, 162, 163, *174*
Kosonen JM, 122, *144*
Kouyoumdjian C, 254, *261*
Kovacs JA, 424, *432*
Koziol BJ, 660, 670, *680*
Kraemer M, 596, *612*
Krafft P, 304, *323*
Kragsbjerg P, 720, *740*
Krahenbuhl B, 594, *611*
Kram HB, 697, 705, 706, 718, *733*, *736*
Kramer DJ, 342, *354*, 692, 701, 710, *730*, *734*, *736*
Kramer HG, 670, *683*
Kramer JJ, 125, *144*
Kramer-Johansen J, 122, *143*
Kraning KK, 713, *737*

Krasney JA, 341, *354*
Krasnow F, 655, 665, *678*
Krasnow N, 655, *678*
Krastins IRB, 204, *225*
Krauer R, 91, *115*, 387, 389, *403*
Krausz MM, 294, *301*
Krayer S, 183, *195*
Kreimeier U, 692, *730*
Kreutzer U, 39, 40, *44*, 106, *118*
Kreuzer F, 49, 90, *108*, *114*, 152, 156, *172*, 390, 393, 394, *404*, 470, *518*, 639, *647*
Krishnan B, 558, 559, 560, 571, *574*, *575*
Kroenke K, 192, 193, *198*
Krogh A, 12, *26*, 66, 81, 89, *111*, *113*, *114*, 386, 389, 390, 391, *402*, *404*, 623, 629, *643*, *644*
Krogh M, 81, *113*
Kronenberg RS, 152, *172*, 619, *642*
Kruezer F, 152, *172*
Krugmire RB, 593, *611*
Kruhoffer P, 85, *114*
Kruithoff KL, 101, *117*, 704, *735*
Kruse JA, 428, *433*, 699, 700, 701, *733*, *734*
Kryger M, 209, *226*
Ku DD, 370, *379*
Kubal K, 695, *732*
Kubes P, 344, *355*
Kubler W, 603, *614*
Kubo H, 662, *681*
Kubo K, 46, 72, *108*, 511, 514, *522*, 532, *549*
Kubo S, 212, *227*, 596, *612*
Kubo SH, 583, 586, 587, *607*, *608*
Kuchan MJ, 638, *646*
Kuchinsky W, 437, 440, *445*
Kud CD, 720, *740*
Kuhlmann M, 715, *739*
Kuhn M, 663, *681*
Kuhnle GE, 133, *145*
Kukielka G, 375, *381*
Kumar V, 695, *732*
Kunert MP, 621, 638, *643*
Kung MD, 206, *225*
Kunitomo F, 152, *172*

Author Index 773

Kunkel SL, 375, *381*, 721, *740*
Kuo HS, 720, *740*
Kurdak S, 488, 511, *520*
Kurdak SS, 39, *43*, 389, 392, 393, *404*, 494, 495, 507, 511, *520*, 531, 532, 534, 537, *548*, *549*, 638, *647*
Kurijiaka DT, 385, 386, 399, *401*, *402*, *407*, 494, *520*
Kurita D, 271, *282*, 566, *577*
Kuriyama T, 152, *172*
Kurosawa Y, 593, *611*
Kurtin P, 660, *680*
Kurtz A, 464, *467*
Kurz S, 583, *607*
Kushmerick MJ, 30, 31, 36, *42*, *43*, 387, 388, *403*
Kushner R, 694, 710, *732*
Kusumi F, 691, 703, *729*
Kutsuzawa T, 271, *282*, 566, *577*
Kuvhenguwha A, 705, 706, 707, *736*
Kuwano K, 245, *260*
Kuzil BB, 515, *522*
Kvart C, 184, *195*
Kvetan V, 724, *741*
Kviele L, 185, *196*
Kvietys PR, 93, 94, *115*, 413, *431*

L

La Belle P, 655, 665, *678*
La Canna G, 655, 662, *677*
La Froce RC, 57, 66, *110*
La Manca J, 605, *615*
Labeeuw M, 662, *681*
Laderoute KR, 641, *647*
Laevy J, 701, *734*
Lagerstrand L, 137, *147*, 212, 213, 215, *227*
Lahiri S, 150, 152, 161, *171*, *172*, *173*, 526, 527, *547*
Lahrmann H, 653, *676*
Laine JF, 286, 289, *301*
Lakatos E, 565, *576*
Lake DC, 200, *224*
Laks H, 596, *612*
Lalka D, 707, *736*

Lam C, 375, *380*, 424, 425, *432*, 693, *731*
LaManca J, 598, 599, 600, 601, *613*, *614*
LaManca JL, 105, *118*
Lamarra N, 46, *108*
Lamb G, 716, *739*
Lambalgen AA, 693, *731*
Lambert M, 660, 665, *680*, *682*
Lamm JEM, 73, *112*
Lamm WJ, 122, *143*
Lamm WJE, 57, *110*
Lammer H, 192, *197*
Lammertsma AA, 98, *116*
Lamping KG, 370, *379*
Lampron N, 307, *325*
Lamy M, 304, 305, *323*
Lancaster JR, 633, *645*
Landau L, 200, *224*
Landes RG, 457, *466*
Landes RR, 451, 452, *465*
Landis EM, 544, *551*
Landry G, 480, 484, 485, *519*
Lane LD, 165, *174*
Lang CH, 691, *729*
Lang DJ, 632, *644*
Lange F, 309, *325*
Lange H, 654, 656, 664, 670, *676*, *677*, *678*
Lange HJ, 142, *147*
Lange P, 691, 694, 695, *729*, *732*
Langeron O, 314, 320, 322, *327*, *329*
Langman V, 55, *109*
Langseetmo I, 471, 474, *518*
Lanigan C, 555, *574*
Lankford SP, 452, 458, 463, *465*
Lapidot C, 657, *679*
Lapinsky SE, 321, *329*
Laravuso RB, 76, *112*, 135, *146*, 230, 231, *257*, 263, 276, *281*, 285, *300*, 303, 306, 307, 312, *323*, *324*
Large SR, 241, *259*
Larrabee P, 583, *607*
Larsen LE, 177, 178, *193*
Larssen NA, 96, *116*, 444, 445
Larsson K, 215, *227*
Lasch HG, 319, *328*
Laser M, 583, *606*

Lategola M, 348, *356*
Lategola MT, 131, *145*
Latham LP, 57, 60, 66, *110*
Latini R, 313, *327*, 705, 718, 719, *736*
Lau CP, 658, 670, *679*
Laughlin MH, 337, *353*, 385, 400, *401*, 470, 488, 491, 492, 493, 494, 495, *517*
Lautt WW, 412, *430*
Lauzon AM, 170, *175*
Laver MB, 184, *195*
Law WR, 360, *377*
Lawin P, 191, *197*
Lawler J, 480, 484, 485, *519*
Lawler PGP, 715, *739*
Lawrence F, 192, 193, *198*
Lawson MS, 620, *643*
Laxson DD, 376, *381*
Lazaro RP, 659, *679*
Lazarus NA, 655, *678*
Le Bas JF, 271, *282*, 566, *577*
Le Gall JR, 686, *728*
Leach-Huntoon CS, 166, *174*
Lear S, 456, *466*
Leary WP, 532, *548*
Leasa D, 317, *328*
Leather R, 347, *355*, 427, *433*
Leathers D, 602, *614*
Leaver DG, 560, 562, *575*
Leblanc P, 183, *195*, 271, *283*, 554, 566, *573, 576*
Leddy C, 596, *612*
Ledingham J, 588, 589, 594, *609, 611*
Ledingham JG, 662, 664, *680*, 692, *730*
Lee AP, 602, *614*
Lee DK, 662, *681*
Lee J, 220, *227*
Lee K, 701, *734*
Lee LN, 212, *227*
Lee TS, 705, 706, 718, *736*
Lee TY, 720, *740*
Leeman M, 292, 294, *301, 302*, 310, 311, 312, 320, 321, *326*, 701, *734*
Leeman N, 286, 287, 288, 289, 290, 292, 293, *300*
Leeman P, 221, *228*
Lees DE, 695, *732*
Lefevre G, 359, 361, 373, 374, *377*

Lefevre J, 132, *145*
Leff AR, 424, *432*
Legall JR, 304, 305, *323*
Legge JS, 205, *225*
Legrand A, 566, *575*
Leibowitz AB, 716, 717, *739*
Leichtweiss HP, 451, 452, *465*
Leieth DE, 188, *196*
Leigh JS, 15, *26*, 30, 39, 40, *42, 44*, 497, *521*, 545, *552*, 588, 589, *609*
Leith DE, 55, *109*
LeJemtel T, 585, 605, *608, 615*
LeJemtel TH, 586, 588, 591, *608*, 610
Lejeune P, 221, *228*, 231, 236, *257*, 286, 287, 288, 289, 290, 292, 293, 294, 295, *300, 301, 302*, 310, 312, 320, *326*
LeMahiew I, 98, *116*
Lemaire F, 251, 252, *260, 261*, 286, 290, 291, 292, *300*, 305, 307, 309, 310, 312, 313, 314, 319, 320, 322, *324, 325, 326, 327, 329*
Leman M, 293, 294, *301*
Lemeshow S, 686, *728*
Lemon DJ, 624, *644*
Lenfant C, 540, *550*, 623, *643*, 690, *728*
Lenkinski R, 588, 590, 591, *609, 610*
Lennard ES, 687, *728*
Lenzen N, 192, *198*
Lenzi GL, 98, *116*
Leon M, 701, *734*
Leonhardt KO, 451, 452, *465*
Lerch R, 376, *381*
LeRoy B, 351, *356*
Letac B, 602, *614*
Letbetter WD, 396, *406*
Leung WH, 658, 670, *679*
Levasseru JE, 158, *173*
Levin D, 565, *575*
Levine BD, 165, *174*
Levine BE, 304, 305, *323*
Levine E, 690, *728*
Levine G, 203, 208, *224*
Levine H, 638, *646*
Levine L, 294, *301*
Levine M, 595, 596, *612*
Levine S, 598, 599, 600, 601, 605, *613, 614, 615*

Author Index

Levine SM, 515, *523*
Levine TB, 583, *606*
Levison H, 204, *225*, 555, *574*
Levitzki A, 707, *736*
Lev-Tov A, 397, *407*
Levy MM, 705, *736*
Levy P, 271, *282*, 566, *577*
Levy RD, 515, *523*, 570, *577*
LeWinter MM, 364, *378*
Lewis BM, 57, 66, 85, *110*, *114*
Lewis DH, 98, *116*, 394, *406*
Lewis MK, 691, 694, *729*
Lewis NP, 654, 655, 662, *677*, *678*
Lewis S, 200, *224*
Lewis SF, 106, *118*
Lexell J, 400, *407*
Ley PC, 297, *302*
Lezotte DC, 701, *734*
Li C, 376, *381*
Li H, 588, 589, *609*
Li QQ, 200, *224*
Liang CS, 583, *607*
Liao R, 583, *606*
Liard JF, 621, 638, *643*
Liggins GC, 39, *44*
Light RW, 565, 566, *576*, 638, *646*
Lighton JRB, 29, *42*
Lileinthal JL, 81, *113*
Liljestrand G, 189, *196*, 237, *259*, 318, *328*
Lillehei RC, 457, *466*
Lillie MA, 345, *355*
Lilly RE, 366, *378*
Lim TH, 662, *681*
Lin CJ, 191, *197*
Lin L, 85, *114*
Lind AR, 386, *402*
Lindberg P, 178, *193*
Lindbom L, 373, *380*, 421, *432*, 628, 629, 630, 640, *644*
Lindell P, 192, *197*
Linden GS, 565, 566, *576*
Lindhard J, 66, *111*
Lindner K, 714, *738*
Lindsay WG, 457, *466*
Lindstedt SL, 387, 389, *402*, *403*
Line BR, 263, 269, 278, *280*, *281*

Linehan JH, 57, *110*
Lingnau W, 192, *197*
Linnarsson D, 125, *144*, 471, 481, *518*
Linstedt SL, 544, *551*
Lipkin D, 590, 599, 600, *610*, *614*
Lipkin DP, 597, *613*
Lipowsky HH, 101, *115*
Lippmann M, 286, *300*
Lipton P, 441, *445*
Lipworth BJ, 254, *261*
Lisander B, 394, *405*
Lisbona R, 70, *111*, 166, *174*
Lissoni A, 304, 305, *324*
Lister G, 341, *354*
Little TL, 370, *379*
Liu CC, 345, *355*
Liu F, 101, *117*
Liu KJ, 101, 103, *117*
Liu N, 320, 322, *329*
Livesey J, 539, *550*
Livingston DH, 724, *742*
Lloyd BB, 478, 480, 481, 482, *519*
Lloyd TC, 57, *110*
Lobdell K, 694, 695, *732*
Lobo J, 558, 559, *574*
Lockhart A, 237, *259*, 566, *575*, 599, *614*
Lockhat D, 697, 699, 705, *733*
Lodato RF, 570, *577*
Loeb GE, 397, *407*
Loeffler HD, 665, 666, *682*
Loewy A, 150, *171*
Lofaso F, 252, *261*
Logan MR, 183, *195*
Loh L, 189, *196*
Lohse MJ, 583, *607*
Loisance D, 309, 313, *325*
Loke J, 566, *576*
Long KA, 572, *578*
Long W, 319, *329*
Longhurst J, 587, *608*
Longmore WJ, 319, *329*
Loopez AG, 375, *381*
Lopaschuk GD, 375, *380*
Lopez F, 254, *261*, 310, 312, 320, *326*
Lopez FA, 312, 313, 315, 319, 320, *327*, *329*, 654, 655, *677*
Lopez RA, 130, *145*

Lorenz JN, 388, *404*, 546, *552*
Lorenzana A, 716, *739*
Lorenzi-Fiho G, 305, 313, 321, *324*, *329*
Lorino AM, 307, *325*
Louy C, 544, *551*
Low LW, 101, *117*
Lowe C, 317, 318, *328*
Lowe PG, 142, *147*
Lowensohn HS, 368, 369, *378*
Lowrie EG, 650, 668, *676*
Lowry OH, 387, *403*
Lowry SF, 691, 720, 721, 722, *729*, *740*
Lowson SM, 192, *197*
Lu Y, 312, 317, *327*
Lubbers D, 99, *117*
Lubbers DW, 98, 101, 102, *116*, *117*, 451, 452, *465*
Lucas CE, 693, *730*
Lucas MK, 200, *224*
Luce JM, 426, *433*
Luchtel Dl, 125, *144*
Luciak M, 667, *682*
Lucido D, 587, *608*
Luck JC, 101, *115*
Lucke B, 457, *466*
Lucke JC, 366, *378*
Ludens JH, 671, *684*
Lund MP, 440, *445*
Lund N, 93, 98, *115*, *116*, 350, *356*, 393, 394, 398, 399, *405*, *406*, 425, *432*
Lundberg G, 594, *611*
Lundberg J, 255, *261*
Lundgren O, 410, 413, 418, 427, *430*, *431*, *433*, 703, *735*
Lundh B, 184, *195*
Lundholm G, 714, *738*
Lundin AP, 655, 656, 657, 665, *677*, *678*
Lundquist H, 178, 180, 181, 182, 183, 185, 186, 190, *193*, *194*, *195*, *196*, *197*
Lundvall J, 345, *355*
Lupton H, 470, *518*
Lutch JS, 711, 712, *737*
Luthi P, 539, *550*
Lutz H, 692, *730*
Luz G, 427, *433*
Luzzana M, 622, 624, 625, *643*, *644*

Lynch JP, 303, 305, 307, 309, 310, 311, 312, 313, *323*, *325*, 347, *356*, 427, *433*, 699, 700, *733*
Lyons HA, 202, 204, *224*

M

Maberly DJ, 203, *224*
Maccari F, 660, *680*
Macdonald IC, 500, 509, 513, *521*, *522*
MacDonald VW, 637, 638, *646*
MacDougall IC, 654, 655, 662, *677*, *678*
MacIntosh DJ, 82, *113*
MacIntyre NR, 85, *114*
Mackay CJ, 716, *739*
Mackenzie A, 721, *740*
Mackie BG, 389, 400, *404*
Macklem P, 67, *111*, 209, *226*
Macklem PT, 242, *259*, 570, *577*, 691, 694, *729*
MacLeod P, 203, 208, *224*
Macquin-Mavier I, 251, *260*
MacScarraigh ET, 532, *548*
Madoff RD, 687, *728*
Maeda S, 670, *683*
Maehara K, 487, 507, *520*
Magaldi RB, 321, *329*
Maginniss LA, 342, 344, *354*, 411, 422, *430*
Magistretti PJ, 437, 440, 441, *445*
Mahieu D, 286, 290, 291, 292, *300*
Mahieu O, 91, *115*
Mahler DA, 566, *576*
Mahler M, 469, 470, 471, 472, 474, 475, 476, 482, *517*, *518*, 544, *551*
Mahutte CK, 565, *576*
Mai NTH, 714, *738*
Maier GW, 366, *378*
Maier V, 603, *614*
Mainwood GW, 387, 392, 394, *402*
Mairbaurl H, 665, *682*
Maistre G, 662, 663, 670, *681*
Mak M, 351, *356*, 694, *732*
Maki S, 670, *683*
Makowska M, 163, *174*
Mal H, 310, 312, *326*

Author Index

Malagari K, 701, *734*
Malconian MK, 23, *27*, 136, *146*, 156, 158, 159, 160, 170, *173*, *175*, 529, 530, 531, 532, 533, 537, *548*, *549*
Malem PT, 203, 208, *224*
Malik AB, 289, *301*
Malin F, 204, *225*
Malinski T, 375, *381*
Malinverni C, 603, 605, *615*
Malmkvist G, 189, *197*
Maloiy GMO, 46, *108*
Maloney JE, 166, *175*
Maltais F, 271, *283*, 554, 566, *573*, *576*
Malvin GM, 503, *522*
Mancebo J, 252, *261*
Mancini D, 583, 585, 588, 589, 591, 598, *607*, *609*, *610*, *613*
Mancini DM, 588, 590, 591, 597, 599, 600, 601, 605, *609*, *610*, *612*, *613*, *614*, *615*
Mandel F, 671, *684*
Manfredi F, 566, *577*
Mangalaboyi J, 105, *118*
Manier G, 231, 235, 236, 243, 256, *257*, *258*, *260*, *261*, 285, 286, 290, 291, 292, *300*
Manikis P, 425, *432*, 701, *734*
Mankad S, 701, *734*
Mann D, 464, *467*
Mannal R, 347, *355*, 427, *433*
Manninen DL, 650, 668, *676*
Mannino FL, 318, *328*
Mannix ET, 566, *577*
Manny J, 692, *729*
Mansell A, 204, *225*
Mansell AL, 161, *173*
Manthous CA, 428, *434*, 694, 710, 711, 712, *732*, *737*
Mantz P, 669, *683*
Marades RM, 139, *147*
Marano MA, 691, *729*
Marciniuk D, 565, *576*
Marciniuk DD, 265, 271, 272, 273, 276, 282, *283*, 555, 557, 560, 561, 562, 564, 565, 567, 568, 569, 570, 571, *574*, *575*, *577*
Marcolin R, 304, 305, *323*, *324*

Marconi C, 14, *26*, 397, *407*, 491, *520*
Marcus JH, 557, 565, *574*
Marcus ML, 370, *379*
Maret KH, 150, 170, *171*, *175*, 527, 529, 530, 537, *547*
Margairaz A, 309, 313, *325*
Marik PE, 693, 704, 709, 711, 712, 713, 715, 716, *731*, *735*, *737*, *739*
Marini C, 394, *406*
Marini MA, 637, *645*
Maris J, 588, 589, *609*, 714, *738*
Mark AL, 593, *611*
Markham A, 662, *681*
Markowitz D, 566, *576*
Marks BH, 583, *606*
Maroko PR, 620, *643*
Marouka Y, 375, *381*
Marr C, 347, *355*, 427, *433*
Marrades R, 217, 222, *227*, 515, *523*
Marrades RM, 4, 20, *26*, *27*, 231, 236, 243, *258*, 566, *576*, 659, 662, 663, 664, *679*, *680*
Marsh M, 184, *195*
Marshall BE, 130, 142, *145*, *147*, 184, 189, 190, *195*, *197*, 691, 703, 704, *729*
Marshall H, 73, *112*
Marshall J, 690, *729*
Marshall JC, 686, 687, *727*, *728*
Marshall JM, 588, *608*
Marshall T, 718, *740*
Marshall W, 703, *735*
Marthan R, 235, 236, *258*
Martin AW, 413, *430*
Martin C, 375, *380*, 424, *432*, 690, 693, *729*, *731*
Martin CJ, 73, *112*
Martin CM, 425, *432*
Martin E, 722, *741*
Martin GV, 370, *379*
Martin J, 585, *608*
Martin JG, 570, *577*
Martin JL, 508, *522*, 620, *642*
Martin LD, 311, *326*
Martin Malo A, 667, *682*
Martin NL, 671, *684*
Martin S, 713, *738*
Martin WH, 483, *519*

Martonen TB, 84, *113*
Marty JJ, 206, *225*
Marvidis G, 654, *677*
Marzo K, 599, *613*
Marzo KP, 597, *613*
Mascheroni D, 304, 305, 317, *324, 328*
Mascia L, 313, *327*
Masclans JR, 20, *27*, 515, *523*, 659, 662, 663, 664, *679, 680*
Masin G, 669, *683*
Maskin C, 585, *608*
Maskin CS, 587, *608*
Mason AD, 694, *732*
Mason D, 587, *608*
Mason DT, 581, 584, *606*
Mason R, 715, 717, *739*
Massey KD, 375, *381*
Massie B, 588, 589, *609*
Massie BM, 591, *610*
Masson F, 662, 663, 670, *681*
Mastai R, 264, *281*
Masuyama S, 152, *172*
Matamis D, 307, 312, 313, *324, 325*
Mateo J, 320, *329*
Mates EA, 317, 318, *328*
Matheson GO, 30, 31, 37, *42, 43*
Mathews WR, 671, *684*
Mathieu O, 91, *115*, 387, 389, *403*
Mathieu-Costello O, 289, *301*, 363, *378*, 387, 389, *402*, 500, 501, 502, 509, 513, 515, *521, 522, 523*, 531, 532, *548, 549*
Mathieu-Costello OA, 29, *42*
Matran R, 599, *614*
Matsen FA, 593, *611*
Matsuda H, 641, *647*
Matsuda M, 670, *683*
Matsumura K, 620, *643*
Matsuyama S, 527, *547*
Matthay MA, 426, *433*
Matthay RA, 566, *576*
Matthews JI, 566, *576*
Matthews ME, 132, *145*
Matthys H, 619, *642*
Matuschak GM, 692, *729*
Mauck HP, 158, *173*
Maurer JR, 271, *283*

Maxwell LC, 387, 389, *403*, 411, 417, *430, 431*
Maycock P, 694, *732*
Mayer G, 655, *677*
Maynard N, 715, 717, *739*
Mayoral J, 636, *645*
Mazer CD, 321, *329*
Mazure NM, 641, *647*
Mazzeo RS, 540, *550*
Mazzone R, 311, 313, *326*
Mazzone RW, 286, 290, *301*
Mc Evoy RD, 318, *328*
McAllister RM, 470, 488, 491, 492, 493, 494, 495, *517*
McAlpine W, 362, *377*
Mcavoy JL, 532, *548*
McCammon AT, 722, *741*
McCance A, 591, 597, 603, *610, 613, 614*
McCarthy D, 209, *226*
McCarthy G, 184, *195*
McCarthy M, 591, *610*, 636, *645*
McClaran SR, 386, *401*, 480, *519*
Mcclean PA, 271, *283*
McClement JH, 269, *282*
McCord JM, 724, 725, *741*
McCormack JG, 36, *43*
McCullough RE, 538, 545, *550*
McCullough RG, 538, 545, *550*
McCully K, 30, *42*, 593, *610*
McCully KK, 590, 591, *610*
McCumber TR, 570, *577*
McDevitt DG, 254, *261*
McDonald DM, 526, *547*
McDonald RH, 364, *378*
McEvan A, 594, *611*
McFadden ER, 202, 203, 204, *224, 225*
McFadden M, 161, *173*
McGillivray-Anderson KM, 386, *402*
McGilvery RW, 39, *44*
McGoon D, 595, *611*
McGough E, 98, *116*
McHale P, 585, *607*
McIlroy MB, 483, *519*
McInnes LM, 125, *144*
McIntyre KM, 292, 294, *301*
McKay CB, 638, *646*

Author Index

McKay R, 595, *612*
Mckechnie JK, 532, *548*
McKenna HP, 79, *112*
McKenna TM, 424, *432*
McKenzie DC, 31, *43*
McKenzie DK, 202, *224*
Mckinney S, 125, *144*
McKinney SE, 125, 133, *144*
McKinnis R, 602, *614*
McKneally SS, 541, *551*
McLean RF, 321, *329*
McLean RL, 557, 565, *574*
McMahon TJ, 618, 641, *642*
McMurphy R, 73, *112*, 122, *143*
McMurray RG, 655, 665, *678*
McNeill JR, 412, *430*, 692, *730*
McNutt M, 200, *224*
McParland C, 558, 559, 560, 569, 571, *573*, *574*, *575*
McPhaul JJ, 657, 667, *679*
McRae J, 166, *175*, 207, *226*
Meade MO, 321, *329*
Meadows DA, 396, *406*
Meakins JL, 703, *735*
Meanly JF, 317, 318, *328*
Mears H, 594, *611*
Mecham RP, 131, *145*
Meddeiros DM, 305, 313, 321, *324*, *329*
Medina F, 637, *645*
Medoff B, 566, *576*
Mehdaoui H, 351, *356*
Meherke G, 340, *354*
Mehta JL, 586, 587, *608*
Mehta N, 717, *740*
Meierhenrich R, 656, 664, 670, *678*
Meinen LG, 340, *354*
Melinyshyn M, 344, *355*
Mellemgaard K, 142, *147*
Melot C, 221, *228*, 231, 236, 251, 253, 256, *257*, *260*, *261*, 286, 287, 288, 289, 290, 291, 292, 293, 294, 295, 298, *299*, *300*, *301*, *302*, 310, 311, 312, 320, 321, *326*
Melsom MN, 122, 125, *143*, *144*
Menager P, 105, *118*
Menlove R, 583, *607*
Menon RS, 36, *43*

Mercer RR, 52, *109*
Meredith JW, 704, 709, 715, *735*
Mertens P, 231, *257*
Mertes N, 715, *739*
Mertsola J, 691, 693, 694, *729*
Mertz WR, 692, *730*
Mery JP, 655, *677*
Merzouk T, 663, 664, *682*
Mesaros S, 375, *381*
Messer-Rehak D, 655, 657, *678*
Messina LM, 368, *379*
Messmer K, 692, *730*
Metcalfe J, 620, *643*
Metra M, 655, 662, *677*
Metz KF, 655, *678*
Meusburger S, 427, *433*
Meuwissen SG, 715, 717, *739*
Meyer M, 14, *26*, 397, *407*, 491, *520*
Meyer RA, 30, 31, *42*, 387, 388, *403*
Meyer T, 591, 597, 603, *610*, *613*, *614*
Meyerick B, 426, *433*
Meyer-Lehnert H, 670, *683*
Mhyre JG, 307, 309, 310, 312, 313, *325*
Michaelson ED, 74, *112*
Michelis MF, 655, 665, *678*
Michels DB, 133, *145*, 162, *174*
Michimata H, 531, 532, 534, *548*
Michorowski B, 603, 605, *615*
Michurski SP, 30, *42*
Migliori G, 567, *577*
Milberg JA, 685, *727*
Milic-Emili J, 122, *143*, 164, *174*, 183, *195*, 209, *226*
Millar RA, 142, *147*
Milledge JS, 152, 170, *172*, *175*, 186, *196*, 527, 528, 529, 530, 537, *547*, *552*
Miller CF, 692, *730*
Miller FL, 189, *197*
Miller JM, 152, 156, *172*, 483, *519*
Miller PR, 704, 709, 715, *735*
Miller RG, 49, *108*
Millward DJ, 714, *738*
Milne N, 566, *576*
Mink J, 560, 569, *573*
Mink JT, 84, *113*

Minobe W, 583, *607*
Minor RL, 375, *381*, 593, *611*
Minotti J, 591, *610*
Minshew BH, 687, *728*
Mintz HM, 565, 566, *576*
Mira JP, 711, 712, *737*
Mirhashemi S, 628, 640, *644*
Misley MC, 209, *226*
Mitch WE, 667, *682*
Mitchel AM, 700, *734*
Mitchell BR, 319, *329*
Mitchell CA, 200, *224*
Mitchell H, 106, 107, *118*
Mitchell J, 598, *613*
Mitchell JH, 511, 515, *522*, *523*, 655, 657, 658, 659, 665, 667, *678*, *679*
Mitchell MM, 132, *145*
Mitchell RA, 691, 694, 695, *729*, *732*
Mitchell RW, 424, *432*
Mithoefer JC, 156, *172*, 237, *259*
Mitlehner W, 20, *27*
Mitzner W, 54, *109*
Miyagi K, 590, 597, *610*, *613*
Miyauchi T, 670, *683*
Mohanakrishnan P, 30, *42*
Mohedin M, 693, *731*
Mohsenifar Z, 427, *433*, 554, *573*, 691, 694, 699, 700, 710, *729*, *733*, *737*
Moinard J, 231, *258*
Mokashi A, 152, *172*
Moldaver LL, 691, *729*
Molhoff T, 192, *198*
Moller JT, 177, 178, *193*
Mols P, 231, 236, 256, *257*, *261*, 292, *298*, *299*, *301*, *302*, 310, 311, 312, *326*
Moncada S, 375, *380*, 586, *608*, 632, *645*, 694, *732*
Monge CC, 152, *172*, 541, *550*, *551*, 618, *642*
Monod J, 622, *643*
Monrad ES, 588, *608*
Monrod J, 622, 623, *643*
Monsallier JF, 359, 361, 373, 374, *377*
Montain S, 588, 591, *609*, *610*
Montaner JSG, 427, *433*
Monti JP, 663, 664, *682*

Montserrat JM, 213, 214, 221, *227*, *228*, 231, 234, 235, 243, *257*, *258*, *260*
Moon HA, 136, *146*
Moon RE, 8, *26*, 82, *113*, 136, *146*, 248, *260*, 267, 272, 274, 275, 277, 279, *283*, 530, 537, 544, *548*
Moonen CTW, 692, *730*
Moore EA, 701, *734*
Moore EE, 701, 722, 724, 725, 726, *734*, *735*, *741*, *742*
Moore FA, 701, 722, 724, 725, 726, *735*, *741*, *742*
Moore GE, 515, *523*, 655, 657, 658, 659, 662, 664, 665, 669, *678*, *679*
Moore GL, 637, *645*
Moore JN, 721, *741*
Moore LG, 152, *172*, 619, *642*
Moore R, 602, *614*
Moraine JJ, 292, *301*, 310, 312, 320, *326*
Morais C, 305, 313, *324*
Moran O, 618, *642*
Moreau G, 341, *354*
Moreno A, 566, *576*
Moreno E, 667, *682*
Moreno LF, 427, *433*
Moreno R, 686, 688, *728*
Moreno RH, 245, *260*
Morgan AP, 685, *727*
Morgan-Hughes JA, 662, *681*
Moricca RB, 554, *573*
Morris A, 304, 305, *323*
Morris JB, 692, *730*
Morris JG, 207, *226*, 713, 714, *738*
Morris K, 585, *607*
Morris KP, 655, 662, *677*, *681*
Morris PJ, 663, *681*
Morris PM, 593, 594, *611*
Morris-Jones W, 594, *611*
Morton JW, 83, *113*
Morton NS, 693, *731*
Mosenthal AC, 724, *742*
Moser KM, 296, *302*
Mosher TJ, 598, *613*
Moskowitz MA, 444, *445*
Moss G, 636, *645*, 690, *728*
Moss GS, 638, *646*

Moss M, 341, *354*
Moss ML, 263, *280*
Moss R, 722, *741*
Motin J, 711, 712, *737*
Mountain RD, 202, *224*
Mountain S, 590, *610*
Mountford PJ, 718, *740*
Mouren S, 629, *644*
Mouri T, 662, 663, 670, *681*
Movilli E, 655, 662, *677*
Moxham J, 555, *574*
Moxley MA, 319, *329*
Moyes CD, 29, *42*
Mrak R, 660, *680*
Mudge G, 596, *612*
Mukoyama M, 670, *683*
Mullen J, 588, *609*
Mullen JL, 590, 591, *610*
Muller AE, 55, *109*
Muller C, 125, *144*
Muller F, 150, *171*
Muller T, 654, *676*, *677*
Munzel T, 583, 588, 590, *607*, *609*, *610*
Munzo C, 321, *329*
Murase N, 593, *611*
Mure M, 125, 133, *144*
Murphey MD, 671, *684*
Murray J, 583, *607*
Murray JF, 426, *433*, 711, 712, *737*
Murthy VS, 94, *115*
Musch T, 598, 602, *613*, *614*
Musch TI, 502, 504, 509, 510, 511, 515, *521*, *522*, *523*
Mwangi DK, 55, *109*
Myburgh KH, 665, *682*
Myrhage R, 90, *114*, 396, *406*
Mythen MG, 704, 709, 715, 716, *735*, *739*

N

Nadel JA, 85, *113*, *114*
Naeije N, 256, *261*
Naeije R, 221, *228*, 231, 236, 251, 253, 256, *257*, *260*, *261*, 286, 287, 288, 289, 290, 291, 292, 293, 294, 295,

[Naeije R]
298, *299*, *300*, *301*, *302*, 310, 311, 312, 320, 321, *326*
Nagai A, 238, *259*
Naimark A, 121, *143*, 188, *196*
Nair PK, 624, *644*
Nakano H, 662, *681*
Nakashima T, 101, 103, *117*
Nakatami T, 713, 714, *738*
Nakayama M, 662, *681*
Naqvi F, 663, 667, *682*
Narayana P, 106, *118*
Nascimben L, 583, *606*
Natanson C, 360, 373, 374, *377*, 707, 708, 709, *736*
Nauman PF, 76, *112*, 285, *300*
Naumann A, 583, *606*
Naumann PF, 230, *257*, 263, 276, *281*, 306, *324*
Naumowicz A, 655, 665, *678*
Nauta JJP, 687, *728*
Navajas D, 216, *227*
Nazzaro D, 598, *613*
Neale TJ, 654, *677*
Neclerio M, 347, *355*, 427, *433*
Neely JR, 359, *376*
Negro F, 701, *734*
Neil JM, 49, *108*
Nejadnik B, 204, *225*
Nelson DP, 349, 350, *356*, 360, 361, *377*, 414, 425, 426, *431*, *432*, *433*
Nelson DPG, 693, 695, 697, *731*
Nelson RR, 364, *378*
Nelson WB, 386, *401*, 480, *519*
Neri M, 567, *577*
Nery LE, 555, 557, 558, 565, *574*
Nesbitt K, 344, *355*
Neubauer S, 583, *606*
Neufeld GR, 57, 66, 67, *110*, *111*, 691, 703, 704, *729*
Neuman MR, 345, *355*
Neutze JM, 692, *730*
Newell JC, 427, *433*, 704, 711, *735*, *737*
Newman PJ, 376, *381*
Newnham DM, 254, *261*
Newsham LGS, 67, *111*, 121, 125, *143*, *144*

Newsholme EA, 36, *43*
Newth CJL, 85, *113*
Newton P, 319, *329*
Ng CKY, 136, *147*
Nguyen PD, 87, *114*
Nguyen PH, 470, 476, *517*
Nho K, 636, *645*
Nicholas JA, 655, 665, *678*
Nicholson DP, 209, *226*
Nickele GA, 386, *401*, 480, *519*
Nicklas J, 583, *607*
Nicolau C, 620, *643*
Nicolay K, 39, 40, *44*
Nicolaysen G, 122, 125, 132, *143, 144, 145*
Nicora R, 660, *680*
Niden AH, 229, *257*
Niebauer J, 603, *614*
Nielsen VG, 722, *741*
Niemczyk S, 692, *730*
Niioka T, 583, *606*
Niklansson F, 703, *735*
Nikolic SD, 586, *608*
Nilsson NJ, 418, *431*
Ninomiya I, 364, *378*
Nioka S, 31, 36, *42, 43*
Nishioka T, 375, *380*
Nitemberg G, 711, 712, *737*
Nixon DG, 370, *379*
Nixon JV, 657, 667, *679*
Njinou B, 204, *225*
Noakes TD, 20, *27*, 532, *548*, 657, 660, 662, 665, 669, *678, 679, 680, 682*
Nocoloff DM, 457, *466*
Noe FE, 85, *114*
Noer I, 386, *402*
Nomura T, 620, *642*
Nonnast-Daniel B, 662, *681*
Nordenfelt I, 278, *283*
Norris CP, 413, *430*
Norstrom LA, 364, *378*
Norton L, 685, *727*
Noud G, 638, *646*
Novogrodsky A, 707, *736*
Novotny EJ, 437, *445*
Noyszewski EA, 15, *26*, 39, 40, *44*, 497, *521*, 545, *552*

Nunn JF, 177, 178, 179, 186, 190, *193, 194, 196, 197*, 690, *729*
Nuno DW, 370, *379*
Nusing RM, 456, *466*
Nusse W, 544, *551*
Nuutinen EM, 30, 31, *42*
Nygaard E, 593, *611*
Nyhof RA, 410, 413, *430*
Nylund U, 185, *196*
Nyman G, 184, *195*
Nyquist O, 254, *261*

O

Oblitas D, 350, 352, *356*
Obregon TM, 669, *683*
Ochi H, 341, *354*
O'Connell JB, 583, *607*
O'Connor MF, 425, *432*
Oddis CV, 375, *381*
Odman S, 98, *116*
O'Donnel T, 594, *611*
O'Donnell DE, 571, *578*
Odoroff CL, 373, *380*, 386, 390, 392, 394, 398, *401, 405*, 693, *731*
Oelberg D, 566, *576*
Oelz O, 152, *172*
Offner B, 603, *614*
Ogilvie CM, 83, *113*
Ogoshi Y, 376, *381*
Oh T, 694, *732*
Oh TE, 351, *356*
O'Hara J, 101, 103, *117*
Ohara JA, 101, *117*
Ohqvist G, 190, *197*
Ohsumi A, 692, *730*
Ohta Y, 271, *282*, 566, *577*
Oka R, 591, *610*
Okamoto K, 695, *732*
Okayama M, 220, *228*
Okubadejo AA, 229, *257*
Okubo T, 4, *26*
Olafsson S, 560, *575*
Oldfield MH, 655, 665, *678*
Oldham K, 724, *741*
O'Leary DS, 336, *353*

Author Index

Oliveira R, 321, *329*
Olivier LR, 532, *548*
Olivier NB, 586, 587, *608*
Olley PM, 375, *380*
Olschewski H, 312, 321, *327*
Olsen JS, 544, *551*
Olsen KS, 440, *445*
Olsen TS, 457, *466*
Olson D, 694, 710, *732*
Olson JS, 624, *644*
Olson LE, 125, *144*
Olsson RA, 370, *379*
Olszowka AJ, 127, *145*
Omerod O, 597, 603, *613*, *614*
O'Neil JJ, 55, *109*
Onizuka M, 122, *143*, 670, *683*
Opie LH, 359, *377*
Opitz N, 101, *117*
Orchard R, 558, 559, *574*
Ordway GA, 388, *404*, 511, *522*, 546, *552*
O'Rear EA, 694, *731*
Oren A, 557, 558, 565, *574*
Oriol A, 207, *226*
Ormerod O, 591, *610*
Oropello JM, 716, 717, *739*
Ortner JP, 701, *735*
Oshima A, 703, *735*
Oskarsson HJ, 375, *381*
Ostgaard G, 426, *433*
Otis AB, 66, *111*, 152, *171*, 386, *402*, 526, *547*
Ounjian M, 397, *407*
Ouwerkerk R, 583, *606*
Oveisi F, 663, 667, *682*
Overbeck MC, 318, *328*
Owen CH, 366, *378*
Owens GR, 565, *575*
Owens ML, 722, *741*
Oyama AA, 620, *643*
Oye RK, 687, *728*

P

Paans AMJ, 98, *116*
Pacin J, 428, *434*, 705, 706, *735*

Padro J, 595, *612*
Pagani C, 669, *683*
Paganini EP, 667, *682*
Page RD, 515, *522*
Page TC, 638, *646*
Pagliarello G, 690, *729*
Paianter PL, 659, 664, *679*
Pain J, 106, *118*
Pain MCF, 203, *224*
Painer PL, 655, 657, 659, 665, *678*, *679*
Paintal AS, 264, *282*
Painter CF, 540, *550*
Painter P, 657, 662, 669, *678*
Painter PL, 515, *523*, 650, 651, 657, 665, *676*, *682*
Paiva M, 57, 66, 67, *110*, *111*, 125, *144*, 162, 168, 169, *174*, 208, *226*
Pakron FJ, 566, *576*
Palazzo M, 705, 718, 719, *736*
Palizas F, 428, *434*, 704, 705, 706, 709, 715, *735*
Pallone TL, 450, *465*
Palmer KNV, 203, 205, *224*, *225*
Palmer RM, 694, *732*
Palmer RMJ, 586, *608*, 632, 633, *645*
Palmieri G, 660, *680*
Palot M, 307, *325*
Palou A, 271, *283*
Panas DL, 375, *380*
Pandey P, 668, *682*
Pantely GA, 620, *643*, 710, *736*
Panz T, 101, *117*
Panza JA, 659, *679*
Paoletti P, 229, *256*
Papadakos P, 321, *329*
Papagerogiou I, 376, *381*
Pappagianopoulos P, 271, *283*, 571, 572, *578*
Pappenheimer JR, 544, *551*
Pappert D, 310, 317, *325*, *328*
Paramelle B, 271, *282*, 566, *577*
Pardy RL, 570, *577*
Pare PD, 238, 245, 246, *259*, *260*
Parent A, 318, *328*
Parent AC, 317, *328*
Parikh RK, 192, *197*
Park JS, 662, *681*

Park R, 104, *118*
Park SK, 662, *681*
Parker I, 57, 66, *110*
Parker JC, 122, 125, 133, *143*, *144*
Parker MM, 360, 373, 374, *377*, 424, *432*
Parkhouse WS, 31, 36, *43*
Parks DA, 722, *741*
Parra C, 704, 709, 715, *735*
Parratt JR, 424, *432*
Parrillo JE, 360, 373, 374, *377*, 424, *432*
Parsons B, 515, *523*
Parsons DB, 659, 665, *679*
Parsons W, 8, *26*
Parsons WJ, 668, *682*
Parthsarathi K, 101, *117*
Partnick DA, 724, *741*
Parviainen I, 716, *739*
Parviainen M, 694, *732*
Parviainene I, 715, *739*
Pasalodos J, 667, *682*
Pascoe JR, 532, *548*
Pasquale MD, 724, *742*
Pasternak CA, 713, *738*
Pasternak FL, 655, 665, *678*
Pastores S, 724, *741*
Patel DP, 363, *378*
Patel M, 596, *612*
Paterson D, 598, *613*
Patessio A, 554, 572, *573*
Pathria MN, 671, *684*
Patterson GA, 271, *283*
Patterson JL, 158, *173*
Pattishal EN, 319, *329*
Paul K, 654, *677*
Paul RJ, 441, *445*
Pauletto P, 583, *606*
Paulson OB, 96, *116*
Payen D, 286, 290, 291, 292, *300*, 320, *329*
Payen JF, 271, *282*, 566, *577*
Payne DB, 101, *115*
Payne JR, 397, *407*
Payne WD, 142, *147*
Pean JL, 56, *110*
Pearson RJ, 714, *738*
Pease W, 441, *445*
Pedegana LR, 593, *611*

Pedersen T, 177, 178, 192, 193, *193*, *197*
Pegelow DF, 386, *401*, 480, *519*
Peinado VI, 241, *259*
Peleg H, 460, 461, *467*
Pellegrino M, 567, *577*
Pellerin L, 441, *445*
Pelligrino DA, 444, *445*
Pelosi P, 304, 305, 315, 317, *324*, *328*, 705, 718, 719, *736*
Pendergast D, 14, *26*
Pendergast DR, 397, *407*, 489, 491, *520*
Pennock BE, 565, *575*
Peolis P, 313, *327*
Pepke-Zaba J, 241, 254, *259*, *261*
Percival C, 711, 712, *737*
Perez R, 667, *682*
Perez W, 570, *577*
Permutt S, 168, *175*
Pernerstorfer T, 304, *323*
Pernow B, 591, *610*
Perry MA, 410, 413, *430*
Perutz MF, 622, *643*
Pesce C, 251, *261*
Peschock RM, 106, *118*
Pesenti A, 304, 305, 313, 315, 317, *324*, *327*, *328*, 705, 718, 719, *736*
Peskoff A, 544, *551*
Pessina AC, 583, *606*
Peters RM, 150, 152, 170, *171*, *172*, *175*, 527, 529, 530, 537, *547*
Petitclerc T, 662, 663, 670, *681*
Petitpretz P, 286, 289, *301*
Petro JK, 488, *520*
Petty RKH, 662, *681*
Petty TL, 238, *259*, 271, *283*, 304, 305, *323*
Pham BA, 690, *729*
Phang PT, 349, *356*, 360, 373, *377*, *380*, 414, 423, 425, 428, *431*, *434*, 693, 695, 699, 700, 710, 711, 712, 714, *731*, *733*, *737*
Phu NH, 714, *738*
Picado C, 222, *228*
Pich J, 310, 321, *326*
Pickett CK, 526, *547*
Pickett MH, 166, *174*
Piegors DJ, 593, *611*

Author Index

Pietra GG, 297, *302*
Pietrabissa A, 414, *431*, 710, *736*
Piiper J, 4, 9, 14, *26*, 67, 79, 87, *111*, *112*, *114*, 156, *173*, 397, *407*, 485, 491, *519*, *520*, 527, 528, 535, *547*, 657, 662, *679*, *681*
Pilch J, 312, *327*
Pillay P, 591, *610*
Pillet O, 231, *258*
Pimmel P, 662, *681*
Pinantadosi CA, 618, 641, *642*
Pine RW, 687, *728*
Ping P, 630, *644*
Pinsky MR, 342, *354*, 692, 701, 710, 720, 721, 724, *729*, *730*, *734*, *736*, *740*
Pison U, 130, *145*, 254, *261*, 310, 312, 319, 320, *326*, *329*
Pitaridis MT, 701, *734*
Pitcher WD, 654, *677*
Pitetti KH, 656, *678*
Pitt B, 292, *301*
Pittenger G, 98, 101, *116*, *117*, 704, *735*
Pittman RN, 101, *115*, *117*, 387, 390, 393, 394, 395, *402*, *404*, *406*
Pizzo C, 527, *547*
Pizzo CJ, 150, 152, *171*, *172*, 527, 529, 530, 537, *547*
Planck J, 440, *445*
Pluskwa F, 310, 312, *326*
Podoloski A, 531, 532, 534, *548*
Pohil RJ, 106, *118*
Pohl U, 641, *647*
Pohlman A, 428, *434*, 694, 710, 711, 712, *732*, *737*
Poincelot F, 710, *737*
Pokorski M, 152, *172*
Polenakovic M, 669, *683*
Polissar N, 73, *112*, 122, *143*
Pologe JA, 100, 101, *117*
Polokoff E, 716, 717, *739*
Polu JM, 566, *576*
Poma V, 251, *261*
Ponte J, 555, *574*
Poole DC, 20, *27*, 95, 107, *116*, *118*, 139, *147*, 363, *378*, 388, 392, 397, *404*, 470, 471, 472, 474, 475, 476, 477, 478, 480, 482, 483, 485, 487,

[Poole DC]
488, 489, 492, 494, 495, 496, 500, 501, 502, 503, 504, 505, 507, 508, 509, 510, 511, 513, 514, 515, *517*, *518*, *519*, *520*, *521*, *522*, *523*, 532, 537, 539, *549*, *550*
Poole-Wilson P, 590, 591, *610*
Poole-Wilson PA, 598, *613*
Popat K, 297, *302*
Popat KD, 298, *302*
Popel AS, 56, 90, 92, *109*, *110*, *115*, 387, 388, 390, 391, 393, 394, 395, *403*, *404*, 504, *521*, 638, *646*
Poppius H, 206, *225*
Porszasz J, 487, 507, *520*
Port JD, 583, *607*
Posner J, 593, *610*
Postma DS, 229, *256*
Potter R, 425, *432*
Potter RF, 363, *378*, 500, 509, 513, *521*, *522*
Potter WA, 560, 562, *575*
Potts JT, 106, 107, *118*
Pourrat O, 204, *225*
Powanda MC, 694, *732*
Powell FL, 526, *547*
Powers SK, 480, 484, 485, *519*
Powers SR, 347, *355*, 427, *433*
Power-Vanwart J, 588, *609*
Pranikoff T, 318, *328*
Pratt CA, 397, *407*
Predel HG, 670, *683*
Prediletto R, 139, *147*, 286, 290, 291, 292, *300*, 310, *325*, 478, 492, 494, 505, 511, *519*, 531, *548*
Presenti A, 304, 305, *323*
Presson RG, 57, *110*, 131, *145*
Preston E, 594, *611*
Preston SB, 57, 66, *110*
Price D, 565, *576*
Price HL, 691, 703, 704, *729*
Price SR, 667, *682*
Pride NB, 229, *256*, 560, 562, *575*
Pries AR, 133, *145*
Prikazky L, 596, 599, 600, *612*, *614*
Print CG, 200, *224*
Prinzen FW, 101, *115*

Prisk GK, 122, 123, 125, *144*, 149, 162, 163, 164, 166, 168, 169, 170, *171*, *173*, *174*, *175*
Proemmel DD, 82, *113*
Pruitt BA, 694, *732*
Prutow RJ, 181, 184, *194*, *195*, 318, *328*
Puga F, 582, 584, *606*
Pugh LG, 158, *173*
Pugh LGCE, 514, *522*
Pun KK, 658, 670, *679*
Punch J, 724, *741*
Puranapanda V, 694, *731*
Purcaro A, 605, *615*
Purdy RE, 663, 667, *682*
Puri VK, 428, *433*
Pusajo J, 428, *434*, 705, 706, *735*
Pusajo JF, 704, 709, 715, *735*
Pussard E, 691, 703, *729*
Putensen C, 192, *197*, 305, 306, 310, 312, 313, 314, 315, 320, 321, *324*, *326*, *327*, *329*
Putensen G, 310, 313, 315, *326*, *327*
Putensen-Himmer G, 192, *197*, 310, 321, *326*
Putz G, 314, *327*

Q

Qayyum M, 598, *613*
Qi L, 691, *729*
Quale JL, 671, *684*
Quezado AMN, 707, 708, *736*
Quillen JE, 375, *381*
Qunibi WY, 463, *467*
Quyyumi AA, 659, *679*
Qvist J, 231, 236, 237, *257*
Qvist T, 184, *195*

R

Rachmilewitz D, 456, *466*
Rackow E, 705, *736*
Rackow EC, 699, 700, *733*
Radaelli A, 591, 597, 603, *610*, *613*, *614*
Radda G, 588, 589, 593, 594, *609*, *611*

Radda GK, 583, *606*, 662, 663, 664, *680*, *681*, 692, *730*
Radermacher J, 655, 663, *677*, *681*
Radermacher P, 310, 312, 313, 315, 320, *325*, *326*, *327*
Radford NB, 388, *404*, 546, *552*
Radomski MW, 586, *608*
Rafel E, 659, *679*
Raffestin B, 566, *575*
Raffin TA, 49, *108*
Rahn H, 66, *111*, 150, 152, *171*, 348, 356, 526, *547*
Raichle ME, 440, *445*
Raichvarg D, 359, 361, 373, 374, *377*
Raij L, 310, *326*
Raine JM, 142, *147*
Rajagopalan B, 583, 588, 589, *606*, *609*, 662, *680*
Rakusan K, 363, *378*, 387, 392, 394, *402*
Ralph DD, 307, 311, 312, *324*
Ramanathan M, 79, 85, *112*, *114*, 487, 520
Ramierz J, 231, 246, *258*
Ramirez C, 237, *259*
Ramirez J, 238, 241, 246, *259*, 264, 265, 280, *282*, 560, 565, *575*
Ramis L, 213, 214, *227*, 243, *260*
Ramis LI, 211, 218, *226*
Rampulla C, 271, *283*
Ranieri VM, 251, *261*, 313, *327*
Rao R, 587, *608*
Rapoport J, 687, *728*
Raposa T, 417, *431*
Rapson NT, 720, *740*
Rasanen J, 312, 313, 315, 320, 321, *327*, *329*
Raskin RE, 532, *548*
Rasmussen HH, 460, *467*
Rasmussen I, 703, *735*
Rasmussen K, 669, *683*
Rasmussen R, 583, *607*
Rassidais A, 691, 694, *729*
Ratcliffe PJ, 692, *730*
Rauss A, 252, *261*
Raventos AA, 319, *329*
Ravikant T, 693, *730*
Ray CA, 399, *407*

Rayford CR, 360, 371, *377*
Raymond GM, 370, *379*
Rayos G, 583, 603, 605, *607, 615*
Read J, 166, *175*, 200, 202, 205, 207, 220, *224, 225, 226, 227*
Read RA, 701, *734*
Reardon WC, 85, *114*
Reber A, 185, 189, *196*
Rector T, 596, *612*
Rector TS, 586, 587, *608*
Reddan WG, 152, 156, *172*
Redl H, 701, *734*
Reed JH, 122, *143*
Reed RK, 426, *433*
Reemstma K, 591, *610*
Rees J, 229, *256*
Rees R, 724, *741*
Reese RE, 480, *519*
Reeves JT, 23, *27*, 136, *146*, 156, 158, 159, 160, 170, *173, 175*, 529, 530, 531, 532, 533, 537, 538, 545, *548, 549, 550*
Reggiani C, 567, *577*
Regnard J, 599, *614*
Regnier B, 309, 313, *325*
Rehder K, 166, *174*, 180, 181, 186, *194*
Reichek N, 588, 590, 591, *609, 610*
Reid JV, 370, *379*
Reid LM, 297, *302*
Reid M, 598, *613*
Reid P, 721, *740*
Reinhart CK, 686, 688, *728*
Reisin E, 657, *679*
Reissmann KR, 620, *642*
Reite M, 160, *173*
Reivich M, 436, *445*
Remington Sprague F, 292, *301*
Remmers JE, 156, *172, 173*
Renkin EM, 389, 392, 393, 398, *404, 405*
Renlund DG, 583, *607*
Rennard SI, 263, 269, 278, *281*
Rennie DW, 489, *520*
Rennotte MT, 309, *325*
Renzetti AD, 142, *147*, 269, *282*
Reschke W, 451, 452, *465*
Reutenauer H, 271, *282*, 566, *577*
Revelly JP, 716, 717, *739*

Reybrouk T, 481, 482, *519*
Reyes A, 220, *228*, 236, 253, *259, 261*, 311, 321, *326*
Reynaert M, 309, *325*
Reynolds HY, 263, *280*
Rhodes GR, 427, *433*
Ribando RJ, 92, *115*
Ribas J, 222, *228*
Rice C, 638, *646*
Rich GF, 192, *197*
Rich MW, 460, *467*
Rich S, 297, *302*
Richard M, 599, *614*
Richards D, 200, *224*
Richardson DW, 158, *173*
Richardson RS, 15, *26*, 39, 40, *44*, 130, *145*, 471, 472, 488, 492, 494, 495, 497, 505, 507, 511, 514, *518, 520, 521, 522*, 531, 532, 534, 537, 545, *548, 549, 552*, 638, *647*
Richelsen B, 456, *466*
Richmond FJR, 396, 397, *406, 407*
Richmond S, 708, 709, *736*
Riddervold F, 667, *682*
Riddington DW, 715, 718, *738, 740*
Riede U, 590, 603, *610, 614*
Riede UN, 515, *523*
Riedel GL, 411, 413, 417, *430, 431*
Ries A, 136, *146*
Rigg JR, 161, *173*
Riley RL, 63, 81, 82, *111, 113*, 150, *171*, 269, *282*
Rime A, 351, *356*
Rinaldo JE, 313, 314, *327*
Ringdal N, 222, *228*
Ringnalda BE, 152, *172*
Ringsted C, 177, 178, 192, 193, *193, 197*
Ringsted CV, 231, 236, 237, *257*
Riordan JF, 203, *224*
Ripe E, 254, *261*
Ripley JM, 654, *677*
Ripper RL, 360, *377*
Ritman EL, 122, *143*, 183, *195*
Riverola A, 231, 246, *258*
Rivington RN, 570, *577*
Rivolta M, 304, 305, *323, 324*
Rix LK, 662, 664, *680*

Roach RC, 526, *547*
Robacker K, 441, *445*
Robbins P, 598, *613*
Robert R, 204, *225*
Roberts AM, 370, *379*
Roberts WC, 263, 265, 269, 273, 276, *280*, *281*
Robertson CF, 200, *224*
Robertson CR, 450, *465*
Robertson HT, 73, *112*, 122, 125, 126, 133, *143*, *144*, *145*, *146*, 166, *175*, 290, *301*, 307, 311, 312, 317, *324*, *328*, 655, 660, *678*, *680*
Robertson PC, 67, *111*
Robertson RJ, 655, *678*
Robinson BF, 488, *520*
Robiollo M, 30, 31, *42*
Robotham JL, 716, 717, *739*
Roca J, 4, 20, *26*, *27*, 107, *118*, 134, 135, 139, *146*, *147*, 211, 212, 213, 214, 216, 217, 218, 220, 221, 222, *226*, *227*, *228*, 231, 232, 234, 235, 236, 238, 241, 242, 243, 245, 246, 250, 253, *257*, *258*, *259*, *260*, *261*, 263, 264, 265, 266, 267, 268, 269, 272, 273, 274, 275, 278, 279, 280, *281*, *282*, 306, 307, 311, 312, 320, 321, *324*, *325*, *326*, *327*, *329*, 388, 389, 390, 392, 397, *403*, *404*, 496, 508, 511, 514, 515, *521*, *522*, *523*, 535, 539, 545, *549*, *550*, *551*, 557, 560, 565, 566, *574*, *575*, *576*, 659, 662, 663, 664, *679*, *680*
Rocha R, 599, 600, *614*
Rochester DF, 564, *575*
Rock PB, 23, *27*, 537, *549*
Rock PD, 530, 537, *548*
Rockow EC, 701, *734*
Rodahl K, 470, 474, 476, 488, *517*
Rodarte J, 595, *611*
Rodarte JR, 125, *144*, 180, *194*, 560, 566, 572, *575*, *578*
Rodenstein D, 309, *325*
Rodriguez KS, 177, *193*
Rodriguez RR, 306, 311, 321, *324*, *326*
Rodriguez-Roisin R, 4, 20, *26*, *27*, 139, *147*, 211, 212, 213, 214, 215, 216,

[Rodriguez-Roisin R]
218, 220, 222, *226*, *227*, *228*, 231, 232, 234, 235, 236, 238, 241, 243, 245, 246, 250, 253, 254, *257*, *258*, *259*, *260*, *261*, 263, 264, 265, 266, 267, 268, 269, 272, 273, 274, 275, 278, 279, 280, *281*, *282*, 307, 311, 312, 318, 320, 321, *325*, *326*, *327*, *328*, *329*, 496, 508, 511, 514, 515, *521*, *523*, 539, *550*, 557, 560, 565, 566, *574*, *575*, *576*, 654, 655, 659, 662, 663, 664, *677*, *679*, *680*
Roeseleer J, 309, *325*
Roger N, 231, 234, 235, 246, *258*, 264, *281*, 320, *329*
Roger SA, 122, *144*, 370, *379*
Rogers RM, 313, 314, *327*, 565, *575*, 692, *729*
Rogiers P, 352, *357*, 425, *432*
Rogovein TS, 321, *329*
Rohlfs RJ, 636, 637, *645*, *646*
Rohrer F, 49, 51, *108*
Roissant R, 310, *325*
Rolandelli RR, 714, *738*
Romaldini H, 311, 321, *326*, 654, 655, *677*
Roman A, 699, 700, 714, *733*
Rombeau JL, 714, *738*
Roncella M, 414, *431*, 710, *736*
Ronco JJ, 360, *377*, 427, 428, *433*, *434*, 695, 697, 699, 700, 705, 711, 712, 714, *733*, *737*
Roos T, 192, *198*
Ropars C, 620, *643*
Ros D, 231, 246, *258*
Rosbolt JP, 532, *548*
Rose B, 207, *226*
Rose CP, 371, 373, *380*
Rose PK, 396, *406*
Rose SJ, 701, *735*
Rosen A, 690, *728*
Rosen AL, 636, 638, *645*, *646*
Rosen S, 447, 448, 451, 452, 456, 457, 458, 460, 461, 462, 463, *465*, *466*, *467*
Rosenthal MR, 105, *118*
Rosenzweig D, 597, *612*
Rosina C, 200, *224*

Ross BB, 49, 51, 67, *108*, *111*
Ross BD, 452, *465*
Ross BK, 290, *301*
Ross DL, 656, *678*
Ross J, 363, *378*, 582, 584, *606*
Ross WRD, 67, *111*
Rossaint R, 130, *145*, 254, *261*, 310, 312, 317, 319, 320, *326*, *328*, *329*
Rossen JD, 375, *381*
Rossi A, 243, *260*
Rossi F, 304, 305, *323*, *324*
Rossi G, 304, 305, *324*
Rossi-Bernardi L, 622, 623, 624, 625, *643*, *644*
Rotger M, 217, 222, *227*
Rothen HU, 184, 185, 188, 189, *195*, *196*
Rothen U, 185, *196*
Rothman DL, 437, *445*
Rothman E, 98, *116*
Rothschild HR, 101, *117*, 704, *735*
Rothschild T, 231, *257*
Rothwell NJ, 714, *738*
Roughton FJW, 8, *26*, 55, 85, *109*, *114*
Rouleau J, 369, *379*
Roumen RMH, 701, *734*
Round J, 590, *610*
Roupie E, 305, 314, 320, 322, *324*, *327*, *329*
Roussos C, 570, *577*, 691, 694, 701, *729*, *734*
Rovetto MJ, 359, *376*
Rovira I, 231, 234, 235, 246, *258*, 320, *329*
Rowan AN, 36, *43*
Rowell LB, 336, *353*, 383, 385, 386, 391, *401*, *402*, 470, 472, 480, 487, 488, 489, 490, 491, 492, 494, 495, *517*, *518*, *520*, 537, 538, *549*, 691, 703, 713, *729*, *737*
Roy RR, 396, 397, *406*, *407*
Roy SS, 437, *445*
Royo C, 715, 717, *739*
Rubin S, 597, *613*
Rubinfeld AR, 212, *226*
Rubinstein I, 455, *465*
Rubio R, 360, 370, *377*, *379*
Rude RE, 620, *643*

Rudin-Toretsky E, 583, *607*
Rudloph M, 101, *115*, 203, *224*, 340, *354*
Rudolp AM, 692, *730*
Ruedy J, 427, *433*
Ruff F, 183, *195*
Ruffin R, 200, *224*
Ruhl KH, 619, *642*
Rumsey WL, 30, 31, *42*
Ruokonen E, 691, 693, 694, 715, 716, *729*, *739*
Rupcic V, 655, *677*
Rusic A, 655, *677*
Russell JA, 349, *356*, 360, 373, 374, *377*, 427, 428, *433*, *434*, 686, 687, 689, 695, 697, 698, 699, 700, 704, 705, 710, 711, 712, 714, 715, 717, 719, 720, *728*, *733*, *735*, *737*, *740*
Russo G, 694, 710, *732*
Ruth WE, 620, *642*
Rutledge FS, 692, *730*
Rysz J, 667, *682*

S

Saal K, 515, *523*
Sabba C, 586, 587, *608*
Sack RD, 396, *406*
Sackner MA, 74, 85, *112*, *114*
Sacristan E, 101, *117*, 704, *735*
Saeki A, 375, *380*
Saetta M, 200, *224*, 238, *259*
Safian R, 595, *612*
Safranyos RG, 392, 393, *405*
Sagawa K, 364, *378*
Sahn SA, 202, *224*
Sair M, 350, *356*
Saito D, 370, *379*
Saito M, 670, *683*
Saito Y, 494, *520*, 670, *683*
Sakai O, 662, *681*
Sakai T, 692, *730*
Sakane M, 670, *683*
Sakata S, 620, *643*
Sakko T, 593, *611*
Sala E, 566, *576*

Sala L, 603, 605, *615*
Salak N, 427, *433*
Salem MM, 360, *377*
Salmeron S, 286, 289, *301*
Salome CM, 207, 209, *226*
Saltin B, 31, *42*, *43*, 383, 385, 386, 387, 389, 390, 391, 392, 398, 400, *401*, *402*, 470, 471, 480, 495, 496, 497, 504, 511, 513, 514, *517*, 535, 537, 538, *549*, *550*, 661, *680*
Saltin J, 591, *610*
Saltzman D, 630, *644*
Saltzman HA, 8, *26*, 76, 82, 105, *112*, *113*, *118*, 129, 136, *145*, *146*, 158, *173*, 180, *194*, 248, *260*, 267, 272, 274, 275, 277, 279, *283*, 285, 291, *300*, 530, 537, 544, *548*
Samaja M, 527, 529, 530, 537, *547*, 618, 619, 620, 622, 625, *642*, *643*
Samaja N, 474, *518*
Samii K, 691, 703, *729*
Sampson D, 206, *225*
Samsel RW, 342, 344, 349, 350, *354*, *356*, 360, *377*, 414, 415, 418, 424, 425, 426, 427, 428, *431*, *432*, *433*, *434*, 693, 695, 697, 710, 711, 712, *731*, *736*, *737*
San Roman E, 428, *434*, 705, 706, *735*
Sanchala V, 695, *732*
Sancho M, 667, *682*
Sanders MH, 313, 314, *327*
Sanders WM, 349, *356*, 414, 426, *431*, *433*, 710, *736*
Sanderson M, 317, *328*
Sandmann W, 313, 315, *327*
Sandrini M, 655, 662, *677*
Sands A, 707, *736*
Sandtner W, 701, *734*
Sanii R, 571, *578*
Sanmarco ME, 602, *614*
Santak B, 310, 312, 313, 315, 320, *325*, *326*, *327*
Santolicandro A, 286, 290, 291, 292, *300*
Santos C, 217, 222, 227, 243, 250, *260*, 307, *325*
Santre C, 351, *356*
Saratini A, 655, 665, *678*

Sarelius IH, 391, 392, 393, 394, 395, 397, 400, *405*, *407*, 492, 494, 504, *520*, *521*, *522*
Sarfeh IJ, 704, *735*
Sarnoff SJ, 364, *378*
Sarnquist F, 541, *551*
Sarnquist FH, 527, 529, 530, 537, *547*
Sartene R, 192, *198*
Sartoris DJ, 671, *684*
Sasahara AA, 292, 294, *301*
Sass DJ, 122, *143*
Sassayama S, 590, 597, *610*, *613*
Sato M, 526, *547*
Sato T, 713, 714, *738*
Satta A, 567, *577*
Sauaia A, 701, *734*
Sauerwein HP, 720, *740*
Sauleda J, 271, *283*
Saulnier F, 686, *728*
Saunders KB, 203, *224*
Saunders MJ, 655, 662, *678*
Saupe KW, 484, 485, *519*, 560, *575*
Saura P, 715, 717, *739*
Saus C, 271, *283*
Savica V, 660, *680*
Savitt MA, 366, *378*
Saxen H, 691, 693, 694, *729*
Sayeed MM, 699, 700, *733*
Scano G, 207, 209, *226*, 560, *575*
Scarani F, 304, 305, *323*
Schacterle RS, 92, *115*
Schade UF, 721, *741*
Schaer GL, 360, 373, 374, *377*
Schafer R, 655, *677*
Schaffartzik W, 20, *27*, 107, *118*, 139, *147*, 310, *325*, 388, 392, 397, *404*, 478, 480, 485, 487, 492, 494, 495, 503, 505, 511, *519*, *520*, *521*, 532, *549*
Schaffer J, 662, *681*
Schaffer T, 317, 318, *328*
Schamberger R, 603, 605, *615*
Schantz P, 539, *550*
Schaper W, 363, *378*
Scharenberg AM, 341, *354*
Scharer K, 654, 657, *677*, *679*
Scheid P, 4, 9, *26*, 79, 87, *112*, *114*, 156, *173*, 485, *519*

Scheiffer B, 515, *523*
Schein RM, 686, *727*
Scher AM, 472, 492, 495, *518*, *520*
Scherer PW, 57, 66, 67, *110*, *111*
Scherer RW, 191, *197*
Schermuly R, 310, 312, 319, 321, *326*, *327*, *328*, *329*
Scherston T, 594, *611*
Schettino GP, 305, 313, 321, *324*, *329*
Schiavi E, 428, *434*, 705, 706, *735*
Schieffer E, 515, *523*
Schilling M, 619, *642*
Schlag G, 701, *734*
Schlehe H, 619, *642*
Schlichtig R, 104, *117*, 342, *354*, 692, 710, 716, 717, *730*, *736*, *739*, *740*
Schlierf G, 603, *614*
Schlosser C, 30, 31, *42*
Schlosser T, 39, 40, *44*
Schmartz D, 425, *432*
Schmehl T, 319, *328*
Schmekel B, 213, *227*
Schmetterer L, 641, *647*
Schmid-Schonbein GW, 630, 631, 638, *644*
Schmidt AM, 531, 532, *548*
Schmidt CF, 96, 97, *116*, 342, 344, *354*, 435, 436, *444*
Schmidt GA, 428, *434*, 694, 710, 711, 712, *732*, *737*
Schmidt H, 722, *741*
Schmidt W, 722, *741*
Schnackerz K, 583, *606*
Schneider AM, 132, *145*
Schneider B, 304, *323*, 540, *550*
Schneider RC, 39, *44*
Schneider T, 310, 312, 319, 321, *326*, *327*, *329*
Schneider TJ, 641, *647*
Schobersberger W, 665, *682*
Schoeffel E, 217, *227*
Schoene RB, 152, 170, *172*, *175*, 527, 529, 530, 532, 537, 541, *547*, *549*, *551*
Schoener B, 105, *118*
Schoeppe W, 669, *683*
Schols AMWJ, 567, *577*

Schone RB, 526, *547*
Schonharting MM, 721, *741*
Schork MA, 383, *401*
Schouten BD, 321, *329*
Schrader J, 371, 373, *380*
Schreiner M, 67, *111*
Schreiner RJ, 318, *328*
Schrier RW, 463, *467*
Schrijen F, 566, *576*, 710, *737*
Schroter RC, 52, *109*, 165, *174*
Schuessler GB, 342, 343, *355*
Schuler G, 603, *614*
Schuler HW, 657, *679*
Schultz R, 375, *380*
Schumacker PT, 318, *328*, 342, 344, 349, 350, *354*, *356*, 360, 361, 376, 377, *381*, 411, 414, 415, 418, 422, 424, 425, 426, 427, 428, *430*, *431*, *432*, 433, *434*, 693, 695, 697, 710, 711, 712, *731*, *736*, *737*
Schumaker PT, 360, *377*
Schurek HJ, 451, 462, *465*
Schuster KD, 87, *114*
Schwartz D, 585, 596, *608*, *612*
Schwarz M, 587, *608*
Schwarz MI, 263, 265, 269, 276, *281*
Schweiger C, 603, 605, *615*
Schweitzer I, 690, *729*
Schwerzmann K, 387, *402*
Scocco V, 605, *615*
Scott C, 375, *380*
Scovill W, 427, *433*
Seaman J, 46, 72, *108*, 511, 514, *522*, 532, *549*
Sears MR, 200, *224*
Sears NJ, 315, *327*
Sebert P, 653, *676*
Secher E, 178, *193*
Secher N, 386, *402*
Secomb TW, 390, 395, *404*
Sediame S, 254, *261*
Seed RF, 189, *196*
Seeger W, 310, 312, 319, 321, *326*, *327*, *328*, *329*
Seeherman HJ, 46, *108*
Segal JM, 360, *377*

Segal SS, 385, 386, 391, 394, 395, 396, 397, 398, 399, 400, *401, 402, 404, 405, 406, 407*, 493, 494, 509, *520, 522*
Segil LJ, 360, *377*
Sehgal H, 636, *645*
Sehgal HL, 638, *646*
Sehgal L, 690, *728*
Sehgal LR, 636, 638, *645, 646*
Sekizawa K, 220, *228*
Selinger SL, 692, *730*
Seltzer H, 304, *323*
Sergysels R, 207, 209, *226*, 256, *261*, 560, *575*
Sessler A, 180, *194*
Sessler AD, 181, 186, *194*
Seto H, 597, *613*
Settergren G, 190, *197*
Settle RG, 714, *738*
Severinghaus JW, 131, *145*, 152, *172*, 526, 531, 532, 534, *547, 548*
Severn A, 720, *740*
Sevransky JE, 707, *736*
Sexton WL, 515, *523*
Seyberth HW, 456, *466*
Seymour M, 656, *678*
Sfyras D, 701, *734*
Shaeffer-McCall GS, 515, *522*
Shaffer RA, 93, *115*
Shah D, 427, *433*
Shah DM, 704, *735*
Shah P, 583, *607*
Shah S, 714, *738*
Shahnarian A, 715, 717, *739*
Shaked G, 707, *736*
Shaldon S, 95, *115*
Shalom R, 655, 665, *678*
Shankar H, 636, *645*
Shanley P, 462, *467*
Shao Z, 376, *381*
Shapell SB, 375, *381*
Shapiro JI, 463, *467*, 660, 670, *680*
Shapiro RM, 692, *730*
Sharma GVRK, 292, 294, *301*
Sharma P, 707, *736*
Sharma S, 292, 294, *301*
Sharma VS, 633, *645*

Sharp J, 599, 600, *614*
Sharp JT, 142, *147*
Sharpe SM, 687, *728*
Shaw JP, 515, *522*
Sheard PW, 397, *407*
Shelley D, 596, *612*
Shemin R, 596, *612*
Shenkin A, 720, 721, 724, *740*
Shennib H, 515, *523*
Shepard J, 122, *143*
Shepard JT, 591, *610*
Shepherd AP, 93, *115*, 410, 411, 413, 415, 417, *430, 431*
Shepherd JT, 383, 386, *401, 402*, 694, *732*
Shepro D, 294, *301*, 724, *741*
Sheriff DD, 472, 492, 495, *518*, 520
Sherlock S, 95, *115*, 714, *738*
Sherrington CS, 437, *445*
Shibutani K, 695, *732*
Shied P, 527, 528, 535, *547*
Shigematus T, 662, *681*
Shih DT, 635, *645*
Shima T, 101, *117*
Shimizu S, 620, *643*
Shindell D, 489, *520*
Shiner RJ, 570, *577*
Shioya S, 271, *282*, 566, *577*
Shirakami G, 670, *683*
Shires GT, 691, *729*
Shoemaker JK, 668, *682*
Shoemaker W, 705, 706, 707, *736*
Shoemaker WC, 697, 705, 706, 718, *733, 736*
Shoji T, 375, *381*
Shorr R, 636, *645*
Shottlender J, 428, *434*, 705, 706, *735*
Shoubridge EA, 662, *681*
Shrager RI, 622, 625, *643*
Shrago E, 660, *680*
Shulkin BL, 318, *328*
Shulman RG, 437, *445*
Shyde P, 544, *551*
Siafakas NM, 229, *256*
Siami G, 660, *680*
Sibbald NJ, 692, *730*
Sibbald W, 375, *380*, 424, *432*, 693, *731*

Author Index

Sibbald WJ, 303, 311, 312, 313, *323*, 425, *432*, 686, 687, 711, 712, *727, 737*
Sibinska E, 667, *682*
Side E, 571, 572, *578*
Siegel JH, 713, 714, *738*
Siegel SC, 207, 209, *226*
Siegler DIM, 208, *226*
Siesjo BK, 435, 436, *444*
Silber DH, 668, *682*
Silliman CC, 724, *741*
Sillye G, 691, 694, *729*
Siloaho M, 715, *739*
Silva P, 447, 448, 456, 457, 458, 462, 463, 464, *465, 466, 467*
Silver IA, 483, *519*
Silverman M, 206, *225*
Silverman NA, 376, *381*
Silvers GW, 238, *259*
Simard A, 554, 566, *573*
Simard AA, 271, *283*
Simard C, 271, *283*, 554, 566, *573*
Simmonds HD, 207, 209, *226*
Simmonds RL, 687, *728*
Simmons CW, 593, *611*
Simmons DH, 713, 714, *738*
Simmons M, 596, *612*
Simmons RL, 375, *381*
Simon AB, 583, *606*
Simon C, 131, *145*
Simon RJ, 705, *735*
Simon W, 597, *613*
Simonneau G, 192, *198*, 237, 252, *259, 261*, 286, 289, *301*, 309, *325*
Simonsen S, 667, *682*
Simonson DC, 46, *108*
Sims WR, 315, *327*
Sinclair SE, 125, *144*
Sinclair-Smith CC, 20, *27*, 657, *679*
Singer J, 686, 687, 689, *728*
Singh M, 694, 710, *732*
Sinha MK, 670, *683*
Sinoway LI, 598, *613*, 668, *682*
Siosteen SM, 83, *113*
Sitbon P, 691, *729*
Sjaastad OV, 122, *143*
Sjostrand J, 418, *431*
Sjostrand TA, 83, *113*

Sjostrom M, 400, *407*
Skeleton TD, 152, *172*, 619, *642*
Skerl L, 583, *607*
Skinner JR, 655, 662, *677, 681*
Skinner NS, 338, *353*, 640, *647*
Skrinar GS, 655, *678*
Slama K, 254, *261*, 310, 312, 317, 320, *326, 328*
Sleight P, 588, 589, 591, 597, 603, *609, 610, 613, 614*
Slinker BK, 364, *378*
Sloniger MA, 475, *518*
Slotman G, 705, *736*
Slutsky AS, 321, *329*
Smail N, 352, *357*
Smatresk N, 152, *172*
Smiesko V, 632, *644*
Smith CW, 375, *381*
Smith D, 105, *118*, 539, *550*
Smith DA, 654, *677*
Smith DJ, 724, *741*
Smith FC, 436, *445*
Smith J, 663, 667, *682*
Smith JL, 79, *113*
Smith MB, 598, *613*, 668, *682*
Smith P, 705, *736*
Smith RM, 319, *329*
Smith S, 656, *678*
Smith T, 669, *683*
Smith TF, 203, *224*
Smithies M, 334, 347, 348, 351, *353, 356*, 699, 700, 715, 717, *733, 739*
Sneider MA, 543, *551*
Snell G, 571, 572, *578*
Snell SM, 637, *645*
Snider GL, 177, *193*, 238, *259*
Snow DH, 36, *43*
Soble JS, 710, *737*
Sodal IE, 526, *547*
Solda P, 591, 597, 603, *610, 613, 614*
Solinas E, 136, *147*
Solomon R, 464, *467*
Solomon S, 586, *608*
Somero GN, 29, *41*
Somjen G, 400, *407*
Song H, 340, *354*, 370, *379*, 494, *520*, 693, *731*

Soni N, 348, *356*
Sonneblick E, 585, *608*
Sonneblick EH, 363, *378*, 582, 584, *606*
Sonnenschein RR, 386, *402*
Soparkar GR, 84, *113*
Sorbini CA, 136, *147*
Sorgato G, 669, *683*
Souktani R, 629, *644*
Souverijn JH, 583, *606*
Spagnolatti L, 142, *148*
Spagnoli LG, 660, *680*
Span JF, 582, 584, *606*
Spanavello A, 567, *577*
Spann JA, 360, 368, 369, *377*, *378*
Spapen H, 425, *432*
Sparks HV, 340, *354*, 383, *401*
Sparr H, 427, *433*
Spellman MJ, 526, *547*
Spencer AA, 192, *197*
Sperling J, 660, *680*
Spicer WS, 83, 84, *113*
Spickard RC, 586, 587, *608*
Spiro SG, 557, 559, 565, *574*
Spitzer JJ, 691, *729*
Spitzer WO, 200, *224*
Spokes K, 458, 462, 463, *466*, *467*
Sporre B, 184, 185, 188, 189, *195*, *196*
Spotnitz HM, 363, *378*
Spragg R, 304, 305, 319, *323*, *329*
Spragg RG, 532, *549*
Sprague RS, 192, *197*
Sprung CL, 686, 687, *727*
Sridhar G, 272, 273, 276, *283*, 561, 562, 564, 568, 569, 570, 571, *575*, *577*
Srivastava DK, 36, *43*
St John-Sutton M, 596, *612*
Stahl WM, 705, *735*
Stainsby WN, 337, 345, *353*, *355*, 383, 386, 397, *401*, *402*
Stalenheim G, 213, *227*
Stamler J, 618, 641, *642*
Stamler JS, 617, 618, 621, 624, 625, 626, 627, 632, 633, 634, 641, *642*, *644*
Stampone P, 222, *228*
Standaert TA, 79, *112*
Standiford TJ, 375, *381*
Stanek KS, 39, *44*

Stanford D, 125, *144*
Stanford RE, 238, *259*
Stanley C, 30, 31, 36, *42*, *43*
Stansbury DW, 566, *576*
Stark RD, 412, *430*, 692, *730*
Stary CM, 474, *518*
Stasiw DM, 637, *646*
Statham NJ, 618, *642*
Statts B, 560, 566, *575*
Staub NC, 82, *113*, 122, *143*, 387, *403*
Steele JM, 635, *645*
Steg G, 251, *260*
Stein JC, 620, *642*
Stein PD, 297, *302*
Stein RA, 655, 656, 657, 665, *677*, *678*
Steinberg KP, 319, *329*, 685, *727*
Steinberg S, 707, *736*
Steinhaur H, 583, *607*
Stel HV, 693, *730*
Stelkens H, 670, *683*
Stengraad-Pedersen K, 456, *466*
Stenius B, 206, *225*
Stenmark KR, 131, *145*
Stephen GW, 691, 703, 704, *729*
Sternberg J, 537, *549*
Sterns DA, 598, *613*
Stetler GI, 635, *645*
Stetz CW, 49, *108*
Stevenson L, 596, *612*
Steward PB, 67, *111*
Stewart PB, 121, 125, *143*, *144*
Stewart TE, 321, *329*
Stibolt T, 596, *612*
Stieglitz P, 271, *282*, 566, *577*
Stiksa J, 560, 562, *575*
Stinsby WN, 540, *550*
Stinson EB, 583, *607*
Stipanic S, 655, *677*
Stock MC, 314, *327*
Stock MJ, 714, *738*
Stoclet JC, 424, *432*
Stojcev S, 669, *683*
Stojceva Taneva O, 669, *683*
Stojkovski L, 669, *683*
Stolp BW, 8, *26*, 82, *113*, 248, *260*, 267, 272, 274, 275, 277, 279, *283*, 530, 544, *548*

Stone D, 254, *261*
Stone W, 660, *680*
Story D, 107, *118*, 388, 389, 390, 392, *403*, 515, *522*, 535, *549*
Strachan D, 200, *224*
Strandberg A, 180, 181, 182, 183, 185, 186, 190, *194*, *195*, *196*, *197*
Strandgaard S, 662, *681*
Strange S, 661, *680*
Stratton H, 704, *735*
Stratton HH, 427, *433*, 711, *737*
Straub J, 693, *730*
Straube RC, 321, *329*
Strauss B, 699, 700, *733*
Strauss HW, 341, *354*
Stray-Gundersen J, 511, 515, *522*, *523*, 655, 656, 658, 659, 662, 665, *678*, *679*
Streeter DD, 363, *378*
Strenn K, 641, *647*
Strieter RM, 375, *381*, 721, *740*
Stringer W, 487, 507, *520*
Strobeck JE, 582, 584, *606*
Strom J, 605, *615*
Strom JA, 586, *608*
Stubbs SE, 186, *194*
Stucker O, 637, *646*
Stulbarg MS, 563, *575*
Stummvoll HK, 655, *677*
Stumpe T, 371, 373, *380*
Sturgeon C, 360, *377*
Stuttard E, 36, *43*
Suarez J, 159, 160, *173*
Suarez RK, 29, 39, *41*, *42*, *43*
Sublett E, 376, *381*
Subramanian HV, 31, *42*
Sudlow MF, 165, *174*
Sue D, 268, *282*, 583, 589, *607*, *609*
Sue DY, 272, *283*, 474, 476, 481, 482, *518*, 554, *573*
Suero JT, 564, *575*
Sufficool W, 705, 706, 707, *736*
Suffredini AF, 424, *432*
Suga H, 359, 364, 365, 366, 375, 376, *376*, *378*, *380*, *381*
Suga S, 670, *683*
Sugar AM, 460, *467*
Sugimachi M, 375, *381*

Sugioka K, 105, *118*
Sugishita Y, 670, *683*
Sugita T, 152, *172*, 527, *547*
Suh BY, 205, *225*
Suissa S, 200, *224*
Sullivan K, 623, *643*
Sullivan M, 590, 591, 597, 603, *610*, *612*, *613*, *614*
Sullivan SM, 387, *402*, 640, *647*
Suman OE, 480, *519*
Sun D, 493, *520*, 587, *608*
Sundquist AR, 633, *645*
Suprenant EL, 207, 209, *226*
Surjadhana A, 369, *379*
Sutarik JM, 205, *225*
Suter PM, 686, 688, 692, *728*, *729*
Sutton JR, 23, *27*, 136, *146*, 156, 158, 159, 160, 161, 170, *173*, *175*, 526, 529, 530, 531, 532, 533, 537, *547*, *548*, *549*
Suzuki S, 375, *381*
Svendmyr N, 714, *738*
Svensson G, 278, *283*
Svensson L, 180, 181, 182, 183, *194*, *195*
Swain DP, 101, *117*, 511, *522*
Swanepoel C, 660, *680*
Swartz HM, 101, 103, *117*
Sweeney D, 686, *728*
Sweeney HL, 387, 388, *403*
Sweeney TE, 394, *405*
Sweet M, 713, 714, *738*
Swenberg ML, 622, 625, *643*
Swenson EW, 131, *145*, 287, *301*
Sybbalo N, 554, 571, *574*
Sykes MK, 189, *196*
Symon Z, 458, *466*
Systrom D, 566, *576*
Systrom DM, 271, *283*, 571, 572, *578*
Szabo C, 352, *357*
Szabo D, 444, *445*

T

Tagliabue M, 304, 305, *324*
Tai E, 200, 202, 205, *224*, *225*
Takagaki TY, 305, 313, 321, *324*, *329*

Takahashi K, 662, 663, 670, *681*
Takala J, 686, 688, 691, 693, 694, 715, 716, *728*, *729*, *732*, *739*
Takaoka H, 366, *378*
Takaori M, 692, *730*
Takasago T, 375, *380*
Takeshita A, 375, *381*
Takeuchi M, 366, *378*
Takishima Y, 220, *228*
Takizawa T, 238, *259*
Tall BD, 713, 714, *738*
Tamm C, 376, *381*
Tan S, 722, *741*
Tanabe N, 131, *145*
Tang GJ, 720, *740*
Tang W, 716, 717, *739*
Tania T, 122, *143*
Tapson VF, 292, *301*
Tarczy-Hornoch P, 317, *328*
Tarnow J, 310, 312, 320, *326*
Tarraga S, 271, *283*
Tashkin D, 596, *612*
Tashkin DP, 427, *433*, 699, 700, 713, 714, *733*, *738*
Tatsumi K, 152, *172*
Tauber J, 427, *433*
Tavazzi L, 603, 605, *615*
Tayler CR, 387, 389, *403*
Taylor AA, 375, *381*
Taylor CR, 46, 55, 90, *108*, *109*, *115*
Taylor DJ, 662, *680*
Taylor DR, 200, *224*
Taylor RW, 321, *329*
Teboul JL, 251, *260*
Teerlink JR, 587, *608*
Teisseire B, 286, 290, 291, 292, *300*, 307, 310, 312, 313, *324*, *325*, *326*, 620, 637, *642*, *646*
Teisseire BP, 620, *643*
Templeton D, 635, *645*
Temporelli PL, 603, 605, *615*
Tenney SM, 480, *519*, 541, *551*, 693, *731*
Teplinsky K, 359, 361, 371, *376*, 414, *431*
tePoel M, 632, 633, *645*
Teres D, 686, 687, *728*

Terjung RL, 389, 400, *404*
Theroux JF, 192, 193, *198*
Thews G, 497, 503, *521*
Thiemermann C, 192, *197*, 424, *432*
Thiene G, 200, *224*
Thijs JG, 693, *730*
Thijs LG, 686, 687, 688, 693, *728*, *730*, *731*
Thoden JS, 152, 156, *172*
Thomas AAG, 36, *43*
Thomas GD, 386, *402*, 668, *682*
Thomas JA, 583, *606*
Thomas ML, 707, 708, *736*
Thomas WJ, 30, *42*
Thompson CH, 662, 664, *680*
Thompson JR, 656, 662, *678*
Thompson WJ, 396, *406*
Thornell L, 539, *550*
Thrush DN, 46, 49, *108*
Thum J, 655, *677*
Thuning CA, 394, *406*
Thurlbeck WM, 238, 242, *259*, 263, 265, 269, 276, *281*
Tian R, 583, *606*
Tien YK, 184, *195*
Tighe D, 722, *741*
Tilney NL, 685, *727*
Timmins AC, 705, 718, 719, *736*
Tinelli C, 142, *148*
Tinker J, 348, 351, *356*, 699, 700, *733*
Tobin MJ, 570, *577*
Tocilj J, 654, *677*
Tockics L, 180, 183, *194*, *195*
Todd GJ, 591, *610*
Todd TR, 321, *329*
Todoran TM, 131, *145*
Tognoni G, 313, *327*, 705, 718, 719, *736*
Tokics L, 178, 179, 181, 182, 184, 185, 186, 188, 190, *193*, *194*, *196*, *197*
Tolins JP, 310, *326*
Tomas P, 271, *283*
Tomioka S, 212, *227*
Tomizawa T, 670, *683*
Tomlin PJ, 142, *147*
Tomlin WC, 210, *226*
Tomlinson B, 351, *356*, 694, *732*

Tompkins RG, 692, *730*
Tooley R, 317, 318, *328*
Topuzovic N, 655, *677*
Tornabene VW, 291, *300*
Torre-Bueno J, 8, *26*, 136, *146*, 530, 537, 544, *548*
Torre-Bueno JE, 267, 272, 274, 275, 277, 279, *283*
Torre-Bueno JR, 82, *113*, 248, *260*
Torre-Bueno RE, 136, *146*
Torregrosa JV, 515, *523*, 659, 662, 663, 664, *679*, *680*
Torres A, 213, 220, *227*, 231, 235, 236, 243, 245, 250, *257*, *258*, *259*, *260*, 264, *281*
Torres Filho IP, 618, 625, 628, 638, *642*, *644*
Torvik D, 667, *682*
Toto RD, 658, 668, 669, *679*, *683*
Totsune K, 662, 663, 670, *681*
Toussaint JF, 588, *608*
Townes BD, 541, *551*
Tran DD, 687, *728*
Trap-Jensen J, 386, *402*
Traver DL, 352, *357*
Traystman RF, 692, *730*
Treiwasser JH, 85, *114*
Tremper KK, 100, 101, *117*, 690, *728*
Trinh-Trang-Tan MM, 448, 450, *465*
Trinkle JK, 515, *523*
Trojaborg W, 669, *683*
Troosters T, 566, *576*
Trop D, 122, *143*, 164, *174*
Trouve R, 637, *646*
Trulock EP, 271, *283*
Trump BF, 462, *467*
Truog WE, 79, *112*
Tsai AG, 632, *644*
Tsairis P, 396, *406*
Tsidemiadou PD, 701, *734*
Tskumoto K, 107, *118*
Tsukimoto K, 139, *147*, 388, 392, 397, *404*, 480, 485, 487, 503, *519*, *520*, 531, 532, *548*, *549*
Tsusaki K, 131, *145*

Tuchler M, 588, *609*
Tuchschmidt J, 350, 352, *356*, 705, 707, 720, *736*
Tuder RM, 241, *259*
Tuley MR, 192, 193, *198*
Tuma RF, 373, *380*, 421, *432*, 629, 630, 640, *644*
Tuma SN, 463, *467*
Tumas J, 620, *643*
Turek Z, 152, *172*
Tuxen DV, 204, *225*
Tuzzo D, 305, *324*
Tweeddale M, 690, *729*
Tweeddale MG, 360, *377*, 428, *434*, 695, *733*
Twiss RD, 691, 703, *729*
Tyml K, 340, *354*, 370, 373, 375, *379*, *380*, 392, 393, *405*, 424, *432*, 494, *520*, 693, *731*
Tyron T, 540, *550*

U

Udden MM, 166, *174*
Ueda H, 347, *355*, 427, *433*
Ueng TH, 191, *197*
Ueno O, 107, *118*, 212, *227*, 388, 389, 390, 392, *403*, 515, *522*, 535, *549*
Ugurbil K, 30, *42*
Uhl RR, 76, *112*, 135, *146*, 231, *257*, 303, 306, 307, 312, *323*, *324*
Uhlig PN, 368, *379*
Ulmer HE, 657, *679*
Ulmer WT, 142, *147*
Ulstad VK, 30, *42*
Ultman JS, 46, *108*
Umans JG, 424, 425, *432*
Uncles DR, 192, *197*
Underhill S, 694, *732*
Ungar A, 342, *355*
Ungerer M, 583, *607*
Uren N, 599, 600, *614*
Uren NG, 597, *613*
Urgurbil K, 36, *43*
Usami S, 101, *115*, 637, *646*

Ussetti P, 238, 242, 246, *259*, 311, 321, *326*, 560, 565, *575*
Utley J, 692, *730*
Utsunomiya T, 294, *301*
Uusaro A, 694, *732*

V

Vagelos R, 596, 599, 600, *612*, *614*
Vaisanen O, 716, *739*
Vajda J, 417, *431*
Valdes RJ, 671, *684*
Valentine DD, 315, *327*
Valenza F, 304, *324*
Valeri CR, 724, *741*
Valles E, 667, *682*
Vallet B, 93, 105, *115*, *118*, 346, 350, 351, *355*, *356*, 425, *432*
Vallez MO, 620, *643*
van Aerde JE, 714, *738*
Van Aken H, 191, *197*
Van Beek JHGM, 122, *144*, 421, *431*
van Damme J, 720, 721, 724, *740*
Van De Wiele B, 591, *610*
Van den Eijnde S, 583, *606*
van der Bos GC, 693, *730*, *731*
Van der Laarse A, 583, *606*
Van der Linden P, 345, *355*
van der Meulen J, 687, *728*
van der Poll T, 720, 721, 722, *740*
van Deventer SJH, 720, *740*
Van Dop C, 583, *607*
van Eeden S, 375, *380*
Van Esbroeck G, 98, *116*
van Kraats AA, 693, *730*
Van L, 152, *172*
van Lambalgen AA, 693, *730*
van Liew J, 707, *736*
van Meerhaeghe A, 560, *575*
van Muylem A, 67, *111*
van Schijndel RS, 687, *728*
Van Slyke DD, 49, *108*
Van Trigt P, 515, *522*
Van Wezel HB, 360, *377*
van Zyl Smit R, 20, *27*
van Zyl-Smydt R, 665, *682*

Vandegriff KD, 617, 624, 636, 637, *641*, *644*, *645*, *646*
Vanden Hoek TL, 376, *381*
Vandenbossche JL, 298, *299*, *302*
Vanderhoeft P, 290, 291, 293, 294, *301*
Vandermeer TJ, 428, 429, *434*, 716, *739*
Vandeviviere J, 207, 209, *226*
Vane J, 424, *432*
Vane JR, 192, *197*
Vanhoutte PM, 386, *402*, 694, *732*
Vanner S, 396, *406*
Varene N, 256, *261*
Vary TC, 429, *434*, 713, 714, *738*
Vaziri ND, 663, 667, *682*
Veazey WB, 583, *607*
Veech RL, 31, *42*
Velez RL, 667, *682*
Venegas JC, 131, *145*
Venkatesh B, 718, *740*
Venkatesh KB, 715, *738*
Verbank S, 67, *111*, 126, *144*
Vergroesen I, 360, *377*
Veriter C, 309, *325*
Vermeij CG, 711, 712, *737*
Vermeire P, 229, *256*
Vermeulen F, 289, 291, *301*
Vetere L, 704, 709, 715, *735*
Viale JP, 711, 712, *737*
Viby-Mogensen J, 177, 178, 192, 193, *193*, *197*
Vicaut E, 629, 637, *644*, *646*, 691, *729*
Victor RG, 386, *402*, 658, 668, 669, *679*, *682*, *683*
Viegas C, 221, *228*, 496, 508, 511, 514, *521*, 539, *550*
Viegas CA, 231, 234, 235, *258*
Vigfusson G, 191, *197*
Vigginao R, 560, 566, *575*
Vikerfors T, 720, *740*
Villaschi S, 660, *680*
Villemant D, 359, 361, 373, 374, *377*
Villringer A, 440, *445*
Vincent JL, 104, *118*, 345, 351, 352, *355*, *356*, *357*, 425, *432*, 686, 688, 699, 700, 701, 703, 714, 720, 721, 724, *728*, *733*, *734*, *740*

Vink H, 390, 391, *404*
Vinogradov S, 101, *117*
Vinogradov SA, 15, *26*
Viries N, 691, 694, *729*
Vitale G, 304, 315, 317, *324*, *328*
Vitek V, 701, *734*
Vivien A, 192, *198*
Vizek M, 526, *547*
Vlahakes GJ, 368, *379*
Voelkel NF, 237, 241, *259*
Vogel JA, 158, 159, *173*
Voigt A, 656, 664, 670, *678*
Volkman K, 583, *607*
Vollmer WM, 209, *226*
Vomacka RB, 370, *379*
von Beckerath N, 340, *354*
Von Euler US, 189, *196*, 237, *259*
Von Gal ER, 263, 265, 269, 273, 276, *281*
Von Ritter C, 94, *115*
Von Saalfeld E, 387, *403*
Voter WA, 388, *403*
Vreim CE, 297, *302*
Vugue B, 691, *729*

W

Waagenwoort C, 595, *611*
Waagenwoort N, 595, *611*
Wada O, 597, *613*
Wade OL, 353, *357*
Wagner H, 130, *145*
Wagner HN, 70, *111*, 341, *354*
Wagner P, 170, *175*
Wagner PD, 2, 4, 7, 8, 10, 12, 15, 20, 22, 23, *25*, *26*, *27*, 31, 39, 40, *42*, *44*, 46, 61, 72, 76, 79, 82, 95, 96, 107, *108*, *111*, *112*, *113*, *116*, *118*, 129, 130, 134, 135, 136, 137, 139, 141, *145*, *146*, *147*, 156, 158, 159, 160, 166, 170, *173*, *175*, 179, 190, *194*, 210, 211, 212, 213, 214, 215, 216, 217, 220, 222, *226*, *227*, *228*, 230, 231, 232, 234, 235, 236, 238, 242, 243, 245, 246, 248, 249, 250, 253, *257*, *258*, *259*, *260*, *261*, 263, 264,

[Wagner PD]
265, 266, 267, 268, 269, 272, 273, 274, 275, 276, 277, 278, 279, *281*, *282*, *283*, 285, 286, 290, 291, 296, *300*, *301*, *302*, 303, 306, 307, 310, 311, 312, 313, 318, 321, *323*, *324*, *325*, *326*, *327*, *328*, 388, 389, 390, 392, 393, 397, *403*, *404*, *405*, 470, 471, 472, 475, 476, 477, 478, 480, 484, 485, 486, 487, 488, 492, 494, 495, 496, 497, 503, 504, 505, 507, 508, 509, 511, 514, 515, *517*, *518*, *519*, *520*, *521*, *522*, *523*, 527, 529, 530, 531, 532, 533, 534, 535, 536, 537, 538, 539, 540, 542, 543, 544, 545, *548*, *549*, *550*, *551*, *552*, 557, 560, 565, 566, 568, *574*, *575*, *576*, *577*, 620, 638, *642*, *647*, 654, 655, 659, 662, 663, 664, *677*, *679*, *680*, 686, 687, *727*
Wagner TM, 131, *145*
Wagner WW, 57, 60, 66, *110*, 470, 486, 504, *517*
Wagner WWJ, 131, *145*
Wahba RWM, 182, 183, *194*
Wahren J, 591, *610*
Wain JC, 271, *283*, 571, 572, *578*
Wainsztein N, 428, *434*, 705, 706, *735*
Walden J, 596, *612*
Walder JA, 635, *645*
Walder RY, 635, *645*
Waldron JA, 263, 265, 269, 276, *281*
Walezak T, 101, 103, *117*
Walker SD, 298, *302*
Walker SR, 206, *225*
Walker TA, 352, *357*, 620, *643*
Walker WA, 692, *730*
Wall MA, 209, *226*
Wallace A, 602, *614*
Wallace AG, 602, *614*
Walley KR, 359, 360, 361, 371, 373, 374, *376*, *377*, *380*, 414, 423, 425, 426, 428, *431*, *433*, *434*, 620, *643*, 693, 694, 695, 697, 698, 711, 712, 714, 715, *731*, *733*, *737*
Wallimann T, 39, 40, *44*
Wallwork J, 241, 254, *259*, *261*

Walmrath D, 310, 312, 319, 321, *326, 327, 328, 329*
Walmrath HD, 319, *328*
Walter B, 603, 605, *615*
Walter G, 590, 591, *610*
Walter M, 637, *646*
Walter SE, 530, 537, *548*
Walters BJ, 125, *144*
Walters E, 571, 572, *578*
Wang C, 56, 92, *110*
Wang H, 101, *117*, 428, 429, *434*, 704, 716, *735, 739*
Wang N, 238, *259*
Wang Y, 364, *378*
Wang ZQ, 663, 667, *682*
Wanger PD, 61, 85, *111*
Wanke T, 653, *676*
Wanner A, 222, *228*
Ward MP, 528, *552*
Ward SA, 480, 481, 482, 483, 489, 509, *519, 520*
Ward SM, 222, *228*
Warley AR, 695, *732*
Warltier DC, 376, *381*
Warner DO, 183, *195*
Warner MA, 183, *195*
Warrell DA, 166, *175*
Warringer CB, 371, *380*
Wasserman K, 46, *108*, 268, 272, *282, 283*, 470, 474, 481, 482, 483, 484, 487, 507, *517, 518, 519, 520*, 554, 555, 557, 558, 565, 572, *573, 574*, 583, 589, *607, 609*
Watenpaugh DE, 165, *174*
Watkins SC, 375, *381*
Wats RE, 272, 276, *283*
Watson D, 705, 718, 719, *736*
Watts D, 565, *576*
Watts R, 554, 571, *574*
Waxman K, 705, 706, 718, 724, *736, 741*
Weatherall DJ, 620, *642*
Weathersby PK, 390, 391, 395, *404*, 638, *646*
Weaver LJ, 307, 311, 312, *324*
Webb A, 722, *741*
Webb AR, 704, 709, 715, 716, *735, 739*
Weber ED, 318, *328*

Weber JM, 36, *43*
Weber K, 583, 596, *607, 612*
Weber KT, 364, *378*, 508, *522*
Weber S, 599, *614*
Wedzicha JA, 229, *257*
Weetzels E, 665, 666, *682*
Weg JG, 303, 305, 307, 309, 311, 312, 313, 319, *323, 325, 329*, 347, *356*, 427, *433*, 699, 700, *733*
Wegener G, 36, *43*
Wegenius G, 185, 188, 189, *196*
Wehr KL, 565, 566, *576*
Wei H, 691, *729*
Weibel ER, 2, 4, *26*, 49, 55, 90, 91, *108, 109, 115*, 156, *172*, 385, 387, 389, 390, 391, 394, *401, 402, 403*, 539, *550*
Weightman D, 659, *679*
Weigle GE, 471, 474, *518*
Weil JV, 160, *173*, 203, *224*, 526, *547*
Weil MH, 142, *147*, 699, 700, 701, 716, 717, *733, 734, 739*
Weiner D, 588, 589, *609*
Weiner DH, 588, *609*
Weinstein J, 595, *612*
Weinstein JM, 464, *467*
Weir EK, 310, *326*
Weisbrode SE, 426, *433*
Weisinger JR, 660, 670, *680*
Weisman IM, 313, 314, *327*
Weiss CH, 451, 452, *465*
Weiss RG, 583, *606*
Weissman C, 46, *108*, 694, 710, *732, 736*
Welbourn R, 724, *741*
Welch GH, 364, *378*
Welch HG, 540, *550*
Welch JE, 620, *643*
Weller R, 594, *611*
Wellman H, 436, *445*
Wells FC, 241, *259*
Wells G, 690, *729*
Wells L, 591, *610*
Welsh DG, 386, 399, *401*, 493, 509, *520, 522*
Wendt M, 192, *198*
Werner C, 464, *467*
Werner HA, 360, 373, 374, *377*
Wertz MJ, 687, *728*

Author Index

Wesley RA, 424, *432*
Wesseling GJ, 567, *577*
West GB, 132, *145*
West J, 597, *612*
West JB, 4, 8, 22, 23, *26, 27*, 61, 71, 73, 74, 76, *111, 112*, 121, 122, 129, 133, 134, 135, *143, 144, 145, 146*, 149, 150, 152, 156, 158, 162, 163, 164, 166, 168, 169, 170, *171, 172, 173, 174, 175*, 178, 179, 180, 188, 190, *193, 194, 196*, 204, 209, 210, 212, 222, *225, 226, 227*, 230, 231, 235, 236, 250, *257, 258, 260*, 263, 264, 276, *281*, 285, 289, 291, *300, 301*, 303, 306, 307, 310, 311, 312, 318, 321, *323, 324, 326, 328*, 388, 392, 397, *404, 405*, 500, 511, 514, *521, 522*, 527, 528, 529, 530, 531, 532, 537, 538, 542, 543, 545, *547, 548, 549, 550, 551, 552*, 565, *576*, 618, 619, 620, *642*
Westbrook PR, 186, *194*
Westerhoff HV, 36, *43*
Westerman J, 318, *328*
Westfall JA, 532, *548*
Wetter TJ, 386, *401*
Wetzel RC, 311, *326*
Whalen WJ, 394, *406*
Wheat JD, 532, *548*
Whipp B, 583, 589, *607, 609*
Whipp BJ, 268, 272, *282, 283*, 469, 470, 471, 472, 474, 475, 476, 480, 481, 482, 483, 484, 489, 509, *517, 518, 519, 520*, 555, *574*
Whisler SK, 598, *613*
White F, 180, *194*
White FC, 311, 313, *326*
White NJ, 714, *738*
White TP, 387, 389, 396, *403, 406*
Whitehill TA, 701, *734*
Whitehouse WM, 101, *117*, 704, *735*
Whitmer JT, 359, *376*
Whitsett TL, 694, *731*
Whittembury J, 618, *642*
Whittenberg BA, 543, 545, *551*
Whittenburg JB, 543, 545, *551*
Whittom F, 566, *576*

Whitwell KE, 532, *548*
Whyche MQ, 184, *195*
Widnell C, 713, *738*
Wiedemann HP, 319, *329*
Wiegel JH, 713, 714, *738*
Wiesner R, 271, *283*
Wiggins T, 665, *682*
Wiggs B, 375, *380*, 711, 712, 714, *737*
Wiggs BR, 231, 238, 245, 246, *258, 259, 260*, 360, 373, *377, 380*, 428, *434*, 695, 699, 700, 714, *733*
Wilen M, 596, *612*
Wilford DC, 638, *647*
Wilkins E, 724, *741*
Willats S, 686, 688, *728*
Willems E, 309, *325*
Willford DC, 503, 504, *522*
Williams AJ, 710, *737*
Williams CA, 386, *402*
Williams DA, 400, *407*
Williams G, 347, *355*, 427, *433*
Williams GW, 297, *302*
Williams J, 131, *145*
Williams R, 585, 602, *607, 614*
Williams RE, 586, 587, *608*
Williams RS, 388, *404*, 546, *552*, 602, *614*, 655, 665, *678*
Williams SG, 125, *144*
Williams T, 571, 572, *578*
Williams TJ, 271, *283*
Willis N, 654, *677*
Willis RE, 540, *550*
Wilmore DW, 694, *732*
Wilson AF, 84, *113*, 207, 209, *226*
Wilson BA, 383, 397, *401*
Wilson DF, 15, *26*, 30, 31, *42*, 101, *117*, 414, *431*, 483, *519*
Wilson J, 583, 585, 591, 603, 605, *607, 608, 610, 615*, 655, *677*
Wilson JR, 508, *522*, 588, 589, 590, 591, 596, 597, 598, *609, 610, 612, 613*
Wilson K, 596, 599, 600, *612, 614*
Wilson LB, 106, 107, *118*
Wilson RF, 691, 694, *729*
Wilson TA, 54, *109*, 125, 126, *144, 145*
Wily SW, 360, *377*
Winaver J, 455, *465*

Winlove CP, 350, *356*
Winn MJ, 346, *355*
Winn RR, 569, *577*
Winniford MD, 375, *381*
Winslow NJ, 541, *551*, 622, *643*
Winslow RM, 101, *117*, 152, *172*, 527, 529, 530, 537, 541, *547*, *550*, *551*, 617, 618, 619, 620, 622, 625, 626, 634, 636, 637, 641, *641*, *642*, *643*, *644*, *645*, *646*
Winter JH, 254, *261*
Winterhalter M, 587, *608*
Wise C, 318, *328*
Wiseman RW, 36, *43*
Wittenberg B, 589, *609*
Wittenberg BA, 39, 40, *43*, 388, *403*, 496, *521*, 661, *680*
Wittenberg J, 589, *609*
Wittenberg JB, 388, *403*, 496, *521*, 639, *647*, 661, *680*
Witty LA, 292, *301*
Wizemann B, 662, *681*
Wizemann V, 655, *677*
Wodzinska J, 635, *645*
Woldenburg MJ, 53, *109*
Wolfe D, 540, *550*
Wolfson M, 660, *680*
Wollert KC, 515, *523*
Wollmer P, 213, *227*
Wollschlager H, 375, *381*
Wolter DT, 721, *741*
Woltz M, 641, *647*
Womack W, 94, *115*
Wong CK, 658, 670, *679*
Wong JTF, 636, *645*
Wong SY, 538, 545, *550*
Wood EH, 122, *143*
Wood LDH, 349, 350, *356*, 359, 361, 371, *376*, 414, 425, 426, 428, *431*, *432*, *433*, *434*, 693, 694, 695, 697, 710, 711, 712, *731*, *732*, 737
Wood PR, 715, *739*
Wood SA, 54, *109*
Wood SC, 503, *522*
Woodard RD, 667, *682*
Woodard T, 667, 671, *682*
Woodson RD, 540, *550*, 620, *642*

Woolcock AJ, 207, 209, *226*
Woolf CR, 564, *575*
Worth H, 67, *111*
Wouters EFM, 567, *577*
Wright DL, 386, *402*
Wright GW, 82, *113*
Wright R, 596, *612*
Wright SJ, 165, *174*
Wrigley SM, 392, 393, *405*
Wschar YR, 142, *147*
Wu EY, 487, *520*
Wurst HJ, 310, 312, 320, *326*
Wuyam B, 271, *282*, 566, *577*
Wyabbalo NC, 558, 559, *574*
Wybitul K, 665, 666, *682*
Wylam ME, 424, 425, *432*
Wyler F, 341, *354*, 692, *730*
Wyman J, 543, *551*, 622, 623, *643*
Wyman R, 595, *612*
Wysocki M, 252, *261*, 320, 322, *329*
Wyss CR, 593, *611*
Wyss M, 39, 40, *44*

X

Xaubet A, 263, 264, 265, 266, 267, 268, 269, 272, 273, 274, 275, 278, 279, 280, *281*, *282*, 312, *327*
Xia J, 370, *379*
Xu D, 691, *729*
Xu FD, 526, *547*

Y

Yafe R, 463, *467*
Yaku H, 376, *381*
Yamabayashi H, 271, *282*, 566, *577*
Yamada A, 375, *381*
Yamada K, 662, *681*
Yamada O, 364, 365, *378*
Yamaguchi I, 670, *683*
Yamaguchi K, 87, *114*
Yamamoto K, 662, *681*
Yamamoto Y, 662, *681*
Yamawaki I, 238, *259*

Author Index 803

Yamaya M, 46, 72, *108*
Yamaya Y, 511, 514, *522*, 532, *549*
Yanagisawa M, 670, *683*
Yang BC, 586, 587, *608*
Yang G, 716, 717, *739*
Yang QX, 668, *682*
Yarmush ML, 692, *730*
Yates DM, 200, *224*
Yau EHS, 705, 718, 719, *736*
Yen TC, 720, *740*
Yeoh TK, 583, *607*
Yernault JC, 229, *256*
Yeung DW, 658, 670, *679*
Yien HW, 720, *740*
Yipintsoi T, 363, *377*
Yonce LR, 398, *407*
Yonekawa H, 345, *355*
Yonge R, 588, 589, *609*
Yoshikawa K, 591, *610*
Youker K, 375, *381*
Younes M, 558, 559, 571, *574*, *575*, *578*
Younes MK, 558, 559, 571, *574*
Young I, 286, 290, *301*
Young IH, 207, 209, 217, 222, *226*, *227*
Young P, 596, *612*
Young PM, 23, *27*, 530, 537, *548*, *549*
Yu M, 705, *736*
Yusef S, 583, *607*

Z

Zabel P, 721, *741*
Zabetakis PM, 655, 665, *678*
Zaccerdelli DS, 319, *329*
Zagelbaum G, 570, *577*
Zager RA, 458, *466*
Zaidi SAJ, 701, *734*
Zamel N, 204, *225*, 271, *283*
Zamora R, 632, 633, *645*

Zanaboni S, 554, 572, *573*
Zanjani ED, 152, *172*, 619, *642*
Zapol DG, 39, *44*
Zapol WM, 39, *44*, 251, 254, 255, *260*, *261*, 310, 312, 320, *326*
Zaret BL, 566, *576*
Zaugg RH, 635, *645*
Zavala E, 243, *260*
Zawadzki JV, 241, *259*, 346, *355*, 632, *645*
Zech P, 662, *681*
Zegna AI, 637, *645*
Zeiher AM, 375, *381*
Zelis R, 587, 588, 602, *608*, *609*, *614*
Zeller WP, 713, 714, *738*
Zellis R, 581, 584, *606*
Zera P, 583, *607*
Zerhouni EA, 54, *109*
Zernicke RF, 396, *406*
Zhang H, 351, 352, *356*, *357*, 425, *432*, 701, *734*
Zhou XJ, 663, 667, *682*
Zhu G, 30, *42*
Zhu XH, 437, *445*
Ziegler TW, 654, 655, *677*
Zifko U, 653, *676*
Zimmer SD, 30, *42*
Zimmerman JE, 686, 687, *727*
Zimmerman SW, 655, 657, *678*
Zimmermann JL, 321, *329*
Zintel T, 554, 558, 559, 560, 571, *574*, *575*
Zintel TA, 272, 273, 276, *283*, 561, 562, 564, 565, 568, 569, 570, 571, *575*, *577*
Zohman L, 591, *610*
Zoia MC, 142, *148*
Zujko KJ, 582, 584, *606*
Zuntz N, 150, *171*
Zweifach BW, 630, 631, 638, *644*
Zyl Smit RV, 659, *680*

Subject Index

A

Acclimatization, 151
Acetazolamide, 161
Acetylcholine, 586, 593
　role in skeletal muscle and vascular activation, 493
Acinus, 57
Actin-myosin ATPase, 365
Acute asthma, 201–203, 213
　hypercapnia, 201
　hypocapnia, 201
　mechanical ventilatory support, 201
　ventilatory responsiveness to CO_2, 202
Acute exacerbations, 243–246
　cardiac output, 243
　decrease in $P\overline{v}O_2$, 243
　oxygen consumption, 243
　respiratory muscles, 243
　$\dot{V}_A/\dot{Q}$ inequality, 243
Acute or chronic thromboembolic pulmonary hypertension, 285
Acute tubular necrosis, 457, 463–464
　atrial natriuretic peptide, 463
　diuretics, 463
　dopamine, 463
　furosemide, 463

[Acute tubular necrosis]
　mannitol, 463
　theophyline, 463
Adenosine diphosphate (ADP), 30, 588
Adenosine triphosphatase (ATPase) Na^+/K^+, 672
Adenosine triphosphate (ATP), 29, 30, 37, 359, 582, 663
　as a primary regulator, 36
　buffering, 37
　concentration in the brain, 442
　demand, 36
　muscle levels, 592
　pathways of, 37
　resynthesis, 583
　supply pathways, 36, 37
　turnover rate, 30, 36, 37, 39, 41
β-adrenergic receptors, 583
β-adrenergic blockade, 415
Adult respiratory distress syndrome, 427
Aerobic capacity, 653, 655, 661
Aerobic metabolism, 651
Aerobic power, 661
Aging, 138–142
　kidney, 459
Airflow obstruction, 599, 600

805

Airway
  generation, 51
  measurement of DLCO, 83
Airway closure, 178, 183–184, 207
  closing capacity, 184
  shunt, 184
  ventilation perfusion mismatch, 184
Aldosterone, 583
Allosteric effectors, 617, 621, 622
Altitude, 150, 525, 619
  acclimatization, 526, 539
  arterial carbon dioxide pressure, 514
  cardiac output, 514
  high, 525
  maximum heart rate, 514
  O_2 delivery, 514
  pulmonary vascular response, 532
  respiratory muscles, 526
Alveolar arterial oxygen tension difference, 124, 158, 177, 484, 565
Alveolar arterial oxygen tension gradient, 264
Alveolar capillary block syndrome, 269
Alveolar capillary diffusion limitation, 137, 264
Alveolar gas equation, 597
Alveolar hypoventilation, 181–182
Alveolar plateau, 66
Alveolar ventilation, 526, 554, 557, 655
American Medical Research Expedition to Everest (AMREE), 152–154
Anaerobic threshold (see Lactic threshold)
Anatomical dead space, 182
Andes, 150
Angiogenesis
  muscle capillaries, 539
Apoptosis
  kidney, 458
Arterial carbon dioxide pressure, 564, 565
Arterial oxygen pressure, 121, 122, 564, 565, 617, 641
  during exercise, 484
Arterial respiratory blood gases, 142

Arteriole
  exercise, 488
  vasoconstrictor tone, 488
Asbestosis, 268, 269, 280
Ascaris suum extract, 209
Asthma during provocation challenge, 215–218
  allergic asthma, 215
  DISP R-E*, 216
  exercise challenge, 217
  ipratropium, 217
  mediators, 217
  methacoline challenge, 215
  placebo, 217
  platelet-activating factor, 217
  salbutamol, 217
Astrocytes, 440
Atelectasis, 178, 184–185, 192
  body mass index, 185
  body weight, 185
  chronic obstructive lung disease, 185
  computed tomography (CT) scan, 185
  Hounsfield scale, 184
  ketamine anesthesia, 184
  obese patients, 185
  regression equation, 185
  shunt, 185
  single-photon emission computed tomography, 185
Atherosclerosis, 593, 658
Atrophy
  tubular, 463
Autonomic dysfunction, 669
Autoregulatory escape, 413
Azotemia, 464
  prerenal, 454

B

Baby lung, 305
Bacteremia, 424
Barometric pressure, 150
Base excess, 154
Blood
  microrheological properties, 487

Subject Index

Blood flow (Q̇), 23, 124, 156, 331, 332, 341, 342, 588, 589, 594, 625, 629, 640, 641, 658, 663–665, 671, 673, 918
  adenosine, 454
  altitude, 536
  capillary (*see* Capillary blood flow)
  cathecholamines, 456
  cerebral, 97, 335, 340, 436, 440
  control of, 409
  coronary, 335, 361–363, 368, 369, 371, 376, 409
    corticomedullary redistribution, 453
    distribution, 334, 335
    distribution, heterogeneity, 361, 370, 374
    distribution, microvascular, 361
    distribution, transit times, 373
    microcirculation, 372, 376
    occlusive artery disease, 361, 375, 376
    perfusion pressure, 369
    pressure-flow relationships, 368, 374
    regulation (*see* Regulatory mechanisms)
    Starling resistor, 368, 374
  cyclooxygenase isoenzymes, 455
  distribution, 420
  dopamine, 456
  exercise, 490
  hepatic, 94
  inert gas technique, 96
  kidney, 447, 454
  kinetics during exercise, 472
  leg, 591, 663
  leg blood flow, 663
  local, 332
  medullary, 454
  muscle, 490, 494
  myocardial, 359
  nitric oxide, 455
  peak, 665, 673
  prostaglandines, 456
  regional, 72, 92, 335, 336
  renal, 454
  spatial reconstruction, 73

[Blood flow (Q̇)]
  skeletal muscle, 384–386, 397, 398, 400
    microvascular unit (MVU) (*see* Capillary, skeletal muscle)
    transit time, 393
  skin, 594
  splanchnic, 409
Blood pressure, 657
Blood viscosity, 637
Blood volume, 165
Borh effect, 623, 636
  capillary, 628
Bohr integration, 80
Brain (*see also* Cerebral), 435–444
  glucose extraction, 435, 440
  metabolic active cell, labeling, 106
  oxygen extraction, 435
  respiratory quotient, 435
Breathing pattern, 558, 560
Bronchial system, 49
Bronchoconstriction, 563, 595
Bronchodilation, 563
Bronchodilators, 220–221, 252–253
  acute severe asthma, 220
  aerosol, 220
  β-agonists, 252
  aminophylline, 253
  fenoterol, 253
  hypoxic pulmonary vasoconstriction, 252
  intravenous, 220
  ipratropium bromide, 253
  isoprenaline, 220
  salbutamol, 220, 253
  severe persistent asthma, 220
  terbutaline, 220, 252
  theophylline, 221

C

Calcium metabolism, 667
Capillaroscopy, 594
Capillary
  alveolar, 57
  anastomosis, 90

[Capillary]
  blood flow, 630, 638
  blood volume, 55
  density, 629
  hydrostatic pressure, 629
  numbers/muscle fiber, 593
  perfusion index, 60
  pressure, 594
  skeletal muscle
    capillary recruitment, 386
    functional organization, 393
    functional unit, 393
    hematocrit, 391
    hematocrit heterogeneity, 391
    microvascular unit (MVU), 394, 395, 398, 399, 400
    oxygen delivery, 389, 390
    physical conditioning, 389
    relationships with mitochondria, 389
    transit time, 393
  transit time, 57
Capillary derecruitment, 421, 425
Capillary neogenesis, 513
Capillary/muscle interface, 659, 662, 663
Capillary/myofiber dissociation, 663
Capillary/myofiber distribution, 659
Carbon dioxide, 617
  output (V_{CO_2}), 168, 553, 598
  radioactive labeled, 72
  solubility coefficient, 627
Carbon dioxide tension
  alveolar, 63
  mixed venous, 63
Carbon monoxide diffusing capacity (D_{LCO}), 263, 280
Carbon monoxide oximeter, 48
Carbon monoxide transfer (T_{LCO}), 204–205, 653, 655
  capillary blood volume, 205
  diffusion impairment, 204
Carbon monoxide transfer coefficient (K_{CO}), 278
Cardiac filling pressure, 657
Cardiac frequency, 165
Cardiac heart failure, 528, 581, 592, 593, 594, 599
  adenylyl cyclase activity, 584
  exercise and, 584–585

[Cardiac heart failure]
  norepinephrine in, 583
  peak oxygen consumption in, 584
Cardiac index, 584, 585, 663
Cardiac output, 47, 95, 123, 158, 165, 237, 307–310, 332, 333, 336, 337, 489, 554, 565, 581, 585, 594, 638, 640, 655, 657, 658, 673
  altitude, 537
  responses to exercise, 584
Cardiac transplantation, 595–597
Cardiogenic mixing, 170
Cardiogenic oscillations, 163, 166, 169
Cardiomyopathy, 583, 592
  ischemic, 584, 586
Cardiopulmonary disease, 471, 508
  constant-load, 469
  heavy, 474
  hypoxic, 546
  inactivity, 471
  incremental, 469, 476–478
  moderate intensity, 474
  onset of, 488
  seventy, 470, 481
  single leg, 488, 494, 511
  training, 471, 507–508, 513
  ventilation, 482
Cardiovascular function, 10–15
  anemia, 12
  cardiac output ($\dot{Q}$), 13
  convective flow, 12
  Fick principle, 13
  hypoxia, 12
  magnetic resonance spectroscopy, 14
  metabolic rate ($\dot{V}_{O_2}$), 13
  mixed venous oxygen concentration, 13
  near-infrared spectroscopy, 14
  oxygen transport ($\dot{Q}_{O_2}$), 10
Carnitine, 661, 676
Carotid bodies, 482, 526
Catecholamines
  exercise, 456
Cell viability, 366
Central venous pressure, 165
Challenge testing, 206
  exercise, 206
  exercise-induced asthma, 206

Subject Index

[Challenge testing]
 histamine, 206
 hypertonic saline, 206
 hyperventilation with dry air, 206
 methacholine, 206
 propranolol, 206
 terbutaline, 206
Childhood asthma, 218
 exercise challenge, 218
 histamine challenge, 218
Chronic diseases
 capillary bed, 515
Chronic obstructive pulmonary disease (COPD), 554, 555, 557, 558
 stable, mild, 241–242
 stable, severe, 242
Chronic pulmonary disease, 553
Chronic renal failure, 649–676
Chronic thromboembolic pulmonary hypertension, 296–299
Chronotropic response, 657
Circulation
 cerebral, 435
 splanchnic, 410
Closed environment life-support systems, 162
Closing capacity, 208
Closing volume, 67, 164
Collateral ventilation, 209
Combined selective pulmonary vasodilation and vasoconstriction, 321–322
 NG-monomethyl-L-arginine (L-NMMA), 321
 nitro G-L-arginine-methylesther (L-NAME), 321
Compliance
 dynamic, 564
 static, 564
Computed tomography, 304
 single-photon emission, 180, 207
Conductance for oxygen, 25
Conductance of the vessels, 166, 658
Congenital heart disease
 thermal dilution, 48
Congestive heart failure, 150, 657, 658
Coronary arterial disease, 656, 657
Creatine kinase, 583

Creatine phosphokinase, 30, 37
Creatinine clearance, 650
Critically ill patient, 427
Cryogenic oxygen, 161
Cryptogenic fibrosing alveolitis, 269
Cyclooxygenase, 629
Cytokine production, 567

D

Dead space, 136, 554, 597, 654
 alveolar, 66
Dead space to tidal volume ratio (V_D/V_T), 480, 557, 597
Dead space ventilation and high $\dot{V}_A/\dot{Q}$ units, 311–312
 overdistension of the alveoli, 311
 redistribution of the blood flow, 311
Definitions, 304
 acute respiratory distress syndrome (ARDS), 304
Deflection pressure (P_{def}), 305
Diabetes, 459
Dialysis, 650, 654, 661, 666–670, 673
Diaphragm
 fatigue, 480
Diffusing capacity, 45, 121
Diffusion, 7–10, 526
 altitude, 8
 binding sites, 9
 blood solubility, 9
 carbon monoxide hemoglobin dissociation curve, 10
 diffusional conductance (D), 8
 diffusive equilibration, 8
 Fick's law of diffusion, 8
 hypoxia, 8
 lung diseases, 8
 mixed venous P_{O_2}, 9
 molecular weight of the gas, 8
 muscle, 541
 myoglobin-facilitated, 543
 peak exercise, 7
 peripheral, 543
 pulmonary, 528–529
 rate of flow of blood, 9

810 *Subject Index*

[Diffusion]
  red cell transit time, 8, 9
  slope of the O_2 Hb dissociation curve, 9
  solubility, 8
  thickness of the alveolar-capillary tissue membrane, 8
  vascular volume, 9
  water solubility, 9
Diffusion capacity of the lung for carbon monoxide, 80
Diffusion equations, 23
Diffusion limitation, 22, 122, 158, 182, 270, 312
  altitude, 530
  exercise, 270, 484, 485
  fibrotic stage of ARDS, 312
  muscle, 543
  rest, 270
Diffusion of oxygen, 264
Diffusional capacity, 155, 166, 653
Diffusional conductance, 23, 653–654, 659, 664, 673
Diffusional shunts, 23
Diffusive
  resistance to, 55
Diffusive capacity
  lung, 55, 56
Digestion, 409
2,3-Diphosphoglycerate, 617, 619, 621, 623, 624, 636, 665
Dissociation curve, 49
Distances for oxygen diffusion, 387
  distribution in skeletal muscle, 387
  oxygen uptake, 392
  relationships with capillaries, 389
  respiration, 390
Dobutamine, 585, 597
Dynamic hyperinflation, 563
Dyspnea, 599, 605

E

Edema
  altitude, 531
  gut, 426

Electrode
  carbon dioxide, 99
  oxygen, 98
Electron paramagnetic resonance, 102
End diastolic volume, 582
End expiratory lung volume, 162, 564
End stage renal disease, 649, 650, 657–659, 663, 665–670, 672, 676
End tidal carbon dioxide pressure (P_{CO_2}), 168, 481
End tidal oxygen pressure (P_{O_2}), 168
Endothelial derived relaxing factor (EDRF), 493, 593, 619, 621, 632–634, 637
  nitric oxide, 493
  prostaglandines, 493
Endothelial glycocalyx, 503
Endothelin receptors, 454
Endothelins, 454, 671
Endothelium, 586
  dependent vasodilator, 586
  dysfunction, 587
  function, 602
Endurance training, 539
Erythropoietin, 155, 641, 655, 657, 663, 676
  recombinant human, 655
  response to hypoxia, 464
  synthesis of, 464
Exercise, 246–250, 336, 383
  capacity, 553
  carbon monoxide diffusing capacity, 81, 85
  cardiac output, 249
  diffusion limitation to oxygen, 249
  in healthy subjects, 122
  intolerance, 651, 655, 659
  limitation, 567
  performance, 585
  pulmonary hypertension, 249
  tolerance, 650
  training, 581, 665, 668, 676
    aerobic, 591, 597, 598, 602, 603, 604
    capacity, 591
    in congestive heart failure, 602–605
    endurance, 605

Subject Index 811

[Exercise]
 [training]
  low-intensity, 605
  small muscle mass, 605
  strength, 605
Experimental endotoxemia, 424
Expiratory flow, 560, 570
Expired ventilation, 478–484
Extrapulmonary factors influencing arterial blood gas, 137, 204, 305
 cardiac output, 204
 cor pulmonale, 204
 foramen ovale, 204
 mixed venous oxygen tension, 204
 oxygen consumption, 204
 pulmonary hypertension, 204

F

Fiber atrophy, 590, 659
Fick equation, 489, 511, 658
Fick principle, 22, 48, 49
Finite element modeling, 56, 91
Flow
 internal resistance, 50
 laminar, 50, 54
Flow limitation, 560
Flow probe, 93
Flow volume curves, 560, 569
Fractal analysis, 124, 125, 134–136
Frequency dependence of dynamic compliance, 208
Functional residual capacity, 182–183
 body plethysmography, 183
 residual volume, 183

G

Gas
 driving pressure, 526, 527, 529
Gas exchange
 alveolar, 60
 diffusive, 55
 during exercise, 137

[Gas exchange]
 efficiency, 45
 lung, 45
 periphery, 45
 pulmonary, 138
 surface, 536
Gas reabsorption, 189
 nitrogen, 189
 preoxygenation procedure, 189
 pulse oximeter, 189
 pure oxygen, 189, 190
 vital capacity maneuver, 189
Gas solubility, 23
Gas store
 intrapulmonary, 46
Gastrointestinal system, 409
 blood flow, 410
 metabolic activity, 409
 metabolic control, 413
 oxygen supply, 410
 resistance, 412, 415
 transit time, 420–422
 two-compartment model, 411
Glomerular filtration, 447
Glucose
 brain, 436, 440
 metabolic rate for, 436
Glutaraldehyde, 637
Glutathione, 634
Glycogene
 stores in muscle, 471, 478
Glycolysis, 483
 brain, 440
Glycolytic enzymes, 590, 593, 661
Gravitational models, 134
Gravity, 70, 122, 162
Guanylate cyclase, 633
Gut
 microcirculation, 409, 411–412
 parallel compartments, 411

H

Haldane transformation, 46
Halothane anesthesia, 181
Heart, 340, 359, 376

Heart rate
  peak, 665, 673
Helium-oxygen mixture, 600
Hematocrit, 427, 628
  microvascular, 628
  pulmonary capillary, 487
Heme, 621
Hemodialysis, 650, 651, 654, 667
Hemodynamic response, 273–275
  cardiac dysfunction, 273
  cardiac output, 273
  hypoxic pulmonary vasoconstriction, 273
  patterns of gas exchange response, 273
  peak $\dot{V}_{O_2}$, 273
  pulmonary circulation, 275
  pulmonary hypertension, 273
  right ventricular afterload, 273
Hemoglobin, 617–641, 656, 662
  altitude, 540–542
  cell free, 634–640
  β chains, 621
  conjugated hemoglobins, 636, 637
  cross-linked hemoglobins, 635–636
  deoxyhemoglobin, 622–624
  in NO metabolism, 618
  oxihemoglobin, 622, 623
  saturation, 627
Hemorrhage, 410, 415, 423, 457
  pulmonary, 532
Heterogeneity of $\dot{V}_A/\dot{Q}$ ratios, 22, 124
High frequency ventilation, 318
  acetone, 318
  high $\dot{V}_A/\dot{Q}$ mode, 318
  neonatal respiratory distress syndrome, 318
High $\dot{V}_A/\dot{Q}$ regions, 178
Homeostasis, 29, 37, 41
Hydrogen ion
  allosteric effects, 617, 621
Hypercapnia, 122, 264
Hypercholesterolemia, 658
Hyperkalemia, 598
Hyperoxia, 511
  in the brain, 443
Hyperparathyroidism, 667, 670

Hyperpnea, 480
  cardiodynamic, 481
Hypertrophy
  kidney, 459
  tubular, 462
Hypotension
  gut, 423
Hypoventilation, 22, 565, 653
  altitude, 527
Hypovolemia,
  thermal dilution, 48
Hypoxemia, 121, 121
  in the brain, 443
  during exercise, 484
Hypoxia, 571–572, 588, 619
  alkalosis in, 619
  ambient, 526, 539
  anemic, 419
  anemic or hemodilutional, 340
  damage, 447
  hypobaric, 530
  hypoxic, 340, 341, 419, 619
  inducible factor-1, 464
  insults, repeated or chronic, 462
  kidney, 447
  medula, 451, 459, 460, 463, 464
  role of adenosine, 454
  simulated, 540
  stagnant or ischemic, 340, 342, 419
  ventilatory response, 527
Hypoxic pulmonary vasoconstriction, 189, 237, 310
  barbiturates, 189
  halothane, 189
  isoflurane, 189
  pulmonary hypertension, 190
Hypoxic ventilatory response (HVR), 152, 153, 161

I

Idiopathic pulmonary fibrosis (IPF), 264, 269
Indocyanine green, 94
Inert gas, 46, 139
Inflammatory pathways, 375

Subject Index

[Inflammatory pathways]
  adhesion molecules, 375
  inducible nitric oxide synthase, 375
Inhalation of prostaglandins, 320–321
  interstitial fibrosis, 321
  intravenous PGI_2 and PGE_1, 320
Inhomogeneity of perfusion, 209
Inhomogeneous airway closure, 209
Inspiratory flow, 560, 564, 570
  maximum, 560
Inspiratory oxygen fraction, 307
Inspired ventilation-perfusion ratio, 179
Insulin resistance, 661, 670
Intermittent claudication, 594
Interstitial lung disease, 554, 555, 557, 558
Intestine, 342
Intrapulmonary factors, 305
Intrapulmonary shunting, 264
Invertebrates, 36
Ionizing radiation, 162
Ipratropium, 600
Ischemia, 160
  reflow model, 462
Ischemia-reperfusion
  myocardial injury, 376

J

J-receptor activation, 264
Juxtaglomerular apparatus, 655

K

Kidney, 447–468
  failure, 457, 460–462
  oxygen extraction, 452
Krogh tissue cylinder, 89, 418

L

Labeled microsphere, 73, 93
  measurement errors, 94

Lactate
  flux across tissue, 104
  hepatic dysfunction, 105
  hypoxia, 104, 105
  intracellular concentration, 588
  leg production, 603
  level, 666
  metabolism, 664
  production, 664
  renal dysfunction, 105
  venous, 650, 658
Lactate levels, 341
Lactic acidosis, 476, 597, 598
Lactic threshold, 482
Left ventricular hypertrophy, 656, 657, 663
Limb muscle
  blood flow, 480
Liver, 37
L-NAME, 223
Lobule, 51
Low ventilation-perfusion ratios (low $\dot{V}_A/\dot{Q}$ regions), 178
Luminescence technique, 101
Lung
  capillary transit time
  exercise, 486, 487
  flow dynamics, 49
  mechanics, 560–563
  regional $\dot{V}_A/\dot{Q}_C$, 62
Lymphatic vessels, 595
Lypoxygenase, 629

M

Magnetic resonance spectroscopy, 30, 566
  hydrogen, 589
  ^{31}phosphorus, 583, 588
Maximal expiratory flow rates, 165
Maximal voluntary ventilation, 570, 601
Maximum ventilatory capacity, 560
McArdle disease, 483
Mean capillary oxygen pressure, 496
Mechanical ventilation, 251–252

[Mechanical ventilation]
  controlled mechanical hypoventilation, 252
  dynamic hyperinflation, 251
  external PEEP, 251
  intrinsic PEEP, 251
  noninvasive positive pressure ventilation, 252
  oxygen consumption, 251
  oxygen delivery, 251
  respiratory quotient, 252
  weaning, 251
Metabolic acidosis, 554, 668
Metabolic demand
  renal, 447
Metabolism
  aerobic, 359, 361, 362, 376, 389, 391, 396
  anaerobic, 361, 362
  fatty acids, 359, 374
  glucose, 359
  glycolysis, 359
  ketone bodies, 360, 374
  lactate, 359, 374
  pyruvate, 360
  substrates, 359
Metabolites
  role in exercise vasodilatation, 494
Methoxamine, 599
Microcirculation
  kidney, 447, 450, 454
Minute volume
  expiratory, 46
  inspiratory, 46
Mitochondria, 383, 535, 536, 553, 593
  abnormalities, 593
  content in skeletal muscle, 387, 389
  distribution of, 91
Mixed venous oxygen tension, 237, 310
Mountain sickness, 541
  hemodilution, 541
Mt. Everest, 150
Mucosal acidosis, 429
Multiple inert gas elimination technique, 76–79, 82, 132, 158
  alveolar capillary block, 79
    rebreathing, 85

[Multiple inert gas elimination technique]
  [alveolar capillary block]
    single breath, 81, 83
    slow exhalation, 84
    steady state, 80, 82
    three equation method, 84
  for carbon dioxide, 87
  heavy exercise, 78
  for nitrous oxide, 87
  for oxygen, 81
Multiple inert gas technique, 654
Multiple organ failure, 427
Muscle, 29
  atrophy, 590, 593
  blood flow, 492
  capillary, 500
  chronic disease, 515
  contractility, 651
  deconditioning, 593
  density, 500
  diffusion capacity, 494, 497
  effective surface area, 502
  fatigue, 476, 482
  fiber type, 567
  function, 553
  geometry, 500
  hematocrit, 503
  loss, 590
  mass, 591
  metabolic rate, 29
  metabolism, 30–36
  needle biopsies, 592
  oxidative potential, 593
  oxidative capacity, 602
  oxygenation, 594
  paralysis and mechanical ventilation, 180
  perfusion, 604
  pump, 488, 492
  red blood cell velocity, 507, 509
  resting metabolic rate, 29, 30, 37
  sarcomere length, 509
  strength, 566, 591
  to fiber ratio, 500
  volume, 590
  wasting, 668
  weakness, 659

Subject Index

Myocardial contractility, 159
  hypertrophy, 582
  hypoxemia, 160
  ischemia, 657
Myoglobin, 39, 103, 387, 497, 498, 505, 545, 589
  cryomicrospectroscopy, 103
  gene-knockout model, 545
  mice homozygotus null for myoglobin, 388
  oxygen diffusion, 388
  oxygen saturation, 372
  percentage myoglobin, 39
Myopathy, 572
  mitochondrial myopathy, 659
  uremic myopathy, 659, 661

N

Near-infrared spectroscopy, 594
Neuropathy, 669–670
  autonomic, 669
  phrenic nerve latency, 653
  uremic, 669
Neurovascular coupling, 437, 443
Nicotinamide adenine dinucleotide, reduced (NADH), 590
Nitric oxide, 222, 319–320, 586, 593, 619, 624, 629, 667–668
  allosteric affect, 621
  as endothelium relaxing factor, 632–634
  mediated vasodilation, 664
  outcome, 320
Nitrous oxide, 165
Norepinephrine, 537, 670

O

Obstructive lung disease, 190, 192
  atelectasis, 191
  chronic hyperinflation, 191
  lung surgery, 190
  shunt, 190
  vascular reconstructive surgery, 190

Obstructive uropathy, 459
One-lung ventilation, 191–192
  apneic oxygenation, 191
  nitric oxide, 192
  nitric oxide guanylate cyclase system, 191
  nitric oxide synthase blocker, 192
Open-circuit technique, 46–47
  bias flow, 46
Operation Everest II, 158
Optimized ventilatory support, 313–314
  oxygen delivery, 313
  positive end-expiratory pressure (PEEP), 313
Osmolarity, 154
Oxidate enzymes, 566, 590, 593
Oxidate phosphorylation, 588
Oxidative phosphorylation
  brain, 442
Oxidative enzymes, 661
  mitochondrial, 662
Oxygen, 553, 617
  active transport, 79
  affinity of the hemoglobin, 154
  affinity, 619, 622–624
  after Epo, 656
  altitude, 535
  availability
  binding, 621
  brain, 436, 440
  carrying capacity, 656
  cellular reserve, 590
  central venous partial pressure, 649
  concentration gradient, 625
  concentrators, 161
  consumption (V_{O_2}), 1, 151, 158
    convection, 541
    muscle, 472
    pulmonary, 472
    slow component, 476
  content, 92, 332, 342, 617
    arterial, 332
    arteriovenous difference, 332
    measurement of, 48
    venous, 332, 337

[Oxygen]
  delivery, 39, 158, 597, 618, 620, 621, 624, 625, 629, 640, 649, 650, 651, 653, 657, 662–668, 673, 676
    kidney, 490
    leg, 664
    muscle, 472, 483, 511
    splanchnic, 490
  demand, 331, 336, 337, 625, 629, 640
    heterogeneity, 396
    myocardial, 359, 361–363, 371, 376
    regional differences, 335
    skeletal muscle, 383
    whole-body, 332, 339
  diffusion, 392, 395, 620, 629, 664
    distance between red blood cells and mitochondria, 392
  diffusional conductance, 667
  diffusive transport, 90
  dissociation curve, 487, 513
    availability, 458
    balance, 458
    intracellular concentrations, 40
    intracellular gradients, 40
    kidney, 447, 454
    medulla, 459
    off-loading, 507
    partial pressure, 617, 625, 640
    partial pressure, in the renal parenchyma, 451
    partial pressure, tissue P_{O_2}, 629
    pulse, 566
    signal, 39, 40
    starvation, 414
    transport, 1
    uptake, 158, 168, 619, 620, 624
  exchange, 136
    efficiency, 65
  extraction, 535, 538, 544, 617, 666, 670
  extraction ratio, 332–334, 336, 342, 343, 349
    critical oxygen extraction ratio, 349
    critical oxygen extraction ratio, myocardial, 360, 361, 371
    critical venous oxygen pressure, 371

[Oxygen]
  [extraction ratio]
    gradient driving oxygen diffusion, 391
    myocardial, 361, 374
    myocardial, skeletal muscle, 386
    partial pressure, 617, 625, 640
    regional venous, 335, 395
  gradient diffusion, 620, 626
  kinetics, 555
  metabolic rate for, 440
  molecule, 622
  muscle, 472, 493
  pathological oxygen supply dependency, 349
    regional, 334, 335
    regional differences, 335
    skeletal muscle, 383, 385, 386, 397, 398
  pathways, 652, 662
  peak $\dot{V}_{O_2}$, 655, 656, 661, 663–666, 673, 676
  plasma oxygen concentration, 627
  red blood cells oxygen concentration, 627
  solubility coefficient, 625
  supply, 331, 333, 334, 336, 341, 342, 349, 350, 352, 359, 649, 658, 663–665
    critical level, 334, 341, 342
    dependency, 349
    distribution, 332, 339
    matching with oxygen demand, 337, 339
    matching with oxygen demand, myocardial, 361
    microregional ratios of oxygen supply/demand, 373
    myocardial, 360, 361
  symmorphosis, 91
  transcutaneous partial pressure, 593
  transfer, 618, 662
  transport
    structural limitation, 91
  uptake, 533, 554, 565, 658, 668
    diffusion-limited, 371
    limitation, 334

Subject Index 817

[Oxygen]
  [uptake]
    myocardial, 360, 361, 365–367
    oxygen diffusion limitation, 390, 392
    oxygen supply dependent, 332, 334, 349
    oxygen supply independent, 332, 334
    pathological oxygen supply dependency, 349
    regional, 335
    resting, 334
    skeletal muscle, 383, 391
    whole-body, 333, 334, 336, 339, 343, 352, 359
  $\dot{V}_{O_2}$ max, 533, 662, 672
    conductance, 665
Oxygen breathing, 250–251
  absorption atelectasis, 250
  collateral ventilation, 250
  high inspired oxygen fractions, 250
  increase in shunt, 250
  low inspired oxygen fractions, 251
  release of hypoxic pulmonary vasoconstriction, 250
Oxygen equilibrium curve, 617- 621, 623–625, 640–641
Oxygen extraction
  critical illness, 428
  gut, 414, 415, 419, 420, 425
Oxygen flux, 529, 537
Oxygen flux density, 500
Oxygen free-radical, 587
Oxygen hemoglobin curve, 528, 542
Oxygen pressure gradient, 662, 663
Oxygen venous pressure, 617
Oxygen-carbon dioxide diagram, 152
Oxyhemoglobin content, 440
Oxyhemoglobin spectroscopy, 101

P

Parallel inhomogeneity, 67
Parasympathetic
  abnormalities, 669

[Parasympathetic]
  tone, 657
Partial liquid ventilation, 317–318
  extracorporal lung assist, 318
  liquid PEEP, 317
  perfluorocarbon, 317
Partial ventilatory support, 314
  airway pressure release ventilation (APRV), 314
  biphasic positive airway pressure (BIPAP), 314
  intermittent mandatory ventilation (IMV), 315
  pressure support ventilation (PSV), 314
Patterns of ventilation perfusion ($\dot{V}_A/\dot{Q}$) distributions, 231
  high pattern, 231
  low pattern, 231
Perfusion
  autoregulatory mechanism, 443
  cerebral, 443
  distribution of, 71, 75
  resistance to, 52
Perfusion heterogeneity, 124
Pericardectomia, 511
Periodic breathing, 160
Peripheral chemoreceptors, 482
Peripheral circulation, 587
Peripheral vascular disease, 592–594, 658–659
Peripheral vasculature
  alterations, 592–594
  resistance, 602
Permissive hypercapnia, 314
Persistent asthma, 203, 210–213
  administration of 100% oxygen, 213
  airway resistance, 213
  bimodal distribution, 210
  bimodal ventilation perfusion distribution, 212
  collateral ventilation, 212
  dead space, 210
  dispersion of the blood flow distribution, 122, 210
  dispersion of ventilation, 210
  high $\dot{V}_A/\dot{Q}$ mode, 210

[Persistent asthma]
  hypoxic vasoconstriction, 213
  isotonic saline, 212
  mechanical ventilation, 213
  methacoline, 212
  pores of Kohn, 212
  shunt, 210
pH
  intramucosal, estimation of, 103
Phosphocreatine, 583, 588, 593, 663
  muscle levels, 592
  recovery, 590, 593
Phosphofructokinase, 483
Phrenic nerve conduction, 653
Phrenic nerve latency, 653
Plasma volume
  exercise, 487
Platelet growth factors, 595
Polycythemia, 155
Polyoxyethylene glycol, 636
Positive end-expiratory pressure (PEEP), 186–188, 304
Positron emission, 98
Postaglandins, 641
Postpulmonary shunting, 485
Potassium
  brain, 441
  channels, role in cerebral vasodilatation, 444
  extracellular concentration, 441
Prazosin, 597
Predicted arterial oxygen pressure, 269, 270
Preload, 657, 658
Pressure/volume (P/V) relationship, 305
Primary pulmonary hypertension, 285, 297–299
  diltiazem, 298
  exercise, 297
  forame ovale, 298
  nifedipine, 298
  prostaglandin E$_1$, 298
  vasodilators, 297
Prone position, 315–317
  Houndsfield units, 317
  oleic acid-induced lung injury model, 315

Prostaglandin, 2, 664
Pulmonary capillary blood flow, 84
Pulmonary capillary pressure, 585, 596, 597
Pulmonary edema, 485
Pulmonary embolism, 286–296
  acetylsalicylic acid, 294
  alveolar-arterial oxygen partial pressure [P(A-a)o$_2$], 132, 286
  anticoagulants, 295
  atelectasis, 287
  bronchial tone, 290
  collateral ventilation, 290
  cyclooxygenase inhibition, 294
  dead space, 289–291
  diffusion impairment, 291
  experimental embolic pulmonary hypertension, 293
  extrapulmonary factors, 286, 291–292
  foramen ovale, 289
  hydralazine, 293
  hypocapnia, 286
  hypoxic pulmonary vasoconstriction, 294
  indomethacin, 294
  microembolism, 289
  nitroprusside, 293
  pulmonary edema, 287
  pulmonary hypertension, 292
  pulmonary vascular tone, 292–295
  shunt, 286–289
  thomboxane A$_2$, 294
  thrombolytics, 295
  ventilation-perfusion inequality, 286, 291
Pulmonary endothelium, 654, 655
Pulmonary fibrosis, 654
Pulmonary function test, 596
  in chronic heart failure, 596
Pulmonary gas exchange, 121, 122, 565
Pulmonary hypertension, 310
  aerosolized PGI$_2$ or PGE$_1$, 310
  almitrine bismesylate, 311
  altitude, 531
  diagnosis of, 72
  intravenous vasodilators, 310

Subject Index

[Pulmonary hypertension]
  L-arginine analogs, 310
  nitric oxide, 310
Pulmonary vascular compliance, 279
Pulmonary vascular resistance, 279, 595
Pulmonary vasoconstriction, 321
  almitrine, 321
Pulmonary venous hypertension, 594–595
Pulmonary venous pressure, 594
Pulse oximeter, 99–101

Q

Quality of life, 553, 650, 676
Quality of sleep, 161

R

Radioactive gas
  insoluble, 70
Radioactive xenon 133, 206
Radioiodine, (^{131}I)-labeled macroaggregated albumin, 207
Rapid shallow breathing, 236
Recruitment maneuvers, 188
  baro/volotrauma, 188
  vital capacity maneuver, 188
Red blood cells
  concentration, 155
  flow, 629
Regional distribution of ventilation, 179
Regional radioactive count rate, 70, 71, 74
Regulation
  metabolic, 39
Regulatory mechanisms, 331, 341, 342, 346
  adenosine, 370
  blood flow, 335
  cholinergic, 370
  dopexamine, 351

[Regulatory mechanisms]
  endothelial cells, 370, 374, 375
  endothelial-derived relaxing factor (*see* Nitric oxide)
  epinephrine, 338
  hypoxic vasodilation, 340, 346, 370
  isoproterenol, 345
  local metabolites, 338
  local modulation, 332
  microvascular control, 350
  nitric oxide, 340, 346, 370, 375
  norepinephrine, 338
  oxygen partial pressure, 338
  prostacyclin, 340, 351
  prostaglandin, 338
  sympathetic regulation, 384, 386
  vasoconstrictor, 336–338, 343, 386
  vasodilator, 336–338, 344, 385
  vasoregulatory, 332, 337, 343, 386
Rehabilitation, 651
Renal, 335
Renal transplantation, 650
Renin-angiotensin system, 583
Resistance vessels, 658
Respiratory alkalosis, 153
  altitude, 542
Respiratory compliance, 305
Respiratory exchange ratio, 169, 554
Respiratory frequency, 558
Respiratory gas exchange, 275–277
  capillary transit time, 276
  cardiac output, 276
  distension, 276
  pulmonary vasculature, 276
  recruitment, 276
Respiratory muscle, 598
  accessory, 598
  diaphragmatic work, 600
  dysfunction, 566
  endurance, 601
  fatigue, 600
  function, 563–565
  perfusion, 598–599, 601
  tone, 188
  transdiaphragmatic pressure, 600
  weakness, 600
Respiratory quotient, 63

S

Salbutamol, 600
Sarcoidosis, 269
Sepsis, 361, 374, 376, 424, 426–429
  glycolytic flux, 429
Serotonin, 593
Shock, 457
  septic, 425
Shunt, 136, 178
  arteriovenous vessels, 417
  countercurrent, 417
  diffusive, 417
  gut, 416–420
  postpulmonary, 137
  right-to-left, 122
  venous admixture, 178
Shunt and low ventilation perfusion ($\dot{V}_A/\dot{Q}$) units, 306–311
Single- and multiple-breath inert gas washouts, 163, 208, 209
Single-breath phase 3 slope, 208
Single-breath washings of helium (He) and sulfurhexafluoride (SF6), 169
Single photon emission computed tomography, 97
Skeletal muscle, 334, 336, 339, 340, 341, 343
  blood flow (see Blood flow, skeletal muscle)
  dysfunction, 567, 572
  glycolytic fibers, 387
  isolated in situ, 337
  microvascular unit (MVU) (see Capillary, skeletal muscle)
  motor unit, 396–399
  oxidative fibers, 387
  oxygen demand (see Oxygen demand, skeletal muscle)
  oxygen extraction, 107
  oxygen supply (see Oxygen supply, skeletal muscle)
  oxygen uptake (see Oxygen uptake, skeletal muscle)
  proton magnetic resonance imaging, 106
  response, 566–567

[Skeletal muscle]
  water content, 106
Skeletal muscle dysfunction, 271
Skeletal muscle fatigue, 585
Skin, 335
Sleep, 206
Slope of phase 3, 163
Slope of the dissociation curve, 156
Sludging, 155
Solubility, 156
Space flight on, 162
Spacelabs Life Sciences 1 and 2, 162
SPECT scanning, 223
Splanchic, 335, 342
Spontaneously breathing, 180
Stochastic or fractal inequalities, 166
Stratified inhomogeneity, 67
Strength, 651, 661, 665, 676
Stroke volume, 159, 165, 582, 602, 657
  exercise, 490
Structure-function relationship, 45
Supplemental oxygen, 218–220
  absorption atelectasis, 218
  acute asthma, 218
  mechanical ventilation, 220
  release of hypoxic vasoconstriction, 218
  shunt, 220
Surface area
  alveolar, 55
  capillary, 55
Surfactant replacement, 318–319
  sepsis-induced ARDS, 319
Sympathetic
  abnormalities, 669
  hyperactivity, 669
  overstimulation, 669
Sympathetic nervous system, 631
Systemic vascular resistance, 663, 664, 670

T

Therapy, 205
  adrenaline, 205
  aminophylline, 205

Subject Index

[Therapy]
  hypoxic vasoconstriction, 205
  isoprenaline, 205
  release hypoxic vasoconstriction, 205
  reversal of pulmonary vasoconstriction, 205
  salbutamol, 205
  terbutaline, 205
Thermal dilution, 48, 95
Thoracic gas compression, 562
Thoracotomies, 192
Thromboxane, 663
Tidal volume, 558
  exercise, 480
  peak exercise, 559
Tissue, 23
  cardiac myocites, 371–373
  dysoxia, 334, 340
  mismatch of oxygen supply to demand, 345
  oxygenation 331, 339
  oxygen partial pressure, 345, 350, 370, 386, 394, 395
    cylindric model (Krogh), 390
    skeletal muscle, 390
Tissue oxygen transport and oxygen extraction, 15–21
  central factors, 18
  chronic obstructive pulmonary disease, 20
  diffusive conductance, 17
  diffusive impedance, 15
  exercising muscle physiology, 20
  fraction of inspired oxygen, 20
  heterogeneity of the $\dot{V}_{O_2}/\dot{Q}$ relation, 21
  impedance, 15
  microvascular P_{O_2}, 15
  mitochondria, 15
  mitochondrial oxidative capacity, 20
  muscle capillary network, 20
  peripheral factors, 18
  renal failure, 20
  tissue diffusive conductances, 15
Tissue oxygenation
  near infrared spectroscopy, 105
Tobacco smoking, 192

Training, 572
  endurance, 572
Transit time
  lung capillaries, 529
Transverse abdominal incision, 192
Tubular injury, 457
Tumor necrosis factor alpha (TNF-α) 375, 587

U

Uremia, 650, 651, 670
Uremic toxins, 671

V

Vascular anatomy
  radiological techniques, 54
Vascular endothelial growth factor, 540
Vascular pressure
  gut, 411
Vascular smooth muscle, 587–588
Vascular tone, 492, 629, 630
Vasculature
  kidney, 448, 450
  resistance, 450
Vasoconstrictor(s), 255–256
  almitrine bismesylate, 256
  humoral, 412, 423
  hypoxic pulmonary vasoconstriction, 256
  renal, 460
Vasodilation
  brain, 436
  extraction, 436
Vasodilators, 253–255
  atrial natriuretic factor, 253
  diltiazem, 253
  endogenous, 444
  felodipine, 253
  nifedipine, 253
  nitric oxide (NO), 254
  prostaglandin E_1, 253
Ventilation ($\dot{V}_E$), 3–4, 236, 554, 557, 559, 598

[Ventilation ($\dot{V}_E$)]
  airway cross-sectional area, 4
  alveolar, 51, 54, 68
    distribution of, 49
  convection, 3
  dead space, 51
  diffusion, 3
  distribution of, 66–71
  expiratory, 47
  isocapnic buffering, 482
  Ohm's law, 4
  ventilation/perfusion matching, 4, 128
  uniformity, 67
Ventilation heterogeneity, 127
Ventilation inequality, 208
Ventilation inhomogeneity, 207
Ventilation maldistribution, 209
Ventilation-carbon dioxide production ratio ($\dot{V}_E/\dot{V}_{CO_2}$), 597
Ventilation-perfusion, 654
Ventilation-perfusion ($\dot{V}_A/\dot{Q}$)
  heterogeneity, 14, 531
Ventilation-perfusion ($\dot{V}_A/\dot{Q}$) inequality, 4–7, 22, 121, 122, 139, 169, 200, 653
  arteriovenous difference in O_2 concentration, 6
  cardiac output, 5
  carbon dioxide removal, 6
  convection, 6
  diffusive mixing, 6
  mixed venous blood, 6
  oxygen uptake, 6

[Ventilation-perfusion ($\dot{V}_A/\dot{Q}$) inequality]
  total ventilation, 5
  with age, 139
Ventilation-perfusion ($\dot{V}_A/\dot{Q}$)
  mismatching, 485, 597
Ventilation-perfusion ratio, 54, 73
  pulmonary, 123
  regional, 73
Ventilatory capacity, 45
Ventilatory response, 271–273
  ventilation, 272
  respiratory frequency, 271
  tidal volume, 271
Ventricular filling, 657
Vessels
  exchange, 415
  gut, 415
  resistance, 415
Videomicroscopy, 93
Vital capacity, 559
Volume depletion, 154
V-slope method, 484

W

Work
  myocardial, 359
    pressure-volume area (PVA), 363, 364, 366, 367, 376
  skeletal muscle, 383
Work capacity, 161
Work of breathing, 596, 599, 601